SEVENTH EDITION

Holistic Nursing

A Handbook for Practice

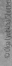

The Pedagogy

Holistic Nursing: A Handbook for Practice, Seventh Edition drives comprehension through various strategies that meet the learning needs of students, while also generating enthusiasm about the topic. This interactive approach addresses different learning styles, making this the ideal text to ensure mastery of key concepts. Examples of the pedagogical aids that appear in most chapters follow:

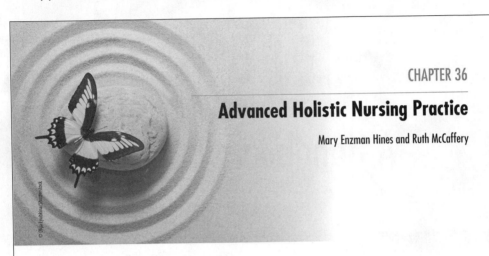

CHAPTER 36

Advanced Holistic Nursing Practice

Mary Enzman Hines and Ruth McCaffery

It has been predicted that the greatest advance in the next decade will not come from technology but from our deeper understanding of what it means to be human, spiritual beings.

—Aburdene, 2007[1]

Nurse Healer Objectives

Theoretical

- Explore the worldview, theories, and models embraced by advanced holistic nurses.
- Discuss the theories and research supporting holistic and integrative care.
- Explore patient-centered care and its components.
- Examine the growth of integrative care models in the U.S. healthcare system.

Clinical

- Explicate the foci of care for advanced holistic nurses.
- Analyze the Consensus Model and its potential effect on advanced holistic nurses.
- Define the key benefits of certification for advanced holistic nurses.
- Analyze the complementary aspects of holistic and integrative care related to patient-centered treatment.
- Define holistic entrepreneurial nursing and discuss its relevance in today's complex healthcare system.

Personal

- Create an integrative/healing model for advanced nursing practice.
- Identify entrepreneurial skills for developing integrative/holistic independent practice.
- Examine areas where you will need assistance to develop a viable holistic/integrative practice and how to obtain resources for the development of this practice.
- Develop short- and long-tern goals implementing and sustaining an advanced holistic nursing practice.

Definitions

Advanced practice holistic nurses: A unique group of nurses weaving a tapestry of bio-psycho-social-spiritual-cultural elements to promote healing within self and others. As advanced practice holistic nurses engage in this healing process, it is a journey of changing and evolving of self and others.

APHN-BC: A certified advanced holistic nurse who synthesizes multiple sources of knowledge and therapies, including patient self-knowledge, when prescribing holistic treatments; develops holistic care plans co-created by partnering with the patient; and prescribes pharmacologic agents based on current knowledge of pharmacology and physiology, clinical indicators, age, holistic

---

Nurse Healer Objectives are divided into three sections: Theoretical, Clinical, and Personal. These objectives provide faculty and students with a snapshot of the key information they will encounter in each chapter and serve as a checklist to help guide and focus study.

Definitions Key words and terms are outlined and defined at the start of every chapter.

- Deep breathing helps to replenish the oxygen and energy of the body and helps the body heal, relax, restore, and renew.
- As the client relaxes, she or he may experience a release of emotional life issues, which can surface in the conscious mind. Be alert for signs of emotional discomfort or letting go, such as tears or a change in breathing to deeper, faster breaths. If such a sign occurs, ask gentle questions (e.g., "Can you put those feelings into words and express them safely?"), and allow time for the client to express and deal with the material before continuing with or concluding the session. (See the earlier sections relating to cryptotrauma and trauma for more information on helping clients stay grounded if they tap into emotion-laden material.) Often, clients in a deeply relaxed state gain insight into how to resolve problems or which direction to take in their lives.

At the end of the session:

- Bring the client gradually into a wakeful state by suggesting that she or he take deep, energizing breaths, begin to move hands and feet, and stretch; orient the client to the room, talking with the client about the comfort she or he created.
- Have the client reevaluate, on the scale of 0 to 10 used earlier, the level of comfort or severity of the parameter previously selected to be changed. Record the level. Take vital signs again and readings on any biofeedback equipment and record postrelaxation practice readings to monitor any psychophysiologic changes pre- and postpractice.
- Allow time for discussion of the experience, including the techniques that seemed especially effective and the client's physical, emotional, and energy awareness. Invite the client to express his or her experience by writing, making a journal entry, or drawing. Different clients will prefer different methods, such as creating an abstract drawing, offering a story, or writing poetry, to express their experience.
- Ensure that medication changes, if indicated, are appropriately monitored.

- Engage the client in continuing practice on an individually assigned basis until the next session.
- Help the client choose supportive mea[...] for practicing his or her relaxation skil[...]
- Review a log or journal in which th[...] ent records relaxation practice, symp[...] medications, time, and results.

Case Study (Implementation)

Case Study 1

Setting: Outpatient; multidisciplinary holistic healthcare center

Client: S. D., a 47-year-old African American man with family history of stroke

Medical diagnosis: Progressive essential hypertension, unresponsive to any antihypertensive therapy

Current medications: Catapres (clonidine), Lasix (furosemide), Valium (diazepam), Minipress (prazosin), potassium chloride

Patterns/Challenges/Needs:

1. Altered physical regulation (essential hypertension)
2. Anxiety
3. Fear
4. Powerlessness
5. Ineffective coping related to anxiety, job stress, and parenting of five children
6. Self-esteem disturbance, situational

S. D. had been diagnosed with severe uncontrollable essential hypertension. He scrupulously took his antihypertensive medications and had an extensive clinical workup to rule out any secondary causes. S. D. was very frustrated because his father had died of a stroke, and S. D. did not want to have a stroke or "die young." He and his wife cared for their five children. He worked at a job that required him to perform physical labor and walk up and down three flights of stairs.

His physician sent him to learn biofeedback-assisted relaxation as an adjunctive therapy. His blood pressure at rest while on medication ranged from 160/100 to 200/120 mm Hg. To reduce S. D.'s fear and feeling of powerlessness, the nurse explored his lived experience of his condition and used healthcare teaching and stress therapies; (2) clinical safety, efficacy, and treatment outcomes of holistic modalities; and (3) the interactive nature of body-mind-spirit."[1] The EBP supports a culture of best practices across multiple settings within a holistic nursing framework to improve health care, client outcomes, and systems. It is essential for holistic nursing to adopt EBP as a culture in education, practice, and research for the ultimate purposes of improving the quality of health care and patient outcomes, as well as empowering holistic nurses to implement best practices, which result in a higher level of professional care and personal satisfaction. Future directions for EBP in holistic nursing practice include the understanding and application of EBP into CER for health policy changes at the national and global levels.

Directions for Future Research

Directions for Future Research

Think critically about the material in each chapter. Using the thought-provoking questions and activities that conclude each chapter, work individually or in a group to engage the material in new ways.

1. Using the evidence-based practice (EBP) process, evaluate holistic, complementary, alternative, integrative, and folk therapies that may promote healthy lifestyles based on client preferences in specific client populations.

2. Using the EBP process, synthesize evidence from literature searches on such topics as body-mind-spirit healing modalities to determine statistically significant and clinically meaningful best practices.

3. Implement quantitative and/or qualitative studies of nurse retention, satisfaction, creativity, and well-being in clinical settings that have and have not implemented system-wide EBP.

4. Implement quantitative and/or qualitative studies of patient and family satisfaction, well-being, and outcomes in clinical settings that have and have not implemented system-wide EBP.

5. Examine the quality of health care, healthcare delivery, and health outcomes from a global perspective as EBP becomes utilized by nurses around the globe as the gold standard for best practices.

6. Develop a working knowledge of ways in which EBP and comparative effectiveness research (CER) work in concert to make policy changes at the national and global levels, taking into consideration the needs and preferences of diverse populations.

7. Determine ways in which complementary, alternative, and integrative approaches to holistic care may be implemented as culturally responsive evidence-based practice programs for individuals, families, communities, and organizations to promote health and reduce healthcare costs.

Nurse Healer Reflections

Nurse Healer Reflections

Reflect on the material presented in the chapter. How might you apply this to your self-development personally and as a holistic nurse?

After reading this chapter, the nurse healer will be able to answer or to begin a process of answering the following questions:

- What is my role in establishing an evidence-based holistic nursing practice?
- How do I feel about the importance of EBP in advancing holistic nursing practice?
- What are my personal and clinical barriers to adopting EBP, and what can I do to reduce these barriers?
- What are my personal and clinical strengths that would support EBP, and what can I do to enhance these strengths?
- Which models are suited to my private or clinical practice, and how can I facilitate the interweaving of a model to improve holistic clinical care?
- How can I become more involved in EBP?
- How can I become more involved in CER to effect policy change?

NOTES

1. American Holistic Nurses Association, "What Is Holistic Nursing?" (2014). www.ahna.org /AboutUs/WhatisHolisticNursing/tabid/1165 /Default.aspx.

2. Sigma Theta Tau International, "Evidence-Based Nursing Position Statement" (2014). www .nursingsociety.org/aboutus/PositionPapers /Pages/EBN_positionpaper.aspx.

3. A. A. Schultz, "Evidence Based Practice: Listening with an Inquiring Mind" (presentation at the Maine Medical Center Outreach Program, Portland, May 25, 2003).

SEVENTH EDITION

Holistic Nursing

A Handbook for Practice

AUTHORS

Barbara Montgomery Dossey, PhD, RN, AHN-BC, FAAN, HWNC-BC

Co-Director, International Nurse Coach Association (INCA)
Co-Director, Integrative Nurse Coach Certificate Program (INCCP)
North Miami, Florida
International Co-Director, Nightingale Initiative for Global Health (NIGH)
Washington, DC and Neepawa, Manitoba, Canada
Director, Holistic Nursing Consultants
Santa Fe, New Mexico

Lynn Keegan, PhD, RN, AHN-BC, FAAN

Director, Holistic Nursing Consultants
Port Angeles, Washington
Co-Director, Golden Room Advocates
Partner, Absolutely Business and Personal Strategic Consulting, LLC
Indianapolis, Indiana
Past President
American Holistic Nurses Association

EDITORS

Cynthia C. Barrere, PhD, RN, CNS, AHN-BC, FAAN

Chair of Faculty Development and Professor of Nursing
School of Nursing
Quinnipiac University
Hamden, Connecticut
Director, Research & Quality
Improvement Consultation Program
American Holistic Nurses Association

Mary A. Blaszko Helming, PhD, APRN, FNP-BC, AHN-BC

Professor of Nursing and Family Nurse Practitioner
School of Nursing
Quinnipiac University
Hamden, Connecticut

Deborah A. Shields, PhD, RN, CCRN, QTTT, AHN-BC

Associate Professor of Nursing
Capital University
Columbus, Ohio

Karen M. Avino, EdD, MSN, AHN-BC, HWNC-BC

Assistant Professor of Nursing
Integrative Nurse Coach
School of Nursing
University of Delaware
Newark, Delaware

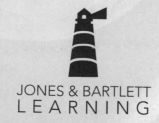

JONES & BARTLETT
LEARNING

World Headquarters
Jones & Bartlett Learning
5 Wall Street
Burlington, MA 01803
978-443-5000
info@jblearning.com
www.jblearning.com

Jones & Bartlett Learning books and products are available through most bookstores and online booksellers. To contact Jones & Bartlett Learning directly, call 800-832-0034, fax 978-443-8000, or visit our website, www.jblearning.com.

08246-3

Production Credits

VP, Executive Publisher: David D. Cella
Executive Editor: Amanda Martin
Associate Acquisitions Editor: Rebecca Myrick
Editorial Assistant: Lauren Vaughn
Production Editor: Sarah Bayle
Marketing Communications Manager: Katie Hennessy
VP, Manufacturing and Inventory Control:
   Therese Connell

Composition: Cenveo Publisher Services
Cover Design: Scott Moden
Rights and Media Research Coordinator:
   Ashley Dos Santos
Cover Image: © Olga Lyubkina/Shutterstock
Printing and Binding: Edwards Brothers Malloy
Cover Printing: Edwards Brothers Malloy

Library of Congress Cataloging-in-Publication Data
Holistic nursing (Dossey)
   Holistic nursing : a handbook for practice / edited by Barbara Dossey, Lynn Keegan, Deborah Shields, Mary Helming, Cynthia Barrere, and Karen Avino. -- Seventh edition.
      p. ; cm.
   Includes bibliographical references and index.
   ISBN 978-1-284-07267-9
   I. Dossey, Barbara Montgomery, editor. II. Keegan, Lynn, editor. III. Shields, Deborah, editor. IV. Helming, Mary A., editor. V. Barrere, Cynthia, editor. VI. Avino, Karen, editor. VII. Title.
   [DNLM: 1. Holistic Nursing. WY 86.5]
   RT42
   610.73--dc23
                    2014045458

6048

Printed in the United States of America
22 21 20 19 18   10 9 8 7 6 5 4 3

The Flame of
Florence Nightingale's Legacy

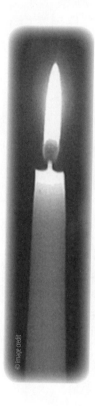

Today, our world needs healing and to be rekindled with Love.
Once, Florence Nightingale lit her beacon of lamplight
   to comfort the wounded
And her Light has blazed a path of service across a Century to us,
Through her example and through the countless Nurses and Healers
   who have followed in her footsteps.

Today, we celebrate the flame of Florence Nightingale's Legacy.
Let that same Light be rekindled to burn brightly in our hearts.
Let us take up our own Lanterns of Caring, each in our own ways.
To more brightly walk our own paths of service to the World.
To more clearly share our own Noble Purpose with each other.

May Human Caring become the Lantern for the 21st Century.
May we better learn to care for ourselves,
   for each other and for all Creation.
Through our Caring, may we be the Keepers of that Flame.
That Our Spirits may burn brightly
To kindle the hearts of our children and great-grandchildren
As they too follow in these footsteps.

Deva-Marie Beck, PhD, RN
International Codirector, Nightingale Initiative for Global Health
Washington, DC and Ottawa, Ontario, Canada
www.NightingaleDeclaration.net

To Our Colleagues in Nursing

When a nurse
Encounters another
Something happens
What occurs
Is never a neutral event

A pulse taken
Words exchanged
A touch
A healing moment
Two persons
Are never
The same

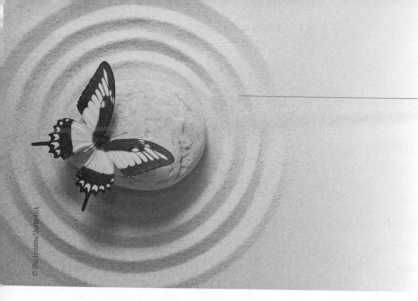

Contents

10   The Psychophysiology of Body–Mind Healing   221

Genevieve M. Bartol

11   Relaxation   239

Jeanne Anselmo

12   Imagery   269

Bonney Gulino Schaub and Megan McInnis Burt

13   Touch and Hand-Mediated Therapies   299

Christina Jackson and Corinne Latini

21 Nurse Coaching 501

Barbara Montgomery Dossey and Susan Luck

22 Applying Cognitive Behavioral Therapy in Everyday Nursing 513

Eileen M. Stuart-Shor, Carol L. Wells-Federman,
and Shanna D. Hoffman

23 Facilitating Change: Motivational Interviewing and Appreciative Inquiry 541

Mary Elaine Southard, Linda Bark, and Darlene R. Hess

27　Evidence-Based Practice　637

Carol M. Baldwin, Alyce A. Schultz, and Cynthia C. Barrere

28　Holistic Nursing Research: Challenges and Opportunities　661

Colleen Delaney, Rothlyn P. Zahourek, and Cynthia C. Barrere

33 Addiction and Recovery Counseling 767

Bonney Gulino Schaub and Megan McInnis Burt

34 Holistic Weight Management 795

Lauren Outland

35 Smoking Cessation 819

Christina Jackson

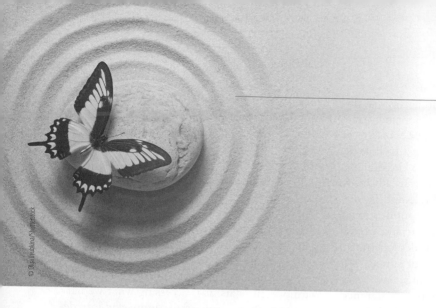

Foreword

The first edition of *Holistic Nursing: A Handbook for Practice*[1] flowed out of the larger questions that had been raised for us in regard to the health or illness of patients/clients and the professional community where we worked, as well as with the family members and friends with whom we lived and played. Each of us had been privileged to work with people who were suffering life-threatening trauma or chronic debilitating disease or illness. Those who taught us the most were people who found ways to transcend challenges with new insights, leading to richer and fuller lives. We continued to explore body-mind-spirit-cultural-environmental connections and healing rituals. Thus, we continue to advocate for a "both/and" instead of an "either/or" approach when interfacing contemporary medical and surgical therapies with healing rituals and complementary modalities. From the beginning we explored three questions:

1. What do we know about the meaning of healing?
2. What can we do each day to facilitate healing?
3. How can we be an instrument in the healing process?

Our fortunate meeting occurred in 1981 through the founding of the American Holistic Nurses Association (AHNA). We immediately recognized that we were each working from our soul's purpose and were seeking new ways of knowing, doing, and being. It was thrilling to find a professional soul mate with an expanded worldview and big vision for challenging nursing's traditional role. This led to our deep friendship; in 1985, we began Bodymind Systems, our holistic nursing business, with our first coauthored title, *Self-Care: A Program to Improve Your Life*.[2]

In 1986, Lynn Keegan, AHNA president, gave a keynote address at the AHNA Sixth Annual Conference at the University of British Columbia in Vancouver. Following her keynote, Lynn was greeted by William Burgower, editorial director of Aspen Publishers in Rockville, Maryland, who briefly described his vision and inquired about her interest in authoring a holistic nursing textbook. He suggested inviting Barbara Dossey to the discussion, knowing of her authorship of *Critical Care Nursing: Body, Mind, Spirit*[3] and *Cardiovascular Nursing: Bodymind Tapestry*.[4] To conceptualize the first holistic nursing textbook, Barbara and Lynn invited nursing colleagues Cathie E. Guzzetta and Leslie G. Kolkmeier to join them as coauthors. In 1988, the first edition of *Holistic Nursing: A Handbook for Practice* was launched at the AHNA Eighth Annual Conference in Estes Park, Colorado.

The AHNA endorsed the first edition in 1988, as well as the following five editions (published in 1995, 2000, 2005, 2009, and 2013). For this seventh edition of *Holistic Nursing: A Handbook for Practice*, AHNA awarded the book with its newly developed Seal of Distinction—the first time this prestigious Seal of Distinction has been offered.

The AHNA Seal of Distinction indicates that the book is aligned with AHNA's mission and vision and with *Holistic Nursing: Scope and Standards of Practice, Second Edition*;[5] is of interest to holistic nurses and of significant value to the nursing profession; provides knowledge that advances holistic nursing; is timely and relevant; is consistent with relevant historical publications; is scientifically and technically accurate; and is authored by individuals with demonstrated expertise in the field of the work submitted.

By the late 1980s, Barbara and Lynn were being invited as holistic nursing conference speakers and consultants at the local, national, and global levels. Many other holistic nurses were also engaging in conversations related to holistic nursing and complementary modalities with colleagues at universities, hospitals, and clinics and in corporations. Holistic nursing courses began to be offered. This led to many nursing organizations also seeking information. In 1993, the American Holistic Nurses Credentialing Corporation began offering holistic nursing certification.

After publication of the third edition of *Holistic Nursing: A Handbook for Practice*, Leslie left the authorship team, followed by Cathie after the fourth edition. During this time, Aspen sold the textbook to Jones & Bartlett Learning. Barbara and Lynn continued as coauthors and also became editors, inviting other holistic nursing contributors for the fourth through the seventh editions. For the sixth edition of *Holistic Nursing: A Handbook for Practice*, Cynthia C. Barrere and Mary A. Helming were invited to join as associate editors. Online programs, an instructor's manual, and CDs were also added, and later PowerPoint slides. With the continued vast influence of holistic nursing in practice, education, research, healthcare policy, and interprofessional collaboration, Barbara and Lynn, along with Cynthia and Mary, invited Karen Avino and Deborah A. Shields to join the project, with Cynthia and Mary as full editors for the seventh edition.

Our vision for the seventh edition of *Holistic Nursing: A Handbook for Practice* continues the exploration of healing that is the lifelong journey into understanding the wholeness of human existence. Along this journey, our lives mesh with those of patients/clients, families, and other interprofessionals where moments of new meaning and insight emerge in the midst of crisis. Healing occurs when we help patients/clients, families, others, and ourselves to embrace what is feared most. It occurs when we seek harmony and balance.

Healing is learning how to open what has been closed so that we can expand our inner potentials. It is the fullest expression of oneself that is demonstrated by the light and shadow and the male and female principles that reside within each of us. It is accessing what we have forgotten about connections, unity, and interdependence. With a new awareness of these interrelationships, healing becomes possible, and the experience of the nurse as an instrument of healing and as a nurse healer becomes actualized. A nurse healer is one who facilitates another person's growth toward wholeness (body-mind-spirit) or who assists another with recovery from illness or transition to peaceful death. Healing is not just curing symptoms. Rather, it is the exquisite blending of technology with caring, love, compassion, and creativity.

As we have explored new meanings of healing in our work and lives, we have interwoven the many diverse threads of knowledge from nursing as well as from other disciplines. This integration has engendered a more vivid, dynamic, and diverse understanding of the nature of holism, healing, and its implications for nursing.

Health care in the 21st century requires a radically different type of nurse who understands relationship-centered care and human flourishing. Holistic, integral, and integrative nursing, along with nurse coaching,[6, 7] are guiding behavioral change strategies, health promotion, health maintenance, and disease prevention. These perspectives and strategies provide a wide range of choices for individuals that are efficient and effective, and that reduce costs. This is fundamental to transforming health care from a disease model of care to one that focuses on health and wellness.

The first priority of nursing is devotion to human health—of individuals, of communities, and of the world. Nurses are educated and prepared—physically, emotionally, mentally, and spiritually—to accomplish the activities with the care team for the health of people.[7, 8] An increasingly severe global nursing shortage is threatening nursing's ranks in almost every nation in the world. The health and happiness of people everywhere in the global community are the only common ground for a secure and sustainable, prosperous future. Yet a healthy world still requires nurses' knowledge, expertise, wisdom, and dedication.

If today's nurses, midwives, and allied health professionals are nurtured and sustained in innovative ways, they can become, like Florence Nightingale, effective voices calling for and demonstrating the healing, leadership, and global action required to achieve a healthy world.[9] This can strengthen nursing's ranks and help the world to value and nurture nursing's essential contributions.

The seventh edition of *Holistic Nursing: A Handbook for Practice* challenges nurses to explore the inward journey toward self-transformation and to identify the growing capacity for change and healing. This exploration creates the synergy for and rebirth of a compassionate power to heal us and to facilitate healing within others. This inner healing allows us to return to our roots of nursing where healer and healing have always been understood and to carry Florence Nightingale's vision for healing, leading, and global action forward into the 21st century.[9, 10] As she said, "My work is my must."[10] By her shining example, she invites each of us to find and know our "must" and to explore our own meaning, purpose, and spirituality.

Barbara Montgomery Dossey
Lynn Keegan

NOTES

1. B. M. Dossey, L. Keegan, C. E. Guzzetta, and L. G. Kolkmeier, *Holistic Nursing: A Handbook for Practice* (Rockville, MD: Aspen, 1988).

2. L. Keegan and B. M. Dossey, *Self-Care: A Program to Improve Your Life* (Temple, TX: Bodymind Systems, 1987).

3. C. V. Kenner, C. E. Guzzetta, and B. M. Dossey, *Critical Care Nursing: Body, Mind, Spirit* (Boston: Little, Brown, 1982).

4. C. E. Guzzetta and B. M. Dossey, *Cardiovascular Nursing: Bodymind Tapestry* (St. Louis, MO: Mosby, 1984).

5. American Holistic Nurses Association and American Nurses Association, *Holistic Nursing: Scope and Standards of Practice*, 2nd ed. (Silver Spring, MD: Nursesbooks.org, 2013).

6. B. M. Dossey, S. Luck, and B. G. Schaub, *Nurse Coaching: Integrative Approaches for Health and Wellbeing* (North Miami, FL: International Nurse Coach Association, 2015).

7. International Nurse Coach Association, "Supporting Nurse Coaches" (2013). http://inursecoach.com/about-inca/.

8. Nightingale Initiative for Global Health, "Why NIGH? Why Now?" (2013). www.nightingaledeclaration.net/about-nigh.

9. B. M. Dossey, *Florence Nightingale: Mystic, Visionary, Healer*, Commemorative ed. (Philadelphia: F. A. Davis, 2010).

10. B. M. Dossey, L. C. Selanders, D. M. Beck, and A. Attewell, *Florence Nightingale Today: Healing, Leadership, Global Action* (Silver Spring, MD: Nursesbooks.org, 2005).

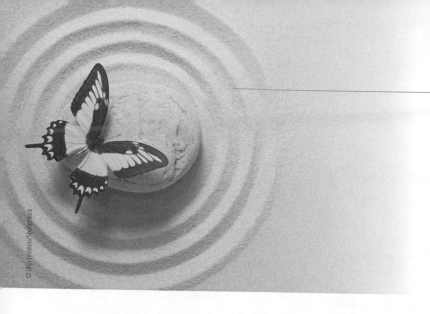

Preface

Holistic Nursing: A Handbook for Practice is a wonderful resource for holistic nurses. We, the editors of this seventh edition, were thrilled to collaborate in the creation of this newest version of what has always been a steadfast, excellent compilation of information designed to deepen the readers' knowledge of the art and science of holistic nursing. From the outset we moved in unison, ever humbled by the day-to-day unfolding of this amazing project. As four nurses brought together by their beloved mentors, Barbara Montgomery Dossey and Lynn Keegan, we grew together through times of joy, sadness, challenge, complexity, and shining light. We learned so much during this process. Developing the seventh edition created the space where four holistic nurse educators worked well together as editors and became lifelong friends. We subsequently invited talented contributors to widen this circle of collegiality, expanding the evidence and clearly articulating that holism is, indeed, the essence of nursing. In the seventh edition of *Holistic Nursing: A Handbook for Practice*, the authors, Barbara Montgomery Dossey and Lynn Keegan; the editors, Cynthia C. Barrere, Mary A. Helming, Deborah A. Shields, and Karen M. Avino; and the contributors have broadened the knowledge base for holistic nursing by delineating holistic nursing as *the* foundational essence of all nursing. The purposes of this book are to (1) expand the readers' understanding of a holistic, integral, and integrative worldview, healing, and the nurse as an instrument of healing; (2) explore the unity and relatedness of nurses,

clients, and others; (3) develop caring, healing interventions that strengthen and support healing of the whole person; and (4) envision basic and advanced holistic nursing practice as integral to health care within local and international communities.

Holistic nursing is recognized as a specialty by the American Nurses Association (ANA). The coauthored American Holistic Nurses Association (AHNA) and ANA publication *Holistic Nursing: Scope and Standards of Practice, Second Edition*,[1] provides the unique scope of knowledge and the standards of practice and professional performance of a holistic nurse. As clinicians, authors, educators, and researchers, we have successfully used these holistic concepts and interventions in acute, outpatient, and community settings, as well as in corporations and the classroom. We view our patients as individuals and co-participants in all phases of care. The challenge is to integrate all textbook concepts into clinical practice and daily life. To support readers in meeting these challenges, each chapter begins with *Nurse Healer Objectives* to direct readers' learning within the theoretical, clinical, and personal domains; includes *Definitions* for quick, easy references; presents *Directions for Future Research* that offer ideas and suggestions for research questions that are timely and in need of scientific exploration; and ends with beautiful *Nurse Healer Reflections* to nurture the reader and spark a special self-reflective experience of bodymindspirit and the inward journey toward self-discovery and healing.

This book is organized according to the five core values of holistic nursing contained within the AHNA and ANA *Holistic Nursing: Scope and Standards of Practice, Second Edition*:

Core Value 1: Holistic Philosophy, Theories, and Ethics

Core Value 2: Holistic Caring Process

Core Value 3: Holistic Communication, Therapeutic Healing Environment, and Cultural Diversity

Core Value 4: Holistic Education and Research

Core Value 5: Holistic Nurse Self-Reflection and Self-Care

Core Value 1 presents the philosophic concepts that explore what occurs when the nurse honors, acknowledges, and deepens his or her understanding of inner knowledge and wisdom. Relationship-centered care is also discussed. *Holistic Nursing: Scope and Standards of Practice, Second Edition* relevant to both basic and advanced practice are reviewed in depth. Trends and issues in holistic nursing are identified, along with opportunities to practice interprofessionally. This section also addresses major issues that affect health care and holistic nursing today and identifies the changes needed to promote health, wellness, well-being, and healing. The effect of the Affordable Care Act on healthcare delivery is elucidated. The foundation for transpersonal human caring and the art of holistic nursing provide insight into how people create change and sustain these new health behaviors related to wellness, values clarification, and motivation theory. Holistic nursing theorists and the grand and midrange theories that guide holistic nurses are discussed, and examples of their application in practice are offered. Holistic ethics are addressed in both personal and professional arenas. Spirituality involves an individual's search for understanding the meaning of life events and relationships. Thus, the chapter examining the importance of attending to one's spiritual health and the positive health outcomes that can result from this exploration was moved from Core Value 4 in the sixth edition to Core Value 1 in this new edition, in alignment with this core value's focus on inner understanding.

Core Value 2 describes how holistic nursing plays a vital role in promoting the 2015 National Patient Safety Goals. The holistic caring process expands the discussion of the more linear nursing process to the circular holistic caring process, a way of thinking about the six steps of the process (assessment, patterns/challenges/needs, outcomes, therapeutic care plan, implementation, and evaluation) as potentially occurring at once and realizing that the nurse may be attending to multiple needs simultaneously. In the seventh edition, a new and exciting way of viewing the holistic caring process is introduced. Based on the Four Quadrants as delineated by Wilber and utilized by Dossey in her Theory of Integral Nursing, the authors posit a "four-quadrant" perspective in order for nurses to better understand the interrelationship between the physical, psychological, cultural, and social dimensions of a person. This approach is sure to influence nursing practice.

The remaining chapters addressing Core Value 2 move the reader from more expansive thoughts of our universal connection to the science of bodymind healing to more specific complementary/integrative therapeutic approaches. The Psychophysiology of Body–Mind Healing chapter, which discusses the immune system, neuropeptides, and brain responses relevant to understanding various complementary/integrative therapies, was moved to this section and lays the groundwork for this exploration. The chapter on Energy Healing adds a brief glimpse of the volumes of history underlying contemporary healing energy therapies; in addition, the discussion of physics and evidence that supports complementary/integrative therapies has been expanded. Relaxation, Imagery, Touch and Hand-Mediated Therapies, and Aromatherapy continue as individual chapters and include new, exciting initiatives. A new chapter, Creative Expressions in Healing, has been developed as an experiential activity in which the reader is invited to explore various aesthetic, reflective activities for self and others through walking in a labyrinth. The authors are excited about this innovative approach to sharing. Another new chapter, Herbs and Dietary Supplements, provides the reader with an excellent, detailed guide to knowledgeably and safely use these substances; presented in succinct tables, the information is readily available and easy to navigate.

Core Value 2 ends with a wonderful chapter about the sacredness of care at the end of life, offering holistic nurses a compendium of ideas and resources that can be applied in their practice as they walk with patients and families.

Core Value 3 explores therapeutic communication and the art and skills of helping. The necessary steps to creating an external and internal healing environment are expanded to help nurses recognize that each person's environment includes everything surrounding the individual, both the external and the internal, as well as patterns not yet understood. Environmental health is an integral part of this core value. The holistic communication approaches that are addressed include also nurse coaching, cognitive therapy, appreciative inquiry, and motivational interviewing. Relationships evolve based on various forms of communication, and therefore the chapter on relationships was relocated to Core Value 3.

Concepts related to cultural diversity are presented so that the nurse can recognize each person as a whole bodymindspirit being. Such recognition facilitates the development of a mutually co-created plan of care that addresses the cultural background, health beliefs, sexual orientation, values, and preferences of each unique individual.

Core Value 4 is intended to provide meaningful resources to prepare nurses as holistic leaders, educators, and researchers who advocate for practicing holistic nursing based on the evidence. A new leadership chapter focuses on how holistic nurses effect positive changes in the provision of holistic care to improve the health of individuals and communities. Additional education strengthens the ability of nurses to understand and provide holistic care. A chapter devoted to education is included that describes forms of simulation as an effective holistic pedagogy; the chapter also provides suggestions on ways to include holistic content in undergraduate curricula and offers ideas for graduate nursing curricula as well. The Holistic Nursing Research chapter discusses the growing need for research studies that provide evidence of the positive health-related outcomes associated with holistic nursing care. It includes solid step-by-step ideas that are designed to support nurses who want to develop a research project. Providing evidence for and outcomes measures

of the practice of holistic nursing is needed to mirror national efforts in these areas. Increased attention in both arenas was expanded to include practical information about evidence-based practice and quality improvement in a blended chapter. Evidence-based holistic nursing practice models the conscientious use of the best available evidence combined with the clinician's expertise and judgment and the patient's preferences and values to arrive at the best decision that leads to quality outcomes.

Core Value 5 explores the importance of self-care through a new chapter on integral holistic self-development and a chapter on self-assessment. These chapters address nurse self-healing strategies as well as offer new ways to teach others to participate in their own healing. Expanded strategies for enhancing healing are featured in individual chapters: Nutrition, Exercise and Movement, Addiction and Recovery Counseling, Holistic Weight Management, and Smoking Cessation. These essential strategies of healing highlight the role of holistic nursing in improving health care in accordance with national prevention and health promotion efforts. Holistic self-care illuminates the importance of holistic nursing in teaching self-care practices and self-responsibility.

Advanced Holistic Nursing

Two exciting new chapters make up this new section of the seventh edition of *Holistic Nursing: A Handbook for Practice*: Advanced Holistic Nursing Practice, and Advanced Integrative Health and Well-Being Practice. Certification is available for both basic- and advanced-level practitioners, including the newest certification for nurse practitioners (APHN-BC), through the American Holistic Nurses Credentialing Corporation. The importance of advanced holistic practice is increasingly recognized. Schools of nursing teach holistic concepts relevant to both basic and advanced levels of practice. Therefore, an increased focus on advancing holistic nursing practice is given with the development of this new section.

The Advanced Holistic Nursing Practice chapter explores the importance of the evolving role of the advanced practice nurse and helps readers envision and provide information to develop a holistic independent practice. The Advanced Integrative Health and Well-Being Practice chapter shares stories by advanced holistic nurses and demonstrates how the special skills and core values of holistic practice are integrated into their roles. It is our hope that with this beginning focus we can continue to advance the knowledge to practice holistic nursing to its fullest.

The seventh edition of *Holistic Nursing: A Handbook for Practice* is intended for all nurses, students, clinicians, educators, and researchers who desire to expand their knowledge of holism, healing, and spirituality. The philosophic and conceptual frameworks are beginner, intermediate, and advanced. Therefore, the reader can approach this book as a guide for learning basic content or for exploring advanced concepts. The specific "how to" for implementing holistic interventions into clinical practice has both basic and advanced levels. Some advanced interventions may require additional training that can be obtained in practicums under mentors or in elective or continuing education courses. Many chapters present case studies or examples that illustrate how to use and integrate the interventions into clinical practice.

The radical changes necessary in healthcare reform are occurring rapidly. These changes provide us with a greater opportunity to integrate caring and healing into our work, research, and lives. It is up to us as nurses to help determine what these new changes will be. We challenge you to capture your essence and emerge as true healers as we navigate the ebbs and flows in this dynamic period in health care. Best wishes to you in your healing work and life.

Cynthia C. Barrere
Mary A. Blaszko Helming
Deborah A. Shields
Karen M. Avino

NOTES

1. American Holistic Nurses Association and American Nurses Association, *Holistic Nursing: Scope and Standards of Practice*, 2nd ed. (Silver Spring, MD: Nursesbooks.org, 2013).

RESOURCES

For more information on the American Holistic Nurses Association and the its continuing education programs and home study courses, contact:

American Holistic Nurses Association (AHNA)
100 SE 9th Street, Suite 3A
Topeka, KS 66612
1-800-278-2462
info@ahna.org
www.ahna.org

For information on holistic nursing certification and nurse coach certification, contact:

American Holistic Nurses Credentialing Corporation (AHNCC)
811 Linden Loop
Cedar Park, TX 78613
1-877-284-0998
ahncc@flash.net
www.ahncc.org

On December 17, 2014, the National Institutes of Health announced that the agency with primary responsibility for research on promising health approaches that are already in use by the American public had a new name: the National Center for Complementary and Integrative Health, formerly known as the National Center for Complementary and Alternative Medicine (NCCAM). This revision was mandated as part of the omnibus budget measure signed by President Obama. For more information about research related to the use of complementary and integrative therapies, contact:

National Center for Complementary and Integrative Health (NCCIH)
9000 Rockville Pike
Bethesda, MD 20892
1-888-644-6226
nccih.nih.gov

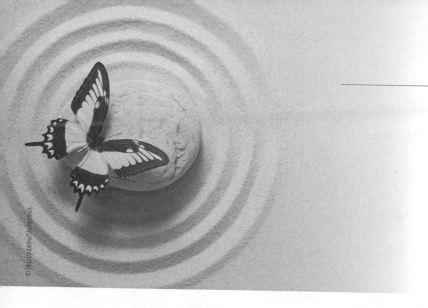

Contributors

Mary Grace Amendola, PhD, RN
Assistant Professor
Rutgers School of Nursing
Newark, New Jersey

Marjorie S. Anderson, MS, RN, PMH-CNS BC
Consultant, Heart of Healing, Inc.
Columbus, Ohio

Veda L. Andrus, EdD, MSN, RN, HN-BC
Vice President, Education and Program
    Development
The BirchTree Center for Healthcare
    Transformation
Florence, Massachusetts

Jeanne Anselmo, BSN, RN, BCIAC-SF, HNB-BC
Holistic Nurse Educator/Consultant
Sea Cliff, New York
Cofounder, Contemplative Urban Law Program
City University of New York School of Law
Queens, New York
Faculty
Merton Contemplative Initiative
Iona Spirituality Institute
Iona College
New Rochelle, New York
Dharma Teacher
Order of InterBeing
Plum Village Tradition of Vietnamese Zen
    Master Venerable Thich Nhat Hanh
Green Island Sangha: Community of Mindful
    Living
Long Island, New York

Karen M. Avino, EdD, MSN, AHN-BC, HWNC-BC
Assistant Professor of Nursing
Integrative Nurse Coach
School of Nursing
University of Delaware
Newark, Delaware

Carol M. Baldwin, PhD, RN, CHTP, CT, NCC, AHN-BC, FAAN
Associate Professor, Southwest Borderlands
    Scholar
Director, Center for World Health Promotion
    and Disease Prevention
Affiliate Faculty, Southwest Interdisciplinary
    Research Center of Excellence
College of Nursing and Health Innovation
Arizona State University
Phoenix, Arizona

Linda Bark, PhD, RN, MCC, NC-BC
Founder and CEO, Wisdom of the Whole
    Coaching Academy
Alameda, California
Adjunct Faculty, Integrative Health Coaching
    Masters Program, University of Minnesota,
    Center for Spirituality and Healing
Minneapolis, Minnesota
Adjunct Faculty, Wellcoaches
Wellesley, Massachusetts

Cynthia C. Barrere, PhD, RN, CNS, AHN-BC, FAAN
Chair of Faculty Development and Professor of Nursing
School of Nursing
Quinnipiac University
Hamden, Connecticut
Director, Research & Quality Improvement Consultation Program
American Holistic Nurses Association

Genevieve M. Bartol, EdD, RN, AHN-BC
Professor Emeritus, School of Nursing
The University of North Carolina, Greensboro
Greensboro, North Carolina

Jane Buckle, PhD, RN
Director, R. J. Buckle Associates, LLC
Hazlet, New Jersey

Margaret A. Burkhardt, PhD, FNP, AHN-BC
Associate Professor Emerita, Robert C. Byrd Health Sciences Center
West Virginia University School of Nursing, Charleston Division
Charleston, West Virginia
Past President, American Holistic Nurses Association

Megan McInnis Burt, MS, RN, PMHBC, CARN, NPD-BC, NC-BC
Faculty, Huntington Meditation and Imagery Center
Huntington, New York

Denise Coppa, PhD, FNP-C, FAANP
Coordinator, Family Nurse Practitioner Program
White Hall
University of Rhode Island
Kingston, Rhode Island

Mary Ann Cordeau, PhD, RN
Nurse Historian
Associate Professor of Nursing
Quinnipiac University School of Nursing
Hamden, Connecticut

Colleen Delaney, PhD, RN, AHN-BC
Associate Professor, School of Nursing
University of Connecticut
Mansfield, Connecticut

Barbara Montgomery Dossey, PhD, RN, AHN-BC, FAAN, HWNC-BC
Co-Director, International Nurse Coach Association
Core Faculty, Integrative Nurse Coach Certificate Program
North Miami, Florida
International Co-Director, Nightingale Initiative for Global Health
Washington, DC, and Neepawa, Manitoba, Canada
Director, Holistic Nursing Consultants
Santa Fe, New Mexico

Carole Ann Drick, PhD, RN, AHN-BC
Director, Conscious Awareness
Director, Golden Room Advocates
Austintown, Ohio
President, American Holistic Nurses Association

Joan C. Engebretson, DrPH, RN, AHN-BC, RN, FAAN
Judy Fred Professor in Nursing, University of Texas Health Science Center
Houston, Texas

Mary Enzman-Hines, APRN, PhD, CNS, CPNP, APHN-BC
Professor Emeritus, University of Colorado, Colorado Springs
Certified Pediatric Nurse Practitioner
Metro Community Provider Network
Englewood, Colorado

Noreen Cavan Frisch, PhD, RN, FAAN
Professor, University of Victoria
British Columbia, Canada
Past President, American Holistic Nurses Association

Kathleen Gareth, RN, MSN, FNP
Center for Integrative Health
Wilmington, Delaware

Jennifer Gaughan, MS, RN, CPNP-PC
Pediatric Nurse Practitioner at Rocky Mountain Pediatrics
Lakewood, Colorado

Francie Halderman, MSN, RN, AHN-BC
Board of Directors Chair-Elect, American
    Holistic Nurses Credentialing Corporation
Cedar Park, Texas
President, Center for Integrative and Holistic
    Nursing Leadership

Mary Anne Hanley, PhD, RN
Education Consultant
Research Trustee, Therapeutic Touch
    International Associates
Delmar, New York
Secretary, Therapeutic Touch Dialogues, Inc.
Whitefish, Montana
Adjunct Faculty, University of Texas
    Permian Basin
Odessa, Texas
Adjunct Faculty, Sul Ross State University
Alpine, Texas

Mary A. Blaszko Helming, PhD, APRN, FNP-BC, AHN-BC
Family Nurse Practitioner
Professor of Nursing, Quinnipiac University
Hamden, Connecticut

Darlene R. Hess, PhD, RN, AHPN-BC, PMHNP-BC, ACC, HWNC-BC
Psychiatric/Mental Health Nurse Practitioner,
    Nurse Coach, Consultant
Brown Mountain Visions
Los Ranchos, New Mexico
Assistant Professor, Northern New
    Mexico University
Española, New Mexico
Practitioner Faculty, University of Phoenix
Phoenix, Arizona

Shanna D. Hoffman, RN, MSN
Simulation and Clinical Education Coordinator
Clinical Center for Education and Research
College of Nursing and Health Sciences
University of Massachusetts, Boston
Boston, Massachusetts

Christina Jackson, PhD, APRN, AHN-BC, CNE
Professor, Eastern University
St. Davids, Pennsylvania

Lynn Keegan, PhD, RN, AHN-BC, FAAN
Director, Holistic Nursing Consultants
Director, Golden Room Advocates
Port Angeles, Washington
Past President, American Holistic Nurses
    Association

Dorothy Larkin, PhD, RN
Professor
The College of New Rochelle School of Nursing
Coordinator/Faculty for the Clinical Specialist
    in Holistic Nursing Program
Private Practice in Psychiatric and Holistic
    Nursing

Corinne Latini, MEd, BSN, RN-BC, CSN
Reiki Master and Healing Touch Level II
Nursing Clinical Resource Laboratory
    Coordinator
Adjunct Faculty, Eastern University
St. Davids, Pennsylvania

Jackie D. Levin, RN, MS, AHN-BC, NC-BC, CHTP
Leading Edge Nursing, Jefferson Healthcare
Port Townsend, Washington

Susan Luck, RN, BS, MA, HNC, CCN, HWNC-BC
Co-Director, International Nurse Coach
    Association
Founder and Director, Earthrose Institute for
    Environmental Health
Certified Clinical Nutritionist, Holistic Nurse
    Educator, and Integrative Nurse Coach
Faculty, Integrative Nurse Coach Certificate
    Program
Miami, Florida

Carla Mariano, EdD, RN, AHN-BC, FAAIM
Faculty, Holistic Nursing Program
Pacific College of Oriental Medicine
New York, New York
Adjunct Associate Professor, New York
    University
New York, New York
Consultant, Holistic Nursing Education
Past President, American Holistic Nurses
    Association

Ruth McCaffrey, DNP, FNP-BC, GNP-BC, FAAN
Sharon Raddock Professor, Christine E. Lynn
    College of Nursing
Florida Atlantic University
Boca Raton, Florida

Kathleen McCarthy, CNM MSN
Co-Owner of The Birth Center Holistic
    Women's Health Care LLC
Wilmington, Delaware

Sharon Murnane, RN, HNB-BC, HTCP
Specialized Senior Care Case Management,
    Inner Wisdom Healing and Healthy By
    Choice
Lead Nurse, Sharp Memorial Cushman Wellness
    Center
San Diego, California

Karen M. Myrick, DNP, APRN, FNP-BC, ANP-BC
Assistant Professor of Nursing, Joint
    Appointment Frank Netter School of
    Medicine
Quinnipiac University
Hamden, Connecticut

Mary Gail Nagai-Jacobson, RN, MSN
Community Health Consultant
San Marcos, Texas

Lauren Outland, DrPH, MSN, RN
Associate Professor, School of Nursing
California State University, Dominguez Hills
Carson, California

Pamela J. Potter, DNSc, RN, CNS-BC
Associate Professor, School of Nursing
University of Portland
Portland, Oregon

Janet F. Quinn, PhD, RN, FAAN
Director, HaelanWorks
Lyons, Colorado

Jennifer Reich, PhD, MA, RN, NC-BC
Part-Time Faculty, School of Nursing
Northern Arizona University
Flagstaff, Arizona

Abby Robin, MSN, Holistic CNS
Westchester Medical Center
Valhalla, New York

Bonney Gulino Schaub, RN, MS, PMHCNS-BC, NC-BC
Co-Director, Huntington Meditation and
    Imagery Center
Director, Transpersonal Coaching Certificate
    Program
Consulting and Coaching
Founder, Florence Press
Steering Committee, Association for the
    Advancement of Psychosynthesis
Huntington, New York

Alyce A. Schultz, RN, PhD, FAAN
Consultant, Clinical Research and Evidence-
    Based Practice
Bozeman, Montana

Marie M. Shanahan, MA, BSN, RN, HN-BC
President and CEO, The BirchTree Center for
    Healthcare Transformation
Florence, Massachusetts

Deborah A. Shields, PhD, RN, CCRN, QTTT, AHN-BC
Associate Professor of Nursing
Capital University
Staff Nurse
Doctors Hospital OhioHealth
Private Practice Therapeutic Touch
Holistic Education and Practice Consultant
Heart of Healing
Columbus, Ohio

Mary Elaine Southard, DNP, RN, APHN-BC, HWNC-BC
Integrative Health Consulting and Coaching,
    LLC
Scranton, Pennsylvania

Sharon Stout-Shaffer, PhD, RN
Professor Emeritus, Department of Nursing
Capital University
Holistic Nursing Education Consultant
Columbus, Ohio

Eileen M. Stuart-Shor, PhD, ANP-BC, FAHA, FAAN
Associate Professor, University of
    Massachusetts, Boston
Nurse Practitioner, Cardiology/Anesthesia/
    Critical Care
Beth Israel Deaconess Medical Center
Boston, Massachusetts

Lucia Thornton, ThD, MSN, RN, AHN-BC
Developer and Author, Whole-Person Caring:
    An Interprofessional Model for Healing and
    Wellness
Consultant, Holistic Nursing Education
Fresno, California
Past President, American Holistic Nurses
    Association

Carol L. Wells-Federman, MEd, MSN, RN
Northwest Regional Coordinator
Reach Out and Read Colorado
Denver, Colorado

Debra Rose Wilson, PhD, MSN, RN, IBCLC, AHN-BC, CHT
Tennessee State University
Nashville, Tennessee
Walden University
Minneapolis, Minnesota

Rothlyn P. Zahourek, PhD, RN, PMHCNS-BC, AHN-BC
Adjunct Clinical Professor, School of Nursing
University of Massachusetts, Amherst
Amherst, Massachusetts

Holistic Philosophy, Theories, and Ethics

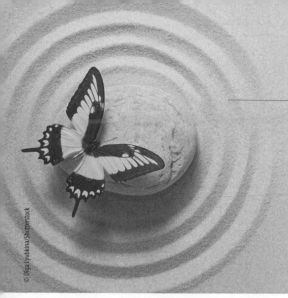

CHAPTER 1

Nursing: Holistic, Integral, and Integrative—Local to Global

Barbara Montgomery Dossey

Nurse Healer Objectives

Theoretical

- Explore global nursing and the effects of decent care and the post-2015 Sustainable Development Goals on health—local to global.
- Link Florence Nightingale's legacy of healing, leadership, global action, and her work as a nurse and citizen activist to 21st-century holistic, integral, and integrative nursing.
- Analyze relationship-centered care and its three components.
- Examine optimal healing environments and their four domains.
- Explore the Theory of Integral Nursing and its application to holistic nursing.

Clinical

- Apply relationship-centered care principles and components in your practice.
- Compare and contrast the three eras of medicine.
- Examine the Theory of Integral Nursing, and begin the process of integrating the theory into your clinical practice.
- Determine whether you have an integral worldview and approach in your clinical practice and other education, research, hospital policies, and community endeavors.

Personal

- Create an integral self-care plan.
- Examine ways to enhance integral understanding in your personal endeavors.
- Develop short- and long-term goals related to increasing your commitment to an integral developmental process.

Definitions

Global health: The area of practice, research, and study that places a priority on improving health and achieving health equity worldwide, reducing health disparities, and providing protection from global health threats (e.g., Ebola) that disregard borders.

Holistic nursing: All nursing practice that has healing the whole person as its goal and honors relationship-centered care and the interconnectedness of self, others, nature, and spirituality; focuses on protecting, promoting, and optimizing health and wellness; incorporates integrative modalities/complementary and alternative modalities (CAM) as appropriate (see Chapter 2 definitions).

Integral nursing: A comprehensive, integral worldview and inclusive way to organize multiple phenomena of human experience related to four perspectives of reality: (1) the individual interior (personal/intentional), (2) individual exterior (physiology/behavioral), (3) collective interior (shared/cultural), and (4) collective exterior (systems/structures); integrative and holistic theories and other paradigms are included; this integral process and integral worldview enlarges our understanding of body-mind-spirit-cultural-environmental connections and our knowing, doing, and being to more comprehensive and deeper levels; incorporates integrative modalities/complementary and alternative modalities (CAM) as appropriate (see the Integral definitions in Table 1-5).

Integrative nursing: A whole-person/whole-system approach that is relationship-centered care where human beings are seen as inseparable from their environments and have an innate capacity for health and well-being. It can be practiced with all patient populations and in all clinical settings and has the potential to strengthen and invigorate the profession; incorporates integrative modalities/complementary and alternative modalities (CAM) as appropriate.

Relationship-centered care: A process model of caregiving that is based in a vision of community in which the patient–practitioner, community–practitioner, and practitioner–practitioner relationships, as well as the unique set of responsibilities of each, are honored and valued.

Nursing: Holistic, Integral, and Integrative

In the future, which I shall not see, for I am old, may a better way be opened! May the methods by which every infant, every human being will have the best chance at health—the methods by which every sick person will have the best chance at recovery, be learned and practiced. Hospitals are only an intermediate stage of civilization, never intended, at all events, to take in the whole sick population. . . .

May we hope that, when we are all dead and gone, leaders will arise who have been personally experienced in the hard, practical work, the difficulties, and the joys of organizing nursing reforms, and who will lead far beyond anything we have done! May we hope that every nurse will be an atom in the hierarchy of ministers of the Highest! But she [or he] must be in her [or his] place in the hierarchy, not alone, not an atom in the indistinguishable mass of thousands of nurses. High hopes, which shall not be deceived!"[1]

These words from Florence Nightingale (1893) empower nurses in their mission of service. In 2010, the Institute of Medicine's landmark report, *The Future of Nursing*, presented four key messages:[2]

1. Nurses should practice to the full extent of their education and training.
2. Nurses should achieve higher levels of education and training through an improved education system that promotes seamless academic progression.
3. Nurses should be full partners, with physicians and other healthcare professionals, in redesigning health care in the United States.
4. Effective workforce planning and policymaking require better data collection and information infrastructure.

Nurses are engaged as change agents to focus on increasing the "health span" of individuals rather than focusing on the length of life span. To accomplish their mission, nurses use the terms *holistic nursing*, *integral nursing*, and *integrative nursing*, all of which are part of nurses raising their voices toward healthy people living on a healthy planet.

Holistic nursing is all nursing practice that has healing the whole person as its goal and honors the interconnectedness of self, others, nature, and spirituality and focuses on protecting, promoting, and optimizing health and wellness.[3] (See Chapter 2 definitions.) Holistic nursing is now officially recognized by the American Nurses Association as a nursing specialty with a defined scope and standards of practice.

Integral nursing can be described as a comprehensive, integral worldview and process that includes holistic theories and other paradigms; holistic nursing practice is included (embraced) and transcended (goes beyond). This integral process and integral worldview enlarge our holistic understanding of body-mind-spirit connections and our knowing, doing, and being to more comprehensive and deeper levels.[4, 5] (See the section on Theory of Integral Nursing later in this chapter for a full discussion.)

Integrative nursing is defined as a whole-person/whole-system approach that is relationship-centered care where human beings are seen as inseparable from their environments and possess healing capacities.[6] It can be practiced with all patient populations and in all clinical settings, and it has the potential to strengthen and invigorate the profession.

Holistic, integral, and integrative nursing all incorporate traditional treatment/protocols and integrative modalities/complementary and alternative modalities (CAM) as appropriate. Nurses must articulate holistic, integral, and integrative nursing with traditional and nontraditional healthcare professionals, healers, disciplines, and organizations to achieve desired outcomes toward health and well-being. Our work is to strengthen the importance of the relationship between practitioner and patient, the focus on the whole person, and to be informed by evidence to achieve optimal health and healing. The next section provides an overview of how we can globally integrate and translate integral, integrative, and holistic nursing concepts.

Global Health, Decent Care, and the Nightingale Declaration

Global Health

Global health is the area of practice, research, and study that places a priority on improving health and achieving health equity worldwide, reducing health disparities, and providing protection against global health threats (e.g., Ebola) that disregard borders.[7, 8] Severe health needs exist in almost every community and country. With globalization and global warming, no natural or political boundaries stop the spread of disease.

The health and well-being of people everywhere can be seen as common ground to secure a sustainable, prosperous future for everyone. Nurses play a major role in mobilizing new approaches to education, healthcare delivery, and disease prevention. Global health requires new leadership models in communication, negotiation, resources, management, work–life balance, mentor–mentee models, and relationships.

Currently, there are an estimated 35 million nurses and midwives engaged in nursing and providing health care around the world.[9] Together, we are collectively addressing human health—the health of individuals, of communities, of environments (interior and exterior), and of the world as our first priority. We are educated and prepared—physically, emotionally, socially, mentally, and spiritually—to accomplish effectively the activities required to create a healthy world. Nurses are key in mobilizing new approaches in health education and healthcare delivery in all areas of nursing. Solutions and evidence-based practice protocols can be shared and implemented around the world through dialogues, the Internet, and publications, all of which are essential as we address the global nursing shortage.[10]

We are challenged to act locally and think globally and to address ways to create healthy environments. For example, we can address global warming in our own personal habits at home as well as in our workplace (using green products, using energy-efficient fluorescent bulbs, turning off lights when not in the room) and simultaneously address our own personal health and the health of the communities where we live. As we expand our awareness of individual and collective states of healing consciousness, as well as holistic, integral, and integrative dialogues, we can explore integral ways of knowing, doing, and being.

We can unite 35 million nurses (**Figure 1-1**) and midwives, along with concerned citizens through the Internet to create a healthy world through many endeavors, such as signing the Nightingale Declaration (at www.nightingaledeclaration.net), as shown in **Figure 1-2**.[11] In the next section, decent care is explored to further our global nursing endeavors at a high level.

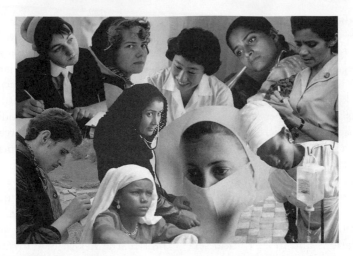

FIGURE 1-1 Global Nurses Collage

Source: Global Nurses Collage from the World Health Organization (WHO).

Photo Credits: Site, Source, Photographer; clockwise from upper left: Switzerland, WHO, John Mohr; Finland, WHO, John Mohr; Japan, WHO, T. Takahara; India, WHO, T. S. Satyan; Brazil, WHO, L. Nadel; Niger, WHO, M. Jacot; Sweden, WHO, John Mohr; Afghanistan, Wikimedia, Ben Barber of USAID; India, Wikimedia, Oreteki; Morocco, WHO, P. Boucas. All World Health Organization (WHO) photos used with attribution as required. Wikimedia Commons: Afghanistan, in the public domain; India, used under the terms of the GNU Free Documentation License.

Nightingale Declaration for A Healthy World

"We, the nurses and concerned citizens of the global community, hereby dedicate ourselves to achieve a healthy world by 2020.

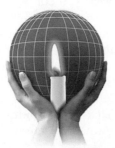

We declare our willingness to unite in a program of action, to share information and solutions and to improve health conditions for all humanity—locally, nationally and globally.

We further resolve to adopt personal practices and to implement public policies in our communities and nations—making this goal achievable and inevitable by the year 2020, beginning today in our own lives, in the life of our nations and in the world at large."

www.NightingaleDeclaration.net

FIGURE 1-2 Nightingale Declaration for a Healthy World by 2020

Source: Used with permission, Nightingale Initiative for Global Health (NIGH), http://www.nightingaledeclaration.net

Decent Care

Nurses extend their nursing in communities to reach the underserved to deliver decent care that is about health for all that leads to human flourishing.[11] Human flourishing begins with building healthy people, neighborhoods, communities, and nations.

Decent care is a comprehensive care continuum approach that is holistic, integral, and integrative.[12, 13] It is inclusive in that individuals are afforded dignity and a destigmatized space to take control of their own destinies. It considers the care and health-related services (physical, preventive, therapeutic, economic, emotional, and spiritual) as well as the person's (includes family, significant others) needs, wants, and expectations. Decent care has the following six key values that parallel the integral perspective discussed later in this chapter:

(1) Agency and (2) Dignity—*individual level.*
(3) Interdependence and (4) Solidarity—*social level.*
(5) Subsidiarity and (6) Sustainability—*systemic level.*

Agency comes from the Latin verb *agere*, which means to drive, lead, act, or do. Agency is the heart of decent care. Without providing the space for, acknowledging, and responding to and respecting the agency of the individual, care is not decent. It is crucial to anyone in a position of vulnerability to own their individual response(s). This means that every person has the capacity to direct her or his own care. *Dignity* represent the humanity of decent care. Without honoring the unique individuality and worth of the "lifeworld" the individual has constructed—her or his needs, desires, relationships, and values—care is not decent.

Interdependence represents the reciprocity of decent care. Without actively participating in our own caring process and in the caring process of others, care is not decent. *Solidarity* represents the communal spirit of decent care. Without being actively responsible for one another's well-being and advocating for one another's needs, care is not decent.

Subsidiarity instructs that people closest to where the care is being offered should allocate resources responsibly. *Sustainability* is the future and legacy of decent care. Without careful stewardship of resources, as well as short- and long-term planning to ensure the ongoing regeneration and evolution of care processes, care is not decent.

Nurses are aware of the challenges of a changing world of individuals' unmet healthcare needs. Three basic questions shape the nurse's approach, the course, and the purpose of decent care in nurse coaching endeavors:[12, 13]

1. What do (I/you/we) need now?
2. How do (I/you/we) live in the face of life/death/wellness/disease?
3. How might (I/you/we) flourish?

With an awareness of the decent care model, nurses can further advance the health framework—local to global. Nurses have an approach to "be with," and they do not tell clients/patients and others what to do. There is a balance of power between the nurse and the client/patient—between those receiving care and those providing care. In the next section, the United Nations Millennium Development Goals and Sustainable Development Goals are discussed to further prepare nurses for global nursing endeavors.

United Nations Millennium Development Goals and Sustainable Development Goals

During the year 2000, world leaders convened a United Nations Millennium Summit to establish eight Millennium Development Goals (MDGs) to be achieved by 2015 in order for the 21st century to progress toward a sustainable quality of life for all of humanity.[14, 15] These goals were an ambitious agenda for improving lives worldwide. Of these eight MDGs, three—Reduce Child Mortality, Improve Maternal Health, and Combat HIV/AIDS, Malaria, and Other Diseases—are directly related to health and nursing. The other five goals—Eradicate Extreme Poverty and Hunger, Achieve Universal Primary Education, Promote Gender Equality and Empower Women, Ensure Environmental Sustainability, and Develop a Global Partnership for Development—are factors that determine the health or lack of health of people.

For each goal, one or more targets, which used the 1990 data as benchmarks, are set to be achieved by 2015. *Health* was the common thread running through all eight MDGs. The goals were directly related to nurses as they worked to achieve them at grassroots levels everywhere while sharing local solutions at the global level.

The MDG framework was a key tool to increase development and concern for development with a time frame that was limited to only 15 years. Thus, it was recognized at the United Nations MDG Summit convened in 2010 that a new and longer framework—the Post-2015 Development Agenda—would need to be implemented.[16] As well, at the Rio+20 Summit convened in the same year, ideas to establish a new set of United Nations Sustainable Development Goals—to be achieved by 2030—were proposed. The combination of these two sets of plans for this agenda resulted in a series of global discussions in several formats and involved—beyond UN-member governments—representatives from nongovernmental organizations, including civil society, philanthropic organizations, academia, and the private sector.

The influence of nursing is global. Nurses, midwives, and allied health professionals must be nurtured and sustained in innovative ways to become like Nightingale—effective voices calling for and demonstrating the healing, leadership, and global actions required to achieve a healthy world. This can strengthen nursing's ranks and help the world to value and nurture nursing's essential contributions. As Nightingale said, "We must create a public opinion, which must drive the government instead of the government having to drive us, . . . an enlightened public opinion, wise in principle, wise in detail."[17] Nurses are initiating new approaches and connecting the dots by empowering both individuals and groups to revisit Nightingale's legacy in 21st-century terms, as discussed next.

Philosophical Foundation: Florence Nightingale's Legacy

Florence Nightingale (1820–1910) (see **Figure 1-3**), the philosophical founder of modern secular nursing and the first recognized nurse theorist, was an integralist. An *integralist* is a person

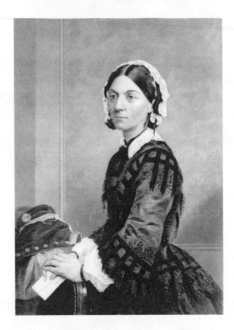

FIGURE 1-3 Florence Nightingale (1820–1910)
Source: Courtesy of the National Library of Medicine.

who focuses on the individual and the collective, the inner and outer, human and nonhuman concerns. Nightingale was concerned with the most basic needs of human beings and all aspects of the environment (clean air, water, food, houses, etc.)—local to global.[18, 19] She also experienced and recorded her personal understanding of the connection with the Divine as an awareness that something greater than she—the Divine—was a major connecting link woven into her work and life.[18]

Nightingale was a nurse, educator, administrator, communicator, statistician, and environmental activist.[18, 19] Her specific accomplishments include establishing the model for nursing schools throughout the world and creating a prototype model of care for the sick and wounded soldiers during the Crimean War (1854–1856). She was an innovator for British Army medical reform that included reorganizing the British Army Medical Department, creating an Army Statistical Department, and collaborating on the first British Army medical school, including developing the curriculum and choosing the professors.

Nightingale revolutionized hospital data collection and invented a statistical wedge diagram equivalent to today's circular histograms or circular statistical representation. In 1858, she became the first woman admitted to the Royal Statistical Society. She developed and wrote protocols and papers on workhouses and midwifery that led to successful legislation reform. She was a recognized expert on the health of the British Army and soldiers in India for more than 40 years; she never went to India but collected data directly from Army stations, analyzed the data, and wrote and published documents, articles, and books on the topic.

In 1902, in addition to her numerous other recognitions, she was the first woman to receive the Order of Merit. She wrote more than 100 combined books and official Army reports. Her 10,000 letters now make up the largest private collection of letters at the British Library, with 4,000 family letters at the Wellcome Trust in London.[18]

Today, we recognize Nightingale's work as global nursing: She envisioned what a healthy world might be with her integral philosophy and expanded visionary capacities. Her work included aspects of the nursing process (see Chapter 7) as well; it has indeed had an influence on nurses today and will continue to affect us far into the future. Nightingale's work was social action that demonstrated and clearly articulated the science and art of an integral worldview for nursing, health care, and humankind. Her social action was also sacred activism, the fusion of the deepest spiritual knowledge with radical action in the world.

In the 1880s, Nightingale began to write that it would take 100 to 150 years before educated and experienced nurses would arrive to change the healthcare system. We are that generation of 21st-century Nightingales who have arrived to transform health care and carry forth her vision of social action and sacred activism to create a healthy world.

Nightingale was ahead of her time. Her dedicated and focused 40 years of work and service still inform and influence our nursing work and our global mission of health and healing for humanity today. Table 1-1 lists the themes found in her *Notes on Hospitals* (1860),[20] in her *Notes on Nursing* (1860),[21] in her formal letters to her nurses (1872–1900),[22] and in her article

"Sick-Nursing and Health-Nursing" (1893).[1] **Table 1-2** shows Nightingale's themes recognized today as total healing environments. The next section presents an overview of the eras of medicine and application of this information to integral, integrative, and holistic nursing.

Eras of Medicine

Three eras of medicine currently are operational in Western biomedicine (see **Table 1-3**).[23] Era I medicine began to take shape in the 1860s, when medicine was striving to become scientific. The underlying assumption of this approach is that health and illness are completely physical in nature. The focus is on combining drugs, medical treatments, and technology for curing. A person's consciousness is considered a by-product of the chemical, anatomic, and physiologic aspects of the brain and is not considered a major factor in the origins of health or disease.

In the 1950s, Era II therapies began to emerge. These therapies reflected the growing awareness that the actions of a person's mind or consciousness—thoughts, emotions, beliefs, meaning, and attitudes—exerted important effects on the behavior of the person's physical body. In both Era I and Era II, a person's consciousness is said to be "local" in nature—that is, confined to a specific location in space (the body itself) and in time (the present moment and a single lifetime).[24]

Era III, the newest and most advanced era, originated in science.[25] Consciousness is said to be nonlocal in that it is not bound to individual bodies. The minds of individuals are spread throughout space and time; they are infinite, immortal, omnipresent, and, ultimately, one. Era III therapies involve any therapy in which the effects of consciousness create bridges between different persons, as with distant healing, intercessory prayer, shamanic healing, so-called miracles, and certain emotions (e.g., love, empathy, compassion). Era III approaches involve transpersonal experiences of being. They raise a person above control at a day-to-day material level to an experience outside his or her local self.

TABLE 1-1   Florence Nightingale's Legacy and Themes for Today

Themes Developed in *Notes on Hospitals* (1860, 1863)

The hospital will do the patient no harm. Four elements essential for the health of hospitals:

- Fresh air
- Light
- Ample space
- Subdivision of sick into separate buildings or pavilions

Hospital construction defects that prevented health:

- Defective means of natural ventilation and warming
- Defective height of wards
- Excessive width of wards between the opposite windows
- Arrangement of the bed along the dead wall
- More than two rows of beds between the opposite windows
- Windows only on one side, or a closed corridor connecting the wards
- Use of absorbent materials for walls and ceilings, and poor washing of hospital floors
- Defective condition of water closets
- Defective ward furniture
- Defective accommodation for nursing and discipline
- Defective hospital kitchens
- Defective laundries
- Selection of bad sites and bad local climates for hospitals
- Erecting of hospitals in towns
- Defects of sewerage
- Construction of hospitals without free circulation of external air

Themes Developed in *Notes on Nursing* (1860)

Understand God's laws in nature

- Understanding that, in disease and in illness, nursing and the nurses can assist in the reparative process of a disease and in maintaining health

Nursing and nurses

- Describing the many roles and responsibilities of the nurse

Patient

- Observing and managing the patient's problems, needs, and challenges and evaluating responses to care

Health

- Recognizing factors that increase or decrease positive or negative states of health, well-being, disease, and illness

Environment

- Both the internal (within one's self) and the external (physical space). (See the specifics listed in the next 12 categories.)

Bed and bedding

- Promote proper cleanliness.
- Use correct type of bed, with proper height, mattress, springs, types of blankets, sheets, and other bedding.

Cleanliness (rooms and walls)

- Maintain clean room, walls, carpets, furniture, and dust-free rooms using correct dusting techniques.
- Release odors from painted and papered rooms; discusses other remedies for cleanliness.

Cleanliness (personal)

- Provide proper bathing, rubbing, and scrubbing of the skin of the patient as well as of the nurse.
- Use proper handwashing techniques that include cleaning the nails.

Food

- Provide proper portions and types of food at the right time and a proper presentation of food types: eggs, meat, vegetables, beef teas, coffee, jellies, sweets, and homemade bread.

Health of houses

- Provide pure air, pure water, efficient drainage, cleanliness, and light.

Light

- Provide a room with light, windows, and a view that is essential to health and recovery.

Noise

- Avoid noise and useless activity such as clanking or loud conversations with or among caregivers.
- Speak clearly for patients to hear without having to strain.
- Avoid surprising the patient.
- Read to a patient only if it is requested.

Petty management

- Ensure patient privacy, rest, a quiet room, and instructions for the person managing care of patient.

TABLE 1-1   Florence Nightingale's Legacy and Themes for Today (*continued*)

Themes Developed in *Notes on Nursing* (1860) (*continued*)

Variety

- Provide flowers and plants and avoid those with fragrances.
- Be aware of effects of mind (thoughts) on body.
- Help patients vary their painful thoughts.
- Use soothing colors.
- Be aware of positive effect of certain music on the sick.

Ventilation and warming

- Provide pure air within and without; open windows and regulate room temperature.
- Avoid odiferous disinfectants and sprays.

Chattering hopes and advice

- Avoid unnecessary advice, false hope, promises, and chatter of recovery.

- Avoid absurd statistical comparisons of patient to recovery of other patients, and avoid mockery of advice given by family and friends.
- Share positive events; encourage visits from a well-behaved child or baby.
- Be aware of how small pet animals can provide comfort and companionship for the patient.

Observation of the sick

- Observe each patient; determine the problems, challenges, and needs.
- Assess how the patient responds to food, treatment, and rest.
- Help patients with comfort, safety, and health strategies.
- Intervene if danger to patients is suspected.

Themes Developed in Letters to Her Nurses (1872–1900)

All themes above in *Notes on Hospitals* and *Notes on Nursing* plus:

Art of nursing

- Explore authentic presence, caring, meaning, and purpose.
- Increase communication with colleagues, patients, and families.
- Build respect, support, and trusting relationships.

Environment

- The environment includes the internal self as well as the external physical space.

Ethics of nursing

- Engage in moral behaviors and values and model them in personal and professional life.

Health

- Integrate self-care and health-promoting and sustaining behaviors.
- Be a role model and model healthy behaviors.

Personal aspects of nursing

- Explore body-mind-spirit wholeness, healing philosophy, self-care, relaxation, music, prayers, and work of service to self and others.
- Develop therapeutic and healing relationships.

Science of nursing

- Learn nursing knowledge and skills, observing, implementing, and evaluating physicians' orders combined with nursing knowledge and skills.

Spirituality

- Develop intention, self-awareness, mindfulness, presence, compassion, love, and service to God and humankind.

Themes Developed in "Sick-Nursing and Health-Nursing" (1893 Essay)

All themes above in *Notes on Nursing* and *Florence Nightingale to Her Nurses* (1872–1893) plus:

Collaboration with others

- Meet with nurses and women at the local, national, and global level to explore health education and how to support each other in creating health and healthy environments.

Health education curriculum and health missioners education

- Include all components discussed in *Notes on Nursing*.
- Teach health as proactive leadership for health.

Source: Used with permission. B. M. Dossey, "Florence Nightingale's Tenets: Healing, Leadership, Global Action," in *Florence Nightingale Today: Healing, Leadership, Global Action,* eds. B. M. Dossey et al. (Silver Spring, MD: Nursesbooks.org, 2005).

TABLE 1-2   Total Healing Environments Today: Holistic and Integral

Internal Healing Environment

- Includes presence, caring, compassion, creativity, deep listening, grace, honesty, imagination, intention, love, mindfulness, self-awareness, trust, and work of service to self and others.
- Grounded in ethics, philosophies, and values that encourage and nurture such qualities as are listed above and in a way that:
  - Engages body-mind-spirit wholeness
  - Fosters healing relationships and partnerships
  - Promotes self-care and health-promoting and sustaining behaviors
  - Engages with and is affected by the elements of the external healing environment (below)

External Healing Environment

Color and texture

- Use color that creates healing atmosphere, sacred space, moods, and that lifts spirits.
- Coordinate room color with bed coverings, bedspreads, blankets, drapes, chairs, food trays, and personal hygiene kits.
- Use textural variety on furniture, fabrics, artwork, wall surfaces, floors, ceilings, and ceiling light covers.

Communication

- Provide availability of caring staff for patient and family.
- Provide a public space for families to use television, radio, and telephones.

Family areas

- Create facilities for family members to stay with patients.
- Provide a comfortable family lounge area where families can keep or prepare special foods.

Light

- Provide natural light from low windows where patient can see outside.
- Use full-spectrum light throughout hospitals, clinics, schools, public buildings, and homes.
- Provide control of light intensity with good reading light to avoid eye strain.

Noise control

- Eliminate loudspeaker paging systems in halls and elevators.
- Decrease noise of clanking latches, food carts and trays, pharmacy carts, slamming of doors, and noisy hallways.
- Provide 24-hour continuous music and imagery channels such as Healing Healthcare Systems Continuous Ambient Relaxation Environment (www.healinghealth.com), Aesthetic Audio Systems (www.aestheticaudiosystems.com), and other educational channels related to health and well-being.
- Decrease continuous use of loud commercial television.
- Eliminate loud staff conversations in unit stations, lounges, and calling of staff members in hallways.

Privacy

- Provide a Do Not Disturb sign for patient and family to place on door to control privacy and social interaction.
- Position bed for view of outdoors, with shades to screen light and glare.
- Use full divider panel or heavy curtain for privacy if in a double-patient room.
- Secure place for personal belongings.
- Provide shelves to place personal mementos such as family pictures, flowers, and totems.

TABLE 1-2   Total Healing Environments Today: Holistic and Integral (*continued*)

Thermal comfort
- Provide patient control of air circulation, room temperature, fresh air, and humidity.

Ventilation and air quality
- Provide fresh air, adequate air exchange, rooftop gardens, and solariums.
- Avoid use of toxic materials such as paints, synthetic materials, waxes, and foul-smelling air purifiers.

Views of nature
- Use indoor landscaping, which may include plants and miniature trees.
- Provide pictures of landscapes that include trees, flowers, mountains, ocean, and the like for patient and staff areas.

Holistic, integral, and integrative practices

Throughout hospitals, clinics, schools, and all parts of a community:
- Combine conventional medical treatments, procedures, and surgery with complementary and alternative therapies and folk medicine.
- Engage in integral and interdisciplinary dialogues and collaboration that foster deep personal support, trust, and therapeutic alliances.
- Offer educational programs for professionals that teach the specifics about the interactions of the healer and healee, holistic philosophy, patient-centered care, relationship-centered care, and complementary and alternative therapies.
- Develop and build community and partnerships based on mutual support, trust, values, and exchange of ideas.
- Use strategies that enhance the interconnectedness of persons, nature, inner and outer, spiritual and physical, and private and public.
- Use self-care and health-promoting education that includes prevention and public health.
- Provide support groups, counseling, and psychotherapy, specifically for cancer and cardiac support groups, lifestyle change groups, and 12-step programs and support groups, and for leisure, exercise, and nutrition and weight management.
- Use health coaches for staff, patients, families, and community.
- Provide information technology and virtual classroom capabilities.

Source: Used with permission. B. M. Dossey, "Florence Nightingale's Tenets: Healing, Leadership, Global Action," in *Florence Nightingale Today: Healing, Leadership, Global Action*, eds. B. M. Dossey, L. C. Selanders, D. M. Beck, and A. Attewell (Silver Spring, MD: Nursesbooks.org, 2005). Used with permission.

"Doing" and "Being" Therapies

Holistic nurses use both "doing" and "being" therapies. These are also referred to as holistic nursing therapies, complementary and alternative therapies, or integrative and integral therapies throughout this text. Doing therapies include almost all forms of modern medicine, such as medications, procedures, dietary manipulations, radiation, and acupuncture. In contrast, being therapies do not employ things but instead use states of consciousness.[23] These include imagery, prayer, meditation, and quiet contemplation, as well as the presence and intention of the nurse. These techniques are therapeutic because of the power of the psyche to affect the body. They may be either directed or nondirected.[24] A person who uses a directed mental strategy attaches a specific outcome to the imagery, such as the regression of disease or the normalization of blood pressure. In a nondirected approach, the person images the best outcome for the situation but does not try to direct the situation or assign a specific outcome to the strategy. This reliance on the inherent intelligence within oneself to come forth is a way of acknowledging the intrinsic wisdom and self-correcting capacity within.

It is obvious that Era I medicine uses doing therapies that are highly directed in their approach. It employs things, such as medications, for a specific goal. Era II medicine is a

TABLE 1-3 Eras of Medicine			
	Era I	**Era II**	**Era III**
Space–Time Characteristic	Local	Local	Nonlocal
Synonym	Mechanical, material, or physical medicine	Mind–body medicine	Nonlocal or transpersonal medicine
Description	Causal, deterministic, describable by classical concepts of space–time and matter–energy. Mind not a factor; "mind" a result of brain mechanisms.	Mind a major factor in healing within the single person. Mind has causal power; is thus not fully explainable by classical concepts in physics. Includes but goes beyond Era I.	Mind a factor in healing both within and between persons. Mind not completely localized to points in space (brains or bodies) or time (present moment or single lifetimes). Mind is unbounded and infinite in space and time—thus omnipresent, eternal, and ultimately unitary or one. Healing at a distance is possible. It is describable by classical concepts of space–time or matter–energy.
Examples	Any form of therapy focusing solely on the effects of things on the body is an Era I approach, including techniques such as acupuncture and homeopathy, the use of herbs, etc. Almost all forms of "modern" medicine—drugs, surgery, irradiation, CPR, etc.—are included.	Any therapy emphasizing the effects of consciousness solely within the individual body is an Era II approach. Psychoneuroimmunology, counseling, hypnosis, biofeedback, relaxation, therapies, and most types of imagery-based "alternative" therapies are included.	Any therapy in which effects of consciousness bridge between different persons is an Era III approach. All forms of distant healing, intercessory prayer, some types of shamanic healing, diagnosis at a distance, telesomatic events, and probably noncontact therapeutic touch are included.

Source: Table [p.19: "Medical Eras"] from REINVENTING MEDICINE by LARRY DOSSEY, M.D. Copyright © 1999 by Larry Dossey, M.D. Reprinted by permission of HarperCollins Publishers.

classic body–mind approach that usually does not require the use of things, except for biofeedback instrumentation, music therapy, and CDs and videos to enhance learning and experience an increase in awareness of body–mind connections. It employs being therapies that can be directed or nondirected, depending on the mental strategies selected (e.g., relaxation or meditation).

Era III medicine is similar in this regard. It requires a willingness to become aware, moment by moment, of what is true for our inner and outer experience. It is actually a "not doing" so that we can become conscious of releasing, emptying, trusting, and acknowledging that we have done our best, regardless of the outcome. As the therapeutic potential of the mind becomes increasingly clear, all therapies and all people are viewed as having a transcendent quality. The minds of all people, including families, friends, and the healthcare team (both those in close proximity and those at a distance), flow together in a collective as they work to create healing and health.[25]

Rational Versus Paradoxical Healing

All healing experiences or activities can be arranged along a continuum from the rational domain to the paradoxical domain. The degree of doing and being involved determines these domains. Rational healing experiences include those therapies or events that make sense to our linear, intellectual thought processes, whereas paradoxical healing experiences include healing events that may seem absurd or contradictory but are, in fact, true.[23]

Doing therapies fall into the rational healing category. Based on science, these strategies conform to our worldview of commonsense notions. Often, the professional can follow an algorithm that dictates a step-by-step approach. Examples of rational healing include surgery, irradiation, medications, exercise, and diet. On the other hand, being therapies fall into the paradoxical healing category because they frequently happen without a scientific explanation. In psychological counseling, for example, a breakthrough is a paradox. When a patient has a psychological breakthrough, it is clear that there is a new meaning for the person. However, no clearly delineated steps led to the breakthrough. Such an event is called a breakthrough for the very reason that it is unpredictable—thus, the paradox.

Biofeedback also involves a paradox. For example, the best way to reduce blood pressure or muscle tension, or to increase peripheral blood flow, is to give up trying and just learn how to be. Individuals can enter into a state of being, or passive volition, in which they let these physiologic states change in the desired direction. Similarly, the phenomenon of placebo is a paradox. If an individual has just a little discomfort, a placebo does not work very well.

Miracle cures also are paradoxical because there is no scientific mechanism to explain them. Every nurse has known, heard of, or read about a patient who had a severe illness that had been confirmed by laboratory evidence but that disappeared after the patient adopted a being approach. Some say that it was the natural course of the illness; some die and some live.

At shrines such as Lourdes in France and Medjugorje in Yugoslavia, however, people who experience a miracle cure are said to be totally immersed in a being state. They do not try to make anything happen. When interviewed, these people report experiencing a different sense of space and time; the flow of time as past, present, and future becomes an eternal now. Birth and death take on new meaning and are not seen as a beginning and an end.

Premonition literally means "forewarning."[26] Premonitions are a cautioning about something just around the corner, something that is usually unpleasant. It may be a health crisis, a death in the family, or a national disaster. But premonitions come in all flavors. Sometimes they provide information about positive, pleasant happenings that lie ahead—a job promotion, the location of the last remaining parking space, or, in some instances, the winning lottery numbers.

These people go into the self and explore the "not I" to become empty so that they can understand the meaning of illness or present situations. To further integrate these concepts, relationship-centered care is discussed next.

Relationship-Centered Care

In 1994, the Pew Health Professions Commission published its landmark report on relationship-centered care.[27] This report serves as a guideline for addressing the bio-psycho-social-spiritual-cultural-environmental dimensions of individuals in integrating caring and healing into health care. The guidelines are based on the tenet that relationships and interactions among people constitute the foundation for all therapeutic activities.

Relationship-centered care serves as a model of caregiving that is based in a vision of community where three types of relationships are identified: (1) patient–practitioner relationships, (2) community–practitioner relationships, and (3) practitioner–practitioner relationships.[27] Each of these interrelated relationships is essential within a reformed system of health care, and each involves a unique set of tasks and responsibilities that address self-awareness, knowledge, values, and skills.

Patient–Practitioner Relationship

The patient–practitioner relationship is crucial on many levels. The practitioner incorporates comprehensive biotechnologic care with psycho-social-spiritual care. To work effectively within the patient–practitioner relationship, the practitioner must develop specific knowledge, skills, and values.[27] This includes an expanding self-awareness, understanding the patient's experience of health and illness, developing and maintaining caring relationships with patients, and communicating clearly and effectively.

Active collaboration with the patient and family in the decision-making process, promotion of health, and prevention of stress and illness within the family are also part of the relationship. A successful relationship involves active listening and effective communication; integration of the elements of caring, healing, values, and ethics to enhance and preserve the dignity and integrity of the patient and family; and a reduction of the power inequalities in the relationship with regard to race, sex, education, occupation, and socioeconomic status.

Community–Practitioner Relationship

In integral health care, the patient and his or her family simultaneously belong to many types of communities, such as the immediate family, relatives, friends, coworkers, neighborhoods, religious and community organizations, and the hospital community. The knowledge, skills, and values needed by practitioners to participate effectively in and work with various communities include understanding the meaning of the community, recognizing the multiple contributors to health and illness within the community, developing and maintaining relationships with the community, and working collaboratively with other individuals and organizations to establish effective community-based care.[27]

Practitioners must be sensitive to the effect of these various communities on patients and foster the collaborative activities of these communities as they interact with the patient and family. The restraints or barriers within each community that block the patient's healing must be identified and improved to promote the patient's health and well-being.

Practitioner–Practitioner Relationship

Providing integral care to patients and families can never take place in isolation; it involves many diverse practitioner–practitioner relationships. To form a practitioner–practitioner

relationship requires specific knowledge, skills, and values, including developing self-awareness; understanding the diverse knowledge base and skills of different practitioners; developing teams and communities; and understanding the working dynamics of groups, teams, and organizations that can provide resource services for the patient and family.[27]

Collaborative relationships entail shared planning and action toward common goals with joint responsibility for outcomes. There is a difference, though, between multidisciplinary care and interdisciplinary care. Multidisciplinary care consists of the sequential provision of discipline-specific health care by various individuals. Interdisciplinary care, however, also includes coordination, joint decision making, communication, shared responsibility, and shared authority.

Because the cornerstone of all therapeutic and healing endeavors is the quality of the relationships formed among the practitioners caring for the patient, all practitioners must understand and respect one another's roles. Conventional and alternative practitioners need to learn about the diversity of therapeutic and healing modalities that they each use. In addition, conventional practitioners must be willing to integrate complementary and alternative practitioners and their therapies in practice (e.g., acupuncture, herbs, aromatherapy, touch therapies, music therapy, folk healers).[3, 28] Such integration requires learning about the experiences of different healers, being open to the potential benefits of different modalities, and valuing cultural diversity. Ultimately, the effectiveness of collaboration among practitioners depends on their ability to share problem solving, goal setting, and decision making within a trusting, collegial, and caring environment. Practitioners must work interdependently rather than autonomously, with each assuming responsibility and accountability for patient care.

After 20 years of leadership and advocacy for health professions education, the philosophy of relationship-centered care[3, 29, 30] and holistic, integral, and integrative concepts are part of the mission and vision of interprofessional collaboration that are also contained in the *Healthy People 2020* report[31] and the Affordable Care Act.[32] In the next section, core competencies and integrative leadership for interprofessional collaborative practice are discussed.

Core Competencies and Integrative Leadership for Interprofessional Collaborative Practice

The Interprofessional Education Collaborative Expert Panel has identified the necessary core competencies for interprofessional collaborative practice that would be safe, high quality, accessible, and inclusive of patient-centered care.[33] Six organizations comprise the expert panel: American Association of Colleges of Nursing, American Association of Colleges of Osteopathic Medicine, American Association of Colleges of Pharmacy, American Dental Education Association, Association of American Medical Colleges, and Association of Schools of Public Health. To achieve its vision the expert panel showed that health professions students need continuous development of interprofessional competencies as an essential part of their learning process. When this type of education occurs, they are more likely to enter the workforce ready to practice effective teamwork and team-based care.

Each expert panel group contributed its competencies, which resulted in interprofessional collaborative practice competencies identified in the following four domains: (1) values/ethics for interprofessional practice, (2) roles/responsibilities, (3) interprofessional communication, and (4) teams and teamwork.[33]

Teaching of these interprofessional collaborative competencies must extend beyond profession-specific education so that students are more likely to work effectively as members of clinical teams. In teaching interprofessional competencies and collaboration with the goal of practicing relationship-centered care, new theories, such as complexity theories,[34] nurse coaching,[35, 36] and health coaching[37] that includes the underserved,[38] will transform organizations and communities. To cross the patient-centered divide and apply relationship-centered care, interprofessional development must include mindfulness practice, formation, and training in

communication skills. The next section explores several examples of how these concepts are being translated.

Creating Optimal Healing Environments

The Samueli Institute (www.samueliinstitute .org) studies relationship-centered care and ways to transform organizational culture through research and innovative projects that articulate and demonstrate a complete optimal healing environment (OHE) framework of actionable practices and evaluation methods.[39] The institute defines an OHE as one in which "the social, psychological, spiritual, physical and behavioral components of health care are oriented toward support and stimulation of healing and the achievement of wholeness." From this perspective, facilitating healing is thought to be a crucial aspect of managing chronic illness and the basis for sustainable health care.

Key concepts in optimal healing environments are awareness and intention. Awareness is a state of being conscious and "in touch" with one's interior and exterior self that is cultivated through reflective practices (meditation, prayer, mindfulness, spiritual practices, journaling, dialogue, art, etc.). **Table 1-4** shows that an OHE contains four environmental domains: internal, interpersonal, behavioral, and external. Under these four domains are eight constructs that each have several elements. The shading shows how these components, elements, and specific areas are integrated with all others. All aspects of this information are connected, from the internal environment to the outer environments of the individual and the collective. Optimal healing environments always start with the individual, whether it is the practitioner, healer, healee (client/patient), a significant other, and/or the community as an entity. Implementing these steps can lead to more cost-effective, efficient organizations in which the environment truly facilitates healing and where practitioners are fully supported to connect to the "soul of healing" and the mission of caring.

Another innovative organization is Planetree International, a global leader in healing

TABLE 1-4	Optimal Healing Environments

Optimal Healing Environments

Surround the individual with elements that facilitate the innate healing process.

Internal	Interpersonal	Behavioral	External
Healing intention	Healing relationships	Healthy lifestyles	Healing spaces
Personal wholeness	Healing organizations	Integrative care	Ecological sustainability

Making healing as important as curing

Source: © 2013 Used with permission. Samueli Institute for Information Biology, 1737 King Street, Suite 600, Alexandria, VA 23314. www.samueliinstitute.org.

environments and innovative patient-centered care models.[40] In healthcare settings throughout the United States, Canada, and Europe, Planetree demonstrates that patient-centered care is not only an empowering philosophy, it is a viable, vital, and cost-effective model. The Planetree model is implemented in acute and critical care departments, emergency departments, long-term care facilities, outpatient services, as well as in ambulatory care and community health centers. The Planetree model of care is a patient-centered, holistic approach to health care that promotes mental, emotional, spiritual, social, and physical healing. It empowers patients and families through the exchange of information and encourages healing partnerships with caregivers. It seeks to maximize positive healthcare outcomes by integrating optimal medical therapies and incorporating art and nature into the healing environment.

As interprofessional collaboration steadily increases and blends traditional health care with integrative health care and complementary and alternative therapies, the relationship-centered care model that includes compassion can assist traditional and integrative practitioners to achieve the highest level of care. This level of care requires modeling health and healing in personal and professional endeavors along with new educational endeavors.[41-43] An example is

the Penny George Institute for Health and Healing, the largest hospital-based program of its kind in the country. It is setting national standards for enhancing health care through a holistic and integrative health approach as follows:[44]

- Blending complementary therapies, integrative medicine, and conventional Western medicine
- Providing services to inpatients and outpatients
- Educating healthcare professionals
- Teaching community members about health promotion and self-healing practices
- Conducting research to identify best practices of integrative health and the effects of these services on healthcare costs

In the next section, the Theory of Integral Nursing is discussed.

Theory of Integral Nursing

Overview

The Theory of Integral Nursing is a grand theory that presents the science and art of nursing. It includes an integral process, integral worldview, and integral dialogues that are praxis— theory in action.[4, 5] Concepts specific to the

Theory of Integral Nursing are set in italics throughout this chapter. Please consider these words as a frame of reference and a way to explain what you have observed or experienced with yourself and others. Definitions specific to the Theory of Integral Nursing are presented in **Table 1-5**.

As you read about the Theory of Integral Nursing, remember that the words *integral* and *integrally informed* are used often because this is a shift to a deeper level of understanding about being human as related to the four dimensions of reality. It is incorrect to substitute the word *holistic* because it does not mean the same thing. Consider where you are now in your life. As a novice, intermediate, or expert nurse, you bring a wealth of experiences that inform you at the professional and personal levels. Begin to explore the integral process in your thinking,

projects, and endeavors. Examine whether your approaches are reductionistic, narrow, or limited, or whether you have an integral awareness and integral understanding that includes the four perspectives of reality.

To decrease further fragmentation in the nursing profession, the Theory of Integral Nursing incorporates existing theoretical work in nursing that builds on our solid holistic and multidimensional theoretical nursing foundation. This theory may be used with other holistic nursing and nonnursing caring concepts, theories, and research; it does not exclude or invalidate other nurse theorists who have informed this theory (see Chapter 5). This is not a freestanding theory because it incorporates concepts and philosophies from various paradigms including holism, multidimensionality, integral, chaos, spiral dynamics, complexity, systems, and many others.

TABLE 1-5   Theory of Integral Nursing: Definitions

Integral: A comprehensive way to organize multiple phenomena of human experience related to four perspectives of reality: (1) the individual interior (personal/intentional), (2) individual exterior (physiology/behavioral), (3) collective interior (shared/cultural), and (4) collective exterior (systems/structures).

Integral dialogue: A transformative and visionary exploration of ideas and possibilities across disciplines where the individual interior (personal/intentional), individual exterior (physiology/behavioral), collective interior (shared/cultural), and collective exterior (structures/systems) are considered as equally important to exchanges and outcomes.

Integral healing process: Contains both nurse processes and patient/family and healthcare worker processes (individual interior and individual exterior), as well as collective healing processes of individuals and systems/structures (collective interior and exterior); an understanding of the unitary whole person interacting in mutual process with the environment.

Integral health: A process through which we reshape basic assumptions and worldviews about well-being and see death as a natural process of living; may be symbolically viewed as a jewel with many facets that is reflected as a "bright gem" or a "rough stone" depending on one's situation and personal growth that influences states of health, health beliefs, and values.

Integral health care: A patient- and relationship-centered caring process that includes the patient, family, and community and conventional, integrative, and integral healthcare practitioners and services and interventions; a process where the individual interior (personal/intentional), individual exterior (physiology/behavioral), collective interior (shared/cultural), and collective exterior (structures/systems) are considered in all endeavors.

Integral nurse: A 21st-century Nightingale who is engaged as a "health diplomat" and an integral health coach who is coaching for integral health.

Integral nursing: A comprehensive, integral worldview and process that includes holistic theories and other paradigms; holistic nursing is included (embraced) and transcended (goes beyond); this integral process and integral worldview enlarges our holistic understanding of body-mind-spirit connections and our knowing, doing, and being to more comprehensive and deeper levels.

Integral worldview: A process where values, beliefs, assumptions, meanings, purposes, and judgments are identified and related to how individuals perceive reality and relationships that include the individual interior (personal/intentional), individual exterior (physiology/behavioral), collective interior (shared/cultural), and collective exterior (systems/structures).

An integral understanding allows us to more fully comprehend the complexity of human nature and healing; it assists nurses in bringing to health care and society their knowledge, skills, and compassion. The integral process and an integral worldview present a comprehensive map and perspective related to the complexity of wholeness and how to simultaneously address the health and well-being of nurses, patients, families and significant others, the healthcare team, the healthcare system/structure, and the world.

The nursing profession asks nurses to wrap around "all of life" on so many levels with self and others that we often can feel overwhelmed. How do we get a handle on "all of life"? The question always arises: "How can overworked nurses and student nurses use an integral approach or apply the Theory of Integral Nursing?" The answer is to start right now. By the time you finish reading this chapter you will find the answers to these questions. Be aware of healing, the core concept in this theory; it is the innate natural phenomenon that comes from within a person and describes the indivisible wholeness, the interconnectedness of all people and all things.

Reflect on this clinical situation. Imagine that you are caring for a very ill patient who needs to be transported to a radiology procedure. The current protocol for transportation between the medical unit and the radiology department lacks continuity. In this moment, shift your feelings and your interior awareness (and believe it!) to: "I am doing the best that I can in this moment," and "I have all the time needed to take a deep breath and relax my tight chest and shoulder muscles." This helps you connect these four perspectives as follows: (1) the interior self (caring for yourself in this moment); (2) the exterior self (using a research-based relaxation and imagery integral practice to change your physiology); (3) the self in relationship to others (shifting your awareness creates another way of being with your patient and the radiology team member); and (4) the relationship to the exterior collective of systems/structures (considering ways to work with the radiology team member and department to improve a transportation procedure in the hospital).

An integral worldview and approach can help each nurse and student nurse increase her or his self-awareness, as well as the awareness of how one's self affects others—the patient, family, colleagues, and the workplace and community. As the nurse discovers her or his own innate healing from within, the nurse can model self-care and how to release stress, anxiety, and fear that manifest each day in this human journey.

All nursing curricula can be mapped to the integral quadrants (see the section on application of the theory later in this chapter). This teaches students to think integrally and to become aware of an integral perspective and how these four perspectives create the whole. Students can also learn the importance of self-care at all times as faculty also remember that they are role models and must model self-care and these integral ideas.

Developing the Theory of Integral Nursing: Personal Journey

As a young nurse attending my first nursing theory conference in the late 1960s, I was captivated by nursing theory and the eloquent visionary words of these theorists as they spoke about the science and art of nursing. This opened my heart and mind to the exploration and necessity to understand and to use nursing theory. Thus, I began my professional commitment to address theory in all endeavors as well as to increase my understanding of other disciplines that could inform me at a deeper level about the human experience. I realized that nursing was neither a science nor an art, but both/and. From the beginning of my critical care and cardiovascular nursing focus, I learned how to combine science and technology with the art of nursing. For example, I gave a patient with severe pain following an acute myocardial infarction pain medication while simultaneously guiding him in a relaxation practice to enhance relaxation and release anxiety. I also experienced a difference in myself when I used this approach combining the science and art of nursing.

In the late 1960s, I also began to study and attend workshops on holistic and mind–body related ideas as well as read in other disciplines such as systems theory; quantum physics; integral, Eastern, and Western philosophy and mysticism; and more. I also read nurse theorists and other discipline theorists who informed my knowing, doing, and being in caring, healing, and holism. My husband, an internist, who was also caring for critically ill patients and their families, was with me on this journey of discovery. As we cared for critically ill patients and their families, some of our greatest teachers, we were able to reflect on how to blend the art of caring, healing modalities with the science of technology and traditional modalities. I joined with a critical care and cardiovascular nursing colleague and soul mate, Cathie Guzzetta, with whom I could also discuss these ideas. We began to write teaching protocols and lecture in critical care courses as well as write textbooks and articles with other contributors.

My husband and I both had health challenges—mine was postcorneal transplant rejection and my husband's was blinding migraine headaches. We both began to take courses related to body-mind-spirit therapies (biofeedback, relaxation, imagery, music, meditation, and other reflective practices) and began to incorporate them into our daily lives. As we strengthened our capacities with self-care and self-regulation modalities, our personal and professional philosophies and clinical practices changed. We took seriously teaching and integrating these modalities into the traditional healthcare setting that today is called *integrative and integral health care*. From then until now, we have found many professional and interdisciplinary healthcare colleagues with whom to discuss concepts, protocols, and approaches for practice, education, and research.

In 1981, I was a founding member of the American Holistic Nurses Association (AHNA). In November 2006, with Lynn Keegan, Cathie Guzzetta, and many other colleagues, we obtained recognition by the American Nurses Association (ANA) of our collective holistic nursing endeavors as the specialty of holistic nursing. The AHNA and ANA *Holistic Nursing: Scope and Standards of Practice* was first published in June 2007 and revised in 2013.[3] I now believe that the important specialty of holistic nursing can be expanded by using an integral lens.

Beginning in 1992 in London during my Florence Nightingale primary historical research studying and synthesizing her original letters,

army and public health documents, manuscripts, and books, I deepened my understanding of Nightingale's relevance to holistic nursing. Nightingale was indeed an integralist. This revelation led to my Nightingale authorship[18] and my collaborative Nightingale Initiative for Global Health and the Nightingale Declaration,[11] the first global nursing Internet signature campaign. My current professional mission is to articulate and use the integral process and integral worldview in my nursing, in integrative nurse coaching (see Chapter 21), and healthcare endeavors and to explore rituals of healing with many.

My sustained nursing career focus with nursing colleagues on wholeness, unity, and healing and my Florence Nightingale scholarship have resulted in numerous protocols and standards for practice, education, research, and healthcare policy. My integral focus since 2000 and my many conversations with Ken Wilber[45-50] and the integral team and other interdisciplinary integral colleagues have led to my development of the Theory of Integral Nursing. It is exciting to see other nurses expanding the holistic process and incorporating the integral model as well.

Theory of Integral Nursing Intentions and Developmental Process

The intention (purpose) in a nursing theory is the aim of the theory. The Theory of Integral Nursing has three intentions: (1) to embrace the unitary whole person and the complexity of the nursing profession and health care; (2) to explore the direct application of an integral process and integral worldview that includes four perspectives of realities—the individual interior and exterior and the collective interior and exterior; and (3) to expand nurses' capacities as 21st-century Nightingales, health diplomats, and integral health coaches who coach for integral health—local to global.

The Theory of Integral Nursing develops the evolutionary growth processes, stages, and levels of humans' development and consciousness to move toward a comprehensive integral philosophy and understanding. This can assist nurses to more deeply map human capacities that begin with healing to evolve to the transpersonal self and connection with the Divine, however defined or identified, and their collective endeavors to create a healthy world.

The Theory of Integral Nursing development process at this time is to strengthen our 21st-century nursing endeavors. We can expand personal awareness of our holistic and caring, healing knowledge and approaches with traditional nursing and health care.

Nursing and health care are fragmented. Collaborative practice has not been realized because only portions of reality are seen as being valid within health care and society. Often, there is a lack of respect for one another. We also do not consistently listen to the pain and suffering that nurses experience within the profession, and neither do we consistently listen to the pain and suffering of the patient and family members or of our colleagues.

Self-care is a low priority. Time is not given or valued within practice settings for nurses to address basic self-care such as short breaks for personal needs and meals; this is made worse by short staffing and overtime. Professional burnout is extremely high, and many nurses are very discouraged. Nurse retention is at a crisis level throughout the world. As nurses integrate an integral process and integral worldview and use daily integral life practices, they will be healthy and model health more consistently and understand the complexities of healing. This will then enhance nurses' capacities for empowerment, leadership, and being change agents for a healthy world.

Integral Foundation and the Integral Model

The Theory of Integral Nursing adapts the work of Ken Wilber (1949–), one of the most significant American new-paradigm philosophers, to strengthen the core concept of healing. Wilber's integral model is an elegant, four-quadrant model that has been developed over 35 years. In his eight-volume *Collected Works of Ken Wilber*,[45-50] Wilber synthesizes the ideas and theories of the best-known and most influential researchers and theorists to show that no individual or discipline can determine reality or have all of the answers.

Many concepts within this integral nursing theory have been researched or are in very

formative stages and exploration within integral medicine, integral healthcare administration, integral business, integral healthcare education, integral psychotherapy, integral coaching, and more. Within the nursing profession, other nurses are also exploring integral and related theories and ideas.[51-58] The Theory of Integral Nursing combines Nightingale's philosophical foundation as an integralist with the integral process and integral worldview. When nurses consider the use of an integral lens they are more likely to expand nurses' roles in interdisciplinary dialogues, explore commonalities, and examine differences and how to address these across disciplines. Our challenge in nursing is to increase our integral awareness as we increase our nursing capacities, strengths, and voices in all areas of practice, education, research, and healthcare policy.

Content, Context, and Process

To present the Theory of Integral Nursing, Barbara Barnum's framework to critique a nursing theory provides an organizing structure that is most useful.[59] Her approach, which examines content, context, and process, highlights what is most critical to understand a theory, and it avoids duplication of explanations within the theory. In the next section, the Theory of Integral Nursing philosophical assumptions are provided. The reader is encouraged to integrate the integral process concepts and to experience how the word *integral* expands one's thinking and worldview. To remove the word *integral* or to substitute the word *holistic* diminishes the effect of the expansiveness of the integral process and integral worldview and its implications, as previously stated. The philosophical assumptions of the Theory of Integral Nursing are listed in **Table 1-6**.

Content Components

Content of a nursing theory includes the subject matter and building blocks that give a theory form. It comprises the stable elements that are acted on or that do the acting. In the Theory of Integral Nursing, the subject matter and building blocks are as follows: (1) healing, (2) the metaparadigm of nursing theory, (3) patterns

TABLE 1-6   Theory of Integral Nursing: Philosophical Assumptions

1. An integral understanding recognizes the wholeness of humanity and the world that is open, dynamic, interdependent, fluid, and continuously interacting with changing variables that can lead to greater complexity and order.

2. An integral worldview is a comprehensive way to organize multiple phenomena of human experience and reality and identifies these phenomena as the individual interior (subjective, personal), individual exterior (objective, behavioral), collective interior (intersubjective, cultural), and collective exterior (interobjective, systems/structures).

3. Healing is a process inherent in all living things; it may occur with curing of symptoms, but it is not synonymous with curing.

4. Integral health is experienced by individuals as well as groups, communities, nations, cultures, and ecosystems as wholeness with development toward personal growth and expanding states of consciousness to deeper levels of personal and collective understanding of one's physical, mental, emotional, social, spiritual, relational, sexual, and psychodynamic dimensions.

5. Integral nursing is founded on an integral worldview, using integral language and integral knowledge that are enacted in these integral life practices and skills.

6. Integral nursing has the capacity to include all ways of knowing and knowledge development.

7. Integral nursing is applicable in any context, and its scope includes all aspects of human experience.

8. An integral nurse is an instrument in the healing process and facilitates healing through her or his knowing, doing, and being.

Source: Data from Barbara Dossey.

of knowing, (4) the four quadrants that are adapted from Wilber's integral theory (individual interior [subjective, personal/intentional], individual exterior [objective, behavioral], collective interior [intersubjective, cultural], and collective exterior [interobjective, systems/structures]), and (5) "all quadrants, all levels, all lines" that are adapted from Wilber.[45]

Content Component 1: Healing

The first content component in the Theory of Integral Nursing is healing, which is illustrated as a diamond shape and shown in **Figure 1-4**.

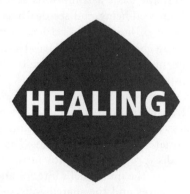

FIGURE 1-4 Healing

Source: Data from Barbara Dossey.

The Theory of Integral Nursing enfolds the central core concept of healing. It embraces the individual as an energy field that is connected with the energy fields of all humanity and the world. Healing is transformed when we consider four perspectives of reality in any moment: (1) the individual interior (personal/intentional), (2) individual exterior (physiology/behavioral), (3) collective interior (shared/cultural), and (4) collective exterior (systems/structures). Using our reflective integral lens of these four perspectives of reality assists us to grasp the complexity that emerges in healing.

Healing includes knowing, doing, and being and is a lifelong journey and process of bringing aspects of oneself at deeper levels into harmony and stages of inner knowing that lead to integration.[5] This healing process places us in a space to face our fears, to seek and express self in its fullness, and to learn to trust life, creativity, passion, and love. Each aspect of healing has equal importance and value and leads to more complex levels of understanding and meaning.

We are born with healing capacities. It is a process inherent in all living things. No one can take healing away from life, although we often get stuck in our healing or forget that we possess it because of life's continuous challenges and perceived barriers to wholeness. Healing can take place at all levels of human experience, but it may not occur simultaneously in every realm. In truth, healing most likely does not occur simultaneously or even in all realms, and yet the person may still have a perception of healing having happened.

Healing is not predictable; it may occur with curing of symptoms, but it is not synonymous with curing. Curing may not always happen, but the potential for healing to occur is always present, even at one's last breath. Intention and intentionality are key factors in healing. *Intention* is being in the present moment with a conscious action. *Intentionality* is holding the heartspace with compassion in our knowing, doing, and being while performing an action.[60, 61]

Content Component 2: Metaparadigm of Nursing Theory

The second content component in the Theory of Integral Nursing is the recognition of the metaparadigm in a nurse theory—nurse, person, health, and environment (society), shown in **Figure 1-5**. These concepts are important to the Theory of Integral Nursing because they are encompassed within the quadrants of

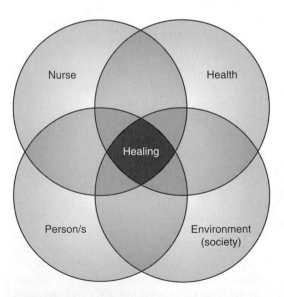

FIGURE 1-5 Healing and Metaparadigm of Nursing Theory

Source: Data from Barbara Dossey.

human experience, as shown in content component 4. Starting with healing at the center, a Venn diagram surrounds healing and implies the interrelated and interdependent effects of these domains as each informs and influences the others; a change in one creates a degree of change in the others, thus affecting healing at many levels.

An *integral nurse* is defined as a 21st-century Nightingale who serves as a health coach while coaching for health that implies engagement in social action and sacred activism, that is working from soul's purpose. As nurses strive to be integrally informed, they are more likely to move to a deeper experience of a connection with the Divine or Infinite, however defined or identified. Integral nursing provides a comprehensive way to organize multiple phenomena of human experience in the four perspectives of reality. The nurse is an instrument in the healing process. She or he brings the whole self into relationship with the whole self of another or a group of significant others, and this reinforces the meaning and experience of oneness and unity.

A *person* is defined as an individual (patient/client, family member, significant other) who engages with a nurse in a manner that is respectful of a person's subjective experiences of health, health beliefs, values, sexual orientation, and personal preferences. A person also can be an individual nurse who interacts with a nursing colleague, other healthcare team members, or a group of community members or other groups.

Integral health is the process through which nurses reshape basic assumptions and worldviews about well-being and see death as a natural process of living. Integral health implies connecting body-mind-spiritual-cultural-environment while striving to reach one's highest potential.

It may also be imagined as a spiral or a symbol of transformation to higher states of consciousness where we can more fully understand the essential nature of our Beingness as energy fields and expressions of wholeness.[61-66] This acknowledges the individual's interior and exterior experiences and the shared collective interior and exterior experiences where authentic power is recognized within each person.

Disease and illness at the physical level may manifest for many reasons. It is important not to equate physical health with mental health or spiritual health because they are not the same. Each is a facet of the jewel of integral health.

An *integral environment* has both interior and exterior aspects. The interior environment includes the individual's feelings; meanings; mental, emotional, and spiritual dimensions; and a person's brain stem, cortex, and other anatomic parts that are internal (inside) aspects of the exterior self. The interior environment also acknowledges the patterns that may not be understood but that may manifest related to various situations or relationships, including those related to living and nonliving people and things, such as the memory of a deceased relative or animal, or a lost precious object stimulated by a current situation (for example, a touch may bring forth past memories of abuse or suffering). Insights gained through dreams and other reflective practices that reveal symbols, images, and other connections also influence one's interior environment. The exterior environment includes objects that can be seen and measured and that are related to the physical and social in any of the gross, subtle, and causal levels that are discussed in component 4.

Content Component 3: Patterns of Knowing

The third content component in the Theory of Integral Nursing is the recognition of the patterns of knowing in nursing, as shown in **Figure 1-6**. These six patterns of knowing are personal, empirics, aesthetics, ethics, not knowing, and sociopolitical. As a way to organize nursing knowledge, Carper,[67] in her now classic 1978 article, identifies the four fundamental patterns of knowing (personal, empirics, ethics, aesthetics), which was followed by the introduction of the pattern of not knowing in 1993 by Munhall,[68] and the pattern of sociopolitical knowing by White in 1995.[69] All of these patterns continue to be refined and reframed with new applications and interpretations. These patterns of knowing assist nurses in bringing themselves into the full expression of being present in the moment with self and others to integrate aesthetics with science and to develop the flow of ethical experience with thinking and acting. (As all patterns of knowing in the Theory of Integral Nursing are superimposed on Wilber's four quadrants in Figure 1-6, these patterns will primarily be positioned as shown; however, they may also appear in one, several, or all quadrants and inform all other quadrants.)

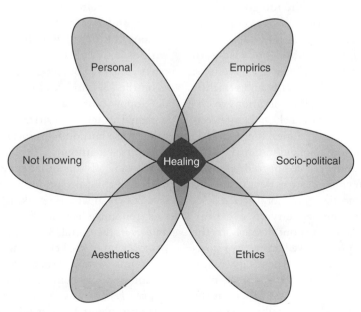

FIGURE 1-6 Healing and Patterns of Knowing in Nursing

Source: Modified from B. Carper (1978), Fundamental Patterns of Knowing in Nursing, Advances in Nursing Science 1(1).

Personal knowing is the nurse's dynamic process and awareness of wholeness that focuses on the synthesis of perceptions and being with self. It may be developed through art, meditation, dance, music, stories, and other expressions of the authentic and genuine self in daily life and nursing practice.

Empirical knowing is the science of nursing that focuses on formal expression, replication, and validation of scientific competence in nursing education and practice. It is expressed in models and theories and can be integrated into evidence-based practice. Empirical indicators are accessed through the known senses and are subject to direct observation, measurement, and verification.

Aesthetic knowing is the art of nursing that focuses on how to explore experiences and meaning in life with self or another that includes authentic presence, the nurse as a facilitator of healing, and the artfulness of a healing environment. It is the combination of knowledge, experience, instinct, and intuition that connects the nurse with a patient or client to explore the meaning of a situation about the human experiences of life, health, illness, and death. It calls forth resources and inner strengths from the nurse to be a facilitator in the healing process. It is the integration and expression of all of the other patterns of knowing in nursing praxis.

Ethical knowing is the moral knowledge in nursing that focuses on behaviors, expressions, and dimensions of both morality and ethics. It includes valuing and clarifying situations to create formal moral and ethical behaviors intersecting with legally prescribed duties. It emphasizes respect for the person, the family, and the community that encourages connectedness and relationships that enhance attentiveness, responsiveness, communication, and moral action.

Not knowing is the capacity to use healing presence, to be open spontaneously to the moment with no preconceived answers or goals to be obtained. It engages authenticity, mindfulness, openness, receptivity, surprise, mystery, and discovery with self and others in the subjective space and the intersubjective space that allows for new solutions, possibilities, and insights to emerge.

Sociopolitical knowing addresses the important contextual variables of social, economic, geographic, cultural, political, historical, and other key factors in theoretical, evidence-based practice and research. This pattern includes informed critique and social justice for the voices of the underserved in all areas of society along with protocols to reduce health disparities.

Content Component 4: Quadrants

The fourth content component in the Theory of Integral Nursing, as shown in **Figure 1-7**, examines four perspectives for all known aspects of reality, or, expressed another way, it is how we look at and describe anything. The Theory of Integral Nursing core concept of healing is transformed by adapting Ken Wilber's integral model.[45]

Starting with healing at the center to represent our integral nursing philosophy, human capacities, and global mission, dotted horizontal and vertical lines are shown to illustrate that each quadrant can be understood as permeable and porous, with each quadrant experience integrally informing and empowering all other quadrant experiences.

Within each quadrant we see "I," "We," "It," and "Its" to represent four perspectives of realities that are already part of our everyday language and awareness. (When working with various cultures, it is important to know that within many cultures the "I" comes last or is never verbalized or recognized because the focus is on the "we" and relationships. However, this development of the "I" and awareness of one's personal values are critical to a healthy nurse to decrease burnout and increase nurse renewal and nurse retention.)

Virtually all human languages use first-, second-, and third-person pronouns.[45] First person is "the person who is speaking," which includes the pronouns *I*, *me*, *mine* in the singular and *we*, *us*, *ours* in the plural. Second person means "the person who is spoken to," which includes the pronouns *you* and *yours*. Third person is "the person or thing being spoken about," such as *she*, *her*, *hers*, *he*, *him*, *his*, or *they*, *it*, *their*, and *its*. For example, if I am speaking about my new car, "I" am first person, and "you" are second person, and the new car is third person. If you

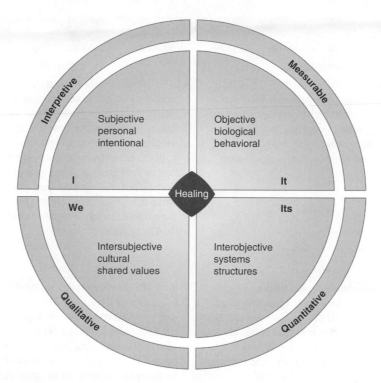

FIGURE 1-7 Healing and the Four Quadrants (I, We, It, Its)

Source: Adapted with permission from Ken Wilber. www.kenwilber.com.

and I are communicating, the word *we* is used to indicate that we understand one another. *We* is technically first person plural, but if·you and I are communicating, then your second person and my first person are part of this extraordinary *we*. We can simplify first, second, and third person as *I*, *we*, *it*, and *its*.

These four quadrants show the four primary dimensions or perspectives of how we experience the world; these are represented graphically as the Upper-Left, Upper-Right, Lower-Left, and Lower-Right quadrants. It is simply the inside and the outside of an individual and the inside and the outside of the collective. It includes expanded states of consciousness where one feels a connection with the Divine and the vastness of the universe and the infinite that is beyond words. Integral nursing considers all of these areas in our personal development and any area of practice, education, research, and healthcare policy—local to global. Each quadrant, which is intricately linked and bound to one another, carries its own truths

and language. The specifics of the quadrants are described as follows and are shown in **Table 1-7**.

On the outside of Figure 1-7, the left-hand quadrants (Upper Left, Lower Left) describe aspects of reality as interpretive and qualitative. In contrast, the right-hand quadrants (Upper Right, Lower Right) describe aspects of reality as measurable and quantitative. When we fail to consider these subjective, intersubjective, objective, and interobjective aspects of reality, our endeavors and initiatives are fragmented and narrow and we often fail to reach identified outcomes and goals. The four quadrants are a result of the differences and similarities in Wilber's investigation of the many aspects of identified reality.[45] The model describes the territory of our own awareness that is already present within us and an awareness of things outside of us. These quadrants help us connect the dots of the actual process to understand more deeply who we are and how we are related to others and all things. See Chapter 8 to explore the steps of the holistic caring process through the four quadrants of Integral Theory.

TABLE 1-7 Integral Model and Quadrants	
Upper Left In this "I" space (subjective; the inside of the individual) can be found the world of the individual's interior experiences. These are the thoughts, emotions, memories, perceptions, immediate sensations, and states of mind (imagination, fears, feelings, beliefs, values, esteem, cognitive capacity, emotional maturity, moral development, and spiritual maturity). Integral nursing requires development of the "I."	*Upper Right* In this "It" (objective; the outside of the individual) space can be found the world of the individual's exterior. This includes the material body (physiology [cells, molecules, neurotransmitters, limbic system], biochemistry, chemistry, physics), integral patient care plans, skill development (health, fitness, exercise, nutrition, etc.), behaviors, leadership skills, and integral life practices (see the section on Process), as well as anything that we can touch or observe scientifically in time and space. Integral nursing with our nursing colleagues and healthcare team members includes the "It" of new behaviors, integral assessment and care plans, leadership, and skills development.
Lower Left In this "We" (intersubjective; the inside of the collective) space can be found the interior collective of how we can come together to share our cultural backgrounds, stories, values, meanings, visions, languages, relationships, and how to form partnerships to achieve a healing mission. This can decrease our fragmentation and enhance collaborative practice and deep dialogue around things that really matter. Integral nursing is built on "We."	*Lower Right* In this "Its" space (interobjective; the outside of the collective) can be found the world of the collective, exterior things. This includes social systems/structures, networks, organizational structures, and systems (including financial and billing systems in health care), information technology, regulatory structures (environmental and governmental policies, etc.), and any aspect of the technological environment and in Nature and the natural world. Integral nursing identifies the "Its" in the structure that can be enhanced to create more integral awareness and integral partnerships to achieve health and healing—local to global.

Source: Modified from Ken Wilber, Integral Psychology: Consciousness, Spirit, Psychology, Therapy (Boston: Shambhala, 2000). Table adapted with permission from Ken Wilber. http://www.kenwilber.com.

Content Component 5: AQAL (All Quadrants, All Levels)

The fifth content component in the Theory of Integral Nursing is the exploration of Wilber's "all quadrants, all levels, all lines, all states, all types" or AQAL (pronounced ah-qwul), as shown in **Figure 1-8**. These levels, lines, states, and types are important elements of any comprehensive map of reality. The integral model simply assists us in further articulating and connecting all areas, awarenesses, and depths in these four quadrants. Briefly, these levels, lines, states, and types are as follows:[45]

- *Levels.* Levels of development that become permanent with growth and maturity (e.g., cognitive, relational, psychosocial, physical, mental, emotional, spiritual) that represent increased organization or complexity. These

levels are also referred to as waves and stages of development. Each individual possesses the masculine and feminine voice or energy. Neither masculine nor feminine is higher or better; they are two equivalent types at each level of consciousness and development.

- *Lines.* Developmental areas that are known as multiple intelligences: cognitive line (awareness of what is); interpersonal line (how I relate socially to others); emotional/affective line (the full spectrum of emotions); moral line (awareness of what should be); needs line (Maslow's hierarchy of needs); aesthetics line (self-expression of art, beauty, and full meaning); self-identity line (Who am I?); spiritual line (where spirit is viewed as its own line of unfolding and not just as ground and highest state); and values line (what a person considers most

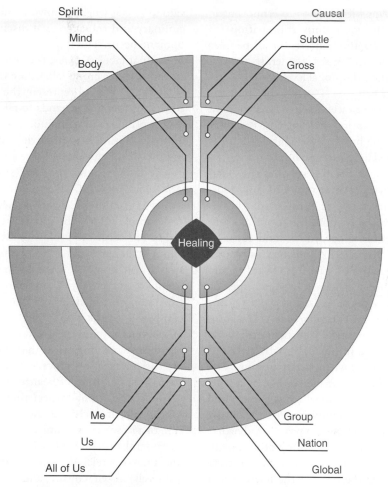

FIGURE 1-8 Healing and AQAL (All Quadrants, All Levels)

Source: Adapted with permission from Ken Wilber. www.kenwilber.com. Copyright © 2007, B. Dossey.

important; studied by Clare Graves and brought forward by Don Beck[70] in his Spiral Dynamics Integral, which is beyond the scope of this chapter).

- *States.* Temporary changing forms of awareness: waking, dreaming, deep sleep, altered meditative states (resulting from meditation, yoga, contemplative prayer, etc.), altered states (resulting from mood swings, physiology, and pathophysiology shifts with disease, illness, seizures, cardiac arrest, low or high oxygen saturation, or drugs), peak experiences (triggered by intense listening to music, walks in Nature, love making, mystical experiences such as hearing the voice of God or the voice of a deceased person, etc.).

- *Types.* Differences in personality and masculine and feminine expressions and development (e.g., cultural creative types, personality types, enneagram).

This part of the Theory of Integral Nursing, as shown in Figure 1-8, starts with healing at the center surrounded by three increasing concentric circles with dotted lines of the four quadrants. This aspect of the integral theory moves to higher orders of complexity through personal growth, development, expanded stages of consciousness (permanent and actual milestones of growth and development), and evolution. These levels or stages of development can also be expressed as being self-absorbed (such as a child or infant), which evolves to ethnocentric (centers on group, community, tribe, nation), to worldcentric (care and concern for all peoples regardless of race, color, sex, gender, sexual orientation, creed), to the global level.

In the Upper Left, the "I" space, the emphasis is on the unfolding awareness from body to mind to spirit. Each increasing circle includes the lower as it moves to the higher level. This quadrant is further explained in the section on process.

The Upper Right, the "It" space, is the external of the individual. Every state of consciousness has a felt energetic component that is expressed from the wisdom traditions as three recognized bodies: gross, subtle, and causal.[45] We can think of these three bodies as the increasing capacities of a person toward higher levels of consciousness. Each level is a specific vehicle that provides the actual support for any state of awareness. The *gross body* is the individual physical, material, sensorimotor body that we experience in our daily activities. The *subtle body* manifests when we are not aware of the gross body of dense matter but of a shift to light, energetic, emotional feelings and fluid and flowing images. Examples are a shift during a dream, during different types of bodywork, during walks in Nature, or during other experiences that move us to a profound state of bliss. The *causal body* is the body of the infinite that is beyond space and time. Causal also includes all aspects of Era III medicine and nonlocality where minds of individuals are not separate in space and time.[25]

When this is applied to consciousness, separate minds behave as if they are linked regardless of how far apart in space and time they may be. Nonlocal consciousness may underlie phenomena such as remote healing, intercessory prayer, telepathy, premonitions, as well as so-called miracles. Nonlocality also implies that the soul does not die with the death of the physical body— hence, immortality forms some dimension of consciousness.[25] Nonlocality can also be both an upper- and lower-quadrant phenomenon.

The Lower Left, the "We" space, is the interior collective dimension of individuals who come together. The concentric circles from the center outward represent increasing levels of complexity of our relational aspect of shared cultural

values. This is where teamwork and the interdisciplinary and transpersonal disciplinary development occur. The inner circle represents the individual labeled as *me*; the second circle represents a larger group labeled *us*; the third circle is labeled *all of us* to represent the largest group consciousness that expands to all people. These last two circles may include people as well as animals, Nature, and nonliving things that are important to individuals.

The Lower Right, the "Its" space, the exterior social system and structures of the collective, is represented with concentric circles. An example within the inner circle might be a group of healthcare professionals in a hospital clinic or department or the complex hospital system and structure. The middle circle expands in increased complexity to include a nation; the third concentric circle represents even greater complexity to the global level where the health of all humanity and the world is considered. It is also helpful to emphasize that these groupings are the physical dynamics such as the working structure of a group of healthcare professionals versus the relational aspect that is a lower-left aspect, and the technical and informatics structure of a hospital or a clinic.

Integral nurses strive to integrate concepts and practices related to body, mind, and spirit (all levels) in self, culture, and Nature (all quadrants). The individual interior and exterior—"I" and "It"—as well as the collective interior and exterior—"We" and "Its"—must be developed, valued, and integrated into all aspects of culture and society. The AQAL integral approach suggests that we consciously touch all of these areas and do so in relation to self, to others, and to the natural world. Yet to be integrally informed does not mean that we have to master all of these areas; we just need to be aware of them and choose to integrate integral awareness and integral practices. Because these areas are already part of our being-in-the-world and cannot be imposed from the outside (they are part of our makeup from the inside), our challenge is to identify specific areas for development and find new ways to deepen our daily integral life practices.

Wilber uses the term *holon* to describe anything that is itself whole or part of some other whole that creates structures, from the very smallest to the largest, with increasing complexity.[45] The upper half of the model represents the individual holons, or the "micro world." The lower quadrants represent the social or communal holons, or the "macro world." These holons create a holarchy of natural evolutionary processes. As one progresses up a holarchy, the lower levels of holons are transcended and included and thus are foundational. All of the entities or holons in the right-hand quadrants possess simple location. These are things that are perceived with our senses such as rocks, villages, organisms, ecosystems, and planets. However, none of the entities or holons in the left-hand quadrants possess simple location. One cannot see feelings, concepts, states of consciousness, or interior illumination. They are complex experiences that exist in emotional space, conceptual space, spiritual space, and our mutual understanding space. The development of one's individual consciousness as part of self-care is primary to the development of all other quadrants and integral thinking, application, and integration.

This aspect of the Theory of Integral Nursing helps us understand coherence and resilience.[71] *Coherence* is the quality of being logically integrated, consistent, and intelligible (as a coherent statement). It implies correlations, connectedness, consistency, efficient energy utilization, wholeness, and global order. A *coherent state* is an increase in physiologic efficiency, and alignment of the mental and emotional systems accumulates resilience (energy) across all four energetic domains. *Resilience* is related to self-management and efficient utilization of energy resources across four domains: physical, emotional, mental, and spiritual. High-level resilience helps us recover from challenging situations and prevents unnecessary stress reactions (frustration, impatience, anxiety) that deplete physical and psychological resources. *Physical resilience* is reflected in physical flexibility, endurance, and strength. *Mental resilience* is reflected in attention span, mental flexibility, optimistic worldview, and ability to integrate multiple points of view. *Emotional resilience* is related to one's ability to self-regulate the degree of emotional flexibility, positive emotions, and relationships. *Spiritual resilience* is related to commitment to core values, intuition, and tolerance of others' values and beliefs.

Structure

The structure of the Theory of Integral Nursing is shown in **Figure 1-9**. All content components are overlaid to create a mandala to symbolize wholeness. Healing is placed at the center, and then the metaparadigm of nursing (integral nurse, person, integral health, integral environment), the patterns of knowing (personal, empirics, aesthetics, ethics, not knowing, sociopolitical), the four quadrants (subjective, objective, intersubjective, interobjective), and all quadrants and all levels of growth, development, and evolution. (Note: Although the patterns of knowing are superimposed as they are in the various quadrants, they can also fit into other quadrants.)

Using the language of Ken Wilber[45] and Don Beck[70] and his Spiral Dynamics Integral, individuals move through primitive, infantile consciousness to an integrated language that is considered first-tier thinking. As they move up the spiral of growth, development, and evolution and expand their integral worldview and integral consciousness, they move into what is considered second-tier thinking and participation. This is a radical leap into holistic, systemic, and integral modes of consciousness. Wilber also expands to a third-tier stage of consciousness that addresses an even deeper level of transpersonal understanding that is beyond the scope of this chapter.

Context

Context in a nursing theory is the environment in which nursing acts occur and the nature of the world of nursing. In an integral nursing environment, the nurse strives to be an integralist, which means that she or he strives to be integrally informed and is challenged to further develop an integral worldview, integral life practices, and integral capacities, behaviors, and skills. An integral nurse values, articulates, and models the integral process and integral worldview, as well as integral life practices and

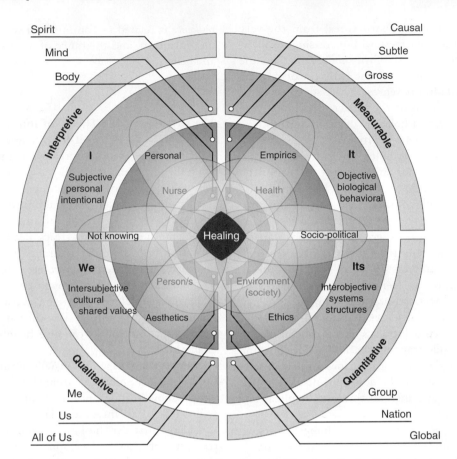

FIGURE 1-9 Theory of Integral Nursing (Healing, Metaparadigm, Patterns of Knowing in Nursing, Four Quadrants, and AQAL)

Source: Adapted with permission from Ken Wilber. www.kenwilber.com.

self-care in nursing practice, education, research, and healthcare policies.

The term *nurse healer* is used to describe a nurse as an instrument in the healing process and a major part of the exterior healing environment of a patient, family, or another. Nurses assist and facilitate individuals with accessing their own healing process and potentials; the nurses do not do the actual healing. An integral nurse also recognizes self as part of the exterior healing environment interacting with a person, family, or colleague and enters into a shared experience (or field of consciousness) that promotes healing potentials and an experience of well-being.

A key concept in an integral healing environment, both interior and exterior, is meaning, which addresses that which is indicated, referred

to, or signified.[72] *Philosophical meaning* is related to one's view of reality and the symbolic connections that can be grasped by reason. *Psychological meaning* is related to one's consciousness, intuition, and insight. *Spiritual meaning* is related to how one deepens personal experience of a connection with the Divine. This may occur by whatever mechanism or modalities an individual uses to feel a sense of oneness, belonging, and a feeling of connection in this human journey of life.

Process

Process in a nursing theory is the method by which the theory works. An integral healing process contains both nurse processes and patient, family, healthcare workers' processes (individual interior and individual exterior), as well as collective healing processes of individuals and of systems/structures (collective interior and exterior). This is the understanding of the unitary whole person interacting in mutual process with the environment.

There are many opportunities to increase our integral awareness, application, and understanding each day. Reflect on all that you do each day in your work and life—analyzing, communicating, listening, exchanging, surveying, involving, synthesizing, investigating, interviewing, mentoring, developing, creating, researching, teaching, and creating new schemes for what is possible. Before long you will realize how these four quadrants and realities fit together. You will also discover whether you are completely missing a quadrant, thus an important part of reality.

As we address and value the individual interior and exterior, the "I" and "It," as well as the collective interior and exterior, the "We" and "Its," a new level of integral understanding emerges, and we may find that there is also

more balance and harmony each day. By incorporating the integral nursing principles discussed next, we may assist others to discover their own healing path. The reader is referred to Figure 1-9 and Table 1-7 for specific components of each quadrant. **Figure 1-10** provides examples of Florence Nightingale's integral ideas as related to each integral nursing principle.

Integral Nursing Principle 1: Nursing Requires Development of the "I"

Integral nursing principle 1 recognizes the interior individual "I" (subjective) space. Each of us must value the importance of exploring one's health and well-being, starting with our own personal exploration and development on many levels.

Nightingale saw nursing first as a calling that was very individual and personal. Throughout her life and nursing career, she reflected carefully on her own thoughts, motives, and desires,

From "Sick-Nursing and Health-Nursing" 1893

Subjective "I"   **Objective "It"**

"What is it to feel a calling for anything? Is it not to do our work in it to satisfy the high idea of what is right and best and not because we shall be found out if we don't do it?" [p.193] She distinguished "calling" as the creation of a life of caring, that deep desire to serve with an involvement of one's whole being – physically, emotionally, mentally and spiritually.

Florence Nightingale addressed her concerns for health by reminding her readers of their responsibilities as citizens. Speaking from her own long experience with informing the public about health issues, she asked her readers to join her: "You must form public opinion.... Officials will only do what you make them. You, the public, must make them do what you want." [p.191]

She called for an "espirit de corps" to forge new methods, collaborations and foster bridge-building in her time. She noted that "the health of the unity of is the health of the community. Unless you have the health of the unity, there is no community health." and called people together secure the best air, the best food, and all that makes life useful, healthy and happy." [p.197]

Her definition of health was "not only to be well, but to be able to use well every power we have." [p.186] She reminded her readers that nursing addressed such "stupendous issues as life and death, health and disease." [p.187] She noted that — as we address these issues, at both micro and macro levels — ultimately "health is [our] only capital." [p.191]

(a)   Intersubjective "We"   **Interobjective "Its"**

FIGURE 1-10 Florence Nightingale's Integral Ideas

Source: Used with permission from the Nightingale Initiative for Global Health (NIGH), Ottawa, Ontario, Canada, and Washington, DC, and B. M. Dossey, L. C. Selanders, D. M. Beck, and A. Attewell, *Florence Nightingale Today: Healing, Leadership, Global Action* (Silver Spring, MD: Nursesbooks.org, 2005).

Subjective "I"   Objective "It"

"Nursing work must be quiet work— an individual work — anything else is contrary to the whole realness of the work. Where am I, the individual, in my utmost soul? What am I, the inner woman, called 'I'? That is the question." (1896)

When we obey all God's laws as to cleanliness, fresh air, pure water, good habits, good dwellings, good drains, food and drink, work and exercise, health is the result: when we disobey, sickness.... No epidemic can resist thorough cleanliness and fresh air." (1876)

"Let us run the race where all may win: rejoicing in their successes, as our own and mourning their failures, wherever they are, as our own. We are all one Nurse... The very essence of all good organization is, that everybody should do her [and his] own work in such a way as to help and not hinder every one else's work." [1873]

"Nursing takes a whole life to learn. We must make progress every year... Nursing is not an adventure, as some have now supposed.... It is a very serious, delightful thing, like life, requiring training, experience, devotion not by fits and starts, patience, a power of accumulating, instead of losing all these things. We are only on the threshold of training. [1897]

(b) *Intersubjective "We"*   *Interobjective "Its"*

FIGURE 1-10   Florence Nightingale's Integral Ideas (*continued*)

Source: Used with permission from the Nightingale Initiative for Global Health (NIGH), Ottawa, Ontario, Canada and Washington, DC and B. M. Dossey, L. C. Selanders, D. M. Beck, and A. Attewell, *Florence Nightingale Today: Healing, Leadership, Global Action* (Silver Spring, MD: Nursesbooks.org, 2005).

as well as her own knowledge, skills, and conduct. In her 1888 address, she wrote:

> Nursing work must be quiet work— an individual work. Anything else is contrary to the whole realness of the work. Where am I, the individual, in my utmost soul? What am I, the inner woman [man], called "I"? That is the question.[73]

This development of the individual "I" supports each nurse in deeply understanding one's interior as well as developing the qualities of nursing presence, the aesthetic knowing of nursing as art, and much more. As Nightingale wrote in 1868:

> Nursing is an art; and if it is to be made an art, it requires as exclusive a devotion, as hard a preparation, as any painter's or sculptor's work; for what is the having to do with dead canvas or cold marble, compared with having to do with the living spirit—the temple of God's spirit? It is one of the Fine Arts; I had almost said, the finest of the Fine Arts.[74]

As nurses continually address their stress, burnout, suffering, and soul pain, as discussed in the next principle, this can assist us to understand the necessity of personal healing and self-care directly related to nursing as art, where we develop qualities of nursing presence and inner reflection. Nurse presence is also a way of approaching a person that respects and honors the person's essence; it is relating in a way that reflects a quality of "being with" and "in collaboration with," as discussed in the next principle.

Our own inner work also helps us to hold deeply a conscious awareness of our own roles in creating a healthy world. We recognize the importance of addressing one's own shadow that, as described by Jung,[75] is a composite of personal characteristics and potentials that have been denied expression in life and of which a person is unaware; the ego denies the characteristics because they are in conflict and incompatible with a person's chosen conscious attitude.

In this "I" space, integral self-care is valued, which means that integral reflective practices are integrated and can be transformative in our developmental process. We become more integrally conscious in our knowing, doing, and being and in all aspects of our personal and professional endeavors.[76]

Mindfulness is the practice of giving attention to what is happening in the present moment, such as our thoughts, feelings, emotions, and sensations. To cultivate the capacity of mindfulness practices one may include mindfulness meditation, centering prayer, and other reflective practices, such as journaling, dream interpretation, art, music, or poetry, that lead to an experience of nonseparateness and love; it involves developing the qualities of stillness and being present for one's own suffering, which also allows for full presence when with another.

In our personal process, we recognize conscious dying, where time and thought are given to contemplate one's own death.[77] Through a reflective practice, one rehearses and imagines one's final breath to practice preparing for one's own death. This integral practice prepares us to not be so attached to material things, to not spend so much time thinking about the future but living in this moment as often as we can and living fully until death comes. We are more likely to participate and fully engage with deeper compassion in the death process with others and ultimately with self. Death is seen as the mirror in which the entire meaning and mystery of life are reflected—the moment of liberation. Within an integral perspective, the state of transparency—the understanding that there is no separation between our practice and our everyday life—is recognized. This is a mature practice that is wise and empty of a separate self.

Integral Nursing Principle 2: Nursing Is Built on "We"

Integral nursing principle 2 recognizes the importance of the "We" (intersubjective) space where nurses come together and are conscious of sharing their worldviews, beliefs, priorities, and values related to enhancing integral self-care and integral health care. It includes being fully present and focused with intention to understand what another person (patient, family, colleague, or other) is expressing, or not expressing. Deep listening is valued. When we listen authentically to a client share her or his story, whether it is about illness or other life challenges that include the person's cultural worldviews and rituals, we assist them to transform crisis into wisdom and helplessness into hope that increases body-mind-spirit healing.

This focus begins an energy flow—by setting an intention for the healing of the client/patient—that moves from the gross body (physical), to the subtle body (light, energy, emotional feelings), to the causal body (the infinite formless state) where realization of not being separate from others is experienced. This energy healing is used to describe the subtle flow of energy within and around a person—creating a field that is experienced by the individual. This is the ability to open one's heart, to be present for all levels of suffering, such that suffering may be transformed for others, as well as for self. This describes what is known as bearing witness and being present for things as they are—a state achieved through reflective and contemplative practice that leads to an experience of nonseparateness. It involves developing the quality of stillness to be present for suffering and the sufferer.

Within nursing, health care, and society, there is much suffering, moral suffering, moral distress, and soul pain, as shown in **Table 1-8.** We are often called on to "be with" these difficult human experiences and to use our nursing presence. Our sense of "We" supports us in recognizing the phases of suffering—"mute" suffering, "expressive" suffering, and "new identity" in suffering.[78, 79] When we feel alone, as nurses, we experience mute suffering; this is an inability to articulate and communicate with others one's own suffering. Our challenge in nursing is to more skillfully enter into the phase of "expressive" suffering where sufferers seek language to express their frustrations and experiences such as in sharing stories in a group process. Outcomes of this experience often move toward new identity in suffering through new meaning-making where one makes new sense of the past, interprets new meaning in suffering, and can envision a new future.

A shift in one's consciousness allows for a shift in one's capacity to be able to transform her or his suffering from causing distress to finding some new truth and meaning in it. As we create times for sharing and giving voice to our concerns, new levels of healing may happen.

> **TABLE 1-8   Suffering, Moral Suffering, Moral Distress, and Soul Pain**
>
> **Suffering:** An individual's story around pain where the signs of suffering may be physical, mental, emotional, social, behavioral, and/or spiritual; it is an anguish experienced—internal and external—as a threat to one's composure, integrity, and the fulfillment of intentions.
>
> **Moral suffering:** Occurs when an individual experiences tensions or conflicts about what is the right thing to do in a particular situation; it often involves the struggle of finding a balance between competing interests or values.
>
> **Moral distress:** Occurs when an individual is unable to translate moral choices into moral actions and when prevented by obstacles, either internal or external, from acting upon them.
>
> **Soul pain:** The experience of an individual who has become disconnected and alienated from the deepest and most fundamental aspects of one's self.
>
> *Source:* Used with permission. J. Halifax, B. M. Dossey, and C. H. Rushton, *Being with Dying: Compassionate End-of-Life Training Guide* (Santa Fe, NM: Prajna Mountain Press, 2007). Adapted from A. Jameston, *Nursing Practice: The Ethical Issues* (Englewood Cliffs, NJ: Prentice Hall, 1984) and M. Kearney, *Mortally Wounded* (New York: Scribner, 1996).

Nightingale consistently realized the value of collaborating well with others, especially nursing colleagues. She focused on what "we" as nurses can do together as a team. She saw that sustainable nursing practice constantly requires strong nursing teamwork, as she expressed in 1883:

> Let us run the race where all may win, rejoicing in their successes, as our own, and mourning their failures, wherever they are as our own. . . . We are all one Nurse. The very essence of all good organizations is that everybody should do her [or his] own work in such a way as to help and not hinder every one else's work.[80]

An integral nurse considers transpersonal dimensions. This means that interactions with others move from conversations to a deeper dialogue that goes beyond the individual ego; it includes the acknowledgment and appreciation for something greater that may be referred to as spirit, nonlocality, unity, or oneness.[25] Transpersonal dialogues contain an integral worldview and recognize the role of spirituality, which is the search for the sacred or holy that involves feelings, thoughts, experiences, rituals, meaning, value, direction, and purpose as valid aspects of the universe. Spirituality is a force that can unify a person with all that is—the essence of Beingness and relatedness that permeates all of life and is manifested in one's knowing, doing, and being; it is usually, though not universally, considered the interconnectedness with self, others, Nature, and God/Life Force/Absolute/Transcendent.

From an integral perspective, spiritual care is an interfaith perspective that takes into account dying as a developmental process and a natural human process that emphasizes meaningfulness and human and spiritual values.[72] Religion is recognized as the codified and ritualized beliefs, behaviors, and customs that take place in a community of like-minded individuals involved in spirituality.[72] Our challenge is to enter into deep dialogue to more fully understand religions different from our own so that we may be tolerant where there are differences.

In this "We" space, nurses come together and are conscious of sharing their worldviews, beliefs, priorities, and values related to working together in ways that enhance integral self-care and integral health care. Deep listening is valued; this is being present and focused with intention to understand what another person is expressing or not expressing. Bearing witness to others, the state achieved through reflective and mindfulness practices, is also valued. Through mindfulness one can achieve states of equanimity, the stability of mind that allows us to be present with a good and impartial heart no matter how beneficial or difficult the conditions; it is being present for the sufferer and suffering just as it is while maintaining a spacious mindfulness in the midst of life's changing conditions.

Compassion is bearing witness and loving kindness, which is manifest in the face of suffering. The realization of the self and another as not being separate is experienced; it is the ability to open one's heart and be present for all levels of suffering so that suffering may be transformed for others, as well as for the self. A useful phrase to consider is "I'm doing the best that I can." Compassionate care assists us in living as well as being with the dying person, the family, and others. We can touch the roots of pain and become aware of new meaning in the midst of pain, chaos, loss, and grief.

Integral action is the actual practice and process that creates the condition of trust where a care plan is co-created with the patient, and care can be given and received. Full attention and intention to the whole person, not merely the current presenting symptoms, illness, crisis, or tasks to be accomplished, reinforce the person's meaning and experience of community and unity. Engagement between an integral nurse and a patient, family member, or colleague is done in a respectful manner; each patient's subjective experience about health, health beliefs, and values are explored. We deeply care for others and recognize our own mortality and that of others.

The integral nurse uses intention, which is the conscious awareness of being in the present moment with self or another person, to help facilitate the healing process; it is a volitional act of love. The nurse is also aware of the role of intuition, which is the perceived knowing of events, insights, and things without a conscious use of logical, analytical processes; it may be informed by the senses to receive information. Intuition is a type of experience of sudden insight into a feeling, solution, or problem where time and things fit together in a unified experience, such as understanding about pain and suffering, or a moment in time with another. This is an aspect within the pattern of unknowing. Integral nurses recognize love as the unconditional unity of self with others. This love generates loving kindness, the open, gentle, and caring state of mindfulness that assists one's nursing presence.

There is an awareness of integral communication that is a free flow of verbal and nonverbal interchange between and among people and pets and significant beings such as God/Life Force/Absolute/Transcendent. This type of sharing leads to explorations of meaning and ideas of mutual understanding and growth and loving kindness.

Integral Nursing Principle 3: "It" Is About Behavior and Skill Development

Integral nursing principle 3 recognizes the importance of the individual exterior "It" (objective) space. In this "It" space of the individual exterior, each person develops and integrates her or his integral self-care plan. This includes skills, behaviors, and action steps to achieve a fit body through strength training and stretching, as well as the conscious eating of healthy foods. It is also modeling integral life skills. For the integral nurse and patient, this is also the space where the "doing to" and "doing for" occur. However, the integral nurse also combines her or his nursing presence with nursing acts to assist the patient to access personal strengths, to release fear and anxiety, and to provide comfort and safety. There is the awareness of conscious dying to assist the dying patient who wishes to have minimal medication and treatment to stay as alert as possible while receiving comfort care until she or he makes the death transition.

Nightingale saw nursing as an integral and spiritual practice where each nurse blends knowledge with ongoing observations to develop and refine nursing practice—to continually combine the external observations of the body and behaviors and, thus, to develop new skills and behaviors. About this dynamic, Nightingale eloquently observed and wrote in 1876:

> When we obey all God's laws as to cleanliness, fresh air, pure water, good habits, good dwellings, good drains, food and drink, work and exercise, health is the result: when we disobey, sickness. 110,000 lives are needlessly sacrificed every year in this kingdom by our disobedience, and 22,000 people are needlessly sick all year round. And why? Because we will not know, will not obey God's simple health laws. No epidemic can resist thorough cleanliness and fresh air.[81]

Within this integral nursing principle, integral nurses with nursing colleagues and healthcare team members compile the data around physiologic and pathophysiologic assessment, nursing diagnosis, outcomes, and care plans (including medications, technical procedures, monitoring, treatments, protocols, implementation, and evaluation). This is also the space that includes patient education and evaluation. Integral nurses co-create care plans with patients when possible, combining caring, healing interventions and modalities and integral life practices that can interface with and enhance the success of traditional medical and surgical technology and treatment. Some common interventions are relaxation, music, imagery, massage, touch therapies, stories, poetry, healing environments, fresh air, sunlight, flowers, soothing and calming pictures, pet therapy, and more.

Integral Nursing Principle 4: "Its" Is Systems and Structures

Integral nursing principle 4 recognizes the importance of the exterior collective "Its" (interobjective) space. In this "Its" space, integral nurses and the healthcare team come together to examine their work, their priorities, use of technologies, and any aspect of the technological environment. They also create exterior healing environments that incorporate Nature and the natural world when possible such as with outdoor and indoor healing gardens, use of green materials with soothing colors, and sounds of music and Nature. Integral nurses identify how they might work together as an interdisciplinary team to deliver more effective patient care and coordination of care.

Nightingale saw nursing as a profession where continual progress with self and others required attention, and she wrote about this in 1897:

> Nursing takes a whole life to learn. We must make progress in it every year. . . . It has been recorded that the three principles which represent the deepest wants of human nature, both in the East and the West, are the principles of discipline, of religion (or the tie to God), of contentment. . . . Nursing is not an adventure, as some have now supposed: "Where fools rush in where angels fear to tread." It is a very serious, delightful thing, like life, requiring training, experience, devotion not

by fits and starts, patience, a power of accumulating, instead of losing—all these things. We are only on the threshold of training.[82]

Application

This section offers examples of how to apply the Theory of Integral Nursing to practice, education, research, healthcare policy, and global nursing.

Practice

The Theory of Integral Nursing can be used in any clinical situation to explore aspects of integral awareness within all quadrants. The following example illustrates this point. Following a shopping trip with her husband and daughter, a woman had a seizure as she sat in her car. She lost consciousness but regained a conscious and alert state within several minutes. The husband immediately drove her to an emergency room. In this situation, which is more important? Is it the patient's brain (Upper Right—neural pathways and brain seizure focal areas) or the patient's and family's mind (Upper Left—emotions, meaning, thoughts, perceptions, fears)? Is it the nurse (Upper Left) or the nurse with the neurologist working together (Lower Left) or the emergency room (Lower Right)?

In an integral approach, the answer is that all of these questions are equally important to prevent this individual from further seizures and potential complications. When all quadrants are addressed, a collaborative, integral treatment plan can be developed. It is also important to ensure that the patient and the family are kept aware of what is happening and that the patient flow in the emergency room is kept at a safe and effective pace. Each quadrant represents an equal quarter of reality, of the totality of our being and existence. This model helps us touch and link all aspects of reality, including the importance of the nurse addressing her or his own needs.

The Theory of Integral Nursing provides a conceptual framework for nurses in the integration of complementary and alternative therapies (CAT) into the routine care of patients receiving rehabilitation services. Juliann Perdue developed

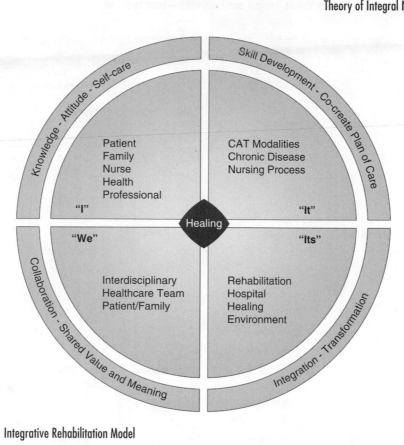

FIGURE 1-11 Integrative Rehabilitation Model

Source: Used with permission. Copyright © 2011. Juliann S. Perdue, DNP, RN, FNP, Assistant Professor & Clinical Site Coordinator, California Baptist University, School of Nursing, Riverside, California.

the Integrative Rehabilitation Model, shown in **Figure 1-11**, as a foundation for the integration of complementary and alternative therapies in integrative rehabilitation that occurs in many settings: general hospital, inpatient rehabilitation facility, outpatient rehabilitation clinic, and skilled nursing facilities or long-term care.[83]

The model also depicts the core aspects of rehabilitation nursing's research agenda, which includes (1) nursing and nursing-led interdisciplinary interventions to promote function in people of all ages with disability and/or chronic health problems, (2) experience of disability and/or chronic health problems for individuals and families across the life span, (3) rehabilitation in the changing healthcare system, and (4) the rehabilitation nursing profession.

The Integrative Rehabilitation Model correlates well with the metaparadigm of nursing and the four quadrants of reality. **Table 1-9** outlines the interconnectedness of the nurse, person,

health, and environment with the realities of "I," "It," "We," and "Its." Through true presence and effective dialogue, the nurse establishes a safe environment for open communication regarding personal use and disclosure of CAT, as well as the sharing of knowledge and attitudes toward CAT.

The integral perspective is incorporated into the 6-month Integrative Nurse Coach Certificate Program.[84] (See Chapter 21.) Another use of integral theory is by Diane Pisanos in her health coaching practice with individuals and groups, as shown in **Figure 1-12**.[85]

Education

The Theory of Integral Nursing can assist educators to be aware of all quadrants while organizing and designing curricula, continuing education courses, health education presentations, teaching guides, and protocols. Most curricula focus minimally on the individual subjective "I" and the

TABLE 1-9   Metaparadigm of Nursing and the Four Quadrants of Reality
Integrative Rehabilitation Model correlates well with the metaparadigm of nursing and the four quadrants.

		Metaparadigm of Nursing			
		Nurse	Person	Health	Environment
Quadrants of Reality	"I" Individual Exterior	Self	Patient Family Healthcare professional	Self-care	Knowledge Attitude Values and beliefs
	"It" Individual Exterior	Nursing process ■ Assessment ■ Diagnosis ■ Outcomes ■ Planning ■ Implementation ■ Evaluation	Chronic disease Disability	CATs Skill development Co-create care plan	Patient room/unit Therapeutic space
	"We" Collective Interior	Nursing profession ■ Certified Rehabilitation Registered Nurse	Interdisciplinary team Patient/family	Relationship-centered care	Collaboration Shared meaning
	"Its" Collective Exterior	Theory of Integral Nursing	Rehabilitation professionals Vision and mission of organization CAT practitioners	Integral health care	Rehabilitation hospital Healing environment Transformational health care

Source: Used with permission. Copyright © 2011. Juliann S. Perdue, DNP, RN, FNP, Assistant Professor & Clinical Site Coordinator, California Baptist University, School of Nursing, Riverside, California.

collective intersubjective "We"; the emphasis is on passing an examination or learning a new skill or procedure, and, thus, the learner retains only small portions of what is taught. Before teaching any technical skills, the instructor might guide a student or patient in a relaxation and imagery rehearsal of the event to encourage the person to be in the present moment.

The reader is referred to Olga Jarrin, who explores integral theory and related definitions for nursing.[52] Cynthia Barrere and her nurse educator colleagues have also used concepts from the Theory of Integral Nursing in selected student engagement learning activities.[86] (See Chapter 36.)

Darlene Hess designed an RN-to-BSN curriculum based on the Theory of Integral Nursing (see **Table 1-10**).[87] The RN-to-BSN Program at Northern New Mexico College is a truly integral holistic nursing education program that offers registered nurses the opportunity to delve deeply into integral theory and holistic nursing while completing requirements for a bachelor's of science degree in nursing.

The program prepares registered nurses to assume leadership roles as integral nurses at the

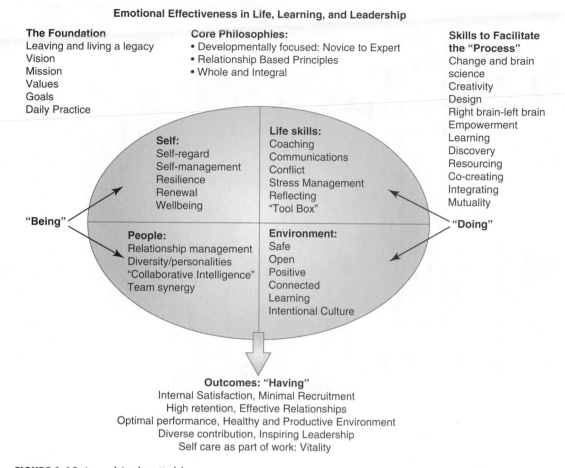

Emotional Effectiveness in Life, Learning, and Leadership

The Foundation
Leaving and living a legacy
Vision
Mission
Values
Goals
Daily Practice

Core Philosophies:
• Developmentally focused: Novice to Expert
• Relationship Based Principles
• Whole and Integral

**Skills to Facilitate
the "Process"**
Change and brain
science
Creativity
Design
Right brain-left brain
Empowerment
Learning
Discovery
Resourcing
Co-creating
Integrating
Mutuality

Self:
Self-regard
Self-management
Resilience
Renewal
Wellbeing

Life skills:
Coaching
Communications
Conflict
Stress Management
Reflecting
"Tool Box"

"Being"

"Doing"

People:
Relationship management
Diversity/personalities
"Collaborative Intelligence"
Team synergy

Environment:
Safe
Open
Positive
Connected
Learning
Intentional Culture

Outcomes: "Having"
Internal Satisfaction, Minimal Recruitment
High retention, Effective Relationships
Optimal performance, Healthy and Productive Environment
Diverse contribution, Inspiring Leadership
Self care as part of work: Vitality

FIGURE 1-12 Integral Coaching Model

Source: Used with permission. Copyright © 2001, 2009. Diane Pisanos, RNC, MS, AHN-BC, NNP, Integrative Health Care Consulting, Denver, CO. E-mail: dpisanos1@aol.com.

bedside, within an organization, in the community, and in the profession, as well as to provide holistic, intentional, relationship-centered care that addresses individual and collective health. This integral holistic model emphasizes self-care and personal development for the nursing student and for faculty who teach in the program. Program learning outcomes, course competencies, and assignments are linked to the Theory of Integral Nursing. Expected outcomes for the RN-to-BSN program are listed in **Table 1-11**. An example is provided in **Table 1-12** that shows how integral nursing principles are explicitly embedded in an assignment.

In its short history this innovative program has achieved national accreditation through the Commission on Collegiate Nursing Education

and has been endorsed by the American Holistic Nurses Credentialing Corporation (AHNCC). To date, 12 students have graduated from the program. Three graduates have been accepted into graduate school, and several students have obtained, or are in the process of applying for, national holistic nurse certification through AHNCC. More information about the program is available at www.ncmc.edu.

Research

Evidence-based practice too often connotes a research-based approach to care, rather than the more complete definition of evidence-based practice that includes practitioner expertise and patient preferences. Useful evidence is derived from many sources, and the utilization of

TABLE 1-10　Curriculum for RN-to-BSN Program Using the Theory of Integral Nursing

Course Title	NURS 343 & 344 Pathophysiology (6 Cr)	NURS 400 Nursing in Transition (2 Cr)	NURS 401 Integral Nursing Theory (3 Cr)
Course Description	This two-part course addresses pathophysiological responses and adaptation of the physical body to an insult. Analysis of pathological alterations in health at the cellular and systems level and implications for nursing care are emphasized. Students focus on multisystem interaction of the body to an illness or injury. The pathophysiological basis of addictions and behavioral disorders is explored. Students are introduced to the biology of belief.	This course examines the expanded role of the baccalaureate-prepared nurse in today's healthcare systems. Historic, contemporary, and future roles of the nurse are addressed. Skills in scholarly exposition and the use of technology are developed.	This course examines the Theory of Integral Nursing. Holistic nursing theories are explored. The concept of praxis is introduced. Florence Nightingale's legacy and philosophical foundation are included. Students develop skills related to self-awareness, self-care, relationship-centered care, and reflective practice. The use of conscious intention is emphasized.
Course Topics	Cellular biology Genetic disease Immunity Inflammation Stress and disease Psychoneuroimmunology Neurologic system Endocrine system Reproductive system Hematologic system Cardiovascular and lymphatic system Pulmonary system Renal and urologic system Digestive system Musculoskeletal system Integumentary system Multiple organ dysfunction Pathophysiology of addictions Pathophysiology of behavioral disorders Biology of belief	Role of the baccalaureate-prepared nurse Scholarly writing and use of scholarly resources Critical thinking Ethics Evolution of holistic nursing Principles of holistic nursing Standards of care Professional nursing organizations Working in groups Technology and informatics Advanced nursing education The nurse of the future	Integral nursing/integral health Holistic nursing Integrative nursing practice Healing Nursing metaparadigm concepts Patterns of knowing Relationship-centered care Self-care Reflective practice Intention Florence Nightingale Spirituality Therapeutic use of self Holistic nursing theories Self-confidence Nurse as environment Holistic caring process

TABLE 1-10 Curriculum for RN-to-BSN Program Using the Theory of Integral Nursing (*continued*)

	NURS 410 An Integral Approach to Evidence-Based Practice (3 Cr)	**NURS 420 Integral Health Assessment (3 Cr)**	**NURS 430 Complementary and Alternative Therapies in Nursing (3 Cr)**
Course Title			
Course Description	This course examines research methodologies utilized in nursing research. Emphasis is on utilization of research findings to establish evidence-based nursing interventions. Students analyze research findings aimed at selected health concerns. Students explore definitions of evidence-based practice and examine how worldviews influence research.	This course emphasizes development of skills in health assessment of (allopathic) human systems. Alternative systems (e.g., Ayurveda, Native American, Chinese Oriental Medicine, Intuitive) are introduced. Skills in interviewing, history taking, physical examination, and documentation and use of assessment data in planning care are developed. Laboratory and selected clinical settings are used to practice skill development. The Theory of Integral Nursing is explored as a model to frame data collection, organization, and synthesis into a cohesive whole.	This course provides an introduction to evidence-based complementary and alternative approaches to health care. Students acquire knowledge related to alternative and complementary healing modalities that can be incorporated into professional nursing practice and self-care practices. Students experience and develop beginning skills in the provision of CAM modalities as they interact with practitioners in selected clinical settings.
Course Topics	Historical evolution of nursing research Quantitative research Qualitative research Ethics in nursing research Theory and research frameworks Outcomes research Statistics Using research in an integral nursing practice Alternative philosophies of science	Presence Active listening, deep listening Centering Therapeutic interviewing Health history Nutritional assessment Spiritual assessment Cultural assessment Physical examination Mental status examination Documentation Synthesis of clinical information	NICAM Whole medical systems Mind–body interventions Energy therapies Biologically based therapies Manipulative and body-based therapies Therapeutic environment Arts and healing

(continues)

TABLE 1-10	Curriculum for RN-to-BSN Program Using the Theory of Integral Nursing (*continued*)		
Course Title	**NURS 440 Health Issues, Policy, and Politics in Health Care (3 Cr)**	**NURS 450 Community and Global Health I (3 Cr)**	**NURS 451 Community and Global Health II (4 Cr)**
Course Description	This course emphasizes empowering students with knowledge, skills, and attitudes to effect change in health policy to improve healthcare delivery. Students analyze contemporary healthcare issues of concern to nursing and learn strategies for effective involvement in policymaking decisions and policy implementation. Students examine work environments and the influence of organizational systems on the quality of care. Students apply the Theory of Integral Nursing to a current health policy issue in a position paper expressed orally to a group.	This first of a two-part course provides an overview of contemporary community health nursing practice. The influence of culture on healthcare beliefs and practices is emphasized. Health problems of selected populations within New Mexico are examined. Public Health Nursing Competencies are linked with the Theory of Integral Nursing to form the basis for student learning experiences in community settings.	This second of a two-part course examines global health issues in relationship to local, regional, and international nursing practice. In this course, students select and focus on a global health issue relevant to local community nursing practice. A service-learning project based on the selected issue provides the focus of clinical experience.
Course Topics	Current healthcare trends	Cultural diversity	Global warming
	Healthcare delivery systems	Cultural competence	Sustainability
	Healthcare financing	Spiritual diversity	Immigration
	Complexity and change theory	Community partnerships	Bioterrorism
	Empowerment	Community as client	Hazardous waste
	Effective patient advocacy	Population-focused care	Pollution
	Navigating the legislative process	Epidemiology	Aging
	Healthcare reform	Demographics	Disaster management
	Communicating the essence of nursing/developing a nursing voice	Health promotion	Vulnerable populations
		Health prevention	Poverty and homelessness
		"Upstream thinking"	Migrant health issues
		Communicable disease risk prevention	Mental health issues
		Case management	Violence
			Role of the nurse in community and global health

TABLE 1-10 Curriculum for RN-to-BSN Program Using the Theory of Integral Nursing *(continued)*

Course Title	**NURS 460 Integral Communication and Teaching (2 Cr)**	**NURS 470 Transformational Leadership in Nursing (4 Cr)**	**NURS 480 Integral Nursing Capstone Course (2 Cr)**
Course Description	This course examines communication techniques, counseling, coaching, and teaching strategies to enhance and facilitate cognitive and behavioral change. Students integrate principles of integral communication, integral health coaching, motivational interviewing, and nonviolent communication.	This courses focuses on the principles of transformational leadership as applied to the nurse leader at the bedside, within an organization, in the community, and in the profession. The student is introduced to complexity science, appreciative inquiry, and emotional intelligence. Career advancement through lifelong learning is emphasized.	This course provides the student an opportunity to critically examine in-depth a personally relevant topic in preparation for an expanded role as an integral nurse. Students develop learning objectives, a learning contract, and criteria for evaluation of project outcomes.
Course Topics	Motivational interviewing Educational theory Fundamentals of health coaching Helping others create healthy lifestyles Helping others navigate the healthcare system Nonviolent communication Presence Learning styles Instructional design methods Counseling Ways of knowing	Transformational model Leadership development Complexity science Professional ethics Interdisciplinary leadership Appreciative inquiry Emotional intelligence Spiritual intelligence Conflict resolution/mediation Delegation Client/customer needs and expectations Visioning and strategic planning Care management Quality and performance management Human resources management	

Total Nursing Credit Hours: 38

Source: Used with permission. Copyright © 2014. Darlene Hess, PhD, RN, AHN-BC, PMHNP-BC, ACC, Brown Mountain Visions, Los Ranchos, NM 87101. http://www.brownmountainvisions.com

---

TABLE 1-11   Expected Outcomes for RN-to-BSN Program Using the Theory of Integral Nursing

1. Use the Theory of Integral Nursing and the American Holistic Nurses Association and the American Nurses Association *Holistic Nursing: Scope and Standards of Practice* (2013) to provide integral and holistic nursing care in a variety of settings. (See Integral Principles 1–4, on pages 33–38).

2. Demonstrate critical thinking skills from an "I," "It," "We," "Its" perspective.

3. Communicate effectively from a relationship-centered care perspective involving patient–practitioner, community–practitioner, and practitioner–practitioner relationships.

4. Conduct integral holistic health assessments in relation to client needs.

5. Apply concepts of integral nursing to a personal plan for holistic self-care.

6. Integrate and apply knowledge to support individual and collective health.

7. Analyze the links between and among individual, community, and global health issues from an integral worldview.

8. Analyze and utilize research findings to facilitate individual and collective health.

9. Demonstrate the role of the integral nurse as change agent in regard to current health policy issues.

10. Utilize integral coaching strategies in relation to client-centered goals.

11. Apply transformational leadership principles to professional nursing practice.

12. Integrate selected complementary/alternative health practices into professional nursing practice.

13. Demonstrate commitment to lifelong learning to facilitate personal and professional development.

Source: Used with permission. Copyright © 2014. Darlene R. Hess, PhD, AHN-BC, PMHNP-BC, ACC, Brown Mountain Visions, Los Ranchos, NM 87107, www.brownmountainvisions.com

---

research findings is but one aspect of delivering safe, accurate nursing care. An intentional approach to evaluating and using diverse evidence from varied sources supports holistic care.

Knowing how to elicit patient preferences is an essential clinical skill.

The Theory of Integral Nursing can assist nurses to consider the importance of qualitative

---

TABLE 1-12   Example of Integral Nursing Principles Explicitly Embedded in a Course Assignment

Community Health Issue Scholarly Paper (See Integral Nursing Principles 1–4, on pages 33–38).

Each student will select and define a community health issue to investigate. Identify your personal relationship to the issue (INP 1, 2) and why this issue is important to nursing (INP 2). Relate the issue to *Healthy People 2020* goals (www.healthypeople.gov/2020/About-Healthy-People) (INP 4). Identify and evaluate relevant data pertinent to the issue from a variety of sources. Determine populations affected by this issue (INP 3). Include at least one nursing research article related to this issue. Summarize the information relevant to the issue and identify gaps in the information that is available. Determine if/how you will incorporate your learning about this issue into your self-care plan (INP 3).

Identify at least one agency or program that provides health promotion or health prevention services that address the selected issue (INP 4). State the mission and goals of the agency or program. Determine how the agency or program is funded. Describe the agency or program's emergency response plan (if it has one). Determine how the agency or program monitors and evaluates outcomes.

Compile the data into an organized and scholarly paper that will be discussed with your nurse classmates (INP 3). Solicit classmate perspectives regarding the selected issue, your findings, and their experiences (INP 1, 2).

Source: Used with permission. Copyright © 2014. Darlene R. Hess, PhD, AHN-BC, PMHNP-BC, ACC, Brown Mountain Visions, Los Ranchos, NM 87107, www.brownmountainvisions.com

and quantitative research.[88] (See Chapter 28.) Often among scientists, researchers, and educators there are arguments as to whether qualitative or quantitative research is more important. Wilber often uses the term *flatland thinking and approaches* to describe the thinking of individuals who use a reductionistic perspective that can be situated in any quadrant or explanations of both the interior and exterior dimensions through only quantitative methodologies that focus on empirical data.

Our challenges in integral nursing are to consider the findings from both qualitative and quantitative data and always consider triangulation of data when appropriate. We must always value introspective, cultural, and interpretive experiences and expand our personal and collective capacities of consciousness and intentionality as evolutionary progression toward achieving our goals. In other words, knowledge does emerge from all four quadrants. This helps us to understand more about the unitary paradigm of consciousness and intentionality, particularly with the World Wide Web and other technological advances.

Healthcare Policy

The Theory of Integral Nursing can guide us to consider many areas related to healthcare policy.[7, 8] Compelling evidence in all of the healthcare professions shows that the origins of health and illness cannot be understood by focusing only on the physical body. Only by expanding the equations of health, exemplified by an integral approach or an AQAL approach, to include our entire physical, mental, emotional, social, and spiritual dimensions and interrelationships can we account for a host of health events. Some of these include, for example, the correlations between poor health and shortened life span, job dissatisfaction and acute myocardial infarction, social shame and severe illness, immune suppression and increased death rates during bereavement, and improved health and longevity as spirituality and spiritual awareness increase.

Global Nursing

Our challenge as integral and holistic nurses is that we see global health imperatives as common concerns of humankind; they are not isolated problems in far-off countries. Like Nightingale, we must see prevention and prevention education as important to the health of humanity.[7, 8]

We can explore all aspects of the Theory of Integral Nursing and apply them to our endeavors in underserved communities and populations. Often in the developed world of health care we believe that decent care is having access to technology, procedures, tests, or surgery when we need it and as quickly as we want. However, the majority of the world does not have access as do those in wealthy, developed nations. And this is still a limited view of what integral or even holistic health care is because primary prevention such as self-care is rarely given its just due in healthcare initiatives.

Consider the World Health Organization's call for "decent care" for HIV/AIDS patients and their families throughout the world as previously discussed.[12, 13] Decent care implies the comprehensive ideal that the medical, physiologic, psychological, and spiritual needs of others are addressed. This includes universal access to treatment with utilization and enforcement of universally accepted precautionary measures for healthcare practitioners, along with adequate supplies and equipment, safe food, free access to clean water, autoclaves, laundries, and safe methods for sterilizing and disposing of infected materials in incinerators.

An example of the Theory of Integral Nursing that has been applied to global nursing is the Nightingale Initiative for Global Health (NIGH),[11] of which I am a founding NIGH board member and co-director. The NIGH is a catalytic grassroots-to-global movement, envisioned in 2000 and officially established in 2003, to honor and extend Florence Nightingale's timeless legacy. The NIGH's twin purposes are, first, to increase global public awareness about the priority of health and, second, to empower nurses, nursing students, and concerned citizens to address the critical health issues of our time. Since the beginning of NIGH's development, these interrelated approaches have been developed intentionally, keeping Nightingale's deep and broad integral legacy in mind.

As NIGH's vision was articulated, we understood what Wilber[45] meant when he noted that omitting the focus of any one of the integral quadrants would cause "hemorrhaging" in attempts to achieve work represented by the other three integral quadrants. Without focusing on strengthening and sustaining individuals, groups of individuals cannot thrive (individual and collective interior). Without focusing on the worldviews underlying all situations in any society, the structures we live and work within cannot be properly understood and sustained (individual and collective exterior). Without first populating an understanding of the nature of these worldviews—with real people in real groups with real needs in mind—structures can quickly become limited and worldviews irrelevant. Without understanding the value of envisioning and proposing structures from worldviews that can make a difference in the world, people and groups tend to drift away from purposeful efforts to actually ever make a difference.

By using the Theory of Integral Nursing, we realized how Wilber's integral modeling would help us to present NIGH's whole picture, as well as the pieces of the whole and—perhaps most important—the relationships among these pieces.[5] Using this jigsaw puzzle metaphor, NIGH's team has recently shaped a related series of NIGH Integral Models. **Figure 1-13** shows the NIGH Integral Models and the outcomes we are envisioning. The Upper-Left "I" quadrant is named "among Individuals"; the Lower-Left "We" quadrant is named "within Groups"; the Upper-Right "It" quadrant is named "at Grassroots Levels"; and the Lower-Right "Its" quadrant is named "at Global Levels."

Nursing's first priority is devotion to human health—of individuals, of communities, and of the world. An integral perspective can assist nurses who are educated and prepared—physically, emotionally, mentally, and spiritually—to effectively accomplish the activities required for healthy people and healthy environments.[7, 89, 90]

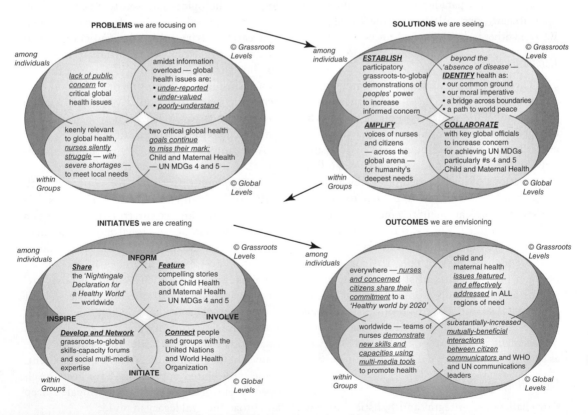

FIGURE 1-13 The Nightingale Initiative for Global Health's Four "Integral" Models

Source: Used with permission, Nightingale Initiative for Global Health (NIGH), http://www.nightingaledeclaration.net

Conclusion

Nursing includes many holistic, integral, and integrative philosophies, principles, and theories. This chapter has focused on global health and the application of decent care and the post-2015 Sustainable Development Goals. My Theory of Integral Nursing was developed to address how we can increase our integral awareness, our wholeness, and heal and strengthen our personal and professional capacities to be more fully open to the mysteries of life's journey and the wondrous stages of self-discovery for ourselves and others. Our time demands a new paradigm and a new language in which we integrate the best of what we know in the science and art of nursing that includes holistic and human caring theories and modalities.

With an integral approach and worldview we are in a better position to share with others the depth of nurses' knowledge, expertise, critical-thinking capacities, and skills for assisting others in creating health and healing. Only by paying attention to the heart of nursing—*sacred* and *heart* reflect a common meaning—can we generate the vision, courage, and hope required to unite nursing in healing. This will help us as we engage in healthcare reform to address the challenges in these troubled times—local to global. This is not a matter of philosophy but of survival.

Directions for Future Research

1. Examine the components of relationship-centered care for clinical practice, education, research, and healthcare policy.
2. Analyze the Theory of Integral Nursing and its application in holistic nursing practice, education, research, and healthcare policy.

Nurse Healer Reflections

After reading this chapter, the nurse healer will be able to answer or to begin a process of answering the following questions:

- How can I apply more of the components of relationship-centered care each day?

- In what ways can the Theory of Integral Nursing inform my personal and professional endeavors?
- Which integral awarenesses and practices may I consider for development in my personal and professional life?

NOTES

1. F. Nightingale, "Sick-Nursing and Health-Nursing," in *Florence Nightingale Today: Healing, Leadership, Global Action*, eds. B. M. Dossey, L. C. Selanders, D. M. Beck, and A. Attewell (Silver Spring, MD: Nursesbooks.org, 2005): 296–297.
2. Institute of Medicine, *The Future of Nursing: Leading Change, Advancing Health* (Washington, DC: National Academies Press, 2010).
3. American Holistic Nurses Association and American Nurses Association, *Holistic Nursing: Scope and Standards of Practice*, 2nd ed. (Silver Spring, MD: Nursesbooks.org, 2013).
4. B. M. Dossey, "Theory of Integral Nursing," *Advances in Nursing Science* 31, no. 1 (2008): E52–E73.
5. B. M. Dossey, "Barbara Dossey's Theory of Integral Nursing," in *Nursing Theories and Nursing Practice*, 4th ed., eds. M. E. Parker and M. C. Smith (Philadelphia: F. A. Davis, 2015): 207–232.
6. M. J. Kreitzer, "Whole-Systems Healing: A New Leadership Path," in *Integrative Nursing*, eds. M. J. Krietzer and M. Koithan (New York: Oxford University Press, 2014): 47–55.
7. D. M. Beck, B. M. Dossey, and C. H. Rushton, "Global Activism, Advocacy, and Transformation: Florence Nightingale's Legacy for the Twenty-First Century," in *Integrative Nursing*, eds. M. J. Kreitzer and M. Koithan (New York: Oxford University Press, 2014): 526–537.
8. D. M. Beck, B. M. Dossey, and C. H. Rushton, "Integral Nursing and the Nightingale Initiative for Global Health (NIGH): Florence Nightingale's Integral Legacy for the 21st Century—Local to Global." *Journal of Integral Theory and Practice* 6, no. 4 (2011): 71–92.
9. World Health Organization, *Global Standards for the Initial Education of Professional Nurses and Midwives* (Geneva, Switzerland: World Health Organization, Department of Human Resources for Health, 2009).
10. International Council of Nurses, *The Global Shortage of Registered Nurses: An Overview of Issues and Action* (Geneva, Switzerland: International Council of Nurses, 2004).

11. Nightingale Initiative for Global Health, "Nightingale Declaration for a Healthy World" (2013). www.nightingaledeclaration.net.

12. J. T. Ferguson, T. Karpf, M. Weait, and R. Y. Swift, *Decent Care: Living Values, Health Justice and Human Flourishing*, World Health Organization Summative Report to the Ford Foundation (Geneva, Switzerland: World Health Organization, 2010).

13. T. Karpf, J. T. Ferguson, R. Y. Swift, and J. Lazarus, *Restoring Hope: Decent Care in the Midst of HIV/AIDS* (London: Palgrave Macmillan, 2008).

14. United Nations, *United Nations Millennium Development Goals* (New York: United Nations, 2000).

15. J. McDermott-Levy and K. Huffling, "Global Earth Caring Through the Millennium Development Goals and Beyond," *International Journal of Human Caring* 18, no. 2 (2014): 9–17.

16. United Nations, "Millennium Development Goals and Post-2015 Development Agenda," (2014). www.un.org/en/ecosoc/about/mdg.shtml.

17. F. Nightingale, *Letter to Sir Frederick Verney*. 23 November 1892, Add. Mss. 68887 ff102–05.

18. B. M. Dossey, *Florence Nightingale: Mystic, Visionary, Healer*, Commemorative ed. (Philadelphia: F. A. Davis, 2010).

19. L. McDonald, *The Collected Works of Florence Nightingale*, Vols. 1–16 (Waterloo, Ontario: Wilfreid Laurier Press, 2001–2012).

20. F. Nightingale, *Notes on Hospitals*, 3rd ed. (London: Longman, Green, Longman, Roberts, and Green, 1860).

21. F. Nightingale, *Notes on Nursing: What It Is, and What It Is Not* (London: Harrison, 1860).

22. F. Nightingale, "Letter from Miss Nightingale to the Probationer-Nurses in the 'Nightingale Fund' at St. Thomas's Hospital, and the Nurses Who Were Formerly Trained There, 1888," in *Florence Nightingale Today: Healing, Leadership, Global Action*, eds. B. M. Dossey, L. C. Selanders, D. M. Beck, and A. Attewell (Silver Spring, MD: Nursesbooks.org, 2005): 203–285.

23. L. Dossey, *Recovering the Soul: Scientific and Spiritual Search* (New York: Bantam Books, 1989).

24. L. Dossey, *Healing Words: The Power of Prayer and the Practice of Medicine* (San Francisco: HarperSanFrancisco, 1993).

25. L. Dossey, *One Mind: How Our Individual Mind Is Part of a Greater Mind and Why It Matters* (Carlsbad, CA: Hay House, 2013): xxviii–xxix.

26. L. Dossey, *Premonition: How Knowing the Future Can Shape Our Lives* (New York: Dutton, 2009).

27. C. P. Tresolini and Pew-Fetzer Task Force, *Health Professions Education and Relationship-Centered Care* (San Francisco: Pew Health Professions Commission, 1994).

28. Consortium of Academic Health Centers for Integrative Medicine, "Definition of Integrative Medicine" (2009). www.imconsortium.org/about/home.cfm.

29. V. L. Andrus, "Person-Centered Care: Enhancing Patient (Person) Engagement," *Beginnings* 34, no. 1 (2014): 18–21.

30. C. A. Drick, "At Last: Moving into Person-Centered Care," *Beginnings* 34, no. 1 (2014): 6–9.

31. U.S. Department of Health and Human Services, "About Healthy People" (2014). www.healthypeople.gov/2020/about/default.aspx.

32. Patient Protection and Affordable Care Act (PPACA) 42 U.S.C. § 18001 et seq. (2010). http://housedocs.house.gov/energycommerce/ppacacon.pdf.

33. Interprofessional Education Collaborative Expert Panel, *Core Competencies for Interprofessional Collaborative Practice: Report of an Expert Panel* (Washington, DC: Interprofessional Education Collaborative, 2011).

34. A. W. Davidson, M. A. Ray, and M. C. Turkel, *Nursing, Caring, and Complexity Science: For Human-Environment Wellbeing* (New York: Springer, 2011).

35. B. M. Dossey, S. Luck, and B. G. Schaub, *Nurse Coaching: Integrative Approaches for Health and Wellbeing* (North Miami, FL: International Nurse Coach Association, 2015).

36. D. M. Hess, B. M. Dossey, M. E. Southard, S. Luck, B. G. Schaub, and L. Bark, *Professional Nurse Coach Role: Defining Scope of Practice and Competencies* (in press).

37. M. Jordan, *How to Be a Health Coach: Integrative Wellness Approaches* (San Raphael, CA: Global Medicine Enterprises, 2013).

38. M. Jordan, "Health Coaching for the Underserved," *Global Advances in Health and Medicine* 2, no. 3 (2013): 75–82.

39. Samueli Institute, "Optimal Healing Environments" (2014). www.samueliinstitute.org/research-areas//optimal-healing-environments.

40. Planetree International, "About Us" (n.d.). http://planetree.org/about/planetree/.

41. A. Perlman, B. Horrigan, E. Goldblatt, V. Maizes, and B. Kligler, "The Pebble in the Pond: How Integrative Leadership Can Bring About Transformation," *EXPLORE: The Journal of Science and Healing* 10, no. 5S (2014): S1–S14.

42. L. L. Ewoldt, "Healthcare Reform: Resolve to Increase Your Knowledge in 2014," *American Nurse Today* 9, no. 1 (2014): 9–11.

43. M. Guarneri, "The Science of Connection," *Global Advances in Health and Medicine* 3, no. 1 (2014): 5–7.

44. Penny George Institute for Health and Healing, *Penny George Institute for Health and Healing: Overview and Outcomes Report 2010* (Minneapolis, MN: Penny George Institute for Health and Healing, 2010).

45. K. Wilber, *Integral Psychology: Consciousness, Spirit, Psychology, Therapy* (Boston: Shambhala, 2000).

46. K. Wilber, *The Collected Works of Ken Wilber*, Vols. 1–4 (Boston: Shambhala, 1999).

47. K. Wilber, *The Collected Works of Ken Wilber*, Vols. 5–8 (Boston: Shambhala, 2000).

48. K. Wilber, *Integral Operating System* (Louisville, CO: Sounds True, 2005).

49. K. Wilber, *Integral Life Practice* (Denver, CO: Integral Institute, 2005).

50. K. Wilber, *Integral Spirituality: A Startling New Role for Religion in the Modern and Postmodern World* (Boston: Shambhala, 2007).

51. L. Shea and N. C. Frisch, "Application of Integral Theory in Holistic Nursing Practice," *Holistic Nursing Practice* 28, no. 6 (2014): 344–352.

52. O. F. Jarrin, "The Integrality of Situated Caring in Nursing and the Environment, "*Advances in Nursing Science* 35, no. 1 (2012): 14–24.

53. C. S. Clark, "An Integral Nursing Education Experience: Outcomes from a BSN Reiki Course," *Holistic Nursing Practice* 27, no. 1 (2013): 13–22.

54. C. S. Clark and G. Pellicci, "An Integral Nursing Education: A Stress Management and Life Balance Course," *International Journal of Human Caring* 15, no. 1 (2011): 13–22.

55. B. M. Dossey, "Theory of Integrative Nurse Coaching," in *Nurse Coaching: Integrative Approaches for Health and Wellbeing*, eds. B. M. Dossey, S. Luck, and B. G. Schaub (North Miami, FL: International Nurse Coach Association, 2015): 29–49.

56. J. F. Quinn, M. Smith, C. Ritenbaugh, K. Swanson, and M. J. Watson, "Research Guidelines for Assessing the Impact of the Healing Relationship in Clinical Nursing," *Alternative Therapies in Health and Medicine* 9, no. 3S (2003): A65–A79.

57. J. F. Quinn, "The Integrated Nurse: Wholeness, Self-Discovery, and Self-Care," in *Integrative Nursing*, eds. M. J. Kreitzer and M. Koithan (New York: Oxford University Press, 2014): 17–32.

58. J. F. Quinn, "The Integrated Nurse: Way of the Healer," in *Integrative Nursing*, eds. M. J. Kreitzer and M. Koithan (New York: Oxford University Press, 2014): 33–46.

59. B. S. Barnum, *Nursing Theory: Analysis, Application, Evaluation*, 6th ed. (Philadelphia: Lippincott Williams & Wilkins, 2005).

60. W. Rosa, "Holding Heartspace: The Unveiling of the Self Through Being and Becoming," *International Journal of Human Caring* 18, no. 4 (2014): 59.

61. W. Rosa, "Reflections on Self in Relation to Other: Core Community Values of a Moral/Ethical Foundation," *Creative Nursing* 20, no. 4 (2014): 242–247.

62. C. Johns, *Becoming a Reflective Practitioner*, 4th ed. (Hoboken, NJ: Wiley-Blackwell, 2013).

63. K. Richards, E. Sheen, and M. C. Mazzer, *Self-Care and You: Caring for the Caregiver* (Silver Spring, MD: Nursesbooks.org, 2014).

64. R. Schaub and B. G. Schaub, *Transpersonal Development: Cultivating the Human Resources of Peace, Wisdom, Purpose and Oneness* (Huntington, NY: Florence Press, 2013).

65. B. L. Seaward, *Managing Stress: Principles and Strategies for Health and Wellbeing* (Burlington, MA: Jones & Bartlett Learning, 2015).

66. Z. R. Wolf, *Exploring Rituals in Nursing: Joining Art and Science* (New York: Springer, 2014).

67. B. A. Carper, "Fundamental Patterns of Knowing in Nursing," *Advances in Nursing Science* 1, no. 1 (1978): 13–23.

68. P. L. Munhall, "Unknowing: Toward Another Pattern of Knowing in Nursing," *Nursing Outlook* 41, no. 3 (1993): 125–128.

69. J. White, "Patterns of Knowing: Review, Critique, and Update," *Advances in Nursing Science* 17, no. 2 (1995): 73–86.

70. D. Beck, "Spiral Dynamics Integral" (n.d.). www.spiraldynamics.net.

71. R. McCraty and D. Childre, "Coherence: Bridging Personal, Social, and Global Health," *Alternative Therapies in Health and Medicine* 16, no. 4 (2010): 10–24.

72. L. Dossey, "Samueli Conference on Definitions and Standards in Healing Research: Working Definitions and Terms," *Alternative Therapies in Health and Medicine* 9, no. 3 (2003): A11.

73. F. Nightingale, "To the Probationer-Nurses in the Nightingale Fund School at St. Thomas's Hospital from Florence Nightingale, 16th May 1888 (Privately Printed)," in *Florence Nightingale Today: Healing, Leadership, Global Action*, eds. B. M. Dossey, L. C. Selanders, D. M. Beck, and A. Attewell (Silver Spring, MD: Nursesbooks.org, 2005): 274.

74. F. Nightingale, "Una and the Lion," *Good Words*, June (1868), 362, in *Florence Nightingale: Mystic, Visionary, Healer*, B. M. Dossey (Philadelphia: Lippincott Williams & Wilkins, 2000): 294.

75. C. G. Jung, *The Archetypes and the Collective Unconscious*, 2nd ed., Vol. 9, Part I (Princeton, NJ: Bollingen, 1981).

76. W. Rosa, "Caring Science and Compassion Fatigue: Reflective Inventory for the Individual Processes of Self-Healing," *Beginnings* 34, no. 4 (2014): 18–20.

77. W. Rosa, "Conscious Dying and Cultural Emergence: Reflective Systems Inventory for the

Collective Processes of Global Healing," *Beginnings* 34, no. 5 (2014): 20–22.

78. J. Halifax, B. M. Dossey, and C. H. Rushton, *Being with Dying: Compassionate End-of-Life Training Guide* (Santa Fe, NM: Prajna Mountain Press, 2007).

79. W. T. Reich, "Speaking of Suffering: A Moral Account of Compassion," *Soundings* 72, no. 1 (1989): 83–108.

80. F. Nightingale, "To the Nurses and Probationers Trained Under the 'Nightingale Fund,' 1883, Privately Printed" (London: Spottiswoode), in *Florence Nightingale Today: Healing, Leadership, Global Action*, eds. B. M. Dossey, L. C. Selanders, D. M. Beck, and A. Attewell (Silver Spring, MD: Nursesbooks.org, 2005): 267.

81. F. Nightingale, "Address from Miss Nightingale to the Probationer-Nurses in the 'Nightingale Fund' at St. Thomas's Hospital, and the Nurses Who Were Formerly Trained There, Privately Printed, 1876" (London: Spottiswoode), in *Florence Nightingale Today: Healing, Leadership, Global Action*, eds. B. M. Dossey, L. C. Selanders, D. M. Beck, and A. Attewell (Silver Spring, MD: Nursesbooks.org, 2005): 251.

82. F. Nightingale, "To the Probationer-Nurses in the Nightingale Fund School at St. Thomas' Hospital from Florence Nightingale 16th May 1897, Privately Printed," in *Florence Nightingale Today: Healing, Leadership, Global Action*, eds. B. M. Dossey, L. C. Selanders, D. M. Beck, and A. Attewell (Silver Spring, MD: Nursesbooks.org, 2005): 283.

83. J. S. Perdue, "Integration of Complementary and Alternative Therapies in an Acute Rehabilitation Hospital: A Readiness Assessment" (unpublished doctoral dissertation, Western University of Health Sciences, Pomona, CA, 2011).

84. International Nurse Coach Association, "Integrative Nurse Coach Certificate Program" (2015). www.iNurseCoach.com.

85. Personal communication. Diane Pisanos, June 15, 2012.

86. C. C. Barrere, "Teaching Future Holistic Nurses: Integration of Holistic and Quality Safety Education for Nurses (QSEN) Concepts," in *Holistic Nursing: A Handbook for Practice*, 6th ed., eds. B. M. Dossey and L. Keegan (Burlington, MA: Jones & Bartlett Learning, 2013): 815–824.

87. Personal communication. Darlene R. Hess, September 12, 2014.

88. S. Esbjörn-Hargens, "Integral Research: A Multi-Method Approach to Investigating Phenomena," *Constructivism in the Human Sciences* 11, nos. 1–2 (2006): 79–107.

89. D. Harper, K. S. Davey, and P. N. Fordham, "Leadership Lessons in Global Nursing and Health from the Nightingale Letter Collection at the University of Alabama at Birmingham," *Journal of Holistic Nursing* 32, no. 1 (2014): 45–53.

90. D. M. Beck, B. M. Dossey, and C. H. Rushton, "Florence Nightingale: Connecting Her Legacy with Local-to-Global Health Today" (2014). http://ce.nurse.com/course/ce598/florence-nightingale/.

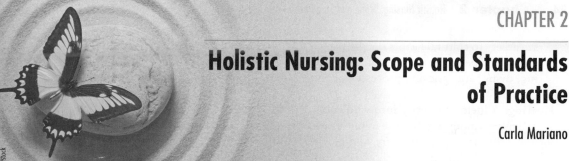

Holistic Nursing: Scope and Standards of Practice

Carla Mariano

Nurse Healer Objectives

Theoretical

- Describe the scope of holistic nursing.
- Describe the standards of holistic nursing.
- Discuss the five core values of holistic nursing.

Clinical

- Integrate the principles of holistic nursing into practice.
- Identify how you implement the standards of holistic nursing in your practice.
- Discuss *Holistic Nursing: Scope and Standards of Practice, Second Edition*, with colleagues.

Personal

- Reflect on your worldview and how it is similar to or different from the philosophy of holism.
- Explore how the concepts of holistic nursing apply to your personal life.

Definitions *

Allopathic/conventional therapies: Medical, surgical, pharmacological, and invasive and noninvasive diagnostic procedures; those interventions most commonly used in allopathic, Western medicine.

Complementary/integrative modalities (CIM)/Complementary/alternative modalities (CAM)**: A broad set of healthcare practices, therapies, and modalities that address the whole person—body, mind, emotion, spirit, and environment, not just signs and symptoms—and that may replace or be used as complements to or in conjunction with conventional Western medical, surgical, and pharmacological treatments.

Critical thinking: An active, purposeful, organized cognitive process involving creativity, reflection, problem solving, both rational and intuitive judgment, an attitude of inquiry, and a philosophical orientation toward thinking about thinking.

Cultural competence: The ability to deliver health care with knowledge of and

---

Note: This chapter is derived from *Holistic Nursing: Scope and Standards of Practice, Second Edition* (2013), C. Mariano, primary contributor. Printed with permission of the American Holistic Nurses Association (AHNA) and the American Nurses Association (ANA).

---

*Many of the definitions in this chapter were adapted from *Holistic Nursing: Scope and Standards of Practice, Second Edition* (2013), with permission, and from Dossey and Keegan (2013).

**For the remainder of the chapter, this will be referred to as "CAM."

sensitivity to cultural factors that influence the health behavior and the curing, healing, dying, and grieving processes of the person.

Healing: A lifelong journey into wholeness, seeking harmony and balance in one's own life and in family, community, and global relations. Healing involves those physical, mental, social, and spiritual processes of recovery, repair, renewal, and transformation that increase wholeness and often (though not invariably) order and coherence. Healing is an emergent process of the whole system bringing together aspects of one's self and the body, mind, emotion, spirit, and environment at deeper levels of inner knowing, leading toward integration and balance, with each aspect having equal importance and value. Healing can lead to more complex levels of personal understanding and meaning and may be synchronous but not synonymous with curing.

Healing process: A continual journey of change and the evolving of one's self through life that is characterized by the awareness of patterns that support or that are challenges or barriers to health and healing and that may be done alone or in a healing community.

Healing relationships: The quality and characteristics of interactions between one who facilitates healing and the person in the process of healing. Characteristics of such interactions involve empathy, caring, love, warmth, trust, confidence, credibility, competence, honesty, courtesy, respect, sharing expectations, and good communication.

Healing system: A true healthcare system in which people can receive adequate, nontoxic, and noninvasive assistance in maintaining wellness and healing for body, mind, emotion, and spirit, together with the most sophisticated, aggressive curing technologies available.

Health: An individually defined state or process in which the individual (nurse, client, family, group, or community) experiences a sense of well-being, harmony, and unity such that subjective experiences about health, health beliefs, and values are honored; a process of becoming an expanding consciousness.

Health promotion: Activities and preventive measures to promote health, increase well-being, and actualize the human potential of people, families, communities, society, and ecology; such activities and measures include immunizations, fitness and exercise programs, breast self-exam, appropriate nutrition, relaxation, stress management, social support, prayer, meditation, healing rituals, cultural practices, and promoting environmental health and safety.

Holistic communication: A free flow of verbal and nonverbal interchange between and among people and significant beings such as pets, nature, and God/Life Force/Absolute/Transcendent that explores meaning and ideas leading to mutual understanding and growth.

Holistic ethics: The basic underlying concept of the unity and integral wholeness of all people and of all nature, identified and pursued by finding unity and wholeness within the self and within humanity. In this framework, acts are not performed for the sake of law, precedent, or social norms, but rather from a desire to do good freely to witness, identify, and contribute to unity.

Holistic healing: A form of healing based on attention to all aspects of an individual—physical, mental, emotional, sexual, cultural, social, spiritual, and energetic. The manifestation of right relationship at one or more levels of the body-mind-spirit-environment-energy system.

Holistic nurse: A nurse who recognizes and integrates body-mind-emotion-spirit-environment principles and modalities into daily life and clinical practice, creates a caring, healing space within herself or himself that allows the nurse to be an instrument of healing, shares authenticity of unconditional presence that helps to remove the barriers to the healing process, facilitates another person's growth (body-mind-emotion-spirit-environment-energetic connections), and assists with recovery from illness or transition to peaceful death.

Holistic nursing practice process: An iterative and integrative process that involves six steps that can occur simultaneously: (1) assessing; (2) diagnosing or identifying patterns, challenges, needs, and health issues; (3) identifying outcomes; (4) planning care; (5) implementing the care plan; and (6) evaluating.

Honor: An act or intention indicating the holding of self or another in high respect, esteem, and dignity, including valuing and accepting the humanity of people with regard for the decisions and wishes of another.

Human caring: The moral ideal of nursing in which the nurse brings one's whole self into a relationship with the whole self of the person being cared for to protect that person's vulnerability, preserve her or his humanity and dignity, and reinforce the meaning and experience of oneness and unity.

Human health experience: That totality of human experience including each person's subjective experience about health, health beliefs, values, sexual orientation, and personal preferences that encompasses health-wellness-disease-illness-death.

Illness: A subjective experience of symptoms and suffering to which the individual ascribes meaning and significance; not synonymous with disease; a shift in the homeodynamic balance of the person to disharmony and imbalance.

Intention: The conscious awareness of being in the present moment to help facilitate the healing process; a volitional act of love; conscious alignment of essence and purpose allowing the highest good to flow through a healing intervention.

Interdisciplinary/interprofessional: Conversation or collaboration across disciplines where knowledge is shared that informs learning, practice, education, and research; it includes individuals, families, community members, and various disciplines.

Meaning: That which is signified, indicated, referred to, or understood. More specifically, philosophical meaning is meaning that depends on the symbolic connections that are grasped by reason. Psychological meaning is meaning that depends on connections that are experienced through intuition or insight.

Patient-centered care: Care that is respectful of and responsive to individual patient preferences, needs, and values, and that ensures that patient values guide all clinical decisions. Patient-centered care encompasses identifying, respecting, and caring about patients' differences, values, preferences, and expressed needs; relieving pain and suffering; coordinating continuous care/listening to, clearly informing, communicating with, and educating patients; sharing decision making and management; and continuously advocating disease prevention, wellness, and promotion of healthy lifestyles, including a focus on population health.[1]

Person: An individual, client, patient, family member, support person, or community member who has the opportunity to engage in interaction with a holistic nurse.

Person-centered care: The human caring process in which the holistic nurse gives full attention and intention to the whole self of a person, not merely the current presenting symptoms, illness, crisis, or tasks to be accomplished, and that also includes reinforcing the person's meaning and experience of oneness and unity; the condition of trust that is created in which holistic care can be given and received.

Presence: The essential state or core of healing; approaching an individual in a way that respects and honors her or his essence; relating in a way that reflects a quality of being with and in collaboration with rather than doing to; entering into a shared experience (or field of consciousness) that promotes healing potential and an experience of well-being.

Relationship-centered care: A process model of caregiving that is based on a vision of community where three types of relationships are identified: (1) patient–practitioner relationship, (2) community–practitioner relationship, and (3) practitioner–practitioner relationship. Each of these interrelated relationships is essential within a reformed integrative healthcare delivery system in a hospital, clinic, or community, or in the home. Each component involves a unique set of responsibilities and tasks that addresses the three areas of knowledge, values, and skills.[2]

Spirituality: The feelings, thoughts, experiences, and behaviors that arise from a search for meaning; that which is generally considered sacred or holy; usually, though not universally, considered to involve a sense of connection with an absolute, imminent, or transcendent spiritual force, however named, as well as the conviction that meaning, value, direction, and purpose are valid aspects of the individual and universe; the essence of being and relatedness that permeates all of life and is manifested in one's knowing, doing, and being; the interconnectedness with self, others, nature, and God/Life Force/Absolute/Transcendent; not necessarily synonymous with religion.

Transpersonal: A personal understanding that is based on one's experiences of temporarily transcending or moving beyond one's usual identification with the limited biological, historical, cultural, and personal self at the deepest and most profound levels of experience possible; that which transcends the limits and boundaries of individual ego identities and possibilities to include acknowledgment and appreciation of something greater. From this perspective the ordinary, biological, historical, cultural, and personal self is seen as an important, but only a partial, manifestation or expression of this much greater something that is one's deeper origin and destination.

Wellness: Integrated, congruent functioning aimed toward reaching one's highest potential.

Scope and Standards of Holistic Nursing Practice

Extraordinary changes have occurred in health care and nursing in the past decade. During this time, holistic nurses recognized that not only were they practicing a unique specialty within nursing, but that they needed to develop and publish standards of practice to document and define that specialty practice. Holistic nursing was officially recognized as a distinct specialty within the discipline of nursing by the American Nurses Association (ANA) in November 2006.

Holistic Nursing: Scope and Standards of Practice, Second Edition,[3] articulates the scope and standards of the specialty practice of holistic nursing and informs holistic nurses, the nursing profession, other healthcare providers and disciplines, employers, third-party payers, legislators, and the public about the unique scope of knowledge and the standards of practice and professional performance of a holistic nurse. *Holistic Nursing: Scope and Standards of Practice, Second Edition,** is the foundational document and resource for holistic nursing education at all levels (undergraduate, graduate, continuing education) and for holistic nursing practice, research, advocacy, and certification.

Function of the Scope of Practice Statement of Holistic Nursing

The scope of practice statement describes the *who, what, where, when, why,* and *how* of the practice of holistic nursing.[3, 4] The answers to these questions provide a picture of that specialty nursing practice, its boundaries, and its membership.

Nursing: Scope and Standards of Practice, Second Edition (2010), applies to all professional registered nurses engaged in practice, regardless of specialty, practice setting, or educational preparation.[4] Along with the *Guide to the Code of Ethics for Nurses: Interpretation and Application*[5] and *Nursing's Social Policy Statement: The Essence of the Profession,*[6] it forms the foundation of practice for all registered nurses. The scope of holistic nursing practice is specific to this specialty, but

---

*To obtain a complete copy of *Holistic Nursing: Scope and Standards of Practice, Second Edition* (2013), or most recent copy, contact the American Holistic Nurses Association (AHNA), 100 SE 9th Street, Suite 3A, Topeka, KS, 66612; 1-800-278-2462 or 1-785-234-1712; www.ahna.org or info@ahna.org.

it builds on the scope of practice expected of all registered nurses.

Function of the Standards of Holistic Nursing

"The Standards of Professional Nursing Practice are authoritative statements of the duties that all registered nurses, regardless of role, population, or specialty, are expected to perform competently."[4, p. 2]

> Standards reflect the values and priorities of the profession. Standards provide direction for professional nursing practice and a framework for evaluation of this practice. Written in measurable terms, these standards define the nursing profession's accountability to the public and the outcomes for which registered nurses are responsible.[7, p. 1]

The standards of holistic nursing practice are specific to this specialty but build on the standards of practice expected of all registered nurses.

Competencies accompany each standard of holistic nursing and articulate the "expected and measureable level of nursing performance that integrates knowledge, skills, abilities, and judgment, based on established scientific knowledge and expectations for nursing practice."[4, p. 64]

Holistic Nursing: Scope and Standards of Practice, Second Edition, presents a differentiation between practice at the basic and advanced practice levels. The *Scope and Standards* are organized according to the ANA criteria used to recognize a nursing specialty area and build on nursing knowledge, skills, and competencies required for licensure.[8, 9] *Holistic Nursing: Scope and Standards of Practice, Second Edition*, provides a blueprint for holistic practice, education, and research. It includes the philosophical beliefs, principles, and practices, as well as new developments and advancements in the field of holistic nursing. The standards guide clinicians, educators, researchers, nurse managers, and administrators in professional activities, knowledge, and performance that are relevant to holistic nursing basic and advanced practice, education, research,

management, and advocacy. Because holistic nursing emphasizes that human experiences are subjectively described and that health and illness are determined by the view of the individual, *Holistic Nursing: Scope and Standards of Practice, Second Edition*, is derived from values that are central to the specialty and are consistent with the philosophies and theories of holism.

Evolution of Holistic Nursing

Holism in health care is a philosophy that emanates directly from Florence Nightingale, who believed in care that focused on unity, wellness, and the interrelationship of human beings, events, and environment. Even Hippocrates, the father of Western medicine, espoused a holistic orientation when he taught doctors to observe their patients' life circumstances and emotional states. Socrates stated, "Curing the soul; that is the first thing." In holism, symptoms are believed to be an expression of the body's wisdom as it reacts to cure its own imbalance or disease.

The root of the word *heal* comes from the Greek word *halos* and the Anglo-Saxon word *haelan*, which means to be or to become whole. The word *holy* also comes from the same source. Healing means "making whole"—or restoring balance and harmony. It is movement toward a sense of wholeness and completion. Healing, therefore, is the integration of the totality of the person in body, mind, emotion, spirit, and environment.

One of the driving forces behind the holistic nursing movement in the United States was the formation of the American Holistic Nurses Association (AHNA). In 1981, founder Charlotte McGuire and 75 founding members began the national organization in Houston, Texas. The national office is now located in Topeka, Kansas. The AHNA's mission is to advance the philosophy and practices of holistic nursing and unite nurses in healing with a focus on holistic principles of health, preventive education, and the integration of allopathic and complementary caring and healing modalities to facilitate care of the whole person and significant others. From its inception in 1981, the AHNA has been the leader in developing and advancing holistic principles, practices, and guidelines. The association predicted that holistic principles, caring and healing, and the integration of complementary and alternative therapies would emerge into mainstream health care.

The AHNA, the definitive voice for holistic nursing, has as its vision "a world in which nursing nurtures wholeness and inspires peace and healing." The mission of the AHNA is to advance holistic nursing through community building, advocacy, research, and education. It is committed to promoting wholeness and wellness in individuals, families, communities, nurses themselves, the nursing profession, and the environment. Through its various activities, AHNA provides vision, direction, and leadership in the advancement of holistic nursing; integrates the art and science of nursing into the profession; empowers holistic nursing through education, research, and standards; encourages nurses to be models of wellness; honors individual excellence in the advancement of holistic nursing; and influences policy to change the healthcare system to a more humanistic orientation.

The goals and endeavors of AHNA have continued to map conceptual frameworks and the blueprint for holistic nursing practice, education, and research, which is the most complete way to conceptualize and practice professional nursing. The relevance and validity of holistic nursing as a science and practice have been increasingly demonstrated in recent years.

> While becoming more popular and more highly regarded, holism and holistic nursing have contributed to enhancing the human condition in many ways. Holism as a philosophy, concept, theory, and practice has been used to expand our understanding of human wellness and illness. Holistic nursing has become more systematized, refined, and diversified as strategies and practices have been shown to have an impact on health and well-being. Holistic nursing . . . has progressed . . . through the development of standards, endorsement of programs, and certification of beginning and

advanced practitioners. Holistic nursing's contributions to human welfare have been increasingly recognized . . . , as evidenced in their current standing in health care and appreciation by society. . . . Holism as a perspective and holistic nursing as a response may offer the world something that counteracts the fragmentation and isolation that exists so predominantly in our society. . . . Holistic nursing . . . provides a context in which nurses can consider, understand, and appreciate all the aspects of human experience that contribute to patterns of life, health, and illness.[10, p. 5]

Scope of Holistic Nursing

Holistic nursing is defined as "all nursing practice that has healing the whole person as its goal."[11] Holistic nursing is a specialty practice that draws on nursing knowledge, theories of nursing and wholeness, expertise, and intuition to guide nurses in becoming therapeutic partners with people in strengthening human responses to facilitate the healing process and achieve wholeness. Holistic nursing focuses on protecting, promoting, and optimizing health and wellness; assisting healing; preventing illness and injury; alleviating suffering; and supporting people to find peace, comfort, harmony, and balance through the diagnosis and treatment of human response.

Holistic nursing care is healing oriented and centered on the relationship with the person in contrast to an orientation toward diseases and their cures. Holistic nursing emphasizes practices of self-reflection and self-care, intentionality, presence, mindfulness, and therapeutic use of self as pivotal for facilitation of healing and patterning of wellness in others. In some sense, all nursing practice can be comprehensive—that is, all nursing practice may have a biopsychosocial perspective. What makes holistic nursing practice a specialty is that there is a philosophy, a body of knowledge, and an advanced set of nursing skills applied to practice that recognize the totality of the human being and the interconnectedness of body, mind, emotion, spirit, energy, society, culture, relationships, context, and environment. Philosophically, holistic nursing is a worldview, a way of being in the world, not just a modality. This philosophy honors the unique humanness of all people regardless of who and what they are. Knowledge for holistic nursing practice derives not only from nursing but from theories of wholeness, energy, and unity as well as from other healing systems and approaches. Holistic nurses incorporate both conventional nursing and complementary/integrative modalities and interventions into practice.

Through unconditional presence and intention, holistic nurses create environments conducive to healing, using techniques that promote empowerment, peace, comfort, and a subjective sense of harmony and well-being for the person. The holistic nurse acts in partnership with the individual or family in providing options and alternatives regarding health and treatment. In addition, the holistic nurse assists the person to find meaning in the health and illness experience.

Holistic nursing focuses on simultaneously integrating as an iterative process all of these realms: a philosophy of being and living, using theories of nursing and wholeness with related knowledge and skills, focusing on the unity and totality of humans, incorporating healing approaches, creating healing environments, partnering with and empowering individuals, and assisting in the exploration of meaning in the care of people. In holistic nursing, the nurse is the facilitator of healing, honoring that the person heals himself or herself. The holistic nurse assists individuals in identifying themselves as the healer and accessing their own innate healing capacities.

The practice of holistic nursing requires nurses to integrate self-care and self-responsibility into their own lives and to serve as role models for others. Holistic nurses strive for an awareness of the interconnectedness of individuals to the human and global community. Thus, holistic nurses also attend to the health of the ecosystem.

Holistic nurses are instruments of healing and facilitators in the healing process. They honor the individual's subjective experience of health, health beliefs, and values. To become therapeutic partners with individuals, families, communities, and populations, holistic nurses draw on nursing knowledge, theories, research, expertise, intuition, and creativity, incorporating the roles of clinician, educator, consultant, coach, partner, role model, and advocate. Holistic nursing practice encourages peer review of professional practice in various clinical settings and provides care based on current professional standards, laws, and regulations that govern nursing practice. The major phenomena of concern to holistic nursing are listed in **Exhibit 2-1**.

Core Values of Holistic Nursing: Integrating and the Art and Science of Nursing

Holistic nursing emanates from five core values summarizing the ideals and principles of the specialty. These core values are listed here and then are discussed:

1. Holistic Philosophy, Theory, and Ethics
2. Holistic Caring Process
3. Holistic Communication, Therapeutic Healing Environment, and Cultural Diversity
4. Holistic Education and Research
5. Holistic Nurse Self-Reflection and Self-Care

Core Value 1: Holistic Philosophy, Theory, and Ethics

Holistic nurses recognize the human health experience as a complicated, dynamic relationship of health, illness, and wellness, and they value healing as the desired outcome of the practice of nursing. Their practice is based on scientific foundations (theory, research, evidence-based/informed practice, critical thinking, reflection) and art (relationship, communication, creativity, presence, caring). Holistic nursing is grounded in nursing knowledge and skill and guided by nursing theory. Florence Nightingale's writings are often referenced as a significant precursor of the development of holistic nursing. Although each holistic nurse chooses which nursing theory to apply in any individual case, the nursing theories of Jean Watson (Theory of Human Caring and Caring Science), Martha Rogers (Science of Unitary

---

EXHIBIT 2-1   Phenomena of Concern to Holistic Nursing

- The caring, healing relationship
- The subjective experience of and meanings ascribed to health, illness, wellness, healing, birth, growth and development, and dying
- The cultural values and beliefs and folk practices of health, illness, and healing
- Spirituality in nursing care
- The use and evaluation of complementary/alternative/integrative modalities in nursing practice
- Comprehensive health promotion, disease prevention, and well-being
- Self-care processes
- Physical, mental, emotional, and spiritual comfort, discomfort, and pain
- Empowerment, decision making, and the ability to make informed choices
- Social and economic policies and their effects on the health of individuals, families, and communities
- Diverse and alternative healthcare systems and their relationships to access and quality of health care
- The environment, ecosystem, and prevention of disease
- Healing environments

Human Beings), Margaret Newman (Health as Expanding Consciousness), Madeleine Leininger (Theory of Cultural Care Diversity and Universality), Rosemarie Rizzo Parse (Human Becoming School of Thought), Josephine Paterson and Loretta Zderad (Humanistic Nursing Theory), and Helen Erickson, Evelyn Tomlin, and Mary Ann Swain (Modeling and Role-Modeling) are most frequently used to support holistic nursing practice. There has been significant development in the evolution of holism, healing, and caring conceptualization and theory, owing in large part to holistic nurses. Prominent among those are Barbara Dossey (Theory of Integral Nursing), Marlaine Smith (Theory of Unitary Caring), Marilyn Anne Ray (Theory of Bureaucratic Caring), Rozzano Locsin (Technological Competency as Caring and the Practice of Knowing Persons in Nursing), Mary Jane Smith and Patricia Liehr (Story Theory), and Joanne Duffy (Quality Caring Model).

In addition to nursing theory, holistic nurses use other theories and perspectives of wholeness and healing to guide their practice. These scientific theories and philosophies present a worldview of connectedness. Examples include the following:

- Theories of Consciousness
- Systems Theory
- Complexity Science
- Chaos Theory
- Energy Field Theory
- C. Pribram's Holographic Universe
- D. Bohm's Implicate/Explicate Order
- Psychoneuroimmunology
- K. Wilber's Integral Theory of Consciousness
- Spirituality
- Alternative medical systems such as Traditional Oriental Medicine, Ayurveda, Native American, and indigenous healing
- Eastern contemplative orientations such as Zen Buddhism and Taoism

Holistic nurses further recognize and honor the ethic that the person is the authority on his or her own health experience. The holistic nurse is an "option giver" and helps the person develop an understanding of alternatives and implications of various health and treatment options. The holistic nurse first ascertains what the individual thinks or believes is happening to him or her, and then assists the person to identify what will help the situation. The assessment begins from where the individual is. The holistic nurse then discusses options, including the person's choices across a continuum and the possible effects and implications of each. For instance, if a person diagnosed with cancer is experiencing nausea caused by chemotherapy, the individual and nurse may discuss the choices and effects of pharmacologic agents, imagery, homeopathic remedies, and so on, or a combination of these. The holistic nurse acts as partner and coprescriber versus sole prescriber. The relationship is a copiloting of the individual's health experience where the nurse respects the person's decision about his or her own health. It is a process of engagement versus compliance.

Client narratives, whether they arise from individuals, families, or communities, provide the context of the experiences and are used as an important focus in understanding the person's situation. Holistic nurses hold the belief that people, through their inherent capacities, heal themselves. Therefore, the holistic nurse is not the healer but the guide and facilitator of the individual's own healing.

In the belief that all things are connected, the holistic perspective espouses that an individual's actions have a ripple effect throughout humanity. Holism places the greatest worth on individuals' developing higher levels of human awareness. This, in turn, elevates the whole of humanity. Holistic nurses believe in the sacredness of one's self and of all nature. One's inner self and the collective greater self have stewardship over not only one's body, mind, and spirit but also the planet. Holistic nurses focus on the meaning and quality of life deriving from their own character and from their relationship to the universe rather than that imposed from without.

Holistic nurses hold to a professional ethic of caring and healing that seeks to preserve the wholeness and dignity of the self and others. They support human dignity by advocating and adhering to the Patient Bill of Rights,[12] the ANA *Guide to the Code of Ethics for Nurses: Interpretation and Application*,[5] and the AHNA *Position Statement on Holistic Nursing Ethics*.[13]

Core Value 2: Holistic Caring Process

Holistic nurses provide care that recognizes the totality of the human being (the interconnectedness of body, mind, emotion, spirit, society, culture, relationships, context, and environment). This is an *integrated* as well as a comprehensive approach. Although physical symptoms are treated, holistic nurses also focus on how the individual cognitively perceives and emotionally deals with the illness; the illness's effect on the person's family, social relationships, and economic resources; the person's values and cultural and spiritual beliefs and preferences regarding treatment; and the meaning of this experience to the person's life. In addition, holistic nurses may also incorporate several modalities (e.g., cognitive restructuring, stress management, visualization, aromatherapy, therapeutic touch) with conventional nursing interventions. Holistic nurses focus on care interventions that promote healing, peace, comfort, and a subjective sense of well-being for the person.

The holistic caring process involves six often simultaneously occurring steps: assessment, diagnosis (pattern, problem, need identification), outcomes, therapeutic care plan, implementation, and evaluation. Holistic nurses apply the holistic caring process in all settings with individuals and families across the life span, population groups, and communities.

Holistic nurses incorporate a variety of roles into their practice, including expert clinician and facilitator of healing; consultant, coach, and collaborator; educator and guide; administrator, leader, and change agent; researcher; and advocate. Holistic nurses strongly emphasize partnership with individuals throughout the entire decision-making process. Holistic assessments include not only physical, functional, psychosocial, mental, emotional, cultural, and sexual aspects but also the spiritual, transpersonal, and energy field assessments of the whole person. Energy assessments are based on the concept that all beings are composed of energy. Congestion or stagnation of energy in any realm creates disharmony and disease. Spiritual assessments glean not only religious beliefs and practices but query a person's meaning and purpose in life and how these may have changed because of the present health experience. Holistic nurses use understanding of energy anatomy and electromagnetic fields in both their assessments and the healing process. Spiritual assessments also include questions about an individual's sense of serenity and peace, what provides joy and fulfillment, and the source of strength and hope.

Holistic assessment data are interpreted into patterns, challenges, and needs from which meaning and understanding of the health and disease experience can be mutually identified with the person. Holistic nurses first ask an individual, "What do you think is going on (happening) with you?" and then, "What do you think would help?" Another important responsibility of the holistic nurse is to help the person identify risk factors such as lifestyle, habits, beliefs and values, personal and family health history, and age-related conditions that influence health, and then to find and use opportunities to increase well-being. The focus is on the individual's goals, not the nurse's.

Therapeutic plans of care respect the person's experience and the uniqueness of each healing journey. The same illness may have very different manifestations in different individuals. A major aspect of holistic nursing practice, in addition to competence, is intention. That is, the nurse intends for the wholeness, well-being, and highest good of the person in every encounter and intervention. This intention honors and reinforces the innate capacity of people to heal themselves. Therefore, holistic nurses respect that outcomes may not be those expected and may evolve differently based on the person's individual healing process and health choices. Holistic nurses endeavor to detach themselves from the outcomes. The nurse does not produce the outcomes; the individual's own healing process produces the outcomes, and the nurse facilitates this process. An important focus of the holistic nurse is on guiding individuals and significant others to use their inner strength and resources through the course of healing.

Holistic nurses consistently provide appropriate and evidence-based information (including current knowledge, practice, and research) regarding the health condition and various treatments and therapies and their side effects. Holistic care always occurs within the scope and standards of practice of registered nursing and in accordance with state and federal laws and regulations.

Holistic nurses integrate CAM into clinical practice to treat people's physiologic, psychological, and spiritual needs. Doing so does not negate the validity of conventional medical therapies but serves to complement, broaden, and enrich the scope of nursing practice and to help individuals access their greatest healing potential. Holistic nurses advocate for integration rather than separation. The National Center for Complementary and Alternative Medicine has categorized CAM approaches, and these are identified in **Exhibit 2-2**.

Therapies frequently incorporated into holistic nursing practice include the following interventions: meditation; relaxation therapy; breath work; music, art, and aroma therapies; energy-based touch therapies such as therapeutic touch, healing touch, and Reiki; acupressure; massage; guided imagery; hypnosis; animal-assisted therapy; biofeedback; prayer; reflexology; diet; herbology; and homeopathy. Other interventions frequently employed in holistic nursing practice in addition to conventional nursing interventions include anxiety reduction and stress management, calming techniques, emotional support, exercise and nutrition promotion, smoking cessation, patient contracting, resiliency promotion, forgiveness facilitation, hope installation, presence, journaling, counseling, cognitive therapy, self-help, spiritual support, coaching, health education, consultation and referral, community health development, and environmental management.

Because many of today's healthcare problems (80% of all U.S. healthcare issues) are stress related, holistic nurses empower individuals by teaching them techniques to reduce their stress. Many interventions used in holistic nursing elicit the relaxation response (e.g., breath work, meditation, relaxation, imagery, aromatherapy and essential oils, and diet). People can learn these therapies and use them without the intervention of a healthcare provider. This allows people to take an active role in the management of their own health care. Holistic nurses also can teach families and caregivers to use these techniques for loved ones who may be ill (e.g., simple foot or hand massage for older clients with dementia).

EXHIBIT 2-2   Categories of CAM Therapies

In the context of this chapter, these descriptive categories encompass generally, but not exhaustively, those therapies described as alternative or complementary.

Natural products. This area includes substances found in nature such as a variety of herbal medicines (also known as botanicals), vitamins, minerals, whole diet therapies, and other "natural products." Many are sold over the counter as dietary supplements. (Some uses of dietary supplements—e.g., taking a multivitamin to meet minimum daily nutritional requirements or taking calcium to promote bone health—are not thought of as CAM.) CAM "natural products" also include probiotics—live microorganisms (usually bacteria) that are similar to microorganisms normally found in the human digestive tract and that may have beneficial effects. Probiotics are available in foods (e.g., yogurts) or as dietary supplements.

Mind–body medicine. Mind–body practices focus on the interactions among the brain, mind, body, and behavior, with the intent to use the mind to affect physical functioning and promote health. Many CAM practices embody this concept—in different ways. Some techniques that were considered CAM in the past have become mainstream (e.g., patient support groups, psychotherapy, cognitive behavioral therapy, stress management). Mind–body techniques include meditation, relaxation, imagery, hypnotherapy, yoga, biofeedback, and tai chi. Other therapies are autogenic training, spirituality, prayer, mental healing, and therapies that use creative outlets such as art, music, dance, or journaling. Acupuncture is considered to be a part of mind–body medicine, but it is also a component of energy medicine, manipulative and body-based practices, and Traditional Chinese Medicine.

Manipulative and body-based practices. Manipulative and body-based practices focus primarily on the structures and systems of the body, including the bones and joints, soft tissues, and circulatory and lymphatic systems. Commonly used therapies fall within this category: spinal manipulation including chiropractic or osteopathic manipulation, massage, and reflexology.

Movement therapies. CAM also encompasses movement therapies—a broad range of Eastern and Western movement-based approaches used to promote physical, mental, emotional, and spiritual well-being. Examples include Feldenkrais method, Alexander technique, Pilates, Rolfing Structural Integration, Trager psychophysical integration, and dance therapy.

Practices of traditional healers. Traditional healers use methods based on indigenous theories, beliefs, and experiences handed down from generation to generation. Examples include Native American healer/medicine man, African, Middle Eastern, Tibetan, Central and South American, and Curanderismo.

Energy therapies. Some CAM practices involve manipulation of various energy fields to affect health. Such fields may be characterized as veritable (measurable) or putative (yet to be measured). Practices based on veritable forms of energy include those involving electromagnetic fields (e.g., magnet therapy, light therapy, or alternating-current or direct-current fields). Practices based on putative energy fields (also called *biofields*) generally reflect the concept that human beings are infused with subtle forms of energy. Some forms of energy therapy manipulate biofields by applying pressure, such as acupressure, and manipulating the body by placing the hands in or through these fields. Examples include qi gong, Reiki, therapeutic touch, and healing touch.

Whole medical systems. Complete systems of theory and practice that have evolved over time in different cultures and apart from conventional or Western medicine may be considered CAM. Examples of ancient whole medical systems include ayurvedic medicine and Traditional Chinese Medicine. More modern systems that have developed in the past few centuries include homeopathy and naturopathy.

Source: National Center for Complementary and Alternative Medicine, National Institutes of Health (2012). http://nccam.nih.gov.

In addition, individuals are taught how to evaluate their own responses to these modalities.

Holistic nurses prescribe as legally authorized. They instruct individuals regarding drug, herbal, and homeopathic regimens, and, just as important, they consult on the side effects and interactions between medications and herbs.

They consult, collaborate, and refer, as necessary, to both conventional allopathic providers and to holistic practitioners. They provide information and counseling to people about alternative, complementary, integrative, and conventional healthcare practices. Very important, holistic nurses facilitate negotiation of services as they guide individuals and families between conventional Western medicine and alternative systems. Holistic nurses, in partnership with the individual and others, evaluate whether care is effective and whether changes in the meaning of the health experience occur for the individual.

Holistic nurses also take a lead in incorporating a holistic caring perspective and integrating healing strategies into practice and system-wide programs and organizations.

Core Value 3: Holistic Communication, Therapeutic Healing Environment, and Cultural Diversity

The holistic nurse's communication ensures that each individual experiences the presence of the nurse as authentic, caring, compassionate, and sincere. This is more than offering therapeutic techniques such as responding, reflecting, summarizing, and so on. This is deep listening, or as some say, "Listening with the heart and not just the ears." It is done with conscious intention and without preconceptions, busy-ness, distractions, or analysis. It takes place in the "now" within an atmosphere of shared humanness—human being to human being. Through presence or "being with in the moment," holistic nurses provide each person with an interpersonal encounter that the individual can experience as a connection with one who is giving undivided attention to his or her needs and concerns. Using unconditional positive regard, holistic nurses convey to the individual receiving care the belief in his or her worth and value as a human being, not solely as a recipient of medical and nursing interventions.

The holistic nurse recognizes the importance of context in understanding the person's health experience. Space and time are allowed for exploration. Each person's health encounter is truly seen as unique and may be contrary to conventional knowledge and treatments. Therefore, the holistic nurse must be comfortable with ambiguity, paradox, and uncertainty. This requires a perspective that the nurse is not "the expert" regarding another's health and illness experience but is actually a "learner."

Holistic nurses have a knowledge base of the use and meanings of symbolic language and use interventions such as imagery, creation of sacred space and personal rituals, dream exploration, narrative, story, journaling, and aesthetic therapies such as music, visual arts, and dance. They encourage and support others in the use of prayer, meditation, and other spiritual and symbolic practices for healing purposes.

A cornerstone of holistic nursing practice is assisting individuals to find meaning in their experience. Regardless of the person's condition, the meaning that individuals ascribe to their situation can influence their response to it. Holistic nurses attend to the subjective world of the individual. They consider meanings such as the person's concerns in relation to health and family economics, as well as deeper meanings related to the person's purpose in life. Regardless of the technology or treatment, holistic nurses address the human spirit as a major force in healing. Each person's perception of meaning is related to all factors in health-wellness-disease-illness.

Holistic nurses realize that suffering, illness, and disease are natural components of the human condition and have the potential to teach us about ourselves, our relationships, and our universe. Every experience is valued for its meaning and lesson.

Holistic nurses have a particular obligation to create a therapeutic healing environment that values holism, caring, social support, and integration of conventional and CAM approaches to healing. They seek to create caring cultures and environments where individuals, both clients and staff, feel connected, supported, and respected. A particular perspective of holistic nursing is the nurse as the "healing environment" and "an instrument of healing." Holistic nurses shape the physical environment (e.g., light, fresh air, pleasant sounds or quiet, neatness and order, healing smells, earth elements). And they provide a relationship-focused environment by creating sacred space through presence and intention where another can feel safe, can unfold, and can explore the dimensions of self in healing. Nationally, holistic nurses have been integral in the movement to transform organizational cultures by creating optimal healing environments.

Culture, beliefs, and values are inherent components of a holistic approach. Concepts of health and healing are based in culture and often influence people's actions to promote, maintain, and restore health. Culture also may provide an understanding of a person's concept of illness or disease and appropriate treatment. Holistic nurses possess knowledge and understanding of numerous cultural traditions and healthcare practices from various racial, ethnic, and social backgrounds. However, holistic nurses honor the individual's understanding and articulation of his or her own cultural values, beliefs, and health practices rather than relying on stereotypical cultural classifications and descriptions. The nurse then uses these understandings to provide culturally competent care that corresponds with the beliefs, values, traditions, and health practices of people. Holistic nurses ask individuals, "What do I need to know about you culturally in caring for you?"

Holistic healing is a collaborative approach. Holistic nurses take an active role in trying to remove the political and financial barriers to the inclusion of holistic care in the healthcare system. Of particular importance to holistic nurses is the human connection with ecology. Holistic nurses actively participate in building an ecosystem that sustains the well-being of all life. This includes raising the public's consciousness about environmental issues and stressors that affect not only the health of people but the health of the planet.

Core Value 4: Holistic Education and Research

Holistic nurses possess an understanding of a wide range of norms and healthcare practices, beliefs, and values concerning individuals, families, groups, and communities from a variety of racial, ethnic, spiritual, and social backgrounds. This rich knowledge base reflects their formal academic and continuing education preparation. Their knowledge also includes a wide diversity of practices and modalities outside of conventional Western medicine. Because of this, holistic nurses have a significant effect on people's understanding of healthcare options and alternatives, thus serving as both educators and advocates.

In addition, holistic nurses provide much-needed information to individuals on health promotion, including such topics as healthy lifestyles, risk-reducing behaviors, preventive self-care, stress management, living with changes secondary to illness and treatment, and opportunities to enhance well-being.

Holistic nurses value all the ways of knowing and learning. They assess health literacy and individualize learning, appreciating that science, intuition, introspection, creativity, aesthetics, and culture produce different bodies of knowledge and perspectives. They help others to know themselves and access their inner wisdom to enhance growth, wholeness, and well-being.

Holistic nurses often guide individuals and families in their healthcare decisions, especially regarding conventional allopathic and complementary/alternative practices. Therefore, holistic nurses must be knowledgeable about the best evidence available for both conventional and CAM therapies. In addition to developing evidence-based practice using research, practice guidelines, and expertise, holistic nurses strongly consider the person's values and healthcare practices and beliefs in evidence-informed practice decisions.

Holistic nurses look at alternative philosophies of science and research methods that are compatible with investigations of humanistic and holistic occurrences, that explore the context in which phenomena occur and the meaning of patterns that evolve, and that take into consideration the interactive nature of the body, mind, emotion, energy, spirit, and environment.

Holistic nurses conduct and evaluate research in such diverse areas as follows:

- Outcome measures of holistic therapies such as therapeutic touch, prayer, and aromatherapy
- Instrument development to measure caring behaviors and dimensions, presence and intention, spirituality, self-transcendence, cultural competence, and so forth
- Client responses to holistic interventions in health/illness/wellness
- Explorations of clients' lived experiences with various health/illness/life phenomena

- Theory development in healing, well-being, caring, intentionality, social and cultural constructions, empowerment, and so forth
- Healing relationships and environments
- Teaching and evaluation of holism

Further, research that advances the work of holistic nursing theories (Watson, Rogers, Newman, Parse, Erickson, and Leninger) helps to build the knowledge base of nursing and advance the nursing science of holism. The AHNA has incorporated an active research agenda by assisting and mentoring members in research endeavors, granting research awards, identifying and reporting on research that focuses on holistic healing phenomena and modalities, and applying research in practice.

Core Value 5: Holistic Nurse Self-Reflection and Self-Care

Self-care as well as personal awareness and continual focus on being an instrument of healing are significant requirements for holistic nurses. Holistic nurses reflect on action to become aware of values, feelings, perceptions, and judgments that may affect actions, and they also reflect on their experiences to obtain insight for future practice. Holistic nurses value themselves and mobilize the necessary resources to care for themselves. They endeavor to integrate self-awareness, self-care, and self-healing into their lives by incorporating practices such as self-assessment, meditation, yoga, good nutrition, energy therapies, movement, creative endeavors, support, and lifelong learning. Holistic nurses honor their unique patterns and the development of the body, the psychosocial and cultural self, the intellectual self, the energetic self, and the spiritual self. Nurses cannot facilitate healing unless they are in the process of healing themselves. Through continuing education, practice, and self-work, holistic nurses develop the skills of authentic and deep self-reflection and introspection to understand themselves and their journey. It is seen as a lifelong process.

Holistic nurses strive to achieve harmony and balance in their own lives and assist others to do the same. They create healing environments for themselves by attending to their own well-being, letting go of self-destructive behaviors and attitudes, and practicing centering and stress-reduction techniques. By doing this, holistic nurses serve as role models to others, be they clients, colleagues, or personal relations.

Holistic nurses have played instrumental roles in creating and implementing self-care programs to increase health and well-being for clients and families, communities, healthcare staff, and nurses themselves.

Standards of Holistic Nursing Practice
Overarching Philosophical Principles of Holistic Nursing

Holistic nurses express, contribute to, and promote an understanding of the following: a philosophy of nursing that values healing as the desired outcome; the human health experience as a complex, dynamic relationship of health, illness, disease, and wellness; the scientific foundations of nursing practice; and nursing as an art. Holistic nursing is based on the following overarching philosophical tenets that are embedded in every standard of practice; these principles underlie holistic nursing.

Person

- There is unity, totality, and connectedness of everyone and everything (body, mind, emotion, spirit, sexuality, age, environment, society, culture, belief systems, relationships, and context).
- Human beings are unique and inherently good.
- People are able to find meaning and purpose in their own lives, experiences, and illnesses.
- All people have an innate power and capacity for self-healing. Health and illness are subjectively described and determined by the view of the individual. Therefore, the person is honored in all phases of his or her healing process regardless of expectations or outcomes.
- Various people are the recipients of holistic nursing services: clients, patients, families, significant others, populations, or

communities. They may be ill and within the healthcare delivery system or well, moving toward personal betterment to enhance well-being.

Healing and Health

- Health and illness are natural and a part of life, learning, and movement toward change and development.
- Health is seen as balance, integration, harmony, right relationship, and the betterment of well-being, not just the absence of disease. Healing can take place without cure. The focus is on health promotion, disease prevention, health restoration, and lifestyle patterns and habits as well as symptom relief.
- Illness is considered a teacher and an opportunity for self-awareness and growth as part of the life process. Symptoms are respected as messages.
- Healing is multidimensional, can occur at any level of the human system, and is creative, unfolding, and unpredictable.
- As active partners in the healing process, people are empowered when they take some control of their own lives, health, and well-being, including personal choices and relationships.
- Treatment is a process that considers the root of the problem/illness/issue and does not merely treat the obvious signs and symptoms.

Practice

- Practice is a science using critical thinking, reflection, evidence, research, theory; practice is also an art requiring intuition, appreciation, creativity, presence, and self-knowledge.
- The values and ethics of holism, caring, moral insight, dignity, integrity, competence, responsibility, accountability, and legality underline holistic nursing practice.
- Intention for the well-being and highest good of the care recipient is the cornerstone of all holistic practice.
- Any and all interventions affect the whole.

- There are various philosophies and paradigms of health, illness, and healing and approaches and models for the delivery of health care both in the United States and in other countries that must be understood and utilized.
- Older adults represent the predominant population served by nurses.
- Public policy and the healthcare delivery system influence the health and well-being of society and professional nursing.

Nursing Roles

- The holistic nurse is part of the healing environment, using warmth, compassion, caring, authenticity, respect, trust, and relationship as instruments of healing in and of themselves.
- The holistic nurse uses conventional nursing interventions as well as holistic, complementary, alternative, and integrative modalities that enhance the body-mind-emotion-spirit-environment connectedness to foster the healing, health, wholeness, and well-being of people.
- The holistic nurse collaborates and partners with all constituencies in the health process including the person receiving care and his or her family, significant others, community, colleagues, and individuals from other disciplines; this is accomplished using the principles and skills of cooperation, alliance, consensus, and respect, as well as honoring the contributions of all.
- The holistic nurse participates in the change process to develop more caring cultures in which to practice, learn, and live.
- The holistic nurse assists nurses to nurture and heal themselves.
- The holistic nurse participates in activities that contribute to the improvement of local and global communities, the environment, and the betterment of public health.
- The holistic nurse acts as an advocate for the rights of and equitable distribution and access to health care for all persons, especially vulnerable populations.
- The holistic nurse participates in the positive transformation of systems.

- The holistic nurse honors the ecosystem and our relationship with and need to preserve it.

Self-Reflection and Self-Care

- Self-reflection—the turning inward to examine one's thoughts, values, beliefs, experiences, behaviors, and inner wisdom—enhances self-understanding and facilitates reflective practice.
- Holistic nurses' self-reflection and self-assessment, self-care, healing, and personal development are necessary for service to others and for growth and change in their own well-being and for understanding of their personal journey.
- Holistic nurses value themselves and their calling to holistic nursing as a life purpose.

Holistic nursing practice is guided by the holistic caring process, whether used with individuals, families, population groups, or communities. This process involves assessment, diagnosis, outcome identification, planning, implementation, and evaluation. It encompasses all significant actions taken in providing culturally competent, ethical, respectful, compassionate, and relevant holistic nursing care to all persons.

Standards of Holistic Nursing Practice*

There are 16 standards in *Holistic Nursing: Scope and Standards of Practice, Second Edition*, 6 for practice and 10 for professional performance.[3] Each standard addresses competencies for both the registered nurse and the graduate-level prepared and advanced practice registered nurse. Because each standard has numerous competencies, only

*The complete and comprehensive statement of standards of holistic nursing practice are contained in *Holistic Nursing: Scope and Standards of Practice, Second Edition* (2013), which can be obtained from the American Holistic Nurses Association (AHNA), 100 SE 9th Street, Suite 3A, Topeka, KS, 66612; 1-800-278-2462 or 1-785-234-1712; www.ahna.org or info@ahna.org.

one or two competency examples per standard are included here.

***Standard 1. ASSESSMENT:** The holistic registered nurse collects comprehensive data pertinent to the person's health and/or the situation.*

The holistic registered nurse:

1. Collects comprehensive data including but not limited to physical, functional, psychosocial, emotional, mental, sexual, cultural, age-related, environmental, spiritual, transpersonal, economic, and energy field assessments in a systematic and ongoing process while honoring the uniqueness of the person.
2. Elicits the person's health and cultural practices, values, beliefs, preferences, meanings of health, illness, well-being, lifestyle patterns, family issues, and risk behaviors and context.

The holistic graduate-level prepared or advanced practice registered nurse:

1. Initiates and interprets diagnostic procedures relevant to the person's current status.
2. Explores the meanings of the symbolic language expressing itself in areas such as dreams, images, symbols, sensations, or prayers that are a part of the individual's health experience.

***Standard 2. DIAGNOSIS:** The holistic registered nurse analyzes the assessment data to determine the diagnosis or issues expressed as actual or potential patterns/problems/needs.*

The holistic registered nurse:

1. Derives the diagnosis or health issues from holistic assessment data.
2. Assists the person to explore the meaning of the health/disease experience.

The holistic graduate-level prepared or advanced practice registered nurse:

1. Utilizes complex data and information obtained during interview, examination, and diagnostic procedures in identifying diagnoses.

Standard 3. *OUTCOMES IDENTIFICATION: The holistic registered nurse identifies outcomes for a plan individualized to the person or the situation. The holistic nurse values the evolution and the process of healing as it unfolds. This implies that specific unfolding outcomes may not be evident immediately because of the non-linear nature of the healing process so that expected, anticipated, evolving, and emerging outcomes are considered.*

The holistic registered nurse:

1. Defines outcomes in terms of the person's values, beliefs, and preferences; culture; age; spiritual practices; ethical considerations; environment; or situation. Consideration is given to associated risks, benefits and costs, current scientific evidence, trajectory of the condition, and clinical expertise.
2. Partners with the person to identify realistic goals based on the person's present and potential capabilities and quality of life.

The holistic graduate-level prepared or advanced practice registered nurse:

1. Identifies outcomes that incorporate healthcare consumer satisfaction, the person's understanding and meanings in his or her unique patterns and processes, quality of life, cost, clinical effectiveness, and continuity and consistency among providers.

Standard 4. *PLANNING: The holistic registered nurse develops a plan that prescribes strategies and alternatives to attain expected outcomes.*

The holistic registered nurse:

1. Develops in partnership with the person, family, and others an individualized plan considering the person's characteristics or situation including but not limited to values, beliefs, knowledge, spiritual and health practices, preferences, choices, developmental level, coping style, culture, environment, and access to technology.
2. Establishes the plan in conjunction with the person, family, significant others, and caregivers, as appropriate.

3. Establishes practice settings and safe space and time for both the nurse and person, family, and significant others to explore suggested potential and alternative options.

The holistic graduate-level prepared or advanced practice registered nurse:

1. Identifies assessments, diagnostic strategies, therapeutic interventions, therapeutic effects, and side effects that reflect current evidence, data, research, literature, expert clinical knowledge, and the person's experiences.
2. Uses linguistic and symbolic language including but not limited to word associations, dreams, storytelling, and journals to explore with individuals possibilities and options.

Standard 5. *IMPLEMENTATION: The holistic registered nurse implements the identified plan in partnership with the person.*

The holistic registered nurse:

1. Partners with the person, family, significant others, and caregivers to implement the plan in a safe, realistic, and timely manner while honoring the person's choices and unique healing journey.
2. Uses self as an instrument of healing.

The holistic graduate-level prepared or advanced practice registered nurse:

1. Facilitates utilization of systems, organizations, and community resources to implement the plan.
2. Incorporates new knowledge and strategies to initiate change in nursing care practices if desired outcomes are not achieved.

Standard 5A. *COORDINATION OF CARE: The holistic registered nurse coordinates care delivery.*

The holistic registered nurse:

1. Organizes the components of the plan.
2. Assists the person to identify options for alternative care.

The holistic graduate-level prepared or advanced practice registered nurse:

1. Provides leadership in the coordination of interprofessional health care for integrated delivery of person-centered services across continuums, settings, and over time.

Standard 5B. HEALTH TEACHING AND HEALTH PROMOTION: The holistic registered nurse employs strategies to promote holistic health, wellness, and a safe environment.

The holistic registered nurse:

1. Provides health teaching to individuals, families, and significant others or caregivers that enhances the mind–body emotion-spirit-environment connection.
2. Uses health promotion and health teaching methods appropriate to the situation and the individual's values, beliefs, health practices, age, developmental level, learning needs, readiness and ability to learn, language preference, spirituality, culture, and socioeconomic status.
3. Assists others to access their own inner wisdom that may provide opportunities to enhance and support growth, development, and wholeness.

The holistic graduate-level prepared or advanced practice registered nurse:

1. Synthesizes empirical evidence on risk behaviors, decision making about life choices, learning theories, behavioral change theories, motivational theories, epidemiology, and other related theories and frameworks when designing holistic health education information and programs.

Standard 5C. CONSULTATION: The holistic graduate-level prepared or advanced practice registered nurse provides consultation to influence the identified plan, enhance the abilities of others, and effect change.

The holistic graduate-level prepared or advanced practice registered nurse:

1. Facilitates the effectiveness of a consultation by involving all stakeholders, including the individual, in decision making and negotiating role responsibilities.

Standard 5D. PRESCRIPTIVE AUTHORITY AND TREATMENT: The holistic graduate-level prepared or advanced practice registered nurse uses prescriptive authority, procedures, referrals, treatments, and therapies in accordance with state and federal laws and regulations.

The holistic graduate-level prepared or advanced practice registered nurse:

1. Prescribes evidence-based treatments, therapies, and procedures and practice considering the person's comprehensive healthcare needs and holistic choices.
2. Uses advanced knowledge of pharmacology, psychoneuroimmunology, nutritional supplements, herbal and homeopathic remedies, and a variety of complementary and alternative therapies in prescribing.
3. Evaluates therapeutic and potential adverse effects of pharmacologic and non-pharmacologic treatments including but not limited to drug, herbal, and homeopathic regimens as well as their side effects and interactions.

Standard 6. EVALUATION: The holistic registered nurse evaluates progress toward attainment of outcomes while recognizing and honoring the continuing holistic nature of the healing process.

The holistic registered nurse:

1. Conducts a holistic, systematic, ongoing, and criterion-based evaluation of the outcomes in relation to the structures and processes prescribed by the plan and the indicated timeline.
2. Evaluates in partnership with the person the effectiveness of the planned strategies in relation to the person's responses and the attainment of the expected and unfolding outcomes.

The holistic graduate-level prepared or advanced practice registered nurse:

1. Uses the results of the evaluation analyses to make or recommend process or structural changes, including policy and procedure or protocol documentation, as appropriate to improve holistic care.

Standard 7. ETHICS: The holistic registered nurse practices ethically.

The holistic registered nurse:

1. Uses the ANA *Guide to the Code of Ethics for Nurses: Interpretation and Application*[5] and the AHNA *Position Statement on Holistic Nursing Ethics*[13] to guide practice and articulate the moral foundation of holistic nursing.
2. Advocates for equitable consumer health care, particularly regarding the rights of vulnerable, repressed, or underserved populations.

The holistic graduate-level prepared or advanced practice registered nurse:

1. Actively contributes to creating an ecosystem that supports well-being for all life.

Standard 8. EDUCATION: The holistic registered nurse attains knowledge and competence that reflect current nursing practice.

The holistic registered nurse:

1. Seeks experiences and formal and independent learning activities to develop and maintain clinical and professional skills and knowledge and personal growth.

The holistic graduate-level prepared or advanced practice registered nurse:

1. Uses current healthcare research findings and other evidence to expand clinical knowledge, skills, abilities, and judgment; to enhance role performance; and to increase knowledge of professional issues and changes in national standards for practice and trends in holistic care.

Standard 9. EVIDENCE-BASED PRACTICE AND RESEARCH: The holistic registered nurse integrates evidence and research into practice.

The holistic registered nurse:

1. Utilizes the best available evidence, including current evidence-based knowledge, theories, and research findings, to guide practice.
2. Actively and ethically participates, as appropriate to educational level and position, in the formulation of evidence-based practice through research activities related to holistic health.

The holistic graduate-level prepared or advanced practice registered nurse:

1. Contributes to nursing knowledge by conducting or synthesizing research that discovers, examines, and evaluates current practice, knowledge, theories, philosophies, context, criteria, and creative approaches to improve holistic healthcare outcomes.
2. Disseminates research findings through activities such as presentations, publications, consultations, and journal clubs for a variety of audiences, including nursing, other disciplines, and the public, to improve holistic care and further develop the foundation and practice of holistic nursing.

Standard 10. QUALITY OF PRACTICE: The holistic registered nurse contributes to quality nursing practice.

The holistic registered nurse:

1. Participates in quality improvement activities for holistic nursing practice.
2. Uses creativity and innovation to enhance holistic nursing care.

The holistic graduate-level prepared or advanced practice registered nurse:

1. Evaluates the practice environment and quality of holistic nursing care rendered in relation to existing evidence and feedback from individuals and significant others, identifying opportunities for the generation and use of research.

Standard 11. COMMUNICATION: The holistic registered nurse communicates effectively in a variety of formats in all areas of practice.

The holistic registered nurse:

1. Conveys information to individuals, families, significant others, the interprofessional team, and others in communication formats that promote accuracy, respect, authenticity, and trust.

2. Uses intention, centering, presence, caring, intuition, and deep listening to create and maintain healing and person-centered communication.

The holistic graduate-level prepared or advanced practice registered nurse:

1. Establishes practice environments that recognize and value holistic communication as fundamental to holistic care.

Standard 12. LEADERSHIP: The holistic registered nurse provides leadership in the professional practice setting and the profession.

The holistic registered nurse:

1. Mentors colleagues for the advancement of holistic nursing practice, the profession, and quality holistic health care.
2. Engages in local, state, national, and international levels to expand the knowledge and practice of holistic nursing and awareness of holistic health issues.

The holistic graduate-level prepared or advanced practice registered nurse:

1. Influences decision-making bodies to improve holistic, integrative care, the professional practice environment, and holistic healthcare consumer outcomes.
2. Articulates the ideas underpinning holistic nursing philosophy and places these ideas in a historical, philosophical, and scientific context while projecting future trends in thinking.

Standard 13. COLLABORATION: The holistic registered nurse collaborates with the healthcare consumer, family, and others in the conduct of holistic nursing practice.

The holistic registered nurse:

1. Communicates with the person, family, significant others, caregivers, and interdisciplinary healthcare providers regarding the person's care and the holistic nurse's role in the provision of that care.

2. Engages in teamwork and team-building processes.

The holistic graduate-level prepared or advanced practice registered nurse:

1. Facilitates the negotiation of holistic, complementary, integrative, and conventional healthcare services for continuity of care and program planning.

Standard 14. PROFESSIONAL PRACTICE EVALUATION: The holistic registered nurse evaluates his or her own nursing practice in relation to professional practice standards and guidelines, relevant statutes, rules, and regulations.

The holistic registered nurse:

1. Reflects on his or her practice and how his or her own personal, cultural, and spiritual beliefs; experiences; biases; education; and values may affect care given to individuals, families, and communities.
2. Engages in self-evaluation of practice on a regular basis, identifying areas of strength, as well as areas in which professional development and personal growth would be beneficial.

The holistic graduate-level prepared or advanced practice registered nurse:

1. Engages in a formal process, seeking feedback regarding his or her own practice from individuals receiving care, peers, professional colleagues, and others.

Standard 15. RESOURCE UTILIZATION: The holistic registered nurse utilizes appropriate resources to plan and provide nursing services that are holistic, safe, effective, and financially responsible.

The holistic registered nurse:

1. Assists the person, family, significant others, and caregivers as appropriate in identifying and securing appropriate and available services to address needs across the healthcare continuum.
2. Identifies discriminatory healthcare practices and their impact.

The holistic graduate-level prepared or advanced practice registered nurse:

1. Utilizes organizational and community resources to formulate interprofessional plans of care.

Standard 16. ENVIRONMENTAL HEALTH: The holistic registered nurse practices in an environmentally safe and healthy manner.

The holistic registered nurse:

1. Promotes a practice environment that reduces environmental health risks for workers and healthcare consumers.
2. Communicates environmental health risks and exposure reduction strategies to healthcare consumers, families, colleagues, and communities.

The holistic graduate-level prepared or advanced practice registered nurse:

1. Analyzes the impact of social, political, and economic influences on the environment and human health exposures.
2. Contributes to conducting research and applying research findings that link environmental hazards and human response patterns.

Educational Preparation and Certification for Holistic Nursing Practice

Holistic nurses are registered nurses who are educationally prepared for practice from an approved school of nursing and are licensed to practice in their individual state, commonwealth, or territory. The holistic registered nurse's experience, education, knowledge, and abilities establish the level of competence. *Holistic Nursing: Scope and Standards of Practice, Second Edition*, identifies the scope of practice of holistic nursing and the specific standards and associated measurement criteria of holistic nurses at both the basic and advanced levels.[3] Regardless of the level of practice, all holistic nurses integrate the previously identified five core values.

A registered nurse may prepare for the specialty of holistic nursing in a variety of ways. Educational offerings range from associate degree, baccalaureate, and graduate courses and programs to continuing education programs with extensive contact hours.

Basic Practice Level

The education of all nursing students preparing for registered nurse (RN) licensure includes basic content on physiological, psychological, emotional, and some spiritual processes with populations across the life span and conventional nursing care practices within each of these domains. In addition, basic nursing education incorporates experiences in a variety of clinical and practice settings from acute care to community. However, the educational focus is most frequently on "specialties" often emanating from the biomedical disease model and cure orientation. In holistic nursing, the individual across the life span is viewed in context as an integrated totality of body, mind, emotion, environment, society, energy, and spirit, with the emphasis on wholeness, well-being, health promotion, and healing using both conventional and complementary/alternative practices. Because of the lack of intentional focus on integration, unity, and healing, the educational exposure of most nursing students is not adequate preparation for assuming the specialty role of a holistic nurse.

Increasingly, schools of nursing are embracing holistic nursing practices and CAM and adding them to their curricula, responding to consumer use of CAM and consumer demand for health professionals who are knowledgeable about holistic practices. The new *Essentials of Baccalaureate Education for Professional Nursing Practice*[14] includes language on preparing the baccalaureate generalist graduate to practice from a holistic, caring framework; engage in self-care; develop an understanding of complementary and alternative modalities; and incorporate patient teaching and health promotion, spirituality, and caring, healing techniques into practice. This acknowledges that nursing recognizes the importance of healing principles and practices in health care and the need for nurses to learn them in the educational process.

Advanced Practice Level

As with the basic level, there are a variety of ways through both academic and professional development that registered nurses can acquire the additional specialized knowledge and skills that prepare them for advanced holistic nursing practice. These nurses are expected to hold a master's or doctoral degree and demonstrate a greater depth and scope of knowledge, a deeper integration of information, increased complexity of skills and interventions, and notable role autonomy. They provide leadership in practice, teaching, research, consultation, advocacy, and policy formation in advancing holistic nursing to improve the holistic health of people. Several schools of nursing that offer graduate programs in holistic nursing have a stable or growing number of applicants. Current advanced practice nurses are increasingly gaining specialized knowledge preparing them as holistic nurses through postmaster's programs, continuing education offerings in holistic nursing care, and certificate programs throughout the country that focus on specific modalities and on the essence of holism.

Continuing Education for Basic and Advanced Practice Levels

The AHNA is a provider and approver of continuing education and is recognized by the American Nurses Credentialing Center (ANCC). Continuing educational programs, workshops, and lectures in holistic nursing and CAM have been popular nationwide, with AHNA or other bodies granting continuing education units.

The AHNA endorses certificate programs in specific areas. These include Holistic Integrative Healing, Reflexology, Imagery, Aromatherapy, Healing Touch, Spirituality, Craniosacral Therapy, Holistic Stress Management, Integrative Healing Arts, Coaching, Whole Health Education, and RN Patient Advocate. It also approves

continuing education offerings in holistic nursing as well as giving the AHNA home study course, Foundation of Holistic Nursing. Other programs in distinct therapies such as acupuncture, Reiki, homeopathy, massage, imagery, healing arts, holistic health, Chinese Oriental Medicine, nutrition, Ayurveda, therapeutic touch, healing touch, herbology, chiropractic, and so on are given nationally as degrees, certificates, or continuing education programs by centers, specialty organizations, or schools.

Certification

Competency mechanisms for evaluating holistic nursing practice as a specialty exist through a national certification/recertification process overseen by the American Holistic Nurses Certification Corporation (AHNCC). The AHNCC offers four certifications: *Holistic Nurse, Board Certified* (HN-BC), which requires a minimum of a diploma or associate degree in nursing from an accredited school; *Holistic Baccalaureate Nurse, Board Certified* (HNB-BC), which requires a baccalaureate degree in nursing from an institution regionally accredited by the Association of Schools and Colleges (ASC); and *Advanced Holistic Nurse, Board Certified* (AHN-BC) and *Advanced Practice Holistic Nurse* (APHN-BC, APRN), which require a master's degree in nursing from an institution regionally accredited by ASC. Further, the AHNCC provides endorsement for schools of nursing meeting the specifications put forth in *Holistic Nursing: Scope and Standards of Practice, Second Edition*.[3] In addition, holistic nurses often are certified in specific CAM modalities such as imagery, Reiki, aromatherapy, healing touch, biofeedback, and reflexology.

Settings for Holistic Nursing Practice

Holistic nurses practice in numerous settings, including but not limited to ambulatory outpatient settings; acute care hospitals; long-term and extended care facilities, nursing homes, and assisted living; home care settings;

complementary/integrative care centers; women's health and birthing centers; hospice palliative care; psychiatric mental health facilities; private practitioner offices; schools; rehabilitation centers; religious parishes; community health and primary care centers; student and employee health clinics; managed care organizations; independent self-employed private practice; telehealth and cyber care services; correctional facilities; international and travel nursing; military; professional nursing and healthcare organizations; informatics; administration; staff development; and universities and colleges.

There are increasing numbers of holistic nurses who hold leadership roles as clinicians, educators, authors, and researchers in university-based schools of nursing, practice environments, nursing, and other professional organizations. Holistic nursing practice also occurs when there is a request for consultation or when holistic nurses advocate for care that promotes health and prevents disease, illness, or disability for individuals, communities, or the environment. A holistic nurse may choose not to work in a critical care setting but provide consultation regarding self-care or stress management to nurses practicing in that area. Or holistic nurses may practice in preoperative and recovery rooms instituting a "Prepare for Surgery" program for individuals who are going to have surgery that teaches them meditation and positive affirmation techniques for both before and after surgery while incorporating a homeopathic regimen for trauma and cell healing. Employment or voluntary participation of holistic nurses also can influence civic activities and the regulatory and legislative arenas at the local, state, national, or international levels.

Because holistic nursing focuses on wellness, wholeness, and development of the whole person, holistic nurses also practice in health enhancement settings such as spas, gyms, and wellness centers. With all populations and in any setting, nurses can empower patients/clients/families by teaching them self-care practices for a healthier lifestyle. In addition, there are numerous entrepreneurial possibilities for holistic nurses to develop integrative care programs in hospitals, home care, primary care practices, occupational and school settings, and the community.

Because holistic nursing is a worldview, a way of being in the world, and not just a modality, holistic nurses can practice in any setting and with individuals throughout the life span. As the public increasingly requests holistic and CAM/integrative services and a comprehensive, humanistic emphasis on the whole person, there will be a greater need for holistic nurses in a wider array of settings. Holistic nursing takes place wherever healing occurs.[15]

Conclusion

The specialty practice of holistic nursing is generally not well understood. Therefore, each holistic nurse must educate other nurses, healthcare providers and disciplines, and the public about the role, value, and benefits of holistic nursing, whether it be in direct practice, education, management, or research. Holistic nurses articulate the ideas underpinning the holistic paradigm and the philosophy of the caring, healing relationship. Jean Watson reminds us that society and the public are searching for something deeper in terms of realizing self-care, self-knowledge, and self-healing potentials. Nurses need to acknowledge the human aspects of practice—attending to people and their experience rather than just focusing on the biomedical orientation and disease. Watson concludes that "nurses have a covenant with the public to sustain caring. It is our collective responsibility to transform caring practices into the framework that identifies and gives distinction to nursing as a profession."[16, p. 12] *Holistic Nursing: Scope and Standards of Practice, Second Edition*, is a means through which holistic nurses are educating the profession and others about the values, principles, and practice requirements of the specialty.

Directions for Future Research

1. Explore research modalities and approaches that are congruent with the holistic paradigm.

2. Examine how the standards of holistic nursing practice are being implemented in healthcare settings.

Nurse Healer Reflections

After reading this chapter, the holistic nurse will be able to answer or to begin a process of answering the following questions:

- What attributes do I have that reflect the core values of holistic nursing?
- What contributions can I make as a holistic nurse to the wholeness and betterment of humankind?

NOTES

1. Institute of Medicine, *Crossing the Quality Chasm: A New Health System for the 21st Century* (Washington, DC: National Academies Press, 2001).
2. C. P. Tresolini and Pew-Fetzer Task Force, *Health Professions Education and Relationship-Centered Care* (San Francisco: Pew Health Professions Commission, 1994).
3. American Holistic Nurses Association and American Nurses Association, *Holistic Nursing: Scope and Standards of Practice*, 2nd ed. (Silver Spring, MD: Nursesbooks.org, 2013).
4. American Nurses Association, *Nursing: Scope and Standards of Practice*, 2nd ed. (Silver Spring, MD: Nursesbooks.org, 2010).
5. American Nurses Association, *Guide to the Code of Ethics for Nurses: Interpretation and Application* (Silver Spring, MD: Nursesbooks.org, 2010).
6. American Nurses Association, *Nursing's Social Policy Statement: The Essence of the Profession* (Silver Spring, MD: Nursesbooks.org, 2010).
7. American Nurses Association, *Nursing: Scope and Standards of Practice* (Silver Spring, MD: Nursesbooks.org, 2004).
8. American Nurses Association, *Recognition of a Nursing Specialty, Approval of a Specialty Nursing Scope of Practice Statement, and Acknowledgement of Specialty Nursing Standards of Practice* (Washington, DC: American Nurses Association, 2010).
9. C. Mariano, *Proposal for Recognition of Holistic Nursing as a Nursing Specialty* (New York: Unpublished

document submitted to the American Nurses Association, 2006).
10. R. W. Cowling, "Holism as a Sociopolitical Enterprise," *Journal of Holistic Nursing* 29, no. 1 (2011): 5–6.
11. American Holistic Nurses Association, *Description of Holistic Nursing* (Flagstaff, AZ: American Holistic Nurses Association, 1998).
12. "Patient Bill of Rights," in *Accreditation Manual for Hospitals* (Oakbrook Terrace, IL: Joint Commission on Accreditation of Healthcare Organizations, 1992).
13. American Holistic Nurses Association, *Position Statement on Holistic Nursing Ethics* (Flagstaff, AZ: American Holistic Nurses Association, revised and approved 2012).
14. American Association of Colleges of Nursing, *The Essentials of Baccalaureate Education for Professional Nursing Practice* (Washington, DC: American Association of Colleges of Nursing, 2008).
15. C. Mariano, "Holistic Nursing: Every Nurse's Specialty," *Beginnings* 29, no. 4 (2009): 4–6.
16. C. Mariano, "Caring for Our Future: An Interview with Jean Watson," *Beginnings* 25, no. 3 (2005): 12–14.

RESOURCE LIST

American Holistic Nurses Association (AHNA)
100 SE 9th Street, Suite 3A
Topeka, KS 66612
Phone: 1-800-278-2462
info@ahna.org
www.ahna.org

American Holistic Nurses Certification Corporation (AHNCC)
811 Linden Loop
Cedar Park, TX 78613
Phone: 1-877-284-0998
AHNCC@flash.net
www.ahncc.org

National Center for Complementary and Integrative Health (NCCIH)
900 Rockville Pike
Bethesda, MD 20892
Phone: 1-888-644-6226
http://nccam.nih.gov

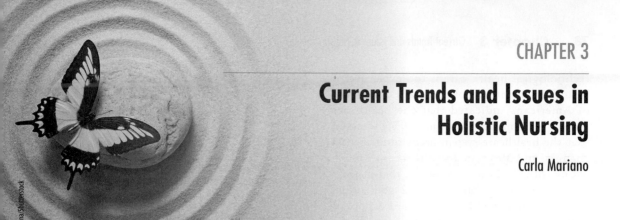

CHAPTER 3

Current Trends and Issues in Holistic Nursing

Carla Mariano

Nurse Healer Objectives

Theoretical

- Describe the major issues in health care and holistic nursing today.
- Identify changes needed in health care to promote health, wellness, well-being, and healing.
- Discuss recommendations of the Institute of Medicine (IOM) report *The Future of Nursing*.

Clinical

- Evaluate how current trends in health care will affect clinical nursing practice.
- Discuss with other health professionals the unique and common contributions of one another's practice.

Personal

- Become a member of the American Holistic Nurses Association (AHNA) to participate in improving holistic health care for society.

The American public increasingly calls for health care that is compassionate and respectful, able to provide a variety of options, economically feasible, and grounded in holistic ideals. A shift is occurring in health care where people desire to be more actively involved in health decision making. They have expressed their dissatisfaction with conventional (Western allopathic) medicine and are calling for a care system that encompasses health, quality of life, and a relationship with their providers. The National Center for Complementary and Alternative Medicine's *Third Strategic Plan 2011–2015*[1] and *Healthy People 2020*[2] prioritize enhancing physical and mental health and wellness, preventing disease, and empowering the public to take responsibility for their health. The vision of *Healthy People 2020* is "A society in which all people live long, healthy lives" and its goals are as follows:[2]

- Attain high-quality, longer lives free of preventable disease, disability, injury, and premature death.
- Achieve health equity, eliminate disparities, and improve the health of all groups.
- Create social and physical environments that promote good health for all.
- Promote quality of life, healthy development, and healthy behaviors across all life stages.

Health Care in the United States

Western medicine is proving ineffective, wholly or partially, for a significant proportion of common chronic diseases. Furthermore, highly technological health care is too expensive to be universally affordable. In a 2011 poll, 55% of Americans indicated that the healthcare system has major problems, 50% indicated that the healthcare system needs fundamental changes, and 36% stated that there is so much wrong with the healthcare system that it needs to be completely rebuilt.[3] A 2012 poll, *Sick in America*,[4] conducted by the Harvard School of Public Health and Robert Wood Johnson Foundation, indicated that more than half of Americans (57%) think there is a serious problem with the quality of the nation's health care. However, their concern about the quality of health care is lower than their concern about the cost of care in the nation. Most Americans (87%) see the cost of care as a "very serious" (65%) or a "somewhat serious" (22%) problem for the country. Furthermore, nearly two-thirds believe that the cost of U.S. health care has gotten worse over the last 5 years (65%). One-quarter of sick Americans report that a doctor, nurse, or other health professional did not provide all of the needed information about their treatment or prescriptions (25%), or they had to see multiple medical professionals, and no one doctor understood or kept track of all of the different aspects of their medical issues and treatments (23%). Nearly three-quarters of sick Americans want their doctor to spend time with them discussing other, broader health issues that might affect their long-term health (72%), as opposed to just talking about their specific medical problem (21%).

> Although medical advances have saved and improved the lives of millions, much of medicine and health care have primarily focused on addressing immediate events of disease and injury, generally neglecting underlying socioeconomic factors, including employment, education, and income and behavioral risk factors. These factors, and others, impact health status, accentuate disparities, and can lead to costly, preventable diseases. Furthermore, the disease-driven approach to medicine and health care has resulted in a fragmented, specialized health system in which care is typically reactive and episodic, as well as often inefficient and impersonal.[5]

Chronic diseases—such as heart disease, cancer, hypertension, diabetes, and depression—are the leading causes of death and disability in the United States. About half of all adults (117 million people) have one or more chronic health conditions. One in four adults has two or more chronic health conditions. Chronic diseases account for 70% of all deaths in the United States, which is 1.7 million deaths each year. These diseases also cause major limitations in daily living for almost 1 out of 10 Americans, or about 25 million people.[6]

Stress accounts for 80% of all healthcare issues in the United States. "*SuperStress*" is a

> result of both the changing nature of our daily lives and our choices in lifestyle habits, as well as a series of unfortunate events. Extreme chronic stress . . . has silently become a pandemic that disturbs not only how we perceive our quality of life but also our health and mortality. . . . The APA [American Psychological Association] issued a report on stress, revealing that nearly half of all Americans were experiencing stress at a significantly higher level than the previous year and rated its level as extreme.[7, p. 7]

Healthcare costs have been rising for several years. Expenditures in the United States for health care surpassed $2.7 trillion in 2011, more than three times the $724 billion spent in 1990, and more than eight times the $255 billion spent in 1980.[8] In May 2014, healthcare expenditures were $3.02 trillion and are projected to be $4.3 trillion by 2017.[9]

In 2013, U.S. healthcare spending was about $8,508 per resident and accounted for 17.5% of the nation's gross domestic product (GDP); this is among the highest of all industrialized countries. Total healthcare expenditures continue to outpace inflation and the growth in national income. The U.S. healthcare system is the most expensive in the world and pays about twice as much per capita on health care as our peers in other advanced nations, but it yields worse results than the systems in Britain, Canada, Germany, France, Japan, Australia, and New Zealand. U.S. residents with below-average incomes are more likely than their counterparts in other countries not to have received needed care because of cost. It is projected that healthcare expenditures will climb to 22% of GDP by 2038.[8]

Healthcare costs for a family of four rose again in 2014, with employees paying a much larger share of the growing expense. The total cost of health care for a typical family of four is $23,215, an increase of 5.4% over 2010. This is double the cost families had to pay in 2004 ($11,192). As costs continue to grow, the cost for health care constitutes a larger and larger portion of the household budget. And what are families paying for? The 2014 Milliman Medical Index indicates that professional services represent 31% of the overall health costs; hospital inpatient costs account for 31%; outpatient costs, 19%; pharmacy, 15%; and other expenses, such as medical equipment, about 4%.[10]

Recently published data from the National Health Interview Study indicate that more than 1 in 4 families in the United States experienced financial burden of medical care. Almost 1 in 6 families had problems paying medical bills in the past 12 months, and 1 in 10 families had medical bills that they were unable to pay at all.[11]

In addition, workers paid 73% more in 2014 than they did in 2007 for the health coverage they get through their jobs, while their wages have increased only 18%. Employers, in contrast, pay 52% more toward their employees' health insurance than they did 5 years ago. Premiums for employer-sponsored health insurance have risen from $9,068 in 2003 to $16,351 in 2013, with the amount paid by workers rising by 89%.[12]

In addition to the rising costs, there is disparity in the number of Americans insured for health coverage. The 2010 U.S. Census Bureau cited the number of uninsured Americans at 50.7 million, 16.7% of the population or almost 1 in 6 U.S. residents.[13] According to the July 2014 Gallup-Healthways Index, the uninsured rate has decreased to 13.4% since the Affordable Care Act's requirement for most Americans to have health insurance went into effect at the

beginning of 2014.[14] The number of underinsured remains a problem at 60% or 25 million.[15] The reasons for both categories include workers losing their jobs in the recession, companies dropping employee health insurance benefits, and families going without coverage to cut costs—primarily as a result of the high costs of health care. In addition, in 2013, around 80 million or 43% of America's working-age adults did not access needed medical services because of the cost. According to the Commonwealth Fund's Biennial Health Insurance Survey, nearly 3 in 10 adults said they did not visit a doctor or clinic when they had a medical problem, while more than a quarter did not fill a prescription or skipped recommended tests, treatment, or follow-up visits. One in five said they did not get needed specialist care.[16]

The Kaiser Family Foundation identified the following forces driving healthcare costs:[17]

- *Technology and prescription drugs.* Because of development costs and generation of consumer demand for more intense, costly services, even if they are not necessarily cost effective.
- *Chronic disease.* Chronic disease accounts for more than 75% of national healthcare expenditures and places tremendous demands on the system, particularly the increased need for treatment of ongoing illnesses and long-term services. One-quarter of Medicare spending is for costs incurred during the last year of life.
- *Aging of the population.* Health expenses rise with age. Baby boomers began qualifying for Medicare in 2011 and many of their costs will shift to the public sector.
- *Administrative costs.* At least 7% of healthcare expenditures are for marketing, billing, and other administrative costs. Overhead costs and large profits are fueling healthcare spending.

The foundation also offered the following proposals to contain costs:[17]

- *Invest in information technology.* Make greater use of technology such as electronic medical records. This is a major component of the health reform plan.

- *Improve quality and efficiency.* Decrease unwarranted variation in medical practice and unnecessary care. Experts estimate that 30% of health care is unnecessary.
- *Adjust provider compensation and increase comparative effectiveness research.* Ensure that fees paid to physicians reward value and health outcomes rather than volume of care, and determine which treatments are most effective for given conditions.
- *Increase government regulation in controlling per capita spending.*
- *Increase prevention efforts.* Provide financial incentives to workers to engage in wellness and to decrease the prevalence of chronic conditions. Improve disease management to streamline treatment for common chronic health conditions.
- *Increase consumer involvement in purchasing.* Encourage greater price transparency and use of health reimbursement accounts.

Much has been written about the current healthcare crisis: the high cost of health care, the lack of universal access to health care and the resulting 13.4% rate of uninsured Americans, the insurance morass and that industry's control of healthcare spending, the disenchantment and disempowerment of healthcare providers, the frustration of clients/patients and healthcare consumers, the lack of incentive for practitioners or insurers to foster prevention and health promotion, and the startling lack of measures being taken for high-quality healthcare outcomes. Hyman states that the national healthcare dialogue omits discussions about the nature and quality of care:

> We speak of evidence-based medicine, not quality-based medicine. Although evidence is important, it is not enough, particularly when the evidence is limited mostly to what is funded by private interests or grounded in the pharmacologic treatment of disease. The fundamental flaw in our approach to the discussion about evidence-based medicine versus quality-based medicine is the lack of focus on prevention and wellness and the lack of funding and research on comparative approaches to chronic healthcare problems. . . .

> Though it is still a matter of public debate, there is ample evidence that lifestyle therapies equal or exceed the benefits of conventional therapies. Nutrition, exercise, and stress management no longer can be considered alternative medicine. They are essential medicine, and often the most effective and cost-effective therapies to treat chronic disease, which has replaced infectious and acute illnesses as the leading cause of death in the world, both in developed and developing countries. . . .

> Hopefully, then, the next 10 years will see a focus on not just the mechanisms of complementary and integrative therapies, but also on measuring their role in improving overall healthcare quality and reducing healthcare costs. Hopefully, the discourse begun by the IOM report will spur policy makers to refocus federal efforts and funding on quality, disease prevention, and health promotion and will help us find the right medicine, regardless of its origin.[18, pp. 18–20]

Use of Complementary Alternative Medicine (CAM)/Complementary Integrative Medicine (CIM)* in the United States

The American public has pursued alternative, complementary, integrative care at an ever-increasing rate. The most recent survey, the 2007 National Health Interview Survey,[19] indicates that 38.3% of adults in the United States aged 18 years and older (almost 4 of 10 adults) and nearly 12% of children aged 17 years and younger (1 in 9 children) used some form of CAM within the previous 12 months. Use among adults remained relatively constant from previous surveys. The 2007 survey provides the

---

*For the remainder of the chapter, this will be referred to as "CAM."

first population-based estimate of children's use of CAM. Americans spent $33.9 billion out of pocket on CAM during the 12 months prior to the survey. This accounts for approximately 1.5% of total U.S. healthcare expenditures and 11.2% of total out-of-pocket expenditures. Nearly two-thirds of the total out-of-pocket costs that adults spent on CAM were for self-care purchases of CAM products, classes, and materials ($22.0 billion), compared with about one-third spent on practitioner visits ($11.9 billion). Despite this emphasis on self-care therapies, 38.1 million adults made an estimated 354.2 million visits to practitioners of CAM.[20]

Barnes and colleagues found that people who use CAM approaches seek ways to improve their health and well-being, attempt to relieve symptoms associated with chronic or even terminal illnesses or the side effects of conventional treatments, have a holistic health philosophy or desire a transformational experience that changes their worldview, and want greater control over their health.[19] The majority of individuals using CAM do so to complement conventional care rather than as an alternative to conventional care. Other findings include the following:[19]

- CAM therapies most commonly used by U.S. adults in the past 12 months were nonvitamin, nonmineral natural products (17.7%), deep breathing exercises (12.7%), meditation (9.4%), chiropractic or osteopathic manipulation (8.6%), massage (8.3%), and yoga (6.1%).
- CAM therapies with increased use were deep breathing exercises, meditation, yoga, acupuncture, massage therapy, and naturopathy.
- Adults used CAM most often to treat a variety of musculoskeletal problems, including back pain or problems (17.1%), neck pain or problems (5.9%), joint pain or stiffness or other joint condition (5.2%), arthritis (3.5%), and other musculoskeletal conditions (1.8%).
- CAM therapies used most often by children were for back or neck pain (6.7%), head or chest colds (6.6%), anxiety or stress (4.8%), other musculoskeletal problems (4.2%), and

attention-deficit hyperactivity disorder or attention-deficit disorder (2.5%).

- CAM use was more prevalent among women, adults aged 30 to 69 years, adults with higher levels of education, adults who were not poor, adults living in the West, former smokers, and adults who were hospitalized in the last year.
- CAM usage was positively associated with number of health conditions and number of doctor visits in the past 12 months; however, about one-fifth of adults with no health conditions and one-quarter of adults with no doctor visits in the past 12 months used CAM therapies.
- When worry about cost delayed the receipt of conventional medical care, adults were more likely to use CAM than when the cost of conventional care was not a worry. When unable to afford conventional medical care, adults were more likely to use CAM.

The most recent survey of consumer use of CAM by the American Association of Retired Persons (AARP) and the National Center for Complementary and Alternative Medicine (NCCAM) found that people 50 years of age and older tend to be high users:[21]

- More than one-half (53%) of people 50 years and older reported using CAM at some point in their lives, and nearly as many (47%) reported using it in the past 12 months.
- Herbal products or dietary supplements were the type of CAM most commonly used, with just more than one-third (37%) of respondents reporting their use, followed by massage therapy, chiropractic manipulation, and other bodywork (22%); mind–body practices (9%); and naturopathy, acupuncture, and homeopathy (5%).
- Women were more likely than men to report using any form of CAM.
- In most cases, the use of CAM increased with educational attainment.
- The most common reasons for using CAM were to prevent illness or for overall wellness (77%), to reduce pain or treat painful conditions (73%), to treat a specific health condition (59%), or to supplement conventional medicine (53%).

Chronically and terminally ill persons consume more healthcare resources than the rest of the population. The great interest in CAM practices among those who are chronically ill, those with life-threatening conditions, and those at the end of their lives suggests that increased access to some services among these groups could have significant implications for the healthcare system. With the number of older Americans expected to rise dramatically over the next 20 years, alternative strategies for dealing with the elderly population and end-of-life processes will be increasingly important in public policy. If evaluations show that some uses of CAM can lessen the need for more expensive conventional care in these populations, the economic implications for Medicare and Medicaid could be significant. If safe and effective CAM practices become more available to the general population, special and vulnerable populations should also have access to these services, along with conventional health care. CAM would not be a replacement for conventional health care but would be part of the treatment options available. In some cases, CAM practices may be an equal or superior option. CAM offers the possibility of a new paradigm of integrated health care that could affect the affordability, accessibility, and delivery of healthcare services for millions of Americans.

A significant aspect of the AARP/NCCAM study was that respondents were asked if they had discussed CAM use with any of the healthcare providers they see regularly:[21]

- More than two-thirds (67%) of respondents reported that they had not discussed CAM with any healthcare provider.
- If CAM was discussed at a medical appointment, it was brought up by the patient 55% of the time, by the healthcare provider 26% of the time, or by a relative/friend 14% of the time. Respondents were twice as likely to say that they raised the topic rather than their healthcare provider.
- The main reasons that respondents and their healthcare providers do not discuss CAM are as follows: the provider never asks (42%), respondents did not know that they

should bring up the topic (30%), there is not enough time during a visit (17%), the provider would have been dismissive or told the respondent not to do it (12%), or the respondent did not feel comfortable discussing the topic with the provider (11%).
- People aged 50 years and older who use CAM get their information about it from a variety of sources: from family or friends (26%); the Internet (14%); their physician (13%, or 21% for all healthcare providers); publications, including magazines, newspapers, and books (13%); and radio or television (7%).

It is clear that people aged 50 years and older are likely to be using CAM. It is also clear that this population frequently uses prescription medications. Common use of CAM as a complement to conventional medicine—and the high use of multiple prescription drugs—further underscores the need for healthcare providers and clients, patients, and families to have an open dialogue to ensure safe and appropriate integrated medical care. The lack of this dialogue points to a need to educate both consumers and healthcare providers about the importance of discussing the use of CAM, how to begin that dialogue, and the implications of not doing so.

Nondisclosure raises important safety issues, such as the potential interactions of medications with herbs used as part of a CAM therapy. In addition, a majority of adults who use CAM therapies use more than one CAM modality and do so in combination with conventional medical care. In the literature, there are limited data about the extent to which use of a CAM therapy may interfere with compliance in the use of conventional therapies. It is not known whether clients/patients use products as directed or even for the purpose recommended. Such information is important. Even if a therapy is efficacious, it may have little or no effect if it is taken or used incorrectly. Furthermore, medicines and other CAM products and procedures may be the source of iatrogenic health problems if they are used incorrectly. Clients/patients who believe that herbal medicines are harmless may be more willing to self-regulate their medication in unsupervised ways.

Healthcare Reform and Integrative Health Care

On March 23, 2010, President Obama signed comprehensive health reform, the *Patient Protection and Affordable Healthcare Act (HR 3590)*, into law. This law and subsequent legislation focus on provisions to expand health coverage, control health costs, and improve the healthcare delivery system. They also incorporate a more integrative approach to healthcare delivery. Discussion of the specifics of this legislation is beyond the scope of this chapter; however, sections that will shape policy relative to integrative healthcare practices in the future are discussed here.[22]

1. *Inclusion of Licensed Practitioners Insurance Coverage* (SEC. 2706. NON-DISCRIMINATION IN HEALTH CARE). Providers: A group health plan and a health insurance issuer offering group or individual health insurance coverage shall not discriminate with respect to participation under the plan or coverage against any healthcare provider who is acting within the scope of that provider's license or certification under applicable state law.

2. *Inclusion of Licensed Complementary and Alternative Medicine Practitioners in Medical Homes* (SEC. 3502. ESTABLISHING COMMUNITY HEALTH TEAMS TO SUPPORT THE PATIENT-CENTERED MEDICAL HOME). The Secretary of Health and Human Services shall establish a program to provide grants to or enter into contracts with eligible entities to establish community-based interdisciplinary, interprofessional teams (referred to as health teams) to support primary care practices. Such teams may include medical specialists, nurses, pharmacists, nutritionists, dietitians, social workers, behavioral and mental health providers, doctors of chiropractic, and licensed complementary and alternative medicine practitioners.

3. *Integrative Health Care and Integrative Practitioners in Prevention Strategies* (SEC. 4001. NATIONAL PREVENTION, HEALTH PROMOTION AND PUBLIC HEALTH COUNCIL). This council will provide coordination and leadership at the federal level, and among all federal departments and agencies, with respect to prevention, wellness, and health promotion practices, the public health system, and integrative health care in the United States; develop a national prevention, health promotion, public health, and integrative healthcare strategy that incorporates the most effective and achievable means of improving the health status of Americans and reducing the incidence of preventable illness and disability in the United States; and propose evidence-based models, policies, and innovative approaches for the promotion of transformative models of prevention, integrative health, and public health on individual and community levels across the United States.

4. *Dietary Supplements in Individualized Wellness Plans* (SEC. 4206. DEMONSTRATION PROJECT CONCERNING INDIVIDUALIZED WELLNESS PLAN). A pilot program will be established to test the effect of providing at-risk populations who utilize community health centers funded under this section an individualized wellness plan that is designed to reduce risk factors for preventable conditions. An individualized wellness plan prepared under the pilot program under this subsection may include one or more of the following as appropriate to the individual's identified risk factors:
   (i) Nutritional counseling
   (ii) A physical activity plan
   (iii) Alcohol and smoking cessation counseling and services
   (iv) Stress management
   (v) Dietary supplements that have health claims approved by the Secretary

5. *Licensed Complementary and Alternative Providers and Integrative Practitioners in Workforce Planning* (SEC. 5101. NATIONAL HEALTH CARE WORKFORCE COMMISSION). The term *healthcare workforce* includes all healthcare providers with direct patient care and support responsibilities, such as

physicians, nurses, nurse practitioners, primary care providers, preventive medicine physicians, optometrists, ophthalmologists, physician assistants, pharmacists, dentists, dental hygienists, and other oral healthcare professionals, allied health professionals, doctors of chiropractic, community health workers, healthcare paraprofessionals, direct care workers, psychologists and other behavioral and mental health professionals, social workers, physical and occupational therapists, certified nurse midwives, podiatrists, the emergency medical services (EMS) workforce, licensed complementary and alternative medicine providers, integrative health practitioners, and public health professionals.

6. *Experts in Integrative Health and State-Licensed Integrative Health Practitioners in Comparative Effectiveness Research* (SEC. 6301. PATIENT-CENTERED OUTCOMES RESEARCH). National priorities will be identified for research, taking into account factors of disease incidence, prevalence, and burden in the United States (with emphasis on chronic conditions); gaps in evidence in terms of clinical outcomes, practice variations, and health disparities in terms of delivery and outcomes of care; the potential for new evidence to improve patient health, well-being, and the quality of care; the effect on national expenditures associated with a healthcare treatment, strategy, or health conditions, as well as patient needs, outcomes, and preferences; the relevance to patients and clinicians in making informed health decisions. An advisory panel will consist of practicing and research clinicians, patients, and experts in scientific and health services research, health services delivery, and evidence-based medicine who have experience in the relevant topic, and, as appropriate, experts in integrative health and primary prevention strategies.

FON Therapeutics lists more than 430 integrative medicine centers in the United States alone.[23] This demonstrates the increasing acceptance and legiticimacy of integrative health care in the nation.

Trends

In addition to the data already cited, several trends affect and will continue to affect the health of society, delivery, and holistic practices.

Workplace Clinics

Interest has intensified in recent years (particularly with the newly enacted healthcare reform law) as employers move beyond traditional occupational health and convenience care to offering clinics that provide a full range of wellness, health promotion, and primary care services. This is seen as a tool to contain medical costs, such as specialist visits, nongeneric prescriptions, emergency department visits, and avoidable hospitalizations, boost productivity, reduce absenteeism, prevent disability claims and work-related injuries, and enhance companies' reputations as employers while attracting and retaining competitive workforces. Types of clinical services for new workplace programs can include traditional occupational health; acute care ranging from low-acuity episodic care to exacerbations of acute chronic conditions; preventive care including immunizations, lifestyle management, mind–body skills, and screenings; wellness assessments and follow up, health coaching, and education; and disease management for chronic conditions.[24]

Many of the nation's largest employers are focusing on prevention and disease management by adopting an integrative medicine approach. At present, the Corporate Health Improvement Program members include the Ford Motor Company, IBM, Corning, Kimberly Clark, Dow Chemical, Medstat, Nestlé, NASA, Canyon Ranch Resorts, and American Specialty Health. Walmart will open health clinics at approximately 400 U.S. stores over the next 3 years and at 2,000 stores in the next 5 to 7 years. CVS Health has more than 720 clinic locations across the United States and it continues to rapidly expand its retail care business. The clinics offer preventive and routine care. More than half of the people visiting the existing workplace clinics lack health insurance, and 15% said they would have to go to an emergency department if the clinics were unavailable. Some evidence suggests that retailers and other new players are taking business away from traditional care providers, potentially irrevocably shifting the flow of healthcare dollars.[25]

Primary Care

The Institute for Alternative Futures, funded by the Kresge Foundation, forecasts the following aspects of the future of primary care in 2025:[26]

- *Focus on primary prevention.* Primary prevention will be the major focus of primary care in 2025 and will be community focused.
- *Continuously improving health.* Health will be continually assessed and worked on along multiple dimensions in 2025 so that the physical, medical, nutritional, behavioral, psychological, social, spiritual, and environmental conditions are measured and improved for all covered by primary care.
- *Patient/client–provider relationships.* Trusting relationships between providers and patients/clients will be the basis of primary care's capacity for promoting health and managing disease. Health provider education will support this capacity. The primary care team members will work to instill caring, joy, love, faith, and hope into their relationship with each person. Once trust has been established, usually through in-person contact, effective communications using responsive and empathic email, phone calls, and avatar-based "cyber care" will reinforce this personal relationship.
- *Primary care team.* Primary care team members will include the patient/client/family, nurse practitioners, physicians, psychologist, pharmacist, a health information technician, and community health workers. "Visits" most often will be phone calls, televisits, or virtual visits, though in some cases the visit will be in the clinic. Besides a strong relationship among the patient/client and some of the primary care team members, most patients/clients will have a relational agent or personal health avatar made available (or enhanced) by their healthcare provider. This virtual agent will provide health education, coaching, and reinforcement, driven by the person's biomonitoring data and advanced care protocols.

- *Focus on behavioral change.* Primary care routinely will work with individuals to understand how to move choices from the limbic system of the brain that unconsciously controls emotionally directed behaviors to the frontal areas of the cognitive brain, which controls conscious behaviors. This should result in more effective behavioral change.
- *Focus on quality and safety.* The chronic care model will evolve to the expanded care model and beyond. By 2025, quality in primary care will include the triple aims of excellent healthcare experience, lower per capita costs, and improved population health.
- *Genome and epigenetic data use.* By 2025, most individuals' genomes will be mapped and documented in their electronic health record (EHR), with secure access available from anywhere according to established permissions.
- *Broadened vital signs.* The nature of vital signs and their collection will evolve to include a wider range of biophysical, mental/neurological, and place/environmental measures.
- *Personal and community vital signs.* In 2025, primary care will be nearly inseparable from community health. Providers will network with neighborhoods and share their data (with appropriate privacy and security protections) with public health officials who coordinate activities to improve population health.
- *Person-centered care.* In 2025, the individual or person involved in and receiving primary care will not be considered the "patient" except when he or she is in "inpatient care" or having care for acute episodes. Individuals will be doing enhanced self-care. Patient-centered primary care will have evolved to person- and family-centered primary care. The whole person will be the focus of care.
- *Integrative encounters in primary care.* Integrative encounters will address all dimensions of health by bringing the knowledge of conventional, unconventional, complementary, alternative, traditional, and integrative medicine disciplines to bear across the many different cultural traditions of persons cared for.

- *24/7 healthcare access.* By 2025, health care will be available anytime and everywhere. People seldom will need to be evaluated in the primary care clinic. People will have 24/7 access to their relational agent and access by phone, email, or televisit to some human member of the primary care team much of the time.

Health Care

PricewaterhouseCoopers identified the following top healthcare issues of the day:[25]

1. Healthcare organizations are reinventing themselves and bluring traditional lines of demarcation.
2. Cash-rich corporations seeking growth opportunities invade the healthcare venture capital space.
3. Employers explore new options with private exchanges.
4. The health industry feels the push to meet growing consumer and employer demands for transparency.
5. Health organizations fuse social, mobile, analytics, and cloud technologies to change the way they do business.
6. Providers befriend technology to meet growing demand and deliver better care.
7. In the face of funding pressures and new competition, failure becomes the saving grace for stagnating healthcare innovation.
8. Alternative care delivery models emerging as traditional care delivery gives way to alternative models outside of physicians' offices and hospitals. There also will be an increase in number and scope of services by work sites, retail health clinics, home health services, and technology-enabled delivery—for example, email, telehealth, and remote monitoring.
9. Community health becomes a new social reality with a major boost in funding from the government.
10. Threats from imitation medicines prompt new rules to protect the nation's drug supply.

Research demonstrates that 74% of all U.S. adults use the Internet, and 61% have looked for health or medical information on the Internet. In addition, 49% have accessed a website that provides information about a specific medical condition or problem.[27]

Health Workforce

HealthLeaders Media projects that job growth will continue in the healthcare sector. The Bureau of Labor Statistics reports that with the healthcare reform bill mandating insurance for another 30 million Americans and the graying of the U.S. population at an unstoppable pace, the healthcare sector will have a hiring resurgence. Census Bureau data show that the ambulatory services sector accounts for nearly one-half of new hires in health care and for the past 3 years has generated more revenues than hospitals have.[28] The slow growth in hospital employment and fast growth in ambulatory care services have been the trend. This trend has been driven by the move away from high-cost, high-risk hospital care and toward more convenient, lower-cost ambulatory care. In recent years this trend has been driven by development of new technologies that have allowed patients who previously required hospital care to be treated in ambulatory settings, such as the use of stents for many people who previously required bypass surgery. Bureau of Labor Statistics preliminary data for August 2014 show that the healthcare sector, which includes hospitals, nursing homes, ambulatory surgery centers, clinics, and physicians' offices, created 32,700 new jobs, which represents 20% of new jobs created in the entire economy for the month.[29]

In addition, recently published research reports that U.S. providers are making significant progress in adopting electronic health record EHR technology, with the number of hospitals using EHR nearly tripling since 2010. Forty-four percent of hospitals report EHR use, with physicians close behind at 38%. All Medicare providers will be required to comply with meaningful use standards by 2015 or face penalties.[30]

Holistic Health

Holistic leader Bill Manahan offered "eight transitions that will bring light and balance to healthcare," including the following transitions:[31]

- From health care being a business to also being a calling
- From the Dominator Model ("What is good for me?") to the Partnership Model ("What is good for all of us?")
- From health care being a science to also being an art—from material, mechanistic, and scientific worldviews to consciousness, mindfulness, and spirit
- From a focus on individual health to a focus on community health—a balance of these two paradigms
- From unrealistic expectations of the medical system to more realistic expectations—a true understanding of what medical care and pharmaceuticals can and cannot do for people
- From Type II medical malpractice (doing the wrong thing the right way) to no malpractice or only Type I medical malpractice (doing the right thing the wrong way) and decreasing the number of unnecessary and inappropriate procedures, tests, and treatments that are not evidence based
- From living in fear of illness and death to acceptance of illness and death as normal parts of life
- From single-causality mentality to an understanding and acceptance of the multiple causality of disease

The preceding driving forces will propel mainstream health care into the future. Access to healthcare providers who possess knowledge and skills in the promotion of healthful living and the integration of holistic/integrative modalities is a critical need for Americans. Holistic nurses are professionals who have knowledge of a wide range of complementary, alternative, and integrative modalities; health promotion and restoration and disease prevention strategies; and relationship-centered, caring ways of healing. They are in a prime position to meet this need and provide leadership in this national trend.

Recommendations

Recommendations from the Robert Wood Johnson Foundation Commission to Build a Healthier America were released in 2014 and include the following suggestions:[32]

1. Making investments in America's youngest children a high priority and launching major new initiatives to help families and communities build a strong foundation in early years for a lifetime of good health.
2. Fully integrating health into community development as neighborhoods are revitalized.
3. Seeking a more health-focused approach to healthcare financing and delivery that will help health professional and healthcare institutions broaden their missions beyond treating illness to helping people lead healthier lives.

The White House Commission on CAM Policy *Final Report* stated that people have come to recognize that a healthy lifestyle can promote wellness and prevent illness and disease and that many individuals have used CAM modalities to attain this goal.[33] Wellness incorporates a broad array of activities and interventions that focus on the physical, mental, spiritual, and emotional aspects of one's life. The effectiveness of the healthcare delivery system in the future will depend on its ability to use all approaches and modalities to contribute to a sound base for promoting health. Early interventions that promote the development of good health habits and attitudes could help modify many of the negative behaviors and lifestyle choices that begin in adolescence and continue into old age. The report recommended the following items, which are equally if not more important today than when the report was first published:

- Include more evidence-based teaching about CAM approaches in the conventional health professions schools.
- Emphasize the importance of approaches to prevent disease and promote wellness for the long-term health of the American people.
- Increase in importance teaching the principles and practices of self-care and provide lifestyle counseling in professional schools so that health professionals can, in turn, provide this guidance to their patients as well as improve their own health.

- Provide those in the greatest need, including those with chronic illnesses and those with limited incomes, access to the most accurate, up-to-date information about which therapies and products may help and which may harm.
- Design the education and training of all practitioners to increase the availability of practitioners' knowledgeable in both CAM and conventional practices. The report was based on the guiding principles shown in **Exhibit 3-1**.

Similarly, the Institute of Medicine (IOM) report *Complementary and Alternative Medicine in the United States* recommended the following, which necessitate attention in today's healthcare context:[34]

- Health professionals take into account a patient's individuality, emotional needs, values, and life issues; implement strategies for reaching those who do not ask for care on their own, including healthcare strategies that support the broader community; and enhance prevention and health promotion.
- Health professions schools (e.g., medicine, nursing, pharmacy, allied health) incorporate sufficient information about CAM into the standard curriculum at the undergraduate, graduate, and postgraduate levels to enable licensed professionals to competently advise patients about CAM.
- National professional organizations of all CAM disciplines ensure the presence of training standards and develop practice guidelines. Healthcare professional licensing boards and crediting and certifying agencies (for both CAM and conventional medicine) should set competency standards in the appropriate use of both conventional medicine and CAM therapies, consistent with practitioners' scope of practice and standards of referral across health professions.
- Needed is a moral commitment of openness to diverse interpretations of health and healing, a commitment to finding innovative ways of obtaining evidence, and an expansion of the knowledge base relevant and appropriate to medical practice. One way to honor social pluralism is in the recognition of medical pluralism, meaning the broad differences in preferences and values expressed through the public's prevalent use of CAM modalities. Medical pluralism should be distinguished from the co-optation of CAM therapies by conventional medical practices. The hazard of integration is that certain CAM therapies

---

EXHIBIT 3-1   The White House Commission on Complementary Alternative Medicine Policy Guiding Principles

1. A wholeness orientation in healthcare delivery.
2. Evidence of safety and efficacy.
3. The healing capacity of the person.
4. Respect for individuality.
5. The right to choose treatment.
6. An emphasis on health promotion and self-care.
7. Partnerships as essential for integrated health care.
8. Education as a fundamental healthcare service. Education about prevention, healthful lifestyles, and the power of self-healing should be made an integral part of the curricula of all healthcare professionals and should be made available to the public at all ages.
9. Dissemination of comprehensive and timely information.
10. Integral public involvement. The input of informed consumers and other members of the public must be incorporated in setting priorities for health care and healthcare research, and in reaching policy decisions, including those related to CAM, within the public and private sectors.

may be delivered within the context of a conventional medical practice in ways that dissociate CAM modalities from the epistemological framework that guides the tailoring of the CAM practice. The proper attitude is one of skepticism about any claim that conventional biomedical research and practice exhaustively account for the human experiences of health and healing.

- Research aimed at answering questions about outcomes of care is crucial to ensuring that healthcare professionals provide evidence-based, comprehensive care that encourages a focus on healing, recognizes the importance of compassion and caring, emphasizes the centrality of relationship-based care, encourages patients to share in decision making about therapeutic options, and promotes choices in care that can include complementary and alternative medical therapies when appropriate.
- The National Institutes of Health (NIH) and other public and private agencies sponsor research to compare the outcomes and costs of combinations of CAM and conventional medical treatments and develop models that deliver such care.
- The U.S. Congress and federal agencies, in consultation with industry, research scientists, consumers, and other stakeholders, amend the current regulatory scheme for dietary supplements.

A recent initiative, Wellness Initiative for the Nation (WIN),[35] was created to proactively prevent disease and illness, promote health and productivity, and encourage the well-being and flourishing of the U.S. population. WIN also plays an important role in preventing the looming fiscal disaster in the healthcare system by addressing preventable chronic illness and creating a productive, self-care society. This may be the only long-term hope for changing a system that costs too much and is delivering less health and little care to fewer people. WIN, focusing on promotion of health through lifestyle change and integrative health practices, would be overseen by the White House, with a director and staff to guide relevant aspects of health reform. It would establish a network of Systems

Wellness Advancements Teams (SWAT) with national and local leaders in health promotion and integrative practices; establish educational and practice standards for effective, comprehensive lifestyle and integrative healthcare delivery; create an advanced information tracking and feedback system for personalized wellness education; and create economic incentives for individuals, communities, and public and private sectors to develop and deliver self-care training, wellness products, and preventive health practices. The components of human health behavior and productivity optimization identified by WIN include stress management and resilience, physical exercise and sleep, optimum nutrition and substance use, and social integration and the social environment.

In September 2010, the Surgeon General convened the National Prevention and Health Promotion Council to create the *National Prevention Strategy*.[36] The vision of this strategy is working together (state, local, and territorial governments, businesses, health care, education and community faith-based organizations) to improve the health and quality of life for individuals, families, and communities by moving the nation from a focus on sickness and disease to one based on wellness and prevention. The strategic directions are Healthy and Safe Communities, Clinical and Community Preventive Services, Empowered People, and Elimination of Health Disparities. The goals are to create community environments that make the healthy choice the easy and affordable choice, to implement effective preventive practices by creating and recognizing communities that support prevention and wellness, to connect prevention-focused health care and community efforts to increase preventive services, to empower and educate individuals to make healthy choices, and to eliminate disparities in traditionally underserved populations. The strategic priorities (e.g., active lifestyles, countering alcohol/substance misuse, healthy eating, healthy physical and social environment, injury- and violence-free living, reproductive and sexual health, mental and emotional well-being) are designed to address ways to prevent significant causes of death and disability by focusing on the factors that underlie their causes.

In February 2009, the Institute of Medicine (IOM) IOM and the Bravewell Collaborative convened the Summit on Integrative Medicine and the Health of the Public that brought together more than 600 participants from numerous disciplines to examine the practice of integrative health care, its scientific basis, and its potential for improving health.[5] The summit sessions covered overarching visions for integrative medicine/health care, models of care, workforce, research, health professions education needs, and economic and policy implications. Participants assessed the potential and the priorities and began to identify elements of an agenda to enhance understanding, training, and practice to improve integrative medicine's contributions to better health and health care. Recurring themes of the summit are identified in **Exhibit 3-2**.

Several considerations for healthcare reform were articulated:

- *The progression of many chronic diseases can be reversed and sometimes even completely healed through lifestyle modifications.* Lifestyle modifications programs have been proven not only to improve people's overall health and well-being but also to mitigate cardiac disease and prostate cancer, among other chronic conditions.

- *Genetics is not destiny.* Recent research shows that gene expression can be turned on or off by nutritional choices, levels of social support, stress reduction activities such as meditation, and exercise.

- *The environment influences health.* Mounting evidence suggests that the environment outside one's body rapidly becomes the environment inside the body.

- *Improving the primary care and chronic disease care systems is paramount.* The U.S. primary care system is in danger of collapse and we must retool how both primary and chronic disease care are delivered. The new system must focus on prevention and wellness and put the patient at the center of care.

- *The reimbursement system must be changed.* The current reimbursement system rewards procedures rather than outcomes, and changes are needed that incentivize healthcare providers to focus on the health outcomes of their patients/clients.

- *Changes in education will fuel changes in practice.* Implementation of an integrated approach to health care requires changes in health provider education. All healthcare

---

EXHIBIT 3-2   Themes of the Summit on Integrative Medicine and the Health of the Public

- *Vision of optimal health:* Alignment of individuals and their health care for optimal health and healing across a full life span
- *Conceptually inclusive:* Seamless engagement of the full range of established health factors—physical, psychological, social, preventive, and therapeutic
- *Life span horizon:* Integration across the life span to include personal, predictive, preventive, and participatory care
- *Person-centered:* Integration around, and within, each person
- *Prevention-oriented:* Prevention and disease minimization as the foundation of integrative health care
- *Team-based:* Care as a team activity, with the patient as a central team member
- *Care integration:* Seamless integration of the care processes, across caregivers and institutions
- *Caring integration:* Person- and relationship-centered care
- *Science integration:* Integration across scientific disciplines, and scientific processes that cross domains
- *Integration of approach:* Integration across approaches to care—for example, conventional, traditional, alternative, complementary—as the evidence supports
- *Policy opportunities:* Emphasis on outcomes, elevation of patient insights, consideration of family and social factors, inclusion of team care and supportive follow up, and contributions to the learning process

practitioners should be educated in team approaches and the importance of compassionate care that addresses the biopsychosocial dimensions of health, prevention, and well-being. Core competencies need to be redefined and new categories explored.

- *Evidence-based medicine/health care is the only acceptable standard.* Health care should be supported by evidence. Further research and testing to expand the evidence base for integrative models of care requires attention.
- *Research must better accommodate multifaceted and interacting factors.* Research must clarify the nature by which biological predispositions and responses interact with social and environmental influences. Projects are needed to identify effective integrated approaches that demonstrate value, sustainability, and scalability.
- *A large demonstration project is recommended.* Because funding for research on the effectiveness of specific models of care is difficult to obtain from standard grant channels, participants voiced support for pursuing a demonstration project funded by the government that would fully exhibit the effectiveness of the integrative approach to care.

In 2014, the IOM Global Forum on Innovation in Health Professional Education convened a forum on Establishing Transdisciplinary Professionalism for Improving Health Outcomes. The forum defined transdisciplinary professionalism (TP) as

> an approach to creating and carrying out a shared social contract that ensures multiple health disciplines, working in concert, are worthy of the trust of patients and the public *in order to improve the health of patients and their communities.*[37]

The two-day forum explored how a transdisciplinary model of professionalism and health and wellness could be integrated into practice and education, the ethical implications of TP, how leadership is taught and practices from a TP perspective, the barriers to TP, and the effect of an evolving TP context on patients, students, and others in the healthcare system.[37]

Issues in Holistic Nursing

In December 2006, holistic nursing was officially recognized by the American Nurses Association (ANA) as a distinct nursing specialty with a defined scope and standards of practice, acknowledging holistic nursing's unique contribution to the health and healing of people and society. This recognition provides holistic nurses with clarity and a foundation for their practice and gives holistic nursing legitimacy and voice within the nursing profession and credibility in the eyes of the healthcare world and the public. *Holistic Nursing: Scope and Standards of Practice, Second Edition*, was published in 2013.[38]

Yet several issues exist or will emerge in the future for holistic nursing. Acceptance of holistic nursing's philosophy, influence, and contribution, both within nursing and within other disciplines, continues as one of the most pressing matters. Other concerns can be categorized into the areas of education, research, clinical practice, and policy. It is important to note that because holistic nursing as well as nursing in general and other disciplines face many of the same issues, an interdisciplinary/interprofessional approach is imperative for success in achieving the desired outcomes.

Education

There are several educational challenges in the holistic arena. With increased use of complementary/alternative/integrative therapies by the American public, both students and faculty need knowledge of and skill in their use. One urgent priority is the integration of holistic, relationship-centered philosophies and integrative modalities into nursing curricula. Core content appropriate for both basic and advanced practice programs must be identified, and models for integration of both content and practical experiences into existing curricula are necessary. An elective course is not sufficient to imbue future practitioners of nursing with this knowledge.

On a positive note, in 2008, the AHNA worked with the American Association of Colleges of Nursing (AACN) on the revision of *The Essentials of Baccalaureate Education for Professional Nursing Practice*.[39] Included in these new *Essentials* is language on preparing the baccalaureate generalist graduate to practice from a holistic, caring framework; engage in self-care; develop an understanding of complementary and alternative modalities; and incorporate patient teaching and health promotion, spirituality, and caring, healing techniques into practice. Holistic nurses will need to continue to work with the accrediting bodies of academic degree programs to ensure that this content is included in educational programs.

The National Educational Dialogue, an outgrowth of the Integrated Healthcare Policy Consortium (IAHC), sought to identify a set of core values, knowledge, skills, and attitudes necessary for all healthcare professional students. The Task Force on Values, Knowledge, Skills, and Attitudes, chaired by Carla Mariano, identified the following core values:[40]

- Wholeness and healing—interconnectedness of all people and things with healing as an innate capacity of every individual
- Clients/patients/families as the center of practice
- Practice as a combined art and science
- Self-care of the practitioner and commitment to self-reflection, personal growth, and healing
- Interdisciplinary collaboration and integration embracing the breadth and depth of diverse healthcare systems and collaboration with all disciplines, clients, and families
- Responsibility to contribute to the improvement of the community, the environment, health promotion, healthcare access, and the betterment of public health
- Attitudes and behaviors of all participants in health care demonstrating respect for self and others, humility, and authentic, open, courageous communication

There is a definitive need for increased scholarship and financial aid to support training in all of these areas. Faculty development programs also are necessary to support faculty in understanding and integrating holistic philosophy, content, and practices into curricula.

A major report by the IOM in 2010, *The Future of Nursing: Leading Change, Advancing Health*,[41] will have a significant effect on the nursing profession. The report recommends that *nurses should achieve higher levels of education and training through improved educational systems* by increasing the proportion of nurses with a baccalaureate degree to 80% by 2020, doubling the number of nurses with a doctorate by 2020, and ensuring that nurses engage in lifelong learning. Nurses need more education and preparation to adopt new roles quickly in response to rapidly changing healthcare settings and an evolving healthcare system. Competencies are especially needed in community, geriatrics, leadership, health policy, system improvement and change, research and evidence-based practice, and teamwork and collaboration. *The Future of Nursing: Campaign for Action* has determined indicators to measure progress toward achievement of the IOM's report recommendations and has established a dashboard to evaluate where nursing is gaining ground and areas that require additional emphasis.

To improve the competency of practitioners and the quality of services, holistic and CAM education and training needs to continue beyond basic and advanced academic education. Continuing education programs at national and regional specialty organizations and conferences may assist in meeting this need. Working with practitioners in other areas of nursing to increase their understanding of the philosophical and theoretical foundations of holistic nursing practices (e.g., consciousness, intention, presence, centering) will also be a role of holistic nurses.

Research

Research in the area of holistic nursing will become increasingly important in the future. Three areas of research seem to be widely proposed: whole systems research, exploration of healing relationships, and outcomes of healing interventions, particularly in the areas of health promotion, disease prevention, and wellness.

There is a great need for an evidence base to establish the effectiveness and efficacy of complementary/alternative/integrative therapies and interventions. Formidable tasks for nurses will be to identify and describe outcomes of CAM and holistic therapies, such as healing, well-being, and harmony, and to develop instruments to measure these outcomes to provide for evidence-informed practice. The IOM report on CAM in the United States recommends qualitative and quantitative research to examine the following:[34]

- The social and cultural dimensions of illness experiences, the processes and preferences of seeking health care, and practitioner–patient interactions
- How often users of CAM, including patients and providers, adhere to treatment instructions and guidelines
- The effects of CAM on wellness and disease prevention
- How the American public accesses and evaluates information about CAM modalities
- Adverse events associated with CAM therapies and interactions between CAM and conventional treatments
- Accessing information about CAM, such as the following:
  - Where the public goes to search for information about CAM modalities
  - Which sources of information they commonly find and access
  - The effect of CAM advertising on the methods of seeking health care
  - Which types of information are deemed credible, marginal, and spurious
  - How risks and benefits are understood and how such perceptions inform decision making
  - What the public expects their providers to tell them

The current mission of the National Center for Complementary and Alternative Medicine (NCCAM) is developing evidence requiring support across the continuum of basic science (How does the therapy/modality work?), translational research (Can it be studied in people?), efficacy studies (What are the specific effects?), and outcomes and effectiveness research (How well does the CAM/CIM practice work in the general population or healthcare settings?). The NCCAM's *Third Strategic Plan, Exploring the Science of Complementary and Alternative Medicine: 2011–2015*[1] identifies five strategic objectives:

1. Advance research on mind and body interventions, practices, and disciplines.
2. Advance research on natural products.
3. Increase understanding of real-world patterns and outcomes of CAM use and its integration into health care and health promotion.
4. Improve the capacity of the field to carry out rigorous research.
5. Develop and disseminate objective, evidence-based information on CAM interventions.

These objectives address the three long-range goals of (1) advancing the science and practice of symptom management; (2) developing effective, practical, personalized strategies for promoting health and well-being; and (3) enabling better evidence-based decision making regarding CAM use and its integration into health care and health promotion.[1]

Presently, most outcome measures are based on physical or disease/pathology symptomatology. However, methodologies need to be expanded to capture the wholeness of the individual's experience because the philosophy of these therapies rests on a paradigm of wholeness.

> Integrative health care is *derived from lessons integrated across scientific disciplines, and it requires scientific processes that cross domains.* The most important influences on health, for individuals and society, are not the factors at play within any single domain—genetics, behavior, social or economic circumstances, physical environment, health care—but the dynamics and synergies across domains. Research tends to examine these influences in isolation, which can distort interpretation of the results and hinder application of results. The most value will come from broader, systems-level approaches and redesign of research strategies and methodologies.[5, p. 7]

The Patient Protection and Affordable Care Act created a Patient-Centered Outcomes Research Institute (PCORI) to act as a nonprofit organization to assist patients, clinicians, purchasers, and policymakers in making informed health decisions by carrying out research projects that provide high-quality, relevant evidence on how diseases, disorders, and other health conditions can effectively and appropriately be prevented, diagnosed, treated, monitored, and managed. Patient-Centered Outcomes Research (PCOR) helps people make informed healthcare decisions and allows their voices to be heard in assessing the value of healthcare options. This research answers patient-focused questions, such as the following:[42]

1. "Given my personal characteristics, conditions, and preferences, what should I expect will happen to me?"
2. "What are my options and what are the benefits and harms of those options?"
3. "What can I do to improve the outcomes that are most important to me?"
4. "How can the healthcare system improve my chances of achieving the outcomes I prefer?"

To answer these questions, PCOR:[42]

- Assesses the benefits and harms of preventive, diagnostic, therapeutic, or health delivery system interventions to inform decision making, highlighting comparisons and outcomes that matter to people;
- Is inclusive of an individual's preferences, autonomy and needs, focusing on outcomes that people notice and care about such as survival, function, symptoms, and health-related quality of life;
- Incorporates a wide variety of settings and diversity of participants to address individual differences and barriers to implementation and dissemination; and
- Investigates (or may investigate) optimizing outcomes while addressing burden to individuals, resources, and other stakeholder perspectives.

The *Journal of Alternative and Complementary Medicine* collaborated with the International Society for Complementary Medicine Research to sponsor a forum on the research issues for whole systems. Participants underscored the political and economic challenges of getting research funded and published if researchers look at the practices and processes that typify whole-person treatment. What is clear is that whole practices, whole systems, and related research need professional and organizational attention.

> Today researchers are being challenged to look at alternative philosophies of science and research methods that are compatible with investigations of humanistic and holistic occurrences. We also need to study phenomena by exploring the context in which they occur and the meaning of patterns that evolve. Also needed are approaches to interventions studies that are more holistic, taking into consideration the *interactive* nature of the body-mind-emotion-spirit-environment. Rather than isolating the effects of one part of an intervention, we need more comprehensive interventions and more sensitive instruments that measure the interactive nature of each client's biological, psychological, sociological, emotional, and spiritual patterns. In addition, comprehensive comparative outcome studies are needed to ascertain the usefulness, indications, and contraindications of integrative therapies. Further, researchers must evaluate these interventions for their usefulness in promoting wellness as well as preventing illness.[43, p. 26]

Investigations into the concept and nature of the placebo effect also are needed because one-third of all medical healings are the result of the placebo effect.[44]

It will be imperative for nurses to address how to secure and maintain funding for their holistic research. They need to apply for funding from National Institutes of Health (NIH) centers and institutes in addition to the National Institute of Nursing Research (NINR) and particularly the National Center for Complementary and

Alternative Medicine (NCCAM). Hand in hand with this is the need for nurses to be represented in study sections and review panels to educate and convince the biomedical and NIH community about the value of nursing research; the need for models of research focusing on health promotion and disease prevention, wellness, and self-care instead of only the disease model; and the importance of a variety of designs and research methodologies, including qualitative studies, rather than sole reliance on randomized controlled trials.

An area of responsibility for advanced practice holistic nurses is the dissemination of their research findings to various media sources (e.g., television, newsprint, social media) and at nonnursing, interdisciplinary/interprofessional conferences. Publishing in nonnursing journals and serving on editorial boards of nonnursing journals also broadens the appreciation in other disciplines for nursing's role in setting the agenda and conducting research in the area of holism and CAM.

Clinical Practice

Clinical care models reflecting holistic assessment, treatment, health, healing, and caring are important in the development of holistic nursing practice. Implementing holistic and humanistic models in today's healthcare environment will require a paradigm shift for the many providers who subscribe to a disease model of care. Such an acceptance poses an enormous challenge. Loretta Ford identified actions that nurse leaders might consider in advancing integrative health:[45, p. 82]

- Create a culture of innovation and involve staff in alternative practices.
- Review the institution's philosophy, mission, policies, programs, and practices for opportunities to include alternative therapies.
- Influence clinical practice for recognition of patients' personal usage of integrative therapies.
- Collaborate and encourage collaboration with other professionals involved in integrative practices.

- Support (financially and otherwise) and guide programs of staff recruitment, preparation, and training in integrative care.
- Publish nursing programs, studies, and reports on alternative therapy outcomes, issues, and challenges.

Holistic nurses, with their education and experience, are the logical leaders in integrative care and must advance that position.

Licensure and credentialing provide another challenge for holistic nursing. As complementary/alternative/integrative health care has gained national recognition, state boards of nursing began to attend to the regulation issues. The 2010 IOM report *The Future of Nursing*[41] notes that regulations defining scope-of-practice limitations vary widely by state. Some states have kept pace with the evolution of the healthcare system by changing their scope-of-practice regulations, but the majority of state laws lag behind in this regard. As a result, what nurse practitioners are able to do once they graduate can vary widely and is often not related to their ability, education or training, or safety concerns but to the political decisions of the state in which they work. The IOM recommends that *nurses should practice to the full extent of their education and training* and that *scope-of-practice barriers should be removed*. The IOM also recommends that *nurse residency programs should be implemented*.

The AHNA conducted a preliminary survey to ascertain the number of state boards of nursing that accepted and recognized holistic nursing and/or permitted holistic practices with its regulations and/or the state's nurse practice act. Of the 39 states that responded, 8 states include holistic nursing in their nurse practice act. The findings from a review of actual state practice acts further revealed that 47 of 51 states/territories have some statements or positions that include holistic wording such as *self-care, spirituality, natural therapies*, and/or specific complementary/alternative therapies under the scope of practice.

It will be important in the future to monitor state boards of nursing for evidence of their recognition and support of holistic, integrative nursing practice and requirements that include CAM. Finally, holistic nursing has the challenge of working with the state boards to incorporate this content into the National Council Licensure Examination, thus ensuring the credibility of this practice knowledge. The 2012 AHNA *Position on the Role of Nurses in the Practice of Complementary and Alternative Therapies* describes the necessity for integration of CAM therapies into a comprehensive holistic nursing practice.[38]

Addressing the nursing shortage in this country is crucial to the health of our nation. Multiple surveys and studies confirm that the shortage of registered nurses (RNs) influences the delivery of health care in the United States and negatively affects patient outcomes. According to the American Hospital Association, the United States is, by all accounts, in the midst of a significant shortage of RNs that is projected to last well into the future. The Tri-Council for Nursing cautions stakeholders about declaring an end to the nursing shortage. Although the shortage has eased in the United States, most analysts believe this development to be temporary. The council expressed serious concerns about slowing the production of RNs given the projected demand for nursing services, particularly in light of healthcare reform. The ANA notes that the United States will need to produce 1.1 million new RNs by 2022 to fill newly created jobs and replace a legion of soon-to-be retirees. The ANA is recommending specific actions in regard to federal funding, nursing education, and hiring practices to ensure a sufficient nursing workforce to meet the demand.[46] Peter Buerhaus and coauthors found that the U.S. nursing shortage is projected to grow to 260,000 RNs by 2025, which would be twice as large as any nursing shortage experienced in the United States since the mid-1960s. Because the demand for RNs will increase as large numbers of RNs retire, a sizeable and prolonged shortage of nurses is expected to hit the United States in the latter half of the next decade.[47]

According to the AACN's report *2012–2013 Enrollment and Graduations in Baccalaureate and Graduate Programs in Nursing*, in 2010, U.S. nursing schools turned away 79,659 qualified applicants from baccalaureate and graduate nursing programs because of insufficient number of faculty, clinical sites, classroom space, clinical preceptors, and budget constraints. Almost two-thirds of the nursing schools responding to the survey pointed to faculty shortages as a reason for not accepting all qualified applicants into their programs, thus constraining schools' ability to expand enrollment to alleviate the nursing shortage.[47]

In addition, there are some distressing statistics regarding nursing: In the United States, 41% of nurses are dissatisfied with their present job. Nationally, nurses give themselves burnout scores of 30% to 40%, and 17% of nurses are not working in nursing. Moreover, 13% of newly licensed RNs had changed principal jobs after 1 year, and 37% reported that they felt ready to change jobs. Nurses often change jobs or leave the profession because of unhumanistic and chaotic work environments and professional and personal burnout. Research shows that reduction of perceived stress is related to increased job satisfaction. Holistic nurses, through their knowledge of self-care, resilience, caring cultures, healing environments, and stress management techniques, have an extraordinary opportunity to influence and improve the healthcare milieu, both for healthcare providers and for clients and patients.[48]

Policy

Four major policy issues face holistic nursing in the future: leadership, reimbursement, regulation, and access. The IOM report *The Future of Nursing*[41] recommends that *nurses should be full partners with physicians and other health professionals in redesigning health care in the United States.* Nurses should be prepared and enabled to lead change in all roles—from the bedside to the boardroom—to advance health. Nurses should have a voice in health policy decision making and be engaged in implementation efforts related to healthcare reform, particularly regarding quality, access, value, and patient-centered care. Nurses must view policy as something they can shape rather than as something that happens to them.

Public or private policies regarding coverage and reimbursement for healthcare services play a crucial role in shaping the healthcare system and will play a crucial role in deciding the future of wellness, health promotion, and CAM in the nation's healthcare system. According to the most recent *Complementary and Alternative Medicine Survey of Hospitals* conducted by the American Hospital Association and Samueli Institute, hospitals across the nation are responding to patient demand and integrating CAM services with conventional services. More than 42% of hospitals in the survey indicated that they offer one or more CAM therapies, up from 37% in 2007 and 26.5% in 2005. Eighty-five percent of responding hospitals cited patient demand as the primary rationale in offering CAM services, and 70% stated clinical effectiveness as their top reason.[49] Often, however, holistic modalities are offered as a supplemental benefit rather than as a core or basic benefit, and many third-party payers do not cover such services at all. In the CAM *Survey of Hospitals*, 69% of CAM services were paid for out of pocket by patients. Coverage and reimbursement for most CAM services depend on the provider's ability to legally furnish services within the scope of practice. The legal authority to practice is given by the state in which services are provided.

Reimbursement of advanced practice registered nurses also depends on appropriate credentials. Holistic nurses will need to work with Medicare and other third-party payers, insurance groups, boards of nursing, healthcare policymakers, legislators, and other professional nursing organizations to ensure that holistic nurses are appropriately reimbursed for services rendered. Another issue regarding reimbursement is the fact that the effectiveness of CAM is influenced by the holistic focus and integrative skill of the provider. Consequently, reimbursement must be included for the process of holistic and integrative care, not just for providing a specific modality.

There are many barriers to the use of holistic therapies by potential users, providing yet another challenge for holistic nurses. Barriers include lack of awareness of the therapies and their benefits, uncertainty about their effectiveness, inability to pay for them, and limited availability of qualified providers. Access is more difficult for rural populations; uninsured or underinsured populations; special populations, such as racial and ethnic minorities; and vulnerable populations, such as older adults and

those with chronic or terminal illnesses.[33] Holistic nurses have a responsibility to educate the public more fully about health promotion, complementary/alternative/integrative modalities, and qualified practitioners and to assist people in making informed choices among the array of healthcare alternatives and individual providers. Holistic nurses also must actively participate in the political arena as leaders in this movement to ensure quality, an increased focus on wellness, and access and affordability for all.

By developing theoretical and empirical knowledge as well as caring and healing approaches, holistic nurses will advance holistic nursing practice and education and contribute significantly to the formalization and credibility of this work. They will lead the profession in research, the development of educational models, and the integration of a more holistic approach in nursing practice and health care.

Conclusion

This chapter concludes with the thoughts and reflections of various leaders in the field of holistic health care and holistic nursing.

> We need to balance the acquisition of knowledge with a deepening in wisdom. That has to happen throughout the education of all healthcare professionals. There has to be a balance between wisdom and knowledge. And we've lost it. That depth has to do with knowing yourself as a human being as well as a practitioner and healer, being yourself and experiencing yourself and your own struggles and possibilities. There are four things: wisdom balancing knowledge, a community of healers, self-care as the heart of all health care, and health care as a right to which everyone is entitled. If we have these, then the whole health system changes, and all of us—our health and the way we look at the world—will change and improve.[50, p. 72]
>
> —James Gordon, MD

Nurses are exceedingly well positioned to become leaders in integrative health. Nurses constitute the nation's largest group of health professionals [more than 3 million]. . . . Nightingale described the nurse's work as helping a patient attain the best possible condition so that nature can act and self-healing may occur. Nurses go beyond fixing or curing to ease the edges of patients' suffering. They help people return to day-to-day functioning, maintain health, live with chronic illness, and/or gracefully move through stages of dying into death. Nurses are experts in symptom management, care coordination, chronic disease management, and health promotion. In addition to caring for people from birth to death, nurses currently manage care for communities, conduct research, lead health systems, and address health policy issues.[45, p. 80]

—Mary Jo Kreitzer, PhD, RN, FAAN

Our work—nursing—is a calling, not only to serve but to deepen our humanity. It is a spiritual practice. . . . The tasks of *Nursing* are the tasks of *Humanity*: healing and relationship with self, others, the planet; developing a deeper understanding of human suffering; expanding and evolving an understanding of life itself; deepening an understanding of death and the sacred cycle. . . . We must revisit the foundations of our work. Caring is an ethic—it forces us to pay attention. Pause and realize that this one moment with this one person is the reason we are here at this time on this planet. When we touch their body, we touch their mind, heart, and soul. When we connect with another's humanity even for a brief moment, we have purpose in our life and work.[51]

—Jean Watson, PhD, RN, AHN-BC, FAAN

Directions for Future Research

1. Identify the strengths and limitations of different research approaches and methods to studying holistic phenomena.
2. Explore research findings on various CAM/CIM therapies.

Nurse Healer Reflections

After reading this chapter, the holistic nurse will be able to answer or to begin a process of answering the following questions:

- What is my vision of a caring, healing, holistic healthcare system?
- What are my beliefs, values, and assumptions about my contributions and other healthcare disciplines' contributions to the health of society?

NOTES

1. National Center for Complementary and Alternative Medicine, *Exploring the Science of Complementary and Alternative Medicine: Third Strategic Plan 2011–2015* (Washington, DC: U.S. Department of Health and Human Services, National Institutes of Health, 2011).
2. U.S. Department of Health and Human Services, *Healthy People 2020* (Washington, DC: U.S. Department of Health and Human Services, 2010).
3. Public Agenda, "Half of Americans Say the Health Care System Has Major Problems" (May 11, 2011). www.publicagenda.org/charts /half-americans-say-health-care-system-has -major-problems-and-most-say-it-needs-be -fundamentally-changed-or.
4. Robert Wood Johnson Foundation, "Sick in America: Topline Findings" (May 21, 2012). www.rwjf.org/en/research-publications/find -rwjf-research/2012/05/sick-in-america.html.
5. Institute of Medicine, *Summit on Integrative Medicine and the Health of the Public* (Washington, DC: National Academies Press, 2009): 1–2.
6. Centers for Disease Control and Prevention, "Chronic Diseases and Health Promotion" (May 9, 2014). www.cdc.gov/chronicdisease/overview /index.htm#ref1.

7. R. Lee, "The New Pandemic: SuperStress?" *EXPLORE: The Journal of Science and Healing* 6, no. 1 (2010): 7–10.

8. Peter G. Peterson Foundation, "Americans Spend Over Twice as Much Per Capita on Healthcare as the Average Developed Country Does," *OECD Health Statistics 2014* (June 2014). http://pgpf.org /Chart-Archive/0006_health-care-oecd.

9. Altarum Institute, "Health Spending Growth Appears More Modest Than Previously Estimated," *Spending Brief #14-07* (June 27, 2014). http://altarum.org/sites/default/files/uploaded -related-files/CSHS-Spending-Brief_June%20 2014_0.pdf.

10. C. S. Girod, L. W. Mayne, S. A. Weltz, and S. K. Hart, *2014 Milliman Medical Index* (May 20, 2014). http://us.milliman.com/insight/Periodicals /mmi/2014-Milliman-Medical-Index/.

11. R. A. Cohen and W. K. Kirzinger, "Financial Burden of Medical Care: A Family Perspective," *NCHS Data Brief No. 142* (January 2014). www .cdc.gov/nchs/data/databriefs/db142.pdf.

12. Kaiser Family Foundation, "2014 Employer Health Benefits Survey" (September 10, 2014). http://kff.org/private-insurance/report/2014 -employer-health-benefits-survey/.

13. R. Wolf, "Number of Uninsured Americans Rises to 50.7 Million," *USA Today* (September 18, 2010). http://usatoday30.usatoday.com/news /nation/2010-09-17-uninsured17_ST_N.htm.

14. J. Levy, "In U.S., Uninsured Rate Sinks to 13.4% in Second Quarter," *Gallup, Inc.* (July 10, 2014). www.gallup.com/poll/172403/uninsured-rate -sinks-second-quarter.aspx.

15. HealthCareProblems.org, "Health Care Statistics" (2014). www.healthcareproblems.org /health-care-statistics.htm.

16. T. Luhby, "Millions Can't Afford to Go to the Doctor," *CNNMoney* (April 26, 2013). http:// money.cnn.com/2013/04/26/news/economy /health-care-cost.

17. Kaiser Family Foundation, "U.S. Health Care Costs: Background Brief" (March 2010). www .kaiseredu.org/Issue-Modules/US-Health-Care -Costs.

18. M. A. Hyman, "Quality in Healthcare: Asking the Right Questions in the Next Ten Years: The Role of CAM in the 'Quality Cure,'" *Alternative Therapies* 11, no. 3 (2005): 18–20.

19. P. M. Barnes, B. Bloom, and R. L. Nahin, "Complementary and Alternative Medicine Use Among Adults and Children: United States, 2007," *National Health Statistics Reports* No. 12 (December 10, 2008). www.cdc.gov/nchs/data /nhsr/nhsr012.pdf.

20. National Center for Complementary and Alternative Medicine, "Americans Spent $33.9 Billion Out-of-Pocket on Complementary and Alternative Medicine" (July 30, 2009). http://nccam.nih .gov/news/2009/073009.htm.

21. American Association of Retired Persons and National Center for Complementary and Alternative Medicine, *Complementary and Alternative Medicine: What People Aged 50 and Older Discuss with Their Health Care Providers* (Washington, DC: U.S. Department of Health and Human Services, 2011).

22. J. Weeks, "Reference Guide: Language and Sections on CAM and Integrative Practice in HR 3590/Healthcare Overhaul," *Integrator Blog* (May 12, 2010). http://theintegratorblog.com/site /index.php?option=com_content&task=view&id =658&Itemid=2.

23. FON Therapeutics, "Integrative Medicine Centers" (2014). http://fontherapeutics.com /resources/integrative-medicine-centers/.

24. H. T. Tu, E. R. Boukus, and G. R. Cohen, "Workplace Clinics: A Sign of Growing Employer Interest in Wellness," *HSC Research Brief No. 17* (December 2010). www.hschange.com /CONTENT/1166/.

25. PricewaterhouseCoopers, "Top Health Industry Issues of 2014," *PWC Research Institute* (2014). www.pwc.com/us/en/health-industries/top -health-industry-issues/index.jhtml.

26. C. Bezold, "Alert: Major Study on Future of Primary Care Seeks Input on IM Therapies and CAM Practitioners," *Integrator Blog* (April 25, 2011). http://theintegratorblog.com/index .php?option=com_content&task=view&id=744 &Itemid=189.

27. R. A. Cohen and P. F. Adams, "Use of the Internet for Health Information: United States, 2009," *NCHS DATA Brief* No. *66* (July 2011). www.cdc.gov/nchs/data/databriefs/db66.pdf.

28. J. Commins, "Eight Healthcare HR Trends for 2010," *HealthLeaders Media* (January 4, 2010). www.healthleadersmedia.com/content /HR-244371/Eight-Healthcare-HR-Trends-for -2010.html.

29. HealthLeaders Media, "Percent Change in Employment" (2014). www.healthleadersmedia .com/slideshow.cfm?content_id=296068.

30. UnitedHealthcare, "*Health Affairs* Reports Electornic Health Record (EHR) Progress" (July 12, 2013). http://uhc.com/united_for _reform,_resource_center/news.

31. B. Manahan, "Revisioning Healthcare in 2009: Eight Transitions That Will Help Bring Light and Balance to Healthcare," *Integrator Blog*

(January 14, 2009). www.theintegratorblog.com/site/index.php?option=com_content&task=view&id=519&Itemid=1.

32. Robert Wood Johnson Foundation, *Time to Act: Investing in the Health of Our Children and Communities: Recommendations from the Robert Wood Johnson Foundation Commission to Build a Healthier America* (Princeton, NJ: Robert Wood Johnson Foundation, 2014).

33. White House Commission on Complementary and Alternative Medicine Policy, *Final Report* (Washington, DC: U.S. Government Printing Office, 2002).

34. Institute of Medicine, *Complementary and Alternative Medicine in the United States* (Washington, DC: National Academies Press, 2005).

35. Samueli Institute, *A Wellness Initiative for the Nation* (Alexandria, VA: Samueli Institute, 2009).

36. National Prevention Council, *National Prevention Strategy: American's Plan for Better Health and Wellness* (Washington, DC: U.S. Department of Health and Human Services, Office of the Surgeon General, 2011).

37. Institute of Medicine, *Establishing Transdisciplinary Professionalism for Improving Health Outcomes: Workshop Summary* (Washington, DC: National Academies Press, 2014): 2.

38. American Holistic Nurses Association and American Nurses Association, *Holistic Nursing: Scope and Standards of Practice*, 2nd ed. (Silver Spring, MD: Nursesbooks.org, 2013).

39. American Association of Colleges of Nursing, *The Essentials of Baccalaureate Education for Professional Nursing Practice* (Washington, DC: American Association of Colleges of Nursing, 2008).

40. Academic Consortim for Complementary and Alternative Health Care, *Clinicians' and Educators' Desk Reference on the Licensed Complementary and Alternative Healthcare Professions* (Seattle, WA: Academic Consortium for Complementary and Alternative Health Care, 2013).

41. Institute of Medicine, *The Future of Nursing: Leading Change, Advancing Health* (Washington, DC: National Academies Press, 2010).

42. Patient-Centered Outcomes Research Institute, *Patient-Centered Outcomes Research Definition Revision: Response to Public Input* (Washington, DC: Patient-Centered Outcomes Research Institute, 2012): 1.

43. C. Mariano, "Contributions to Holism Through Critique of Theory and Research," *Beginnings* 28, no. 2 (2008): 12–13, 26–27.

44. C. Mariano, "Research in Holism: A Nursing Perspective" (keynote address, Lexington, KY, March 2011).

45. M. Mittelman, S. Alperson, P. Arcari, G. Donnelly, L. Ford, M. Koithan, and M. J. Kreitzer, "Nursing and Integrative Health Care," *Alternative Therapies* 16, no. 5 (2010): 74–84.

46. American Nurses Association, "Nurse Training Act 50th Anniversary: Increased Investment Needed to Head Off Nursing Shortage," *Nursing World* (September 2, 2014). www.nursingworld.org/HomepageCategory/NursingInsider/Archive-1/2014-NI/Sept-2014-NI/Increased-Investment-Needed-to-Produce-11-Million-RNs.html.

47. American Association of Colleges of Nursing, "Nursing Shortage," *AACN Fact Sheet* (April 24, 2014). www.aacn.nche.edu/media-relations/fact-sheets/nursing-shortage.

48. C. Mariano, "The Nursing Shortage: Where Are the Nurses?" (presentation at the Integrative Health Care Symposium, New York, NY, March 2013).

49. Health Forum and Samueli Institute, *2010 Complementary and Alternative Medicine Survey of Hospitals: Summary of Results* (Alexandria, VA: Samueli Institute, 2011).

50. K. Gazella and S. Snyder, "James S. Gordon, MD: Connecting Mind, Body, and Beyond," *Alternative Therapies* 12, no. 2 (2006): 72–73.

51. J. Watson, "Human Caring and Holistic Healing: The Path of Heart and Spirit" (keynote address at the American Holistic Nurses Association Annual Conference, Colorado Springs, CO, 2010).

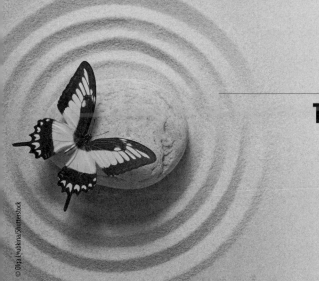

CHAPTER 4

Transpersonal Human Caring and Healing

Janet F. Quinn

Nurse Healer Objectives

Theoretical

- Define transpersonal human caring.
- Define healing.
- Compare and contrast the processes of healing and curing.
- Discuss the nature of "right relationship" as it relates to healing.

Clinical

- Apply the elements of a "caring occasion" to facilitate healing.
- Describe examples of healing at the body, mind, and spirit levels of human experience that you have observed in practice.
- Begin to imagine how your own clinical practice setting might evolve to become a "Habitat for Healing."

Personal

- Imagine what right relationship would look like and feel like when applied to something you want to heal in yourself.

Portions of this chapter have been published as: J. Quinn, "Healing: A Model for an Integrative Health Care System," *Advanced Practice Nursing Quarterly* 3, no. 1 (1997): 1–7, by permission of Aspen Publishers.

- Identify ways in which you can create your own healing environment.

Definitions

Habitats for Healing: Healthcare practice environments that provide a context of caring, for the purpose of healing, which may include curing.[1]

Healing: The emergence of right relationship at one or more levels of the bodymindspirit system.[2]

Healing system: A true healthcare system in which people can receive adequate, nontoxic, and noninvasive assistance in maintaining wellness and in healing for body, mind, and spirit, together with the most sophisticated, aggressive curing technologies available.

Human caring: The moral ideal of nursing in which the nurse brings his or her whole self into relationship with the whole self of the patient or client, to protect the vulnerability and preserve the humanity and dignity of the one caring and the one cared for.[3]

Right relationship: A process of connection among or between parts of the whole that increases energy, coherence, and creativity in the bodymindspirit system.

Transpersonal: That which transcends the limits and boundaries of individual ego identities and possibilities to include acknowledgment and appreciation of something greater. *Transpersonal* may refer to consciousness, intrapersonal dynamics, interpersonal relationships, and lived experiences of connection, unity, and oneness with the larger environment, cosmos, or Spirit.

Theory and Research

Within the discipline of nursing, there is widespread acceptance of the concept of caring as central to practice. However, there is no widespread consensus as to what caring is.[4-8] Morse and her colleagues, in their now classic paper, reported that five basic conceptualizations, or perspectives, on caring can be identified in the nursing literature: (1) caring as a human trait, (2) caring as a moral imperative or ideal, (3) caring as an affect, (4) caring as an interpersonal relationship, and (5) caring as a therapeutic intervention.[9]

The term *transpersonal human caring* is most often associated with Jean Watson's theory of nursing as the art and science of human caring.[10-12] Watson defines human caring as the moral ideal of nursing, in which the relationship between the whole self of the nurse and the whole self of the patient or client protects the vulnerability and preserves the humanity and dignity of the patient or client. This emphasis on the whole self—the whole person of both nurse and patient—requires the addition of the term *transpersonal* in Watson's framework and in the discussion of human caring as it relates to holistic nursing practice. Within a transpersonal perspective, people are more than the body physical and the mind as contained in that body. A transpersonal perspective acknowledges that all people are body, mind, and spirit or soul, and that interactions between people engage each of these aspects of the self. A nurse with a transpersonal perspective recognizes that this is a fact of human interaction, not an optional event. A holistic nurse recognizes, as Watson suggests, that there is something beyond the personal, separate selves of the nurse and the patient involved in the act of caring.

When nurses enter into caring, healing relationships with patients, bringing with them

an acknowledgment and appreciation of the body, mind, and spirit dimensions of their own human existence, they are engaged in a transpersonal human caring process. In this type of relationship, they know themselves to be interconnected with the patient and with the larger environment and cosmos. They know that they are walking on sacred ground when they walk this path with their patients, and they recognize that neither one will be the same afterward. For that moment, they are joined with the other who is patient or client, and so become part of something larger than either alone. In this transpersonal healing process, they are each changed.[12]

Watson calls these healing encounters "caring occasions" and suggests that they actually transcend the bounds of space and time.[13] The field of consciousness created in and through the caring, healing relationship has the potential to continue healing the patient long after the physical separation of nurse and patient. Moreover, the nurse, following engagement in a true caring occasion, will also continue to benefit from the mutual process. When nurses are able to engage their full, caring selves in the art of nursing, it is both energizing and satisfying.

It is often assumed that nurses burn out as a result of caring too much. However, today's nurses are far more likely to burn out for a different reason: the difficulty in finding the time to care for patients with their whole selves within healthcare systems that do not value caring.[2]

Healing: The Goal of Holistic Nursing

Although caring is the context for holistic nursing, healing is the goal. The origin of the word *heal* is the Anglo-Saxon word *haelan*, which means to be or to become whole. Defining what it means to be or to become whole is a challenging task. For example, is wholeness a goal, an end point that is something to work toward but is rarely achieved? Is wholeness a state of perfection of body, mind, and spirit? Is wholeness something that people either have or do not have, something that people can obtain and hold on to, or something that comes and goes?

Is it a state or a process? Is wholeness dependent on the structure and functioning of the body? Can one ever be not whole; that is, can one ever be other than wholly who or what one is at any point in space and time? If one cannot be not whole, then how is it possible to talk about becoming whole? Each holistic nurse is invited to spend some time thinking about what this means to her or him because a nurse's perspective on wholeness will influence everything that she or he does.

Healing as the Emergence of Right Relationship

Wholeness is frequently described as harmony of body, mind, and spirit, while harmony is defined as an ordered or aesthetically pleasing set of relationships among the elements of the whole. This simple definition illustrates the implications of associating harmony with healing. First, wholeness involves more than the intactness of physical structure and function, or the status of isolated parts of a person. Second, if healing is about harmony, it is necessary to expand the ways of knowing about healing to include the aesthetic as well as the scientific.

Synonyms for the word harmony include *unity*, *integrity*, *connection*, *reconciliation*, *congruence*, and *cohesion*. Taken together, these terms begin to suggest that wholeness is not necessarily a state of any kind but a process that is fundamentally about relationship. Wholeness is about the relationship of the parts of a system to one another and to the larger systems of which they are a part. When the theoretical physicist David Bohm was asked, "How can anything become more whole if everything is already part of the indivisible wholeness of the implicit order of the universe?" he responded with one word. "Coherence," he said, creating no doubt that wholeness was not about adding and subtracting parts, but about how those parts related to one another.[14] Increasing the wholeness of a system is about establishing a pattern of relationships among its elements that is more and more coherent.[15]

Healing, if it is a process of being or becoming whole, must be an emerging pattern of relationships among the elements of the whole person that leads to greater integrity, connection, and cohesion of the whole system. This pattern of relationships can be called *right relationship*. Thus, healing is the emergence of right relationship at or between or among any and all levels of the human experience. It is a process rather than a state. It is dynamic, and it always affects the whole person, no matter at which level the shift actually occurs. Key to an understanding of the effects of a shift into right relationship at any level are theories about how systems, particularly living systems, work.[16-20] The new sciences are

> known collectively as the sciences of complexity, including general systems theory (Bertalanffy, Weiss), cybernetics (Wiener), nonequilibrium thermodynamics (Prigogine), cellular automata theory (von Neumann), catastrophe theory (Thom), autopoietic system theory (Maturana and Varela), dynamic systems theory (Shaw, Abraham), and chaos theories, among others.[21, p. 14]

Within a systems perspective, human beings are simultaneously autonomous wholes and parts of larger wholes. Each "holon" is embedded in an "irreversible hierarchy of increasing wholeness, increasing holism, increasing unity and integration."[22]

Several principles related to the nature of systems are fundamental to all of these theories and have direct implications for the understanding of healing. The first and most basic is that a system is more than and different from the sum of its parts. It is "more than" its parts because the pattern of relationships among the parts of the whole gives the system its own unique identity. "A pattern of organization [is] a configuration of relationships characteristic of a particular system."[23, p. 80]

A second principle is that a change in the part always leads to a change in the whole. Because human beings are living systems governed by these principles, any shift, no matter how small or at which level it appears, will always affect the whole bodymindspirit. Furthermore, because every person is simultaneously a part of the larger whole of family, society, the ecosystem, and the universe, a change in an individual bodymindspirit leads to a change in all of these as well. This awareness is, of course, part of the teaching of virtually every spiritual tradition, and it affirms that nurses' individual healing work matters to far more than just the nurses.

The third principle that relates directly to healing is that the nature of the change in the whole cannot be predicted by the nature of the change in the part. "The new state [of a system] is decided neither by initial conditions in the system nor by changes in the critical values of environmental parameters; when a dynamic system is fundamentally destabilized, it acts indeterminately."[24]

Human beings as living systems are complex, adaptive, self-organizing systems, capable of—indeed, striving toward—order, self-transcendence, and transformation.[16, 25] "We are beginning to recognize the creative unfolding of life in forms of ever-increasing diversity and complexity as an inherent characteristic of all living systems."[23, p. 222] Thus, the healing process itself is inherent within the person. This urge toward healing, toward right relationship, when manifested, may be thought of as the "haelan effect."[26, p. 553]

In the context of these principles, right relationship is not a moral judgment, a statement about right and wrong, good or bad. Rather, it is a way of understanding a particular quality of pattern and organization. The inherent tendency of any living system, as part of the evolutionary process, is toward actualizing its "deep structure"[21, p. 40] (i.e., an acorn "wants" to actualize its inherent tree nature). The consequence of not being in right relationship is the tendency toward "self-dissolution."[21, p. 44] Right relationship may be thought of as any pattern of organization within the system that supports, encourages, allows, or generates actualization and self-transcendence—at any or all levels. Thus, consistent with the tendencies inherent in all living systems healing, the emergence of right relationship at any level of body, mind, or spirit:

- Increases coherence of the whole bodymindspirit
- Maximizes free energy in the whole bodymindspirit
- Maximizes freedom, autonomy, and choice in the whole

- Increases the capacity for creative unfolding of the whole bodymindspirit

Because of its inherently creative nature, true healing is always a process of emergence into something new, rather than a simple return to prior states of being.[27] Holistic nurses do not limit the focus of their care to recovery alone, but rather expand their focus to helping patients integrate their illness experience and transcend their former selves toward new patterns of self-actualization. This is the growth process of nature. Nightingale's statement that the goal is to put the patient in the best condition so that nature can act on him or her may refer to this natural, forward-moving tendency toward wholeness.

Healing as the emergence of right relationship may occur at any level of the bodymindspirit. For example, when an organ is transplanted, the emergence of right relationship between the new organ and the surrounding cells and tissues of the recipient's bodymindspirit signals healing. If that right relationship does not occur, if the cells of the new organ do not become integrated into the existing bodymindspirit, if rejection rather than acceptance happens, then the patient may die from a lack of right relationship, and thus healing, at the cellular level. When broken bones knit together, or when the edges of a wound begin to approximate, right relationship is emerging at the physical level. Each of these emerging right relationships has an affect on the whole, as noted earlier.

The effects on the whole person of a shift toward right relationship at the emotional level are evident in a moment of forgiveness or a release of a long-held resentment. At such a time, the way in which a person stands in relationship to an event or a person from the past changes. The letting go of resentment carries with it an often overwhelming release of energy for new growth and an expanded consciousness. The bodymindspirit of one who is experiencing forgiveness moves toward integration and transcendence of previous patterns and forms. Forgiveness of one's self or another has profound effects at every level of being.

Sometimes right relationship emerges at the spiritual level before it manifests itself anywhere else. In moments of deep love—such as grati-tude, or the sudden awareness that one is not alone but in fact connected to everything and everyone else in the cosmos—individuals have come into right relationship with the transcen-dent dimensions of life: God, the One, Ultimate Reality, the Ground of Being. The language is not as important as the recognition of change. Those who have this experience are more whole, more coherent, more free to become who they are most deeply meant to be, more healed.

Healing vs. Curing

Healing and curing are different processes. Curing is the elimination of the signs and symptoms of disease, which may or may not correspond to the end of the patient's disease or distress. The diagnosis and cure of disease pro-vide the focus of the modern healthcare (sick-ness–cure) system. This is not a wrong focus, only an incomplete one. When it is estimated that 85% of health problems are either self-limit-ing or chronic, it becomes clear that something in addition to a focus on the curing of diseases is required. That something is healing, which is different from curing in several key ways.

Healing may occur without curing. The per-son dying of acquired immune deficiency syn-drome (AIDS) who reconciles with his parents after a long separation is healing. The person who has become quadriplegic and uses this as an opportunity to recommit to living a life of meaning and service is healing. The mother of young children who consents to radical, inva-sive surgery for an otherwise incurable cancer is healing by aligning with her highest values and making choices based on her commitment to live for her children. The surgery may not cure her disease, but the choice to undergo the sur-gery is a healing choice. Curing is almost always focused on the person as a physical entity, a body. If the body cannot be fixed, if the physi-cal disease state or state of disability cannot be cured, then there is "nothing more we can do for you." Healing is multidimensional. It can occur at the physical level, but it can also occur at each of the other levels of the human system—emo-tion, mind, and spirit.

Curing may or may not be possible, but heal-ing is always possible. Many of the diseases of our time are, in fact, not curable, and people who are living with chronic illnesses make up a large percentage of the caseload of any primary care provider. In contrast, because healing is the emergence of right relationship at any or all lev-els of the human system, it can happen even when there is no possibility for physical cure. The potential for healing exists within every human being by the very fact that, as humans, we have a multidimensional, self-reflective nature. Indeed, for some people, the very fact that they are facing an incurable disease or sit-uation provides enough instability in the sys-tem to catalyze tremendous healing shifts,[28] an "escape to a higher order" in the language of Prigogine's model of dissipative structures.[29]

Although curing follows a usual or pre-dictable path, healing is always creative and unpredictable in both process and outcome. In textbooks on curing, the events that will be probable parts of recovery and the timeline are described, and the actual progress of the patient is measured against these referents. The mis-application of this information is increasingly apparent as patients in the modern sickness–cure system are being told exactly how many days of care they are permitted for cure to occur. The nature and the direction of a heal-ing change cannot be predicted, however. Fur-thermore, because the direction of healing is always toward self-transcendence, something new is emerging, and the whole that was before becomes a part of the new, larger (or deeper) whole. This unidirectional unfolding toward increasing complexity and diversity is also, of course, a fundamental premise of the Science of Unitary Human Beings proposed by Rogers.[30] The end point of a healing process cannot be predicted ahead of time. It can only be observed as it emerges.

Death is seen as a failure in the sickness–cure system but as a natural process in the healing system. Death is seen as the enemy, that which is to be avoided at all costs, even at the expense of the humanity and personhood of the one being treated in the sickness–cure system. The increas-ingly widespread use of "living wills"—formal, legal documents that are required to allow death without the heroic battle waged in sickness–cure institutions—provides abundant evidence of this observation. Rather than being a failure, however, death is part of the natural unfolding of the life process. All living systems eventually die. In some spiritual traditions, death itself is viewed as the ultimate healing because it releases the eternal soul from the limitations, pain, and suffering of embodiment. This, of course, is a matter of individual belief.

The Healer

> It is often thought that medicine is the curative process. It is no such thing; medicine is the surgery of functions as surgery proper is that of limbs and organs. Neither can do anything but remove obstructions; neither can cure. Nature alone cures.[31]

This same perspective applies to healing.

Healing is completely unique and creative and may not be coerced, manipulated, or controlled, even by the one healing. The nurse healer is a facilitator of this process—a sort of midwife—but is not the one doing the healing. Neither is the locus of the healing an isolated part of the patient (i.e., the mind or the spirit). All healing emerges from within the totality of the unique bodymindspirit of the patient, sometimes with the assistance of therapeutic interventions but not because of them. Therapeutics (drugs, surgery, complementary therapies) may be necessary for the patient to be cured or healed, but they are not sufficient causes. Every nurse has cared for patients who "should have" gotten better but did not, as well as patients who "should have" died but went on to live long, healthy lives.

The assumption that the patient accomplishes all healing and curing does not mean that the patient controls all healing and curing. The causes of illness and cure are so complex and multifaceted that no simple statement of cause and effect is appropriate to describe either. Nurses can participate knowledgeably in the healing process, formulating a healing intention and doing what they believe is best in the situation, but the outcome of that process remains indeterminate. At least part of the healing process will always be an unfolding mystery. Believing otherwise may contribute to a sense of failure for patients when they are unable to cure themselves of disease and for the nurses who care for them. True caring is a moral commitment to protect the vulnerability of self and other, not add to it.

A True Healing Healthcare System

As noted previously, the current healthcare system continues to focus almost exclusively on the curing process, thus making it more akin to a sickness–cure system, despite 2010 reforms, which were primarily about access to the existing system and not a fundamentally changed system. Although necessary and excellent in its own right, this system is incomplete. The use of new tools of care, including alternative, holistic, or complementary therapies, without a fundamental shift in the philosophy of care with which they are used will not transform the sickness–cure system into a true, healing healthcare system, however. This error of confusing the tools of care with the philosophy of care may lead to serious consequences for both healthcare practitioners and their patients.

The fundamental orientation of a holistic practitioner is toward an appreciation of and attention to the wholeness and uniqueness of every person. Holistic nurses remember that, in effect, there is nothing that is not holistic. There is no intervention that does not affect the whole bodymindspirit of the patient because the bodymindspirit is integral and cannot be divided. There are natural and nonnatural modalities, for example, but both affect the whole bodymindspirit. There are invasive and noninvasive interventions, but both affect the whole bodymindspirit. There are interventions that start in the body (e.g., medications, surgery, exercise, movement therapy), the mind (e.g., autogenic training, hypnotherapy, guided imagery), or the spirit (e.g., meditation, prayer, gratitude practice, loving kindness). None of these interventions is inherently more holistic than the other, however, because all roads lead to the bodymindspirit; all interventions affect the whole.

For this reason, simply adding new tools of care will not transform the sickness–cure system. The way in which practitioners use the tools available, whether the tools are conventional or complementary, and their willingness to become a midwife to nature rather than the hero of success stories, make the care holistic or integrative. The true healthcare system will emerge when both curing and healing processes are equally valued, sought after, and facilitated for all, and when the full range of curing, caring, and healing modalities is available to all. Holistic nurses have a key role to play in facilitating this level of change in the existing systems and in revisioning/recreating hospitals and clinics, wellness centers, and hospices as "Habitats for Healing," optimal healing environments in which nurses thrive and patients heal. Habitats for Healing are characterized by autonomy of the nursing staff; a holistic, caring/healing/relationship-centered framework that guides practice; and the integration of complementary and alternative healing modalities into regular nursing care.[1]

Integration of the Masculine and the Feminine

The Western sickness–cure system is characterized almost exclusively by attributes usually ascribed to the masculine principle and usually carried by men. This is a natural consequence of the fact that men have been the principal creators of that system and continue to be the dominant culture of the system. These attributes are extremely useful in the treatment of acute injury and disease, but without the attributes usually ascribed to the feminine principle, they provide an incomplete foundation for a true, integrative healing healthcare system.

Exhibit 4-1 suggests another perspective on these different attributes. A perspective that sees the goal as "getting the job done" can be associated with the sickness–cure model, while one that focuses on "holding sacred space" can facilitate healing of the whole bodymindspirit.[32, p. 33]

EXHIBIT 4-1	Ways of Being with People Seeking Help

"Getting the Job Done"

Authority vested in the external "expert"

Source of healing: what the expert provides

Gathering, collecting, taking in information

Problem solving/fixing

Making "something" happen, where "something" is:

- Defined by the external "expert"
- Defined ahead of time
- Meeting the goal

Directing/taking over to make it happen

Doing to or for

Leading

Power over

Expert is accountable and responsible for outcome

Failure is the nonachievement of predetermined outcome

"Holding Sacred Space"

Authority vested in the individual client(s)

Source of healing: the bodymindspirit of the client(s)

Receiving information

Life unfolding/facilitating

Allowing "something" to happen, where "something" is:

- Defined mutually
- Defined in the moment
- Emergence of mystery

Guiding/helping to allow it to happen

Being with

Walking with

Power with

Facilitator is accountable and responsible for competent practice

Failure is giving up on the unfolding process

Nurse as Healing Environment

One of the most powerful tools for healing is the presence of the nurse in the patient's environment. In fact, the nurse has the greatest effect of all the elements in the patient's environment. Simply by virtue of the role, a nurse has all the ritual power of the shaman of other cultures. The nurse is guardian of the patient's journey through illness and healing; the keeper and bestower of information, medicines, and treatments; and the mediator of the system and the comings and goings of others in the system.

In recent years there has been a rapidly growing increase in research about the placebo effect, called the "haelan effect" earlier in this chapter, particularly as it relates to the therapeutic relationship. In reviewing more than 200 papers published between 1995 and 2013, Jubb and Bensing suggest that "it is the quality of the patient–practitioner interaction that accounts for a sizeable chunk of the effect seen in placebo responses."[33, p. 2712] Aspects of holistic nursing, such as delivering therapies in a warm and caring way; incorporating reassurance, relaxation, suggestion, and anxiety reduction; listening; providing empathy and understanding; and touching the patient have all been identified as having the potential to elicit patients' innate healing capabilities and thus enhance the effects of all therapies.[34]

In a model of the universe that includes the nonlocal nature of consciousness[35, 36] or the possibility for the existence of a human energy field that extends beyond the skin,[37] the nurse is not simply part of the patient's environment, but rather the nurse is the patient's environment.[32]

The healing environment of the patient may be optimized when the nurse intentionally shifts consciousness into a centered or meditative state. The interconnectedness of the energy fields of the nurse and the patient can facilitate relaxation, rest, or healing in the patient. When a nurse is centered in the present moment and has the intention to be a healing environment, he or she may carry this intention in the energy field and manifest it in the voice, the eyes, and the quality of touching. Nurses should ask themselves:

- Do patients hear in my voice that I care? That I have time for them? That they are safe with me?
- What is the quality of my facial expression? Of my eyes? Do they communicate care and compassion, or are they perfunctory and distant? Does the patient feel seen by me, or overlooked? If the eyes are the windows to the soul, what is my soul saying to the soul of my patient? What is the patient's soul saying?
- Am I focused on the task at hand and simply touching the patient to get the job done? Or does my touch convey care, support, nurture, and competence? Does my touch communicate that I know I am touching this person's spirit as I contact his or her skin, because where else is the spirit located but in the body? Do I speak of love and kindness and respect through my hands?

Learning how to shift consciousness into a healing state is a basic skill for the holistic nurse. Nurses are not simply separate selves "doing to" the patient but an integral part of the patient's environment, "being with" them on the healing journey. The quality of the energy with which the patient is interacting is part of what nurses attend to, and this means attending to their own state of consciousness and well-being before, during, and after their interactions with patients. Thus, taking time for themselves to learn and practice relaxation, meditation, centering, or other self-care strategies becomes essential in this model and serves both nurses and patients.[7, 38-44] Nurses are not being selfish by taking this time. They are recognizing that unless they are energized, relaxed, and centered, they will be trying to give what they do not have to give. This results in less than optimal care for the patients and burnout for the nurses.

Conclusion

Transpersonal human caring provides the context for holistic nurses to facilitate healing—the emergence of right relationship—in patients and clients. Through the use of centering and intentionality, the holistic nurse may become a healing environment and participate in the creation of a true, healing healthcare system that integrates both masculine and feminine attributes. "Holding sacred space" for healing is an additional skill of the holistic nurse. This skill does not replace "getting the job (of curing) done," but it enhances it.

Directions for Future Research

1. Collect personal stories and narratives that provide exemplars of "caring occasions."
2. Conduct interviews with patients who see themselves as healing, even in the absence of curing, to search for patterns that may facilitate this shift for other patients.
3. Explore the relationship between job satisfaction in nurses and the practice of centering and holding sacred space.
4. Explore the effects of caring, healing relationships on both nurses and patients.[45]

Nurse Healer Reflections

After reading this chapter, the holistic nurse will be able to answer or to begin a process of answering the following questions:

- How do I feel when I am engaged in a "caring occasion"?
- How do I know when healing is happening in my patients? In myself?
- Which small changes could I make in my practice to begin to transform my work environment into a Habitat for Healing?

NOTES

1. J. F. Quinn, "Habitats for Healing: Healthy Environments for Health Care's Endangered Species," *Beginnings* 30, no. 2 (2010): 10–11.
2. J. F. Quinn, "The Integrated Nurse: Way of the Healer," in *Integrative Nursing*, M. J. Kreitzer and M. Koithan (New York: Oxford University Press, 2014): 34.
3. J. Watson, *Nursing: Human Science and Human Care* (New York: National League for Nursing Press, 1988): 54.
4. H. Covington, "Caring Presence: Delineation of a Concept for Holistic Nursing," *Journal of Holistic Nursing* 21, no. 3 (2003): 301–317.
5. W. R. Cowling and D. Taliaferro, "Emergence of a Caring-Healing Perspective: Contemporary Conceptual and Theoretical Directions," *Journal of Theory Construction and Testing* 8, no. 2 (2004): 54–59.
6. P. Pearcey, "'Caring? It's the little things we are not supposed to do anymore,'" *International Journal of Nursing Practice* 16, no. 1 (2010): 51–56.
7. A. Ranheim and K. Dahlberg, "Expanded Awareness as a Way to Meet the Challenges in Care That Is Economically Driven and Focused on Illness—A Nordic Perspective," *Aporia* 4, no. 4 (2012): 20–24.
8. A. Ranheim, A. Kärner, and C. Berterö, "Caring Theory and Practice—Entering a Simultaneous Concept Analysis," *Nursing Forum* 47, no. 2 (2012): 78–90.
9. J. Morse, S. Solbert, W. Neander, J. Bottorff, and J. Johnson, "Concepts of Caring and Caring as a Concept," *Advances in Nursing Science* 13, no. 1 (1990): 1–14.
10. J. Watson, *Caring Science as Sacred Science* (Philadelphia: F. A. Davis, 2005).
11. J. Watson, *Human Caring Science: A Theory of Nursing*, 2nd ed. (Burlington, MA: Jones & Bartlett Learning, 2012).
12. K. Sitzman and J. Watson, eds., *Caring Science, Mindful Practice: Implementing Watson's Human Caring Theory* (New York: Springer, 2014).
13. Watson Caring Science Institute, "Caring Science Theory and Research" (2014). http://watsoncaringscience.org/about-us/caring-science-definitions-processes-theory/.
14. D. Bohm, response to a question raised at the International Transpersonal Association meeting, Prague, Czechoslovakia, 1992.
15. D. J. Siegel, *Pocket Guide to Interpersonal Neurobiology* (New York: Norton, 2012).
16. M. Koithan, I. R. Bell, K. Niemeyer, and D. Pincus, "A Complex Systems Perspective for Whole Systems of CAM Research," *Forsch Komplementmed* 19, Suppl 1 (2012): 7–14.
17. L. Skyttner, *General Systems Theory* (River Edge, NJ: World Scientific, 2002).
18. E. Morin, *On Complexity: Advances in Systems Theory, Complexity, and the Human Sciences* (New York: Hampton Press, 2008).
19. C. Lindberg, S. Nash, and C. Lindberg, *On the Edge: Nursing in the Age of Complexity* (Bordentown, NJ: Plexus Press, 2008).
20. A. W. Davidson, M. A. Ray, and M. C. Turkel, *Nursing, Caring and Complexity Science* (New York: Springer, 2011).
21. K. Wilber, *Sex, Ecology and Spirituality: The Spirit of Evolution* (Boston: Shambhala, 1996).
22. K. Wilber, *The Marriage of Sense and Soul* (New York: Random House, 1998): 67.
23. F. Capra, *The Web of Life* (New York: Anchor Books, 1996).

24. E. Laszlo, *Evolution: The Grand Synthesis* (Boston: Shambhala, 1987): 36.

25. L. M. Holden, "Complex Adaptive Systems: Concept Analysis," *Journal of Advanced Nursing* 52, no. 6 (2005): 651–657.

26. J. F. Quinn, "On Healing, Wholeness and the Haelan Effect," *Nursing and Healthcare* 10, no. 10 (1989): 552–556.

27. D. McElligott, "Healing: The Journey from Concept to Nursing Practice," *Journal of Holistic Nursing* 28, no. 4 (2010): 251–259.

28. D. Zucker, "An Inquiry into Integral Medicine," *Journal of Integral Theory and Practice* 6, no. 4 (2011): 131–136.

29. I. Prigogine, *Order Out of Chaos* (New York: Bantam Books, 1984).

30. M. E. Rogers, "The Science of Unitary Human Beings: Current Perspectives," *Nursing Science Quarterly* 7, no. 1 (1994): 33–35.

31. F. Nightingale, *Notes on Nursing: What It Is and What It Is Not* (New York: Dover, 1969): 133.

32. J. Quinn, "Holding Sacred Space: The Nurse as Healing Environment," *Holistic Nursing Practice* 6, no. 4 (1992): 26–36.

33. J. Jubb and J. M. Bensing, "The Sweetest Pill to Swallow: How Patient Neurobiology Can Be Harnessed to Maximise Placebo Effects," *Neuroscience Biobehavioral Review* 37, no. 10 Pt 2 (2013): 2709–2720.

34. H. Walach and W. Jonas, "Placebo Research: The Evidence Base for Harnessing Self-Healing Capacities," *Journal of Alternative and Complementary Medicine* 10, Suppl 1 (2004): S-103–S-112.

35. L. Dossey, *Healing Words* (San Francisco: Harper San Francisco, 1993): 43.

36. P. van Lommel, "Non-Local Consciousness: A Concept Based on Scientific Research on Near-Death Experiences During Cardiac Arrest," *Journal of Consciousness Studies* 20, nos. 1–2 (2013): 7–48.

37. M. Rogers, "Nursing: Science of Unitary, Irreducible, Human Beings: Update 1990," in *Visions of Rogers' Science-Based Nursing*, ed. E. A. M. Barrett (New York: National League for Nursing, 1990).

38. C. Fearon and M. Nicol, "Strategies to Assist Prevention of Burnout in Nursing Staff," *Nursing Standard* 26, no. 14 (2011): 35–38.

39. S. A. Senzon, "Five Keys to Real Transformation in Health Care," *Journal of Alternative and Complementary Medicine* 17, no. 11 (2011): 1085–1089.

40. Oncology Nursing Society, "Manage Anxiety and Depression in Patients and Nurses," *ONS Connect* (May 2011): 16S.

41. S. Letvak, C. J. Ruhm, and T. McCoy, "Depression in Hospital-Employed Nurses," *Clinical Nurse Specialist* 26, no. 3 (2012): 177–182.

42. S. Letvak, C. J. Ruhm, and S. N. Gupta, "Nurses' Presenteeism and Its Effects on Self-Reported Quality of Care and Costs," *American Journal of Nursing* 112, no. 2 (2012): 30–38.

43. J. Muhammad, "Promoting the Healthy Nurse: Diagnosis and Plan for Self-Care," *Nevada RNformation* (May 2012): 4.

44. J. Maben, R. Peccei, M. Adams, G. Roberts, A. Richardson, T. Murrells, and E. Morrow, *Exploring the Relationship Between Patients' Experiences of Care and the Influence of Staff Motivation, Affect and Wellbeing. Final Report* (Southampton, England: National Institute for Health Research Service Delivery and Organisation Programme, 2012).

45. J. F. Quinn, M. Smith, C. Ritenbaugh, K. Swanson, and M. J. Watson, "Research Guidelines for Assessing the Impact of the Healing Relationship in Nursing," *Alternative Therapies in Health and Medicine* 9, no. 3 Suppl (2003): A65–A79.

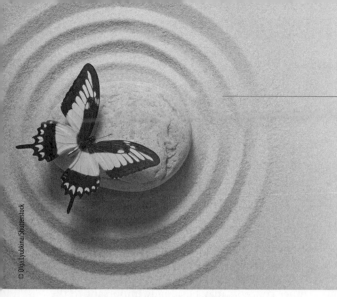

CHAPTER 5

Nursing Theory in Holistic Nursing Practice

Noreen Cavan Frisch and Pamela Potter

Nurse Healer Objectives

Theoretical

- Understand the current use and nonuse of nursing theory in the discipline.
- Describe the elements of holistic nursing and explain why the use of theory is one of the elements.
- Familiarize oneself with the following established nursing theories: Nightingale's Theory of Environmental Adaptation; Erickson, Tomlin, and Swain's Modeling and Role-Modeling Theory; Watson's Theory of Transpersonal Caring; Rogers's Science of Unitary Human Beings; Newman's Theory of Health as Expanding Consciousness; and Parse's Theory of Human Becoming.
- Identify the use of midrange theories as supportive of holistic nursing practice, particularly Kolcaba's Theory of Comfort.
- Identify how nonnursing theoretical perspectives, Complexity Theory, and Integral Theory can support holistic nursing thinking.
- Appreciate the Theory of Integral Nursing as a consequence of nursing's examination and exploration of new ideas.

Clinical

- Apply the nursing theories and a theoretical perspective in the clinical setting.

- Determine how theory can influence nursing care and the evaluation of that care.

Personal

- Select a nursing theory or theories that provide a framework and philosophy consistent with your own view.
- Use the theory or theories and evaluate their effect on your personal worldview.

Definitions

Concept: An abstract idea or notion.

Conceptual model: A group of interrelated concepts described to suggest relationships among them.

Framework: A basic structure; the context in which theory is developed; the structure that permits theory to be understood.

Grand theory: A theory that covers a broad area of the discipline's concerns.

Metaparadigm: Concepts that identify the domain of a discipline.

Metatheory: Theory about theory development; theory about theory.

Midrange theory: A focused theory for nursing that deals with a portion of nurses' concerns or that is oriented to patient outcomes.

Model: A representation of interactions between and among concepts.

Nursing theory: A framework; a set of interrelated concepts that are testable; a way of seeing the factors that contribute to nursing practice and nursing thought.

Worldview: A perspective; a way of viewing, perceiving, and interpreting one's experience.

Nursing Theory: Background and Current Challenges

By definition and by history, nursing is a holistic practice. Nursing's work is concerned with the restoration and promotion of health, the prevention of disease, and the supports necessary to help the client gain a subjective sense of peace and harmony. As a profession, nursing has never focused solely on the physical body or the disease entity. Rather, taking into account the holistic nature of all persons, nursing is concerned with clients' experiences of their conditions. In addition, nurses attend to the environmental influences that promote recovery as well as the social and spiritual supports that promote a sense of well-being for clients. Nurses have found that nursing theories help to articulate the nature of nursing practice and guide nursing interventions to meet client needs.

Nursing Theory Defined

A nursing theory is a framework from which professional nurses can think about their work. Theory is a means of interpreting one's observations of the world and is an abstraction of reality. For example, most nurses have studied developmental theory, which provides a framework for viewing the childhood behaviors expected with various ages and phases of child growth. Consequently, when nurses observe a toddler crying when his mother must leave him alone with nurses in the hospital, nurses interpret the child's crying as separation anxiety, an expected and predicted toddler behavior according to developmental theory. The theory provides a means of understanding behavior that otherwise might seem random and, therefore, is a framework from which to understand the child's actions. Thus, "a theory suggests a direction in how to view facts and events."[1, p. 4]

In the past, four basic ideas (or concepts) were common to all nursing theories—the concepts of nursing, person, health, and environment. These concepts were thought to compose the core content of the discipline—the "metaparadigm" of nursing. As the discipline has matured, authors in the 1990s and 2000s suggested that the four concepts were too restrictive for development of nursing knowledge,[2] and some recommended additions to the four. Full discussion of this debate is outside the scope of this chapter; however, it is important to recognize the belief that other concepts may be equally important to the core of nursing.[3] For example, concepts such as caring, healing, energy fields, development, adaptation, consciousness, or nurse–client relationships may be as important to describing and understanding nursing as the concept of health.

Challenges to the Use of Nursing Theory

Currently, however, there are three developments in nursing that consign nursing theories to a tenuous or vulnerable place. These are (1) omission or lack of emphasis of nursing theory in many nursing curricula, accompanied by a view from some that theory is obsolete; (2) a move toward interdisciplinary and interprofessional practice; and (3) the attention given to quality, safety, and nursing outcomes that has focused more on the "doing" of nursing than the reflection on practice that theory demands. Each of these will be discussed.

Omission of Nursing Theory from Curricula

In 21st-century practice, the use of nursing theories has very likely declined. A group of nursing educators has raised concerns that nursing theory is no longer taught in many programs and that other content required in curricula (quality, safety, evidence-based practice, research methodologies, and interdisciplinary collaborations) may be taking precedence over nursing theory.[4] These authors provide a sound rationale for maintaining nursing theory: that an understanding and ability to reflect on the discipline is essential for the development of nursing scholars, that knowledge of one's own disciplinary approach is a prerequisite for interdisciplinary practice, and that theory assists professionals to learn that there are many ways of developing new knowledge for nursing and of understanding evidence. Nonetheless, omission or lack of emphasis on nursing theory should give pause to holistic nurses everywhere as there has not been a full consideration of what might be lost in the process.

Nursing and Interdisciplinary Practice

The move in all health care toward truly interprofessional practice leaves those who ascribe to nursing theory without a core group of team members who even understand the use and meaning of theory-based practice. Nursing has been alone in the health professions in regard to its theory development. Nurses have identified (through the writings of theorists such as Jean Watson) that professional practice *is* reflective practice. Other health professionals have simply not had that perspective and do not have a history of identifying philosophical underpinnings and theoretical frameworks for their healthcare practice. This development leaves many nurses in positions where they could be the lone nurse member of a healthcare team with the ability to express theory-to-practice applications. In addition, many nurses may be working in a health system where their immediate supervisor is a nonnurse health professional, creating predictable communication challenges.

Theory in an Era of Safety, Quality, and Evidence

With the publication of the Institute of Medicine's *To Err Is Human*[5] and *Health Professions Education*,[6] the entire healthcare system in the United States and beyond has appropriately given priority attention to ensuring safe practice, providing control over errors, confirming quality assurance (as defined by enacting clinical practice guidelines based on best evidence and/or professional consensus), and reducing regional variation on practices known to be effective. While there is nothing in this movement that prohibits the use of nursing theory, use of theory is not the priority of this focus. It would seem that theory that addressed interprofessional communication (as a contributing factor to errors), and theory that addressed health professional–patient interactions, might gain more purchase than theory perceived to be one held by nurses only. Nonetheless, the very important focus on quality, safety, prevention of complications, and movement toward care outcomes has trumped any use of theory or reflection, now viewed as of lesser importance.

Is There Still a Need for Theory?

Nurses committed to holism are kind and compassionate nurses who share a philosophy that emphasizes a balance between self-care and the ability to care for patients using the interconnectedness of body, mind, and spirit. Theory suggests—in fact, demands—that nurses reflect on philosophy and consider how their practice is working (or not working) to achieve holistic ideals. Reed and Rolfe write that use of theory requires reflection and is a precondition for professional practice: Theory is understood as "a purposeful form of abstract thinking essential to a discipline and, by definition, a characteristic of the professional nurse."[7 p. 120]

The description of holistic nursing developed by the American Holistic Nurses Association states, "Holistic nursing practice draws on knowledge, theories, expertise, intuition, and creativity."[8] All five elements are necessary for the nurse to function in an ideal way: Nursing knowledge is essential for the understanding of health and disease states and the various regimens required to achieve health. Theories enable one to reflect on practice and to consider carefully all alternatives of care. Expertise is necessary to perform nursing skills and for the ability to make accurate assessments and decisions about care. Intuition is needed to understand the client and to appreciate the subjective experiences of others. Creativity is helpful in solving care problems that seem insurmountable; it provides the nurse with novel ideas and ways of being with clients. Each one of these elements is as important as the others. Knowledge and theory are cognitive tools that help the nurse understand and reflect on practice. Expertise is an experiential tool that comes from practice and a significant number of encounters in nurse–client situations. Intuition and creativity are affective tools that lead the nurse to feel, experience, and follow inner guidance when working with clients.

Professional practice requires that nurses use these five elements to achieve the best possible results. A holistic nurse can move back and forth between intuitive knowing and logical reasoning, between a creative approach to care and a standard care protocol, and between a hunch of what to do and a considered direction grounded in the predictions of a theory. All of the elements of practice come only by learning how to use them. **Table 5-1** presents a summary of the five elements of holistic nursing practice.

Once a nurse adapts a holistic way of thinking, embraces the complexities of the lived experiences of clients, and accepts ways of knowing that include aesthetics, personal and ethical knowledge, and empirical knowledge, that nurse needs a means of assembling the ideas, concepts, thoughts, and feelings that originate from practice in a way that is coherent and personally meaningful. It is through use of theory that the nurse can accomplish this. Theory provides the nurse with a framework from which to understand and make meaning out of complex experiences. Theory also provides guidance in practice—guidance to consider alternate explanations for what is observed and alternate ways of addressing concerns. At a time of emphasis on evidence, quality, safety, and outcomes, theory could not be more important to address the parts of practice—comfort, sense of security, creation, and maintenance of a supportive external environment for the patient—that most influence care outcomes. Further, a nurse who is a lone member of an interdisciplinary team might well benefit from communication theories and leadership theories that help in establishing the perception that nursing knowledge is a valuable contributor to the patient and family experience and care outcome. For the holistic nurse today, ignoring theory is as unacceptable as ignoring evidence.

Theory Development

Theories develop over time as a theorist defines concepts, suggests relationships between concepts, tests and evaluates the relationships, and modifies the theory based on research findings. When the theorist provides definitions of the concepts and suggests possible relationships, the work is called a *conceptual model*. Some writers find the distinction between a theory and a conceptual model irrelevant.[7] It is important, however, for nurses to understand that theories develop and mature and that they pass through the following stages, each serving increasingly complex purposes:

1. *Description.* The theory provides definitions of concepts, suggests a way of looking at the world, and provides a framework for describing the phenomena of nursing.
2. *Explanation.* The theory suggests relationships between and among various concepts and gives the nurse a means of explaining observed events.
3. *Prediction.* The theory has research findings that establish clear relationships between aspects of nursing, and the nurse is able to predict outcomes.

TABLE 5-1	Five Elements of Holistic Nursing Practice	
Element	**Domain**	**Use in Practice**
Knowledge	Cognitive	Understanding health and disease states; interpreting regimens of care
Theory	Cognitive	Reflection; considered judgments
Expertise	Experiential	Skilled performance
Intuition	Affective	Subjective knowing
Creativity	Affective	Spontaneity; solving problems or challenges

4. *Prescription.* The theory is well developed and permits a nurse to prescribe nurse or client actions with confidence in the outcomes.

Most nursing theories are developed to the stage of description and explanation, and theorists and researchers are currently developing nursing theories to the stages of prediction and prescription. Concepts and relationships of a theory can be evaluated and tested through research. For example, if a theory states that a person is a human energy field and suggests that there is an exchange of energy between two persons, research can be designed to evaluate such an exchange. For a theory to reach the stages of prediction and prescription, a considerable body of research is needed.

Theories are divided into two main categories: grand theories, which are broad in scope and apply to all of nursing, and midrange theories, which apply to specific specialty areas or particular aspects of care. Most of the theories that are presented as nursing theories are grand theories (Watson's Theory of Transpersonal Caring, Parse's Theory of Human Becoming, or Erickson, Tomlin, and Swain's Modeling and Role-Modeling Theory). Examples of midrange theories include theories of comfort, maternal-role attainment, self-transcendence, and the synergy model for critical care.

A recent nursing textbook presents 16 theories for professional nursing practice. Adding some of the midrange theories could easily provide a list of nearly 30 theories. Full description of these theories is beyond the scope of this chapter; however, **Table 5-2** presents a summary of the theories used most frequently in holistic nursing practice.

Interdisciplinary Theories of Interest to Nursing

Today, there are two wide-reaching interdisciplinary theories that have proven useful in thinking about the changing modern environment where a nurse can feel lost in the middle of fast-paced action, uninterpretable observations, and situations of great human need. These two theories are Complex Adaptive Systems Theory (or simply Complexity Science) and Ken Wilber's Integral Theory. These theories present important ideas and concepts that are being brought into nursing thought and have already made contributions to nursing theory development. These theories may provide holistic nurses with a framework to articulate care needs and processes to other members of the healthcare team, as these theories may have more acceptance in team interactions than something perceived as "nursing." In addition, both of these theories permit a nurse to enter dialogue and thinking with other health team members about theory in general and may be an entrée to discussing nursing-specific theoretical perspectives that affect the care situations at hand. For these reasons, each is discussed briefly.

Complexity Science is defined as the study of complex adaptive systems.[10] This is a science that addresses diverse or multifaceted elements that are able to change, react, and adapt and that are interconnected in some way. As in Systems Theory, the elements studied from this theory adapt independently and affect the whole. However, Complexity Science focuses on systems that have a "densely connected web of interacting agents, each operating from its own schema,"[11, p. 255] addressing structures that are self-organized, unpredictable, and ever changing. This theory is useful when working within a structure that faces challenges of uncertainty, the need to act, the lack of a predictable outcome, and a level of complexity in which even complicated techniques such as model building and forecasting are inadequate to take into account all contingencies. Modern healthcare organizations are a perfect example of the type of system requiring a new way of thinking. Complexity Science suggests that, when organizations face uncertainty, managers can best operate by distributing (rather than centralizing) control and supporting individual parts (or people) of the organization who are trying to develop solutions.

Complexity Science postulates that, in an uncertain environment, freedom to innovate, coupled with qualities of intelligence and resourcefulness, will produce best outcomes. Astin and Forys suggest that following the

TABLE 5-2   Summary of Selected Nursing Theories Used in Holistic Nursing Practice

Theory	Theorist	Date of First Publication	Major Concepts or Ideas	Current Uses
Theory of Environmental Adaptation	Florence Nightingale Louise Selanders	1860 1998[9]	Providing external supports for healing to take place. Emphasizing the health properties of the environment (cleanliness, fresh air, light, warmth, and order). Compelling nurses to care for nutritional needs and emotional comfort.	Healthcare facility design. Nurse's control of external environment to support health and prevent complications.
Modeling and Role-Modeling	Helen Erickson Evelyn Tomlin Mary Ann Swain	1983	Adaptation (striving for equilibrium) and assessment of Adaptive Potential. Five aims of intervention: build trust, promote positive orientation, promote perceived control, promote strengths, and set mutual health-directed goals. Modeling the client's world (building a model of the world from the client's perspective). Role-modeling healthy behaviors from within the client's worldview.	Used in all practice areas and settings. Particularly useful in environments where the expectation is that the client will be in charge of his or her own health decisions.
Theory of Transpersonal Caring and Caring Science	Jean Watson	1979	Caring relationships between nurse and client. Multiple truths, physical and nonphysical realities, relativity of time and space. Caring ethic as foundational to all health care. Postmodern organization of healthcare settings.	Used in all practice settings. Helpful in the evaluation of caring as a measure of professional nursing.
Science of Unitary Human Beings	Martha Rogers	1970	Unitary Human Beings. Human energy field/environmental energy field. Evolution of people in a way that is irreversible and unidirectional.	Used in all practice settings. Provides a framework and explanation of energy-based modalities.

TABLE 5-2   Summary of Selected Nursing Theories Used in Holistic Nursing Practice (*continued*)

Theory	Theorist	Date of First Publication	Major Concepts or Ideas	Current Uses
Theory of Health as Expanding Consciousness	Margaret Newman	1994	Health is expanding consciousness that includes an individual's total pattern. Nursing is caring—a moral imperative. People are open systems. Health–illness as a unitary process. Research is praxis.	Used in all practice settings. Work within this theory focuses on the meaning and purpose of living with illness.
Theory of Human Becoming	Rosemarie Rizzo Parse	1981	A person is a unitary whole. Nurses guide clients to make choices concerning health. Nurses offer authentic presence. Health is a process of becoming, a personal commitment, and a process related to lived experiences.	Used in all practice settings. Work within this theory focuses on intersubjective dialogue and the client's lived experiences. Nurse and client co-create reality.
Theory of Comfort	Katherine Kolcaba	1991	Comfort as a holistic phenomenon. Comfort reflects holistic well-being. Comfort is described as feelings of relief, ease, and transcendence.	A midrange theory applied to many practice settings. Comfort measures are assessed by the client as being in a state of comfort or having been comforted.

principles of Complexity Science permits order and creativity to emerge.[12] Complexity Science is undoubtedly useful to healthcare leaders and administrators and is perhaps especially helpful to holistic nurse managers who may already recognize the requirement to give over the control of actions and outcomes. Geary and Schumacher provide an example of pairing complexity theory with transition theory in the practice of discharging patients from hospital to home.[13] These authors suggest that complexity theory gives nurses new tools to account for the unpredictable nature of the patient discharge situation and the multiple interacting agents that come into play simultaneously. Kramer and colleagues illustrated how newly licensed registered nurses enter practice thinking that that their actions result in more predictable outcomes than is realistic.[14] These authors report that expanding nurses' thinking to encompass complexity provides room for innovation and creates a more supportive environment in which to work. The essence of applying Complexity Science is the ability to trust the process and the people to make the right choices and decisions and to be accountable for their actions.

James speaks to all holistic nurses when she suggests that nurses can and should lead healthcare systems at the system level and become "healers of a very fragmented and siloed health care system."[15, p. 137] She goes on to advise that "A machine can be fixed with a replacement part, while an organic system must be cared for as a whole."[15, p. 139] Complexity Science draws nurses to a systems level and a leadership role within the healthcare system. This may well be a first step in nurses' ability to influence the establishment of theoretic perspectives focusing on individual patient care as well.

Integral Theory draws on ideas, concepts, and theories from many traditions to integrate views that interpret world and life experiences from seemingly irreconcilable differences.[16] Essentially, this theory divides "all that is" into four quadrants—the four corners of the universe—each quadrant representing a domain, a view of reality, or a dimension of "what is." The quadrants are the interior dimensions of individuals (feelings, meanings, beliefs), the interior dimensions of the collective (cultural beliefs, shared worldviews), the exteriors of individuals (the body, its organs and tissues, behaviors), and the exteriors of the collective (social structures). Wilber embraces the notion that the domains of each quadrant represent four true realities, each that can be understood through differing methods of study, sources of data, and worldviews. Thus, to understand human experience, one must understand all four dimensions. His theory can be easily applied to holistic health because it addresses the need for a comprehensive approach to treating illness and providing care to people.[16] Integral approaches treat the illness, the person, and the healthcare provider—going beyond the mind–body perspective and taking a panoramic look at all modes of inquiry. This theory can be considered a metatheory (and is so considered by Wilber and his followers) because it is so encompassing it can incorporate the perspectives of many of our existing nursing theories and other psychological theories into a framework of the quadrants, identifying how each contributes to a panoramic whole.[17]

In addition, Integral Theory examines a "chain of pathologies" that causes illness rather than attempting to identify a singular cause. Holistic nurses understand the need for multiple modes of inquiry and multiple realities. Wilber's theory provides a scholarly framework from which to embrace new understandings of nursing's work. Clark has used the theory in her teaching and explains that this model has helped students to care deeply for patients and to experience nursing's art as transformative.[18] In using the integral model as a framework to view the complexities of the healthcare system in which we work, one observes that the current system is dominated by thinking in the physical and social domains and requires attention in the individual and collective internal domains. The integral model calls for a more comprehensive understanding of the health–illness, caring, healing, mind-emotion-body, and individual-cultural group relationships than are accounted for in daily practices. Because holistic nurses are at the forefront of much of the scholarship related to the internal domains, the integral model applied to nursing practice and published in the literature provides a call for translating nursing knowledge beyond the profession of nursing.[19] See Chapter 8 for a description of the use of Wilber's four quadrants as a way to understand the enactment of the holistic caring process. Other writings provide examples of application of Integral Theory to an individual case study of a surgical patient.[20]

Theory of Integral Nursing

In 2008, Barbara Dossey first presented her work on the development of a grand theory of nursing that would incorporate Wilber's theory, particularly the use of the quadrants in understanding the dimensions of how we perceive the world, coupled with Carper's theory of how we come to know what we know.[21] Dossey's Theory of Integral Nursing (TIN) is meant to address very broad areas of the discipline's concerns. The TIN has shifted the paradigm in nursing to expand our notions of whom and what we are. The reader is referred to the discussion in this text of integral and holistic nursing, from local to global, for a description of the TIN theory and its application to nursing (see Chapter 1). Dossey's work is a creative blending of worldviews that include how we define, know, experience, and react to our realities and how our new understandings of our realities can influence ourselves and our work. She provides a framework for application of integral principles with practice domains of direct care, education, and research. As scholars and practitioners take up this theory, there will be more learnings as a consequence of Dossey's expansion of our notions of nursing. Specific concepts within our nursing worldviews will be challenged; for example, Wilber's work includes concepts of human development in stages of growth that have been rejected by unitary nursing scholars who adhere to an evolutionary model of human change. Other issues will undoubtedly arise as nursing scholarship proceeds. The TIN provides an exciting opportunity to move nursing's work and holistic nursing in entirely new directions that we do not yet fully understand.

Conclusion

A theory provides a means of interpreting and organizing information. Nursing theories give nurses the tools to ensure that nursing assessments are comprehensive and systematic and that care is meaningful. While some nurses do not use a theory at all, holistic nurses will use theories to provide a base for that "reflective" and "cognitive" part of practice that is so important in holism. Because there are several theories, each nurse must decide which theory to use and when to use an alternative perspective. In selecting a theory, a nurse should ask two questions: What theory is most comfortable for me? What theory is most comfortable for my client? The perspective selected must be comfortable for both. Many clients, as well as nurses, have strong feelings and opinions about what nursing is and the type of care they wish to receive. If the theory's perspective is not comfortable for the client, the nurse is ethically obligated to change her or his perspective and adopt a framework that is compatible with the client's needs.

Lastly, holistic nurses ought to give careful consideration to theories of practice, such as Complexity Science and Integral Theory, that take our thinking to a systems level or a higher

level of abstraction than existent nursing theories. These two perspectives are being used in healthcare practice and not only provide the holistic nurse with tools for leadership and innovation but may well establish enough interest in theory in general for nurses to bring other nursing theories into practice as well.

Directions for Future Research

1. Holistic nurses should consider what is and is not known about any theory being applied to practice and evaluate the next steps needed to develop the theory in their own area of practice.
2. Evaluate theories related to the identification of specific outcomes of care.

Nurse Healer Reflections

After reading this chapter, the holistic nurse will be able to answer or to begin a process of answering the following questions:

- Which of the nursing theories can I use in my practice?
- How will I determine if the theory I am using is acceptable to my clients?
- In what ways am I able and willing to become a nursing leader, using my background to "heal" the system?
- What is my personal plan for studying new theories and learning to apply them to my professional work?

NOTES

1. J. S. Hickman, "An Introduction to Nursing Theory," in *Nursing Theories: A Base for Professional Practice*, 6th ed., ed. J. George (Upper Saddle River, NJ: Prentice Hall, 2011): 1–22.
2. V. M. Malinski, "Notes on Book Review of Analysis and Evaluation of Nursing Theories: Response," *Nursing Science Quarterly* 8 (1995): 59.
3. M. E. Parker, *Nursing Theories and Nursing Practice*, 2nd ed. (Philadelphia: F. A. Davis, 2006).
4. P. Donnahue-Porter, M. O. Forbes, and J. H. White, "Nursing Theory in Curricula Today: Challenges for Faculty at All Levels of

Education," *International Journal of Nursing Education Scholarship* 8, no. 1 (2011): article 14. doi:10.2202/1548-923X.2225.

5. Institute of Medicine, *To Err Is Human: Building a Safer Health System* (Washington, DC: National Academies Press, 2000).

6. Institute of Medicine, *Health Professions Education: A Bridge to Quality* (Washington, DC: National Academies Press, 2003).

7. P. G. Reed and G. Rolfe, Nursing Knowledge and Nurses' Knowledge: A Reply to Mitchell and Bournes. *Nursing Science Quarterly*, 19 (2006): 120–123.

8. American Holistic Nurses Association and American Nurses Association, *Holistic Nursing Practice: Scope and Standards of Practice* (Silver Spring, MD: Nursesbooks.org, 2007).

9. J. George, ed., *Nursing Theories: The Base for Professional Practice*, 6th ed. (Upper Saddle River, NJ: Prentice Hall, 2011).

10. B. J. Zimmerman, "Complexity Science: A Route Through Hard Times and Uncertainty," *Health Forum Journal* 42, no. 2 (1999): 44–46, 96.

11. J. W. Begun, B. Zimmerman, and K. J. Dooley, "Health Care Organizations as Complex Adaptive Systems," in *Advances in Health Care Organization Theory*, eds. S. S. Mick and M. E. Wyttenback (San Francisco: Jossey Bass, 2003): 253–288.

12. J. A. Astin and K. Forys, "Psychosocial Determinants of Health and Illness: Integrating Mind, Body, and Spirit," *Advances in Mind-Body Medicine* 20, no. 4 (2004): 14–21.

13. C. R. Geary and K. L. Schumacher, "Integrating Transition Theory and Complexity Science

Concepts," *Advances in Nursing Science* 35, no. 3 (2012): 236–248.

14. M. Kramer, B. Brewer, D. Halfer, P. Maguire, S. Beausoliel, K. Claman, M. Macphee, et al., "Changing Our Lens: Seeing the Chaos of Professional Practice as Complexity," *Journal of Nursing Management* 21, no. 4 (2013): 690–704.

15. K. M. James, "Incorporating Complexity Science into Nursing Curricula," *Creative Nursing* 16, no. 3 (2010): 137–142.

16. K. Wilber, "Foreword to *Integral Medicine: A Noetic Reader*" (2007). http://wilber.shambhala.com /html/misc/integral-med-1.cfm.

17. O. Jarrin, "An Integral Philosophy and Definition of Nursing," *AQAL: Journal of Integral Theory and Practice* 2, no. 4 (2007): 79–101.

18. C. S. Clark, "An Integral Nursing Education: Exploration of the Wilber Quadrant Model," *International Journal for Human Caring* 10, no. 3 (2006): 22–29.

19. K. Fiandt, J. Forman, M. E. Megel, R. A. Pakieser, and S. Burge, "Integral Nursing: An Emerging Framework for Engaging the Evolution of the Profession," *Nursing Outlook* 51, no. 3 (2003): 130–137.

20. L. Shea and N. C. Frisch, "Application of Integral Theory in Holistic Nursing Practice," 28, no. 6 (2014): 344–352.

21. B. M. Dossey, "Theory of Integral Nursing," *Advances in Nursing Science* 31, no. 1 (2008): e52–e73.

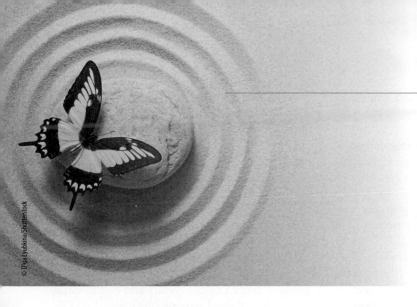

CHAPTER 6

Holistic Ethics

Margaret A. Burkhardt

Nurse Healer Objectives

Theoretical

- Review the classic principles of ethics.
- Synthesize the basic tenets from the work of traditional ethical theorists.
- Explore the concept of holistic ethics.
- Discuss Earth ethics as an integral component of holistic ethics.

Clinical

- Relate ethical theory to clinical situations.
- Discuss nursing considerations related to advance directives and informed consent.
- Describe processes for ethical decision making in clinical situations.
- Discuss ethical imperatives for nurses involved in research.

Personal

- Discuss daily choices as opportunities to make a positive influence on the world.
- Clarify personal values and ideas.
- Describe moral courage.

Definitions

Being: The state of existing or living.

Consciousness: A state of knowing or awareness.

Earth community: Includes all beings of the Earth, nonhuman as well as human.

Earth ethics: A code of behavior that incorporates the understanding that the Earth community has core value in and of itself and includes ethical treatment of the nonhuman world and the Earth as a whole. This code influences the way that we individually and collectively interact with the environment and all beings of the Earth.

Ethical code: A written list of a profession's values and standards of conduct.

Ethics: The study or discipline concerned with judgments of approval and disapproval, right and wrong, good and bad, virtue and vice, and desirability and wisdom of actions, as well as dispositions, ends, objects, and states of affairs; disciplined reflection on the moral choices that people make.

Holistic: Concerned with the interrelationship of body, mind, and spirit in an everchanging environment.

Holistic ethics: The basic underlying concept of the unity and integral wholeness of all people and of all nature, which is identified and pursued by finding unity and wholeness within one's self and within humanity. In this framework, acts are not performed for the sake of law, precedent, or social norms, but rather from a desire to do good freely, to witness, identify, and contribute to unity.

Informed consent: A process by which patients or participants in research studies are informed of the purpose, possible outcomes, alternatives, risks, and benefits of treatment or the research protocol; individuals are required to freely give their consent for the treatment or participation in the study.

Moral courage: The willingness to stand up for personal core values and ethical beliefs, even when one stands alone or risks other consequences such as ridicule or threat of job loss.

Morals: Standards of right and wrong that are learned through socialization.

Nursing ethics: A code of values and behavior that guides the way nurses work with those in their care, with one another, with society, and with the whole Earth community.

Personal ethics: An individual code of thought, values, and behavior that governs each person's actions.

Values: Concepts or ideals that give meaning to life and provide a framework for decisions and actions.

The Nature of Ethical Problems

Because ethical issues reflect diverse values and perspectives, they are extremely complex. Ethical questions arise from all areas of life. The ramifications of life-sustaining technology, the population explosion, assisted suicide, euthanasia, genetic engineering, environmental degradation, equitable access to health care for all people, and allocation of increasingly scarce resources are only a few examples of a host of controversial ethical issues. Ongoing developments in our society such as advances in medical technology, greater recognition of patients' rights, limited access to health care for some populations, malpractice cases, court-ordered treatment, and end-of-life decisions call nurses to increase their ethical awareness. Another factor that becomes increasingly important in holistic ethics is the ethical treatment of the other than human world, indeed the Earth as

a whole, the health of which is intricately connected to human health.

Unfortunately, ethical dilemmas are usually characterized by the fact that there is no right answer. There are often two or more unsatisfactory answers or conflicting responses. In addition, nurses often find that the expectations of employers, physicians, patients, or other nurses are sources of conflict.[1] Changes in the knowledge that forms the basis of our values and advances in health care are leading to new sources of ethical dilemmas. For example, technologies related to computers and communications have affected patient confidentiality. Life support technology may prolong living but may also increase suffering and prolong the dying process. In the midst of dealing with sophisticated technology, nurses often find that their focus is more on the machines than on the patient. Such advances have opened the doors to new possibilities for extending or prolonging life, but they also prompt a critical ethical question: Does having the technology always mean it should be used?

Morals and Principles

Ethical principles serve as a guide for dealing with ethical issues. These principles are basic and obvious moral truths that offer guidance for both deliberation and action. Principles found in major ethical theories include autonomy, beneficence, nonmaleficence, veracity, confidentiality, justice, and fidelity. All of these ethical principles presuppose respect for persons. These principles represent many obligations: to respect the wishes of competent persons, to not harm others, to take actions that benefit others, to produce a net balance of benefits over harms, to distribute benefits and harms fairly, to keep promises and contracts, to be truthful, to disclose information, and to respect privacy and protect confidential information.[1, 2]

Orentlicher, a physician, lawyer, and ethicist, thinks that there are, at root, only two ways to guide proper behavior: rules and precedents. He notes that rules are designed to support underlying values (e.g., speed limits are set to promote public safety). Rules are attractive because they provide seemingly clear lines of conduct that prevent metaphorical slippery slopes. They also can help to avoid the capriciousness of personal discretion and the obtrusiveness of governmental intrusion in decision making. However, Orentlicher is concerned with the unintended consequences of rules and cites, as an example, the case of mandating pregnant women to undergo certain medical procedures to prevent harm to their fetuses. Another moral concern is the political difficulty of having explicit rules where life-and-death decisions are being made, such as the allocation of scarce organs. Here, society tends to adopt a system of vague precedents that operate under the guise of rules. The appearance of objectivity, which is inherent to general rules, can hide the vagueness of the processes that actually are being used.[3]

Orentlicher argues that rules sometimes work to the detriment of the value that prompted implementation of the rule in the first place. In fact, this phenomenon is widely considered a kind of natural law: the law of unintended consequences. For example, a medicolegal question might ask whether pregnant women should be forced to undergo treatment to help their fetuses. If forced treatments were endorsed, then some women might avoid prenatal care, thus—and here is the unintended consequence—harming their fetuses. The answer might depend on whether forced treatment would help more fetuses than would be harmed by women who would be driven away from prenatal care. This is but one example of the complexity of ethical decision making.[3]

Within natural law ethics, the principle of double effect has special importance for nurses. Often, nurses are involved in actions that have untoward consequences. For example, administering a drug to relieve a cancer patient's pain may shorten the patient's life. In double effect situations, four conditions must be met before an act can be justified:[4]

1. The act itself must be morally good, or at least indifferent.
2. The good effect must not be achieved by means of the bad effect.
3. Only the good effect must be intended, even though the bad effect is foreseen and known.

4. The good effect intended must be equal to or greater than the bad effect.

Moral problems incorporate a mix of values, risks, benefits, and harms. They are as complex as they are important, include elements of uncertainty and conflict, and defy easy solutions. One must take care with moral decision making because many such decisions are irreversible. Ethics addresses different types of moral problems:

- Moral uncertainty (i.e., unsureness about moral principles or rules that may apply, or the nature of the ethical problem itself)
- Moral dilemma (i.e., conflict of moral principles that support different courses of action)
- Moral distress (i.e., inability to take the action known to be right because of external constraints)
- Practical dilemmas (i.e., a situation where moral claims compete with nonmoral claims)[1]
- Moral courage (i.e., willingness to stand up for personal and professional ethical values even when this stance is unpopular and may mean standing alone)[5, 6]

Ethical debate helps to relieve moral uncertainty by clarifying questions and illuminating the ethical features of a situation. Discussion and reflection help to clarify moral dilemmas by revealing general and specific obligations and values. Adhering to ethical obligations and personal values and facing fears related to standing up for what is ethically right in spite of consequences supports the ability to act with moral courage. Many factors contribute to the complexity of ethical problems:

- Context (i.e., a person's unique life circumstances)
- Uncertainty (i.e., a lack of predictability of the outcome of a given act)
- Multiple stakeholders with potentially strong and diverse preferences
- Power imbalance within the healthcare institution
- Variables outside of the direct patient care setting, such as institutional policies

- Urgency (i.e., situations in which a decision must be made before one has a chance to deliberate as much as one would like)[1]

Holistic nurses need to know the language of ethics and have the courage to act ethically and participate fully in ethical decision making. This requires using principles and theory to deal with issues of relationships as well as healthcare concerns. A holistic approach to ethical problems incorporates both thinking and feeling as credible ways of knowing and recognizes a legitimate role for both in ethical decision making. Heart and mind, reason and emotion need to be attended to when making ethical decisions, appreciating that what one feels in relation to the circumstances of the situation is as important as what one thinks is right or wrong.

Traditional Ethical Theories

Many nurse clinicians turn away in frustration when confronted with the details of ethical theories. Perhaps this is because in the past it has been difficult to see how these historical, philosophical theories relate to contemporary clinical situations. To make these theories meaningful to the work setting, it is helpful to think of situations in which they may apply to current clinical practice.

Several ethical theories have played a role in Western civilization and have laid the foundation for the development of contemporary nursing ethics. Aristotelian theory is based on the individual manifesting specific virtues and developing his or her own character. Aristotle (384–322 BCE) believed that an individual who practices the virtues of courage, temperance, integrity, justice, honesty, and truthfulness will know almost intuitively what to do in a particular situation or conflict.[5, 7, pp. 59–63] The system of Immanuel Kant (1724–1804) formulated the historical Christian idea of the Golden Rule: "So act in such a way as your act becomes a universal for all mankind."[7, p. 273] Kant was very much concerned with the "personhood" of human beings and persons as moral agents.

Other theories that are helpful in understanding a holistic approach to ethics include the Utilitarianism Theory of Jeremy Bentham (1748–1832) and John Stuart Mill (1806–1873), the Natural Rights Theory of John Locke (1632–1714), and the Contractarian Theory of Thomas Hobbes (1588–1679). Briefly stated, the consequentialist, or utilitarian, view of Bentham and Mill is that the consequences of our actions are the primary concern, that the means justify the ends, and that every human being has a personal concept of good and bad. The Natural Rights Theory of Locke was the forerunner of the U.S. Declaration of Independence because it included the tenet that individuals have inalienable rights and that other individuals have an obligation to respect those rights. The Contractarian Theory of Hobbes contends that morality involves a social contract indicating what individuals can and cannot do.[7, pp. 163–169]

Another way of viewing ethics is in terms of the two traditional forms: the deontologic style (from a Greek root meaning knowledge of that which is binding and proper) and the teleologic style (from a Greek root meaning knowledge of the ends). The former assigns duty or obligation based on the intrinsic aspects of an act rather than its outcome, meaning that action is morally defensible on the basis of its intrinsic nature. The latter assigns duty or obligation based on the consequences of the act, meaning that action is morally defensible on the basis of its extrinsic value or outcome.

Development of Holistic Ethics

Ethics is the study of the paths of practical wisdom. It is concerned with judgments of good and bad and right and wrong, based on a philosophic view of the nature of the universe. The holistic view of reality reopens vistas of thought that were dominant in the pretechnologic era, when people were generally closer to their environment and the Earth. The allure of new science and technology sidetracked many of us into primarily linear, rational, unidirectional thought. Furthermore, although technology has provided conveniences and easy solutions, it has also contributed to a tendency to objectify the universe.

Holistic ethics is a philosophy that couples both reemerging and rapidly evolving concepts of holism and ethics that reflect elements of Eastern and Western philosophies and spiritual and ethical beliefs of people from contemporary and indigineous cultures. It involves a basic underlying concept of the unity and integral wholeness of all people, and of all nature, which is identified and pursued by finding unity and wholeness within one's self, within humanity, and within the larger Earth community. Within the framework of holistic ethics, acts are not performed solely for the sake of law, precedent, or social norms; they are performed from a desire to do good freely, to witness, identify, and contribute to unity of the self and of the universe, of which the individual is a part. Encompassing traditional ethical views, the holistic view is characterized by the balance and integration evident in the Eastern monad of the yin-yang mode and in the Western concept of masculine-feminine.

Holistic ethics originates in the individual's own character and in the individual's relationship to the universe. In some way, the universe is present totally in each individual; paradoxically, the person is just a small part of that same universe. Gregorios believed that wisdom is a condition in which the self and the world are in communion with one another, within the larger communion, and with the infinite totality of being in its integrity.[8] A holistic view takes into account the relationship of unity of all beings. Albert Einstein, in the course of a serious illness, was asked if he feared death. He replied, "I have such a feeling of solidarity with every living being, that it does not matter to me where the individual begins and ends."[9]

Holistic ethics is grounded or judged not so much in the act performed or in the distant consequences of the act as in the conscious evolution of an enlightened individual who performs the act. Understanding that all things are connected, the primary concern is the effect of the act on the individual and his or her larger self (i.e., that unity of which the individual is a part, including the entire Earth community). Unethical acts are those that degrade or brutalize the individual who performs the act and that detract from his or her conscious evolution, which, in turn, degrades the whole. The effect of an unethical act is to make us aware of the deprivation of divinity within humanity and of humanity itself. The unethical act dissolves the unity of matter and takes away wholeness. Acts must be judged in this setting to determine whether they promote wholeness and integration of either an individual or the collective whole. As each of us evolves our own individual consciousness, we assess and direct the evolution of the consciousness of our species and contemplatively examine our relationship with the universal being.

An a priori belief for a holistic person is likely, "I believe in being," or even more simply, "I am." In this belief system, no act, principle, or person is independent, but all are interrelated; all are "I." Each and every action is a moral action, either contributing to the unity of being or diminishing it. It is the enlightened and completely expanded "I" that creates a holistic view of ethics.

Moral acts may be judged not solely in terms of their intrinsic nature nor solely in terms of their ends, but in both ways. The act may affect the nature of the person performing the act (the "I") and his or her relationships, as well as affect the object of the act and the object's relationships. In addition, it can be helpful to explore the relationship of the act to the present and future of humanity and the Earth as a whole. Through this construct, holistic ethics is both deontologic and teleologic. Holistic ethics is specifically teleologic in questioning the meaning and quality of life.

As a philosophic design for living, holistic ethics is a system for the individual. It appeals to the emotions, senses, aesthetic appreciation, and the inner self as revealed by meditative techniques. Such techniques may be active (e.g., the body movements of tai chi or jogging), passive (e.g., a sitting, meditative posture), or traditional prayer.

The educative process of holistic ethics is not merely a matter of memorizing facts or historical perspectives but is instead a process of developing an attitude of awareness of the sacredness of ourselves and of the entire Earth community. It is a process in which there is an expanded view that, for both internal and external transformation, our inner self and the collective greater self have stewardship not only of our bodies, minds, and spirits but also of our planet and the total universe.

Based on this emergent ethical theory, the American Holistic Nurses Association (AHNA) developed a position statement on holistic nursing ethics (**Exhibit 6-1**).

Holistic ethics embraces and strives for the fusion between self and others. In the process,

---

EXHIBIT 6-1   American Holistic Nurses Association Position Statement on Holistic Nursing Ethics

Code of Ethics for Holistic Nurses

We believe that the fundamental responsibilities of the nurse are to promote health, facilitate healing and alleviate suffering. The need for nursing is universal. Inherent in nursing is the respect for life, dignity and right of all persons. Nursing care is given in a context mindful of the holistic nature of humans, understanding the body-mind-spirit. Nursing care is unrestricted by considerations of nationality, race, creed, color, age, sex, sexual preferences, politics or social status. Given that nurses practice in culturally diverse settings, professional nurses must have an understanding of the cultural background of clients in order to provide culturally appropriate interventions.

Nurses render services to clients who can be individuals, families, groups or communities. The client is an active participant in health care and should be included in all nursing care planning decisions.

In order to provide services to others, each nurse has a responsibility toward him/herself. In addition, nurses have defined responsibilities towards the client, coworkers, nursing practice, the profession of nursing, society and the environment.

Nurses and Self

The nurse has a responsibility to model health behaviors. Holistic nurses strive to achieve harmony in their own lives and assist others striving to do the same.

Nurses and the Client

The nurse's primary responsibility is to the client needing nursing care. The nurse strives to see the client as a whole, and provides care that is professionally appropriate and culturally consonant. The nurse holds in confidence all information obtained in professional practice, and uses professional judgment in disclosing such information. The nurse enters into a relationship with the client that is guided by mutual respect and a desire for growth and development.

Nurses and Coworkers

The nurse maintains cooperative relationships with coworkers in nursing and other fields. Nurses have a responsibility to nurture each other, and to assist nurses to work as a team in the interest of client care. If a client's care is endangered by a coworker, the nurse must take appropriate action on behalf of the client.

Nurses and Nursing Practice

The nurse carries personal responsibility for practice and for maintaining continued competence. Nurses have the right to utilize all appropriate nursing interventions, and have the obligation to determine the efficacy and safety of all nursing actions. Wherever applicable, nurses utilize research findings in directing practice.

Nurses and the Profession

The nurse plays a role in determining and implementing desirable standards of nursing practice and education. Holistic nurses may assume a leadership position to guide the profession toward holism. Nurses support nursing research and the development of holistically oriented nursing theories. The nurse participates in establishing and maintaining equitable social and economic working conditions in nursing.

Nurses and Society

The nurse, along with other citizens, has responsibility for initiating and supporting actions to meet the health and social needs of the public.

Nurses and the Environment

The nurse strives to manipulate the client's environment to become one of peace, harmony, and nurturance so that healing may take place. The nurse considers the health of the ecosystem in relation to the need for health, safety and peace of all persons.

Source: Courtesy of the American Holistic Nurses Association, Topeka, KS.

it becomes a cosmic ecology, a flowing with the universal tide of events, and a co-creator of celestial harmony. All events and ethical decisions become part of the unfolding of a harmonious order and a realization of potentials. Even tragic events can be analyzed within this harmonious spectrum with full realization of the fusion of relationships. One's own actions can become courageous; full of truth, being, and beauty; assured; detached; and virtuous.

Earth Ethics

Ethical discussions and deliberations most often refer to principles and practices related to human experiences, values, and ways of being in the world. Such discussions seldom include consideration of ethical treatment of the nonhuman world. Our sense of relationship with the natural world flows from our worldview or cosmology. The worldview that underlies the Western scientific perspective holds that there is a radical distinction between humans as subjects and the natural world as object.[10] A sense that the human experience is separate from and in opposition to nature has engendered and permitted a destructive attitude toward Earth and a belief that all species and resources of the Earth have been put here primarily for human use. A shift, which began emerging in the 17th century, from an organic understanding of reality in which everything is alive, to a mechanistic view of reality, engendered the belief that humans have a right to do anything they want with nature. This attitude promotes little sense of ethical responsibility toward the nonhuman world. Instead, it has allowed us to turn a blind eye to our complicity in the exploitation of the planet. After several centuries of demoting the natural world to a collection of material objects available for human exploitation, we are now realizing that this complete disregard for the realities of ecological systems and the limited capacity of the natural world to sustain this exploitation and destruction are contributing to the ill health of humans and to the planet itself.

There is an urgent need for holistic nurses and all of humanity to move beyond a human-centered focus in ethical concerns and begin to relate to all parts of the Earth community as having core value. We need to incorporate Earth ethics into our understanding and practice of holistic ethics. Remembering that we are part of the interconnected web of life, we recognize that what we do to the Earth we do to ourselves. Indigenous peoples, mystics of many traditions, and contemporary scholars teach us that the world is a seamless garment in which there is no separation between humans and nature, the sacred and the secular. We cannot have healthy minds, bodies, spirits, or communities without healthy land and environment. When we destroy the source of our life and sustenance, our health (physical, mental, emotional, and spiritual) suffers. When we understand that, as humans, we are only one part of the interconnected Earth community, and we recognize the interdependence and unity of all in the natural world, we appreciate that all species have an intrinsic right to exist. Within this understanding, our ethical principles must address the integrity and health of the entire community of life. The moral imperative of holistic ethics then directs us to apply principles of beneficence, nonmaleficence, and justice to our treatment of the whole Earth community, not only to its human members.

Development of Principled Behavior

Healthcare providers with a holistic ethics perspective and high standards of principled behavior are best prepared to analyze clinical dilemmas. Nathaniel asserts that principled behavior flows from personal values that guide and inform one's responses, behaviors, and decisions in all areas of one's life.[11] Holistic nurses need to be aware of personal values and know how these values influence relationships with oneself, others, and the Earth community.

Values Clarification

Values develop over time and have cultural, familial, environmental, and educational components. Values clarification is a never-ending process in which an individual becomes increasingly aware of what is important and just—and why. Understanding and openly discussing different views in a given situation helps us to appreciate the truth inherent in the various perspectives. Values clarification within groups and organizations requires conscious identification of spoken and written (i.e., overt) values as well as those values that are unspoken or unwritten (i.e., covert) values. Identifying the underlying values of an organization enables us to determine whether our personal and professional values are congruent with those of the organization. This awareness serves as a basis for determining whether we can work in a particular environment or support a particular organization.

Often, patients must clarify their values to participate fully in ethical decision making. Holistic nurses can assist patients in this process in a variety of ways. One way is for nurses to listen carefully and reflect back what they hear patients say that is personally important to them. Another might be to list several health behaviors or values, such as happiness, good relationships with family, health, and independence, and ask patients to rank them or to identify how they incorporate them into their lives.

Integrity and Empowerment

Personal integrity and sense of empowerment are cornerstones of ethical behavior that are espoused throughout *Holistic Nursing: Scope and Standards of Practice, Second Edition*.[12] Both are grounded in self-awareness and personal reflection and are essential to the holistic caring process. Identifying personal values strengthens the ability to make choices that reflect these values. Integrity implies trustworthiness, wholeness, consistency of values, emotions, and behaviors, as well as adherence to moral norms over time. Empowerment implies having the ability to choose, being responsible and accountable for personal actions, having the courage to take risks, and having the desire, ability, and resources to make decisions. When faced with ethical issues, personal empowerment enables us to be true to ourselves, make choices based on our core values, and allow our actions to flow from our essence. Having the moral courage to do what is right in spite of fear of reprisal, such as risks of rejection, ridicule, anxiety, shame, and even potential unemployment, reflects a high degree of personal integrity and empowerment.

Self-care is a reflection of personal integrity and empowerment. Being honest with and caring for ourselves and treating ourselves with respect are ways we demonstrate congruence between our values and behavior. Knowing that the energy of the self is interconnected with the energy of the Earth community, holistic nurses understand that the growth of personal strength and power unfolds within the context of love and respect for all forms of life.

Legal Aspects

Healthcare providers must adhere to the law. All nurses are responsible and accountable to comply with the Nursing Practice Act as well as the rules and regulations of the board of nurse examiners in the state where they are licensed and work. Standards of professional nursing practice require that each nurse practice to the level of his or her knowledge and skills. In this regard, holistic nurses need to be familiar with and adhere to the standards of practice for holistic nurses.[12] Whatever an individual nurse's personal ethic, he or she must still adhere to the standards of practice and to the law.

Ethical Decision Making

Nurses are confronted daily with the need to make personal and professional ethical decisions, yet many of them feel unprepared to be equal participants in ethical decision making. Some decisions nurses face are minor, and others are fraught with long-term multifaceted ramifications. To make decisions appropriately, holistic nurses need to be grounded in an understanding of the integral wholeness of all beings and do their best to articulate and examine their core values and their relationship to nursing and institutional standards. Participation in decision-making groups necessitates that nurses become fluent in the language of nursing and bioethics and that they learn to appreciate the diverse moral perspectives of patients and colleagues. It is necessary as well that nurses operate from a set of principles and have facility with processes that help sort out and classify the elements of the problem. There are many well-established guidelines for analyzing individual cases in ethics that may be helpful to nurses. Two such processes are summarized here.

Burkhardt and Nathaniel approach ethical decision making from a nursing problem-solving frame of reference that includes sensitivity to the human story.[1] They suggest that, although the steps of an ethical problem-solving process may seem linear on paper, the process is nonlinear in practice. They note that the ethical decision-making process overlays other dynamic biological, psychological, and social processes— layer on layer. Because nothing in the human sphere is static, nurses need to appreciate that physical conditions and opinions change, knowledge evolves, and time passes. In light of the changing nature of human experience, these authors describe a decision-making process in which key facets are revisited from an evolving perspective as one moves toward a decision or resolution. They present a framework for entering a decision-making process that is spiral in nature. This process requires an ongoing evaluation and assimilation of information, with each step being revisited as often as is required and molded by the dynamics of changing facts, evolving beliefs, unexpected consequences, and participants who move in and out of the process. They have formed a five-step process of ethical decision making with the following components: (1) articulating the problem, (2) gathering data and identifying conflicting moral claims, (3) exploring strategies, (4) implementing the strategy, and (5) evaluating outcomes of the action.

1. Articulating the Problem

Ethical decision making begins when there is concern that a moral problem exists. Clearly articulating and identifying the undesirable situation enables one to also clarify the goal because a problem consists of a discrepancy between the current situation and a desired state or goal. A goal must be identified before moving toward strategies, which is Step 3 of this model.

2. Gathering Data and Identifying Conflicting Moral Claims

Clarify the issues by gathering information that provides evidence of conflicting goals, obligations, principles, duties, rights, loyalties, values, or beliefs. In this process, nurses must pay attention to the societal, religious, and cultural values and beliefs of all involved. Data gathering should include information about facts as well as feelings that seem important, such as expectations, preferences, quality-of-life issues, understanding of the situation, relationships and supports, and projected outcomes of available options. Gaps in the information also need to be identified. Key participants (which include healthcare providers) need to be identified, including who is affected and how; who is legitimately empowered to make the decision; issues of conflict and agreement among participants and what is most important to each; the level of competence of the person most affected; and the rights, duties, authority, and capabilities of all participants. These data can help those involved to understand the ethical components, principles of concern, and the various perceptions of issues and principles of all involved in the situation.

3. Exploring Strategies

Through the assessment process, possible alternative strategies that address the desired outcomes begin to emerge. In consideration of legal and other consequences, participants need to determine which alternatives best meet the identified goals and fit their basic beliefs, lifestyles, and values. By reviewing options with both head and heart, participants need to eliminate unacceptable alternatives and begin the process of listing, weighing, prioritizing, and sensing the energy of those that are considered acceptable, recognizing that there is rarely a perfect solution. Once an option is chosen, the decision makers must be willing to act on the choice.

4. Implementing the Strategy

Although taking action is a major goal of the process, it can be one of the most difficult parts of the process. Emotions laced with both certainty and doubt about the rightness of the decision often emerge. Empowering patients and families to make difficult decisions requires special attention to the emotions that often manifest at this point of the process.

5. Evaluating Outcomes of the Action

Once the action step is taken, participants begin a process of response and evaluation that sheds light on the effectiveness and validity of the process. In evaluating the action in terms of the effects on those involved, it is important to determine whether the original ethical problem has been effectively resolved and whether other problems have emerged related to the action. As new data emerge and the situation changes, participants may identify subsequent moral problems that require adjusting the course of action based on both new information and responses to the previous decision.

Jonsen and colleagues divided the ethical case analysis process into four components: (1) medical indications, (2) patient preferences, (3) quality of life, and (4) contextual issues.[13] Present in every clinical, ethical case, these four topics are necessary for a thorough analysis. The holistic approach adds relationship questions: Who am I? What is my relationship to others and to the whole? What other factors are contributing to my decisions? Am I wise and courageous enough to perceive and respect others' differences and honor them as I would honor my own beliefs?

Medical Indications

The underlying ethical principles in considering medical indications is beneficence—be of benefit—and do no harm. Discussion should focus on discerning the relationship between the pathophysiology and the diagnostic and therapeutic interventions (both conventional and integrative) available to remedy the patient's pathologic condition. Questions regarding the overall goal of the care are important considerations in this component. For example, for the patient who is terminally ill, there may be discussions about the time to switch from further medical treatment to palliative care.

Patient Preferences

In all interventions, patient preferences are relevant. There are many questions to be asked: What does the patient want? Does the patient comprehend his or her choices? Is the patient being coerced? In some cases, there is no certainty because the patient is incapable of self-expression. Whenever possible, it is essential to ensure that the patient's right to self-determination based on his or her personal values and evaluation of risks and benefits is honored. However, it is necessary to be clear about what is realistically feasible in relation to the patient's wishes.

In the case of a child, nurses must ask the questions: Do the parents understand the situation? Do the parents appear to have the best interests of the child at heart? Are the parents in agreement or discord? At which level can a child have input into the discussion?

Quality of Life

A patient enters a health crisis situation with an actual or potential reduction in quality of life, manifested by the signs and symptoms of the illness. The objective of healthcare interventions is to improve quality of life. In each case, multiple questions surround quality-of-life issues: What does quality of life mean, in general? In particular? How are others responding to their perceptions of it? How do particular levels of quality impose obligations, if any, on providers? This component may be a difficult part of the analysis of clinical problems, but it is indispensable.

Contextual Issues

Every case has a patient at its center. The patient exists in a social, psychological, spiritual, economic, and relational environment. To be relevant, all decisions must be considered in the light of this expanded conceptual and holistic view of personhood and personality. The major factors affected are psychological, emotional, financial, legal, scientific, educational, and spiritual.

Advance Directives

Many ethical dilemmas arise surrounding end-of-life care options and choices. Supporting a patient's right and ability to make choices is an essential element of holistic nursing practice and holistic ethics. The Patient Self-Determination Act, effective December 1, 1991, requires that all individuals receiving medical care also receive written information about their right to accept or refuse medical or surgical treatment and their right to initiate advance directives. Advance directives are instructions that indicate healthcare interventions to initiate or withhold, or that designate someone who will act as a surrogate in making such decisions in the event that decision-making capacity is lost. Advance directives support people in making decisions on their own behalf and help to ensure that patients have the kind of end-of-life care they want. Advance medical directives are of two types: treatment directives (often referred to as living wills) and appointment directives (often referred to as powers of attorney or health proxies). A living will specifies the medical treatment that a patient wishes to refuse in the event that he or she is terminally ill and cannot make those decisions. A durable power of attorney for health care appoints a proxy or surrogate, usually a relative or trusted friend, to make medical decisions on behalf of the patient if he or she can no longer make such decisions. It has broader applications than a living will and can apply to any illness or injury that causes the patient to lose decision-making capacity temporarily or long term. The authority of the surrogate is effective only for the duration of the loss of decision-making capacity.

An advance directive applies only if a patient is incapacitated. It may not apply if, in the opinion of two physicians, the patient can make decisions. Individuals can cancel advance directives at any time. An advance directive may be simple or complex. Individuals should give a copy of the advance directive to their family members and physician and should carry a copy if and when hospital admission is necessary.

As part of patient assessment, a holistic nurse may consider asking the following questions:

- Have you discussed your end-of-life choices with your family and/or designated surrogate and healthcare team workers?
- Do you have basic information about advance medical directives, including living wills and durable powers of attorney?
- Do you wish to initiate an advance medical directive?
- If you have already prepared an advance medical directive, can you provide it now?

Ethical Considerations in Practice and Research

Because nursing is inherently a moral endeavor, nurses may encounter challenges in making the right decisions and taking the right actions in both nursing research and nursing practice. An important consideration for nurses in ensuring legal and ethical protection of a patient's right to personal autonomy is the process of informed consent. Obtaining informed consent from patients is important both in relation to medical and other treatments and to participation in research studies. The process of informed consent for medical and other treatments provides the opportunity for the patient to choose a course of action regarding plans for health care, including the right to refuse medical recommendations and to choose from available therapeutic alternatives. An informed consent must include the following:

1. The nature of the health concern and prognosis if nothing is done
2. Description of all treatment options, even those that the healthcare provider does not favor or cannot provide
3. The benefits, risks, and consequences of the various treatment alternatives, including nonintervention

The issue of informed consent with complementary/alternative modalities (CAM) raises some important questions. Because listing alternative treatments is one of the elements of an informed consent, nurses must consider whether it is an ethical duty for practitioners of bioscientific medicine to include CAM in discussion of therapeutic alternatives. Nurses also need to ask whether practitioners of other healing modalities should ensure that their clients are aware of biomedical alternatives. Holistic nurses who offer CAM therapies should explain the intervention and discuss risks, expected effects and benefits, and treatment options prior to initiating therapy. Because CAM therapies may affect conventional interventions in varying ways, it is important to inform other health team members of the use of these therapies.

Research expands the unique body of knowledge of nursing and provides an organizing framework for nursing practice. Although participating in research is important and rewarding, it can also present dilemmas for the nurse and nurse researcher in both research institutions and clinical realms. Adding to nursing's knowledge and understanding is the expected motivation for conducting research. However, other motivating factors such as personal or institutional gains related to grant funding, prestige, or promoting a product may challenge principled behavior in regard to research.

The principles that underlie the ethical conduct of research include respect for human dignity (i.e., the rights to full disclosure and self-determination or autonomy), beneficence (i.e., the right to protection from harm and discomfort, as in balancing between the benefits and risks of a study), and justice (i.e., the rights of fair treatment and privacy, including anonymity and confidentiality). These principles provide the basis for informed consent related to participation in research studies.[14] Informed consent in research refers to freely choosing to participate in a research study after the research purpose, expected commitment, risks and benefits, any invasion of privacy, and ways that anonymity and confidentiality will be addressed have been explained. Nurses who work in clinical areas where research is being conducted must ensure that these principles are followed.

Nurses who assist with research or who work on units where research is being conducted need to be familiar with elements of informed consent and attentive to ensuring that informed consent is obtained from research participants. A particular area of concern is protection of human rights in research studies focused on vulnerable populations such as children; persons with disabilities; persons who are challenged, institutionalized, or incarcerated; older adults; pregnant women; and those who are dying. Nurses who are involved in research are accountable to professional standards for reporting research findings. An important consideration in this regard is the ethical treatment of data, which demonstrates the integrity of research protocols and honesty in reporting data.

Cultural Diversity Considerations

Cultural values and beliefs guide our way of being in the world and our reaction to life experiences in patterned ways. Patterns influenced by culture that are significant in providing holistic health care include beliefs about health and practices related to health and healing. These beliefs and practices manifest in both direct and subtle ways, and sensitivity to them can affect patient outcomes and satisfaction with the care. The increasing cultural diversity in modern society may present challenges in transcultural ethical decision making for healthcare workers. Such transcultural issues arise when nurses, patients, and families are guided by different moral paradigms and hold differing views of what is important or necessary regarding health, recovery, illness, or the dying process. Ethical or legal dilemmas may arise from lack of understanding of language, procedures, expectations, and other elements of the culture that lead to miscommunication, unclear decisions, and a sense of powerlessness or lack of control. Dealing with transcultural issues requires self-awareness on the part of the nurse. A good starting point for becoming sensitive to the culture of another is to understand one's own culture and its influence on personal perceptions and behaviors. Similarly, incorporating cultural assessment into care with patients facilitates better understanding of sometimes overlooked factors that influence a patient's health behaviors and decisions. Nurses who are sensitive and knowledgeable about the cultural perspective of individual patients acknowledge an individual's cultural background and consider the characteristics of different cultures when planning the patient's care. This facilitates the process of ethical decision making.

Culture guides choices regarding when and where to go for health care, what kind of care to seek, and how long to participate in care. When considering definitions of health and values such as autonomy, beneficence, justice, or the right to self-determination, it is important to ask from whose perspective these values are understood—that of the nurse or that of the patient. For example, some cultures place a higher emphasis on loyalty to the group than on Western values of individual autonomy. Healthcare decisions in these cultures may require input and agreement from groups such as the family, community, or society, rather than relying primarily on the individual. Cultural assessment provides insight into the congruence, or lack thereof, between patients' and nurses' values and understandings of health.

Flowing from the concept of the unity and integral wholeness of all people, holistic ethics must encompass a global perspective. This perspective includes cultural competence and cultural humility that enable the nurse to acknowledge and respect multiple ethical paradigms. Nursing care and research require awareness of, respect for, and congruence with the culture and needs of individuals and the community that are the focus of services or research.[15] Broad principles and concepts that can guide holistic nursing practice and research with cultures other than one's own include respect for persons and for communities, honoring the unity and wholeness of all beings, beneficence, justice, respect for human rights, contextual caring, and fidelity to one's professional code of ethics.

Conclusion

The holistic view of reality reopens vistas of thought that were dominant in the pretechnologic era, when people were generally closer to their environment and the Earth. Holistic ethics is a philosophy that couples both reemerging and rapidly evolving concepts of holism and ethics. It involves a basic underlying concept of the unity and integral wholeness of all people, and of all nature, that is identified and pursued by finding unity and wholeness within the self, within humanity, and within the Earth community. The complexity of ethical issues relates to the diverse values and perspectives involved. Skills in cultural assessment can help nurses to more effectively deal with ethical issues. Understanding the nature of ethical problems requires holistic nurses to be familiar with traditional ethical theories and concepts and aware of other ethical paradigms and to be able to integrate this knowledge with holistic theory and practice. An increasingly important factor in holistic ethics is the ethical treatment of the nonhuman world and the Earth as a whole, the health of which is intricately connected to human health. Awareness of personal values, beliefs, and understanding of health grounds the ability to deal effectively with ethical situations. The principles and processes of holistic ethics apply to research as well as to clinical practice situations. Holistic nurses need to know the language of ethics, be familiar with processes of ethical decision making, be attentive to cultural differences, and have the courage to participate fully in ethical decision making. This requires using principles, theory, and cultural competence and incorporates both thinking and feeling as credible ways of knowing in ethical decision making.

Directions for Future Research

1. Determine how and where the theory of holistic ethics fits into the continuum of emerging ethical theories.
2. Develop a process of clinical case analysis based on the process of holistic ethics.
3. Examine specific clinical situations and research protocols through a process of holistic ethics.
4. Analyze the application of holistic ethics to planetary ethical issues.

Nurse Healer Reflections

After reading this chapter, the nurse healer will be able to answer or to begin a process of answering the following questions:

- What new insights do I have about the process of ethics?
- How do I incorporate ethics into my clinical practice?
- How does my response to morally troubling situations reflect personal integrity and empowerment?
- How am I involved in ethical decision making within my work setting?
- How do my ethical values influence my day-to-day personal life?
- Am I ready to look at planetary issues from a holistic ethical perspective?

NOTES

1. M. A. Burkhardt and A. K. Nathaniel, *Ethics and Issues in Contemporary Nursing*, 4th ed. (Albany, NY: Delmar, 2014).
2. S. T. Fry, R. M. Veatch, and C. R. Taylor, *Case Studies in Nursing Ethics*, 4th ed. (Sudbury, MA: Jones & Bartlett Learning, 2011).
3. D. Orentlicher, *Matters of Life and Death: Making Moral Theory Work in Medicine and the Law* (Princeton, NJ: Princeton University Press, 2001).
4. A. McIntyre, "Doctrine of Double Effect," *Stanford Encyclopedia of Philosophy*, ed. E. N. Zalta (Winter 2014). http://plato.stanford.edu/entries/double-effect.
5. A. Gallagher, "Moral Distress and Moral Courage in Everyday Nursing Practice," *Online Journal of Issues in Nursing* 16, no. 2 (2011).
6. V. D. Lachman, "Strategies Necessary for Moral Courage," *Online Journal of Issues in Nursing* 15, no. 3 (2010).
7. H. Sidgwick, *Ethics* (Boston: Beacon Press, 1960).
8. P. M. Gregorios, *Science for Sane Societies* (New York: Paragon House, 1987).
9. M. Born, *The Born–Einstein Letters: Friendship, Politics and Physics in Uncertain Times* (New York: Macmillan Press, 1971): 91.
10. B. Swimme and M. E. Tucker, *Journey of the Universe* (New Haven, CT: Yale University Press, 2011).
11. A. K. Nathaniel, "Moral Reckoning in Nursing," *Western Journal of Nursing Research* 28, no. 4 (2006): 419–438.
12. American Holistic Nurses Association and American Nurses Association, *Holistic Nursing: Scope and Standards of Practice*, 2nd ed. (Silver Spring, MD: Nursesbooks.org, 2013).
13. A. R. Jonsen, M. Siegler, and W. J. Winslade, *Clinical Ethics: A Practical Approach to Ethical Decisions in Clinical Medicine*, 7th ed. (New York: McGraw-Hill, 2010).
14. U.S. Department of Health and Human Services, "Office for Human Research Protections (OHRP)" (n.d.). www.hhs.gov/ohrp.
15. J. N. Harrowing, J. Mill, J. Spieres, J. Kulig, and W. Kipp, "Culture, Context, and Community: Ethical Considerations for Global Nursing," *International Nursing Review* 57, no. 1 (2010): 70–77.

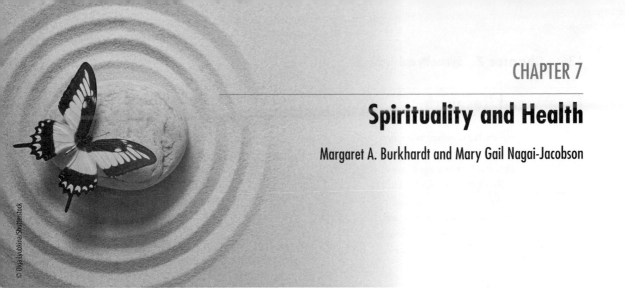

CHAPTER 7

Spirituality and Health

Margaret A. Burkhardt and Mary Gail Nagai-Jacobson

Nurse Healer Objectives

Theoretical

- Describe spirituality.
- Compare and contrast spirituality and religion.
- Discuss common elements of spirituality and their varying manifestations in different people.
- Recognize mystery, suffering, love, hope, forgiveness, peace and peacemaking, grace, and prayer as spiritual issues.
- Differentiate between spiritual issues and psychological issues.

Clinical

- Explore the efficacy and place of prayer in healing.
- Discuss listening as intentional presence.
- Identify approaches to spirituality assessment integral to holistic care.
- Discuss the use of story in spirituality assessment and care.
- Describe approaches for responding to spiritual concerns.

Personal

- Explore the need for nurses to nurture their own spirits and ways to do so.

- Discuss ways in which ritual, rest, leisure, play, and creativity relate to spirituality.
- Explore ways of naming and nurturing important connections.

Definitions

Religion: An organized system of beliefs regarding the cause, purpose, and nature of the universe that is shared by a group of people, and the practices, behaviors, worship, and ritual associated with that system. Religion connects persons through shared beliefs, values, and practices, making clear particular belief systems that are different from other belief systems, thus defining differences between groups of persons.

Spirituality: The essence of our being. It permeates our living in relationships and infuses our unfolding awareness of who we are, our purpose in being, and our inner resources. Spirituality is active and expressive. It shapes—and is shaped by—our life journey. Spirituality informs the ways we live and experience life, the ways we encounter mystery, and the ways we relate to all aspects of life. Inherent in the human condition, spirituality is expressed and experienced through living our connectedness with the Sacred Source, the self, others, and nature.

Theory and Research

We join spokes together in a wheel,
but it is the center hole
that makes the wagon move.
We shape clay into a pot,
but it is the emptiness inside
that holds whatever we want.
We hammer wood for a house,
but it is the inner space
that makes it livable.
We work with being,
but non-being is what we use.[1]

Spirituality is perhaps the most basic, yet least understood, aspect of holistic nursing. Spirituality often eludes the cognitive mind because it is intangible in many ways and defies quantification. A definition of spirituality is a starting point, appreciating that the mystery and experience of spirituality cannot be fully captured by any definition. Language for expressing the experience of spirit or soul is limited, thus people speak of spirituality however they can, often with symbols, metaphor, and story.[2] The term *spirituality* derives from the Latin *spiritus*, meaning breath, and relates to the Greek *pneuma*, or breath, which refers to the vital spirit or soul. Spirituality is the essence of who we are and how we are in the world and, like breathing, is integral to our existence as human beings.

All people are spiritual. By virtue of being human, all persons, at all ages, are bio-psycho-social-spiritual beings. Attending to spirituality across the life span implies an understanding of the developmental aspects of spirituality, particularly an awareness that expressions of spirituality may vary with age. Some people describe themselves or others as not spiritual because they do not attend religious services or believe in God. This reflects the common practice of describing spirituality in terms of religious beliefs and practices. Nurses and other healthcare providers often link spiritual caregiving with determining a patient's religious affiliation and understanding the health-related beliefs, norms, and taboos of that religion. Although such knowledge is important for holistic nursing, spiritual caregiving requires an understanding that spirituality is broader than religion and a recognition that, although some people may not be religious, everyone is spiritual.

Relationship Between Spirituality and Religion

Holistic nurses appreciate that spirituality and religion are not synonymous. *Spirituality* is the essence of one's being and is integral to all persons. Spirituality is a manifestation of each person's wholeness and being that is not subject to choice but simply is. Being spiritual is integral to the human experience in the same way that being physical, emotional, and sexual are part of being human. Religion per se is not essential to existence. Religion is chosen. Spirituality is expressed and experienced in many ways, both within and beyond the context of religion.

Religion refers to an organized system of beliefs shared by a group of people and the practices related to that system. Ritual, worship, prayer, meditation, style of dress, and dietary observances are examples of such practices. Because culture influences a person's values and beliefs, religious and other spiritual expressions often relate to personal culture. Religions reflect particular approaches to, and understandings of, spirituality. Religious precepts and practices often assist persons in attending to their spiritual selves; at times, however, these actions do little to nurture a person's true spirituality. Life issues that are spiritual in nature may or may not relate to religion. Knowledge of the histories, symbols, beliefs, practices, and languages of various religious traditions increases the nurse's ability to hear, recognize, and address the religious needs of patients; however, information alone about religious affiliation and practices offers only a glimpse into a person's spiritual self.

Because religion offers a particular structure for expressing spirituality, nurses may be more comfortable discussing spiritual concerns when they arise within an identifiable religious context than when they occur within a broader perspective of spirituality. Satisfying the rites and rituals of a particular religion may or may not meet all of a patient's spiritual needs. Spiritual care and interventions need to be individualized and reflect the patient's personal and cultural perspectives and worldview.[3] This is of particular concern when a patient's spirituality is not expressed through an affiliation or alignment with the practices of a particular religion, and when the patient's culture and spiritual perspective are different from that of the nurse. Holistic nursing practice recognizes that religion and spirituality are different and honors the unique ways in which people express, experience, and nurture their spiritual selves.

Understanding Spirituality

One of the barriers to incorporating spirituality into holistic nursing care is the paucity of language within Western societies for discussing and expressing matters of the spirit or soul. This difficulty with the language of spirituality is evident in the nursing literature. In Western cultures, the language used for describing and expressing spirit is generally that of science or of religion derived from the Judeo-Christian tradition. Although research related to spirituality in different cultures has increased in past years, much of the discussion of spirituality within nursing and other healthcare literature continues to reflect Judeo-Christian values and perspectives regarding the Divine, relationships with others and the world, experience of suffering, prayer, and the like. Understandings of spirituality and language describing spiritual values and experience may be different for many people in the world who do not adhere to the Judeo-Christian tradition. Because spirituality is the essence of every person and is not limited to a particular religious perspective, nurses strive to be open to, or to create a language that allows room for, each person's unique expression of spirituality.

Approaching spirituality primarily from a Western cultural perspective can lead to misinterpretation of spiritual expression and concerns. Engebretson notes that not all assumptions of Western Judeo-Christian-Islamic traditions (e.g., monotheism, transcendence, dualism) are shared with Eastern and Nature religious traditions.[4] Monotheism is a belief in one God that is above and beyond Nature, contrasted with a belief in the existence of many gods (polytheism) or the existence of the sacred in all living things (pantheism) found in Eastern and Nature religions. Transcendence, which means to exist above material existence, is implied in the Western view of God as separate from humanity. People from such Western traditions often seek connection with the Divine by focusing outward through ritual and prayer. Eastern and Nature traditions focus on immanence, the experience of the Divine within each person. Looking inward through meditation and spiritual exercises is a way of connecting with the Divine in these traditions. Dualism (the separation of spirit and matter) is a familiar concept in Western traditions, while reality is conceived as a unified whole in Eastern metaphysical traditions of monism. The polarization of science and religion found in the West reflects the impact of the assumptions of dualism on perceptions, definitions, and expectations of the spiritual experience within health care. Of special concern is the labeling of spiritual issues as pathology, or not recognizing them at all because they do not fit a familiar paradigm.

Elements of Spirituality

Increased interest in spirituality and health over the past two decades has generated many definitions and descriptions of spirituality within the healthcare literature. In many ways, however, trying to define spirituality is like trying to lasso the wind. The wind can be felt and its effect on things seen, but it cannot be contained within imposed boundaries, conceptual or otherwise. This somewhat elusive nature of spirituality poses a particular challenge for minds that feel more at home with phenomena that can be categorized, quantified, and measured. Understanding spirituality requires opening to many ways of knowing, including cognitive, intuitive, aesthetic, experiential, and deep inner sensing or knowing.

The healthcare literature provides no single agreed-upon understanding of spirituality. Elements of spirituality found in broad descriptions of the concept include the essence of being, a unifying and animating force, the life principle of each person, a sense of meaning and purpose, and a commitment to something greater than the self.[2, 5-10] Spirituality permeates life, shapes our life journey, and is vital to the process of discovering purpose, meaning, and inner strength. Although matters of spirit transcend culture, a person's cultural perspective influences personal expressions of spirituality. Personal values are rooted in and flow from spirituality and are reflected in a cultural perspective. Spirituality helps to ground one's sense of place and fit in the world. Because it is practical and relevant to daily life, people experience spirituality in the mundane as well as in the profound, the secular as well as the sacred.

A sense of trust that people have or are given the resources needed for dealing with whatever comes their way—expected or not—is a manifestation of spirituality. These resources include both strength and guidance from within and support from sources beyond themselves. Through encountering obstacles along their life path, learning through experiences, and developing new awarenesses, people gain appreciation for the ways that spirituality shapes and gives meaning to their unfolding life journey. To reach this point, people may find it necessary to reconcile new experiences with previously held values, resulting in new values and understandings. Often, the pattern of the journey and the meaning of life events become clear only in retrospect.

A sense of peace, often described as inner peace, is a spiritual attribute. Peace in this context implies a deep confidence and an ability to remain calm in the midst of the storm, to know somehow that all is well. Spiritual peace is experienced in the space of the heart and may not make sense to the cognitive mind. In the Judeo-Christian tradition, references to "a peace which passeth understanding" flow from an awareness of life beyond immediate circumstances and unbounded by the past. In the Zen tradition, practices of mindfulness foster connection with the peace that is available in every moment within every life experience. Peace is a product of living in relationship with the Sacred Source, others, and all creation in a way that acknowledges and nurtures the soul in the midst of all that life brings.

Connectedness with the Sacred Source

Research continues to demonstrate that people express and experience spirituality in the context of relationships with the Sacred Source, Nature, others, and the self.[2, 6, 8, 9] The Sacred Source may be experienced as a person, a presence, or a mystery that is beyond words. The inadequacy of language is especially apparent when we try to discuss or describe that power that is greater than us and that is within, among, and yet beyond us. From before the beginning of recorded history, humanity has searched and sought to understand the mystery of the Sacred Source. Various cultures, faith traditions, individuals, and groups use names such as Life Force, Source, God, Allah, Lord, Goddess, Absolute, Higher Power, Spirit, Vishnu, Inner Light, Tao, Great Mystery, Tunkasila, the Way, Universal Love, and the One with No Name to refer to that in which we live, move, and have as part of our being. For this discussion, this Being or Sacred Mystery is referred to as God or the Sacred Source.

A connection with the Sacred Source is at the heart of one's being. Our rational minds cannot think or grasp God, and any descriptions or words used to speak of the Sacred Source are lacking. God is far more than anything the human mind can conceptualize. Words and descriptions are, however, tools of the rational mind that can point us toward God or the Sacred Source. Concepts of God developed by the rational mind may be personal or shared within a group. Persons find and name the Sacred Source in ways that are authentic to them, using terms and language that reflect their experiences and perspectives. Connecting with the Sacred Source may involve such things as prayer, ritual, reconciliation, and stillness. Teachings of various religious traditions offer their own perspectives and guidance on how to be in relationship with the Sacred Source. Understanding how persons seek and experience connection with the Sacred Source and the obstacles they may encounter is important in spiritual caregiving.

The concept of reverence is associated with many understandings of the Sacred Source. Reverence arises from a deep appreciation of human limitations and a sense of awe in relation to what is beyond understanding and outside our control—God, truth, the natural world, even death. Awareness that the sacred is intrinsic and omnipresent engenders reverence toward the Sacred Source and all of life.[11] Reverence acknowledges that we are in and of God, yet, as Woodruff notes, it also keeps human beings from trying to act like gods.[12] Some persons do not claim a religion or give a name to that which they hold most sacred. However, they may experience a sense of reverence in their recognition of that which is beyond and greater than their own understanding, but with which they experience an often mysterious relationship.

Connectedness with Nature

Spirituality is frequently expressed and experienced in and through a sense of connectedness with Nature, the environment, and the universe. Relationship with creatures of the Earth, both wild and domesticated, provides meaning and joy for people of all ages and cultures. Awareness of all beings of the Earth, and their belonging within the natural order, is a way of connecting with the spiritual in all of life.[13] Beavers at work on a dam, red rock canyons, or bees among the flowers all illustrate the wonder of various life forms that may provide deeply spiritual experiences.

Awareness of a connectedness with the Earth and, indeed, the entire cosmos is particularly evident within indigenous spiritual traditions. A speech attributed to Chief Seattle emphasizes that all things are connected.[14] Individuals are not the weavers of the web of life; rather, each is a strand in the web. What they do to the web they do to themselves. Thus, what happens to the Earth and the environment affects them, and conversely, their choices and actions in all levels of their being affect the Earth.[11, 15] Understanding the interconnectedness of spirit and matter is basic to some traditions and known at some level in all spiritual traditions, particularly among the mystics.

Many people, particularly those who live close to the land, experience a sense of connection with the Sacred Source through Nature, regardless of their religious background. Paying close attention to the natural world and living in conscious relationship with the other-than-human beings of the world is a way of attuning more to one's own soul and spirit. People often express a particular feeling of closeness to their spiritual selves while walking on a beach, sitting by their favorite tree, viewing a sunset, listening to flowing water, watching a fire, caring for plants, and otherwise experiencing the natural order. Nature can be a source of strength, inspiration, and comfort, all of which are attributes of spirituality. A sense of awe at the wonder of life and a feeling of connectedness with all things, with or without a belief in a divine being, is an experience of spirituality. For some, connection with Nature flows from a sense of finding God in all things; many experience a relationship with the Earth and all of its creatures at an energetic level. Appreciating, respecting, and caring for the Earth and its inhabitants are elements of spirituality.

Connectedness with Others

Spirituality is known and experienced in and through relationships, with the comfort, support, conflict, and strife that mark those connections. People express and experience spirituality through an appreciation of a common bond with all humanity and in their particular relationships with others. Spirituality is shaped and nurtured within one's experience of community, beginning with one's family. The many communities, both formal and informal, in which people live provide a context for spiritual expression and development. Communities provide an opportunity for sharing spiritual journeys.

People often speak of their spirituality in terms of their relationships, both harmonious and discordant. The formation, work, nurture, and healing of relationships are an important part of one's spirituality. Being with others in loving and supportive ways is an expression of spirituality, as is struggling with painful and difficult relationships with family, friends, and acquaintances. Relationships that need healing are as important to spirituality as those that provide support and comfort. Spirituality embraces both the joys and sorrows of relationships and prompts reconciliation where connections have been frayed. Lack of connections often produces a dispiriting sense of aloneness and isolation and may lead to spiritual crisis.

Spiritual connectedness with others involves both giving and receiving. Receptive openness to Love, Light, Life, and the Sacred Source is a spiritual stance. Although it is common to think of spirituality in terms of doing for another, being able to receive from others, both the gift of themselves and the things that they do or say, is also an expression of spirituality. Indeed, the genuine presence that someone shares with another, with its implicit loving honesty and intimacy, is a manifestation of spirituality.[16-19] Spirituality is evident in both common experiences of daily living and special times shared with others: times of joy, sorrow, ritual, loving sexuality, prayer, play, encouragement, anger, reconciliation, and concern. Relationships as a source of growth and change are integral to spirituality.

Advances in technology have brought both individuals and distant and isolated countries and cultures together into a world community. Social media provides instant contact with others, including family, friends, and many strangers as well. As a result, understanding factors that create and support community has become essential. The ability to connect with people around the globe enables better understanding of how personal and collective decisions affect the larger human family. Social structures that provide a context for relationships with others often are instrumental in nurturing the spiritual dimensions of community life. Structures such as health care, educational institutions, faith-based services, social organizations, informal affiliations, social media, and Internet links with others are often places that mediate and support the spiritual dimensions of life.

Connectedness with Self

Spirituality infuses the ever-unfolding awareness of who one is—of self-becoming. The ability to be in the place of awareness that flows from spirit or soul is a pivotal element of connectedness with self. Awareness opens people to the experience of living in the moment, present to their own bodymindspirit, and allows them to receive all aspects of themselves without judgment. They experience awareness through Being, the art of stillness and presence with self, others, the Sacred Source, and Nature. Being simply is. Being includes experiencing the present moment more deeply, aware from the physical experience of all levels of one's bodymindspirit energetic self in interaction with all in the environment. Being is bringing one's whole self—alert and aware—to an experience, allowing one to pay attention to the quiet place inside and find inner peace, synchrony, harmony, and openness. Attentiveness to being allows a person to attune to sources of inner strength and deepest knowing.

Spirituality manifests and is experienced in knowing, which includes cognitive, intuitive, and energetic dimensions. Knowing provides ways of understanding our multidimensional nature and our relationships to the Sacred Source, self, others, Earth, and the cosmos. Knowing flows from a stance of openness and attuning to an inner source. It involves actively seeking knowledge and insights and maintaining an openness and receptivity to the lessons life offers. Spirituality reflected in one's knowing includes appreciation of life as a gift and a sense of connectedness to all creation.

From being and knowing flows doing, the outward and more visible aspect of spirituality. Because doing is more tangible and measurable, it is the manifestation of spirituality that is most often addressed in healthcare literature. Generally, the concept of doing brings to mind activities such as attendance at religious services or ceremonies, scripture study, prayer or meditation, participation as student or teacher in religious education, and spiritual reading. Spirituality can be demonstrated as well through actions such as assisting others, gardening, becoming involved in environmental concerns, attending to the sick, caring for family, spending time with friends, taking a walk, taking time to nurture one's own spirit, and creating sacred space for self and others.

The concept of sacred space applies both to one's inner being and to places in one's environment. Although to "create" sacred space suggests doing something, inner sacred space is often the result of being in awareness and stillness. Buildings such as religious edifices or monuments represent sacred space for many. Special places in Nature are often experienced as sacred. Any place can become sacred space if one intentionally brings awareness of the spirit into the setting. Words, actions, sounds, scents, colors, and objects may shape such spaces. A sacred space is a home for the spirit, providing rest, stillness, nurture, and opportunities for opening to various connections. A special plant in a sunlit space, a garden or workshop, a room for prayer or meditation, a corner of a porch with a rocking chair, family surrounding a loved one in a hospital bed—each space touched by the intention of those who arrange it—are examples of sacred spaces.

Spirituality and the Healing Process

In a holistic paradigm, bodymindspirit is an intertwined and interpenetrating unity; thus, every human experience has bodymindspirit components. In considering spirituality and healing, it is useful to remember that the words *healing*, *whole*, and *holy* derive from the same root: Old Saxon *hal* or *haelan*, meaning whole. This suggests that, by its nature, healing is a spiritual process that attends to the wholeness of a person. The work of healing requires recognition of the spiritual dimension of each person, including the healer, and an awareness that spirituality permeates every encounter. The shared relationship acknowledging the common humanity and connectedness between the caregiver and the receiver, which is basic to healing, is a manifestation of spirituality.

Spiritual View of Life Issues

Spiritual issues are core life issues that often draw people to look into the deepest places in their beings. These issues are not quantifiable and are more authentically expressed as questions, tentative definitions, or as mysteries that cannot be fully explained. They challenge the individual to experience life at its highest heights and deepest depths. Considerations of mystery, love, suffering, hope, forgiveness, peace and peacemaking, grace, and prayer are all inherent in the spiritual domain.

Mystery

Discovering with others the personal and unique ways that mystery is encountered on their spiritual journeys is an important part of spiritual care. Mystery is inherent to human experience and thus is inherent to spirituality. Mystery may be described as a truth that is beyond understanding and explanation. Many life experiences prompt questions of why and wonderings about what if. Appreciation of the mystery inherent in life events often sustains people in the unknowing. As people encounter that which is troubling and unexplainable, spirit recognizes mystery and helps them survive the unknowing. Spirituality supports and encourages them in the questioning and seeking that often emerge when they are faced with such mystery. The spiritual self helps them embrace both the darkness and the light, enabling them to appreciate the challenges and gifts of both.

Love

Loving presence is a key component of spiritual care. Love, which is the source of all life, fuels spirituality, prompting each person to live from the heart, the center where the ego is detached from outcomes. Love, like the spirit, is nonlocal, transcending place and time, enabling its energy to be shared for healing at many levels. The relationship of love to healing is a continuing source of exploration and wonder.[16, 20-21] In its truest sense, love is a mystery that involves both choice and emotion. It often underlies acts of courage and compassion that defy explanation. Love is both personal and universal and is experienced and expressed in both giving and receiving care. Flowing from and prompting interconnectedness, love includes dimensions of self-love, divine love, love for others, and love for all of life.

Suffering

In both its presence and its meaning, suffering is one of the core issues and mysteries of life. It occurs on physical, mental, emotional, and spiritual levels. People throughout the ages have struggled to understand the nature and meaning of suffering. Their attempts to make sense of suffering have shaped cultural and religious traditions. Suffering may be a transformative experience, the nature of the transformation varying with each individual. For some, suffering enhances spiritual awareness; for others, suffering appears meaningless and engenders feelings of anger and frustration. One interpretation of burnout among healthcare professionals is that it represents the inability to find ways to tend the spirit as one suffers the suffering of another.

Sociocultural, religious, familial, and environmental factors influence an individual's response to suffering. Thus, having knowledge of personality, culture, religious traditions, and family background is helpful in understanding the nature and meaning of suffering for a particular person. In the same vein, nurses who are aware of their own responses to and understanding of suffering are less likely to confuse their perceptions with those of the patient. This awareness enables nurses to be more fully present in an intentional, healing way with those who are suffering. Such presence allows nurses to discern whether honoring another's suffering requires action, presence, absence, or a combination of these. The ability to be with another who is suffering is crucial, particularly when nurses confront suffering that cannot be alleviated and must simply be borne. Such presence supports a person's spiritual journey toward discovering transcendent meaning within the experience.[21] Listening with one's whole being as another wonders aloud and expresses deep feelings regarding some of life's unanswered questions is a critical part of being with those who suffer.

Hope

Hope, a desire accompanied by an expectation of fulfillment, goes beyond believing or wishing. Hope is future oriented yet grounded in the present moment. The saying "hope springs eternal" reflects this energy of the spirit and prompts the anticipation that tomorrow things will be better, or at least different. There are two levels of hope: The first, specific hope, implies a goal or desire for a particular event or outcome. The second is a more general sense of hope that the future is somehow in safekeeping. Hope is

a significant factor in overcoming illness and in living through difficult situations.[22,23] It helps people deal with fear and uncertainty and enables them to envision positive outcomes.

Forgiveness

Ultimately a matter of self-healing, forgiveness is a deep need and hunger of the human experience. Religious beliefs, cultural traditions, family upbringing, and personal experience all help to shape an individual's attitudes about forgiveness, both given and received. Beliefs about the nature of God or the Sacred Source influence one's ability to offer and receive forgiveness. Difficulties with forgiving others, forgiving oneself, and accepting forgiveness from others often relate to a misunderstanding of the nature of forgiveness. Forgiveness is something one does for oneself, not for others. Forgiveness does not necessarily mean forgetting, condoning, absolving, or sacrificing; rather, it is a process of extending love and compassion to self and others.[24-26] An act of the heart, forgiveness is an internal process of releasing intense emotions attached to incidents from the past, releasing any need to carry grudges, resentments, hatred, self-pity, or desire to punish people who have done hurtful acts, and accepting that no punishment of others will promote internal healing. Forgiveness, a sign of positive self-esteem, allows a person to put the past in proper perspective, free energy once consumed by grudges and resentments, nurse unhealed wounds, and use this energy for opening to healing and moving on with life.

Self-forgiveness—releasing the desire or need to berate or punish oneself for past actions—is an important part of forgiveness and is essential for spiritual growth and healing. Self-forgiveness is not about regret or guilt but rather concerns acknowledgment of responsibility for one's choices and actions. Self-forgiveness is a gift to oneself that provides an opportunity to remove the energetic consequences from past actions and thoughts. Through acknowledgment of personal responsibility for past thoughts and actions, and the willingness to let go of any energetic attachment to these thoughts and actions, the cumulative energy of these actions is released so that they will not adversely affect the self. The notion of free will—that the actual or energetic result of one's actions and thoughts cannot be bypassed by God or the universe—is basic to self-forgiveness. The following analogy illustrates the self-forgiveness process: If you go for a walk and along the way get a sharp pebble in your shoe, every step from that point on is painful. The more you walk, the more it hurts. The pebble will cause pain and potential harm to the foot as long as it is in the shoe. Healing cannot take place as long as the pebble is irritating the foot; however, once the pebble is removed, the body can begin the healing process. Self-forgiveness, like taking the pebble out, enables the natural self-healing energy that is a part of the universe to begin and gives all of God's grace room to provide comfort.

Peace and Peacemaking

Peace, for many people, is inseparable from justice. Inner peace reflects a way of being, a space from which one is able to live and be in ways that nurture and heal. This peace does not depend on external circumstances; it flows from the connections that sustain us. Spiritual practices from many traditions sustain people and help them align with an inner peace in the midst of trials and hardships. Today as in the past, many people throughout the world are experiencing brutal trials. Living as peacemakers in times and places of uncertainty, fear, injustice, and war is a spiritual challenge facing all citizens of the world, and it demands courageous and creative solutions. The work of peacemaking is grounded in the awareness that:

> There is an inherent power in rightness, in goodness in love, and in love of peace, and that if even a single individual chooses to act rightly and truthfully and peacefully in the midst of tempting and contrary choices, the power of that act and aspiration can change the world. By extension, if untold numbers of single individuals love peace enough, seek peace enough, stand for peace enough, are themselves persons of peace, the ideal of peace will become the world's transforming reality.[27]

As persons appreciate and live in the reality of their connection with others and all creation across distance, time, and space, the possibility of peace with justice grows.

Grace

Experiences of grace contain elements of surprise, awe, mystery, and gratitude. Grace is often experienced as a support that is unplanned and unexpected. An experience of grace may touch one's spirit in deep and profound ways and may be life changing. Grace opens one's awareness to the experience of wholeness, healing, and connectedness. Grace is reflected in statements such as the following:

- He just showed up at the door right when I needed him.
- I didn't know how I was going to pay for everything; then, this check arrived.
- I don't know why my spirits lifted that morning; perhaps it was the rain after such a long drought.
- I didn't think I could stand another bout of chemotherapy, but my friend said she will go with me and we'll take one day at a time.
- My CT scan was clear for the third time, something that the doctors didn't expect and that I didn't dare hope for.

Although some see such happenings as coincidence or chance, others sense something deeper that connects persons within the web of life and enables us to find acceptance, courage, peace, and endurance beyond our own making or understanding. Grace is often spoken of as a gift from the Sacred Source, or from Life itself, that enables, assists, and empowers a person in the midst of difficult and sometimes seemingly overwhelming circumstances. The experience of grace as a blessing that comes into one's life unearned calls forth a response of gratitude.

Prayer

An expression of the spirit, prayer is a deep human instinct that flows from the core of one's being where the longing for and awareness of one's connectedness with the source of life are blended. Prayer represents a longing for communion or communication with God or the Sacred Source. The most fundamental, primordial, and important language that humans speak, prayer is an endeavor that starts and ends without words. In this understanding, prayer flows from yearnings of the soul that rise from a place too deep for words and move to a space beyond words.

Forms and expressions of prayer are as varied as the people who pray. Prayer, which is intrinsic to many religious traditions and rituals, may be public or private, individual or communal. It is not always a fully conscious activity. Speaking (sometimes silently), singing, chanting, listening, waiting, moaning, being attuned to what is going on in the present moment, and being silent can all be elements of prayer. Prayer includes petition, intercession, confession, lamentation, adoration, invocation, thanksgiving, being, and showing care and concern for others. Some people incorporate processes and techniques such as relaxation, quieting, breath awareness, focusing, imagery, and visualization into their prayer. Movement such as walking, dancing, or drumming may be expressions of prayer. A reminder of our nonlocal, unbounded nature, prayer is infinite in space and time. It is divine, the universe's affirmation that we are not alone.[28]

That prayer is an appropriate consideration for nursing is grounded in the writings of Florence Nightingale.[29, 30] Research affirms the truth that people have known for ages: Prayer can affect healing.[31-34] Both directed prayer, which focuses on a specific outcome, and nondirected prayer, which focuses on the greatest good of the organism, can affect healing and other outcomes, although nondirected prayer may be more effective. Even at a distance, prayer alters processes in a variety of organisms, including plants and people. Furthermore, the observed effects of prayer do not depend on what the one prayed for thinks. In his book *Be Careful What You Pray For*, Dossey reminds us that prayer is a potent force that is best used thoughtfully, with care and discernment.[35]

Spiritual and Psychological Dimensions

The term *psyche* means soul or spirit, reflecting the relationship between the spiritual and the psychological that is evident even in the spoken language. Before the time of Freud, phenomena of the sentient realm that could not be explained physically often were considered matters of the spirit and viewed in religious terms. With the advent and ongoing development of psychology, matters of the soul often have been subsumed into psychological theory and frequently interpreted as pathology. Within a holistic paradigm, spiritual and psychological elements are interconnected because the bodymindspirit is an integrated whole. Failing to differentiate the spiritual and psychological dimensions, however, can lead nurses to miss cues regarding spiritual concerns and thus inappropriately label spiritual issues as psychopathology. Consider, for example, a 90-year-old deeply spiritual man who was active and independent until sustaining a compression fracture of his lower spine. He exhibits obvious distress related to pain and his limited mobility. When he says he is praying for God to take him home, a holistic nurse recognizes the need to differentiate between spiritual concerns related to meaning, purpose, and suffering, and psychological concerns such as depression or even suicide risk. Although spiritual awakenings and deepenings may be accompanied by elements of psychological distress, the "dark night of the soul" may be a significant aspect of the process of moving to greater awareness, enlightenment, and healing. Fortunately, many contemporary psychological models address the spiritual dimension.

Unlike Eastern and indigenous traditions around the world, Western traditions have only a limited familiarity and comfort with the spiritual nature of different levels of awareness. The misinterpretation of behaviors, emotions, and reactions associated with individual experiences and expressions of the spiritual is keenly evident in the life of Florence Nightingale and the many interpretations of her life.[30, 36, 37] Some have interpreted the behaviors and health concerns evident throughout her life after her return from the Crimea as psychological pathology, such as anxiety, neurosis, malingering, depression, and stress burnout. Approaching Nightingale's life from a spiritual as well as psychological perspective, however, allowed Dossey to recognize Nightingale for the mystic that she was.[30, 36] In a similar vein, appreciating the difference between spiritual and psychological domains enables nurses to assess spiritual cues and spiritual crises more effectively, as well as to recognize opportunities to foster spiritual growth.

Spirituality in Holistic Nursing

Nurturing the Spirit

The way that nurses care for and nurture themselves influences their ability to function effectively in a healing role with another. The spiritual path is a life path. Attentiveness to one's own spirit is a key component of living in a healing way and is foundational to integrating spirituality into clinical practice. Care of their spirit or soul requires nurses to pause to reflect on and absorb what is happening within and around them; to take time for themselves, for relationships, and for other things that animate them; and to be mindful about nourishing their spirits. The many ways nurses nurture their spirits and respond to their spiritual concerns are the same as those that they suggest to their patients.

Care of the spirit is a professional nursing responsibility and an intrinsic part of holistic nursing. Within a holistic perspective, providing spiritual care is an ethical obligation, which, if ignored, deprives patients of their dignity as human beings. As an interpersonal, intuitive, altruistic, and integrative expression, spiritual caregiving draws on the nurse's awareness of the transcendent dimension and is grounded in the patient's reality.[8, 38] Nurses must become competent and confident with spiritual caregiving, expanding their skills in assessing the spiritual domain and developing and implementing appropriate interventions. A persistent barrier to incorporating spirituality into clinical practice is the fear of imposing particular religious values and beliefs on others. Nurses who integrate spirituality into their care of others recognize that although each person acts out of and is informed by her or his own spiritual perspective, acting from this foundation is not the same as imposing these beliefs and values on another. In fact, many practitioners believe that the more they are grounded in an awareness of

their own spiritual journey, the less likely they are to impose their values and beliefs on others.

Assessing and Investigating Spirituality in Practice and Research

The literature reflects attempts to make sense of spirituality within a scientific frame of reference, and clinicians and researchers continue to struggle with the inherent difficulties of assessing and measuring a phenomenon that defies definition. Many researchers approach the study of spirituality primarily through examining religious beliefs and practices. This approach can be problematic, however, in that many people do not express their spirituality within a religious tradition; conversely, religious practices do not necessarily indicate a person's true spirituality. Using assessment scales in research on spirituality that reflect a strong bias toward particular traditions or beliefs may suggest that those who do not ascribe to these traditions may not be spiritual. Cultural sensitivity is an essential part of spirituality assessment in both practice and research.

Developing credible quantitative instruments for spiritual inquiry may facilitate a more formal integration of spirituality assessment into health care by including such instruments in a patient's medical record. However, attempts to quantify spirituality, even with more broadly applicable scales, are at best a reflection of a particular perspective of spirituality as understood through the lens of the concepts included in the scale. Appreciating the elusive nature of spiritual phenomena, nurses recognize that an individual's spiritual journey may have many facets and meanings that are not captured within the limitations of a particular scale. Providing opportunities to explore personal meaning and understanding with patients is essential to effective spirituality assessment. A goal of holistic nursing is to know a person in the fullness and complexity of her or his wholeness. Knowledge obtained about a person through any process of assessment is not an end in itself; rather, it is useful inasmuch as it contributes to understanding and knowing more of the essence of the person. Listening and intentional presence are key to exploring individual meanings associated with a patient's spiritual journey.

Listening and Intentional Presence

Attentive listening and focused presence are at the heart of caring for the spirit, and they are essential in any approach to spirituality assessment. This concept is simple in many ways but requires intention and conscious attention. Good therapeutic communication skills facilitate the exploration of spiritual issues. Broad, open-ended questions are often useful. Questions and statements such as "Tell me more about . . . ," "Help me to understand what you need," "I don't understand what you are trying to say," and "What was that like for you?" are useful as nurses seek a deeper understanding of their patients. Creating a sacred space in which spirituality can be expressed and being clear about one's own spiritual perspective enhance a nurse's facility with spirituality assessments. Practicing spiritual disciplines such as prayer, centering, awareness, and meditation make it easier for nurses to be fully present, available to be with and listen to another. In the face of distractions from within and without, the nurse's healing presence is enhanced by the ability to focus on the relationship with a particular person in a particular moment.

One of the gifts of intentional, active listening is that the client, in sharing with an openhearted and fully present listener, often hears herself or himself with greater clarity and understanding. Such a listener provides a safe space for expression of negative as well as positive feelings and experiences and time for complexities to be pondered. The contradictions, pains, questions, and struggles are heard without judgment or advice. As the richness and complexity of the situation are taken in more fully, the person moves into the future with increased awareness.

Holistic nurses assess their own abilities as listeners and consider barriers to intentional listening that are part of their personal journeys. There may be topics that make one uncomfortable. Although discomfort alone need not make one an unsuitable listener, being aware of one's discomfort, and its source and manifestations, is an important part of a self-evaluation. Recognizing how external distractions such as the environment or time pressures affect their ability to listen may help nurses become more conscious listeners. Awareness of how body posture conveys presence and attention enables nurses to be more present in the moment. A hospice patient illustrated an experience of intentional listening and presence in describing his relationship with one of the hospice workers on his team:

> feel good to see him come in. One day he and I both fell asleep, kind of took a nap for a bit. He probably knows as much about me as anyone—because he's the kind of guy who's interested in everything I talk about, my family, my worries, my sickness. Sometimes he asks a question, but mostly he just listens—but I mean really listens, like he wants to know about whatever is on my mind.

Intentional listening and presence foster authenticity in the nursing process. Such listening and presence demand a recognition of both verbal and nonverbal cues in communication, and the validation by the patient of any of the nurse's interpretations. In reflecting on personal experiences of intentional listening, nurses might ask themselves the following questions: When have I been intentionally present for another, listening with my whole being and with an open heart? Which factors, internal and external, help me to listen attentively or make that difficult for me? When have I been in the presence of one who was fully present for me? How did I recognize that full presence? How did that affect me?

The core of active listening and healing presence lies in the intention and attention of the nurse who recognizes all persons as spiritual beings. **Exhibit 7-1** lists important considerations for nurses as they strive to listen in healing ways to their clients. According to Bruchac, "It all begins with listening. There are stories all around us, but many people don't notice those stories because they don't take the time to listen."[39]

Using Story and Metaphor in Spiritual Care

Recognizing all persons, including themselves, as ongoing and unfolding stories offers nurses a valuable perspective from which to approach

---

EXHIBIT 7-1   Listening in Healing Ways

- Be intentionally present.

- Maintain focus on the patient/client as a whole person.

- Set aside the need to fix, answer, or correct.

- Learn to be with another in silence.

- Interrupt as little as possible, recognizing that even what is not said at a particular time has meaning and that the way and sequence in which a story is told are part of the story.

- View the other as embodied spirit, an ongoing and unfinished story.

- Hear the journey, the relationships, and the meanings in the story.

- Listen with all your senses.

- Do not prematurely diagnose.

- Let the conversation flow, being with silence as well as words.

- Breathe!

Source: M. G. Nagai-Jacobson and M. Burkhardt, © 1997.

---

spiritual caregiving.[2, 40, 41] Story and metaphor often provide a language and form for conveying the richness of one's spirituality when factual statements of experience fail to do so. Stories bring people enjoyment, teach them to solve problems, help them form identities, and are wonderful teachers. Sharing stories helps people to understand themselves and their world. Through the vehicle of story, people learn to know one another and themselves from many perspectives. Stories reveal experiences of relationships, emotions, conflicts, struggles, and responses that are at once personal and universal. Nurses become part of the life stories of those for whom they care. Nurses' own life stories inform and form them, and understanding those stories deepens the awareness with which they hear another's story.

Listening and encouraging people to share their stories can be both assessment and intervention in spiritual care. Stories make it possible to move beyond physical symptoms, diagnoses, and theoretical constructs, which may be similar for any number of patients. Attentiveness to story allows nurses another glimpse into the wholeness and uniqueness of each person and the particular way in which he or she fits into the family and community. As an assessment

approach, story and metaphor provide insight into spiritual concerns such as supportive and disruptive relationships, questions of meaning, values and purpose, issues of forgiveness, hope and hopelessness, and experiences of grace. Listening is a reminder that life stories are ongoing and unfinished.

The sharing of story and metaphor can also be a nursing intervention. In sharing with a fully present listener, patients hear their own stories with new insights and appreciation for their own lives—affirmations and validations, conflicts and struggles, questions of meaning and dark times—life in its variety and fullness. In a safe space, patients can express fears and perceived failures, hopes and wonderings, disappointments and achievements, as they consider pages of their life stories. Through this process, patients come to see themselves more clearly and, in an atmosphere of acceptance, accept themselves in their full humanity. From such a stance, patients are able to participate more consciously in the present situation. The case of Mr. M. is an example of the power of the story:

> Mr. M. has been diagnosed with probable cancer of the lungs and is scheduled for exploratory surgery in a few

days. Several times he has asked the nurse, "How serious do you think this is?" After he asks once again, the nurse says, "Mr. M., you seem to be asking me more than how serious this is. Can you tell me more about what is concerning you?" He responds, "Well, to be honest, I've been thinking about telling the kids . . . especially my son in Chicago. You see, we haven't been on very good terms." And so begins an important story for Mr. M. to tell and for the nurse to hear. The medical information about Mr. M.'s illness is but one piece of the greater fabric of his life as a family man and father. The nurse now hears Mr. M. talk about his concerns for his family and the relationships within the family as his upcoming surgery and uncertain future affect them. In telling his story, Mr. M. participates in both the assessment and intervention related to his spiritual care. The nurse learns about his relationships and his concerns surrounding them, and Mr. M. begins to understand what the most important aspects of his situation are from his unique perspective. With that understanding, he can begin to plan what he will do and what help he will seek. The nurse becomes a partner in his plan, which will be revised and updated as his story continues to unfold.

Sharing a story brings the listener face to face with quandaries, insights, struggles, joy, suffering, pain, and healing moments. Stories may make the listener feel helpless in the face of perceived hopeless situations or help the listener recognize the hope that lies in such a situation. Stories challenge nurses to understand the wholeness of a person and to listen for the meaning of a life. One nurse commented:

> I used to think that people who told me stories about their lives were just wasting my time and theirs, but now I realize that they are telling me about what is really important. I've learned to listen and to use what they say to help

them see who they really are, what they can really do. Even when they tell me things that are really hard to hear, or even to understand, it seems like they just want me to know that it is part of their life, too.

Stories help the nursing process fit the patient rather than requiring the patient to fit the process.

Some shared wonderings and questions that may help others tell their stories include the following:

- If you were writing your life story, what would be the title?
- What is the title of the current chapter?
- Who are some of the heroines and heroes of your story?
- How would you like this chapter to turn out?
- Tell me more about how you handled your child's accident.
- I wonder where you get your spunk.
- I wonder what it's like to live with your physical limitations.
- You've mentioned several times that your sister is ill, and you seem worried.

Nurses can affirm the sharing of stories through statements such as "Your sharing has helped me see this in a different light." As nurses encourage clients to share their stories, it is helpful to encourage the significant people in the clients' lives to participate in the process. The exercises presented in **Exhibit 7-2** may increase attentiveness to story, both among nurses themselves and with clients.

Using Guides and Instruments to Facilitate Spirituality Assessment

Different approaches to assessing spirituality are available to facilitate the integration of spirituality into holistic care. When incorporated into a clinical setting, spirituality assessment guides are a means of gaining a deeper understanding of a person from a holistic perspective. Rather than considering the completion of an instrument to be an end point, nurses can use the questions of an assessment guide

---

EXHIBIT 7-2   Exercises to Facilitate Awareness of Story

1. Take a few moments to become quiet, perhaps using some breath awareness. In this quiet space, allow yourself to remember, in as much detail as possible, something about yourself, some event or incident that comes to mind. How has this experience or event become a part of who you are? What meaning does it have for your life at this moment?

2. Keep a journal in which you record events, feelings, experiences, insights, and questions in your life. Periodically review your writings, noting themes flowing through your story. Reflect on your story as it keeps evolving.

3. Think about books, stories, songs, fairy tales, movies, plays, or works of art that have special meaning for you. Take time to consider why and how they hold that meaning for you. Think about the images, characters, colors, and sounds that are found in each of these and how they are reflective of your own story. What meanings do you find that provide insight into your own unfolding journey?

4. Write an autobiography for your eyes only. Take your time. Reread and reflect on it. Are there parts you want to share? With whom would you share? What new awareness and insights into yourself and your life journey have come to you?

5. Look at some old family photos or photos of friends. What story do they tell? What memories and feelings come with these pictures? Do you want to tell someone else about them? What do you want to say? Would you like to hear someone else's story about these same photos?

Source: M. Burkhardt and M. G. Nagai-Jacobson, © 1997.

---

as openings or reference points for discussing spirituality with patients and thus come to know and understand them better as unique persons. Furthermore, nurses can adapt the various guides to the specific situation and person. Assessing a person's understanding of spirituality and ways of expressing spirituality includes exploring the role and influence of important connections in the present circumstances; issues related to meaning and purpose; important beliefs, values, and practices; prayer or meditation styles; and desire for connection with religious groups or rituals. Many instruments and approaches for assessing spirituality have been developed in recent years. The discussion that follows highlights a few examples of different approaches to assessing spirituality developed from a nursing perspective.

The Spiritual Assessment Tool (see **Exhibit 7-3**) is based on a conceptual analysis of spirituality

---

EXHIBIT 7-3   Spiritual Assessment Tool

To facilitate the healing process in clients/patients, families, significant others, and yourself, the following reflective questions assist in assessing, evaluating, and increasing awareness of the spiritual process in yourself and others.

Meaning and purpose: These questions assess a person's ability to seek meaning and fulfillment in life, manifest hope, and accept ambiguity and uncertainty.

- What gives your life meaning?
- Do you have a sense of purpose in life?
- Does your illness interfere with your life goals?
- Why do you want to get well?
- How hopeful are you about obtaining a better degree of health?
- Do you feel that you have a responsibility in maintaining your health?
- Will you be able to make changes in your life to maintain your health?

(continues)

EXHIBIT 7-3   Spiritual Assessment Tool (*continued*)

- Are you motivated to get well?
- What is the most important or powerful thing in your life?

Inner strengths: These questions assess a person's ability to manifest joy and recognize strengths, choices, goals, and faith.

- What brings you joy and peace in your life?
- What can you do to feel alive and full of spirit?
- What traits do you like about yourself?
- What are your personal strengths?
- What choices are available to you to enhance your healing?
- What life goals have you set for yourself?
- Do you think that stress in any way caused your illness?
- How aware were you of your body before you became sick?
- What do you believe in?
- Is faith important in your life?
- How has your illness influenced your faith?
- Does faith play a role in regaining your health?

Interconnections: These questions assess a person's positive self-concept, self-esteem, and sense of self; sense of belonging in the world with others; capacity to pursue personal interests; and ability to demonstrate love of self and self-forgiveness.

- How do you feel about yourself right now?
- How do you feel when you have a true sense of yourself?
- Do you pursue things of personal interest?
- What do you do to show love for yourself?
- Can you forgive yourself?
- What do you do to heal your spirit?

These next questions assess a person's ability to connect in life-giving ways with family, friends, and social groups and to engage in the forgiveness of others.

- Who are the significant people in your life?
- Do you have friends or family in town who are available to help you?
- Who are the people to whom you are closest?
- Do you belong to any groups?
- Can you ask people for help when you need it?
- Can you share your feelings with others?
- What are some of the most loving things that others have done for you?
- What are the loving things that you do for other people?
- Are you able to forgive others?

These next questions assess a person's capacity for finding meaning in worship or religious activities and a connectedness with a divinity or universe.

- Is worship important to you?
- What do you consider the most significant act of worship in your life?

EXHIBIT 7-3   Spiritual Assessment Tool (*continued*)

- Do you participate in any religious activities?
- Do you believe in God or a higher power?
- Do you think that prayer is powerful?
- Have you ever tried to empty your mind of all thoughts to see what the experience might be like?
- Do you use relaxation or imagery skills?
- Do you meditate?
- Do you pray?
- What is your prayer?
- How are your prayers answered?
- Do you have a sense of belonging in this world?

These next questions assess a person's ability to experience a sense of connection with all of life and Nature, an awareness of the effects of the environment on life and well-being, and a capacity or concern for the health of the environment.

- Do you ever feel at some level a connection with the world or universe?
- How does your environment have an impact on your state of well-being?
- What are your environmental stressors at work and at home?
- Do you incorporate strategies to reduce your environment stressors?
- Do you have any concerns for the state of your immediate environment?
- Are you involved with environmental issues such as recycling environmental resources at home, work, or in your community?
- Are you concerned about the survival of the planet?

Source: Based on M. Burkhardt, "Spirituality: An Analysis of the Concept," *Holistic Nursing Practice* 3, no. 3 (1989): 69.

derived from Burkhardt's critical review of the literature.[42] This instrument poses open-ended, reflective questions that assist nurses in developing awareness of spirituality for themselves and others. These questions are meant to be prompts to focus on pertinent spiritual concerns. Similar types of questions are equally appropriate. Some areas may be addressed more fully than others, depending on a particular client's needs. This instrument is meant to be a guide for nurses, to support and enhance their comfort and skills with spirituality assessment, and is not designed as a self-administered survey.

Howden's Spirituality Assessment Scale (SAS), presented in **Exhibit 7-4**, is a 28-item instrument based on a conceptualization of spirituality as a phenomenon represented by four critical attributes.[43] These attributes and the corresponding items on the scale are as follows:

1. *Purpose and meaning in life.* The process of searching for or discovering events or relationships that provide a sense of worth, hope, or reason for existence (Items 18, 20, 22, 28)
2. *Innerness or inner resources.* The process of striving for or discovering wholeness, identity, and a sense of empowerment, manifested in feelings of strength in times of crisis and calmness or serenity in dealing with uncertainty in life, a sense of being guided in living and being at peace with oneself and the world, and feelings of ability (Items 8, 10, 12, 14, 16, 17, 23, 24, 27)
3. *Unifying interconnectedness.* The feeling of relatedness or attachment to others, a

EXHIBIT 7-4   Spirituality Assessment Scale

DIRECTIONS: Please indicate your response by circling the appropriate letters indicating how you respond to the statements.
MARK:

SA	if you STRONGLY AGREE
A	if you AGREE
AM	if you AGREE MORE than DISAGREE
DM	if you DISAGREE MORE than AGREE
D	if you DISAGREE
SD	if you STRONGLY DISAGREE

There is no right or wrong answer. Please respond to what you think or how you feel at this point in time.

1. I have a general sense of belonging.	SA	A	AM	DM	S	SD
2. I am able to forgive people who have done me wrong.	SA	A	AM	DM	S	SD
3. I have the ability to rise above or go beyond a physical or psychological condition.	SA	A	AM	DM	S	SD
4. I am concerned about destruction of the environment.	SA	A	AM	DM	S	SD
5. I have experienced moments of peace in a devastating event.	SA	A	AM	DM	S	SD
6. I feel a kinship to other people.	SA	A	AM	DM	S	SD
7. I feel a connection to all of life.	SA	A	AM	DM	S	SD
8. I rely on an inner strength in hard times.	SA	A	AM	DM	S	SD
9. I enjoy being of service to others.	SA	A	AM	DM	S	SD
10. I can go to a spiritual dimension within myself for guidance.	SA	A	AM	DM	S	SD
11. I have the ability to rise above or go beyond a body change or body loss.	SA	A	AM	DM	S	SD
12. I have a sense of harmony or inner peace.	SA	A	AM	DM	S	SD
13. I have the ability for self-healing.	SA	A	AM	DM	S	SD
14. I have an inner strength.	SA	A	AM	DM	S	SD
15. The boundaries of my universe extend beyond usual ideas of what space and time are thought to be.	SA	A	AM	DM	S	SD
16. I feel good about myself.	SA	A	AM	DM	S	SD
17. I have a sense of balance in my life.	SA	A	AM	DM	S	SD
18. There is fulfillment in my life.	SA	A	AM	DM	S	SD
19. I feel a responsibility to preserve the planet.	SA	A	AM	DM	S	SD
20. The meaning I have found for my life provides a sense of peace.	SA	A	AM	DM	S	SD
21. Even when I feel discouraged, I trust that life is good.	SA	A	AM	DM	S	SD
22. My life has meaning and purpose.	SA	A	AM	DM	S	SD
23. My innerness or an inner resource helps me deal with uncertainty in life.	SA	A	AM	DM	S	SD
24. I have discovered my own strength in times of struggle.	SA	A	AM	DM	S	SD

EXHIBIT 7-4	Spirituality Assessment Scale (*continued*)						
25. Reconciling relationships is important to me.		SA	A	AM	DM	S	SD
26. I feel a part of the community in which I live.		SA	A	AM	DM	S	SD
27. My inner strength is related to belief in a Higher Power or Supreme Being.		SA	A	AM	DM	S	SD
28. I have goals and aims for my life.		SA	A	AM	DM	S	SD

Source: Judy W. Howden, Development and Psychometric Characteristics of the Spirituality Assessment Scale, Copyright © 1992, Judy W. Howden. Texas Women's University.

sense of relationship to all of life, a feeling of harmony with self and others, and a feeling of oneness with the universe or Universal Being (Items 1, 2, 4, 6, 7, 9, 19, 25, 26).

4. *Transcendence.* The ability to reach or go beyond the limits of usual experience; the capacity, willingness, or experience of rising above or overcoming body or psychic conditions; or the capacity for achieving wellness or self-healing (Items 3, 5, 11, 13, 15, 21)

The SAS is a 6-point response-rating scale that uses the following numerical rating: strongly disagree (SD) = 1; disagree (D) = 2; disagree more than agree (DM) = 3; agree more than disagree (AM) = 4; agree (A) = 5; strongly agree (SA) = 6. There is no neutral option. It is scored by summing the responses to all 28 items; subscale scores may be obtained by summing the responses to subscale items.

Another quantitative assessment, the Spirituality Scale (SS), shown in **Exhibit 7-5**, was developed by Delaney as a way to holistically assess beliefs, practices, lifestyle choices, intuitions, and rituals that represent the human spiritual dimension.[44] The SS is a 23-item questionnaire designed to measure the essence of spirituality and guide spiritual interventions in diverse nursing settings. The SS focuses on three domains of spirituality: self-discovery—related to meaning and purpose in life (4 items); relationships—connections with others based on respect and reverence for life (6 items); and eco-awareness—connection with Nature based on the belief that Earth is sacred (13 items). Delaney suggests that the scores of the SS (range 23–138) indicate the relative importance of

spirituality to the person, with high scores suggesting that spirituality is more evident in the person's life.

The usefulness of numerical scores derived from quantitative spirituality assessment instruments may be more apparent within the context of a research study. In a clinical setting, however, scales such as the SAS or SS can enable a nurse to gain an overall sense of a person's spirituality, either when administering the instrument or when discussing it with a client who has already completed it. The pattern of responses to individual items, more than a numerical score, provides nurses with insights into areas of spiritual strengths and concerns, enabling them to support the strengths and address the concerns. For example, discovering that a person may be experiencing a lack of kinship with others and a lack of connection to life enables the nurse to explore these concerns further and plan appropriate interventions. In the clinical arena, nurses need to remember that a quantitative measure should be an adjunct to, but not a replacement for, listening presence.

Barker offers another approach to spirituality assessment in her Personal Spiritual Well-Being Assessment (PSWBA) and Spiritual Well-Being Assessment (SWBA), presented in **Exhibit 7-6**.[45, 46] These instruments, which originate in her clinical experiences and research, were developed initially as a short process for assessing spiritual well-being among cancer patients. The SWBA is intended for use by clinicians as they elicit information about the patient's place in the spiritual walk. The PSWBA was originally intended for use by clinicians in determining and clarifying their own spiritual well-being prior to addressing the spiritual well-being of

EXHIBIT 7-5   Spirituality Scale

Please indicate your level of agreement with the following statements by circling the appropriate number that corresponds with the answer key.

KEY

1. Strongly disagree
2. Disagree
3. Mostly disagree
4. Mostly agree
5. Agree
6. Strongly agree

1. I find meaning in my life experiences.	1	2	3	4	5	6
2. I have a sense of purpose.	1	2	3	4	5	6
3. I am happy about the person I have become.	1	2	3	4	5	6
4. I see the sacredness in everyday life.	1	2	3	4	5	6
5. I meditate to gain access to my inner spirit.	1	2	3	4	5	6
6. I live in harmony with nature.	1	2	3	4	5	6
7. I believe there is a connection between all things that I cannot see but can sense.	1	2	3	4	5	6
8. My life is a process of becoming.	1	2	3	4	5	6
9. I believe in a Higher Power or Universal Intelligence.	1	2	3	4	5	6
10. I believe that all living creatures deserve respect.	1	2	3	4	5	6
11. The earth is sacred.	1	2	3	4	5	6
12. I value maintaining and nurturing my relationships with others.	1	2	3	4	5	6
13. I use silence to get in touch with myself.	1	2	3	4	5	6
14. I believe that nature should be respected.	1	2	3	4	5	6
15. I have a relationship with a Higher Power or Universal Intelligence.	1	2	3	4	5	6
16. My spirituality gives me inner strength.	1	2	3	4	5	6
17. I am able to receive love from others.	1	2	3	4	5	6
18. My faith in a Higher Power or Universal Intelligence helps me cope during challenges in my life.	1	2	3	4	5	6
19. I strive to correct the excesses in my own lifestyle patterns/practices.	1	2	3	4	5	6
20. I respect the diversity of people.	1	2	3	4	5	6
21. Prayer is an integral part of my spiritual nature.	1	2	3	4	5	6
22. At times, I feel at one with the universe.	1	2	3	4	5	6
23. I often take time to assess my life choices as a way of living my spirituality.	1	2	3	4	5	6

Note: Those interested in using the Spirituality Scale for clinical or research purposes are asked to contact Dr. Colleen Delaney, RN, PhD, AHN-BC, Associate Professor, University of Connecticut, 231 Glenbrook Rd., Storrs, CT 06269-2026, Colleen.Delaney@uconn.edu.

Source: © Copyright 2003, C. Delaney.

EXHIBIT 7-6   Spiritual Well-Being Assessment Instruments

Personal Spiritual Well-Being Assessment

Relationship to Self

Overall, in the last month, I feel _____ about myself.

Overall, this feeling is _____.

Overall, my "well" feels _____.

Relationship to God/Creative Source

Overall, in the last month, my sense of connection to God/my Creative Source is

_____.

Overall, I feel a purpose to being where I am today _____.

Overall, I feel _____ about my place in the world.

Relationship to Others

I feel most connected to _____.

This connection feels _____.

Overall, my relationships are _____.

I have one intimate relationship _____.

This relationship brings me _____.

Relationship to Nature

My favorite part of creation is _____.

The last time I was able to experience this part of creation was _____.

When I experienced this part of creation, I felt _____.

Spiritual Well-Being Assessment

What is (the illness or other concern) _____ like for you?

What do you do to cope with (the illness or other concern)? _____

What makes you smile? _____

If you could be anywhere, where would you be? _____

What relationships are most important to you? _____

How can I help? _____

Source: E. R. Barker, Copyright © 1996.

---

others, but it may be useful with patients as well. The respondent is asked to verbalize thoughts regarding the key guiding questions. Each instrument uses four broad facets of spiritual well-being: relationship to self, relationship to God/Creative Source, relationship to others, and relationship to Nature. Although this type of assessment format can be self-administered, a greater depth of information and insight can be gained from an interactive process that allows for an exploration of responses.

Barker cautioned nurses to be aware of certain barriers related to spiritual well-being assessment. These barriers include believing that there is not enough time to do the assessment, being embarrassed about asking the questions, thinking that doing the assessment means that the nurse has to solve all of the patient's problems (rescue fantasy), doubting that the nurse can make a difference in the patient's life, feeling responsible for the patient's place in the cosmos, and accepting responsibility for the patient's choices. When experiencing such reactions, nurses can utilize the PSWBA or other processes to explore their own understanding of spirituality, to develop the necessary skills, and to become comfortable with this area of holistic nursing care.

Burkhardt's Care and Nurture of the Spiritual Self—Personal Reflective Assessment (PRA) is derived from qualitative research and broad study of spirituality.[2] This assessment process is designed for personal and clinical use, offering healthcare professionals and patients an opportunity to reflect on the spiritual nature of their life journeys. The PRA encourages persons to take a deeper look at what gives meaning to their lives and important connections with the self, the Sacred Source, others, Nature, and the balance between rest and activity that shapes their spiritual journey. The questions are designed to assist persons in becoming more aware of and attentive to spiritual needs, concerns, supports, and direction at the present time, acknowledging that responses, needs, and insights to a particular question may vary with each visit. Because it is a reflective process, persons are encouraged to focus on those questions that speak to them at the present time. The following are examples of questions included in the PRA:

- *Purpose and meaning.* Which principles, values, or beliefs guide your life? How are your life choices congruent with what you consider to be your spiritual path?
- *Connection with self.* What helps you become more aware of who you are, your purpose in being, your place in the cosmos? How do you express your spirit through your physical body? How has your intuitive knowing supported your spiritual journey?
- *Connection with the Sacred Source.* What is most sacred for you? How do you seek and

experience relationship with the Divine? What is prayer for you?
- *Connection with others.* Where is forgiveness needed in your life and relationships? How do you nurture your spirit through service to others? Which relationships allow you to be who you are and to receive as well as to give?
- *Balance of rest and recreation.* How do you incorporate Sabbath time—balance between activity and rest—into your life?
- *Connection with Nature.* How is your spirit nurtured through Nature? Which kinds of connection with Nature enliven you?
- *Reflecting on the journey.* As you reflect on your Soul journey, what is the next thing you wish or need to do to support or attune to your wholeness, your self-becoming? How can you make this step real in your life?

The reflective nature of the PRA encourages persons to identify spiritual strengths and supports, as well as needs and concerns, in caring for the spiritual self, and to commit to processes or actions that will assist and support them on the spiritual journey. Nurses can use this process personally and with patients to explore where they are on the spiritual journey, where they feel their path is leading them, where they might like to be going, and what their next step might be in the process.

Each of the assessment guides that have been discussed provides a process for exploring the elements of spirituality. For example, spirituality involves relationships, and each instrument offers a different way in which a nurse may enhance the patient's awareness of significant relationships. The Spiritual Assessment Tool addresses the area of harmonious interconnectedness; Howden's work asks the patient to consider questions related to unifying interconnectedness; Delaney's scale asks about nurturing relationships with others; Barker asks which relationships are most important to the patient; and Burkhardt explores relationships that need mending as well as those that provide support. As nurses become more at home with the concept of spirituality and its language, they will form their own questions and make their own observations in understanding another person as a whole being whose essence is spirit.

Holistic Caring Process Considerations

Spiritual caregiving requires an understanding of the integrative holistic caring process in which assessment and intervention may well be the same process, and where description is more useful than labeling. Identification of needs in the area of spirituality does not necessarily indicate pathology or impairment, rather it provides a way of understanding a person in his or her wholeness and a glimpse into what provides meaning. Research on spirituality and health continues to highlight the importance of describing the human spirit in the language of each person's unique experience and expression and exploring individual meaning within the context of the person's life story. Holistic nurses recognize that spirituality is an important dimension of any health concern, and they use the evolving nursing diagnoses regarding spirituality appropriately. Nurses collaborate with clients and their families in determining appropriate outcomes, developing a plan, and organizing overall care to ensure the incorporation of each person's selfhood, values, and worldview. Nurses facilitate this process when they promote an atmosphere that is accepting and encouraging of spiritual expression in its many and varied forms.

Tending to the Spirit

Care of the spirit, a fundamental aspect of holistic nursing care, takes place in the context of the significant connections in a person's life. The nurse, for a time, enters the patient's world and, through intentional presence in this relationship, may facilitate healing. Assessment, diagnosis, planning, and intervening are all experienced within a unique and particular relationship. Recognizing that all persons are spiritual beings provides the basis for being alert to the many and varied ways in which persons express their spirituality. Often, simply hearing and validating questions and concerns of the

spirit are not only part of the assessment but part of the intervention as well. Simply giving clients the opportunity to discuss and reflect on spiritual concerns enables them to become more aware of their spirituality and personal spiritual journeys.

Awareness of and care for self as a spiritual being constitute an important aspect of holistic nursing care. Spiritual co-counseling among colleagues who also deal with spiritual issues and consciously pursue a spiritual path can nurture a nurse's spirit. Forming spiritual companionship, mentoring, or support groups within the work environment, even with one or two colleagues, can help nurses maintain their spirits in the midst of the daily demands on their energies.

Regular practices of prayer, centering, mindfulness, meditation, or starting the day with intention assist nurses in both maintaining and drawing from their own wholeness and ground their practice of intentional presence with each patient encounter. With intentionality and consciousness, busy nurses can use common activities as processes or rituals for leaving past situations behind to be more fully present in a current client encounter. For example, when washing hands between patients, nurses can release the concerns of the previous patient and, thus, be more open to those of the next patient. Similarly, by consciously taking a breath before entering an examination room, nurses can clear themselves of other distractions so as to focus on the person to be seen. Pausing to center and focus; "stepping back" from a confusing, distressing situation to reenter from a point of calmness; and being silent as one listens deeply are skills that develop as nurses attend to spirit. With awareness and creativity, nurses can use almost any activity as a way to foster spiritual presence.

Touching

Physical contact through touch in its myriad forms may foster connection. Sensitivity to the meaning of touch for each person is essential in using touch therapeutically. When appropriate, a hand on the shoulder can provide support, a handclasp can convey understanding and presence, an arm around the waist can literally and figuratively give a lift. One patient described a nurse's support in saying, "When the doctor came in to give me the news, she was standing beside me and I could feel her hand on my arm the whole time he was talking. I was so glad that she was just there with me." At times when words cannot be found, or in circumstances where persons are more comfortable with physical expression than with words, touch is a powerful expression of spirit and an instrument of healing.

Fostering Connectedness

Relationships are a major aspect of spirituality. Awareness and an appreciation of important relationships in the patient's life enable the nurse to help strengthen meaningful and supportive bonds. Some family members may need encouragement and guidance in visiting and calling. Patients may need assistance in sharing some aspects of their situation with others— even when they very much want to explain what is happening to them and express their feelings about it. Nurses can remind patients of their network of care and support by recognizing and affirming the support of significant others. Statements such as "You seem especially close to Marta" may provide an opportunity for sharing about a special relationship. Photographs, artwork, and memorabilia of loved ones provide reminders of connections beyond the confines of illness or injury. Pictures or discussions of special places or pets are evidence of other special connections. Visits from pets may be as spiritually uplifting for some people as those from human companions. Using imagery, pictures, and stories can help persons connect with important places, people, and experiences.

Contact with persons from religious, social, business, neighborhood, school, hobby, or interest groups may provide reminders of connections with and participation in the larger community and world. In some healthcare settings, such as intensive care or long-term care facilities, bonds of mutual caring develop among various patients, families, and caregivers. These networks of support can become very significant in the lives of all involved. Holistic care implies a recognition of the healing potential in such relationships and impels nurses to foster the development of such relationships.

The client's sense of connection with the environment may be an important source of comfort and strength. For persons to be able to feel the wind, see the stars, smell the flowers, touch the trees, and simply to experience the world may be a significant aspect of healing. Is there a window with a view of Nature? Can the patient spend some time outside, perhaps in a healing garden? Is there a photograph of a scene from Nature on the wall or one of a special place that can be placed at the bedside? Would the patient enjoy a plant, a bouquet of flowers, or a single rose? Some people enjoy audiotapes of music or of nature sounds. Spiritual uplifting can occur when visitors share the progress of the vegetable garden, the news of a recent fishing trip, or reflect on the weather conditions.

Spirituality often calls to mind one's relationship with the sacred. People have unique and personal understandings and experiences of the sacred, and language may pose a problem when talking about this aspect of spirituality. Those who are comfortable with the Judeo-Christian tradition of God or Lord, or the Islamic Allah, may find themselves less comfortable with understandings expressed as Higher Power, Tao, Universal Light, or Absolute. The reverse may also be true. For some people, "new age" is a relevant term that connotes spiritual growth and expansion; for others, however, anything "new age" is suspect and can be spiritually distressing. Listening beyond specific words to hear what is most sacred for this person and how his or her relationship with the sacred may be nurtured is important in addressing spiritual concerns. Are particular words of importance to this person? What is the place of formal religion and a person's own rabbi, priest, shaman, minister, imam, or spiritual leader in his or her spiritual journey? How do music, prayer, sacred texts, books, particular objects, foods, or rituals nurture the spirit of this person?

Sensitivity to and appreciation of persons who profess atheism (i.e., disbelief in the existence of a supreme being) or agnosticism (i.e., doubt surrounding the existence of God or ultimate knowledge) involve moving beyond what is not believed. Instead, the nurse listens for that which gives meaning and purpose to the patient's life, including that which brings joy and satisfaction, the nature of hopes and fears, and the recognition of important relationships. How does this particular health crisis fit into the patient's understanding of her or his life, and how is she or he dealing with it? For example, an astronomer who noted that she was not religious and did not believe in God described her understanding and awe in regard to the evolution of the universe as a cause of deep wonder to her that all that had gone before led to this particular time. This sense gave her a feeling "that I belong." The words voiced were not traditionally religious language, but her expressions of appreciation, awe, wonder, and meaning spoke of spirituality.

Nurses who attend to spiritual concerns are willing to be present with mystery, uncertainty, pain, or suffering, seeking not to fix or to answer but to be in the mystery with another. Nurses demonstrate holistic care by letting the client know that they are willing, with their whole being and intention, to stay the course through times of difficulty, pain, and mystery. Patients may feel support when nurses are willing to say, "I don't understand this either." This willingness on the part of the nurses may help family and friends to understand that, when they feel that there is nothing they can do, their presence and expressions of love and care are important and valuable components of their healing support.

As nurses learn to understand the relationships and connections that frame a client's life, they become more aware of recurring themes and concerns. When such themes are noted, the nurse reflects on and validates them with the client. Statements such as "It seems I have often heard you speak of . . . with great concern" gives the client the opportunity to hear the nurse's perceptions and to validate or correct them. In general, it is reassuring to the client to know that the nurse is indeed listening and responding to deep concerns.

Using Rituals to Nurture the Spirit

Rituals serve as reminders to allow sacred time and space in our lives. Both the ritual behavior and the mindfulness that accompanies it are important aspects of ritual. Three phases are common in rituals found in many traditions. The first phase is the symbolic breaking away from routine and everyday busyness. The second phase is the transition phase, which calls for the identification and focus on areas of life that need attention. The third and final phase, referred to as the return phase, is the reentry into everyday life. In essence, ritual gives a person time apart so that he or she may return to the world in a clearer, more centered way. Ritual then can enable nurses to be more intentionally present in healing ways with another.

Either shared with others or highly personalized, rituals are significant aspects of various religious traditions and cultures. Rituals come in many shapes and forms. Routine morning walks, daily prayer time, sharing of the day's experiences with family over dinner, or a soothing bath can all be rituals. Anything done with awareness may serve as a ritual. Rituals provide a rich resource in caring for the spirit, and attending to rituals in one's life can be an important aspect of self-care.

Developing Centering, Mindfulness, and Awareness

Spiritual disciplines are those practices that cause people to pause in the midst of their activities and busyness to attend to matters of the spirit or soul. The practice of spiritual disciplines requires intention and attention. Eastern and many indigenous traditions around the world emphasize the importance of mindfulness and awareness as disciplines that permeate all of life. Similar to the practice of centering prayer in Judeo-Christian traditions, the mystical path of many traditions calls one to quietness. Making the intentional decision to pause and be mindful of the present moment and all that it holds nurtures the ability to be centered and aware. Taking the time to observe what is going on within oneself, without judgment or elaboration, and to note thoughts, feelings, physical sensations, and distractions, provides valuable experiences in the practice of awareness. Observing what is going on in the environment, attending to all senses, and experiencing all sensations enhance a person's full presence in the moment.

Processes of relaxation and imagery facilitate awareness and centering and assist patients in accessing their own Sacred Space. The practice of spiritual disciplines provides access to a centered space from which the nurse and client can work together, confronting significant life experiences in an environment that is often busy and complex. Questions such as "Have you ever tried any particular methods of relaxing?" or "What kinds of activities help you find calm in the middle of a busy day?" may facilitate a person's practice of spiritual disciplines in a more intentional way.

Praying and Meditating

Prayer and meditation are spiritual disciplines practiced in many traditions, both cultural and religious. Appreciating the personal nature of these disciplines, the nurse, with respect and sensitivity, can help patients remember or explore ways in which they reach out to and listen for God or the Sacred Source. Recalling the place and meaning of prayer, and the ways in which they experience the presence of and communion with God or the Sacred Source, provides patients with a rich resource. In the clinical setting, both the nurse's and the patient's understanding of prayer will determine the role of prayer. Clarifying the patient's understanding of and need for prayer is a part of holistic care. Some patients want others to pray with or for them, while others do not believe in prayer. Asking patients if they would like to pray, to whom they wish to pray, and how they pray are important elements of a holistic assessment.[34] Supporting each patient's requests and needs for prayer may mean inviting others to take part in various forms of prayer with and for the patient or simply praying with the patients themselves. The nurse can encourage expression of the patient's desire for shared prayer, for participation in religious worship, or for quiet, uninterrupted periods of time for personal spiritual practices. Facilitating the appreciation and practice of prayer in a patient's life is an important aspect of caring for the spirit.

Exploring as many aspects of the prayer experience as possible enriches both the nurse's and the patient's understanding of the nature and place of prayer for a particular individual. Sacred or inspirational readings, music, drumming, movement, light or darkness, aromas, and time of day are among the many factors that may be important considerations in one's prayer life. The patient's prayer life, in all of its fullness and meaning, nurtures the spirit, and the nurse may be able to support the patient's prayer needs by facilitating changes in the environment or schedule. It is wise to remember that merely the process of listening to and appreciating the prayer life of another nurtures the spirit and acknowledges the spiritual dimension of that person.

Ensuring Opportunities for Rest and Leisure

Rest, leisure, and Sabbath time are integral aspects of holistic living and care of the spirit that enhance growth, creativity, and renewal.[47, 48] Leisure is an attitude of the heart that facilitates connection with the inner self and the Sacred Source and opens one to reflect on and envision a life of doing to allow for more Being. Authentic leisure implies an approach to living that allows one to relax into a level of being that deepens self-awareness, nourishes one's wholeness, and enriches connections with the Sacred Source and other people. Assisting persons to consider the place of rest and leisure in their lives is part of holistic nursing. Taking stock of how they integrate rest and leisure into their own lives is a necessary part of self-care for nurses as well. In an increasingly busy society—where filling each moment is viewed in terms of productivity, where even leisure time is scheduled—the notion of rest and leisure deserves thoughtful consideration.

Holistic nurses try to enhance patients' conscious awareness of how rest and leisure are, or are not, part of their lives. Such awareness makes those areas available for intentional evaluation and, if desired, change. Observations and questions that may be helpful in the exploration of this aspect of spirituality include the following:

- I notice that you read a lot. What does reading do for you?
- You say you just can't rest. When have you been able to rest? Are there things that usually help you to rest?

- What is a real vacation like for you?
- Which time of the day (year, season, week) is most restful or peaceful for you?
- How do you relax?
- Some people just help us to relax; who does that for you?
- Is there something I can do to help you to relax?

Regular exercise, music, imagery, a specific time for rest and quiet, and the commitment to incorporating these experiences into daily life encourage rest and leisure. Validating the importance of rest and leisure and encouraging a commitment to making time for renewal an essential part of one's life are important aspects of holistic care.

Arts and Spirituality

The arts have a role in the life of the spirit. Many people find that various forms of artistic endeavor are doors to and expressions of the spirit. The term *artist* can include anyone who creates—the homemaker who cooks and sews and the carpenter who designs and builds, as well as the more easily recognized persons whose works are heard in symphonies or seen in galleries. As an expression of her or his wholeness, an artist's work is also a reflection of spirituality. L'Engle expresses this well:

> As I listen in the silence, I learn that my feelings about art and my feelings about the Creator of the Universe are inseparable. To try to talk about art and about Christianity is for me one and the same thing, and it means attempting to share the meaning of my life, what gives it, for me, its tragedy and its glory. It is what makes me respond to the death of an apple tree, the birth of a puppy, northern lights shaking the sky, by writing stories.[49]

Literature contains life stories, both real and fictional, to which people relate and from which they learn, gain comfort, and garner encouragement. Poetry contains deep truths, often in a few well-chosen words, a rhythm, and spaces for

silence. Music expresses feelings that are beyond words. Songs bring back memories or capture what people would like to say. Pottery awakens the senses of touch and sight as one forms a vessel or holds a favorite mug. Dance moves people, literally and figuratively, in space and time. Photography connects individuals and sometimes moves their hearts for those known only through the images seen all over the world. Drumming awakens deep, basic yearnings and calls some to worship. Gardens nourish not only the body but also the senses of sight, touch, taste, and smell. Cave drawings are reminders of civilizations past and awaken a sense of wonder.

Providing an atmosphere that, as much as possible, is pleasing to the sensibilities of the patient may promote rest and relaxation. It may also facilitate the use of other interventions, such as imagery. Encouraging and facilitating opportunities for people to engage in or share stories of their creative endeavors is one of the ways that nurses include spirituality in care.

Conclusion

Because all persons, nurses as well as patients, are spiritual beings, care of the spirit is integral to holistic nursing care. Care of the spirit requires the evolution of language to express this dimension of ourselves better and an approach to the nursing process that is integrative rather than linear. Spirituality assessment and intervention, which are often the same process, require intentional listening, presence, and a willingness to hear another's story. Spiritual care is based on a recognition that people express and experience their spirituality in and through relationships with the Sacred Source, others, Nature, and self.

Spiritual care may incorporate "experts," such as representatives of particular religious traditions or other spiritual support people, but nurses need to do more than merely refer matters of the spirit to these persons. Although spiritual matters are both deep and personal, they often come to the forefront of life when health crises cause a person to stop, to take stock, to experience anxieties and fear, and to seek that which is at the heart of his or her life.

Nurses offer spiritual support as they are able to be present with mystery and the life questions of others. Tending to matters of the spirit may include incorporating ritual, prayer, meditation, rest, art, and any activity that enhances awareness of oneself and one's place in the world.

Directions for Future Research

1. Further explore the influence of spirituality in health and illness across cultures and in different age groups, using both qualitative and quantitative methodologies and culturally valid instruments.
2. Explore the role of spirituality in dealing with illness and promoting positive health outcomes.
3. Investigate ways to support nurses in identifying spiritual practices within different populations and in integrating spirituality into clinical practice.

Nurse Healer Reflections

After reading this chapter, the nurse healer will be able to answer or to begin a process of answering the following questions:

- In recognizing my wholeness, how would I describe my relationship with my physical being, my emotional being, and my spiritual being?
- What signals spiritual distress in my own life?
- How do I nurture my spirit?
- How do I nurture and make time for the most important connections in my life?
- Which areas of the spirit need intentional care in my own life, perhaps because of pain or distress, or because there are areas in which I want to focus and grow?
- How have my life experiences contributed to the growth and development of my spirit?
- How have I experienced intentional presence?

NOTES

1. L. Tzu, *Tao Te Ching* (London: Penguin Books, 1988).
2. M. A. Burkhardt and M. G. Nagai-Jacobson, *Spirituality: Living Our Connectedness* (Albany, NY: Delmar, 2002).
3. E. Mok, F. Wong, and D. Wong, "The Meaning of Spirituality and Spiritual Care Among the Hong Kong Chinese Terminally Ill," *Journal of Advanced Nursing* 66, no. 2 (2010): 360–370.
4. J. C. Engebretson, "Cultural Diversity and Care," in *Holistic Nursing: A Handbook for Practice*, 6th ed., eds. B. M. Dossey and L. Keegan (Burlington, MA: Jones & Bartlett Learning, 2013): 677–702.
5. M. A. Burkhardt, "Becoming and Connecting: Elements of Spirituality for Women," *Holistic Nursing Practice* 8, no. 4 (1994): 12–21.
6. L. Lephard, "Spirituality in Men with Advanced Prostate Cancer: 'It's a holistic thing . . . it's a package,'" *Journal of Holistic Nursing* 32, no 2 (2014): 89–101.
7. L. H. Tiew and V. Druey, "Singapore Nursing Students' Perceptions and Attitudes About Spirituality and Spiritual Care Practice," *Journal of Holistic Nursing* 30, no 3 (2012): 160–169.
8. L. Rykkje, K. Eriksson, and M. Raholm, "A Qualitative Metasynthesis of Spirituality from a Caring Perspective," *International Journal for Human Caring* 15, no. 4 (2011): 40–56.
9. H. G. Buck and S. H. Meghani, "Spiritual Experiences of African Americans and Whites in Cancer Pain," *Journal of Holistic Nursing* 30, no. 2 (2012): 107–116.
10. A. Noble and C. Jones, "Getting It Right: Oncology Nurses' Understanding of Spirituality," *International Journal of Palliative Nursing* 16, no. 11 (2010): 565–569.
11. T. Berry and M. E. Tucker, *The Sacred Universe: Earth, Spirituality, and Religion in the Twenty-First Century* (New York: Columbia University Press, 2009).
12. P. Woodruff, *Reverence—Renewing a Forgotten Virtue* (Oxford, England: Oxford University Press, 2001).
13. B. Plotkin, *Nature and the Human Soul* (Novato, CA: New World Library, 2008).
14. S. Jeffers, *Brother Eagle, Sister Sky* (New York: Dial Books, 1991).
15. M. A. Burkhardt, "Healing Relationships with Nature," *Complementary Therapies in Nursing and Midwifery* 6, no. 1 (2000): 35–40.
16. J. Watson, *Human Caring Science*, 2nd ed. (Sudbury, MA: Jones & Bartlett Learning, 2012).
17. L. Thornton, *Whole Person Caring: An Interprofessional Model for Healing and Wellness* (Indianapolis, IN: Sigma Theta Tau International, 2013).
18. E. Yuen, "Spirituality and the Clinical Encounter," *International Journal for Human Caring* 15, no. 2 (2011): 42–46.

19. P. Kimble and A. Bamford-Wade, "The Journey of Discovering Compassionate Listening," *Journal of Holistic Nursing* 31, no. 4 (2013): 285–290.

20. A. Hankey, "The Thermodynamics of Healing, Health, and Love," *Journal of Alternative and Complementary Medicine* 13, no. 1 (2007): 5–7.

21. K. Sitzman and J. Watson, *Caring Science, Mindful Practice: Implementing Watson's Human Caring Theory* (New York: Springer, 2014).

22. S. Johnson, "Hope in Terminal Illness: An Evolutionary Concept Analysis," *International Journal of Palliative Nursing* 13, no. 9 (2007): 451–459.

23. T. B. Pipe, A. Kelly, G. LeBrun, D. Schmidt, P. Atherton, and C. Robinson, "A Prospective Descriptive Study Exploring Hope, Spiritual Well-Being, and Quality of Life in Hospitalized Patients," *MEDSURG Nursing* 17, no. 4 (2008): 247–253, 257.

24. A. C. Recine, J. S. Werner, and L. Recine, "Concept Analysis of Forgiveness with a Multi-Cultural Emphasis," *Journal of Advanced Nursing* 59, no. 3 (2007): 308–316.

25. A. C. Recine, J. S. Werner, and L. Recine, "Health Promotion Through Forgiveness Intervention," *Journal of Holistic Nursing* 27, no. 2 (2009): 115–123.

26. S. Menahem and M. Love, "Forgiveness in Psychotherapy: The Key to Healing," *Journal of Clinical Psychology* 69, no. 8 (2013): 829–835.

27. M. Arnold, B. Ballif-Spanvill, and K. Tracy, eds., *A Chorus for Peace—A Global Anthology of Poetry by Women* (Iowa City: University of Iowa Press, 2002): xv.

28. L. Dossey, *Prayer Is Good Medicine* (San Francisco: Harper, 1996).

29. M. D. Calabria and J. A. Macrae, eds., *Suggestions for Thought by Florence Nightingale: Selections and Commentaries* (Philadelphia: University of Pennsylvania Press, 1994).

30. B. M. Dossey, *Florence Nightingale: Mystic, Visionary, Healer* (Springhouse, PA: Springhouse, 2000).

31. A. Narayanasamy and M. Narayanasamy, "The Healing Power of Prayer and Its Implications for Nursing," *British Journal of Nursing* 17, no. 6 (2008): 394–398.

32. C. French and A. Narayanasamy, "To Pray or Not to Pray: A Question of Ethics," *British Journal of Nursing* 20, no. 7 (2011): 1198–1204.

33. M. B. Helming, "Healing Through Prayer: A Qualitative Study," *Holistic Nursing Practice* 25, no. 1 (2011): 33–44.

34. B. Hubbartt, D. Corey, and D. D. Kautz, "Prayer at the Bedside," *International Journal for Human Caring* 16, no. 1 (2012): 42–47.

35. L. Dossey, *Be Careful What You Pray For* (San Francisco: HarperCollins, 1997).

36. B. M. Dossey, "Florence Nightingale: A 19th-Century Mystic," *Journal of Holistic Nursing* 28, no. 1 (2010): 10–35.

37. B. M. Dossey, "Florence Nightingale: Her Crimean Fever Chronic Illness," *Journal of Holistic Nursing* 28, no. 1 (2010): 38–53.

38. D. R. Hodge and V. E. Horvath, "Spiritual Needs in Health Care Settings: A Qualitative Meta-Synthesis," *Social Work* 56, no. 4 (2011): 306–316.

39. J. Bruchac, *Tell Me a Tale* (New York: Harcourt, Brace, 1997): 1.

40. P. R. Liehr and M. J. Smith, "Story Theory," in *Middle Range Theory for Nursing*, 2nd ed., eds. M. J. Smith and P. R. Liehr (New York: Springer, 2008): 205–224.

41. J. Reich, "Becoming Whole: The Role of Story for Healing," *Journal of Holistic Nursing* 30, no. 1 (2012): 16–23.

42. M. A. Burkhardt, "Spirituality: An Analysis of the Concept," *Holistic Nursing Practice* 3, no. 3 (1989): 69–77.

43. J. W. Howden, "Development and Psychometric Characteristics of the Spirituality Assessment Scale" (unpublished doctoral dissertation, Texas Woman's University, Denton, 1992).

44. C. Delaney, "The Spirituality Scale: Development and Psychometric Testing of a Holistic Instrument to Assess the Human Spiritual Dimension," *Journal of Holistic Nursing* 23, no. 2 (2005): 145–167.

45. E. R. Barker, "Patient Spirituality Assessment: A Tool That Works" (paper presented at the Uniformed Nurse Practitioners Association Meeting, Seattle, WA, November 1996).

46. E. R. Barker, "How to Do Research, Get Finished, and Not Lose Your Balance" (paper presented at the Nursing Research Symposium, San Diego, CA, 1998).

47. W. Mueller, *Sabbath: Restoring the Sacred Rhythms of Rest* (New York: Bantam Books, 2000).

48. P. Heintzman, "Leisure-Spiritual Coping: A Model for Therapeutic Recreation and Leisure Services," *Therapeutic Recreation Journal* 42, no. 1 (2008): 56–73.

49. M. L'Engle, *Walking on Water: Reflecting on Faith and Art* (Wheaton, IL: Harold Shaw, 1980): 16.

CORE VALUE 2

Holistic Caring Process

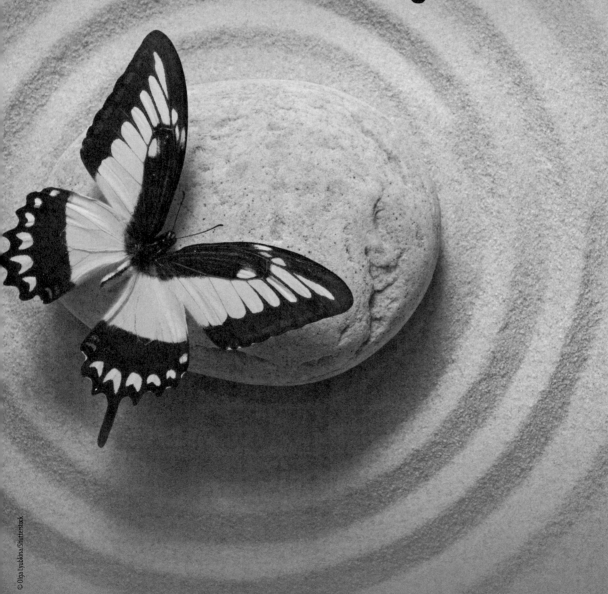

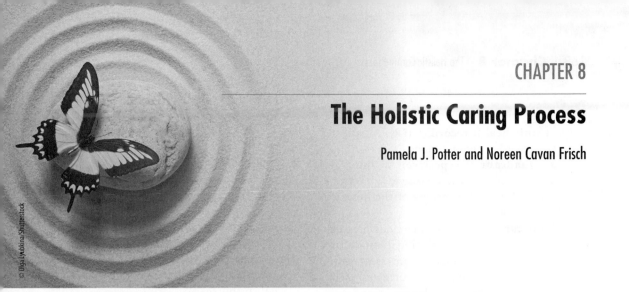
© Olga Lyubkina/Shutterstock

CHAPTER 8

The Holistic Caring Process

Pamela J. Potter and Noreen Cavan Frisch

Nurse Healer Objectives

Theoretical

- Define the terms *nursing process* and *holistic caring process*.
- Outline the steps of the holistic caring process.
- Explore the steps of the holistic caring process through the four quadrants of Integral Theory.
- Discuss the ways in which standards of holistic nursing practice are incorporated into the holistic caring process.

Clinical

- Analyze the assessment tool that you are using in clinical practice to determine whether the tool is consistent with a holistic nursing perspective.
- Explore the ways to document holistic nursing care in a computerized electronic health record through use of standardized terms such as those found in nursing diagnostic taxonomies, the Nursing Interventions Classification, and the Nursing Outcomes Classification.
- Identify the nursing concerns and activities most relevant to your clients.
- Integrate the Four-Quadrant Perspective into mapping nursing diagnosis,

implementation, and outcomes evaluation into the treatment plan.
- Implement *Holistic Nursing: Scope and Standards of Practice, Second Edition*, into your work and life.[1]

Personal

- Observe the pattern appraisal and identification process in your everyday life as you walk into a new situation.
- Identify the four patterns of knowing (empirical, ethical, aesthetic, and personal knowledge) as they guide you within the nurse–person interaction.
- Develop and trust your intuitive thinking processes when assessing clients' conditions.
- Develop and trust your application of research data and quality improvement/quality assurance findings to provide evidence-based and/or evidence-informed practice.
- Evaluate the effect of intuitive thinking in both your professional and personal lives.
- Evaluate the effect of knowledge and data application in your professional and personal lives.
- Explore your own beliefs and values regarding the concepts of holistic nursing.
- Write down specific examples of holistic nursing care while reflecting on your enactment of the holistic caring process.

Definitions

Electronic health record (EHR): A patient care record in digital format.

Four-Quadrant Perspective: An integral map[2] for organizing objective, subjective, and collective dimensions of the holistic caring process.

Holistic caring process: A circular process that involves six steps that may occur simultaneously. These steps are assessment, patterns/challenges/needs, outcomes, therapeutic care plan, implementation, and evaluation.

Holistic nursing: All nursing practice that has healing the whole person as its goal.

Holon: Anything that is itself whole or part of some other whole that creates structures, from the very smallest to the largest, with increasing complexity.[3, 4]

Intuition: The perceived knowing of things and events without the conscious use of rational processes; using all of the senses to receive information.

NANDA-I diagnosis: A multiaxial classification schema for the organization of nursing diagnoses based on functional domains and classes.

Nursing diagnosis (NDx): A clinical judgment about individual, family, group, or community experiences/responses to actual or potential health problems/life processes . . . [and] the basis for selection of nursing interventions to achieve outcomes for which the nurse has accountability.[5]

Nursing Interventions Classification (NIC): A standardized comprehensive classification or taxonomy of treatments that nurses perform, including both independent and collaborative, as well as direct and indirect.[6]

Nursing Outcomes Classification (NOC): A standardized comprehensive taxonomy of frequently identified goals; measurable responses to nursing interventions.[7]

Nursing process: The original model describing the "work" of nursing, defined as steps used to fulfill the purposes of nursing, such as assessment, diagnosis, client outcomes, plans, intervention, and evaluation.

Paradigm: A model for conceptualizing information.

Patterns/challenges/needs: A person's actual and potential life processes related to health, wellness, disease, or illness, which may or may not facilitate well-being.

Person: An individual, client, patient, family member, support person, or community member who has the opportunity to engage in interaction with a holistic nurse.

Standards of practice: A group of statements describing the expected level of care by a holistic nurse.

Holistic Caring Process: Background

Focused on establishing health and well-being, the holistic caring process represents the entire range of activities taking place within the nurse–person relationship. It is, quite simply, the process of nurse and client coming together in a professional interaction. The holistic caring process is not essentially different from the nursing process many nurses learned in school. Naming our work the *holistic caring process* gives attention to the physiologic priorities of care as well as the important intangibles of practice, such as presence, hope, support, caring, and mutuality. Holistic nurses must remember that the nursing process is a framework that gives us the means to reflect on the entire range of nursing activities. These activities are described as the following steps:

1. Assessment
2. Diagnosis, or identification of problems or needs, or pattern recognition
3. Outcomes
4. Care plan
5. Implementation or intervention
6. Evaluation

The original concept of nursing process can be traced to the late 1950s and early 1960s when nurses in the United States sought to identify what they did as a distinct, autonomous profession within health care. Early on, proponents of the nursing process readily saw it as a tool to describe professional activities carried out by nurses that were unnoticed and unrecognized as having important contributions to care and recovery. For example, even very basic nursing activities such as those related to patient comfort (positioning, creating a calming atmosphere), nutrition (timing of meals and presentation of food and fluids), sleep (relaxation, back rubs), or skin integrity (massage, turning, and attention to bed linens) were carried out by nurses but often referred to as "common sense" rather than as professional responses to identified client needs. The concept of a nursing process allowed nurses to use a common language, systematize nursing practice and education, and enhance nursing autonomy.

There have been two definitions of the nursing process: one a linear process for solving problems and the other a circular process for describing our understanding of our encounters with clients.[8] The linear process is a step-by-step depiction of nursing work and mirrors scientific problem solving. Here, the nurse gathers data and assesses the client situation, uses data to make clinical judgments and plan care and interventions, implements the care plan, and evaluates the outcomes. The linear nursing process depicts nursing as if one step is always carried out before the next, as if the nurse attends to one client problem or concern at a time, and as if there is a conscious pattern of moving from one step to the other. Although experienced nurses know that the nursing process is not really linear in the enactment of our work, the linear process was adopted in the 1980s as a foundation for education and practice. It made sense to think in these linear terms to teach students and to guide novice nurses through one step at a time so that they could grasp the connections among nursing assessments, judgments, actions, and outcomes. Further, it made sense to think about nursing in a logical step-by-step fashion to document nursing as separate from medicine and to study outcomes of nursing care. Thus, the linear nursing process provided a framework that helped nurses identify their contributions to care.

In contrast to the linear nursing process, the circular nursing process is a way of thinking about nursing with a full understanding that every step of the nursing process may be happening all at once and that the nurse may be addressing multiple client needs simultaneously. The circular nursing process is more related to the subjective experience of "being a nurse" than is the linear model. A nurse may be assessing while she or he is intervening. A nurse may be evaluating while diagnosing, or she or he may be attending to comfort needs and gathering data related to spiritual needs at the same time. When a nurse walks into a client room, she or he begins the nurse–patient encounter with an intervention—the nursing presence. The circular model is readily understood by experienced nurses. Emphasizing holistic care, Erickson and colleagues supported the circular nursing process model and described the process as "the ongoing, interactive exchange of information, feelings, and behavior between nurse and client(s) wherein the nurse's goal is to nurture and support the client's self-care."[9]

There are some who continue to critique the nursing process, first on the grounds that it is reductionistic and steeped in positivism, second on the grounds that it serves the profession more than it does the clients, and third that its use runs counter to current practice on interdisciplinary teams. These critques have more to do with how the nursing process is enacted than the nursing process itself.

The origins of the nursing process reside within the concept of pattern recognition, an innate tendency found among humans. When nurses encounter a patient for the first time, they observe the state of the person's health. They notice the person's color (pale or cyanotic), affect and eye contact, respiration depth and rate, rate and volume of speech, body odor, scars, wounds, and more. Within 60 seconds, they notice if something is different from the expected and whether any nursing action is necessary. This is pattern appraisal and pattern recognition. Using all of their nursing knowledge, nurses apply the patterns they observe to known patterns, make decisions about those patterns, and then act on those decisions. After doing so, they reappraise and react based on the patient's response.

Because nursing cannot be conceptually separated from the cultural context within which it is practiced, the holistic nurse must consider this context when implementing theory-based practice. For example, although one's theoretical underpinnings for nursing may define nursing as "the practice of presence" within the nurse–person relationship, the culture and the patient may define nursing by activities carried out by the nurse on behalf of the patient. Holistic nurses who work within contemporary healthcare culture must balance formal knowledge and expertise gained from nursing education and practice with philosophies of health that may not yet be fully embraced by mainstream culture.

Reflective Practice Within the Holistic Caring Process

Reflective practice is a mindful process of self-observation in the midst of an experience, as well as after, for the purpose of resolving values and practice contradictions, gaining new self-insights and empowerment, and responding more congruently in future situations.[10] Insights derived from the four patterns of knowing identified by Carper guide the nurse's process within the nurse–person interaction.[11] Empirical or scientific knowledge is based on objective information measurable by the senses and by scientific instrumentation. Ethical knowledge flows from the "basic underlying concept of the unity and integral wholeness of all people and of all nature."[12] Aesthetic knowledge draws on a sense of form and structure and of beauty and creativity for discerning pattern and change. Personal knowledge incorporates the nurse's self-awareness and knowledge (emotional intelligence), as well as the intuitive perception of meanings based on personal experiences, and is demonstrated by the therapeutic use of self. Currently, Dossey's Theory of Integral Nursing (TIN)[4] incorporates Carper's ways of knowing[11] as a means to help nurses reflect on their practice at a deep level to stimulate such questions as: How do we as nurses know what we know? How and when do we act on our knowledge?

The Johns model of reflective practice is placed within Carper's ways of knowing and enables the nurse to "access, understand, and learn through her or his lived experiences and, as a consequence, to take congruent action towards developing increasing effectiveness within the context of what is understood as desirable practice."[13, p. 227]

Intuitive Thinking Within the Holistic Caring Process

The holistic caring process involves collection and evaluation of information from an intuitive, nonverbal (right-brain) mode. Intuitive perception allows one to know something immediately without consciously using reason. Clinical intuition has been described as a "process by which we know something about a client that cannot be verbalized or is verbalized poorly or for which the source of the knowledge cannot be determined."[14, p. 52] It is a "gut feeling" that something is wrong or that we should do something, even if there is no real evidence to support that feeling. Within the caring relationship between nurse and person, intuitive events emerge as the nurse is open and receptive to the person's subtle cues.

Effken describes this perception as the direct detection of environmental information.[15, 16] Intuition, characterized as direct perception, occurs when the holistic nurse perceives in the environment higher-order variables that call for action. Framing intuition as direct perception offers an explanation for how experts who perceive complex higher-order variables cannot report with accuracy underlying lower-order properties, as well as how new information, outside of the nurse's previous experience, may be interpreted intuitively as an opportunity for action. When characterized as direct perception, intuition becomes an "observable, lawful phenomenon that is measurable, potentially teachable, and appropriately part of nursing science."[15, p. 252]

Evidence-Based or Evidence-Informed Practice Within the Holistic Caring Process

Modern health care is informed by evidence, and every clinical practice setting is required to demonstrate practice according to internationally accepted standards of care. These care standards are based on empirical research and epidemiological evidence indicating the approaches to care most likely to result in improved patient outcomes. The holistic Registered Nurse is required to have knowledge of basic and applied research techniques, including statistics and use of concepts of probability and confidence intervals, to make sense of the thinking behind current practice standards and clinical practice guidelines.

Much of medical care, pharmacological recommendations, and treatement of physiological conditions are guided by empirical research findings accumulated through controlled clinical or naturalistic trials. When such data are available, the resulting care recommendations have solid evidence for patient benefit. However, as such data are not available for all conditions and for all patient populations, care recommendations are made on the best evidence and clinical jugement available to the care team. The patient and his or her family often have to make choices with the care providers about actions when evidence is not clear.

The roles of the holistic Registered Nurse in these settings are twofold: First is to have a good understanding of how professionals interpret research findings as applied to patient populations and individual patients, and second is to be able to contribute to care decisions from the perspective of having meaningful interactions with the patient so that patient choices and autonomy are maintained.

The Four-Quadrant Perspective

Integral Theory as delineated by Wilber[2]—and utilized by Dossey[4] in her Theory of Integral Nursing—posits a "four-quadrant" perspective for mapping approaches to understanding interrelationships among physical, psychological, cultural, and social dimensions (see **Figure 8-1**). A four-quadrant map is a useful tool for visualizing the holistic caring process. The Upper-Right Quadrant represents the objective,

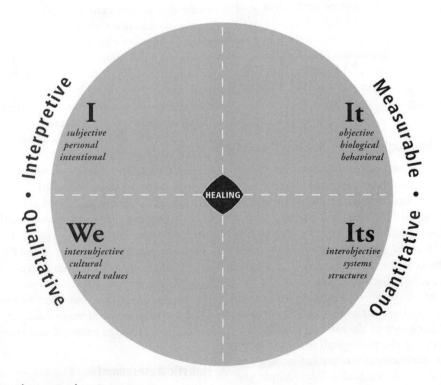

FIGURE 8-1 The Four-Quadrant Perspective.

Source: Adapted with permissionn from Ken Wilber. http://www.kenwilber.com

observable, quantifiable, material external world of the individual—the domain of physiological assessment and care. The Upper-Left Quadrant, expressed through self-knowledge, represents the personal subjective, interpretive, qualitative internal world of the individual—thoughts, feelings, and beliefs that form a person's identity. The Lower-Left Quadrant, expressed through relationships, represents the collective cultural, subjective, interpretive, qualitative internal world of the collective—shared vision, understanding, and meaning within a community. The Lower-Right Quadrant represents the objective, observable, quantifiable external world of the collective—the systems and structures of society.

As nurses, we are educated and usually practice with a focus on physiologic care; we can get lost in the focus on "objective" evidence. As holistic nurses, we stress the importance of also attending to the person who is our patient, to relationship that is informed by cultural context, as well as the bio/behavioral presentation, while considering the system structures that enhance or inhibit care. Our thinking is multidimensional. Viewing the holistic caring process through the Four-Quadrant Model creates an informative and manageable way to acknowledge the many interconnections that influence holistic nursing care.

The Four Quadrants and the Nursing Process

Nurses should recognize that the four quadrants are not absolutes; they provide a structure for looking at a particular focus of interest. Perdue,[17] as described by Dossey[4] in articulating the nursing's metaparadigm from an integral perspective, places the nursing process—as a process that can be objectively observed—in the Upper-Right Quadrant. Because each quadrant is a holon in itself, so too each whole/part within a quadrant will reflect aspects of the greater whole.[2, 18] Each step of the nursing process contains aspects of the four quadrants, and every element of the nursing process can be mapped to one of the four quadrants. For example, the Objective Quadrant (IT) (UR) addresses the client's physiological and behavioral presentation.

The Subjective Quadrant (I) (UL) addresses both the nurse as a person with interior dimensions, as well as the client as a person with interior processes. The Intersubjective Quadrant (WE) (LL) addresses the relationship that must be established between client and nurse and nurse and family. Further, recognition of culture (the client's as well as the nurse's medical culture) is a consideration of this dimension. The Interobjective Quadrant (ITS) (LR) reflects system factors influencing caregiving and receiving, including the nurse's responsibility to the healthcare structure through adequately documenting care. Thus, the Four-Quadrant Perspective not only provides a framework for all of nursing's work, the holistic caring process as carried out by nurses requires considerations or activities in each of the quadrants.

Holistic Caring Process

Nurses who adhere to the holistic caring process focus on the care of the whole unique person: respecting and advocating for the person's rights and choices. Based on a holistic assessment and identification of the person's health patterns, decisions about care flow from collaboration with the person, other healthcare providers, and significant others. The person assumes an active role in healthcare planning and decision making by seeking the professional expertise of the nurse via various nurse–person interactions. Facilitated by the nurse in the healing relationship, the person expresses health concerns and strengths—a unique health pattern—that the nurse identifies and documents in the healthcare record. The person is encouraged to participate as actively as possible, taking responsibility for personal health choices and decisions for self-care. The holistic caring process is presented here within the Four-Quadrant Perspective as a six-step process including holistic assessment, identification of patterns/challenges/needs, outcome identification, therapeutic care plan, implementation, and evaluation. The following sections describe each phase.

Holistic Assessment

The holistic Registered Nurse collects comprehensive data pertinent to the person's health or situation.[1] Assessment is the information-gathering phase in which the nurse and the person identify health patterns and prioritize the person's health concerns. A continuous process, assessment provides ongoing data for changes that occur over time. During assessment the holistic nurse looks for the overall pattern of interrelationships. Each nurse–person encounter provides new information that helps to explain interrelationships and validates previously collected data and conclusions. A key to holistic assessment is to appraise the overall pattern of the responses. Each pattern identification taps into the hologram of the person, contributing to the revelation of the whole. Integral assessment considers all four quadrants (see **Exhibit 8-1**).

Upper Right: Objective. **The nurse gathers physiological and behavioral data.** Assessment from this quadrant perspective is one of identifying objective data. The nurse gleans information about the person's patterns via observations and measurement. Nursing observation relies on information perceived by the five senses (including energy field assessment if grounding one's work in energy-based theory) while measurement provides quantifiable information obtained from instruments (e.g., lab values, vital signs). The nurse uses appropriate empirical data from the literature to support observations.

Upper Left: Subjective. **The nurse gathers data about the internal processes as expressed by the client.** The nurse and the client each bring a personal subjective experience to the health care encounter. The client brings personal life experience, values and beliefs, self-concept, and health perceptions. The client is the primary source and interpreter of the meaning of information obtained by the assessment process. Reflectively, the nurse brings awareness of his or her own self-process; perceptions, feelings, and thoughts about patterns as identified by the person; and intuition and emotional intelligence (the ability to sense and feel beyond appearances). A lack of awareness about one's own personal beliefs and patterns may subtly influence the nurse–client interaction (e.g., communication barriers relative to culture, class, age, gender, sexual orientation, education, or physical limitation) and impede holistic assessment.

Lower Left: Intersubjective. **The nurse gathers data about family processes and cultural meaning.**

Assessment occurs within the nurse–client *relationship*. Relationship, established within the "We" space of the four quadrants, necessitates cultural consideration, honoring how the client makes meaning. Sense of belonging to a community with shared understanding of cultural beliefs necessitates inclusion of family within its cultural milieu in the assessment. Interpersonal interaction with client and family reveals perceptions, feelings, and thoughts. Recognizing that the client is the primary source and interpreter of meaning, the nurse may use motivational interviewing as an approach to discovering patterns/challenges/needs to identify stages of change, readiness to learn, and insights for interventions.

Within the nurse–client relationship, interpersonal interaction reveals perceptions, feelings, and thoughts about health patterns/challenges/needs as identified by the person. Family and significant others bring cultural perspective about factors that may be influencing the client's current health situation. Further, other members of the healthcare team may also contribute to identifying patterns/challenges/needs through supplemental information. The holistic nurse views the person as a whole and listens for the meaning of the current health situation to the person within the environment. While acknowledging his or her own patterns and their potential influence on the healing relationship, the nurse reflects on the person's patterns recognized from the assessment. In response, the person validates the meanings of these identified health patterns. Within the cultural context of negotiation, the assessment phase may be seen as an "exchange of expert knowledge" wherein both the nurse and the person bring expertise to the exchange.[9]

Lower Right: Interobjective. **The nurse gathers data on system factors that may enhance or impinge upon client health.** All pertinent data, including demographic data, are documented in the person's record. The nurse also collects pertinent data from previous client records and other members of the healthcare team, if appropriate. Assessment and documentation are continuous within the nurse–client interaction because changes in one pattern always influence the other dimensions.

EXHIBIT 8-1   Holistic Assessment: Concepts and Assessment Parameters Appropriate for Each Quadrant

Subjective Quadrant

The Nurse's "I" Space

- Nurse reflective process
- Perceptions, feelings, and thoughts about patterns as identified by the person
- Nurse's awareness of own self-processes
- Caring presence
- Intuition
- Emotional Intelligence

The Client's "I" Space

- Self-concept
- Perception of the health situation
- Meaning/effect on role/self-perception
- Feelings about health experience
- Beliefs about current health pattern
- Values

The nurse gathers data about the internal processes as expressed by the client.

Objective Quadrant

The "IT" Space

- Evidence-informed observation through the five senses: touch, taste, smell, sight, hearing
- Physical assessment
- Objective measurements (such as lab values, vital signs, and physiologic indicators)
- Energy field
- Lifestyle risk factors
- Diet patterns
- Mobility status
- Exercise/rest/relaxation patterns
- Medications used: prescribed and over the counter
- Sensory perception
- Behavioral manifestations of stress, comfort, and other feelings

The nurse gathers physiological and behavioral data.

Intersubjective Quadrant

"We" Space: Nurse–Client Relationship

- Interpersonal interaction
- Interviewing techniques (such as motivational)
- Relationship-centered care
- Client role as primary source and interpreter of meaning
- Sense of belonging
- Meaning of death
- Meaning of birth
- Cultural beliefs
- Community share
- Co-creating the healing environment

Other Relationships: Family, Culture, Community

- Family and significant others provide supplemental information
- Family helps to identify the psychosocial conditions and patterns affecting the client's health and well-being
- Interpersonal interaction reveals perceptions, feelings, and thoughts

The nurse gathers data about family processes and cultural meaning.

Interobjective Quadrant

The "ITS" Space: System Factors

- Documented health history
- Client records
- Electronic health record
- Healthcare team
- Organizational protocols
- Translation available
- Healthcare system
- Health insurance
- Economics

Demographics

- Socioeconomic status
- Group memberships
- Family structure
- Social systems
- Ecosystems
- Job/role
- Population health and risk factors

The nurse gathers data on system factors that may enhance or impinge upon client health.

Source: Nursing Process Organized in Four Quadrants Copyright © 2014, Pamela J. Potter, DNSc, RN, CNS-BC.

Identification of Patterns/Challenges/Needs

The holistic Registered Nurse analyzes the assessment data to determine the nursing diagnosis or issues expressed as actual or potential patterns/challenges/needs that are related to health, wellness, disease, or illness.[1]

Within the second step of the holistic caring process, the nurse describes a person's patterns/challenges/needs preferably through use of a standardized language (see **Exhibit 8-2**).* When needed, narrative data also support the meaning of the nurse's thinking. Nursing diagnoses (NDx) describe human responses to health conditions and life processes in an individual, family, group, or community.[5]

Upper Right: Objective. **The nurse identifies nursing diagnoses reflective of the client's physical and behavioral health presentation.** The nurse draws from current literature and practice expertise. Diagnoses in the Upper-Right Quadrant describe the client's physiological and biological processes to be addressed by nursing care. These observable and measurable processes concern the physical body and cognition including genetic, physical, neurological, developmental, and cognition.

Upper Left: Subjective. **The nurse identifies nursing diagnoses reflective of the internal processes expressed by the client.** The *person* of the nurse and the *person* of the client inform identification of patterns associated with the Upper-Left Quadrant. The life and practice experience the nurse brings to the process informs pattern identification. Self-perception of the lived experience informs the client's descriptions of patterns/challenges/needs.

Lower Left: Intersubjective. **The nurse identifies nursing diagnoses reflective of family processes and cultural meaning.** Considering cultural norms and practices, a common language is created within the nurse–client relationship that may bridge the standardized language of health care with the client's language of personal experience. Family is included in articulation of patterns/challenges/needs. In addition to specific patterns reflective of the individual client, some patterns identified may include family processes.

Lower Right: Interobjective. **The nurse includes diagnoses related to system and external factors that may enhance or impinge upon client health (community diagnoses).** The nurse documents NDx in standardized language (NANDA-I) that is understandable to nurses, other healthcare professionals, and the managed care provider. The diagnostic statement describes actual, risk, health promotion/wellness, and syndromes (clusters of diagnoses with interconnected interventions and outcomes). Various diagnoses have applicability in each of the four quadrants as illustrated in **Exhibit 8-3**.

Outcome Identification

The holistic Registered Nurse identifies outcomes for a plan individualized to the person or the situation. This implies that specific outcomes may not be evident immediately because of the nonlinear nature of the healing process so that both expected/anticipated and evolving outcomes are considered.[1]

Outcome identification begins with the process of mutual goal setting. An outcome is a direct statement of a goal identified through the nurse–person relationship that is to be achieved within a specific time frame. Outcomes reflect the goals of the nurse–client intervention. An outcome indicates the maximum level of wellness that is reasonably attainable for the person in view of objective circumstances and the person's perceptions. Outcomes predict the expected intervention effect and describe the tools, tests, and observations (measures) used to determine whether outcomes were achieved, or a change in status indicting that movement toward desired (target) outcomes was observed. Client outcomes direct the care plan (see **Exhibit 8-4**).

Upper Right: Objective. **The nurse chooses nursing outcomes (and appropriate measures) reflective of the client's physical and behavioral health presentation.** Outcomes in the Upper-Right

---

*For the purpose of providing consistent examples NANDA-I diagnoses, the terms *Nursing Intervention Classification* (NIC) and *Nursing Outcomes Classification* (NOC) are used throughout this chapter.

EXHIBIT 8-2 Identification of Patterns/Challenges/Needs: Concepts and Conditions Appropriate for Each Quadrant

Subjective Quadrant

The Nurse's "I" Space

- The life and practice experience the nurse brings informs pattern identification
- Ways of knowing
- Intuition

The Client's "I" Space

- Description of patterns/challenges/needs
- Sense of self
- Consciousness
- Sense of spirit
- Lived experience

The nurse identifies nursing diagnoses reflective of internal processes expressed by the client.

Objective Quadrant

The "IT" Space

- Describes the client's physiological and biological processes to be addressed by nursing care
- Genetics
- Physical
- Neurological
- Developmental

The nurse identifies nursing diagnoses reflective of the client's physical and behavioral health presentation.

Intersubjective Quadrant

"We" Space: Nurse–Client Relationship

- Nurse and client create a common language that may bridge the standardized language of health care with the person's language of personal experience

Other Relationships: Family, Culture, Community

- Family is included in articulation of a common language describing client patterns/challenges/needs
- Cultural considerations
- Cultural practices
- Social norms
- Religion
- Moral values

The nurse identifies nursing diagnoses reflective of family processes and cultural meaning.

Interobjective Quadrant

The "ITS" Space: System Factors

Standardized language that is understandable to nurses, other healthcare professionals, and the managed care provider (e.g., NANDA-I Taxonomy Diagnoses): actual, risk, health promotion, system-level patterns/processes/needs (e.g., community diagnoses; external risks for illness, injury, and iatrogenic illnesses)

The nurse includes diagnoses related to system and external factors that may enhance or impinge upon client health.

Source: Nursing Process Organized in Four Quadrants Copyright © 2014, Pamela J. Potter, DNSc, RN, CNS-BC.

Quandrant describe the expected effect or influence of interventions that address the physiological and biological condition to be achieved within a specific time frame, measured by tools, tests, and observations to demonstrate attainment.

Upper Left: Subjective. **The nurse chooses nursing outcomes (and appropriate observational criteria)**

reflective of internal processes expressed by the client. Informed by practice expertise and personal factors, the nurse brings hopes and expectations for outcomes. The client brings hopes and expectations as well as readiness for change.

Lower Left: Intersubjective. **The nurse chooses nursing outcomes (and appropriate observational criteria) reflective of family processes and cultural**

EXHIBIT 8-3   Four-Quadrant Perspective: Nursing Language Covering the Greater Dimensions of Nursing

Upper Left: Subjective Quadrant
Psycho/spiritual
NANDA-I Dx
- Anxiety r/t inability to breathe effectively, fear of suffocation
- Ineffective coping r/t situational crisis
- Risk for Spiritual Distress r/t discouragement over
- health condition

NOC Outcomes
- Anxiety Self-Control
- Coping
- Hope
- Spiritual Health

NIC Activities
- Anxiety Reduction
- Coping Enhancement
- Spiritual Support

Upper Right: Objective Quadrant
Physiology
NANDA-I Dx
- Ineffective airway clearance
- Ineffective breathing pattern
- Impaired gas exchange
- Risk for Allergy Response

NOC Outcomes
- Respiratory Status: Airway Patency, Gas
- Exchange, Ventilation

NIC Activities
- Airway Management

Behavior
NANDA-I Dx
- Readiness for self health management

NOC Outcomes
- Health-Seeking Behavior
- Health-Promoting Behavior
- Knowledge

NIC Activities
- Anticipatory Guidance
- Mutual Goal Seeking
- Patient Contracting
- Self-Responsibility Facilitation

Lower Left: Intersubjective Quadrant
NANDA-I Dx*
- Disabled Family Coping
- Readiness for enhanced family processes

NOC Outcomes
- Family Normalization
- Family Coping
- Health-Seeking Behavior
- Health-Promoting Behavior
- Client Satisfaction

NIC Activities
- Family Process Maintenance
- Risk Identification

Lower Right: Interobjective Quadrant
NANDA-I Dx
- Risk for contamination r/t air pollution
- Readiness for Enhanced Community Coping

NOC Outcomes
- Community Health Status
- Community Risk Control

NIC Activities
- Environmental Risk Protection
- Health Policy Monitoring
- Health Education
- Program Development

*Culture is addressed in these diagnoses, outcomes, and interventions (Activities).

Source: This article was published in B. J. Ackley and G. B. Ladwigm, *Nursing Diagnosis Handbook: An Evidence-Based Guide to Planning Care*, 9th ed, Pamela J. Potter, DNSc, RN, CNS-BC., Nursing Language Organized in Four Quadrants, Copyright Elsevier 2011.

EXHIBIT 8-4 Outcome Identification: Nurse-Sensitive Outcomes Appropriate for Each Quadrant

Subjective Quadrant

The Nurse's "I" Space

- Hopes and expectations for outcomes

The Client's "I" Space

- Desire for healing
- Readiness for change
- Hopes and expectations for outcomes

The nurse chooses nursing outcomes (and appropriate observational criteria) reflective of internal processes expressed by the client.

Objective Quadrant

The "IT" Space

- Goal statement that addresses the physiological and biological condition to be achieved within a specific time frame
- Reasonably attainable maximum level of wellness
- Measures (tools, tests, observations) to demonstrate movement toward goals
- Expected effect or influence of interventions
- Produces psychophysiologic outcomes

The nurse chooses nursing outcomes (and appropriate measures) reflective of the client's physical and behavioral health presentation.

Intersubjective Quadrant

"We" Space: Nurse–Client Relationship

- Determine reasonably attainable maximum level of wellness
- Goals are established within the nurse–client relationship
- Client helps to establish observable milestones
- Client makes a commitment to move toward personally valued change

Other Relationships: Family, Culture, Community

- Family and significant others may participate in goal setting
- Consider family resources available to support goal achievement
- Consider available community resources

The nurse chooses nursing outcomes (and appropriate observational criteria) reflective of family processes and cultural meaning.

Interobjective Quadrant

The "ITS" Space: System Factors

- Other healthcare practitioners may participate in goal setting
- NOC terminology provides a standardized structure for documenting and assessing achievement of outcomes

System Supporting Patient Outcomes

- Consider available systems to support goal achievement
- Electronic health records that document outcomes
- Healthcare system culture/perspective/requirements
- Computer-codeable language is a systems factor

The nurse includes outcomes (and appropriate measures) related to system factors that may enhance or impinge upon client health.

Source: Nursing Process Organized in Four Quadrants Copyright © 2014, Pamela J. Potter, DNSc, RN, CNS-BC.

---

meaning. If outcomes are to be achieved, the nurse and client may be in a situation where they need to establish them with the assistance of the client and family. Goals are established within the nurse–client relationship. The holistic nurse suggests interventions on the basis of desired outcomes, discussing with the client possible ways for achieving these desired outcomes. The client helps to establish observable milestones for knowing whether desired changes have occurred and makes a commitment to move toward change. Family and significant others

may participate in goal setting and consideration of family recourses available to support goal achievement. The person must be motivated to establish outcomes suggested in the care plan. Assumptions made by the nurse concerning desired outcomes without collaboration with the person impede outcome achievement.

Lower Right: Interobjective. **The nurse includes outcomes (and appropriate measures) related to system factors that may enhance or impinge upon client health.** The nurse documents expected outcomes preferably using standardized language

(NOC) for communicating the effectiveness of nursing actions—a language recognizable by providers, payers, and other healthcare professionals. Outcomes describe the expected effect or influence of the intervention on movement toward the desired result. Within this classification system a *nursing-sensitive client outcome* is a measurable state, behavior, or perception that is responsive to nursing interventions.[7] Nursing outcomes are described along continuums that depict movement toward or away from desired goals, allowing for the measurement of change as positive, negative, or no change in the person's situation, behaviors, or perceptions. Outcome measures can be used as indicators of individual change as well as for quantitative comparison with a greater population when data are aggregated. These outcomes can be organized among the four quadrants depending on the aspect they address. Various outcomes have applicability in each of the four quadrants, as illustrated in Exhibit 8-3.

Therapeutic Care Plan and Interventions

The holistic Registered Nurse develops a plan that identifies strategies and alternatives to attain outcomes.[1] During the planning stage, nurses who use the holistic caring process help the person identify ways to repattern her or his behaviors to achieve a healthier state. The planning process reveals interventions that will achieve outcomes. The plan outlines nursing interventions, which are the specific actions that the nurse performs to help the person solve problems and accomplish outcomes. Nursing interventions direct the implementation of care (see **Exhibit 8-5**). A nursing intervention has been defined as "any treatment, based upon clinical judgment and knowledge, that a nurse performs to enhance client or client outcomes."[19]

Upper Right: Objective. **The nurse chooses appropriate nursing interventions for addressing physical and behavioral health presentation.** Prioritized by urgency and based on clinical judgment, nursing interventions may be independent (autonomous actions initiated by the nurse in response to nursing diagnosis) or collaborative (actions performed by the nurse in collaboration with other healthcare practitioners, responding to both medical and nursing diagnoses and potentially requiring a physician's order).[20] Nursing interventions include conventional and complementary/alternative modalities.

Upper Left: Subjective. **The nurse chooses appropriate nursing interventions for addressing internal processes expressed by the client.** Drawing on experience level (novice to expert) the holistic nurse engages *best thinking* about how to prioritize care. The client reflects internally and—based on ability to actively or receptively carry out the agreement—contracts with self for participation in care. Holistic nurses frequently select complementary/alternative modalities and generally noninvasive nursing interventions to complement standard nursing care. Holistic nurses incorporate complementary modalities into their practice as interventions for treating the body (biofeedback, therapeutic massage), relieving the mind (humor, imagery, meditation), comforting the soul (prayer), and supporting significant interpersonal interaction (healing presence).[21] Therapies such as acupressure, meditation, guided imagery, and therapeutic touch are listed as nursing interventions in the classification.

Lower Left: Intersubjective. **The nurse chooses appropriate nursing interventions reflective of family processes and cultural meaning.** The holistic nurse selects interventions on the basis of desired outcomes, discussing with the client possible ways for achieving these desired outcomes. The holistic nurse chooses interventions based on utility, relationship to the person's patterns/challenges/needs, effectiveness, feasibility, acceptability to the person, and nursing competency. Holistic nursing interventions reflect acknowledgement of the person's values, beliefs, culture, religion, and socioeconomic background.

Lower Right: Interobjective. **The nurse chooses appropriate nursing interventions related to system factors that may enhance or impinge upon client health.** The nurse considers available systems to support access to interventions. When offering complementary/alternative therapies, the nurse should refer to the rules and regulations within state licensure to clarify the legal scope of practice within some jurisdictions.

EXHIBIT 8-5   Therapeutic Care Plan and Interventions: Planned Nursing Activities Appropriate for Each Quadrant

Subjective Quadrant	**Objective Quadrant**
The Nurse's "I" Space	**The "IT" Space**
■ Best thinking about how to prioritize care	■ Nursing interventions, specific actions the nurse performs to help the client accomplish outcomes
■ Nurse presence	■ Prioritized by urgency
■ Novice-to-expert competencies	■ Based on clinical judgment
The Client's "I" Space	■ Independent
■ Client's contract with self	■ Collaborative
■ Ability to carry out the contract (actively or receptively)	■ Conventional
	■ Complementary/alternative
	■ Client engagement in specific actions to accomplish outcomes
The nurse chooses appropriate nursing interventions for addressing internal processes expressed by the client.	*The nurse chooses appropriate nursing interventions for addressing physical and behavioral health presentation.*
Intersubjective Quadrant	**Interobjective Quadrant**
"We" Space: Nurse–Client Relationship	**The "ITS" Space: System Factors**
■ The nurse helps the person identify ways to repattern behaviors to achieve a healthier state	■ Documented in client record through clear language such as the NIC terminology
■ Codefining specific client activities/contract	■ Evaluated and revised as necessary
■ Prioritize in collaboration with client when possible	**System Supporting Culture**
Other Relationships: Family, Culture, Community	■ Consider available systems to support access to interventions
■ Prioritize in collaboration with family as appropriate	
■ Reflect acceptance of the client's values, beliefs, culture, religion, and socioeconomic background	
■ Support family process	
The nurse chooses appropriate nursing interventions reflective of family processes and cultural meaning.	*The nurse chooses appropriate nursing interventions related to system factors that may enhance or impinge upon client health.*

Source: Nursing Process Organized in Four Quadrants Copyright © 2014, Pamela J. Potter, DNSc, RN, CNS-BC.

The therapeutic care plan is documented. Any revision of the plan reflects the person's current status or ongoing changes. In the client's record the nurse documents nursing-identified interventions in the therapeutic care plan using standardized language (NIC) compatible with NANDA-I and NOC terminology. These interventions can be organized among the four quadrants depending on the aspect they address. Various interventions have applicability in each of the four quadrants, as illustrated in Exhibit 8-3.

Implementation

The holistic Registered Nurse implements the identified plan in partnership with the person.[1] Nurses who are guided by a holistic framework approach the implementation phase of care with an awareness that (1) people are active participants in their care; (2) nursing care must be performed with purposeful, focused intention; and (3) a person's humanness is an important factor in implementation (see **Exhibit 8-6**). During this phase, the various persons deemed

Subjective Quadrant

The Nurse's "I" Space

- Nurse's presence within the process
- Nurse coaching

The Client's "I" Space

- Recipient of nursing action
- Client independent action

The nurse implements interventions for addressing internal processes expressed by the client in accordance with the documented care plan.

Objective Quadrant

The "IT" Space

- Nursing care performed with purposeful, focused intention
- Level of client engagement in specific actions to accomplish outcomes

The nurse implements physical and behavioral care in accordance with the documented care plan.

Intersubjective Quadrant

"We" Space: Nurse–Client Relationship

- Clients are active participants in their care
- Nurse implements therapeutic use of self

Other Relationships: Family, Culture, Community

- The nurse, client, family, or another person or agency implements the planned strategies

The nurse implements interventions reflective of family processes and cultural meaning in accordance with the documented care plan.

Interobjective Quadrant

The "ITS" Space: System Factors

- Procedures are carried out according to protocol, best practice guidelines, and best evidence
- Documented in the client's record

System Supporting Culture

- Time factors supporting or inhibiting

The nurse implements interventions related to system factors that may enhance or impinge upon client health in accordance with the documented care plan.

Source: Nursing Process Organized in Four Quadrants Copyright © 2014, Pamela J. Potter, DNSc, RN, CNS-BC.

appropriate—the nurse, the client, the family, or another person or agency—implement the planned strategies.[22]

A holistic nurse's encounter with a client for whatever purpose—talking to the person, touching the person, or taking a blood pressure—produces psychophysiologic outcomes. The encounter changes the consciousness and the physiology of both the nurse and the person. Because human emotions can be translated into physiologic responses, the greatest tool or intervention for helping and healing clients is the therapeutic use of self.[23]

Upper Right: Objective. **The nurse implements physical and behavioral care in accordance with the documented care plan.** Nursing care performed with purposeful, focused intention contributes to physiologic outcomes. Within the holistic framework, anything that produces a physiologic change causes a corresponding psychological, social, and spiritual alteration.

Upper Left: Subjective. **The nurse implements interventions for addressing internal processes expressed by the client in accordance with the documented care plan.** The nurse as coach to support client success expresses personal presence within the process. The client—recipient of nursing action rather than being merely acted upon—is an independent actor with a unique and individual response to care. Interior change within the client produces a psychological change that causes corresponding physiologic, social, and spiritual alteration.

Lower Left: Intersubjective. **The nurse implements interventions reflective of family processes and cultural meaning in accordance with the documented care plan.** Within the nurse–client relationship, the nurse implements therapeutic use of self, thus creating an interpersonal dynamic with the client recipient. People are active participants in their care. The nurse, client, family, or another person or agency implements the planned strategies.

Lower Right: Interobjective. **The nurse implements interventions related to system factors that may enhance or impinge upon client health in accordance with the documented care plan.** Procedures are carried out according to protocol/practice guidelines and documented in the client record. The nurse notes time and resource factors (e.g., staffing) that may support or inhibit implementation

Evaluation

The holistic Registered Nurse evaluates progress toward attainment of outcomes while recognizing and honoring the continuing holistic nature of the healing process.[1] Evaluation is a planned review of the nurse–person interaction to identify factors that facilitate or inhibit expected outcomes (see **Exhibit 8-7**). Within the holistic caring process, evaluation is a mutual process

EXHIBIT 8-7 Evaluation: Outcome Assessments of the Nursing Care Plan Appropriate for Each Quadrant	
Subjective Quadrant **The Nurse's "I" Space** - Reflects on client interaction and on nurse self-performance **The Client's "I" Space** - Satisfaction with outcome achievement - Enhanced self-awareness - Client becomes more aware of connections among previous patterns and sees benefit of repatterning behaviors *The nurse evaluates interventions for addressing internal processes expressed by the client as established in the care plan.*	**Objective Quadrant** **The "IT" Space** - Bio-psycho-social-spiritual status and responses - Related to identified patterns, outcome criteria, and nursing interventions - Assessed and recorded through NOC terminology and/or other tools, tests, and observations *The nurse evaluates physical and behavioral outcomes measures as established in the care plan.*
Intersubjective Quadrant **"We" Space: Nurse–Client Relationship** - Implementation strategies are evaluated to identify successful repatterning behaviors toward wellness - Review of nurse–client interaction to identify factors facilitating or inhibiting outcomes - Mutual process with client - Family is included in the evaluation of client outcomes within the nurse–client relationship *The nurse evaluates interventions reflective of family processes and cultural meaning as established in the care plan.*	**Interobjective Quadrant** **The "ITS" Space: System Factors** - Supportive of full documentation in client record **System Supporting Culture** - The person expresses level of satisfaction with care through client surveys or other means - The system recalibrates accordingly - Short- and long-term effects on healthcare delivery system, physical environment, and greater social context - Evaluation of care has implications for professional practice standards, health policy, environmental policy, achievement of holistic care - Ability to retrieve data for quality-assurance, safety, and research purposes *The nurse evaluates interventions related to system factors that may enhance or impinge upon client health in accordance with the established care plan.*

Source: Nursing Process Organized in Four Quadrants Copyright © 2014, Pamela J. Potter, DNSc, RN, CNS-BC.

between the nurse and the person receiving care. Data about the client's bio-psycho-social-spiritual status and responses are collected and recorded throughout the holistic caring process. The information is related to the person's patterns/challenges/needs, the outcome criteria, and the results of the nursing intervention. The nurse, in collaboration with the person during the course of care, may use measures from the NOC to document the effectiveness of the nursing interventions received.

The goal of evaluation is to determine if outcomes have been successful and, if so, to what extent. The nurse, person, family, and other members of the healthcare team all participate in the evaluation process. Together, they synthesize the data from the evaluation to identify successful repatterning behaviors toward wellness. During the evaluation, the person becomes more aware of previous patterns, develops insight into the interconnections of all dimensions of his or her life, and sees the benefits of repatterning behaviors. For example, does the person understand that his or her current job and level of stress have a direct effect on the current illness?

Upper Right: Objective. **The nurse evaluates physical and behavioral outcomes measures as established in the care plan.** Bio-psycho-social-spiritual status and responses related to identified patterns (NDx), implemented interventions (NIC), and outcome criteria (NOC) are evaluated to demonstrate attainment by comparing objective physiological and behavioral measures pre- and postimplementation.

Upper Left: Subjective. **The nurse evaluates interventions for addressing internal processes expressed by the client as established in the care plan.** The nurse determines satisfaction level with the care implementation by reflecting on self-performance of interpersonal and technical skills and outcome achievement. During the evaluation, the client expresses enhanced self-awareness about previous patterns, develops insight into the interconnections of all dimensions of his or her life, and sees the benefits of repatterning behaviors. For example, the client demonstrates understanding that his or her current job and level of stress have a direct effect on the current illness.

Lower Left: Intersubjective. **The nurse evaluates interventions reflective of family processes and cultural meaning as established in the care plan.** Implementation strategies are evaluated to identify successful repatterning behaviors toward wellness. In mutual processes, the nurse and client review the care trajectory to identify factors facilitating or inhibiting outcomes. The nurse, client, family, and other members of the healthcare team all participate in the evaluation process. Together, they synthesize the data from the evaluation to identify successful repatterning behaviors toward wellness and to reframe the care plan as needed.

Lower Right: Interobjective. **The nurse evaluates interventions related to system factors that may enhance or impinge upon client health in accordance with the established care plan.** Evaluation of the holistic caring process comes full circle with a self-aware appraisal of the entire nursing process by the nurse. From an ecological perspective, the evaluation of the holistic caring process extends beyond the level of the person to include the short- and long-term effects on the healthcare delivery system, the physical environment, and the greater social context. The holistic nurse must also reflect on the greater implications of the holistic caring process for professional practice standards and for health and environmental policy.

Multidimensionality of the Holistic Caring Process

From the Four-Quadrant Perspective, each step of the holistic caring process is multidimensional. The Upper Right contains the objective, physiological, and behavioral observations that can be made about the client, diagnoses reflective of these objective observations, as well as the corresponding outcome norms, interventions, and evaluation measures. The Upper Left contains both the intrapersonal space of the nurse and the client, as well as the corresponding client diagnoses, outcome, intervention, and evaluation measures. The Lower Left contains the interpersonal relationship established between the nurse and the client. This dimension includes consideration of family and culture in the nurse–client relationship. Further, corresponding diagnoses, outcome, intervention, and evaluation measures reflective of family and culture are describable in this quadrant. The Lower Right reflects system factors that influence caregiving and receiving outcomes, organizational structures, policies, and procedures (e.g., staffing levels, documenting care in the electronic health record). This dimension also considers environmental factors that may be contributing to the client's health presentation with corresponding diagnoses, outcome, intervention, and evaluation measures. The Four-Quadrant Perspective gives holistic nurses a framework to honor all ways of knowing and being. The Four-Quadrant Perspective mapped to the holistic caring process provides a means to understand and give voice to care that encompasses all dimensions of nurse–client experiences. The authors, who have been working with the nursing process and the holistic caring process for years, are grateful to the practitioners of Integral Theory who have brought a perspective to our work that adds clarity and offers new directions.

Conclusion

By definition, any nurse in any setting can practice holistic nursing. *Holistic Nursing: Scope and Standards of Practice, Second Edition*[1] (see Chapter 2), can be framed in the universal language of the holistic caring process and may easily be combined with other more physiologically based standards, such as those for cardiovascular and critical care nursing. Thus, *Holistic Nursing: Scope and Standards of Practice, Second Edition*, can be incorporated into all subspecialty standards of care to ensure not only high-quality physiologic care but also high-quality holistic nursing care to these specialty populations.

Holistic Nursing: Scope and Standards of Practice, Second Edition, necessitates the application of a whole new lens to the nursing process. Although standardized language is beneficial for the acknowledgment and documentation of nursing expertise and practice, such labels do not always communicate adequately the person's health situation and need for care. Viewing standardized nursing diagnoses, interventions, and outcomes through a lens of *Holistic Nursing:*

Scope and Standards of Practice, Second Edition, gives nurses a means to refine and enhance their care as well as to describe and document the caring process of nursing.

Directions for Future Research

1. Evaluate each nursing diagnosis, nursing intervention, and nursing outcome for compatibility with holistic nursing practice standards.
2. Explore whether writing nursing diagnoses related to holistic nursing standards (e.g., readiness for enhanced nutrition) improves outcomes.
3. Evaluate the effectiveness and nature of intuitive judgments used by holistic nurses.
4. Investigate whether incorporating the holistic caring process into a four-quadrant perspective positively affects subjective and objective client outcomes.
5. Determine the effects of incorporating the holistic caring process into practice on nurse work satisfaction and turnover.

Nurse Healer Reflections

After reading this chapter, the nurse healer will be able to answer or to begin a process of answering the following questions:

- How am I guided in my everyday life and work by the holistic caring process?
- How can I take an integral perspective, utilizing the four quadrants for organizing my implementation of the holistic caring process?
- How do I reconcile what I know about health and healing to the beliefs and realities that might be held by the people to whom I give care and by my coworkers?
- How can I systematically begin to apply the holistic caring process in terms of standardized nursing taxonomies for diagnoses, interventions, and outcomes?
- How can I cultivate my intuitive processes?
- How do I react when clients indicate that they are not motivated to change health patterns and behavior?

■ How do I feel when I incorporate the principles of holistic nursing into my nursing practice?

NOTES

1. American Holistic Nurses Association and American Nurses Association, *Holistic Nursing: Scope and Standards of Practice*, 2nd ed. (Silver Spring, MD: Nursesbooks.org, 2013).

2. K. Wilber, *A Brief History of Everything* (Boston: Shamabala, 2000).

3. K. Wilber, *Integral Psychology* (Boston: Shambhala, 2000).

4. B. M. Dossey, "Nursing: Integral, Integrative, and Holistic—Local to Global," in *Holistic Nursing: A Handbook for Practice*, 6th ed., eds. B. M. Dossey and L. Keegan (Burlington, MA: Jones & Bartlett Learning): 3–57.

5. NANDA International, *Nursing Diagnoses: Definitions and Classification, 2012–2014*, ed. T. H. Herdman (Oxford, England: Wiley-Blackwell, 2012): 93.

6. G. M. Bulechek, H. K. Butcher, J. M. Dochterman, and C. Wagner, *Nursing Interventions Classification (NIC)*, 6th ed. (St. Louis, MO: Mosby, 2013).

7. S. Moorhead, M. Johnson, M. Maas, and E. Swanson, *Nursing Outcomes Classification (NOC)*, 5th ed. (St. Louis, MO: Mosby, 2013).

8. F. R. Kreuter, "What Is Good Nursing Care?" *Nursing Outlook* 5 (1957): 302–304.

9. H. C. Erickson, E. M. Tomlin, and M A. P. Swahi, *Modeling and Role-Modeling: A Theory and Paradigm for Nursing* (Englewood Cliffs, NJ: Prentice Hall, 1983): 103.

10. C. Johns, *Becoming a Reflective Practitioner*, 2nd ed. (Oxford, England: Blackwell, 2004).

11. B. A. Carper, "Fundamental Patterns of Knowing in Nursing," *Advances in Nursing Science* 1, no. 1 (1978): 13–23.

12. American Holistic Nurses Association, *Position Statement on Holistic Nursing Ethics* (Flagstaff, AZ: American Holistic Nurses Association, 2007). http://www.ahna.org/Resources/Publications/Position-Statements#P2

13. C. Johns, "Framing Learning Through Reflection Within Carper's Fundamental Ways of Knowing in Nursing," *Journal of Advanced Nursing* 22, no. 2 (1995): 226–234.

14. C. E. Young, "Intuition and the Nursing Process," *Holistic Nursing Practice* 1, no. 3 (1987): 52–62.

15. J. A. Effken, "Information Basis for Expert Intuition," *Journal of Advanced Nursing* 34, no. 2 (2001): 246–254.

16. J. A. Effken, "The Informational Basis for Nursing Intuition: Philosophical Underpinnings," *Nursing Philosophy* 8, no. 3 (2007): 187–200.

17. J. S. Perdue, "Integration of Complementary and Alternative Therapies in an Acute Rehabilitation Hospital: A Readiness Assessment" (unpublished doctoral dissertation, Western University of Health Sciences, Pomona, CA, 2011).

18. C. S. Clark, "Beyond Holism: Incorporating an Integral Approach to Support Caring-Healing-Sustainable Nursing Practices," *Holistic Nursing Practice* 26, no. 2 (2012): 92–102.

19. J. Dochterman and G. M. Bulechek, *Classification of Nursing Interventions: Implications for Nursing Diagnoses* (St. Louis, MO: Mosby, 2004): 3.

20. B. J. Ackley and G. B. Ladwigm, *Nursing Diagnosis Handbook: An Evidence-Based Guide to Planning Care*, 10th ed. (Maryland Heights, MO: Mosby, 2014).

21. N. C. Frisch, "Standards for Holistic Nursing Practice: A Way to Think About Our Care That Includes Complementary and Alternative Modalities," *Online Journal for Issues in Nursing* 6, no. 2 (2001).

22. J. Engebretson and L. Y. Littleton, "Cultural Negotiation: A Constructivist-Based Model for Nursing Practice," *Nursing Outlook* 49, no. 5 (2001): 223–230.

23. D. Krieger, *Foundation of Holistic Health Nursing Practice* (Philadelphia: J. B. Lippincott, 1981).

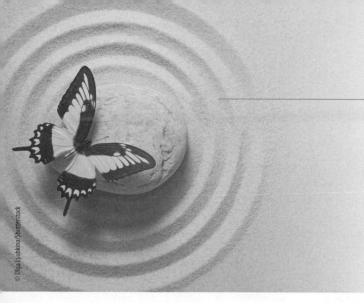

CHAPTER 9

Energy Healing

Deborah A. Shields and Debra Rose Wilson

Nurse Healer Objectives

Theoretical

- Examine the history of energy healing.
- Describe three major energetic structures.
- Discuss one view of chakras.
- Describe electromagnetic induction and entrainment and how they might operate in energy healing.
- Discuss the role of intention in creating healing space.
- Discuss one problem in energy healing research.

Clinical

- Find an expert energy healing practitioner and determine what makes this person an expert. What made you decide this person was an expert? If this person is a nurse practicing energy healing, how is energy healing integrated into his or her nursing practice?

Personal

- Use the experiential exercises included in the online resources to explore auras, chakras, and meridians.
- Experience a laying-on-of-hands modality.
- Explore the effect of your presence.

- Experience an essential oil, flower essence, and/or homeopathic preparation that may be useful for you.
- Experience the effects of music you do not like. Stand a few feet away as you listen to it for a few minutes. Gradually, over several weeks, move closer.

Definitions

Atom: The building block of matter consisting of a nucleus (which is made up of protons and neutrons) surrounded by a swarm of circulating electrons.

Aura: A vague, luminous glow surrounding something. The luminous glow may be an electromagnetic field that contains information.

Chakra: An energy center in the subtle, or energetic, body that is described as a whirling vortex of light. Chakras are believed to be portals for energy and information flowing into and out of a person.

Electromagnetic field: A field is an area in which something can act on or influence something else. An electromagnetic field is a space in which there are charged objects and magnetic fields at the same time. The magnetic field pulls on the charged objects and the objects influence the magnetic field.

Electromagnetic radiation: The energy given off, or that radiates from, an electromagnetic field.

Electron: A negatively charged tiny particle orbiting the nucleus of an atom.

Energy healing: The deliberate process of using an external energy field to induce a change in one's own or another's field for the purpose of physical, mental, emotional, and spiritual healing. Energy healing may involve the presence of a caring person.

Entanglement: Quantum entanglement is one of the central principles of quantum physics. *Entanglement* is a term used to describe the way that particles of energy and matter can become correlated to predictably interact with one another regardless of how far apart they are. This suggests that space is just the construct that gives the illusion that there are separate objects.

Entrainment: The phenomenon of rhythmic processes synchronizing with one another. Synchronization is recognized in pendulum clocks, planets, music, an organism adjusting to the light–dark cycle, brain waves, social groups, and more.

Intention: Choosing to think, act, or be a certain way.

Meridian: Microvolt electrical conduits organized in an electrical mesh that permeates the body and precedes development of vessels and organs. In Eastern philosophies, the meridians are said to conduct *chi*, or universal energy.

Nonlocality: Describes the apparent ability of objects to instantaneously know about one another's state, even when separated by large distances (potentially even billions of light years), almost as if the universe at large instantaneously arranges its particles in anticipation of future events. Nonlocality suggests that the universe is profoundly different from our habitual understanding of it, and that the "separate" parts of the universe are actually potentially connected in an intimate and immediate way. Nonlocality occurs due to the phenomenon of entanglement.

Nucleus: The center of an atom. The nucleus is composed of several structures, including the well-known protons, but also quarks, which include the oddly named Up, Down, Beauty, and Strange. Gluons hold them together to create the nucleus of an atom; once thought to be the smallest piece of mass, impenetrable and unable to ever break into pieces.

Photon: A small packet of light bundled; the smallest part of an electromagnetic force, considered a messenger particle. Einstein conceived of light as being particles that he called photons, or *quanta*, thus quantum physics.

Proton: A positively charged particle found in the nucleus of an atom, made up of three quarks.

Sham healing: A term used for control groups in experimental studies where a pretend energy healing treatment is given.

Subtle energy: Barely noticeable electrical and magnetic fields of living organisms that may be related to internal electrical and magnetic activity.

Energy Healing

In his essay "All Tangled Up: Life in a Quantum World," Larry Dossey reminds readers of the joys and complexities of living during these transformative times.[1] We are, as a society, increasingly aware of and willing to discuss ideas that were once taboo or thought to be out of the realm of possibility. One need only look at publications such as *My Stroke of Insight* to appreciate the speed with which quantum realities are becoming part of the contemporary culture.[2] In this thought-provoking book, Dr. Bolte Taylor recounts her healing journey after experiencing a stroke at the age of 37. Through a description of the events that began with the onset of her symptoms, she shares that on the morning of her stroke "my consciousness shifted into a perception that I was at one with the universe."[2, p. xv] Throughout her story, Dr. Bolte Taylor discusses the effects that people had on her: "I paid very close attention to how energy dynamics affected me. I realized that some people brought me energy while others took it away."[2, p. 77]

One example of new thinking involves the nature of consciousness. The notion that consciousness is situated only in the human brain and body is becoming passé. Several scientists posit that some level of consciousness has been embedded in biological systems since the first organism, and organisms have evolved and adapted to take advantage of it. Animals clearly have consciousness, and studies indicate that they possess a consciousness that is not as highly evolved as that of humans.[1] There is a belief that consciousness is nonlocal and entangled. Dossey suggests that a nonlocal, entangled consciousness would enable humans to act the way we do, whereas another kind of consciousness would not.[1] Radin presents evidence suggesting that consciousness is unrelated to space and time.[3] All of this indicates that we still have much to learn about consciousness—it is not local, it does not respond to the laws of space and time, and it is entangled with our biological structure. Ancient healing traditions such as those found in Eastern cultures have long taught this as truth, and these teachings have become part of wisdom traditions. Energy healing practices evolved in these wisdom traditions and are found in almost every society, as if they are a natural form of healing. These wisdom traditions seem to know what science is just discovering.

Energy practices appear to involve a meshing of consciousness and elements that physicists study, such as electromagnetic fields. This leads to the idea of holism, or the notion that our life cannot be defined only by its bodily parts but also by its interaction with our consciousness. We may not be able to separate ourselves into parts at all. If we are a whole, how does that whole interact with other wholes, other beings? Perhaps the answer is in physics' realm, rather than biology's.

There are several energy therapies, including laying-on-of hands types such as Therapeutic Touch, Reiki, and Healing Touch, to name a few. Evidence suggests that therapies such as these are effective in a variety of situations. Other forms of energy modalities, such as aromatherapy, flower essences, sound, and light, also show positive outcomes.

By expanding the discussion that basic physics principles are involved in energy therapies and integrating this evidence with those qualities that we know are foundational in healing (e.g., compassion, presence, intention, and intuition), a holistic perspective of energy as a healing phenomenon, and possible explanations of how energy healing therapies work, is offered.

History

Historical literature abounds with rich descriptions of the evolution of healing and therapies that support the process. The exploration of energy healing invites holistic nurses to reflect on the foundations of energy as a life force to more clearly understand contemporary energy healing practices. This connection offers the reader a brief glimpse into the energy story and an opportunity to meet some of the trailblazers who have, in many ways, created spaces for the integration of energy therapies into caring for the whole person.

The concept of a life energy that is a vital life force has been a basic philosophy since ancient times.[4] The worldview of traditional societies was one of harmony and communication within and between humans and all that surrounded them. This philosophy included a belief that there was a life force involved in this interchange, and that the balance or imbalance that resulted from this interchange was the source of health or illness.[4-7] This life force is called by different names in different cultures (e.g., Chinese *qi*; Japanese *ki*; Greek *pneuma*; Tibetan *lung*; Native American *oki*, *orenda*, *ton*; Hindu *prana*; and Western *biofield*). Each is described similarly in relation to properties and function with vital energy/life force flowing freely through and between living beings and their environment.

Ancient Healing Traditions

Archeological evidence suggests that indigenous healers and shamans have existed throughout the world for 20,000 years.[7, 8] Healing in shamanic tradition "relies on insight and intuition, on the ability to create and interpret vivid images, and to induce in others altered states of consciousness conducive to self-healing."[7, p. 19] Energy healing, often in the form of the laying on of hands, was a part of everyday life. Pyrenees cave paintings from 15,000 years ago, ancient Egyptian rock carvings from 2700 BC, Ebers Papyrus writings from 1552, and Greek manuscripts from the Aesculapian temples dating to 400 BC describe, through carvings and the written word, the use of energy to help the sick.[4, 7]

Hippocrates (circa 460 BC) established a medical school at the end of the 5th century. He believed in unification and harmony between nature and man and recognized a healing life force present in all organisms. Hippocrates believed that disease was a dual process and that treatments must include both systematic medicine as well as that which activates the patient's own healing. He summed up his extensive healing experience this way: "It has often appeared, while I have been soothing my patients, as if there were some strange property in my hands to pull and draw from the afflicted parts aches and diverse impurities."[9]

The next section will review ancient healing systems that are still practiced today, including Confucianism, considered one of the oldest schools of philosophy in China, and Buddhism and Jainism, which developed about the same time in India. The youngest, Taoism, evolved in China around 200 years before the time of Christ.[10, 11]

Traditional Chinese Medicine

Traditional Chinese Medicine, believed to be 5,000 years old, is derived from Taoist, Buddhist, and Confucian lineage.[12] Within Chinese mythology, it is said that people experimented with certain exercises after work and noticed energy vibrating through their bodies and up and down their extremities. These movements were precursors to the meditation practices of taiji quan and qi gong.[13] As people refined these techniques, they noticed increased mental clarity and vitality, leading to a sense of well-being and relaxation while exercising. This vibrating energy was called *qi*.

The Fire Emperor, Shen Nong (2698–2598 BC), is considered the founder of Chinese herbal medicine. *The Yellow Emperor's Inner Classic*, dated approximately 2700 BC and written by the Yellow Emperor Huang Di, is perhaps the earliest written history of Traditional Chinese Medicine.[14, 15] The goal of Traditional Chinese Medicine is health promotion and quality of life; the emphasis is always on the patient, not the illness. The philosophical belief that there exists a natural order in the universe and an interconnectedness between the body and the cosmos underlies the search for balance and harmony within an environment in constant flux.[14]

Qi is the central concept of Traditional Chinese Medicine; it is life essence, the vital energy that is behind all physiological processes, and flows through animals, plants, people, the Earth, and the sky. Qi is distributed throughout the organism along a network of meridians, which connect all parts of the organism. All life processes are based in the movement of qi. Obstructed, disordered, excess, or deficient qi flow results in problems that are unique to the person and involve disorders of the bodymindspirit.

In Traditional Chinese Medicine, wholeness is a union of opposites.[14] These opposite and complementary aspects are the yin and the yang. Yin and yang are in constant motion and each is a part of the other. Yin represents passivity and restfulness and is associated more with substance than with energy. Yang is activity and aggressiveness and is the energy that directs movement and supports substance. Yin and yang coexist and are dependent on one another. Health and well-being result from a balance of yin and yang energy.

Traditional Chinese Medicine is a complex system in which there is unity and interaction within all human components. It is easiest to understand using the well-known picture of yin and yang and the idea of Tao, or All. The Tao contains two cycles, the Shen and the K'o.

The Tao is represented by a circle containing yin and yang and all opposites; the clockwise flow of this circle forms the Shen cycle. In health, people flow with the Tao. This natural flow is linked to the five seasons, which are each associated with the five elements. The elements are further associated with a color, climate, direction, sound, odor, taste, power, life aspect, time of day, emotion, body and sense organs, and a secretion. The K'o cycle is implicit within the Shen cycle and is considered the cycle of control. It is associated with thoughts, emotions, and behaviors, which also exist as opposites (e.g., joy/sorrow, love/hate).[8] The Chinese believe that "a combination of life force elements makes up the substance and functions of the body, mind, and spirit and that these three are one and the same."[14, p. 62]

Ayurveda

Early Egyptians believed that humans were a "microcosm of the macrocosm, and expected to reflect its order and harmony."[7, p. 20] This was achieved by balancing the divine, the upward movement of Earth energies, and the vital life energies. The vital life energies were believed to be regulated by a spiritual body that enveloped the physical body, and temple healers (priests) "sought to direct these forces by passes over the body."[7, p. 20]

The Egyptian belief in interconnection also underlies the traditional medical system Ayurveda, which has been practiced in India for at least 5,000 years.[7, 14] Ayurveda embraces the philosophy of balance of body, mind, and spirit as well as balance among people, their environment, and the cosmos. Ayurveda is Sanskrit, derived from the roots *ayur* (life) and *veda* (knowledge) and literally translates to "the science of life."[14] The basic concepts of this intricate, complex system are founded on the belief that there is a fundamental connection between the microcosm and the macrocosm—people are created by the universe and contain everything that comprises the surrounding world. To understand people, one must understand the world and vice versa. The interdependence between individuals and society informs health and the quality of life.

Ayurveda views people and nature as composed of five elements (water, air, fire, earth, space), which are both energy and matter. All that exists is related to the interaction of these elements. Ayurveda "sees the body as *doshas* (vital energies), *dhatus* (tissues), and *malas* (waste products)."[14, p. 81] The doshas create body tissues, eliminate unnecessary wastes, and are responsible for all psychological and physiological processes.[14] Health is the balance of each dosha that is right for that individual. When there is balance, there is health in the body, mind, spirit, and environment.

Energy is prana. It is the basic life force, the original creative power, and prana is distributed along the nadis, which are energy pathways of the subtle body. Prana has many meanings, from the physical breath to the energy of consciousness. The five pranas are categorized "according to movement, direction, and body region."[14, p. 85] Energy moves inward, downward, upward, and outward and in so doing involves all of the body and all functions. See the suggested readings at the end of this chapter for more information on pranic energy.

Lifestyle interventions are the major preventive and therapeutic approaches in Ayurveda. These might include nutrition, herbs, exercise, yoga, breathing, meditation, massage, aromatherapy, music, and purification. Each treatment is designed according to the person's dosha, with the goal of returning right balance.

Themes in Eastern Healing Traditions

Similarities between these and other Eastern healing traditions are evident. They all believe that the universe is a subtle energy system reflected within the human body. Energy is distributed along pathways and, when a person is healthy, there is a balanced, harmonious flow of energy along them. People are part of their environment, and it is not possible to "treat" a health challenge without considering a person's environment. Eastern healing systems recognize the importance of a person's inner journey and its role in health; integrating contemplative practices such as meditation or prayer into daily life can create the quiet time needed to listen to those "inner messages." Movement practices, such as taiji quan, qi gong, and yoga, are thought to strengthen the energy pathways. The practitioner's goal is to co-create with the person therapeutic plans that will restore the balanced and harmonious flow of energy.

Western Healing Traditions: 16th Century Through 19th Century

Ancient medical systems are viewed as precursors to modern Western-evolved energy therapies. It is helpful to explore how emerging forces within science and religion influenced healing ideals and practices in the time after the birth of Christianity. In early times, healing was associated with religion and religious leaders. Hands-on healing, along with administering sacraments and preaching, was a part of the Christian ministry. By the 11th century, political power play was increasing between church and state. Church leaders believed that illness was a punishment for sins, and healing was only possible through acts of repentance; healing outside the church was viewed as suspicious. Healers were called witches and their practice was considered to be witchcraft or devil's work. Practitioners were often put to death by burning at the stake, which kept their practice secret. Royalty believed that only they had the power to heal through the laying on of hands, given to them by divine right. Thus came the term we now know as the *royal touch*.[16]

Scrofula (tuberculous cervical lymphadenitis), a disease common in the Middle Ages, was termed the *king's evil*.[16] Scrofula was distressing and created much physical and social suffering in individuals. Interestingly, this scourge was amenable to cure through the king's touch, or royal touch. Thus, healing through the touch of a king's hand became well known and was, in fact, one of the most famed ceremonies in the English monarchy.[16] Roman emperors Vespasian and Hadrian, King Philip I of France, and Edward the Confessor were among those known to possess this ability. King Olaf II of Norway was respected as a compassionate healer; he was canonized and was considered the patron saint of healers.

Interestingly, Valentine Greatrakes (circa 1628), an Irish gentleman, also possessed this ability.[16] Greatrakes, six or seven years after returning home from service in the English army under Oliver Cromwell, experienced a powerful realization that he could heal scrofula, and this transformed his life. He undertook this mission, working with and curing many people with a variety of diseases; he did not request monetary compensation. As his fame grew so did interest in him by the English monarchy: How could a "nonroyal" accomplish these healings?

Two men who used subtle energies to heal have come down in history with varied repute; some believe them to be trailblazers, others charlatans. Theophrastus Bombastus von Hohenheim (Paracelsus), a 16th-century mystic, described *munia*, a magnetic, healing, solar force that swept in waves throughout the universe. Paracelsus believed that munia radiated around the human body in a luminous shield and could be transmitted at a distance. Despite the many healings attributed to him, Paracelsus was not only derided by his peers but also negatively immortalized in the epithet "bombastic," based on his birth name Bombastus.[9] Inspired by Paracelsus, Dr. Franz Anton Mesmer (1734–1815) claimed that a subtle life energy of a magnetic nature was exchanged between healer and patient during the laying on of hands. He was credited with many cures, such as ridding a Munich scientist of paralysis and a professor of blindness, simply by passing his hands over them. When hypnosis was discovered through experimentation with his techniques, Mesmer's cures were dismissed as the power of suggestion. His name was used disrespectfully as "mesmerize," connoting undue influence.[9]

During the period of scientific enlightenment, as medicine moved into the laboratory, a universal energy, often with magnetic properties, was rediscovered many times. Luigi Galvani (1737–1798), an Italian physician and anatomy professor in Bologna, described a life force similar to electricity and magnetism that seemed to radiate from the sun and had an affinity for metal, water, and wood. This life force permeated everything—it pulsated through the human body by means of the breath and streamed from the fingertips. Galvani is credited with the discovery of "animal electricity."[9] Physicians began experimenting with the application of electricity and magnetism for the treatment of disease. During the 19th century there was a widespread interest in electrotherapy devices. It has been estimated that, by 1884, there were 10,000 physicians in the United States using electricity every day for therapeutic purposes.[17]

It is important to note that while this interest in electricity and magnetism was occurring, the scientific model became the gold standard and dominated the world of medicine. Biomedicine was founded on the beliefs of René Descartes (the mind and body are separate) and the principles of physics proposed by Sir Isaac Newton (the universe and everything in it operates in a linear, sequential form).[14] The human body was viewed as a series of smaller and smaller parts, which, in illness, required repair. Health was viewed as the absence of disease, and the focus of care was on symptom eradication and cure rather than on the whole person. Discovery and growth was rapid, and the emphasis shifted from healing to curing. The biomedical paradigm predominated in the Western world, not only in the approach to care but also in the development of educational curricula. The Pure Food and Drug Act of 1906 and the Flexner Report of 1910 strengthened the resolve for science to ground education and practice. The declaration that electrical and other energy therapies were scientifically unsupportable and therefore illegal set the stage for the pharmacological age of the 20th and 21st centuries—and the belief that there would be a "pill for everything."[17]

Early 20th Century

The fascination with electricity as a diagnostic and therapeutic force continued to resonate with researchers despite governmental regulations and taboos.[17] Initially, research focused on electrophysiology and the basis of electrical energy measurements (e.g., electroencephalogram, electrocardiogram) but soon included the healing properties of energy. Nikola Tesla, the inventor of modern alternating current technology (circa 1889), promoted the use of high-frequency coil devices for healing. In these devices, an electric wire was wrapped into a coil through which high-frequency electricity could flow. These coil designs worked by producing a broad spectrum of high-frequency emissions that appeared to create beneficial conditions within living tissues. Tesla's coil designs were often used in the treatment of those living with cancer.

In 1919, Dr. Albert Abrams developed his theory: the Electronic Reactions of Abrams (ERA). According to ERA, all diseases have their own "vibratory rate," which can be measured and treated with unique electronic boxes developed by Abrams. Abrams's theory posited that disease could be cured by "transmitting" back to the diseased tissue the same subtle vibratory rate it was transmitting. This would neutralize the abnormal vibrations and allow the tissue to exhibit healthy vibratory rates, thus potentially eliminating the disease. Abrams also believed that drugs worked when they had the same or similar vibrations as the disease they cured. This approach to disease management was similar to the principles of homeopathy set forth by its founder, Samuel Hahnemann. Abrams's work was one of the first attempts in the 20th century to apply the subtle energy domain to medicine and is said to have contributed to later developments with electromagnetic waves and the principles of vibrational medicine as described by Gerber.[17]

Harold Saxton Burr, a neuroanatomist at the Yale University School of Medicine, investigated energy fields in living systems from 1932 to 1956. He believed that life not only *exhibited* electromagnetic properties but that these same properties were "the organizing principle" that kept living tissue from falling into a chaotic state. Burr demonstrated that all living systems are molded and controlled by invisible electrodynamic force fields that can be measured and mapped with standard voltmeters. He called these basic blueprints of all living things "fields of life" or "L-fields," believing that they reflected physical and mental conditions. In 1937, he began a series of experiments that sought to measure and characterize the "bio-magnetic field" associated with living organisms. Burr believed their voltage could be used to diagnose physical and mental conditions *before* symptoms developed and validated his theory by comparing the L-fields of mice injected with cancer to control groups of healthy mice. He provided evidence with sophisticated electrical measurements and by being the first scientist to demonstrate that the appearance of physical illness (cancer, in this case) occurs *after* a measurable change in the organism's electric field. Burr's work was ahead of its time and contributed to the scientific understanding of the organizing principles animating all life.[18] Sadly, his ideas were dismissed by many scientists; today, however, his work is being revisited and is pivotal in the discoveries occurring in the field of energy healing.[4, 17, 19]

The Paradigm Is Shifting

The logical order of the universe and the mechanistic worldview was dominant until

20th-century physics, relativity, and quantum theory challenged this concept of boundaries. Early scientists who challenged this theory included Faraday and Maxwell and their discovery that light was a rapidly alternating electromagnetic field traveling through space in the form of waves.[20] Einstein's Theory of Relativity (1961) viewed the universe as a dynamic whole whose parts are interrelated and understood as a pattern of process. The idea of absolute time and space was abolished by this theory.

> Radin suggests that Einstein's Special Theory of Relativity proposes that matter and energy are different aspects of the same substance. . . . Entanglement is a property of both matter (as in atoms) and energy (as in photons). This means that the bioelectromagnetic fields around our bodies are entangled with the electromagnetic fields in the local environment and with photons arriving from distant stars.[3, p. 268]

This idea supports the connection and interpenetration of all energetic fields.

Nobel Laureate Albert Szent-Györgyi (1893–1986) developed fundamental ideas about the application of the theories of quantum physics to biochemistry and later to cancer. His research on the subatomic properties of the protein fabric of the body led to the recognition that the living matrix behaved like a semiconductor. Dr. Szent-Györgyi recognized that almost all of the body formed an energetic continuum, with molecules acting as vital "conductors" in the energetic "dance of life." His later work involved research with free radicals and their relationship to cancer and aging; he believed that cancer was an electronic problem at the level of the molecule.

The General Systems Theory of von Bertalanffy (1960) described the world in terms of relationships, emphasizing the basic principle of organization, interconnections, and interdependence of the parts. Systems behave as a collective whole and "the living domain of nature can be regarded as a hierarchy or network of nested systems of organized complexity."[21, p. 705] On the other hand, linear systems are mechanistic, expressing stimulus–response behavior within a system that can be taken apart and rebuilt

and that will behave in the same way. Linear thinking underpins much of the dominant biomedical paradigm as scientists search for cause-and-effect relationships. However, nonlinear systems are irreducible and possess complex patterns of communication, including feedback. Thus, the response is never predictable. This thinking underpins the newer scientific paradigm that recognizes that living systems are, indeed, nonlinear.

Scientific exploration also led to the development of energy field theory. Burr and Northrup proposed that all of life was enveloped in electromagnetic "life" fields.[22] In the 1960s, Bernard Grad, a Canadian biochemist, and Oskar Estebany, a healer, began double-blind studies on wounded mice using the laying on of hands. In the first experiments, skin wounds were made on the backs of mice. The healer, Mr. Estebany, treated the mice by placing them in containers between his hands for two 15-minute periods daily, five-and-one-half days per week. The wounds were healed 20 days after they were made. Control mice were left untreated or placed between the hands of persons who were not healers. The rate of healing was significantly faster in Mr. Estebany's group. In two subsequent experiments, Dr. Grad studied the effect of water "treated" by Mr. Estebany on the growth of plants. Once again, similar results were obtained.[23] The groundwork for future research was in place. Similarly, early nursing research related to energy healing was conducted by Krieger in the 1970s. In three separate research studies she found that sick persons receiving Therapeutic Touch experienced increased hemoglobin levels.

A pivotal shift occurred in the 1950s when Bassett and colleagues at Columbia University rediscovered the use of electricity and magnetism as treatments for the nonunion of fractures. Electrical stimulation, the preferred method of treatment in the mid-1800s, was discontinued along with all other electrotherapies following the Flexner Report of 1910. The discovery by these orthopedic surgeons that one could "jump-start" healing in a bone that had failed to heal for as long as 40 years led to extensive clinical trials under excessively stringent FDA supervision; eventually, pulsing electromagnetic field therapy became an accepted and widely used procedure for treating nonunion of fracture.[4] A few years later, Dr. Norm Shealey introduced the TENS (transcutaneous nerve stimulators) unit for treatment of pain. He, too, experienced a lengthy and difficult interaction with the FDA, but the TENS unit was finally recognized as safe and effective.

The importance of our broadening awareness of culture and traditions that inform caring and healing unfolded during the 20th century as travel opportunities and communication expanded. As we learned about other cultural healing practices, we began to integrate these into our health care. Elmer Green, considered by some to be one of the fathers of biofeedback, was interested in psychic phenomena and psychophysiology. Beginning in 1964 in the research department of the Menninger Foundation in Topeka, Kansas, Elmer and Alyce Green conducted research on the self-regulation skills of yogis, Tibetan trance meditators, and others having this ability. They demonstrated that ordinary people could develop skills in self-regulation much like yogis.[17] About this same time (1979), Kabat-Zinn was introducing mindfulness as a meditative approach to quieting the mind and managing stress.[24] People were becoming more interested in integrating holistic self-care practices into their daily lives. See the suggested readings at the end of this chapter for more information on Kabat-Zinn's Mindfulness-Based Stress Reduction Program.

In 1969, the Conference on Consciousness began exploring hands-on healing. The work was cosponsored by the Menninger Foundation and the Association of Transpersonal Psychology. One of the most significant outcomes of these observations was that people could learn hands-on healing techniques; it was not necessary to be born with this gift. This knowledge contributed to the development of energy therapies (e.g., Therapeutic Touch, Healing Touch).

The ideas of subtle energy in the form of life energy, or qi, began to be more widely appreciated in America after President Richard Nixon's visit to China in 1971. Accompanying President Nixon on his trip was journalist James Reston, who fell ill with appendicitis, had emergency surgery, and was treated postoperatively with acupuncture for pain relief. Reston was impressed by his experience with acupuncture and wrote about it in *The New York Times*.[25] This created interest in acupuncture and Traditional Chinese Medicine. Not long after, Eisenburg and colleagues examined 16 alternative therapies. The results were surprising and included the following:[26]

- One in three adults sought alternative therapies.
- There were more visits to alternative therapists than to primary physicians.
- People spent $14 billion on these therapies, $10 billion out of their own pockets.
- Seventy percent chose not to tell their physicians.
- The typical patient was educated, upper income, aged 25 to 49, and Caucasian.

This study, published in the *New England Journal of Medicine*, created yet another shift in thinking.

Within the rising tides of transformation, individuals emerge who contribute their ideas and visions to change the world. Since the 1970s, there have been an increasing number of researchers active in the field of subtle energies. Our vision has become more expansive as well in the way in which we conduct research. The mid- to late 20th century saw the growing acceptance of research methods that supported the exploration of human experience. Utilizing a variety of methodological approaches that will be explored more fully later, researchers wanted to better understand the meaning—the experiences of healers and patients sharing these interactions.

This journey into the yesteryears illuminates several common themes, points of intersection, and spaces open for deepening exploration. There are many ways to view energy, and different areas of expertise examine the phenomena from various viewpoints. The following section reviews some of the ideas that can lead to a better understanding of energy and its implications in health and healing.

Theory and Research

In an attempt to provide a foundation for the energy field around living organisms, we are required to consider several different theoretical explanations. Cause and effect are not clearly understood. The effects of the energy fields are measurable but the mechanism of action is not. Energy fields involve numerous forces examined by physicists: magnetic fields, electric fields, radiation, sound, electron activity, and particle and wave behavior. There are likely multiple layers of various types of energy wave networks harmoniously involved in functioning, communication between cells, and healing for all living organisms.

Traditionally, following Newton's reductionist thinking, we have examined and studied only the "solid" elements and ignored the "empty space" between. Isaac Newton taught us that everything moved like a mechanical part, with only the solid visible parts relevant. We now know that there are waves of energy interacting with what we once thought of as solids, and even solidity is now questioned. Newtonian physics does not have a wide enough application, and there is a fundamental shift in our understanding of the universe. New ways of thinking about the physics of the world are required.

The Biofield

All objects radiate a hierarchy of unique electric, magnetic, and radioactive fields. Living beings are considered to be complex, open systems, always self-organizing, responding, and adapting to the environment to maintain homeostasis. The biofield–energy field model asserts that a weak electromagnetic/radiation field around living organisms is involved in homeostasis and communication of body functions interacting with cellular health, emotions, social connections, the environment, and healing. The heart, for example, is known to give off electrical, magnetic, chemical, and thermal fields and signals that are uniquely different from all other body tissues and organs.

There is a well-defined range of frequencies of electromagnetic radiation waves (see **Figure 9-1**). These include very low frequencies, such as radio waves on a continuum, up to high-frequency ultraviolet light. The human eye is capable of seeing only a very narrow range of these frequencies, called the *visible spectrum*. The rest of the waves still have an influence on the environment around us, even if we cannot see them.

Electricity and magnetism are different but related and can act separately, but when combined they create an electromagnetic field that is more than either of the two. The biofield includes electromagnetic fields around the living organism that are involved in the organization of structure, function, and health.

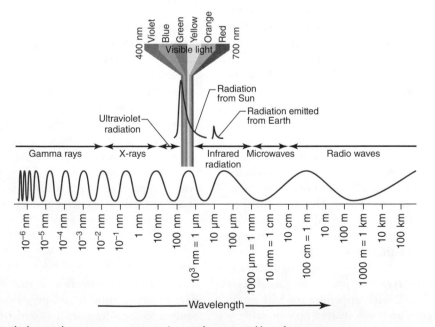

FIGURE 9-1 The known electromagnetic spectrum showing the range visible to the eye.

Electrical

There are numerous fields influenced by electrically charged particles from molecules, cells, and organs of different frequencies that work together harmonically and present as complex waves. Many electric elements of a living organism's energy fields have been carefully measured, including electrocardiography (ECG) and electroencephalogram (EEG). In addition to these well-known tests, the electric field near skin, which has been found to decline with aging, is used to noninvasively assess wound healing.[27] Electricity is also used for healing, as with the TENS stimulation of the nerve, which has been used to effectively treat chronic pain for decades and to repair tissue such as bone fractures.[28] Depression can be treated with electrically stimulating seizure activity.[29] Electricity can also be dangerous, even beyond the electric shocks we have all experienced. There have been links made between the presence of high-voltage power lines and childhood leukemia.[30] We are electrical beings, and we are influenced by waves of electricity.

Magnetic

Like electricity, magnetics has its uses in measurement and treatment, but it also has a dangerous side. Historically, exposure to magnetic fields was not thought to be hazardous. Considerable evidence, however, has emerged on magnetic field exposure and long-term health effects including cancer, fertility difficulty, and numerous other health conditions in various systems of the human body.

The magnetocardiogram (MCG) examines the heart's magnetic field, and the magnetoencephalogram (MEG) provides information on the head's magnetic field. The MEG can measure brain waves and neuronal and thinking activity by magnetic field changes around the head. This is a profound point. Thinking gives off a measurable field around the head. There is much theoretical discussion about how this field of wave activity then influences the cell membrane through a complex communication system of signals.

The MRI (magnetic resonance imaging) produces pictures of the body at the cellular level. The MRI exposes patients and technicians to a magnetic field that influences biology; there is considerable research attention on and study of these effects and potential health risks. Hassan and Abdelkawi researched the effects of short-term exposure to magnetic fields used in security or MRIs on exposed humans and the hemoglobin molecule's electric conductivity.[31] A measurable effect of magnetic fields can be examined in the red blood cells of rats exposed to magnetic fields. The hemoglobin membrane elasticity, permeability, and structure, as well as electrical conductivity, were changed by magnetic pulses similar to levels in an MRI. The protein's charges and molecular weights were altered, and even subtle changes of protein levels have a ripple effect on the body's function, influencing immunity, psyche, and healing.

Magnetic treatments are taking their place alongside the older electrical ones, such as electroconvulsive therapy (ECT). Repetitive transcranial magnetic stimulation (rTMS) has emerged as an alternative treatment for depression using magnetic instead of electrical stimulation of the brain. When treating those with psychotic depression, ECT is more effective than rTMS, but rTMS was just as effective as ECT in those with nonpsychotic depression.[29] Further, rTMS does not have the potential side effect of memory loss associated with ECT.

Low-Dose Radiation

The subtle energies around a living organism include a low-dose radiation given off by electrons circulating the nucleus of each atom of the body. There is considerable evidence that low doses of radiation influence cell structure and function, change ion potential of the membrane, and alter cell permeability, ion gates, and electric potential.[31] There is a ripple effect on illness and health.

Alpha, gamma, photon, and X-rays easily travel through all body tissue, most passing through the body without touching any cells. At an atomic scale, the body is mostly empty space. When rays interact with human tissue, they are able to ionize the atoms, causing energy transfer from the rays to the atoms (usually electrons) of the tissue.

Alpha particles are released when an atom decays, reduces in size, and the remaining atom becomes a new element. Alpha and gamma particles are emitted by radioactive nuclei (e.g., uranium, radium) and are used in the field of radiology for both diagnosing and treating disease. When the three-dimensional cells in human tissue are irradiated for treatment of a tumor, for example, cells outside the area of treatment are influenced. The term *bystander effect* is used to describe cells that have not been exposed to radiation, and are not physically close enough to the irradiation, but are affected by radiation though multiple signaling mechanisms between the cells. This effect, first noted by radiobiologists in the early 1990s, is a plausible mechanism for how electromagnetic fields signal the body to change response to pain, illness, and healing.[32]

The mechanism of action appears to be along the channels of the cell membrane where the ion transfer influences cell shape, function, and electrical conductivity. Oxidative stress follows. Free radicals are electrons released from their atom, bouncing through cells and doing damage at an atomic level.[31] Antioxidants (those found in foods such as blueberries) are compounds of molecules that are lacking an electron, and the free, bouncing radicals are drawn back into an atom system, stable once again. Theoretically, the ionizing radiation subtly changes the biofield, resulting in rebalancing along the ion gradients of every cell of the body. This would aid in the survival of cells that may have died off due to damage from free radicals and waves of radioactive decay.

Possibly, energy healing acts in a similar way to antioxidants. Acupuncture and Reiki were found to reduce the effects of ionizing radiation on human epithelial cells. Acupuncture was found to be effective in preventing and reducing the bystander effect when tissue was exposed to radiation. Reiki was found to have a dose-dependent factor, more treatments reducing damage to the bystander cells. This suggests a strong biological component of energy healing and may have application to accidental or medical radiation exposure.[32]

Resonance

There are rhythms seen in nature that are the foundation of life. These include seasons, circadian rhythms, brain waves, planetary orbit, and

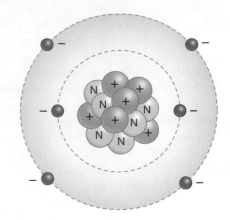

FIGURE 9-2 The atom, a small unit of matter.

electron orbit of a nucleus. Electrons, negatively charged, circle the positively charged nucleus. Electrons usually stay within their own ring (see **Figure 9-2**).

At an atomic level, when an electron moves to a higher level of orbit, a specific quantity and frequency of energy is required, in much the same way that it takes more energy to speed up when passing a slower car. If an electron moves to a lower level of orbit, it radiates energy of the same frequency. This specific frequency is referred to as the resonant frequency in physics.

Resonance is the tendency to vibrate at a specific frequency. A tuning fork creates a field of vibration around it once struck. This vibration energy moves out and influences other tuning forks of the same note. The term *resonance* is used in the field of energy psychology to describe the easy connection between two people, where it seems as if they are on the same *wavelength*. The experience of being close to a positive person is uplifting—can change mood—and the connection is said to have the right *vibe*. Resonance in objects is, perhaps, best known as the effects of sound waves shattering glass, vibrating strings, or pendulum clocks beating in unison. At a specific frequency, a sound wave can shatter glass because the note matched the same resonant frequency as the glass. If you pluck a D string on a guitar, D strings on nearby guitars will vibrate and resonate.

Many energy healing therapies, such as homeopathy, sound, and flower essences, use resonance as the basis for connecting in a healing and therapeutic way. These therapies are discussed later in the section Overview of the Practice of Energy Healing.

Always Interacting

Central to the theoretical understanding of energy in the human is the concept that energy does not stay within the realm of one physical body. From this understanding comes the common quote originating in chaos theory: the *butterfly effect*. The small turbulence created when a butterfly flaps its wings can create a storm in another part of the world. One (of many) interpretations of this is that subtle changes do have a larger influence on bigger, more unstable systems. Released electrons, atoms, waves, and other very subtle and difficult to measure factors of radiation travel to other cells in the environment. The field of radiation biology has changed significantly in the last 10 years, and low-dose radiation is no longer ignored as having no effect.

We are paying more attention to these numerous, subtle energies and discovering that these energies also carry information packages. Einstein's famous relativity equation tells us that energy is made up of mass (stuff that weighs something) times the speed of light (squared). $E = mc^2$ is the recipe for creating the amount of energy necessary to create mass. The very tiniest part of matter appears to be energy influenced by other energy waves in the environment.

The nucleus of the atom was once thought to be the smallest building block of matter, as well as unbreakable. What we find when we break the atom is that it is full of energy—an atomic blast occurs. When we look at the particle (hard stuff) very closely, it is nothing solid; rather, it appears to be waves and swirls of light and energy at the smallest level. Matter, the hard stuff, is made up of waves of light and energy. Matter can no longer be thought of as the fundamental property of physics; rather, energy is. There are waves of energy all around us, coming from us, and mingling with other waves of energy from other sources. Matter is the information packets of stuff used and organized by the energy to create the physical reality around us.

This concept aligns well with Martha Rogers's nursing theory of a unitary energy system continually interacting with others and unifying with a larger universal energy. Organisms are constantly exchanging energy, electrons, and information at multiple levels, and the individual is influenced by and influencing all those around it. Rogers rejected Cartesian dualism in favor of a unitary model. Fields of energy are in continuous process, and through this continuous process the fields are in continuous change—influencing and influenced by one another.

Meridian Lines

The meridians are thought to be energy flow paths marked by polarization of atomic molecules fundamental to development and perhaps preceding nervous and vascular systems.[33, 34] These subtle energies are thought to be magnetic but giving off an electrical field. When energy flow is compromised, illness may result in body parts fed by that tiny energy pathway, estimated to be smaller than a human hair in diameter.

Acupuncture is the best known meridian technique and involves inserting sterile needles into specific acupoints along meridian lines and points. This ancient Chinese healing technique is thought to improve the flow of qi energy through a living organism. In acupuncture, there is no clearly visible anatomical structure as we can see in the circulatory system. Acupressure points do not seem to correlate anatomically to body organs. Thinking in systems, like in Western medicine, really does not work when considering acupuncture. The electric and skin conductance characteristics of acupuncture have been studied, and there is movement toward developing tools to measure skin conductance for assessment and treatment.

However, it is unlikely that an electrical field is the only field functioning in this system. Current theory proposes that the meridian system is liquid collagen aligned along a "crystalline continuum in the connective tissues of the body, with its layers of structured water molecules supporting rapid semi-conduction of protons."[35] These liquid crystals are responsive, can reorder, and can change in response to electric or magnetic waves. It is thought that liquid crystals are part of how the membrane of every cell interacts and exchanges information and matter with the environment.[36] This acts as an interconnection and intercommunication system that functions at the speed of light and carries a charge of energy influencing pH and cell function. The cell membrane is signaled from outside the cell by electro/magnetic/radiation waves and it changes. The cell is governed from outside.

Acupuncture was viewed skeptically by Western medicine for many years, but strong research has solidified evidence for its safe and effective use, and it is currently one of the better researched complementary therapies. It has been found to be effective in providing relief of the symptoms of chronic lower back pain in a meta-analysis of 13 randomized controlled studies of more than 2,600 patients.[37] In a meta-analysis examining 72 randomized controlled studies of acupuncture for greater than 3,200 dysphagia patients, acupuncture was found to reduce difficulty swallowing after a stroke.[38] The World Health Organization recognizes acupuncture as therapeutic for more than 100 different conditions and diseases, many of which are chronic and difficult to treat with Western medicine.[39] There is strong research for its effective use in depression, infertility, posttraumatic stress disorder, chronic diseases, various types of pain, and autoimmune diseases such as fibromyalgia or rheumatoid arthritis (see **Table 9-1**).

Chakras

The word *chakra*, Sanskrit for "wheel of light," describes energy centers of the body. These centers appear to be points where there is a continuous exchange of information between the body and the environment. There are various beliefs about the number of chakras, their location, and how they relate to the Western ideas of nerves, plexus, neurotransmitters, neuroendocrine glands, and organs.

Most commonly, seven major chakras are identified, and there have been analogies to Maslow's hierarchy of needs, as well as energy healing techniques developed based on the seven-chakra system. For examples of how chakras can be interpreted see **Table 9-2** and **Table 9-3**. See also **Figure 9-3**.

TABLE 9-1 Similarities Between Electric Currents and Simple Computers and Meridians

Meridians resemble electric currents and simple computers.

Electrical Devices	**Meridians**
Electric currents exist when electrons flow from areas with lots of electrons to areas with few.	Meridians carry a unidirectional current within a complex mesh that is embedded throughout our body that reaches into every cell.
Some electric currents flow in one direction only. Resistance to an electrical current can occur when the wire is long and narrow. Such an electric current requires periodic boosting to maintain the signal.	Meridians are very long and narrow, 0.5 to 1.5 micron in diameter. Without boosting at regular intervals, the signal dies out.
A current is induced in one electric wire when a current changes in a nearby one.	Meridians are a series of adjacent electrical currents. Each is constantly changing and being changed by the nearby meridians.
The original computers of the 1940s were not able to conduct complex information or carry it as quickly as modern computers. They could not be used to do the complex calculations that computers now can.	Meridians act like our early computers; they carry simple information slowly and do not perform complex logical functions.

Source: Data from Material on electrical components and systems interpreted from P. G. Hewitt, *Conceptual Physics*, 10th ed. (San Francisco: Pearson/Addison Wesley, 2006); P. Xiong-Skiba, personal communication, March–April 2007.

TABLE 9-2   Traditional Chakra Locations, Associated Organs and Nervous Structures, and Attributes

	Chakra		**Nervous System**		
Location	**Structure**	**Function**	**Gland**	**Color**	**Tone**
7 — Crown of head	Pineal gland	Spiritual	Pineal or pituitary	Violet/white	B
6 — Brow	Pituitary gland, carotid plexus	Intuition, insight	Pituitary or pineal	Indigo (red-blue)	A
5 — Throat and shoulders	Pharyngeal plexus	Expression, speak own truth	Thyroid	Blue	G
4 — Heart and knees	Carotid plexus	Heart, love	Thymus	Green	F
3 — Stomach	Solar plexus	Emotions	Adrenals	Yellow	E
2 — Lower abdomen	Pelvic plexus, wrists and ankles	Reproduction, creativity, passion	Lymphatic tissue	Orange	D
1 — Groin	Coccygeal, palms and soles plexus	Survival, security	Gonads	Red	C

Source: Data from B. A. Brennan, *Hands of Light: A Guide to Healing Through the Human Energy Field* (New York: Bantam Books, 1987): 48; R. L. Bruyere, *Wheels of Light: A Study of the Chakras*, Vol. 1 (Sierra Madre, CA: Bon Productions, 1989): 42; R. Gerber, *Vibrational Medicine: New Choices for Healing Ourselves* (Rochester, VT: Bear & Company, 1988): 130; A. Judith, *Wheels of Life: A User's Guide to the Chakra System* (Woodbury, MN: Llewellyn, 1990): 23; Z. F. Lansdowne, *The Chakras and Esoteric Healing* (York Beach, ME: Samuel Weiser, 1978): 56; A. E. Powell, *The Etheric Double* (Wheaton, IL: Theosophical, 1978): 56; C. W. Leadbeater, *The Chakras* (Wheaton, IL: Theosophical, 1927): 40–41.

TABLE 9-3   Four Perspectives of Chakra Functions

	Bruyere	**Brennan**	**Maslow**	**Covey**
7th Chakra	Release, surrender	Integration of total personality, spiritual aspects	Aesthetics needs, wonder, beauty, harmony	
6th Chakra	Inspiration, insight	Visualization, carry out ideas	Need to know and understand	Interdependence
5th Chakra	Expression	Sense of self, taking in and assimilating	Self-actualization, realize one's potential growth, autonomy	
4th Chakra	Secondary feeling (usually contrary to first feeling)	Love, openness to life, ego will	Self-esteem, self-worth, feeling dignity, self-reliance, self-respect, independence	Independence
3rd Chakra	Opinion	Healing who you are in the universe	Love and belonging, intimacy	
2nd Chakra	Feeling	Pleasure, sexual energy	Safety	Dependence
1st Chakra	Concept, original idea	Physical energy, will to live	Survival	

Source: Data from R. L. Bruyere, *Wheels of Light: A Study of the Chakras*, Vol. 1 (Sierra Madre, CA: Bon Productions, 1989): 43; B. A. Brennan, *Hands of Light: A Guide to Healing Through the Human Energy Field* (New York: Bantam Books, 1987): 47–54; A. H. Maslow, *Motivation and Personality* (New York: Harper & Bros., 1954): 35–51; A. H. Maslow, *Psychological Review*, no. 50 (1943): 370–396; S. R. Covey, *The 7 Habits of Highly Effective People: Restoring the Character Ethic* (New York: The Free Press, 2004): 53.

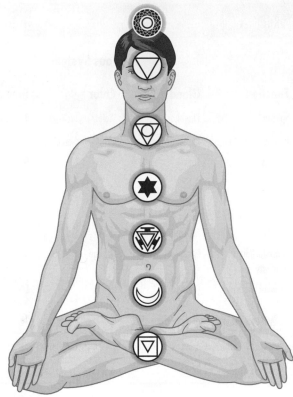

7th Chakra: Sahasrara—Understanding and will; violet; enlightenment, spiritual connectedness

6th Chakra: Ajna (Om)—Imagination; indigo; intuition, understanding

5th Chakra: Visuddha (Ham)—Power; blue; communication, healing

4th Chakra: Anahata (Yam)—Love; green; balance, love

3rd Chakra: Manipura (Ram)—Wisdom; yellow; energy, virility

2nd Chakra: Svadishthana (Lam)—Order; orange; relationships, emotions

1st Chakra: Muladhara (Vam)—Life; red; grounding, security

FIGURE 9-3 Locations and functions of the 7 Chakra system.

Aura

Called the *aura* in some traditions, the biofield resembles the orderly electromagnetic field you can see when sprinkling iron filings near a magnet. Magnetic fields that were not visible to the naked eye can now be seen. One theory about what makes up an aura is that healthy human blood cells contain large amounts of iron in the hemoglobin. The electrical flow of neurons, the pulses along each cell membrane, and a vascular system that distributes iron throughout the core of the body result in electrical flow around an iron core. The result is a body that puts out an electromagnetic field. There are likely numerous other waves of energy that make up the aura around a living being.

Torsion physics is a theory that examines the energy that interacts with the spinning particles and offers another explanation of an aura.[40] Subatomic particles spin; some spin left, some right. Whenever a particle changes its spin processes, a force called *torsion* is produced. One

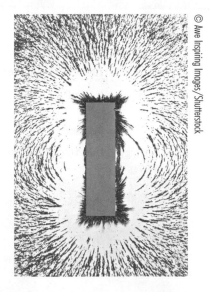

© Awe Inspiring Images/Shutterstock

type of subatomic particle is the photon, or a particle of light. Living beings emit photons in an organized field around the body, and this field of particles of light is theoretically accompanied by torsion forces. Particles in torsion fields travel faster than the speed of light, which traditionally was not thought possible. Torsion waves can be generated, measured, and have been found to influence DNA structure and reproduction at the level of the cell membrane. Through this field, faster than the speed of light, information is exchanged. It is believed that this information exchange is a mechanism in the phenomenon of distance healing.

Intention and Presence

Because we all have an electromagnetic field around us, and likely several more yet to be determined fields, when we enter the biofield of another, we change and are changed. The fields cross and interact, and electrons, energy, and information are exchanged. The mechanism of action of complementary therapies that use energy healing therapies is thought to involve the waves of electromagnetic radiation they emit.

The quantum physics theorem, Kochen-Specker, addresses intention by examining the outcomes of assuming where a photon will be prior to measuring it. The Kochen-Specker Theory proposes that the experimenter's intention changes the results of photon experiments, that guessing where a photon will be before you even measure it alters its course. When an observer just let the photon travel, it went one way; when he guessed where it would be, it went another. As mentioned earlier, the observer is part of the event and changes the result—the Heisenberg effect.

Savva suggests that energy transferred from one to another is more than electromagnetic waves and includes a mental component that carries intention or caring.[41] Current research shows that there are information packages traveling with waves and electrons. This idea aligns with the nursing theorist Watson's identification of caring as a factor in healing. See the suggested readings at the end of this chapter for more information on Watson's Theory of Human Caring.

An understanding of these principles suggests that the *presence* of a nurse is electromagnetic, and that the mere presence of a caring person can be healing. This concept adds to the difficulty of studying energy healing. The presence of another being—an observer, the nurse, a researcher—changes the experience.

Rosemarie Parse's Theory of Human Becoming helps illustrate the importance of this concept to the practice of nursing.[42] We are intersubjective. Personal history and choices are influenced by others. Being in *true presence* with another reflects an experience of engaging with another at a genuine level. True presence is an intentional process, which reflects the belief that clients know their own way. In practice, the nurse enters the client's perception of the world with openness, and in a nonjudgmental, unconditional, and therapeutic way. The nurse's whole attention and being is with the client, focusing on the client's perception of the world. This involves intentionally setting aside the nurse's own values.

Simply, intention is purposefully choosing a direction. In physics, intention has been shown to alter the activity of a particle. In nursing, the nurse intends to alter the condition of the patient. The nurse prepares for true presence with a quiet pause, becoming self-reflective before engaging with the client. The nurse plans to bring some sunshine and hope to the patient behind the door. *Intention is set.* The nurse consciously allows personal worries and concerns to drift into the background while the client's concerns are foremost. The nurse enters the room with intention. The nurse is mindfully aware of the client's words, silences, stillness, and body language. Simultaneously, the client is aware of the nurse's genuine presence by expression of the shared feelings that exude from the nurse with facial expressions, touch, and words. The nurse and client are on the same *wavelength*.

The suggested readings at the end of this chapter include works on physicists' study of consciousness and intention, as well as additional information on Watson's and Parse's work. These resources will provide further insight into these complex physics concepts that seem unrealistic at first glance—and maybe even second glance. We are learning that our reality includes stuff outside the body, something that Watson and Parse and most nurses already knew.

Neural Coupling

Numerous scientifically sound studies have been completed examining communication between the speaker and listener on EEG and functional MRI. There is a growing body of research suggesting that when our brains are engaged there is a highly predictive nature of the listener's brain, and neurologists and language specialists are closely examining this phenomena. When speakers and listeners are truly engaged, there is a correlation found in the functional MRI between the two. Speakers and listeners exhibit similar, synchronized brain activity patterns during successful communication. We are anticipating events in the surroundings, preparing for responses. Looking at neural coupling between a storyteller and a listener, it appears that communication is enhanced the more we are engaged, and we are anticipating what next will be said. The matched brain-wave rhythm between speaker and listener occurs only when there is focus and true presence.[43]

What is interesting about the research on brain waves is the timing of similar waves between people. You would expect the listener to have a delay in brain waves as the speaker thinks about the word then speaks it and the listener hears and processes it, but that is not so. The changes in both people's brain waves are simultaneous.[43, 44] There appears to be either a predictive component to what the listener is experiencing, or there is something else happening that causes the brain waves between two people to allow synchronous waves of energy.

When a nurse enters the attention of a patient and an emotional state is shared, the brain networks between the two synchronize. One study examined how shared emotional states facilitate understanding of intention. When research participants watch movies that elicit a variety of emotions, their brain waves synchronized. Brain activity "ticked together" for participants' brain networks.[45]

Brain-wave studies suggest that empathy is more than a nice concept. Neuroimaging studies have revealed that being empathic with another person's emotions allows the observer to "tune in" or to "get in sync" with the other person. Speaker–listener neural synchronization seen between two speakers on functional MRI enhances communication, comprehension, and an understanding of the emotional state of another.[44, 45]

In the neuroimaging studies of emotional interactions, we can see patterns in the limbic system of one person's brain showing up in the limbic brain of another person, which may result in enhanced contextual understanding. Moreover, empathy can be measured coming off of the body in an EEG. It would appear that the brain-wave synchronization coexists with the person's body releasing empathy.

Quantum Physics

We have traditionally understood the physics of the universe through the work of Newton, but those ideas are no longer adequate to explain wave and particle behavior at an atomic level. The field of quantum physics is still being hotly debated by physicists, and a solid understanding of the theoretical concepts and the multiple nuances require a calculus and physics background. However, the potential applications of quantum physics appear to be boundless within health and human functioning. Discussion of quantum physics in this chapter is not meant to be all inclusive but rather to ignite an interest for further reading.

While some argue that the leap between what is happening on a quantum level and at the level of the cell is theoretical, the gap in our understanding is closing. New, contemporary physics differs profoundly from Newtonian physics, including the theoretical relationship between the mind and matter. In Newtonian physics, they are separate. In contemporary physics, there appears to be a union between them; matter and consciousness are related. The implications from quantum physics for health and human functioning have yet to be explored by most physicists. The suggested readings at the close of this chapter provide background on where this thinking is going.

Quantum Theory

Conventionally, the central idea in classical or Newtonian physics is that the physical universe is made of solid stuff—*matter*. This hard material is subject to "local" laws of physics. While things are made up of tiny jiggling atoms, the object is still localized. Conventional physics purported that matter responds only to things in its immediate environment and is unaware of anything outside its own environment. The basis of modern Newtonian scientific study—that things are localized and respond only to the immediate environment—is an essential belief if you plan to objectively measure and quantify matter.

Heisenberg was the first person to publish the idea that the objective reality that Newtonian physics works with does not exist.[46] Quantum physics has made the idea of a solid reality invalid. We know that, by observing and measuring a phenomenon, we change it. The mathematics of the action of the particle does not tell us about the particle, as we thought; rather, the math reflects what we know about or expect from the particle. As knowledge about the particle changes, precise measurements change.

Conscious thought changes matter. The Heisenberg principle remains the basis of the theories in today's discussion of quantum physics. If there is no real objective view of the world, then how can any study be unbiased? How can measurements be accurate? This paradigm shift came very slowly because scientists have always found math to be objective and finite. Now, to understand atomic phenomena, they would need to abandon their understanding of measurement and mathematics. Einstein said that "the 'macroscopic' and 'microscopic' are so inter-related that it appears impracticable to give up this program [physics focusing on just the matter] in the 'microscopic' alone."[47, p. 674]

The study of quantum physics began with early work in light waves that give off an electromagnetic wave or frequency. This vibration of energy carries a stream of packets of light called photons. We think of light waves, but photons are particles; thus, light is made up of waves and particles. The question became: Can other particles, such as electrons, act like waves? Energy waves carry with them more than just a vibration at an atomic level. They carry packets of information.

Physicist Maxwell Planck identified that light energy comes in small packets, now called photons (or quanta), and came up with Planck's constant: 1.05×10^{-27} grams/cm/second. The amount of energy in a photon, while really tiny (that is $\times 10$ to the negative 27), is dependant on its frequency $E = h \times nu$. There is a finite size of energy that can be lumped together, and a photon is the smallest constituent of an electromagnetic field.

Quantum physics studies how waves of possibility (potentiality) change from energy waves to particles when measured. There is a paradox in this quantum measurement. How can something be a wave of energy and then solid matter? Choosing to measure the wave causes the change. The conscious choice alone is responsible for the collapse of the wave into a particle and back again to a wave.

Consciousness at an Atomic Level

Consciousness has been described in various ways, such as an awareness of a world, as individual, as "looking out" from inside a physical body, and as a function of the brain.[48] Now, quantum theory suggests that we are not just benign observers of the hard stuff out in the world. Consciousness is better thought of as a collection of electrons and energy and very small packets of information, moving about in a special way, interacting with matter. Traditional physics described the world as lumps of matter separated by a void of nothing. Quantum physics describes that void among stuff at macro, microscopic, and atomic levels as alive with wave and particle activity and a grid of shooting protons and electrons. These waves of energy connect us to others and to the world.

Psychologist Carl Jung and physicist Wolfgang Pauli both suggested that there is a universal consciousness of shared information between all conscious things, much like an ocean of information in which all beings swim. Jung believed that archetypical ideas in the shared, collective consciousness guided personal perception and thinking. Jung's ideas fit very well into the discoveries of quantum physics and how we might share energy with one another.

When Jung and Pauli united, they suggested that the concept of synchronicity would help build a bridge between hard science and the subjective experience. Synchronicity is the occurrence of coincidences that seem unrelated but to which people attribute meaning.

Synchronicity reveals an underlying pattern of the universe, a connectedness that does not seem to be influenced by how far apart coincidental events are. Jung and Pauli believed that the world was not just a series of random events but reflected a deeper order, the *Undus mundus* (one connected world). Coincidences seem to happen without geography or distance being an element.

Two Particles Stay in Touch

Quantum's theory of nonlocality implies a connection among objects—synchronized, connected—without distance being part of the equation. This action at a distance theory shows how objects communicate faster than the speed of light.

In the experimental setting, when an atom emits two lumps of light (photons) going opposite ways, these two photons have been shown to still affect one another, even though they seem to be too far apart to exchange information. The effect on one another is instantaneous, faster than the speed of light, regardless of whether they are near or are galaxies apart. This *entanglement* between two particles allows them to produce these nonlocal actions simultaneously. Although entanglement is more commonly portrayed as an algebraic concept, it implies that if we are measuring one of those two particles, the other particle somehow knows and reacts without any obvious way of communicating. The field of torsion physics examines how these particles move information instantaneously as a wave, which moves faster than physicists believed waves could travel. These concepts imply a holistic universe, a concept of wholeness where separated things can act instantaneously on one another regardless of distance.

Relationship of Physics and Healing

There is no consensus on the theoretical constructs of quantum physics and its connection to healing. Some argue that the minute layers of waves are too small and cannot have an effect on the larger macro world and proudly label themselves skeptics. The evidence is unfolding. This "it's too small to have an effect" belief is similar to the cries from "modern scientific minds" of the time against Semmelweis's germ theory in the 1800s. These scientists claimed that "Nothing could be so small, not be seen by the human eye and yet cause disease; hand washing is a superstitious ritual." The microscope was later developed confirming germ theory. (See the suggested readings at the end of this chapter for Morton Thompson's 1949 book *The Cry and the Covenant*.) A type of microscope to show clearly

the atomic-sized world and its influence on living things is a next step.

Biophotonics

Biophotonics is a branch of quantum biology made famous by Fritz-Albert Popp in the 1970s. This field, which is relatively new, examines the connection between the photons' emission and cell function. Photons appear to transmit information to the cells at the speed of light, allowing another communication system for the body. These ultra-small waves of photons are consistent, are stable, and can be seen in the infrared spectrum.

Researchers are just now learning the basics of biophotons, including how they are produced and discharged; how they communicate with and direct metabolism, cells, and biorhythms; and how they might be used in assessing disease. The mechanism of action appears to be the cell membrane, a liquid crystalline continuum, which was discussed earlier, that causes changes in the cell.

Popp characterized this phenomenon as different from thermal radiation, chemical luminescence, or a by-product of metabolism. Because we have been taught to think in a biological model, we think of chemicals as triggers and catalysts for change. The vibrations from the chemical reactions appear to be also relevant. One important role in the emission of these photons has been linked to the function of DNA and the field of epigenetics.

Epigenetics

Epigenetics is the field of study that examines the effect of the environment on genetic expression. Begun in 1990, The Genome Project was launched to discover the makeup of human genes.[49] The project was completed far earlier than anticipated because researchers were expecting to find hundreds and hundreds of thousands of genes, but there appear to be fewer than 30,000 in the human DNA. Because there are so relatively few genes to create such amazing human function and diversity, it is likely that something else is contributing to genetic expression.

Previously, DNA and RNA were thought to be the answer to many health problems; health was thought to be completely prechosen, ruled by DNA. It now appears that genetics is not that predetermined. Genes are not the only things that decide physical fate; they only show a genetic predisposition, a possible blueprint.

Moreover, it is not some random mutation that causes the gene to mutate; stem cells play a part. The body can direct stem cells, which are found in large amounts in placentas and umbilical cords, to increase in quantity and become any number of different kinds of cells depending on need. The proteins of stem cells change shape as a response to positive and negative electric changes along the cell membrane. As they fold themselves up and change shape, they are converted into building blocks appropriate for whatever tissue they will become.

The stem cells receive a signal that contains directions for reproduction. It is the signal that changes the ion or electrical potential of the protein of the cell and thus the shape. It is the signal that causes genetic mutation or healthy cellular growth.

Stem cells are not the only cells that respond to environmental signals. Electric stimulus, particles, light, waves of protons, electricity, electrons, and even sound waves can act as signals across any living cellular tissue, making minute but profound changes. And if the communication and signal are jumbled, disease is the result. It appears that a signal that is sent to the cell's genes is the relevant piece that changes biology.

What is that signal? It appears to be a waveform, similar to the waves measured around the head when thoughts change. There may be many sources of a waveform, including DNA itself, which gives off biophotons. The biophoton from the DNA releases a wave of the torsion force. Like the signals from the outer environment, the biophotons released by DNA may be able to create a genetic mutation.

There are so many questions about this signal, such as what influences it and how it might be influenced. The electric-, magnetic-, radiation-filled environment can change the signal, but what else? Can thoughts change it? Is this how thoughts influence biology? Is this how quantum waves, thoughts, and consciousness influence cellular structure? These questions are hotly debated. It is hoped that some

day individuals will be able to influence that energy signal to heal, rather than having to rely exclusive on pharmaceuticals or surgery. See the suggested readings at the end of this chapter for information on Bruce Lipton's work on cell biology.

Energy Healing Modalities

There are many diverse types of energy healing (biofield) modalities, with Therapeutic Touch, Reiki, and Healing Touch being the most widely known in the medical community.[50] These therapies are used in a variety of healthcare settings including pain clinics, hospitals, hospices, oncology centers, and private practices.[51] The National Center for Complementary and Integrative Health divides all complementary health approaches into two general areas: natural products and mind–body practice.[52] The mind–body practice includes a diverse group of practices such as meditation, tai chi, guided imagery, hypnosis, yoga, and, included in the mind–body list, energy healing.

The educated health consumer's demand for evidence-based, noninvasive, gentle, caring, and affordable interventions has been heard. In a best-evidence synthesis of 66 clinical studies, Jain and Mills found that while not all studies had rigorous methodology, there is strong evidence that biofield/energy healing techniques are effective.[53] Energy healing techniques were found to induce relaxation and reduce intensity and duration of pain. Cancer pain is difficult to manage in 80% of patients, and there are numerous studies that find improvement in quality of life and pain management as a result of energy healing.[51, 53] In patients living with cancer, acute pain was reduced and quality of living was improved in various studies. Patient pain in various populations found relief with energy healing, increased relaxation, and improved quality of life.

The benefits of Reiki, a Japanese biofield therapy, include a sense of relaxation, decreased cortisol levels, and lower blood pressure.[54] Baldwin, Fullmer, and Schwartz examined the efficacy of Reiki and reconnective healing on physical therapy for increasing limited range of arm motion.[55] Reiki is an energy healing technique involving centering and presence. Reconnective healing (RH) is an energy technique using hands to manipulate biofields. This study used a strong sample of 78 participants with a similar shoulder injury, attending physical rehabilitation divided into five groups: physical therapy, Reiki, RH, sham healing, and RH plus physical therapy control groups. The measurement of arm elevation is reported on the scapular plane in degrees and was measured after a 10-minute treatment. Reconnective healing and Reiki were more effective than physical therapy alone. Pain levels were also measured in this study, but there was no significant difference between the groups. The authors postulated that efficacy related to of Reiki and RH (but not sham healing) arose from healing of the muscle and joint, not from reduced pain.

The effect of energy healing modalities on the human brain have been studied. Okada Purifying Therapy (OPT), a Japanese biofield therapy similar to Reiki, was studied in adults. After a 15-minute OPT session, there was an increase in alpha waves of the frontal and central cortex seen on EEG.[56] "In chemistry, a molecule doesn't do anything that isn't allowed by a wave form—an inner image—of one of its virtual states. In life, a human being does nothing that isn't allowed by an inner image of the mind."[57, p. 609]

The Practice of Energy Healing

The holistic nurse weaves together historical, philosophical, theoretical, and research knowledge to create a foundational framework for the practice of energy healing. As personal, ethical, and intuitive knowledge are integrated into the framework, the practice becomes ever expansive and holistic.

Within this, healers and healees come together in relationships, co-creating spaces for healing. Knowing that there exists a universal connection between all, holistic nurses understand that everyone involved in a healing interaction will be forever changed. There is no other option; thus, the nature of this interaction is vitally important in supporting a healing, not necessarily a curing, outcome. We enter into these relationships holding the intention for healing, for the highest good of the other.

Holistic nurses utilize a variety of therapies in the delivery of care. While these may be rooted in varied philosophical traditions or be enacted in diverse approaches, there exists common themes and beliefs that may help us begin to articulate how these therapies facilitate healing.

Overview of the Practice of Energy Healing

Energy exists in many forms (e.g., thermal, kinetic, nuclear, chemical), but in healing we are most involved with electrical, electromagnetic, and subtle energies.[19] The concept that all matter is energy vibrating at different frequencies is basic in understanding energy and energy healing practices. A fundamental assumption of energy healing is that all life is sustained by a universal life energy that moves freely within and without sentient beings and that, in health, it is balanced and harmonious. Energy healing practices, then, are those practices that alter the flow of subtle energy to facilitate healing. Based on a holistic assessment, an energy healing practitioner uses specific techniques to relax, clear, repattern, strengthen, and balance the energy field, thus supporting the flow of energy.

Quantum physicists posit that reality consists of energy fields vibrating at different frequencies. Some are visible (such as you and me) and some not so much so (such as electromagnetic and gravitational fields). Consider this: Can you remember a time when you entered a place and suddenly your mood changed? Perhaps you entered a bit down, but the feelings in the place you entered lifted your spirits. Or maybe you have come upon a situation and experienced a "gut feeling" and later came to know you were right. These intuitive experiences remind us of the sensitivity and power of those unseen forces and how, in the blink of an eye, we affect one another and our environment.

The principles of energy fields describe the human as a physical entity of internal and external energy fields in continuous interaction. Energies are exchanged in human interactions and modulated in the universal field that permeates all matter. Through this perpetual energy exchange, each field is affected and changed.[58-60] In a healthy energy field, there is an unlimited availability of free-flowing energy and synchronicity between the fields. Illness results when there are blockages in flow or disordered patterns. Disruption of energy flow affects all of the fields.

Feinstein and Eden posit that three energy systems work in concert to regulate processes: the biofield, chakras, and meridians.[19] The biofield (vital, etheric) is the field surrounding the body. The biofield corresponds to the aura, that clearly discernible yet intangible field that holds an electromagnetic signal and has been described by numerous researchers. Two cameras are used to show movement within the aura. Polycontrast Interference Photography, invented by Harry Oldfield, shows energy moving around the body. Colored bands depict areas of decreased or blocked energetic flow or leakage. The Electrophotonic Camera, based on Gas Discharge Visualization analysis, allows for viewing of real-time changes in the energy field of humans and other organisms.

The aura is understood as a light surrounding the body, with thickness or density that lessens as you move outward, away from the body. There are different traditional explanations of the aura, but commonalities include the presence of two hemispheres, linked by a band, that store information and transmit it throughout the organism through an integral relationship with the chakras.[59, 61] Slater describes possible ways in which the aura can be damaged, resulting in biopsychosocial challenges that manifest as fatigue, stress, depression, and pain or suffering.[62] Sources of harm include, for example, accidents, trauma, confrontational situations, bottling up thoughts and feelings, and surgery. It is important to be cognizant that memories are stored deeply in the aura and, if not immediately evident, can surface later. Energy healing may be effective in meeting these challenges and at least begin a path to peace and healing.

The local fields, concentrated in specific areas of the body, are the chakras.[19] These vortexes of energy are, in essence, wheels of light that exchange energy with the environment and transform it—process it—in a way that is meaningful to the person. This transformation of interpretation might be the source of intuitive knowing. Kunz emphasized that rhythm and order are integral to chakra functioning.[63]

While there are varied beliefs about the locations and exact functions of the chakras, common themes include that chakras emit colors and tones in an orderly increase in vibratory frequency, that they are organized from the least to the most complex and abstract, and that there is agreement of the general function of each. This suggests that each chakra processes information on a higher frequency than the one below it, creating an information tree; the higher the chakra, the more complex. Each chakra receives only the specific information with which it works, processes it quickly, adds a person's specific choices, and forwards the whole bundle to the next one. It is an intricate process of receiving, adding, processing, and forwarding a complex body of information. Before moving "upward," however, the information in the lower chakra must be processed.

This thinking blends beautifully with Maslow's hierarchy of needs (discussed previously). The reader is referred to Table 9-2 and Table 9-3 to better envision these characteristics of the chakras. Counseling and contemplative practices, in addition to energy healing, are useful in restoring movement and rhythm to the chakras.[62]

Meridians, which carry subtle energy throughout the body, include 12 to 14 pairs of pathways that are considered segments of a continuous energy system.[19, 62] Believed to precede the development of most organs, the meridian system constitutes a mesh network of fine fibers (smaller than a human hair) that diverge into smaller and smaller channels, carrying electromagnetic impulses to all areas within our being.[34] Acupoints along the meridian are pressure- and light-sensitive areas that are believed to regulate the energy in a particular meridian. Meridians are named for organs, but this designation can be misleading because in actuality they influence all of the cells and organs along their path; a disruption or block in flow of qi along the meridian is believed to result in illness.

Motoyama and Becker have long researched meridian flow. The Apparatus for Meridian Identification designed by Motoyama measures the meridians' electrical charge and is currently being used to study the effects of pranic healing. In a study conducted with persons living with breast cancer, Tsuchiya and Motoyama measured changes in the body's energetic conditions through four sessions of non-touch pranic healing.[64] They report that this is the "first observation of Qi-energy changes by means of an electrically measurable variable, which provides strong objective evidence for the reality of Qi-energy manipulation claimed in non-touch energy healing."[64, p. 15] See the suggested readings at the end of this chapter for additional information on Motoyama's work.

The meridian system of information transmission is complete yet slow. Slater reminds us that we must be patient when tuning into information revealed from the meridian as the "gestalt reveals itself."[62, p. 765] Table 9-1, presented earlier in this chapter, offers a visual resource related to the meridians.

Reflecting on energy systems and field theory elucidates the intricacies and complexities of a system designed to gather information and to process, store, and transmit it. Each component is integral to the process, playing a unique role that is interdependent and vital in health and well-being. Beginning within the body and closely surrounding it, the aura holds our history; moving inward, our chakras receive and process information quickly; finally, meridians spread the word, slowly and completely. Moving outward from the biofield, each energy field receives and transmits information, perhaps of a more complex and abstract nature, interpenetrating and connecting with all. This offers a basis for understanding how energy therapies work.

Energy Healing Interactions

While we know that all healing interactions—or interactions of any sort, for that matter—are energetic, some nurses are called to deepen their knowledge and skill in the use of energy healing practices. Within the process of self-development, energy practitioners explore the unique philosophies and core values of the therapy that they are studying. Although universal core beliefs are elusive, energy practitioners tend to agree on some basic assumptions.[65, 66] Energy healing practitioners believe that energy moves within and through living beings and is part of

a universal field, that the energy field is dynamic and can be perceived by another with education and practice, and that imbalances and disorders in energy flow are associated with illness. There also exists the belief that the potential for healing is always possible, and humans possess an innate capability to access inner wisdom and guidance. The nature of the relationship between the energy healing practitioner and the healee is integral and interconnected within the universal field, yet practitioners know and respect energetic boundaries. Energy healing practices are rooted in ethical knowing. Energy healing practitioners know that "the destiny of the patient is not in [our] . . . hands."[63]

Hands-on energy healing practices are often associated with a process that begins with the practitioner quieting his or her mind, bringing the attention inward to a still point in order to focus on the energetic cues revealed during the assessment. There are numerous approaches to this state of focused attention, and energy healing practitioners cultivate that which is effective for them. Throughout this text, readers are introduced to contemplative techniques that they may find helpful.

Whichever path practitioners select, this quiet, still state invites a space for presence and deep listening. It may also alter their electromagnetic field.[62] An early experiment by Zimmerman found that when Therapeutic Touch practitioners entered into the still, healing state, a biomagnetic field emanated from their hands, pulsing within a range of 0.3 to 30 Hertz. In this study, nonpractitioners were unable to produce the biomagnetic pulses.[67] In a different review of physiological effects on practitioners during healing, only 3 of 67 studies examined electrodermal activity, and each of these three found changes. The researchers caution that despite the interest in and research on identifying healing-related biomarkers, "little robust evidence of unique physiological changes has emerged to define the healers' state."[68, p. 159] Energy healing practitioners, however, sense that something different happens during this quiet state, which is why it continues to be a widespread practice. Additional research is needed to fully determine what happens physiologically and electromagnetically in such a state.

Energy Healing Process

The pattern that many energy healing practitioners use in the energy healing process includes self-preparation, assessment of the energy field, intervention, and reassessment. This pattern resembles the well-known nursing process. The second step in this process—assessment—is when the practitioner uses her or his hands and intuitive knowing to search for cues about the state of the healee's energy flow. A balanced energy field is characterized by flow, rhythm, symmetry, and gentle vibration—a pattern indicating a background of implicate order. An unbalanced field is disordered in some way. The energy healing practitioner is able to discern these imbalances and then intervene to begin bringing the energy field back into greater balance.

Energy healing practitioners seek to restore balance and order to the healee's energy field. Techniques to accomplish this vary, but practitioners understand that they serve as facilitators of the energy movement and that energy goes where it is needed. Energy healing practitioners are midwives to the process of healing, not in charge of it. Reassessment and intuitive knowing guide the practitioner in determining when the session is complete. Expert energy healing practitioners understand that completion is not necessarily measured by "fixing" or "totally balancing" the healee's field; rather, wisdom guides them to create space for the healee to rest, integrate the energy, and then plan further sessions.

Although each specific energy practice is unique, the overview of the process offers a general guided description. It would appear that energy healing is a linear process, but that is not true. The holistic caring process is a beautiful circular process of interaction and possibilities; it is, in many ways, a holistic, transformative unfolding.

Energy Healing Practitioner

Cultivating the knowledge and skill necessary to grow as holistic nurses and energy healing practitioners requires commitment and discipline. There is movement, and as we evolve we learn much about the practice and much about ourselves. Krieger reminds us that practitioners must be willing to do the inner work that is necessary for true presence in healing interactions and that, when moving more inward, we learn more and more about our true self.[65] Perhaps this inner journey reveals to us our compassion, a quality that is often said to be the most important. We develop compassion as we open our heart and willingly use our self and our abilities to help another. We stand with others, bearing witness and trusting; we do not judge or pity, but rather we meet people where they are. Our self-compassion and inner wisdom allow us to be with and not own another person's journey.

Healing is facilitated in spaces where the energy healing practitioner is in presence with the healee. Presence was introduced earlier in this chapter and readers are invited to reflect on the meaning that presence has for them. Importantly, we have within us the ability to decide how we will show up—in a healing interaction or in everyday life. It is our choice and, from our knowledge of energy, we know that others will "sense" whether we are present.

There is much discussion about intention and intentionality and the role these play in energy healing practices. Intention, as described earlier, is purposefully choosing a direction. Zahourek differentiates intention and intentionality: Intentionality is "greater than and different from intention. . . . it is the capacity for, and the quality of, intention; it activates intention."[69, p. 347] She describes intentionality as a dynamic, evolving state, unique to a person and contextually informed: "Intention is the care plan; intentionality is how the individual implements the plan."[70, p. 7] In energy healing practices, then, intentionality is a foundational component underlying the framework while reminding energy healing practitioners that healing is an individual experience and that the outcome is not in our hands. If we as energy healing practitioners are present and set the intention for the best (we do not define what is best) for the healee, then intentionality guides our interaction in a fluid, evolving way. We trust that the outcome will be what it is for that person—and we will, through compassionate presence, stay out of the way.

The idea of ritual and technique is of interest to holistic nurses and energy healing practitioners. Bengston, and later Moga and Bengston, studied hands-on healing with mice injected with cancer.[71, 72] These studies give us cause to consider the act of quieting the mind. In early experiments, Bengston did not enter a meditative state but rather thought about 20 things he wanted in life and focused on these during the hands-on healing treatments; all six mice were cured. He repeated this study using four skeptics as the healers and, again, the mice were cured. Bengston suggests that neither belief nor quieting are requisite to healing and that, perhaps, they might interfere with it.[72] It may be, however, that the key is entering the interaction without expectation—remembering that the outcome is not in our hands.

In a grounded theory study, Warber, Deogracia, Straughn, and Kile examined the biofield therapy experience from the perspective of the practitioners.[73] Through interviews, the team discovered that practitioners and clients come together as energetic entities, each with a responsibility to engage in the process of healing. Energy healing practitioners must, as well, meet people where they are psychologically and energetically. In the interaction, the practitioner draws on the universal energy source that flows into the healee. The authors found that the healees' desire to heal surpasses their belief in the therapy. Overall, "the self-portrayal of energy healers evoked here is one of highly sensitive, attuned individuals operating, not as charlatans, but as ethical healing facilitators with specialized knowledge of the world just beyond our ordinary senses."[73, p. 1107] Energy healing practices can be learned. Energy healing practitioners advance their practice by cultivating a discipline of gentle self-development, study, and practice. Interactions with healees are grounded in trust and respect.

Energy Therapies

There are many energy healing practices that use hands-on and -off techniques. Many would say that all therapies, including bed baths and sitting with a patient, are energetic in nature because regardless of what we are doing it is truly our way of being that makes a difference.

Holistic nurses are familiar with several biofield therapies. Therapeutic Touch was the first energy healing therapy introduced in nursing. Developed by Dolores Krieger and Dora Kunz in 1972, Therapeutic Touch is an evidence-based therapy that incorporates the intentional and compassionate use of universal energy to promote balance and well-being; it is a contemporary interpretation of traditional Indian laying on of hands.[74] Older Eastern Asian traditions of laying on of hands include qi gong (China) and Reiki (Japan). Nurses also use newer laying-on-of-hands therapies that originated in the West, including Healing Touch, Hands of Light, Touch for Health, Polarity Therapy, and Quantum Touch. These energy therapies are widely used by nurses and other energy healing practitioners. There are many studies of energy therapies, but results are mixed. In reviewing 66 studies, Jain and Mills found one consistency: Energy therapies have a positive effect on decreasing pain.[53] They also found moderate evidence of decreased agitation in people living with dementia but overall concluded that the majority of studies reported the use of energy therapies for pain.

Existing studies have used such different methodologies that few of the results can be compared. To remedy this problem, Hammerschlag and colleagues convened a panel to identify methodological and scientific issues that have become apparent.[75] Methodologically there needs to be consistency in research design among different studies, including studies of different types of energy modalities, and there must be an ongoing dialogue between energy healing practitioners of the various modalities. Studies need to be conducted to measure the electrical changes in and between the practitioner and the healee of various modalities. Baldwin and Hammerschlag echoed this conclusion with their recommendation to study healing-related biomarkers in energy healing practitioners such as skin changes.[68]

Other Energy Therapies

There are other forms of energy healing that holistic nurses use in their practices. These therapies are powerful healing allies and are often integrated with other therapies in designing a holistic care plan. All matter, living and nonliving, is understood as energy that is organized by waveforms and frequencies. Matter generates electrical and electromagnetic energy fields at precise frequencies and, when the frequencies between two or more sources align, they exist in a state of vibrational/harmonic resonance. Familiar examples of such resonance, or entrainment, are clock pendulums near one another that swing at exactly the same, as if they are one; women living in close proximity who have similar monthly cycles; and musical instruments or crystals that respond to a note from another instrument. Each of these demonstrates vastly different experiences of harmonic resonance.

In health, we are in harmonic resonance within ourselves and with all else; illness generally is associated with lower-frequency and unbalanced vibrations. Perhaps this is part of the reason why when our bodies, minds, and/or spirits hurt, we feel zapped and drained.

Energy therapies, which could also be called *vibrational therapies*, can help people move their state to a higher vibration that can then lead to greater balance and equilibrium. As shown by the example of women's simultaneous menstrual cycles, a person can entrain and resonate to something else. Energy healing therapies, many of which are ancient, are believed to enable a person to change his or her resonance toward greater health.[76]

In an interview, Richard Gerber discussed the diagnostic and healing uses of vibrational medicine.[77] According to Gerber, vibrational therapies work by "injecting selective frequencies of energy into the body that encourage the body's own self-healing systems to do the work." Based on the notion that everything has a unique vibrational energy signature, these therapies work with a person's energetic system to restore vibration and resonance, providing an environment for self-healing. We are familiar with the application of these principles in conventional health care in treatments such as stimulators for bone healing and full-spectrum light therapy use for people living with Seasonal Affective Disorder. Vibrational therapies also include subtle energy therapies such as biofield approaches like Therapeutic Touch, as well as sound, light, color, aromatherapy, flower essences, and homeopathy.

Sound

Most ancient cultures used sound as a form of healing. The Aboriginal people of Australia are the first known culture to heal with sound. Their *yidaki* (modern name *didgeridoo*) has been used as a healing tool for at least 40,000 years. The Aborigines healed broken bones, muscle tears, and illnesses of every kind using the yidaki. Interestingly, the sounds emitted by the yidaki are in alignment with modern sound-healing technology.[78]

Sound as healing was "rediscovered" in the West in the 1930s when experiments conducted by Hans Jenny, a German scientist, revealed that iron filings, sand, and fine powders placed on a flat metal plaque and vibrated with sound waves arranged themselves in intricate patterns.[79] The patterns, known as Chalynadi figures, were most concentrated where the sound was most dense. The study of sound waves and vibrations, called *cymatics*, has shown that iron filings, sand, and fine powders move into different shapes with different frequencies of sound, confirming the idea that form is a function of frequency.[8, 80]

Healing with sound is based on the principles of harmonic resonance (also known as vibrational resonance) and the assumption that specific sound frequencies resonate with specific organs of the body. Using the vibrational energy of tones, music, chants, song, the spoken word, and a variety of sound-producing instruments, sound therapists seek those frequencies that will promote relaxation and healing for an individual. We respond to sounds wholly. Think for a moment about a sound that, for you, is beautiful. Perhaps it is listening to a light breeze rustling through the trees, waves gently washing ashore, a flute symphony, singing Tibetan bowls. Your response to these frequencies creates an energetic pattern of harmonic resonance and healing. You may also recall sounds that are unsettling to you; these, too, have a deep effect and you can almost feel the discomfort on a physical level.

There are several sound therapies that are familiar to holistic nurses. Music therapy is an evidenced-based intervention that is increasingly used in a wide variety of settings. Studies have demonstrated the psychophysiological effects of music such as lowering of blood pressure and heart rate, changes in muscle activity, and a profound sense of relaxation.[8, 14] Music is processed in the deep parts of the brain and activates the amygdala, where memories are stored. People living with cognitive challenges such as dementia show powerful, positive effects, including decreased agitation and restlessness, when hearing music. The Chalice of Repose Project is a long-standing program that gently provides care and support to the dying through prescriptive music (see the suggested readings at the end of this chapter for more information on this project).

Other forms of sound healing may be integrated into a holistic healing practice for self or other. Chanting, toning, Tibetan singing bowls, and drumming are but a few examples. The regular use of sound, combined with intention, may result in faster vibrations at the molecular level. This higher rate of vibration creates larger spaces between the cells, making us less dense and preventing negative or intrusive energies from sticking to us easily.[80] The energy healing practitioner committed to developing knowledge and skills related to the use of sound can create spaces in which people can experience deep, whole healing.

Light

Light is another vibrational energy therapy that has a long history of use in healing. Our well-being and health are deeply affected by light—or the lack of it. Can you imagine life without light? As Popp showed, light may be essential to human functioning. Remember that our DNA continuously produces light—photons—that travels throughout the body.[76, 81]

One source of light, the sun, also seems to be essential. The sun is an important component of the sleep cycle as it tones down melatonin and stimulates serotonin production. When sunlight is in short supply, our biorhythms are affected and we likely feel droopy, sleepy, sad, depressed, and at times unable to rest; indeed, sun may be a vital nutrient.

Light therapy uses light on the eyes, acupuncture and acupressure points, chakras, meridians, reflex zones, and perhaps the pineal gland to restore proper frequencies to the energy field and stimulate self-healing.[81] Seasonal Affective Disorder and skin disorders are both treated with light therapy, utilizing natural and artificial sources. Perhaps the best approach to avoid some of these light-related problems is to sit or walk outside in the sun every day for 20 to 30 minutes.

Color

Color is a form of visible light; color therapy is the use of the different frequencies of light for the purpose of balance and healing. The primary colors (red, orange, yellow, green, blue, indigo, purple) each have a specific frequency and resonate with specific color and light frequencies in living systems. We are all affected by color, both consciously and unconsciously. How do you feel when you enter a room that is painted with bright red walls? With blue ones? Is there a difference?

An energy healing practitioner can apply the principles of light and color using verbal suggestion, visualizations, and other tools such as sensitively placed fabrics to support energy balance. We can also teach healees and their support people to envision a color filling the body—even color a solution such as chemotherapy—to imbue it with healing properties.

Homeopathy

Homeopathy was developed by Samuel Hahnemann, a German physician and chemist, in the late 1800s. The homeopathic system of healing is based on the premise that what we might call symptoms are really the body's attempt to heal itself, so we should support its effort. Homeopaths choose remedies that create the same symptoms as the problem that the person is encountering. It is based on the principle of similars that assumes that substances that, in high doses produce symptoms of sickness in healthy people, will have a curative effect when administered in homeopathic doses to sick people exhibiting similar symptoms.[14, 75]

Through a series of repeated dilutions and vigorous shakings (succussion), remedies are created that have no molecules of the original plant. Succussion is believed to increase the vibratory field of remedies. Lenger posited that homeopathic remedies are photons that are magnetically bound to their carrier substances.[82] She measured the magnetic fields during dilution and succussion and discovered that the resonance frequencies (megahertz) increased with each successive succession.

Aromatherapy and Flower Essences

Aromatherapy is an energy healing therapy (see Chapter 15). Prepared and delivered in a variety of ways, essential oils are used for both their biologic and energetic properties. Essential oils have myriad uses, including their powerful antibiotic and antifungal effects that rapidly heal sunburns, are soothing, can help calm frightened or overly energetic children, and can even neutralize the tobacco smell in closed rooms.

Flower essences are an energetic preparation of highly diluted flowers and plants. Edward Bach developed flower essence therapy in the 1930s; he believed that the early morning dew found on flower petals retained the healing properties of that plant. The practitioner prepares the essences by placing the flower in clean water and then putting this in sunlight for a few hours. When it is removed from the sunlight, the solution is diluted with more water and mixed with a stabilizing substance such as vinegar or brandy. This is the "mother tincture," which can be diluted many times to make multiple doses that one can drink.

The theory is that the sun's electromagnetic frequencies cause the electrical essence of the plant to be transferred to the water. When someone drinks the essence, he or she is believed to be ingesting the flower's energetic pattern, its electromagnetic frequency, which interacts with and can balance the person's energetic state. As with aromatherapies, different flowers produce different results.

Thoughts on Energy Therapies

Energy therapies, whether laying on of hands, sound, light, flower essences, or any type of energy modality, have many followers who are convinced that these approaches not only work but that they occasionally may be more appropriate, and perhaps more successful in some cases, than biological medicine. Even as more and more nurses are studying these approaches, there is little scientific evidence to support the claims of energy healing practitioners or of skeptics.

Because of the movement toward evidence-based treatments, more energy therapies are being subjected to research. Holistic nurses have the opportunity to be trailblazers—to design research studies that contribute to the body of nursing knowledge and, ultimately, to contribute to the art and science of holistic nursing.

Support for the Healer

Regardless of one's experience, collegial support is important to people involved in energy healing practices. There are numerous associations that support those interested in energy healing practices; we will review only three. The American Holistic Nurses Association (AHNA), founded in 1981 by Charlotte McGuire, is a nonprofit membership association for nurses and other holistic healthcare professionals. The AHNA's mission is to advance holistic nursing through community building, advocacy, research, and education. The AHNA envisions a world in which nursing nurtures wholeness and inspires peace and healing. See www.ahna.org.

The International Society for the Study of Subtle Energies and Energy Medicine (ISSSEEM) is an interdisciplinary organization for the study of the basic sciences and medical and therapeutic applications of subtle energies. Founded by Drs. Carol Schneider, T. M. Srinivasan, and Elmer Green, ISSSEEM operated under its own charter until June 2013, when it was placed under the corporate umbrella of Holos University Graduate Seminary. As the International Research Division of Holos, ISSSEEM retains its original name and goals. See http://issseem.org/mission-vision-values.html.

The Institute of Noetic Sciences, founded in 1973 by Apollo 14 astronaut Edgar Mitchell, is a nonprofit research, education, and membership organization whose mission is supporting individual and collective transformation through consciousness research, educational outreach, and engaging a global learning community in the realization of our human potential. See http://noetic.org/.

In addition to these three general organizations, practitioners of energy therapies have developed their own organizations. Whether created for general interest or to support practitioners of a specific energy therapy, these groups enable one to remain abreast of the most current evidence, obtain continuing education, learn about initiatives that inform regulation, and, perhaps most important, connect us to a network of like-minded people. Refer to the suggested readings at the end of this chapter; it is not intended to be a complete list but a place for you to start.

Directions for Future Research

The use of energy healing has gained visibility, credibility, and use in evidence-based practice of nurses, allied healthcare practitioners, and physicians in the last 20 years.[50] At first met with general skepticism, research is emerging that proves efficacy beyond a placebo effect. The best evidence shows that energy therapies are effective for reducing the intensity of postoperative pain, anxiety in a wide variety of situations, and agitation in dementia patients.[53]

Researching energy therapies effectively has been difficult. Recall the problem physicists have studying photons: These tiny particles will go wherever the physicist intends. Applying this to research suggests that whatever the researcher intends will influence the outcome of an experiment. The gold-standard research approach—the experimental/control design—makes the assumption that the people involved will not influence the results, but we now know that is not true. Anytime a laying-on-of-hands modality is studied, the modality must not include a sham provider because that person is likely to have a healing effect. People are not neutral and always have some intention; that intention must be taken into account and, if possible, removed from the experimental protocol.

Another problem is that most research is designed to look at the immediate effect of something. While there are some immediate changes in energy healing therapies, most of the results are cumulative, individual, and, often, complex. Healing can be paradoxical, with unexpected personal growth and transcendence, but experimental/control designs do not look for these.

The energy therapy researcher of the future will need to design novel approaches that provide an entirely new model for researching human–human interactions and for measuring both immediate and long-term results of treatments. This might be done most efficiently by comparing the efficacy and outcomes of energy therapies with traditional therapies. For example, one could study the effects of aromatherapies versus exercise on the agitation level of dementia patients. The possibilities are endless, but designing a study that accurately measures the effect of energy therapies will require the future nurse researcher to be creative.

Nurse Healer Reflections: The Tapestry Revealed

As we bring closure to our exploration of energy, we return to the original question: How does energy healing work? Weaving all ways of knowing into universal truths, we are offered a beginning idea. Energy healing practitioners and healees enter into an energetic relationship with the intention to restore balance and order to the healees' field—they come together in a healing interaction. Empiric knowing guides the energy healing practitioner in the appropriate use of a technique that creates space for electromagnetic induction and entrainment of the higher frequencies needed to effect healing. Personal knowing informs both the energy healing practitioner and the healee, building on life experiences and previous healing encounters. Their interaction is grounded in respect and trust; boundaries are never crossed. Because energy healing practitioners are used to listening to their sixth sense, their intuitive knowing is used throughout the entire healing process. Coming to a still point may be part of an ethical practice as energy healing practitioners are more able to appreciate the energetic boundaries. Ego is not a part of the healing interaction; rather, humility and gratitude are manifest. Aesthetically, energy healing practitioners offer compassionate presence, listening, and the willingness to co-create healing spaces with healees.

NOTES

1. L. Dossey, "All Tangled Up: Life in a Quantum World," *EXPLORE: The Journal of Science and Healing* 7, no. 6 (2011): 335–344.
2. J. Bolte Taylor, *My Stroke of Insight: A Brain Scientist's Personal Journey* (New York: Viking, 2008).
3. D. Radin, *Entangled Minds: Extrasensory Experiences in a Quantum Reality* (New York: Simon & Schuster, 2006).
4. J. L. Oschman, *Energy Medicine: The Scientific Basis* (New York: Churchill Livingstone, 2000).
5. D. Bradley, "Energy Fields: Implications for Nurses," *Journal of Holistic Nursing* 5, no. 1 (1987): 257–263.
6. D. Krieger, "Healing by the 'Laying-on' of Hands as a Facilitator of Bioenergetic Change: The Response of In-Vivo Human Hemoglobin," *Psychoenergetic Systems* 1 (1976): 121–129.
7. H. Graham, *Time, Energy, and the Psychology of Healing* (Philadelphia: Jessica Kingsley, 1990).
8. H. Graham, *Complementary Therapies in Context: The Psychology of Healing* (Philadelphia: Jessica Kingsley, 1999).
9. W. Bengston, "A Brief History of Energy Healing" (December 28, 2010). www.sooperarticles.com/health-fitness-articles/general-health-articles/brief-history-energy-healing-249621.html#ixzz32TC5Rgku.
10. R. C. Solomon and K. M. Higgins, *A Passion for Wisdom: A Very Brief History of Philosophy* (New York: Oxford University Press, 1997).
11. R. Tarnas, *The Passion of the Western Mind: Understanding the Ideas That Have Shaped Our World View* (New York: Ballantine Books, 1991).
12. B. McLean and A. Dworkin, "Understanding Chinese Medicine," *CME Resource* 72, no. 1 (2001): 1–30.
13. D. Ehling, "Oriental Medicine: An Introduction," *Alternative Therapies in Health and Medicine* 7, no. 4 (2001): 71–82.
14. K. L. Fontaine, *Complementary and Alternative Therapies for Nursing Practice*, 3rd ed. (Upper Saddle River, NJ: Prentice Hall, 2011).
15. X. Shen, "The Art of Acupuncture" (lecture at the Anhui College of Traditional Chinese Medicine, 2006).
16. L. Dossey, "The Royal Touch: A Look at Healing in Times Past," *EXPLORE: The Journal of Science and Healing* 9, no. 3 (2013): 121–127.
17. K. Maret, "Energy Medicine in the United States: Historical Roots and the Current Status," (July 2009). www.faim.org/energymedicine/energy-medicine-united-states-historical-roots-current-status.html.
18. R. Matthews, "Harold Burr's Biofields: Measuring the Electromagnetics of Life," *Subtle Energies and Energy Medicine* 18, no. 2 (2007): 55–61.
19. D. Feinstein and D. Eden, "Six Pillars of Energy Medicine: Clinical Strengths of a Complementary Paradigm," *Alternative Therapies in Health and Medicine* 14, no. 1 (2008): 44–54.
20. F. Capra, *The Tao of Physics: An Exploration of the Parallels Between Modern Physics and Eastern Mysticism* (Boston: Shambhala, 1975).
21. B. Rubik, "The Biofield Hypothesis: Its Biological Basis and Role in Medicine," *Journal of Alternative and Complementary Therapies* 8, no. 6 (2002): 703–717.
22. H. S. Burr and F. S. C. Northrup, "An Electro-Dynamic Theory of Life," *Quarterly Review of Biology* 10, no. 3 (1935): 322–333.
23. B. Grad, "The Laying on of Hands: Implications for Psychotherapy, Gentling and Placebo Effect," *Human Dimensions* 5, nos. 1–2 (1965): 40–45.
24. J. Kabat-Zinn, *Coming to Our Senses* (New York: Hyperion, 2006).
25. J. Reston, "Now, About My Operation in Peking; Now, Let Me Tell You About My Appendectomy in Peking," *The New York Times* (July 26, 1971). www.acupuncture.com/testimonials/restonexp.htm.
26. D. M. Eisenberg, R. C. Kessler, C. Foster, F. E. Norlock, D. R. Calkins, and T. L Delbanco, "Unconventional Medicine in the United States: Prevalence, Costs, and Patterns of Use," *New England Journal of Medicine* 328, no. 4 (1993): 246–252.
27. R. Nuccitelli, P. Nuccitelli, C. Li, S. Narsing, D. M. Pariser, and K. Lui, "The Electric Field Near Human Skin Wounds Declines with Age and Provides a Non-Invasive Indicator of Wound Healing," *Wound Repair and Regeneration* 19, no. 5 (2011): 645–655.
28. R. K. Aaron, D. M., Ciombor, S., Wang, and B. Simon, "Clinical Biophysics: The Promotion of Skeletal Repair by Physical Forces," *Annals of the New York Academy of Sciences* 1068, no. 1 (2006): 513–531.
29. J. Ren, H. Li, L. Palaniyappan, H. Liu, J. Wang, C. Li, and P. M. Rossini, "Repetitive Transcranial

Magnetic Stimulation Versus Electroconvulsive Therapy for Major Depression: A Systematic Review and Meta-Analysis," *Progress in Neuropsychopharmacology and Biological Psychiatry* 51 (2014): 181–189.

30. A. A. Feizi and M. A. Arabi, "Acute Childhood Leukemias and Exposure to Magnetic Fields Generated by High Voltage Overhead Power Lines: A Risk Factor in Iran," *Asian Pacific Journal of Cancer Prevention* 8, no. 1 (2007): 69–72.

31. N. S. Hassan and S. A. Abdelkawi, "Changes in Molecular Structure of Hemoglobin in Exposure to 50 Hz Magnetic Fields," *Nature and Science* 8, no. 8 (2010): 236–243.

32. C. Mothersill, R. Smith, M. Henry, and C. Seymour, "Alternative Medicine Techniques Have Non-Linear Effects on Radiation Response and Can Alter the Expression of Radiation Induced Bystander Effects," *Dose Response* 11, no. 1 (2013): 82–98.

33. R. Gerber, *Vibrational Medicine: New Choices for Healing Ourselves* (Santa Fe, NM: Bear & Company, 1988).

34. R. Gerber, *Vibrational Medicine for the 21st Century: A Complete Guide to Energy Healing and Spiritual Transformation* (New York: HarperCollins, 2000).

35. M-W. Ho and D. P. Knight, "The Acupuncture System and the Liquid Crystalline Collagen Fibres of the Connective Tissues: Liquid Crystalline Meridians," *American Journal of Chinese Medicine* 26, nos. 3–4 (1998): 251–263.

36. B. H. Lipton, *The Biology of Belief: Unleashing the Power of Consciousness, Matter, and Miracles* (New York: HayHouse, 2008).

37. M. Xu, S. Yan, X. Yin, X. Li, S. Gao, R. Han, L. Wei, and G. Lei, "Acupuncture for Chronic Low Back Pain in Long-Term Follow-Up: A Meta-Analysis of 13 Randomized Controlled Trials," *American Journal of Chinese Medicine* 41 no. 1 (2013): 1–19.

38. Y. B. Long and X. P. Wu, "A Meta-Analysis of the Efficacy of Acupuncture in Treating Dysphagia in Patients with a Stroke," *Acupuncture in Medicine* 30, no. 4 (2012): 291–297.

39. World Health Organization, "Institutional Repository for Information Sharing" (2014). http://apps.who.int/iris/.

40. D. L. Rapoport, "On the Fusion of Physics and Klein Bottle Logic in Biology, Embryogenesis and Evolution," *NeuroQuantology* 9, no. 4 (2011): 842–861.

41. S. Sava, "Exploring the Biofield Hypothesis," *Shift: At the Frontiers of Consciousness* (2004–2005).http://media.noetic.org/uploads/files/s5_rubik.pdf

42. R. R. Parse, *The Human Becoming School of Thought: A Perspective for Nurses and Other Health Professionals* (Thousand Oaks, CA: Sage, 1998).

43. S. Dikker, L. J. Silbert, U. Hasson, and J. D. Zevin, "On the Same Wavelength: Predictable Language Enhances Speaker–Listener Brain-to-Brain Synchrony in Posterior Superior Temporal Gyrus," *Journal of Neuroscience* 34, no. 18 (2014): 6267–6272.

44. R. Lui and M. Pelowski, "Clarifying the Interaction Types in Two-Person Neuroscience Research," *Frontiers in Human Neuroscience* 8, no. 276 (2014): 1–4.

45. L. Nummenmaa, E. Glerean, M. Viinikainen, I. P. Jääskeläinen, R. Hari, and M. Sams, "Emotions Promote Social Interaction by Synchronizing Brain Activity Across Individuals," *Proceedings of the National Academy of Sciences of the United States of America* 109, no. 24 (2012): 9599–9604.

46. W. Heisenberg, *Physics and Philosophy: The Revolution in Modern Science* (New York: Harper & Row, 1958).

47. A. Einstein, "Einstein's Reply to Criticisms," in *Albert Einstein: Philosopher–Scientist*, ed. P. A. Schilpp (Peru, IL: Open Court, 1949): 665–686.

48. A. Watts, "The Nature of Consciousness" (1960). www.erowid.org/culture/characters/watts_alan/watts_alan_article1.shtml.

49. National Human Genome Research Institute, "All About the Human Genome Project" (March 18, 2014). www.genome.gov/10001772.

50. J. Hart, "Energy Medicine: Advances in the Medical Community," *Alternative and Complementary Therapies* 18, no. 6 (2012): 309–313.

51. J. G. Anderson and A. G. Taylor, "Biofield Therapies and Cancer Pain," *Clinical Journal of Oncology Nursing* 16, no. 1 (2012): 43–48.

52. National Center for Complementary and Integrative Health, "Complementary, Alternative, or Integrative Health: What's in a Name?" (July 2014). http://nccam.nih.gov/health/whatiscam.

53. S. Jain and P. J. Mills, "Biofield Therapies: Helpful or Full of Hype? A Best Evidence Synthesis," *International Journal of Behavioral Medicine* 17, no. 1 (2010): 1–16.

54. L. Diaz-Rodriguez, M. Arroyo-Morales, I. Cantero-Villanueva, C. Fernandez-Lao, M. Polley, and C. Fernandez-de-las-Penas, "The Application of Reiki in Nurses Diagnosed with Burnout Syndrome Has Beneficial Effects on Concentration of Salivary IgA and Blood Pressure," *Latin American Journal of Nursing* 19 (2011): 1132–1138.

55. A. L. Baldwin, K. Fullmer, and G. E. Schwartz, "Comparison of Physical Therapy with Energy

Healing for Improving Range of Motion in Subjects with Restricted Shoulder Mobility," *Evidence-Based Complementary and Alternative Medicine* 2013 (2013): 329–338.

56. S. Uchida, T. Iha, K. Yamaoka, K. Nitta, and H. Sugano, "Effect of Biofield Therapy in the Human Brain," *Journal of Alternative and Complementary Medicine* 18, no. 9 (2012): 875–879.

57. D. V. Ponte and L. Schäfer, "Carl Gustav Jung, Quantum Physics and the Spiritual Mind: A Mystical Vision of the Twenty-First Century," *Behavioral Sciences* 3, no. 4 (2013): 601–618.

58. D. Krieger, *The Therapeutic Touch: How to Use Your Hands to Help or Heal* (New York: Prentice Hall, 1979).

59. D. Kunz and E. Peper, "Human Fields and the Energetics of Healing," in *Spiritual Aspects of the Healing Arts*, ed. D. Kunz (Wheaton: IL: Theosophical): 211–235.

60. R. Weber, "Philosophical Foundations and Frameworks for Healing," in *Therapeutic Touch: A Book of Readings*, eds. D. Borelli and P. Heidt (New York: Springer, 1981): 13–29.

61. B. A. Brennan, *Hands of Light: A Guide to Healing Through the Human Energy Field* (New York: Bantam Books, 1988).

62. V. Slater, "Energy Healing," in *Holistic Nursing: A Handbook for Practice*, 6th ed., eds. B. Dossey and L. Keegan (Burlington, MA: Jones & Bartlett Learning): 751–773.

63. Personal communication. Dora Kunz, 1998.

64. K. Tsuchiya and H. Motoyama, "Study of Body's Energy Changes in Non-Touch Energy Healing 1. Pranic Healing Protocol Applied for a Breast Cancer Subject," *Subtle Energies and Energy Medicine* 20, no. 2 (2009): 15–29.

65. D. Krieger (lecture provided on Therapeutic Touch Dialogues, Whitefish, MT, 2013).

66. J. Levin, "Energy Healers: Who They Are and What They Do," *EXPLORE: The Journal of Science and Healing* 7, no. 11 (2011): 13–26.

67. J. Zimmerman, "The Laying-on-of-Hands, Healing and Therapeutic Touch: A Testable Theory," *BEMI Currents* 2 (1990): 8–17.

68. A. L. Baldwin and R. Hammerschlag, "Biofield-Based Therapies: A Systematic Review of Physiological Effects on Practitioners During Healing," *EXPLORE: The Journal of Science and Healing* 10, no. 3 (2014): 150–161.

69. R. Zahourek, "Intentionality Forms the Matrix of Healing: A Theory," *Alternative Therapies in Health and Medicine* 10, no. 6 (2004): 40–49.

70. R. Zahourek, "Intentionality: The Matrix of Healing Creates Caring, Healing Presence," *Beginnings* 34, no. 2 (2014): 6–9.

71. W. Bengston, "Breakthrough: Clues to Healing with Intention," *EdgeScience* 2 (2010): 5–9.

72. M. Moga and W. Bengston, "Anomalous Magnetic Field Activity During a Bioenergy Healing Experiment," *Journal of Scientific Exploration* 24, no. 3 (2010): 397–410.

73. S. L. Warber, C. Deogracia, J. Straughn, and G. Kile, "Biofield Energy Healing from the Inside," *Journal of Alternative and Complementary Medicine* 10, no. 6 (2005): 1107–1113.

74. D. Kunz and D. Krieger, *The Spiritual Dimension of Therapeutic Touch* (Rochester, VT: Bear & Company, 2004).

75. R. Hammerschlag, S. Jain, A. L. Baldwin, G. Gronowicz, S. K. Lutgendorf, J. L. Oschman, and G. L. Yount, "Biofield Research: A Roundtable Discussion of Scientific and Methodological Issues," *Journal of Alternative and Complementary Medicine* 18, no. 12 (2012): 1081–1086.

76. V. Silver, "Holistic Energy Healing Guide" (2014). www.holistic-mindbody-healing.com/holistic-energy-healing.html.

77. E. Brown, "New Choices for Healing Ourselves: Interview with Richard Gerber" (April 1999). http://share-international.org/archives/health-healing/hh_ebnewch.html.

78. J. Stuart and A. Reid, "Rediscovering the Art and Science of Sound" (2010). www.tokenrock.com/sound_healing/wonders_of_sound.php.

79. H. Jenny, *Cymatics: A Study of Wave Phenomena and Vibration* (Newmarket, NH: MACROmedia, 2001).

80. N. Kornblum, "The Healing Power of Sound and Overtone Chant" (2012). www.globalsoundhealing.net/en/content/healing-power-sound-and-overtone-chant.

81. R. S. Levy, "Healing with Light and Color" (2011). www.energyhealing-quantumhealing.com/healing-with-light-and-color.php.

82. K. Lenger, "Homeopathy—Applied Quantum Physics: Detection of Photons in Homeopathic Remedies" (October 19, 2013). www.comb.cat/cat/colegi/seccions/doc/05%20%20Homeopathy_applied_quantum_physics_detection_of_photons_in_homeopathic_remedies_lenger.pdf.

SUGGESTED READINGS

Websites

Subtle Anatomy: Nadis

www.subtleanatomy.com/Nadis.htm

Center for Mindfulness: History of Mindfulness-Based Stress Reduction Program
www.umassmed.edu/cfm/stress-reduction/history-of-mbsr/

Watson Caring Science Institute and International Caritas Consortium
http://watsoncaringscience.org/about-us/jean-bio/
http://watsoncaringscience.org/about-us/caring-science-definitions-processes-theory/

Bruce Lipton
www.brucelipton.com

Horishi Motoyama: Apparatus for Meridian Identification Device
www.cihs.edu/AMI/ami_articles.asp

Chalice of Repose Project: The Voice of Music-Thanatology
www.chaliceofrepose.org

Rosemarie Rizzo Parse:
http://www.humanbecoming.org/human-becoming.php
http://currentnursing.com/nursing_theory/Rosemary_Pars_Human_Becoming_Theory.html

Books
M. Thompson, *The Cry and the Covenant* (New York: Doubleday, 1949).

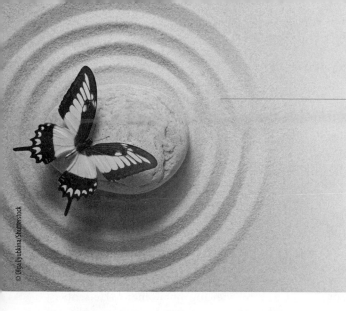

CHAPTER 10

The Psychophysiology of Body–Mind Healing

Genevieve M. Bartol

Nurse Healer Objectives

Theoretical

- Articulate a comprehensive conceptual model of body–mind interactions.
- Interpret the application of selected models, theories, and research in the field of psychoneuroimmunology.
- Explain the interconnections of mind modulation and the autonomic, endocrine, immune, and neuropeptide systems.

Clinical

- Recognize the implications of body–mind interactions for clinical practice.
- Incorporate the knowledge of body–mind interactions in planning nursing interventions.

Personal

- Identify one's own patterns of body–mind interactions as expressed in attitudes, tensions, and images.
- Recognize the implications of one's own body–mind patterns for self-care and self-healing.

Definitions

Allostasis: The adaptation process to maintain homeostasis and well-being.

Allostatic load: Occurs when one experiences overwhelming stress or has inadequate coping skills.

Autopoiesis: The self-organizing force in living systems.

Bifurcation: A point at which transformational change occurs in a complex system; at a fork in the road of life.

Body–mind: A state of integration that includes body, mind, and spirit.

Chaos: The stable and orderly but irregular, unpredictable behavior of a complex system.

Complexity science: The study of systems with many interdependent components.

Cycles: One of the simplest nonlinear behaviors that is periodic and recurrent.

Epigenetics: The study of how genes produce their effect on the phenotype of the organism.

Information Theory: A mathematical model that helps explain the connections between consciousness and body–mind healing.

Limbic-hypothalamic system: The major anatomic modulating link connecting the brain/mind and the autonomic, endocrine, immune, and neuropeptide systems.

Mind modulation: The bidirectional inter-relationships of thoughts and feelings with neurohormonal messengers of the nervous, endocrine, immune, and neuropeptide systems that support body–mind connections.

Network: Interconnected and interrelated system.

Neuropeptides: Messenger molecules produced at various sites throughout the body to transmit body–mind patterns of communication.

Neuroplasticity: The ability of the nervous system to respond to intrinsic and/or extrinsic stimuli by reorganizing its structure, function, and connections.

Neurotransmitters: Chemicals that facilitate the transmission of impulses through nerves in the body.

Psychoneuroimmunology: A branch of science that strives to show the connections among psychology, neuroendocrinology, and immunology.

Receptors: Sites on cell surfaces that serve as points of attachment for various types of messenger molecules.

Self-Regulation Theory: A person's ability to learn cognitive processing of information to bring involuntary body responses under voluntary control.

Traumatic stress response (TSR): Occurs when the normal stress response is altered as a result of overwhelming and/or ongoing stress.

New Scientific Understanding of Living Systems

Developments in science and concomitant advances in technology continue to reveal human beings in new ways. The mechanistic view of the body–mind has given way to a holistic view. The habit of looking at persons from their component parts while ignoring interactions and contexts is misleading and creates problems of its own. The body can no longer be considered a machine powered by the mind to which healthcare practitioners apply assorted therapies to effect healing. Humans are complex, open, highly integrative systems embedded in and supporting other systems. As we free our scientific imagination and increase our knowledge of laws that are the opposite of mechanistic, such as the concepts of nonlocality and superposition of states in quantum physics, our understanding of living systems will continue to change.[1,2] The term *body–mind* includes the body and mind as a unified whole.

Quantum Theory

Discoveries in quantum physics replaced the old ways of viewing phenomena. Heisenberg described the changed world as a complicated tissue of events, in which connections of different kinds alternate, overlap, or combine and thereby determine the texture of the whole.[3] In the past, the properties and behavior of the parts were believed to determine those of the whole. Now it is clear that the whole also defines the behavior of the parts.

The realization that systems are integrated wholes that cannot be understood simply by analysis shattered scientific certitude. No longer was it possible to believe that, given enough time, effort, and money, all questions would have answers. Rather, all scientific concepts and theories have limitations. Scientific explanations do not provide complete and conclusive answers but instead generate other questions.[4] The more we learn, the more we discover how much we do not know. Even one additional piece of data can change the whole configuration. It is important to remain open to all possibilities because absolute certainty is an illusion. Increasingly, scientific findings demonstrate a changing world. Planck found radiant energy was emitted from light sources in discrete amounts, or *quanta*, and that changes in the amount of radiant energy occurred in leaps, not sequential steps.[3] Bohr extended Planck's discovery to the field of subatomic particles and showed that electrons could move from one orbit of energy to another. The behavior of light does not follow one set of rules. Light possesses the qualities of both waves and particles. One explanation is not correct and the other wrong; both interpretations are useful in explaining the behavior of light in different situations.

The world is complex and unified; parts complement one another and participate in the whole. Similarly, all parts of the body work together. Health and illness are indivisible; both are natural and necessary. Hyperpyrexia (fever) may be seen as a sign of illness as well as a sign of the body's healthy response to a threat. Fever indicates that the hypothalamic set point of the body has changed.[5] The alteration occurs in the presence of pyrogens (e.g., bacteria, viruses).

A mild temperature elevation up to 39 degrees Centigrade (102.2 degrees Fahrenheit) stimulates the body's immune system, increases white blood cell production, and reduces the concentration of iron in blood plasma, thereby suppressing the growth of bacteria. Fever also stimulates the production of interferon, which protects the body against viruses. Using medications to lower the body temperature prematurely, particularly in the first 24 hours, may actually interfere with this important defense mechanism.

Systems Theory

The major traits of systems thinking appeared concurrently in several disciplines during the first half of the 20th century, but it was von Bertalanffy's General Systems Theory that established systems thinking as the predominant scientific movement.[6] Resultant theories and models of living systems initiated a radical shift in the understanding of human beings. It is now believed that persons and their environments make up an interconnected dynamic system in which a change at any point may effect changes at other points. The idea that the world is hierarchical, with each level organized separately, has been replaced with a new understanding of relatedness and context.

Human beings are living systems, organizationally closed and structurally open, embedded within the web of life.[7] They are *organizationally closed* because they are self-organizing; that is, they establish their own order and behavior rather than submitting to those imposed by the environment. They are *structurally open* because they engage in a continual exchange of energy and matter with their environment. Words like *feedback*, *integration*, *rhythm*, and *dynamic equilibrium* account for the continually changing components of living systems. These components

do not operate in isolation from one another. A dysfunction in any one system of the body reverberates in the other systems. For example, a dysfunction of the endocrine system referred to as hypothyroidism may manifest itself by thinning hair or clinical depression.[8] Hypothyroidism, in fact, may be secondary to a dysfunction in another organ system and not represent primary failure of the thyroid gland. Thyroid deficiency may occur when the pituitary gland is malfunctioning or when there is damage to the hypothalamus. It is not possible to identify conclusively a single cause of what was formerly named a primary dysfunction. All body systems participate in the biodance; changes in one system result in changes in the other systems and, in circular fashion, changes in itself, just as the pituitary gland increases its secretion of thyroid-stimulating hormone when the thyroid gland is underproducing thyroid hormone.

Theory of Relativity

Einstein developed a system of mechanics that acknowledges the relative character of motion, velocity, and mass, as well as the interdependence of matter, time, and space.[3] This theory is based on the principle that there is no absolute frame of reference independent of the observer. Each person views others from his or her own perspective, including his or her particular biases.

Scientists can no longer describe their work as finding a piece to a puzzle or as adding a building stone to a firm foundation of knowledge. Rather, it has become increasingly apparent that scientific knowledge is a network of concepts and models, none of which is any more fundamental than the other. All things (objects) and events (happenings) in one's life are connected and relative within the whole. The mind and body are inseparably intertwined; thoughts, feelings, and actions influence a person's state of health and illness. Stone reminds us of how the nurses' presence and intention or lack thereof while administering care can positively or adversely influence the patients' experience.[9]

Studies using imaging devices show that mindfulness meditation strengthens the neurological circuits that calm a part of the brain that acts as a trigger for fear and anger and increases the amount of activity in the brain associated with positive emotions. Fear and anger can provoke harmful actions. Happiness and inner balance are crucial to survival.[10, 11]

Principles of Self-Organization

The key ideas of current models of self-organizing systems were refined and extended during the 1970s and 1980s, and a unified theory of living systems emerged.[7, 12] This unified theory encompassed the creation of structures and modes of behavior in the processes of development, learning, and coevolution. In the past, living systems were viewed from two perspectives: in terms of physical matter (structure) and the configuration of relationships (pattern). Structure is concerned with quantities, things weighed and measured. Pattern is concerned with qualities and is expressed by a map of the configuration of relationships. Qualities, such as color or size, were considered accidental characteristics. A bicycle may be red or green, stand 24 or 26 inches high, and have a light or heavy frame, but it remains a bicycle as long as it has the configuration of relationships consistent with a bicycle.

Systems, whether nonliving or living, are configurations of ordered relationships whose attributes are the properties of pattern. The bicycle, a nonliving system, consists of several components arranged to perform a particular function. The various kinds of bicycles (e.g., mountain bicycles, touring bicycles) embody the essential characteristics known as a bicycle. Bicycles have a structure with specific components and operate as bicycles as long as the pattern of relationships that defines them as bicycles remains.[12, p. 85] Living systems, however, are fundamentally different from nonliving systems. Living systems do not function mechanically and are not explained just by physical principles. The components of living systems are interconnected by internal feedback loops in a nonlinear fashion and are capable of self-organization.

Not only is the activity of living systems purposeful, but it also appears to be under the direction of an overall design or purpose.[7, p. 40] The pattern of organization of living systems includes a fundamental self-organizing force known as autopoiesis.[13] If the pattern of a living system is destroyed, the system dies even though all of the components of the system remain intact. A living system cannot be restored simply by recreating the pattern. A nonliving system, like a bicycle, will regain function if the parts are reassembled correctly. Living systems do not rest in a steady state of balance as do nonliving systems but rather operate far from equilibrium.[12] Stability in living systems embodies change. Relationships are not linear but extend in all directions. Bifurcation occurs and generates new feedback loops.[7, pp. 38–39] Living systems regulate and recreate themselves.

Life process (cognition) is the link between pattern and structure in a living system.[13, pp. 150–162] Life process is "the activity involved in the continual embodiment of the system's pattern of organization."[13, p. 162] Life process is related to autopoiesis and may be considered distinct facets of the same phenomenon of life. All living systems are cognitive systems; therefore, cognition indicates the existence of an autopoietic network.[10] Structure, pattern, and process are inextricably intertwined in a living system.

Organisms appear to be under the direction of an overall design or purpose and do not just function mechanically. For example, the symptoms experienced by humans represent attempts to gain health and, therefore, are signals of stability, not breakdown. The human immune system recognizes an invading organism as dangerous and quickly reacts to counter the threat. Symptoms are really signs of the inherent organization and adaptability of a living system. We cannot unerringly predict the outcome of these complex relationships among organisms—one person may become sick while another may be seemingly unaffected and yet infect others with whom he has contact. Even invading organisms, also living systems, learn and adapt. The ability of pathogens to modify themselves and develop resistance to antibiotics is a striking example of the ability of a living system to reorganize. We participate in the web of life, and the changes that we have made are sometimes good (eradicating smallpox) and sometimes bad (autoimmune diseases).

Santiago Theory of Cognition

Derived from the study of neural networks, the Santiago Theory of Cognition is linked to the concept of autopoiesis.[13] Cognition is generally defined as the process of knowing or perceiving; it is associated with the mind, implicitly with the brain and nervous system. The Santiago Theory offers a radical expansion of the traditional concept of cognition. In this new view, cognition involves the whole process of life, including perception, emotion, and behavior. Even the cells that make up the immune system perceive the characteristics of their environment and will, for example, move to the site of a wound and increase in numbers to deal with an invading organism. Despite the absence of a brain, cognition is present; in this event, it can be described as embodied action.[13, p. 268] Perception and action in these cells are inseparable.

A living organism is an interconnected network (system) that undergoes structural change while preserving its pattern of organization as it interacts with other systems.[7] Changes in both autopoietic networks take place. In other words, one living system may trigger an autopoietic network response in the other but does not direct or control the response. A living organism chooses which stimuli from the environment will trigger structural changes. Moreover, not all changes in an organism are acts of cognition; a person who is injured in an accident does not specify and direct those structural changes. Other structural changes (e.g., perception and response of the circulatory system) that accompany the imposed changes are acts of cognition.

Fundamental shifts in our understanding of the human mind help explain how humans receive, generate, and transduce information. New ideas and events evoke body–mind changes; that is, neural pathways and consciousness couple to enable information transduction. For example, a person with asthma that increasingly interferes with her activities may remember that her mother's asthma also became more severe as she aged, and she may begin to become resigned to what she sees as an inevitable decline in her health. Subsequently, she learns how to monitor her asthma. She begins to see a pattern to her attacks, identifies potential triggers, and uses both traditional and holistic interventions to gain more control. The asthma attacks decrease in severity and frequency.

The extent of the interactions that a living system can have with its environment outlines its "cognitive domain."[13 p. 175] Emotions are not just an accompaniment of perception and behavior but are an inherent part of this domain. For example, a fear response to a situation initiates an entire pattern of physiologic processes. Blood goes to the large skeletal muscles, making it easier to run, while the face blanches. Freezing for a moment allows time to assess the situation and determine whether hiding might be a wiser choice. Circuits in the brain's emotional centers trigger a flood of hormones that sounds a general alert. Although experience and culture modify responses, emotions occur simultaneously with and are part of every cognitive act.

Complexity Science

Complexity science is the study of systems with many interdependent components.[14] Nursing is concerned with caring and, therefore, with relatedness and relationships. "Mother" is defined as a female parent. Complexity science uses a relational definition: what a child calls his or her female parent. Nursing is concerned with caring for another; thus, relationship is of vital importance. Nursing science, caring science, unitary and complexity science are integrated into a new whole. Nursing is a complex task that requires a wholistic orientation that allows us to consider the complexity of our environments with the complexity of the individuals and groups we serve based on a unitary model.[15] Too often we view our bodies as vulnerable mechanisms that require constant vigilance and tinkering to prevent disaster. Most things get better by themselves. Bodies are complex and designed to heal themselves. We always need to recognize that any presenting symptom has to be considered in the context of the whole person and may represent the body's efforts to heal itself. Even pain has a positive value because it reminds us that our bodies are self-monitoring. If we simply direct all of our efforts toward eliminating the pain without identifying the mechanisms and context of the pain, we may be doing more harm than good. We need to be always aware of what we choose to ignore.

There is also increasing evidence that we can use psychobiotics to help persons suffering from a variety of psychiatric illnesses. Researchers can now discern which strains of gut bacteria affect the nervous system and even map the exact pathways through which specific gut bacteria influence the brain. For example, people suffering from major depression frequently have elevated levels of the hormone cortisol, which is released in response to stress. A probiotic cocktail of *Lactobaccilus helveticus* and *Bifidobacterium longum* was found to reduce cortisol levels. Deficiency in the neurotransmitter GABA is found with depression. Researchers have identified strains of *Lactobacillus* and *Bifidobacterium* that actively secrete GABA; consuming dark chocolate leads to an increase in both of these gut microbes. *Bifidobacterium infantis* alters the levels of serotonin as does Prozac. We must consider the effects of antibiotics on the helpful bacteria in our gut when we are using them for minor sniffles, when rest and fluids would be sufficient. We have also learned that the appendix is not a vestigial organ. Beneficial organisms retreat to the appendix when we suffer from an attack of dysentery and are known to repopulate the gut when the dysentery subsides. We can no longer consider the other species that reside in our bodies as enemies. We must recognize what remains beneath the surface and how the wild life living in our bodies helps us.[16]

Bell's Theorem

Cause-and-effect thinking, with its before, after, now, and later sequence, is no longer acceptable. According to Bell's Theorem, the whole determines the actions of the parts, and changes occur instantaneously.[7] Experience teaches us that not all people respond in the same way to the same treatment. Peptic ulcers, for example, were once considered the result of excessive production of stomach acid stemming from stress. Treatment was directed toward reducing the stress with rest and counteracting the acid with a special diet. Some patients recovered after

submitting to this regimen; others did not. Did those who recovered do so because of the treatment of diet and rest or did some other intervening factor bring about this change? Surely, for some, the enforced rest increased their stress and exacerbated the ulcer. We have since learned that peptic ulcers are associated with a common bacterium and may be healed with an antibiotic.

There is more than one way to promote healing. Even a fleeting thought can hasten or hinder recovery. Changes do not happen in an orderly, stepwise sequence. Healing is dependent on hope and belief. Beliefs, thoughts, and feelings are all part of the configuration, and each affects the human states of wellness and illness. Individuals have personal preferences for coping with adverse events. Miller classifies people as monitors and blunters.[17] Monitors need information to reduce their stress, whereas blunters prefer distraction. Explaining the details of upcoming surgery to a monitor can be expected to reduce stress and promote healing. Blunters prefer to trust in the skills of the caregiver and do not want to hear how that will be accomplished.

Personality and Wellness

Researchers have unsuccessfully tried to link specific illnesses with particular personality constellations. Yet, for example, individuals with peptic ulcers have as many personality configurations as does the general population. Kabat-Zinn found that healthy attention and meditation helped persons effectively cope with chronic illness and intractable pain.[18] Scientific studies of forgiveness have revealed that whenever people choose to forgive a transgression, areas in the emotional limbic center of the brain are activated.[19] The activity decreases when the person focuses on the unfairness of the situation but increases when the person imagines forgiving the offender. Multifaceted research studies on the relationship of forgiveness and health repeatedly show that forgiveness is good for our physical, mental, and emotional well-being.

There is increasing interest in the benefits of positive emotions on the immune system.[10, 11, 20] Studies suggest that transient positive mood states such as humor and joy are associated with an up-regulation of components of the innate immune system among healthy volunteers. Even though a direct cause-and-effect relationship between any personality factor and health or illness cannot be determined, research suggests that developing personality strengths to protect one from the stresses of living seems to bolster one's defense against illness.

Concern is often expressed that undue emphasis on competition and continuous exposure to violence in video games desensitize us and may provoke us to act violently. McGonigal reminds us that games that engage our imagination can also make us better and help us find solutions—for example, to environmental challenges—that affect our health.[21] Cooperative game play has more benefits than competitive games and offers us creative ways to manage complexity and change health care. Video games are now being used to help children understand and manage their asthma. The games help them to learn about triggers and to develop proper technique for using a controller inhaler. The free video application also helps children cope with stigma by providing a fun, normalizing virtual companion.[22]

Information Theory

Patterns of communication and patterns of organization in organisms can be viewed analogously.[13] Information Theory, a mathematical model, was developed to define and measure amounts of information transmitted through telegraph and telephone lines. The theory was used to explain how to code a message as a signal to determine what to charge customers. A coded message (signal) is essentially a pattern of organization. Information flow (i.e., pattern of communication and pattern of organization) in human beings is able to unify physiologic, psychological, sociological, and spiritual phenomena in a holistic framework. Information flow is the missing piece that makes it possible to transcend the body–mind split because information resides in both the body and the mind. Our emotions and feelings are sources of vital information. Emotions proper are life-regulating phenomena that help maintain our health

by making adaptive changes in our body states and form the basis for feelings. The information generated by these processes is designed to be protective and is more complex than reflexes.

Emotions and the Neural Tripwire

The traditional view in neuroscience has been that the sensory organs transmit signals to the thalamus and from there to the sensory process areas of the neocortex, which translates the signals into perceptions and attaches meanings. The signals then move to the limbic system, which sends the appropriate response to the body. This has all changed, however, with the discovery of a smaller bundle of neurons that leads directly from the thalamus to the amygdala—in addition to those that connect with the neocortex (see **Figure 10-1**). Sensory impulses go directly from the sensory organs to the amygdala, allowing for a faster response. The amygdala triggers an emotional response even before the person fully understands what is happening. Taking immediate action, the amygdala sends impulses through the brain to the body. If the stimulus is traumatic, the amygdala responds with extra strength. Key changes take place in the locus ceruleus, which regulates catecholamines; adrenaline and noradrenaline are released. Other limbic structures, such as the hippocampus and the hypothalamus, respond, and the main stress hormones bring about the typical body responses labeled *fight, flight, faint,* or *freeze.* Changes in the brain opioid system that secretes endorphins prepare the person to meet the danger. Meanwhile, the neocortex processes the impulse and a more considered response follows. Emotions are not dispensable but rather an integral part of the whole.

State-Dependent Memory and Recall

What people learn depends on their mood or feelings at the time of the experience.[23] Feelings are integral to human living, not just an extravagance or an annoyance. The emotion-carrying molecules, or ligands, which accompany all human activity, bind to cellular receptors and

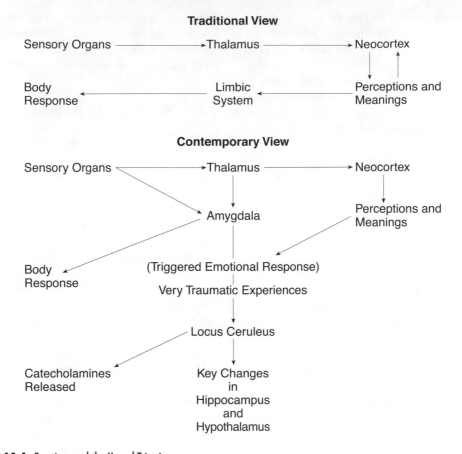

FIGURE 10-1 Emotions and the Neural Tripwire

Copyright © Genevieve Bartol.

send an informational message to the cell where they can be stored as memories.

Feelings and actions are intertwined. People are more likely to help others when they are in a good mood and more likely to hurt others when they are in a bad mood. Likewise, feelings and memories are intertwined. Thoughts that occur throughout daily routines are repeated patterns of memories and their associative emotional connections. Memories are accompanied by emotions that, in turn, are influenced and affected by the context in which they were acquired. A particularly traumatic experience is stamped in the memory with special strength. Subsequent stimuli in new situations and emotional experiences can attach to and reawaken past memories. These reactivated thoughts and emotions direct and shape our actions in the present.

Feelings or mood also play a major role in body–mind healing. Recent work with persons suffering from posttraumatic stress disorder has revealed that relearning is the route to healing. Writing therapy, bibliotherapy, bodywork, art therapy, and even the traditional talk therapies are all ways of releasing a picture frozen in the amygdala that is capable of triggering the fight, flight, freeze, or faint response provoked by seemingly benign stimuli. Because people have network responses with the systems that they contain and those within which they nest, healing can occur from multiple directions.[24]

Location of the Brain Centers

Brain function may be best understood using the model of a hologram. A hologram is a specially processed photographic record that provides a three-dimensional image when a light from a laser is beamed through it. If any part of the hologram should be destroyed, any one of the remaining parts is capable of reconstructing the whole image. This holographic model is congruent with the new understanding of the way in which information is transmitted, received, and stored.

- Memories are not stored in any specific part of the brain but rather in multiple overlapping areas. They can be retrieved in their entirety by a stimulus to more than one area of the brain. Loss of specific memory is related more to the amount of brain damage than to the site of the injury.
- The ability to recall what was lost when gunshot wounds injure the brain, for example, often returns. The brain has the ability to grow whole new neurons.
- Paranormal events, including the transpersonal healing associated with shamanism and other approaches to metaphysical healing, involve communicating information in ways that do not conform to the current understanding of receiving, processing, and sending energy.
- Phenomena such as phantom limb sensations and auras that extend beyond the corpus challenge traditional perceptions of body image, as well as the understanding of the physical boundaries of the body.
- Mechanisms of consciousness, such as the ability of the person to reflect on the self or create and retrieve images, cannot be explained simply in terms of the structure and function of current anatomic models. Experience can change brain structure.

Viewing the brain in a holographic manner reveals its influence on psychophysiologic functioning. People who believe that they do not have the conscious ability to effect a physical change with their imagination do not try to do so. They will not explore memories and patterns formed of past experience and will continue to respond unconsciously as they have in the past. Cognitive therapy is an example of an attempt to modify negative irrational thinking that leads to emotional distress. People are taught strategies that help them evaluate their thoughts, challenge them, and replace them with more rational responses, thereby enhancing health. Furthermore, the revolutionary discovery of the neuroplasticity of the brain is opening new worlds of possibility in human development.[25-27]

Neuroplasticity

It was once believed that the hardware of the brain was fixed and immutable. According to that belief, the brain virtually establishes all of its connections, such as the auditory cortex and the visual cortex, in the first years of life. Depictions of the specific areas and functions of the different parts of the brain were commonly accepted. If an area responsible for one function was injured, it was believed that no other area of the brain assumed its function.

Rehabilitation once focused on forgetting what function was lost and strengthening and compensating with whatever function remained intact. Current rehabilitation efforts are directed toward restoring those abilities. Now we acknowledge that the brain can respond to altered sensory inputs and reprogram itself to resume previous lost functions. Patients, for example, are instructed to move their unaffected arm while looking at the movement in a mirror, which has been found to stimulate movement in the affected arm. At other times, rehabilitation efforts are energized by restricting movement in the unaffected arm with the goal of prompting movement in the affected arm.

Our brain is being continuously rewired in keeping with the world of digital technology and the information revolution. The human brain changes throughout a person's lifetime. The changes are reflected in our new vocabulary. Consider such terms as *digital technology*, *cyberspace*, and *collective intelligence* and how they bring about neural rewiring. Reflect on how Facebook, LinkedIn, and Twitter are changing our communication patterns and making new neural connections in response to the intercultural world of the global society in which we live.[19, 20]

We now know that the immune system can affect the function of the central nervous system (CNS) and even alter cognitive processes. Low-grade chronic neuroinflammation of the microglia that occurs with normal aging may contribute to cognitive deficits. And we know that microglia also promotes regeneration after injury. Any effective treatment must reduce inflammatory activity while safeguarding the microglia's neuroprotective function. Attempts to identify a simple cause-and-effect relationship are not possible. Rather, efforts need to be directed toward discovering factors that reduce neuroinflammation while protecting normal microglia activity in the aging brain. Simple cause-and-effect remedies are not feasible.[20]

Epigenetics

Our genes are not fixed; we are not simply genetically determined. Our genes are modulated by our inner environment—the emotional, chemical, mental, energetic, and spiritual landscape—as well as our outer environment—the social and ecological systems in which we reside. Genes may be activated or deactivated by the meaning we assign to an experience. Truly we are formed and molded by the thoughts that stimulate the formation of neural pathways that either reinforce old patterns or initiate new ones.

The process by which a gene produces a result in the body is well established. Signals pass through the cell membrane to the nucleus, enter the chromosome, and activate a specific strand of DNA. Each strand of DNA is protected by a protein. The protein serves as a barrier between the information contained in the DNA and the rest of the intracellular environment. As long as the DNA is wrapped by the protein, the DNA lies dormant. When a signal arrives, the protein around the DNA unwraps and, with the assistance of RNA, the DNA molecule replicates an intermediate template molecule. At this point, the targeted gene moves into active expression where it creates other actions within the cell by constructing, assembling, or altering products. What was dormant potential is moved into active expression by a signal that comes from outside the cell and not from the DNA. This process may take 1 second or hours.[27-29]

According to McClelland and colleagues, epigenetic mechanisms program gene expression.[27] Key neuronal genes are modified by early life experience and govern learning and memory throughout life. Enriched postnatal experience enhances spatial learning, whereas chronic early life stress may result in persistent deficits in the structure and function of hippocampal neurons. Graff and coauthors note that epigenetic mechanisms are an integral part of a multitude of brain functions, including basic neuronal functions and higher-order cognitive processes.[28] Wright discusses the role of stress in the development of asthma.[29] Evidence suggests that maternal stress influences programming of integrated physiologic systems in the offspring beginning in pregnancy, indicating that stress effects may be transgenerational. Biological, psychological, and social processes clearly interact throughout life to influence the expression of strengths as well as disorders. De Sevo annotates 16 websites for readers who would like additional timely, reliable, genetic, and genomic information.[30]

Mind Modulation

Indirect and direct anatomic and biochemical pathways connect the neuroendocrine, nervous, and immune regulatory systems.[31] Communication among these systems is multidirectional with signal molecules and their receptors regulating the cellular outcomes. Feedback loops, up-regulation, and down-regulation of hormones and receptors function to protect the body.

Stress Response

The stress response is designed to protect against threats to well-being. Threats may be physical, social, psychosocial, real, and/or simply perceived. Biochemical functions of the major organ systems are modulated by the mind.[32] Thoughts and feelings are transduced into chemicals (i.e., neurotransmitters, neurohormones, and peptides) that circulate throughout the body and convey messages to various systems within the body. The stress response illustrates the way in which various systems cooperate to protect an individual from harm.

> A young man is walking to his car alone late at night when a stranger grabs his arm. His immediate response

is one of fear, and his body primes him to manage the danger by preparing him physically. The locus ceruleus (LC), with nerve endings in the forebrain, instantaneously secretes norepinephrine directly into the cortex. At the same time, the sympathetic nervous system (SNS) fibers also extend into the adrenal medulla, stimulating medulla secretion of norepinephrine. The young man's body is now full of norepinephrine, and he feels the effects. Muscular tension results from neural messages and stimulation of the SNS to prepare him for physical challenges. All of this happens even before he is fully aware of any danger.

Quickly, the young man registers what is happening. The hypothalamus secretes corticotropin-releasing factor (CRF) into the hypothalamic-pituitary circulation in the brain. Within approximately 15 seconds, CRF triggers the release of the pituitary hormone adrenocorticotropic hormone. In a matter of minutes, the adrenal cortex releases glucocorticoids. Hypothalamic, pituitary, and adrenal neuropeptides and other substances interact with the immune response, completing the multidirectional circle of communication among the nervous, endocrine, and immune systems. The young man has now experienced a full-blown psychophysiologic stress reaction to the fear of being hurt.

Physiologically, the cascade of changes associated with the stress response manifests as increased heart and respiratory rates, tightened muscles, increased metabolic rate, and a general sense of foreboding, fear, nervousness, irritability, and negative mood. Other physiologic responses include elevated blood pressure, dilated pupils, stronger cardiac contractions, and increased levels of blood glucose, serum cholesterol, circulating free fatty acids, and triglycerides. Although these responses prepare a person for short-term stress, they can lead to structure changes and clinical illness if prolonged. The memory of this experience is stored in the brain and other body cells and has psychological effects. The individual may reexperience the stress reaction in future similar events with less intense stress, such as having a friend brush against his arm as they walk toward the car. Indeed, just thinking about this experience can initiate a stress response. **Table 10-1** contains a review of the effects of sympathetic and parasympathetic stimulation.

When the stress has been dealt with or is no longer a threat, the body returns to its normal, homeostatic state. However, when one experiences a traumatic threat or the threat becomes chronic, the normal stress response is altered, resulting in the traumatic stress response (TSR). Severe traumatic threats range from childhood abuse to a near-death automobile accident while a chronic ongoing threat or stress could be related to caregiving for an elderly spouse with Alzheimer's disease or tense working conditions. Initiation of the stress response that is short lived does not lead to adverse health results, whereas severe and/or long-term chronic stress can lead to adverse health events.[33]

Homeostasis, the body's steady state, is maintained through ongoing changes in response to physical and environmental challenges. Allostasis is the process used to maintain homeostasis and well-being.[34] The general adaptation syndrome, the nonspecific physiologic stress response, is part of allostasis. The number of demands requiring adaptation determines the allostatic load. When an individual experiences overwhelming stress or has inadequate coping skills to deal with the stress, allostatic overload occurs and can lead to structural changes in the body and illness.

Long-term and unremitting stress can influence cardiovascular disease and gastrointestinal problems and lead to depression, drug problems, and accidents. The long-term presence of high levels of cortisol over an extended period of time promotes lipolysis in the extremities and lipogenesis in the face and back, suppresses the inflammatory process, increases the risk of osteoporosis and ulcers, and leads to atrophy of immune system organs. Levels of various reproductive hormones (e.g., progesterone, estrogen,

TABLE 10-1 Effects of Sympathetic and Parasympathetic Stimulation		
Structure	**Sympathetic Stimulation**	**Parasympathetic Stimulation**
Pupil of eye	Dilates	Contracts
Ciliary muscle	Relaxes, accommodates for distance vision	Contracts for close-up vision
Bronchial tubes	Dilates	Constricts
Heart	Accelerates and strengthens actions	Depresses and slows actions
Stomach muscles	Depresses activity	Increases activity
Glands	Alters secretion	Increases secretion
Liver	Stimulates glycogenolysis	
Visceral muscles of the intestine	Depresses peristalsis	Increases peristalsis
Adrenal medulla	Causes secretion of epinephrine	
Sweat glands	Increases activity	Decreases activity
Coronary arteries	Dilates	Constricts
Abdominal and pelvic viscera	Constricts	
Peripheral blood vessels	Constricts	
External genitalia	Constricts blood vessels	Dilates, causing erections

Source: Copyright © Genevieve Bartol.

and testosterone), growth and thyroid hormones, and insulin decline during stress, likely to conserve energy.[35]

The stress response is modulated by disposition, personality, and coping skills. Psychological stressors stimulate a physiologic response and are referred to as a reactive response. Students may have a reactive response when taking an examination. Anticipatory stressors can also elicit the stress response. For example, children who have been abused by a parent may experience a physiologic response when the parent comes near.[35] Perceived stressors begin in the areas of the brain that control cognition and emotions, the cerebral cortex and the limbic system. Quite simply, there are individual differences in hormonal, neuroendocrine, and immunologic responses to stress.[32, 36]

Three major body systems are involved with the stress response and operate in symphony-like ways to protect the body from harm: the nervous system, the endocrine system, and the immune system.

Nervous System

The brain is the cognitive center. It is here that memories are stored, ideas generated, and emotions expressed.[37] Emotions that affect the body originate in the brain; the brain, then, has a powerful influence over the body and is also the link to emotions and the immune system. The interconnectedness of the CNS means that frontal cortex thoughts and images are in intimate communication with the emotion-related limbic center. As the biochemicals transduced from thoughts circulate through the limbic-hypothalamic system, memory cells from past experiences affect their structure. The hypothalamus, the central control center, coordinates the biochemical cascade, integrating neuroendocrine functions by secreting both releasing and inhibiting hormones, as well as stimulating the SNS.[38] The SNS branch of the autonomic nervous system (ANS) is connected to the limbic system, has fibers extending into the adrenal medulla, and includes a pathway of nerves to the thymus, lymph nodes, spleen, and bone marrow. Hence, the connections are not only biochemical but also anatomic. The SNS, with preganglionic fibers that terminate in the adrenal medulla, stimulate the secretion of epinephrine (80%) and norepinephrine (20%) that begin the physiologic stress response and result in increased heart and respiratory rates, elevated blood pressure, and increased blood to skeletal muscle. The effects of epinephrine occur within seconds.[37, 39]

Integration of the stress response occurs in the CNS. Communication is dependent on neuronal pathways among the cerebral cortex, limbic system, thalamus, hypothalamus, pituitary gland, and reticular activating system (RAS).[32] The focus of the cerebral cortex is on cognition, focused attention, and vigilance. The limbic system is the emotional center focused on feelings such as rage, anger, and fear. This system elicits an endocrine response indirectly via stimulation of neural pathways for sensory information and stimulates a central response by direct stimulation of the LC. The thalamus is the relay station. It is in the thalamus that sensory data are sorted and distributed. The hypothalamus is the coordinator of the endocrine and the ANS. The RAS is the modulator of ANS activity, skeletal muscle tone, and mental alertness. The LC, located in the brain stem, has afferent pathways connecting the hypothalamus, hippocampus, limbic systems, and cerebral cortex; it is rich with norepinephrine-producing cells, integrating the ANS response. The entire process is not only complex but also not completely clear.

Understanding the psychophysiologic stress response as it affects the nervous system helps to clarify how the different holistic therapies work. It is possible to interrupt feelings of anxiety by using a relaxation technique to calm the self or a cognitive restructuring technique to change thought patterns. When patients learn to use relaxation, imagery, music therapy, or certain types of meditation, their sympathetic response to stress decreases and the calming effect of the parasympathetic system takes over, leading to body–mind healing. Biofeedback can reduce arousal and tension, and it is so effective that it has become a common intervention for many conditions induced or exacerbated by uncontrolled stimulation of the stress

response. To illustrate, warming the fingers by using biofeedback decreases the discomfort that accompanies Raynaud's disease. Changes in physiology change thoughts and feelings; changes in thoughts and feelings, conversely, change physiology. Of course, it is also possible for misuse to occur—for example, meditation to block the normal sympathetic response that our bodies use to protect us from harm.

Medications are used to treat conditions, such as panic attacks, that consist of a hyper reaction of the SNS. Beta blockers, for example, block the alpha adrenergic receptors, producing lower heart rate and blood pressure. Patients who are taking beta blockers may not exhibit the normal reactions to threat. Older people often have decreased psychophysiologic stress responses because their reactions to SNS stimulation are blunted. Medications may be required with panic attacks, but they may have troublesome side effects. At the same time, the use of mind–body interventions often reduces or eliminates the need for medication.

Endocrine System

The nervous and endocrine systems are so closely connected and interactive that they are referred to as the neuroendocrine system. The specific organs of the endocrine system and the stress response are the pituitary and adrenal glands. Hormones, secreted by the endocrine glands, are the specialized chemical messengers that act to modulate both cellular and systemic responses. They are always present in body fluids, but their concentrations vary. They produce both localized and generalized effects. Furthermore, one hormone can stimulate a variety of effects in different tissues, and a single function may be subject to regulation by more than one hormone. Hormones include amines and amino acids (e.g., norepinephrine, epinephrine, dopamine), peptides, polypeptides, proteins, and steroids.[40]

Each cell has a multitude of receptor molecules that can be modified or altered. Hormones act by binding to their specific receptor on target cell surfaces. Treatment with methadone is effective for heroin addicts, for example, because the methadone binds to the opioid receptor sites. A decrease in hormone levels can increase the number of receptor sites available. This is *up-regulation*. Conversely, an elevated hormone level leads to a decrease in receptors, or *down-regulation*.[40] Also, many of the hormones have a negative feedback loop that maintains the balance in serum hormonal levels. Stimuli such as circadian rhythms, the environment, and emotional and physical stressors influence the secretion of hypothalamic hormones.

The major endocrine hormones in the stress response are epinephrine from the adrenal medulla and glucocorticoids from the adrenal cortex (see next section). Other hormones associated with the stress response include pituitary hormones (growth hormone, prolactin, estrogen, and testosterone). Growth hormone (GH) and prolactin are secreted by the anterior pituitary during stress. The GH affects metabolism of carbohydrates, protein, and lipids. Estrogen may attenuate the hypothalamus-pituitary-adrenal (HPA) axis effects because women tend to respond more to stressors with a greater HPA axis stress response. Decreased testosterone levels occur in men during stressful experiences. The opioids (i.e., endorphins, enkephalins) are synthesized in the pituitary and other parts of the CNS. Opioids have a morphine-like effect with receptors throughout the body. These naturally occurring hormones produce the "runner's high," increase a person's pain threshold, and explain how people can "ignore" their own serious injury to save a loved one. The endorphins are secreted by immune cells during stress, leading to analgesia.[39]

Corticotropin-Releasing Factor

A peptide and neurotransmitter, CRF is part of the neuroendocrine stress response. The CRF is found in the brain stem, hypothalamus, limbic systems, and extra-hypothalamic structures. When released from the hypothalamus, CRF leads to pituitary secretion of adrenocorticotropic hormone (ACTH). The ACTH induces the secretion of glucocorticoid hormones from the adrenal cortex. Cortisone helps to mediate the stress response and has several physiologic outcomes.[38] There is a sympathetic nervous system connection to the blood vessels supplying the immune cells, thereby creating a direct nervous system and immune system pathway.[38]

Cortisol produces similar effects as those of epinephrine, but the effects last from minutes to days. To explain, epinephrine is secreted quickly during the alarm stage and cortisol is secreted for the long term during the resistant and exhaustion stages. Cortisol stimulates gluconeogenesis, increasing blood glucose levels and resulting in protein breakdown. This breakdown leads to loss of muscle, negative nitrogen balance, increased gastrointestinal secretion, and suppression of the immune system.[39]

Immune System

The immune, endocrine, and nervous systems communicate with hormones, neuropeptides, neurotransmitters, and products of immune cells. This communication is bidirectional. Anatomically, the nervous system has direct connections to immune system organs (thymus, bone marrow, lymph nodes, and spleen). Likewise, immune system cells produce messengers that signal the nervous system. There are receptors on the immune system cells for the neurotransmitters such as the opioid peptides, dopamine, catecholamines, and ACTH. The nervous system has direct sympathetic innervation of immune system blood vessels. The SNS pathways of norepinephrine and epinephrine secretion and the HPA axis with glucocorticoid secretion have direct effects on immune system cells. Glucocorticoids suppress the immune system. Cortisol, for example, suppresses white blood cells, and it is even administered to suppress the immune system in people with autoimmune diseases.[37]

Recent findings indicate that CNS and ANS neuropeptides and endocrine hormones stimulated by the nervous system directly affect immune system cells. Receptor sites located on the surface of the T and B lymphocytes have the ability to activate, direct, and modify immune function. For example, CRF suppresses monocytic macrophages and T helper lymphocytes. Lymphocytes produce the stress hormone ACTH and the brain peptide endorphin.[38] Endorphins have both enhancing and suppressing effects on immune system cells, depending on their concentration. They may elevate active T cells, whereas too many endorphins may suppress the immune system.[37, 39] In turn, cytokines—that is, secretions of immune system cells—affect the nervous and endocrine systems.

Interventions to reduce the stress response can have a positive effect on the immune system. Interventions that induce the parasympathetic response have healing effects on the body. Because all systems are interconnected, holistic interventions contribute to health and healing. It is important to remember that there are individual differences in immunologic reactivity, hormonal responses, and autonomic responses to stress.[27] Nakata conducted a review of bibliographic databases (PubMed, PsychINFO, Web of Science, Medline) to identify current knowledge about the possible association between psychosocial job stress and immune parameters in blood, saliva, and urine. Using the snowball method, Nakata found 56 studies that showed high job demands, low job control, high job strain, job dissatisfaction, high effort–reward imbalance, overcommitment, burnout, unemployment, organizational downsizing, and economic recession had a measurable effect on immune parameters (reduced NK cell activity, NK and T cell subsets, CD4+/CD9+ ratio, and increased inflammatory markers). Clearly, the evidence supports that psychosocial job stresses are related to disrupted immune responses.[11] How can these responses that are generated by psychosocial job stress be effectively mitigated? What can be done to help persons effectively manage this stress while finding appropriate solutions to the situations that provoke the stress? Simply reducing or eliminating the stress with medication is not without problems. Earlier observations questioned if child abuse was sometimes increased when a parent was taking a tranquilizer, supposedly because there was a concomitant decrease in concern for the consequences of such behavior. The question remains: Would the same concern apply to other interventions that promote a relaxation response?

Neuropeptides

With their receptors, neuropeptides help further explain body–mind interconnections and the way that emotions are experienced in the body. Circulating throughout the body, neuropeptides are considered the messengers that connect body and mind. The first neuropeptides were discovered in the intestine, which has many receptors; this may help explain those "gut feelings." Neuropeptides can be exchanged and produced by most all body tissues and even from inflammatory cells.[27]

The limbic system and hippocampus are rich with neuropeptide receptors, containing almost all of them and connecting emotions and learning. The concept of emotions as neuropeptides explains why people have trouble remembering and learning when they are experiencing stress. Performance, too, is affected. Those who experience severe anxiety before speaking in public often benefit from relaxation techniques and cognitive restructuring.

Emotions cannot be ignored. Nurses who attend only to the body are not providing holistic care. Interventions to support and enhance coping offer another opportunity to promote healing and wholeness. We are increasingly faced with the challenges of complexity. Persons with heart failure, a major and costly public health concern with high hospitalization and mortality rates, also experience disproportionately high rates of depression. Jimenez and Mills are using neuroimmunologic principals to study how neurohormonal and cytokine activation link these comorbid disorders. Simple cause-and-effect explanations are no longer sufficient.[11] The exploration of the extensive interactions among psychological and behavioral factors, the nervous system, the immune system, the endocrine system, and the environment should help us understand the mechanisms underlying health, wellness, and diseases. Evidence already exists that supports the relationship between unmanaged stress, depression, and inflammation with disorders such as cardiovascular disease, skin diseases, obesity, diabetes, arthritis, and Alzheimer's disease.[14]

Conclusion

New scientific understandings of living systems, such as principles of self-organization and mind modulation of the body–mind systems, provide a theoretical base for holistic healing interventions. Understanding the physiologic principles that are involved in nursing interventions helps nurses design individualized and appropriate holistic care for clients. Nurses, aware of their own wounds and sensitive to the wounds of clients, are strategically placed to lead clients in facilitating health and healing. Walking the talk is about being authentic and congruent, allowing nurses to relate to patients in authentic and congruent ways. Caring for oneself is essential for nurses to model wholeness. Nurses who do not care for themselves are unable to provide holistic care for their patients. The process of becoming authentic makes one sensitive to the needs of others. Modeling is, perhaps, the strongest teaching strategy.

Patients are increasingly knowledgeable about complementary and alternative interventions and have incorporated them with positive results. New scientific information invalidates the idea of the dualism of mind and body. Thoughts, emotions, and consciousness do not reside solely in the brain but are present in various body parts—the brain, the glands, and the immune, enteric, and sexual systems.

The research data overwhelmingly document the body–mind interrelationships. Nurses must continue to incorporate wholeness into their own lives while exploring effective ways to deliver holistically oriented care to their clients. The meaning of the illness, the method of giving the diagnosis, the tone of voice and the touch of the nurse, and the relationships to family and friends are all important. As nurses, we must always be aware of that on which we focus and what we tend to ignore.[41]

Directions for Future Research

1. Develop instruments that accurately measure psychophysiologic responses for particular holistic nursing interventions.
2. Explore the effectiveness of holistic interventions in preventing illness and promoting health.
3. Investigate the effects of holistic nursing practice on nurses.
4. Carry out longitudinal studies to examine the effects of the regular use of holistic nursing interventions.

Nurse Healer Reflections

After reading this chapter, the nurse healer will be able to answer or to begin a process of answering the following questions:

- Do I attend to my own body–mind communication?
- Do I provide time for reflection?
- How do I heighten my awareness of who I am?

NOTES

1. S. K. Leddy, *Integrative Health Promotion: Conceptual Bases for Nursing Practice* (Sudbury, MA: Jones & Bartlett, 2006).
2. L. Dossey, "The Unsolved Mystery of Healing," *Shift: At the Frontiers of Consciousness* (December 2004–February 2005): 25–26.
3. D. Lindley, *Uncertainty: Einstein, Heisenberg, Bohr, and the Struggle for the Soul of Science* (New York: Doubleday, 2007).
4. B. Haisch, "Freeing the Scientific Imagination," *IONS Noetic Science Review* (September–November 2001): 24–29.
5. M. A. Boyd, *Psychiatric Nursing: Contemporary Practice*, 5th ed. (Philadelphia: Lippincott Williams & Wilkins, 2011).
6. L. von Bertalanffy, *General Systems Theory* (New York: George Braziller, 1968).
7. E. Laszlo, *The Systems View of the World: A Holistic Vision of Our Time* (Cresskill, NJ: Hampton Press, 2012).
8. M. C. Porth, *Essentials of Pathophysiology Concepts of Altered Health States*, 3rd ed. (Philadelphia: Lippincott Williams & Wilkins, 2012).
9. J. Stone, *Minding the Bedside: Nursing from the Heart of the Awakened Mind* (Minneapolis, MN: Lagdon Street Press, 2011).
10. R. Ader, ed., *Psychoneuroimmunology*, 4th ed. (New York: Elsevier, 2007).
11. Q. Yan, *Psychoneuroimmunology: Methods and Protocols* (New York: Humana Press, 2012).
12. I. Prigogine, *The End of Certainty* (New York: The Free Press, 1997).
13. F. Capra, *The Web of Life* (New York: Doubleday, 1996).
14. A. W. Davidson, A. Ray, and M. C. Turkel, eds., *Nursing, Caring, and Complexity Science: For Human-Environment Well Being* (New York: Springer, 2011).
15. Y. Bar-Yam, "Foreword," in *Nursing, Caring, and Complexity Science: For Human-Environment Well*

Being, eds. A. W. Davidson, A. Ray, and M. C. Turkel (New York: Springer, 2011): xix–xx.

16. R. Dunn, *The Wild Life of Our Bodies: Predators, Parasites and Partners That Shape Who We Are Today* (New York: HarperCollins, 2011).

17. G. M. Bartol, "Creating a Healing Environment," *Seminars in Perioperative Nursing* 92, no. 7 (1998): 90–95.

18. J. Kabat-Zinn, *Coming to Our Senses* (New York: Hyperion, 2006).

19. V. Simac, "The Challenge of Forgiveness," *Shift: At the Frontiers of Consciousness* no. 13, (December 2006–February 2007): 29–33.

20. K. J. Karren, B. Q. Hafen, N. L. Smith, and K. J. Frandsen, *Mind/Body Health: The Effects of Attitudes, Emotions and Relationships*, 3rd ed. (New York: Pearson, 2006): 251–271.

21. J. McGonigal, *Reality Is Broken: Why Games Make Us Better and How They Can Change the World* (New York: Penguin Books, 2011).

22. National Institutes of Health, "What Is Asthma?" (August 4, 2014). www.nhibinihgovhealth /healthtopics/topics/asthma/.

23. D. Goleman, *Emotional Intelligence*, 10th anniversary ed. (New York: Bantam Books, 2006).

24. N. C. Frisch and L. E. Frisch, *Psychiatric Mental Health Nursing*, 4th ed. (New York: Delmar, 2011).

25. B. Rabin, "Stress: A System of the Whole," in *Psychoneuroimmunology*, 4th ed., Vol. II, ed. R. Ader (New York: Elsevier, 2007): 709–722.

26. S. Begley, *Train Your Mind, Change Your Brain* (New York: Ballantine Books, 2006).

27. S. McClelland, A. Korosi, J. Cope, A. Ivy, and T. Z. Baram, "Emerging Roles of Epigenetic Mechanisms in the Enduring Effects of Early-Life Stress and Experience on Learning and Memory," *Neurobiology of Learning and Memory* 96, no. 1 (2011): 79–88.

28. J. Graff, D. Kim, M. M. Dobbin, and L. H. Tsai, "Epigenetic Regulation of Gene Expression in Physiological and Pathological Brain Processes," *Psychological Reviews* 91, no. 2 (2011): 603–649.

29. R. J. Wright, "Epidemiology of Stress and Asthma: From Constricting Communities and Fragile Families to Epigenetics," *Immunology and Allergy Clinics of North America* 31, no. 1 (2011): 19–39.

30. M. R. De Sevo, "Genetics and Genomics Resources for Nurses," *Journal of Nursing Education* 49, no. 8 (2010): 470–474.

31. M. C. Porth, *Essentials of Pathophysiology: Concepts of Altered Health States*, 4th ed. (Philadelphia: Lippincott Williams & Wilkins, 2010).

32. R. Ader, "Integrative Summary: On the Clinical Relevance of Psychoneuroimmunology," in *Human Psychoneuroimmunology*, eds. K. Vedhara and M. Irwin (Oxford, UK: Oxford University Press, 2005): 343–350.

33. J. R. Piazza, D. M. Almeida, N. O. Dmitrieve, and L. C. Klein, "Frontiers in the Use of Biomarkers of Health in Research on Stress and Aging," *Journal of Gerontology Series B: Psychological Sciences and Social Sciences* 65B (2010): 513–525.

34. R. J. Emerson, "Homeostasis and Adaptive Responses to Stressors," in *Pathophysiology*, 4th ed., eds. L.-E. C. Copstead and J. L. Banasik (St. Louis, MO: Saunders Elsevier, 2010): 14–27.

35. K. R. Wilson, D. J. Hansen, and M. Li, "The Traumatic Stress Response in Child Maltreatment and Resultant Neuropsychological Effects," *Aggression and Violent Behavior* 16, no. 2 (2010): 87–97.

36. K. L. McCance, B. A. Forshee, and J. Shelby, "Stress and Disease," in *Pathophysiology: The Biologic Basis for Disease in Adults and Children*, 5th ed., eds. K. L. McCance and S. E. Huether (St. Louis, MO: Mosby Elsevier, 2006): 51–57.

37. K. J. Karren, B. Q. Hafen, N. L. Smith, and K. J. Frandsen, *Mind/Body Health: The Effects of Attitudes, Emotions, and Relationships*, 5th ed. (Boston: Pearson, 2013).

38. M. C. Porth, *Essentials of Pathophysiology: Concepts of Altered Health States*, 4th ed. (Philadelphia: Lippincott Williams & Wilkins, 2010).

39. L. D. Oakley, "Stress, Adaptation, and Coping," in *Pathophysiology*, 3rd ed., eds. L.-E. C. Copstead and J. L. Banasik (St. Louis, MO: Saunders Elsevier, 2005): 24–45.

40. S. E. Huether, "Mechanisms of Hormonal Regulation," in *Pathophysiology: The Biologic Basis for Disease in Adults and Children*, 5th ed., eds. K. L. McCance and S. E. Huether (St. Louis, MO: Mosby Elsevier, 2006): 121–124.

41. B. S. Barnum, *Spirituality in Nursing: The Challenges of Complexity*, 3rd ed. (New York: Springer, 2011).

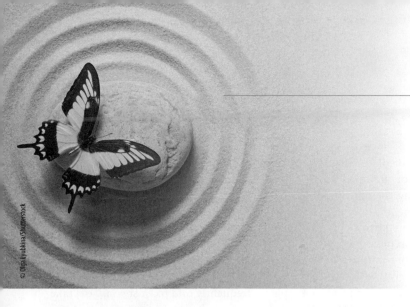

© Olga Lyubkina/Shutterstock

Nurse Healer Objectives

Theoretical

- Define the terms *relaxation* and *self-regulation*.
- Compare and contrast different relaxation exercises.
- List the body-mind-spirit changes that accompany profound relaxation.

Clinical

- Describe three different types of relaxation exercises and their appropriate clinical application.
- Describe the indications and contraindications for two forms of relaxation and/or meditation practices.
- Identify technology or equipment commonly used in your nursing practice, and describe how it can be integrated as a biofeedback instrument.
- Use breathing strategies with a client, and record the subjective and clinical changes that occur with relaxed breathing.

Personal

- Pick one or a combination of relaxation and/or meditation practices and use it as daily self-care practice for a month. See what changes you experience, and experiment with applying your practice to a stressful moment.

- Explore ways that your chosen relaxation and/or meditation practices support your well-being and your ability to respond to and transform stress.
- Identify through focused awareness the areas in your body where you most often accumulate tension.
- Identify three personally meaningful therapeutic suggestions, and use them as reminders to support your self-care relaxation practice and well-being.

Definitions

Autogenic training: Developed by Drs. Johannes Schultz and Wolfgang Luthein 1932, this practice teaches relaxation through the repetition of phrases that influence muscle relaxation by bringing an awareness of sensations and feelings of warmth, heaviness, and relaxation to one's body.

Biofeedback: The use of technology or monitors that augment and feed back usually imperceptible signals from the person's psychophysiologic processes for the purpose of cultivating the ability to influence or change stress-related patterns or symptoms. This self-regulation process, developed in the 1960s, is usually paired with a relaxation practice. Combined, they offer the person an opportunity to be an active participant in his or her own healing and health maintenance.

Hypnosis: A process for focused awareness and expanded consciousness with diminishing perception of peripheral sensations, thoughts, and feelings.

Mantra: A word, short phrase, or prayer that is repeated either silently or aloud as a focus of concentration during the practice of meditation.

Meditation: Originally based in spiritual traditions, the practice of awareness, focus, and concentration while maintaining a passive yet awake attitude; evolves with discipline and practice and is known to provide health benefits as well as being a road to personal and spiritual transformation.

Pain (medical definition): Localized sensation of hurt, or an unpleasant sensory and emotional experience associated with actual or potential tissue damage, or described in terms of such damage.

Pain (nursing definition): A subjective experience including both verbal and nonverbal behavior.

Power: Barrett's theory of Power as Knowing Participation in Change is being aware of what one is choosing to do, feeling free to do it, and doing it intentionally.

Progressive muscle relaxation (PMR): Originally developed by Edmund Jacobson in 1934, it is now found in both its original and modified forms; the process of alternately tensing and relaxing muscle groups to become aware of subtle degrees of tension and relaxation.

Relaxation (psychophysiologic definition): A psychophysiologic experience characterized by parasympathetic dominance involving multiple visceral and somatic systems; the absence of physical, mental, and emotional tension; the opposite of Canon's fight-or-flight response and Selye's general adaptation syndrome.

Relaxation response: An alert, hypokinetic process of decreased sympathetic nervous system arousal that may be achieved in many ways, including through breathing exercises, relaxation and imagery exercises, biofeedback, and prayer. A degree of discipline is required to evoke this response, which increases mental and physical well-being.

Self-hypnosis: An approach for voluntarily fostering a consciousness process for the purpose of influencing one's thoughts, perceptions, behaviors, or sensations.

Stress (psychophysiologic definition): The felt experience of overactivity of the sympathetic nervous system. Stress-related illnesses account for 75% to 80% of illness in modern life.

Theory and Research

People are frequently told to "just relax" or "take it easy" as part of their recovery from illness, as if everyone knew how to practice this skill. Yet the ancients knew that relaxation is a paradox: It is and is not simple. Throughout the ages, in cultures around the world, practitioners of the sacred healing arts and sciences developed and practiced stopping, quieting, and calming on a disciplined and regular basis, offering themselves deep rest to still the bodymindspirit and emotions. They did this not only to access their natural ability to heal, restore, and renew their bodymindspirit but also to open themselves to the divine, the oneness of being, the numinous. As the waves of the mind stilled and the activity of the body quieted into the deep rest and relaxation found within their meditative refuge and relaxation practice, this oneness of being offered itself to these ancient spiritual voyagers.

Today, we continue this voyage to touch shores beyond our unhealthy habit patterns and belief systems through the practice of the ancient arts of relaxation, meditation, yoga, qi gong, and breathing, as well as their modern counterparts: autogenic training, progressive muscle relaxation, hypnosis, biofeedback, self-regulation, relaxation response, and body scanning.

We now understand relaxation to be an ancient art with many modern interpretations, which have been anchored throughout nursing practice from childbirth education to pre- and postoperative teaching. (See the relaxation definitions at the beginning of this chapter.) Relaxation interventions are useful for people in all stages of health and illness: the critically ill, expectant parents attending childbirth preparation classes, taxi drivers learning to regulate blood pressure while weaving through city traf-fic, and nursing students dealing with test anxi-ety. Even in the acute phase of recovery from a myocardial infarction or during an examination in an emergency room after an accident, clients can derive the clinical benefits of relaxation by learning basic breathing and muscle relaxation exercises (see **Exhibit 11-1**).

Over the past four decades, nurses in all areas of practice can be found who offer relaxation and breathing techniques and some form of meditation to their clients. Yet this is not new to nursing. Florence Nightingale counseled her nurses to support patients' rest and well-being by reducing unnecessary noise, not awakening patients out of their first sleep, and protecting patients from unnecessary disturbances such as conversations of doctors or friends within ear-shot and the disturbing rustling of crinolines. She advised in *Notes on Nursing* that "all hurry or bustle is peculiarly painful to the sick."[1] One wonders what Nightingale would say if she were to visit hospitals and healthcare settings today and witness our efforts to follow her legacy in the chaos of our times.

These days, nurses offer relaxation prac-tices in self-care circles for themselves and their colleagues, as well as for clients in hos-pitals, community and adult education pro-grams, outpatient clinics, and homeless shelters, to promote a variety of personal benefits (see **Exhibit 11-2**). Nurses also offer these practices to individuals, families, groups, children in classrooms, clients and families in home care and hospice, and workers and executives in workplaces and corporations.

Cross-Cultural Context

Relaxation practices are found throughout time in all cultures around the world. Whether these practices are mediated through the use of herbs, acupuncture, movement, or prayer, evidence of the power, influence, and impor-tance of relaxation and the use of breath can be seen in shamanic healing, yoga, meditation, Chinese medicine, and other traditions around the globe. Modern research exploring the area of psychoneuroimmunology demonstrates the vital importance of relaxation in improving immune system function. Thus, psychoneuro-immunologic research suggests the importance of this ancient practice for our modern scien-tific world (see Chapter 10 for further informa-tion). Modern psychology uses relaxation as a dimension of systematic desensitization, in which clients learn to relax in the face of mild, then moderate, and then intense stressors. Neuroplasticity research demonstrates that the structure and function of the brain, originally believed to be fixed, is much more changeable and is influenced by relaxation practices such

---

EXHIBIT 11-1   Clinical Benefits of Relaxation

Relaxation training has the following clinical benefits:

- Decreases the anxiety accompanying painful situations, such as debridement or dressing changes
- Eases the muscle tension pain of skeletal muscle contractions
- Decreases fatigue by interrupting the fight-or-flight response
- Provides a period of rest as beneficial as a nap
- Helps the client fall asleep quickly
- Increases the effect of pain medications
- Increases the ability to tolerate pain

EXHIBIT 11-2   Whole-Self Benefits of Relaxation

Relaxation has the following benefits to self:

- Decreases pain
- Decreases anxiety
- Improves immune system function
- Quiets the fight-or-flight sympathetic response
- Facilitates sleep
- Provides rest
- Increases efficacy of pain medications
- Reduces muscle tension and increases blood flow
- Improves sense of well-being
- Offers insight and creativity

as mindfulness practice. This new field demonstrates that cultivating the mind also changes or grows the brain. Practitioners of biofeedback include relaxation practice with their therapy to help clients learn to self-regulate their peripheral temperature, heart rate velocity, muscle activity, and brain-wave frequencies.

Jon Kabat-Zinn, in his original research at the University of Massachusetts, found relaxation breathing and body scanning to be a vital dimension of a mindfulness-based stress-reduction practice used for dealing with pain and depression.[2] Dean Ornish includes relaxation, meditation, breathing, and yoga in his pioneering cardiac rehabilitation program to reverse heart disease.[3] Dolores Krieger and Dora Kunz guided nurses to perform sustained centering and presencing, a practice of meditative inner connection and relaxed awareness, before entering into Therapeutic Touch practice with their clients.[4,5] These modern pioneers all continue to validate the importance of the ancient practice of relaxation through the use of its modern counterparts.

Caring for Ourselves, Caring for Others: A Spiritual Journey

These challenging times of constant change and global uncertainty require nurses to walk a wellness path of self-care, self-healing, and spiritual awareness. Finding and then cultivating a personal relaxation practice can help nurses restore and renew, deepen professional self-development, and avoid burnout, as well as model a personal wellness path for their clients. Living this path and sharing by example give nurses an inner understanding and appreciation of the benefits and challenges their clients face as they start to integrate complementary practice into their everyday lives.

Whether individuals are being with themselves and with "all that is" in meditation; exploring their own past issues, traumas, or painful life experiences in counseling and psychotherapy; or expanding their awareness in intuitive practices and energy healing, a foundation of deep relaxation of the bodymindspirit is a fundamental step on the path (see **Exhibit 11-3**).

The American psyche, poised to do everything with intensity and competitiveness, also enters with us into self-healing and spiritual practices. This intensity and competitiveness can be our undoing, especially if we forget the importance to our bodymindspirit of nondoing, which is different from "doing nothing." Achaan Chah offers us guidance in his wise insight on letting go, peace, and nondoing.[6]

> *Do everything with a mind that lets go,*
> *Do not expect any praise or reward.*
> *If you let go a little, you will have a little peace.*
> *If you let go a lot, you will have a lot of peace.*
> *If you let go completely, you will know complete peace and freedom.*
> *Your struggles with the world will have come to an end.*

Reproduced from J. Levey and M. Levey, *The Fine Arts of Relaxation, Concentration, and Meditation: Ancient Skills for Modern Minds* (Somerville, MA: Wisdom Publications, 2003).

Nurses must reclaim their legacy of caring by cultivating their compassion, wisdom, spirit of

---

EXHIBIT 11-3 Benefits of Relaxation for the Nurse and Holistic Nursing Practice

Relaxation:

- Is an essential element of self-care
- Cultivates a centered, calm presence
- As a self-care practice offers insights into the challenges and benefits that clients will experience
- Offers a vehicle to modulate and self-regulate the nurse's own stress response in stress-filled work settings
- Supports a therapeutic, energetic bond and connectedness when practicing along with clients or colleagues
- Creates opportunity for intuitive exploration, insight, and understanding of self and others, issues, and problems
- Is an excellent vehicle for beginning professional gatherings and staff meetings; offers the opportunity to be present, creative, open, and connected
- Can be done anywhere, without any cost or equipment; is easily teachable and easily practiced
- Can be a spiritual practice for opening ourselves to deeper ways of being

service, and heart-centered health care in their culture. Relaxation is a first step along this path.

The Stress Response

The last decade has brought new awareness to what constitutes an emergency response, both for individuals and for society. Whether we are dealing with a national or international tragedy or disaster or the everyday intense internal reactions we experience when faced with a truck cutting in front of us on the highway, a "code blue" coming over the loudspeaker, or a child darting into the street, we experience what some researchers refer to as an adrenaline rush, the familiar fight-or-flight response. This response is a complex series of psychophysiologic processes that prepare us to deal with the real or perceived emergency. It is important to note that people respond to an imagined threat in the same way that they respond to an actual threat to their well-being. That is why in times of personal threat, such as facing a possible health crisis or the fear of potential terrorism, relaxation practices help us keep balanced or self-regulated.

The following are the generalized stress responses of the body, mind, and energy field:

- Constriction of blood flow to the hands and feet (cool extremities)
- Tightening of the muscles
- Constriction of one's energy field (closing down or blocking flow)
- Increased heart rate
- Increased oxygen consumption
- Increased brain-wave activity
- Increased sweat gland activity
- Increased blood pressure
- Increased anxiety

This stress response readies the bodymindspirit through this instinctive response pattern to prepare for a stress, shock, or trauma. In modern life, the body physically alerts or readies itself far beyond what is needed to deal with a fast-paced, stressful life. Most people know how to turn on this stress response but have little familiarity with how to relax or turn it off. Not only do people not know how to relax, but our society typically has a negative view of relaxed people. The paradox is that masters of ancient practices have learned that, although instinctive responses such as fight or flight can put one on alert to help provide protection in an emergency or a crisis, a more conscious relaxation discipline, practice, and philosophy offers deeper possibilities.

Meditation

Relaxation Response Meditation

This "relaxation response" is a phrase attributed to Herbert Benson and his colleagues at Harvard University, who used a nonreligious form of meditation similar to transcendental meditation to produce the opposite of the fight-or-flight response. Their relaxation response meditation has been applied in a variety of healthcare settings and studies, demonstrating its efficacy in treating hypertension and anxiety. Both transcendental meditation and relaxation response meditation offer a practice consisting of 20 minutes of daily passive concentration focused on a neutral word, such as the Sanskrit word *Om* in transcendental meditation or *one* in relaxation response meditation. In relaxation response meditation, slow repetition of the word with each exhalation has been shown to bring about the same psychophysiologic responses as other deep relaxation processes. Further studies have documented a deep relaxation response when the client focuses on a short, personally meaningful religious statement or quotation, as was found in what Benson termed the *faith factor*.

The changes that occur when an individual reaches a deep level of relaxation are exactly the opposite of those that occur in the fight-or-flight response. Alterations take place in the autonomic, endocrine, immune, and neuropeptide systems as follows:

Deep relaxation increases:
- Peripheral blood flow (warm extremities)
- Electrical resistance of skin (dry palms)
- Production of slow alpha waves
- Activity of natural killer cells (improved immune function)

Deep relaxation decreases:

- Oxygen consumption
- Carbon dioxide elimination
- Blood lactate levels
- Respiratory rate and volume
- Heart rate
- Skeletal muscle tension
- Epinephrine level
- Gastric acidity and motility
- Sweat gland activity
- Blood pressure, especially in hypertensive individuals

The holistic nurse may wish to explore and experience each of the relaxation practices presented in this chapter and write her or his insights and experiences in a journal.

Breathing In and Breathing Out

Conscious awareness of breathing—whether the slow, deep, diaphragmatic breaths of hatha yoga or the mindful awareness of breathing in and out in mindfulness meditation—can be practiced in formal sessions of 20 to 45 minutes once or twice a day. Conscious awareness of breathing also can be practiced informally by breathing with mindfulness during everyday activities.

Jon Kabat-Zinn developed a mindfulness-based stress-reduction program that demonstrates how conscious awareness of breathing can help to relieve chronic pain, depression, and anxiety. Participants in the 8-week program practice mindfulness meditation every day; they also practice body scanning (systematically bringing attention to each part of the body, letting the attention rest there, letting go of any judgment about how it is "supposed to feel," being with this part of the body, and then moving on to the next place in the body) and yoga (performance of meditative asanas or postures combined with breathing to create a union of body, mind, and spirit). Several studies in clinics, communities, and prisons have demonstrated that Kabat-Zinn's program, as well as other modern forms of meditation, can improve quality of life and reduce symptoms.[7–10]

Breathing and Energy Healing Practice

Breathing practice is also an integral dimension of yoga and qi gong. The breath or life force, called *prana* in yoga and *qi* (or *chi* or *ki*) in Chinese energy practice, is the vital force or energy that animates life. Nurses practicing Therapeutic Touch center themselves through conscious meditation on their intention to help or to heal by letting go of outside distractions and by opening themselves to allow the universal life force to flow through them to their clients. They can use their breathing practice to help enhance this sustained centeredness and their openness to this healing life force.

Qi gong practices date back to about 5000 BC. Taoist and Buddhist qi gong masters channeled the flow of qi from nature and the universe through their bodies by practicing simple movements combined with an awareness of breathing and meditation. These ancient Chinese practices, which are one of the dimensions of Traditional Chinese Medicine, have long been renowned for producing health benefits and slowing the aging process. These effects are now being researched and documented in scientific literature (see **Table 11-1**).[12–15]

Other Forms of Meditation

Some say that hundreds of practices can be listed under the heading of meditation. Each practice cultivates a qualitative state of mind that can induce a deep experience of relaxation and calm. In some meditative practices, such as transcendental meditation and relaxation response meditation, the individual focuses on an object of meditation to move away from and minimize thoughts. Other traditions, such as mindfulness meditation, insight meditation, and vipassana meditation, invite practitioners to cultivate greater focus by returning to the breath as sensations, thoughts, and feelings are present.

Centering prayer, a Christian meditation practice developed by Father Thomas Keating, focuses on words or sounds in somewhat the same way that transcendental meditation uses

TABLE 11-1   Research-Based Outcomes of Meditation

Practice	Modern Forms	Adapted by	Clinical Benefits	Researcher
Meditation	Mindfulness, insight meditation, vispassana		See the list of deep relaxation changes in the Relaxation Response Meditation section.	
	Transcendental meditation	Maharashi Mahesh Yogi	Reduced the risk of African American mortality, heart attack, and stroke.	Schneider, Grim, Rainforth, Kotchen, Nidich, Gaylord-King, Salerno, et al. (2012)[7]
	Relaxation response meditation	Herbert Benson (1975)	Decreased hypertension.	Benson, Alexander, and Feldman (1974)[8]
	Mindfulness-based stress reduction	Jon Kabat-Zinn (1977)	Decreased chronic pain.	Kabat-Zinn, Lipworth, Burncy, and Sellers (1987)[9]
			Significant pain reduction for chronic arthritis, back and neck pain; less pain reduction for headache, migraine.	Rosenzweig, Greeson, Reibel, Green, Jasser, and Beasley (2010)[10]
			Reduction in test anxiety and more focused attention in nursing students.	Moriconi and Stabler-Haas (2011)[11]
Prayer	Loving kindness meditation		Self-compassion reduced sympathetic and cardiac parasympathetic anxiety.	Arch, Brown, Dean, Landy, Brown, and Laudenslager (2014)[12]
	Self-compassion practice		Loving kindness meditation over time "increases mindfulness, purpose in life, social support, decreased illness symptoms."[13, p. 1045]	Fredrickson, Cohn, Coffey, Pek, and Finkel (2008)[13]
Moving meditation	Yoga, meditation, stress reduction, nutrition, lifestyle	Dean Ornish	Reversal of heart disease.	Ornish (1990)[3]
	Yoga		Improved back function in chronic/recurrent low back pain.	Tilbrook, Cox, Hewitt, Kang'ombe, Chuang, Jayakody, Aplin, et al. (2011)[14]
	Qi gong, chi kung		Decreased physical pain and emotional distress; improved sleep, concentration, and decision making.	Coleman (2011)[15]
	Therapeutic Touch			Krieger (1993)[4]

mantras (sacred Sanskrit syllables and words such as *Om*).[16] Other meditation practices invite meditators to gaze at the flame of a candle, a sacred image, or a mandala; to chant aloud; or to concentrate on a nondual or unanswerable question (or koan), as in Zen practice.

The purpose of spiritually focused meditation is to awaken to a higher consciousness, to be at one with the sacredness of "All," and to become one with the Divine. Individuals practice such meditation to open the bodymind-spirit to the qualities of compassion, wisdom, forgiveness, skillfulness, no fear, stillness, openness, and interconnectedness. The Center for Contemplative Mind in Society provides a comprehensive list of practices.[17]

Reflect on the following: What would health care be like if nurses, physicians, and other healthcare practitioners began by cultivating a heart of compassion and service? What would the healthcare system be like? Would burnout exist? (See the section on Loving Kindness Meditation later in this chapter.)

Mindful Breathing During Nursing Practice

Nurses who wish to be more present with their clients, to practice self-care, and to awaken to the simple sacredness of everyday nursing practice (e.g., hanging an intravenous bag, writing nursing notes, eating, walking down a hall, feeding a patient) may want to practice mindful breathing each moment, as in the following exercises.

EXERCISE: BREATHING I

Script: Breathing in, I am aware of breathing in. Breathing out, I am aware of breathing out.

Breathing in, I am aware of introducing this healing medication through this intravenous line.

Breathing out, I send my healing intentions along with the medication to help support this patient's healing.

EXERCISE: BREATHING II

Script: Breathing in, I am walking down this hall.

Breathing out, I smile, enjoying my steps.

Breathing in, I am fresh.
Breathing out, I celebrate my aliveness.

Begin with the breath, reminding oneself that to offer self-care in each moment by consciously breathing with each activity is a gift of self-renewal, freshness, and aliveness that deepens with practice. It is a gift nurses can give to themselves every moment.

The Pause

At the Compassionate Care Initiative at the University of Virginia (UVA), Dr. Dorrie Fontaine, along with the UVA nurses and doctors, integrate the self-care practices of yoga, meditation, journaling, and specially developed mindfulness practices for the most challenging of circumstances in hospital life. After the death of a patient, caregivers pause together in silence for 45 seconds to 2 minutes to recenter, reflect, and be, honoring both the human life that has just changed forms and the human care that was offered instead of throwing down their gloves and running to the next emergency.[18]

Mindful Breathing Meditations

Exploring and practicing relaxation and meditation help the nurse gain insight into specific methods and issues that clients may face as they work to integrate these techniques into their daily lives. When choosing a meditation practice to explore, the nurse should commit to that practice for at least 4 to 6 weeks before trying another, while keeping a journal of his or her reflections along the way.

EXERCISE

Mindfulness of the Breath Exercise (Sitting)

In a quiet place, find a comfortable seated position. Either sit on a chair with your feet on the floor and your back supported and straight, or sit on the floor using a meditation cushion (zafu) or a regular pillow folded in half to create a supportive lift under your buttocks. If you are sitting on the floor, find a comfortable way to place your legs, either crossed in lotus or half-lotus position with or without pillows under your knees, Indian style, or straight out in front of you, with a pillow under your knees and your back supported against a reclining support or against the wall. Focus on a point on the floor in front of you and gently lower your eyelids until they are almost closed. Gently bring your attention to your breath.

Script: Breathing in, I am aware of breathing in. Breathing out, I am aware of breathing out.
In.
Out.
Breathing in, I am calm.
Breathing out, I smile.[19]

— *Thich Nhat Hanh*

*Reproduced from T. Nhat Hanh, The Blooming of a Lotus: Guided Meditation Exercises for Healing and Transformation (Boston, MA: Beacon Press, 1993): 17.

Continue to bring your attention to your breath, allowing any thoughts, feelings, or sensations to be gently held by your mindful awareness, as you gently bring your attention back to the breath and the repeated phrase. Practice for approximately 15 to 20 minutes. After your practice, note your experience in your journal.

This practice is an example of using meditation to become aware of our minds and to practice just being, being present in this moment, and nondoing rather than "doing nothing." We get so caught up in believing that we always have to be doing or multitasking that we lose the essence of what is of true value. Mindfulness helps us to get back in touch with what is truly healing within and around us.

As you continue, you may want to note Kabat-Zinn's attitudinal foundations of mindfulness practice, which include nonjudging, patience, trust, nonstriving, the cultivated freshness of seeing everything as new (called *beginner's mind*), acceptance, and letting go.[2]

Walking Meditation

Walking as if one were planting peace with each step—this is the essence of walking meditation.[20] This practice can be especially helpful during times of trauma and crisis and can be done to center oneself in the most challenging and traumatic of circumstances.

To practice, start with the left foot and begin walking slowly by synchronizing the in and out of the breathing meditation practice with each step. Sometimes you may take three steps to the inhale and three steps to the exhale. Play with your practice, exploring how carefully you can become aware of the subtle sensations of slowly lifting, moving, and placing each step as you continue your awareness of breathing.

This practice can be interspersed between sitting practice sessions: 20 minutes of sitting, 10 minutes of walking, 20 minutes of sitting, 10 minutes of walking. This also is a wonderful meditation to practice at a more normal pace of walking at work, as well as going to and from work. "Walking down the hall, I am aware of my footsteps and my breathing. Being in this present moment, I know this is the only moment." Practicing walking meditation often allows the practice to be in our bones so that it is there for us when we need it most.

Cultivating the Heart of Compassion Meditation

Loving Kindness Meditation

This meditation for helping professionals is adapted from Thich Nhat Hanh's loving kindness meditation in *Teachings on Love*.[21] (Also see Kristin Neff's self-compassion practice, which includes the three elements of self-kindness, connecting to our common humanity, and mindfulness,[22] and HeartMath's quick coherence technique at www.heartmath.com/personal-use/quick-coherence-technique.html).

Sitting peacefully, begin as in sitting meditation practice, and then plant each phrase like a healing seed within your heart, following your breath and focusing on your intention to cultivate compassion. Say each line to yourself in your mind, or ask a friend to read this meditation aloud to you, pausing after each line so that you can slowly repeat it silently to yourself. This practice is offered in both the short and long forms.

Part I: May I be peaceful.
May I be happy.
May I be safe.
May I be well.
May I be free.

In Part II of this meditation, repeat the same meditation while imagining that someone you care about or are having difficulty with is sitting in front of you, and center your attention on cultivating and offering compassion while repeating silently in your mind:

> *Part II:* May you be peaceful.
> May you be happy.
> May you be safe.
> May you be well.
> May you be free.

Then, in Part III, imagine offering compassion to all beings on Earth, to the Earth, to all the planets, and to all beings throughout the universe and beyond time and space:

> *Part III:* May all beings be peaceful.
> May all beings be happy.
> May all beings be safe.
> May all beings be well.
> May all beings be free.

For other heart-opening meditations, see the St. Francis prayer and www.Beliefnet.com.

Quiet Heart Prayer

One of the most frequently used traditional nursing spiritual therapies is prayer. Prayer is a way of eliciting the relaxation response in the context of one's deeply held personal, religious, or philosophic beliefs. Benson refers to this as incorporating the "faith factor" into relaxation.[23] Many people are comfortable with prayer as meditation, and it requires only seconds to minutes. In healthcare settings nurses must accommodate the client's spiritual needs, either by calling on his or her personal spiritual and religious background and resources or by enlisting the help of clergy, chaplaincy staff, or the client's family.

Modern Relaxation Methods

Progressive Muscle Relaxation

The body responds to anxious thoughts and stressful events with increased muscle tension; this body-mind-spirit tension further provokes subjective sensations of anxiety. In 1935, Edmund Jacobson detailed a strategy leading to deep muscle relaxation. In progressive muscle relaxation (PMR), the practitioner deliberately tenses muscle groups, focusing on the tightening

sensations, and then slowly releases that tension. In this way, the individual learns to manage levels of muscle tension. The PMR allows the client to deepen the experience of comfort.

Several studies have demonstrated that PMR reduces subjective feelings of anxiety and increases peak expiratory flow rates in asthmatic clients; it also helps clients with insomnia, headaches, ulcers, hypertension, and colitis (see **Table 11-2**).[24-27]

In the original form of PMR, clients learn to relax 16 of the body's muscle groups. They inhale while tensing their muscles and then exhale and relax their muscles very slowly. Variations on PMR, or modified PMR, are integrated into many relaxation practices.

EXERCISE

Progressive Muscle Relaxation Tension Awareness

The purpose of a tension awareness exercise is to help the client identify subtle levels of mental tension and anxiety and the physical tension that accompanies these mental and emotional states. The client who is aware of the internal differences induced by this exercise can move to threshold levels of tension, holding just enough tightness in the muscle group to be aware of beginning tension and then relaxing the group. By moving from strong contractions to very subtle ones, the client becomes aware of the ability to fine-tune the relaxation process.

The PMR exercise requires 10 to 30 minutes depending on how many areas of the body you include. If the client is experiencing pain or difficulty with a particular part of the body, the exercise should begin as far away from the involved area as possible and conclude with the primary area of difficulty. Clients should be coached to breathe throughout the session, thereby avoiding the temptation to hold their breath as they tighten their muscles. Clients may learn to exhale as they tighten muscle groups. Tension in muscles should be held short of true discomfort.

The PMR is particularly effective for clients who are feeling physically tense, anxious, and perhaps agitated. Because it is an active intervention, it may be preferable to other passive exercises, especially early in client training. It should be used with caution in certain clients (e.g., those with ischemic myocardial disease, hypertension, and back pain).

TABLE 11-2 Research-Based Outcomes of Relaxation

Modern Form of Relaxation Practice	Developed by	Clinical Benefits	Researcher
Progressive muscle relaxation (PMR)	Jacobson	Immunocompetence in geriatric population: Those practicing PMR demonstrated better immunocompetence (increased natural killer cell count and herpes antibodies) and decreased stress.	Keicolt-Glaser, Glaser, Williger, Stout, Messick, Sheppard, Ricker, et al. (1985)[24]
		Reduced pain and fatigue in hospitalized cancer patients receiving radiation therapy.	Pathak, Mahal, Kohli, and Nimbran (2013)[25]
PMR, loving kindness meditation (LKM), and mindfulness		Mindfulness helps reduce reactivity to repetitive thoughts more than LKM or PMR.	Feldman, Greeson, and Senville (2010)[26]
PMR and voice characteristics of therapist		Study supports that speaking in a "smooth and quiet, perhaps even monotonous, but not purposely hypnotic"[27, p. 75] tone while pacing the therapist's voice rhythm with the patient's breathing positively effects therapeutic PMR training.	Knowlton and Larkin (2006)[27]
Autogenic training	Schultz and Luthe	Reduced muscle tone, blood pressure, and skin resistance.	Schultz and Luthe (1959)[28]
		Generalized improvement in irritable bowel syndrome.	Shinozaki, Kanazawa, Kano, Endo, Nakaya, Hongo, and Fukudo (2010)[29]
Autogenic training, biofeedback therapy		Reduced idiopathic essential hypertension.	Fahrion (1991)[30]
Biofeedback		Heart rate variability biofeedback plus treatment as usual improved combat-related posttraumatic stress disorder symptoms in veterans.	Tan, Dao, Farmer, Sutherland, and Gevirtz (2011)[31]
		Biofeedback reduced pain and improved mobility and recovery in rehabilitation patients.	Giggins, Persson, and Caulfield (2013)[32]
Biofeedback-assisted relaxation therapy (BART)		Two sessions of heart rate variability and skin temperature using BART resulted in higher reduction of pain and enhanced mood in pain plus anxiety versus only pain or only anxiety in pediatric patients (>8).	McKenna and Gallagher (2014)[33]
		Autogenic training combined with biofeedback skin temperature and pulse reduced physiologic measures of stress response for test anxiety in nursing students.	Prato and Yucha (2013)[34]

Autogenic Training

In 1932, Johannes Schultz and his student, Wolfgang Luthe, developed a series of brief phrases called *autogenic* because of their ability to assist a person in inducing self- (auto) change from within.[28] Although similar to self-hypnosis, autogenic strategies are a specific present-time-oriented means of gaining access to the natural restorative mechanisms of the mind. Autogenic training has been found to be effective in managing disorders in which cognitive involvement is prominent.[29] These self-healing phrases can be combined with PMR as an integrative approach to relaxation to help a broader spectrum of clients. Autogenic training is one of the most widely used approaches in teaching clients to warm their hands during bio-feedback temperature training.[30-34] Table 11-2 includes examples of research-based outcomes of relaxation.

Autogenic training should begin in a warm (75°F to 80°F) room to facilitate sensations of warmth. Clients can progress to cooler environments to generalize their training (to simulate being outside). Using the phrases while the mind is relaxed and receptive allows the peripheral circulation to increase and cardiac and respiratory rates and rhythms to slow and stabilize. Several weeks may be required for the client to feel sensations of heaviness and warmth, although the client usually achieves restful heart rate and respiratory patterning much sooner.

Effects of Relaxation Therapies

Practitioners involved in stress reduction, relaxation training, and biofeedback have questioned whether all of the various techniques elicit a single relaxation response, as hypothesized by Herbert Benson in 1975, or whether specific practices render specific effects. The latter view proposes that specific cognitive effects are produced by the use of cognitively oriented methods (see the section on Autogenic Training earlier in this chapter), autonomic effects are produced by autonomically oriented methods, and muscular effects are produced by muscularly oriented methods (see the section on Progressive Muscle Relaxation earlier in this chapter). **Table 11-3** provides an overview of the hypothesized effects of relaxation techniques.[35-39]

Holistic Nurse Learning Experiment I

One of the most effective tools for understanding relaxation is self-exploration and self-experimentation. Within herself or himself, the nurse is a minilaboratory able to explore these various methods and conduct her or his own inner research. All that is needed is a journal and the commitment to inner exploration and personal and professional self-development.

TABLE 11-3 Hypothesized Effects of Relaxation Techniques		
Relaxation Technique	**Hypothesized Effect**	**Researcher**
Progressive muscle relaxation (PMR)	Modified PMR might be expected to develop muscular skill.	Davidson and Schwartz (1976)[35]
Autogenic training (AT)	AT might generate both cognitive and somatic effects because it emphasizes body awareness through repeated self-suggestion.	Linden (1993)[36]
AT versus PMR	AT is particularly effective in cultivating specific sensations, as indicated in the self-suggestion statements, and has much greater effects in that realm than does PMR.	Lehrer, Atthowe, and Weber (1980)[37] Shapiro and Lehrer(1980)[38]
Relaxation response meditation	The relaxation response elicited is hypothesized to be universal (all relaxation techniques are considered equivalent).	Benson (1975)[39]

A commitment must be made to practice the method for at least 4 to 8 weeks to explore beyond initial positive or negative reactions. Practice each day, following your script or recording of the practice, and keep a journal of your awareness observations (e.g., how you felt in your body before and after the session, any areas of comfort or discomfort you noted before or after the session, and other observations). After practicing, exploring, and journaling about your selected practice, you may want to explore another practice in a similar fashion and compare and contrast their effects.

Another method of exploration is to invite others to join you in experimenting with the same practice or different ones. Holding periodic group meetings to review your observations and your inner laboratory journals can help you to explore variations in experiences with the same practice and compare and contrast differences in and preferences for various practices.

Selecting Relaxation Interventions for Clients

No formula exists for determining which relaxation intervention is best for which client. The approach must be tailored to the individual based on his or her condition, personal preferences, and available time. Some clients may initially resist the idea of relaxation practice in spite of the nurse's best efforts to present it in a positive manner. In this situation, the issue need not be forced, for the client may accept the intervention at a later time. Taking some time to explore the client's experience and the source of the resistance may reveal misconceptions or myths that further dialogue can dispel. Recall your list of descriptors of a relaxed person from the beginning of this chapter and its implications for motivation and client participation.

Online resources, applications, and relaxation CDs and DVDs present relaxation in a nonthreatening, gentle manner. Often accompanied by soothing music (and images), this format can be offered over hospital closed-circuit television, downloaded onto clients' electronic devices, iPods, or MP3 players, from the Internet, or become part of a nursing comfort cart on each floor. The use of such media may hasten acceptance of this intervention. Relaxation CDs/downloads can also be played on the home or business audio system as a gentle background for daily activities. The following are guidelines for the client in the use of relaxation audio or videos:

1. Listen to an exercise at least once (preferably twice) a day.
2. Never listen to a relaxation exercise when you are driving or operating a vehicle.
3. Arrange to have uninterrupted privacy while you listen to the practice.
4. Listen with headphones or earbuds to help block out distracting noises from the environment.
5. Listen or watch in a relaxing position in which your body is supported.

Hypnosis and Self-Hypnosis

Most people misunderstand the use of trance and hypnosis and associate it with stage professionals and entertainment. However, hypnosis and trance have been used for healing and therapeutic purposes from the times of ancient Egypt and Greece.

Hypnosis has been defined in many ways. Nursing expert Dorothy Larkin describes hypnosis as "a process of therapeutic communication, awareness, and behavior within the context of a therapeutic relationship."[40] In hypnosis, attention can be more focused or more mobile, and there is a tendency for greater responsiveness to suggestion. Once the visual, behavioral, and thinking processes and cues associated with hypnosis are understood, they may be seen to occur spontaneously under avariety of circumstances. According to David Cheeks, an expert in the study of trance and hypnosis, "Hypnotic states may occur when people are frightened, disoriented in space, unconscious, very ill, or stammering."[41, p. 140] These are experiences that nurses' patients and clients contend with every day, and thus most nurses first encounter their patients and clients in an already altered process of hypersuggestibility. This naturally occurring trance opens up the client to the influence of nurses' therapeutic presence and therapeutic suggestions.

Recall Cheeks's description of the hypnotic trance of frightened and ill patients, and consider how clients and patients are given the news of their diagnosis and prognosis by their physicians while they are in that state of fear and hypersuggestibility. Many patients today still are told that they have only a few months to live or that nothing can be done for them. This nontherapeutic suggestion is being instilled in a patient's consciousness in a suggestible moment by one of his or her most trusted authorities, the physician. What outcome could be expected? How might the process differ if the client were offered more positive therapeutic suggestions?

Nursing experts have been interested in exploring and integrating hypnosis, trance, and therapeutic suggestions because of the history of hypnosis in healing throughout the cultures of the world, because of its natural availability through client hypersuggestibility during healthcare crises, and because of its ease of use and practicality.[42] Larkin and many other nurse experts in hypnosis have explored ways in which therapeutic suggestion can enhance patient cooperation and comfort.[43] Nurses can recognize a hypnotic experience in clients who have a faraway stare, glazed eyes, or fixed attention. Larkin notes that nurses can utilize this receptive state by offering therapeutic suggestion, reassurance, and health-promoting education. Continual assessment will need to be observed so that, if the subject's attention suddenly shifts, the nurse can concurrently change the offered therapeutic strategy to meet the patient's needs and altered perceptions.[43]

Learning how to use therapeutic suggestion is not foreign to nurses who have used health education to focus clients on healing and health-promoting phrases to help them reframe their experiences. Integrating therapeutic suggestions into our conversations with patients is called *conversational induction*. These can be most helpful in situations of great crisis or trauma when the patient's capacity for other forms of relaxation may be impeded. "The therapeutic use of suggestions, interspersed in daily conversations with patients, can highly augment their sense of comfort and participation in their healing process."[44, p. 380] Learning how to use this skill during usual nursing care embeds it deeply into

our awareness so that it can be easily accessed in times of crisis or trauma.

Therapeutic suggestion is also a vital accompaniment in disbursing medication. For example, the nurse might say, "This medication will help to quiet your nervous system so that you can relax more comfortably into sleep" rather than "This pill is for your insomnia." The former emphasizes the possible comfort response, and the latter focuses on the problem. Suggestion and hypnosis have been used in a wide variety of clinical settings. Hypnosis has been used by nurses in hospice care, palliative care, home care, and critical care, as well as in burn units and oncology, obstetrics, medicine, and surgery units, to name only a few areas.

All nurses can learn to use reframing, conversational inductions, and positive therapeutic suggestion, and to recognize an everyday hypnotic trance process of clients in crisis (see the section on Cryptotrauma later in this chapter). In addition to teaching clients this practice, nurses can also practice self-hypnosis and therapeutic suggestion as part of their personal self-care so that they can continue self-care at home.

Biofeedback

Educating clients about how their bodies respond to stress in the moment, in real time, and teaching them how to react more healthfully is the work of biofeedback. When any device monitoring unitary bodymindspirit is turned so that it acts as a mirror for clients to see its display, and when this information is combined with awareness practices so clients can make therapeutic changes, biofeedback is being practiced.

Recall what has just been explored with regard to therapeutic hypnotic suggestion and reframing, and imagine how this new knowledge and awareness might be used to empower clients as they encounter the monitors and other technical equipment in the healthcare setting. If you can imagine turning the monitors around and teaching clients the positive meaning of the monitors' signals so that they can understand how their bodies respond to thoughts and feelings, then you have already begun to understand the effect and usefulness of biofeedback. With practice, clients can tune their inner awareness to become like the yogis and learn to influence and control these previously imperceptible and seemingly uncontrollable signals.

The most widely used biofeedback monitors include temperature-sensing units for measuring vasodilatation of extremities, electromyographs for monitoring motor neuron activity of the muscles, electroencephalographs for measuring brain-wave frequencies and patterns, and electrodermal response units for measuring electrical activation of the sweat glands. Heart rate variability monitors and blood pressure monitors also are widely used in biofeedback. **Exhibit 11-4** presents the clinical indicators for the use of biofeedback.

Holistic Nurse Learning Experiment II

Biofeedback can offer nurses the opportunity for independent professional practice, whether in private practice or in an institutional setting. Many nurses integrate biofeedback into relaxation therapy, stress management, health counseling, and teaching. Other nurses specialize in neurofeedback for the care of insomnia, depression, addictions, and attention deficit hyperactivity disorder. Another area of particular interest to nurses is heart rate variability, as well as the use of electromyography to help clients manage urinary and fecal incontinence (see **Table 11-4**). All of these areas of specialization require extensive study, practice, and mentoring. However, every nurse can benefit from using simple biofeedback principles and techniques in everyday nursing practice.

Learning to understand these biofeedback principles from the inside out is the purpose of simple biofeedback experiments. One or two psychophysiologic monitors, paper, and a pen are required. Any monitors available—pulse oximetry, blood pressure, heart rate, incentive spirometer—can be used, or an inexpensive temperature-sensing unit can be purchased through resources found at the Association for Applied Psychophysiology and Biofeedback (www.aapb.org). Examine **Exhibit 11-5** to determine whether any of these factors can help to explain your response.

EXHIBIT 11-4   Clinical Indicators for Biofeedback

Neuromuscular disorders
- Chronic muscle contraction
- Movement disorders
- Spasticity

Central nervous system disorders
- Stroke
- Some epilepsies

Vascular disorders
- Raynaud's disease
- Migraine

Pain
- Headache
- Back pain

Gastrointestinal and genitourinary disorders
- Urinary and fecal incontinence
- Urinary and fecal retention

Stress reduction
- Insomnia
- Anxiety
- Phobias
- Alcoholism and addiction
- Attention deficit hyperactivity disorder
- Procedure-related anxiety

Variation A: Client Practice

Try a biofeedback experiment on a client. Use an abbreviated form of the experiment (5 to 10 minutes), taking readings before and after relaxation practice. Explore and explain the meanings of the readings, and invite the client to describe what he or she felt inside and what he or she feels the readings mean. It is important to experiment with yourself first before trying this with a client, as your personal experiences from the inside out will help you understand, relate to, and support the process and the results.

Integrating biofeedback provides an opportunity for healthcare teaching and counseling to move from client compliance to client

---

EXHIBIT 11-5   Important Factors in Relaxation Practice

- *Passive volition.* Letting go, being without doing or striving, allowing, being with the process as it unfolds rather than making it happen; planting a seed in the mind of wanting to relax, and then letting go and watching the process.

- *Attention to the here and now.* Being oriented toward the present, not caught up in what happened or what might happen.

- *Altered perception of time.* Experiencing time as expanded or contracted. Relaxation practice can change the perception of time so that a very short practice session feels like a long time or a long practice session is experienced as a few moments.

- *Enjoyment of practice.* Committing to practice and, even more important, enjoying practice. Most traditional healers and teachers of the restorative arts ask their students if they are enjoying their practice. Finding a practice that helps one weather the storms of life and enhances one's inner connection is a joy.

---

empowerment. Teaching clients how anxiety, worry, and stress can produce higher blood pressure, cooler hands, and tenser muscles, and how relaxation can produce the opposite responses, is an easy way to begin a dialogue, providing clients with insight into the stressors of their lives and how they respond to them.

Variation B: Group Self-Care Experiment

Try relaxation or biofeedback in a group. Start with a group of colleagues rather than a group of clients. (You can begin to introduce this technique to a group of clients later as you gain experience and knowledge with the practice.) Schedule a relaxation break for your unit. Take 15 minutes at the beginning of a staff meeting, or schedule the relaxation practice during a lunch break every week or month.

Special issues for groups include, "I don't have time," "I'm too busy," and "I could be/should be catching up on my work, not relaxing." Sandy O'Brien and Jeanne Anselmo developed a staff wellness project using the practices described previously.[45] The answer they found to the challenge of "I don't have time to practice" is that we cannot afford not to take time to center ourselves and care for ourselves to do the best for our own health while offering the best of care to our clients and families.

Although relaxation practice does take time and commitment, most groups learn to avoid giving in to the work-and-hurry sickness and begin to enjoy the benefits of stopping, calming, and letting go. In fact, according to the Nurses' Health Study from Harvard, the more friends

and social ties nurses had, the less likely they were to develop physical ailments and the more joyous their lives were. Researchers from UCLA demonstrated that women's social ties reduce the risk of heart disease by lowering blood pressure, cholesterol, and heart rate.[46]

Cautions and Contraindications for Relaxation, Meditation, and Biofeedback

Medications

Clients who take insulin, thyroid replacement medication, antihypertensives, cardiac medications, antianxiety agents, and sleep medications must be monitored for a change in their symptoms and medication needs as they learn to deepen their relaxation response. As clients learn to regulate their stress response, their medication requirements may change. Work closely with clients' prescribing providers to ensure that their medications are titrated properly.

Education and Information

Discussing issues and experiences associated with relaxation before and after each session helps to involve clients, positively empower them, and reframe any of the anticipatory anxiety or questions they may have.

Mental Health History

Clients with a history of dissociative experiences, acute psychosis, borderline personality, and post-traumatic stress disorder (PTSD) are best cared for by nurses and professionals skilled in treating such clients. Check your client's mental health history before beginning relaxation practice.

Cryptotrauma

Many patients have experienced undiagnosed physical or psychological trauma. Many times patients are reluctant to disclose these problems, and many times health professionals are unskilled in or uncomfortable with exploring these issues. Domino and Haber report that 66% of women at a multidisciplinary pain center with chronic headaches had a prior history of physical or sexual abuse (61% had experienced physical abuse; 11%, sexual abuse; and 28%, both physical and sexual abuse).[47] The average duration of abuse was 8 years.

The term *cryptotrauma* indicates that the trauma that is the cause of the patient's pain is hidden or has not been revealed. Signals to watch for in clients with PTSD and/or cryptotrauma include the following:[47]

- Hypervigilance
- Difficulty falling or staying asleep
- Irritability or outbursts of rage
- Difficulty concentrating
- Exaggerated startle response
- Dissociation
- Addiction
- Flashbacks
- Numbing
- Panic attacks
- Disturbed self-perception, denigration
- Isolation
- Inability to be comfortable with touch
- Nightmares

Even with the most sensitive and careful history taking and preparations, clients with such disorders can have flashbacks related to the underlying trauma. If this occurs, first, do not panic. Remember your intention to help and support, and trust your therapeutic bond with the client. Second, center and ground yourself. Clients in a panic state related to anxiety or flashback are supersensitive to people around them; centering, calming, and grounding yourself will deeply help them. Third, reassure the client, speak to the client in a calm, soothing voice, and use therapeutic suggestions. Have the client open his or her eyes, feel his or her feet on the

floor, or touch the furniture; if possible, have the client tighten and release the hands and feet and be aware of the body and of being with you in the present. If appropriate, hold the client's hand; use your judgment. Fourth, remember that the information with which the client is getting in touch is important for the client's wholeness and healing. A simple, short statement explaining this to the client helps to reframe the situation and plant therapeutic suggestions during these most open and suggestible moments. Seek appropriate referrals for the client as needed.

PTSD, Cryptotrauma, and Working in Times of Trauma, Natural Disaster, or Major Crisis

Clients who suffer from cryptotrauma or who have sustained one or more major losses around the time of a disaster are at the greatest risk for developing PTSD. Nurses and other helping professionals who are aware of the previously mentioned symptoms for cryptotrauma could be the first line of assistance for assessing, recognizing, and helping a client, colleague, child, or even a neighbor or family member suffering from traumatic grief or PTSD after any major community trauma or crisis. In a time of tragedies, such as school shootings, soldiers and military families coping with their uncertainty or the return of traumatized or wounded soldiers from war, or environmental disasters such as hurricanes, earthquakes, floods, tornados, and tsunamis, understanding lessons learned from the lived experience of our colleagues in communities that have been affected can be a great service to all.

Though everyone grieves differently, and most people recover without much intervention, some will experience traumatic grief and PTSD and will need psychotherapy and medication. In a time of crisis or disaster, all members of the community are needed. Both spiritual and religious helpers and professionals and paraprofessionals are needed to help, and all must be trained to deal with the enormous needs of the community after a disaster.

Evolution of PTSD After a Community Crisis or Disaster

An important lesson professionals learned after disasters such as September 11 was that even while the rest of the city and country began to move on and feel better, symptoms of PTSD continued long after the event. This is because as others move on, those with PTSD actually get worse and feel even more isolated and out of synch with the rest of the community and country. The antithetical dimension of PTSD is that, left untreated, with time the symptoms do not get better but actually get worse.

Those people who suffer an additional loss around the time of a disaster (e.g., job loss, financial crisis, illness or death in the family) are four to five times more likely to develop PTSD than those who do not have any additional loss or trauma. Those who sustain multiple additional losses around the time of the disaster are 47 to 50 times more likely to develop PTSD.[48]

According to a study published in 2007 by Canadian researchers, those with PTSD are significantly more apt to have numerous health conditions including cardiovascular diseases, respiratory diseases, chronic pain, gastrointestinal illnesses, and cancer. Those with PTSD were also more prone to short- and long-term disability, poor quality of life, and suicide attempts.[49, p. 242] Understanding the significance of these data alerts us to the importance of recognizing PTSD in those we serve and getting those suffering from PTSD the appropriate mental, emotional, and physical help and support.

Our human community is learning that we live in a time in which major disaster can strike anywhere, whether rural or urban, and no place or group is immune from such tragedy. Most parts of the world have had to live with trauma and tragedy as part of their reality every day, but even the extraordinary preparedness of the Japanese people was deeply challenged in the face of multiple and concurrent disasters. Currently, North America is experiencing floods, hurricanes, forest fires, mudslides, major snow storms, and tornados on a unprecedented scale, yet this increase is but a small percentage of what others in the world have been challenged by for decades. With awareness, reflection, and insight, these experiences can open, enliven, and enlarge our hearts to experience our shared humanity and vulnerability and grow our understanding, compassion, wisdom, and interconnectedness as a human family living on this precious planet.

As holistic nursing leaders, we exercise true power when we open our awareness to recognize the personal and professional resources, education, and skills we have that are both available and needed to help ourselves and our communities in case of a disaster (see Barrett's Theory of Power in the Holistic Nursing Perspective section later in this chapter, as well as Neff's self-compassion practice[22]).

Living in a mobile society, nurses and helping professionals can also be confronted with a client or patient who immediately moved away from a disaster area or who has friends or family at risk in the disaster and is thereby also at risk for PTSD or vicarious trauma. Recognizing, understanding, and supporting those who evacuated or moved outside of the area where the original crisis or disaster occurred is vital for they are still at risk, and it is important to build a trauma evaluation into our nursing history taking and look for signs of cryptotrauma. Many people have delayed responses and are not immediately diagnosed. The main statement that trauma therapists treating those with PTSD continue to hear is, "I thought I'd be over this by now." Please remember that the more time that elapses from the time of the event, the more distressing the symptoms and reactions become for persons with PTSD.[48]

Caring for Those with PTSD

The PTSD is characterized by avoidance, numbness, and feelings of helplessness and hopelessness. For those suffering from PTSD, conversational induction and therapeutic suggestion may be even more helpful and appropriate than any form of deep relaxation.[49] As stated earlier, conversational induction helps to support a person's defenses while promoting comfort, important qualities to be cultivated for PTSD sufferers, especially in the immediate time during or after a major trauma. As in any clinical situation, professional experience, clinical judgment, and the client's comfort level with the intervention all help to determine the best approach for that client.

Because rescue or relief workers and professionals involved with trauma work of disaster victims may continuously return to the disaster site, thereby reexposing themselves to reexperiencing the crisis, they, too, may experience vicarious traumatization and feel stuck and isolated while other colleagues move on. They also need personal, workplace, and community healing support.

Holistic Nursing Perspectives for Living in a Time of Uncertainty

According to Dr. Elizabeth Barrett*:

> Power, from a Rogerian perspective, is the capacity to participate knowingly in the nature of change characterizing the continuous patterning of the human and environmental field. The observable, measurable pattern manifestations of power are awareness, choices, freedom to act intentionally, and involvement in creating change.[50, p. 4]

What awareness, choices, intentions, and involvement do we want to offer, as holistic nurses, to foster community unitary well-being in times of uncertainty? How do we help to support empowered awareness and choices in times of helplessness or uncertainty?

Our own practices of self-healing, meditation, and relaxation support us during times of illness and stress by helping us to build inner skills, awareness, and resiliency. Similarly, communities also can cultivate our inner resiliency by building our own inner capacities and a more connected interdisciplinary team. Increased training of clergy, child care workers, mental health professionals, teachers, and funeral directors, as well as nurses, social workers, physicians, chiropractors, and nutritionists, to recognize and deal with various forms of trauma and teach self-care practices and group support is one example of developing inner resources of a resilient community. This model of a resilient community fosters a true interdisciplinary team of healers building a lived community of well-being.

Cultivating Wellness Preparedness for Professionals, Communities, and Organizations

As holistic nursing leaders, we can build in preparedness within a wellness and healing framework in which communities focus on self-care and community care as shared values. In this way, when times of crisis or disaster arise, community self-care is already in place. One suggestion is to invite your healthcare community to create self-care practice buddies. Make a pact with colleagues to look out for one another's physical, emotional, and mental health by supporting healing breaks and encouraging one another's self-care practice to help maintain our best ability to be present. Though these breaks may take a different form in a time of great challenge, having positive healing patterns already in place can help build needed resiliency to cope with uncertainty and trauma or disaster.

Restorative Practices

Relaxation practice also brings the gifts of restoring, opening, and renewing.

Yoga

Yoga is a philosophy of living that unites physical, mental, and spiritual health. When practiced for the purpose of relaxation, it involves breathing and stretching exercises and postures. The exercises vary greatly in difficulty. Because yoga starts with very gentle stretches and breathing techniques, it is ideally suited for clients with stiff muscles and decreased activity levels who are attempting to begin an active relaxation and exercise program. Clients need not embrace the philosophy to benefit from the activity.

In restorative yoga, practitioners open themselves more deeply to the healing energies that flow through them in each posture (asana). They accomplish this by supporting their bodies in yoga poses using bolsters, pillows, and blankets.[51] Daily practice of restorative yoga—even 10 to 15 minutes a day—creates energy, restorative rest, spiritual renewal, and calm. Restorative yoga is a wonderful practice to perform during a break at work, and restorative yoga and yoga therapy are evolving as areas of therapeutic practice.[52]

Neurogenic Yoga and Trauma and Tension-Releasing Exercises

Neurogenic yoga is a self-help neurophysiological process accessed by combining the practice of yoga asanas (postures), trauma and tension-releasing exercises (TRE®), and breathing to

---

*Reproduced from E. Barrett, "The Theoretical Matrix for a Rogerian Nursing Practice," Theoria: Journal of Nursing Theory, no. 9 (2000): 4.

activate a healing form of neurogenic tremors called *self-induced therapeutic tremors*.[53] These therapeutic tremors are a part of our body's natural stress discharging system that is built in animals and humans; it is still active in animals but has been suppressed by humans. Self-induced therapeutic tremors are the nervous system's way of discharging long-held tension or unconscious muscle contraction in order to restore the body to wholeness. Based on Dr. Berceli's TRE® technique (see http://trauma prevention.com), simple exercises and practices facilitate the lengthening and relaxation of the psoas muscle and the release of physical and emotional stress and tension. Used with rescue workers as well as those directly affected by trauma or natural disaster, TRE® has been taught worldwide and is easy to learn and integrate into one's self-care regimine.[54] When experiencing TRE® or a neurogenic yoga session, tremors begin in the legs and often spread throughout the entire body. You can view video of neurogenic tremors in animals and humans on YouTube.

Qi Gong

Seasonal qi gong practices restore, renew, center, and open meridians as the energy field and body changes with the seasons. Some techniques of Chinese qi gong have been practiced for at least 5,000 years. Simple movements are combined with breath and meditation in a flow with nature's healing qi. Restoration and healing come from daily practice. Qi gong practices are a part of Chinese medicine, which includes acupuncture, external qi gong (receiving healing energy from a healer or master), herbal medicine, diet, massage, and self-care.

Restorative Gardens and Optimal Healing Environments

"Nature alone heals"[1] is one of Nightingale's most famous quotes. What Nightingale knew, and what gardeners and nature lovers also know, is that nature can heal and cure. Many hospitals and healthcare centers are creating healing gardens, restorative gardens, greenhouses, meditative gardens, and labyrinths in their plazas, lobbies, rooftops, and other inner and outer spaces to help cultivate relaxation, renewal, and peace.

Bringing nature inside the healing environment is not at all new; it dates back to medieval monastic healing sanctuaries. The medieval architectural designs included low windows so that patients could look out at nature's beauty. Simply helping clients to be with nature amid the high-tech healthcare system can improve their well-being, reduce their anxiety, and calm their fears. Nurses themselves can benefit from resting in a garden or creating natural spaces within the healthcare setting.[55]

Many organizations are looking to cultivate optimal healing environments (OHEs). The Samueli Institute recommends development of thefollowing eight domains for an OHE:[56]

1. Developing healing intention
2. Experiencing personal wholeness
3. Cultivating healing relationships
4. Creating healing organizations
5. Practicing healthy lifestyles
6. Applying integrative health care
7. Building healing spaces
8. Fostering ecological sustainability

Whereas restorative gardens focus on cultivating the natural environment and inclusion of healing structures and design for healing, the OHE focuses on both ecologically sustainable, natural healing spaces as well as the personal, professional, and organizational self-care practices needed to sustain vitality, healing, and transformation.[56]

Reflect on the ways that you are currently personally and professionally supporting OHEs and write them in your journal and share with your colleagues. Then learn how the Samueli Institute views nursing's role in creating an OHE online (www.reflectionsonnursingleadership.org/pages/vol36_3_fts_samueliinstitute.aspx).

Holistic Caring Process

Holistic Assessment

In preparing to use relaxation interventions, the nurse assesses the following parameters and lived experiences:

- The client's perception of personal tension levels and need to relax
- The client's readiness and motivation to learn relaxation strategies because relaxation is a subjective and personal endeavor
- The client's past experience with the process of relaxation, hypnosis, or meditation
- The client's personal definition and lived experience of what it means to be relaxed
- The client's ability to remain comfortable in one position for 15 to 30 minutes
- The client's hearing acuity, so that the nurse can speak at an appropriate level while guiding the client in relaxation exercises
- The client's spiritual and religious beliefs, so that the nurse can present the relaxation process in a way that will meld comfortably with the client's belief system
- The client's level of pain or discomfort, anxiety, fear, or boredom
- The client's perception of reality, history of depersonalization states, and locus of control because deep relaxation may exacerbate the symptoms of psychotic and prepsychotic individuals
- The client's medication intake, particularly of medications that may alter response to relaxation or that may need to be titrated as relaxation progresses

A questionnaire can be used to complete the assessment. The information gathered in the questionnaire provides starting points for discussion and further exploration.

Identification of Patterns/ Challenges/Needs

The patterns/challenges/needs (see Chapter 8) compatible with relaxation interventions are as follows:

- Social isolation
- Altered coping; ineffective individual and family
- Activity intolerance, actual or potential
- Deficit in diversional activity
- Powerlessness
- Altered self-concept; disturbance in self-esteem, role performance, personal identity

- Altered sensation and perception: visual, auditory, kinesthetic, gustatory, tactile, olfactory
- Altered thought processes
- Anxiety
- Altered comfort: pain
- Fear
- Potential for violence: self-directed or directed at others

Outcome Identification

Table 11-4 guides the nurse in client outcomes, nursing prescriptions, and evaluations for the use of relaxation as a nursing intervention.

Therapeutic Care Plan and Interventions

Before the session:

- Become personally familiar with the experience of the relaxation intervention before approaching the client.
- If the client has previous positive experience with a particular relaxation intervention, encourage further practice and use of that intervention.
- Review with the client his or her lived experience and gather information from the chart, diaries, and/or verbal self-report concerning pain, anxiety, and activity levels since the last session.

Preparation of the environment (ideal):

- Arrange medical and nursing care to allow for 15 to 45 minutes of uninterrupted time.
- Keep the room warm and ventilated, not cold.
- Shut the door or otherwise decrease extraneous noise and distraction. Place a note on the door indicating a need for privacy until a designated time.
- Turn off the telephone and cell phones or ask a family member or friend to answer the telephone should it ring during the relaxation training session.
- Reduce lighting to a low level.
- Use natural or incandescent lighting if possible; fluorescent lighting can cause headaches in some patients.

TABLE 11-4 Nursing Interventions: Relaxation		
Client Outcomes	**Nursing Prescriptions**	**Evaluation**
The client will demonstrate decreased anxiety, tension, and other manifestations of the stress response as a result of the relaxation intervention.	Guide the client in the relaxation exercise. Evaluate for decrease in anxiety, tension, and other manifestations of the stress response as evidenced by heart rate within normal limits, decreased respiratory rates, return of blood pressure toward normal, resolution of anxious facial expressions and mannerisms, decrease in repetitive talking or behavior, and inability to sleep or restlessness.	The client exhibited decreased anxiety, tension, and other manifestations of the stress response as evidenced by normal vital signs; a slow, deep breathing pattern; and decreased anxious behaviors.
The client will demonstrate a stabilization or decrease in pain as a result of the relaxation intervention.	Evaluate for decrease in pain as evidenced by reduction or elimination of pain control medication and increased activities or mobility.	The client's intake of pain medication stabilized and then decreased with relaxation skills practice. The client began to participate in activities previously limited by pain.
The client will link breathing awareness to a commonly occurring cue and use this combination to reduce tension.	Teach awareness of breathing patterns and habitual linking of relaxing breathing to a cue in the environment.	The client used turning in bed as a cue to take a slow, deep breath and relax jaw muscles.

Client comfort measures:

- Have the client empty his or her bladder before starting the intervention.
- Help the client find a comfortable sitting or reclining position, with hands resting by the sides or on the thighs.
- Ensure the client's comfort by providing a blanket or by adjusting the thermostat to a comfortably warm setting; have small, soft pillows available for positioning.

Timing of the session (ideal):

- Hold the training session before meals or more than 2 hours after the last meal. A full stomach coupled with relaxation may lead to sleep.

Support tools:

- Have recorded music available.
- If the session is to be followed by drawing, have paper, crayons, or colored markers available.
- Tell the client that you may ask simple yes or no questions during the session to check the comfort level of the music or to confirm

the client's understanding of verbal instructions. The client may answer these questions by raising a preestablished "yes" finger or "no" finger or nodding the head.

At the beginning of the session:

- Review briefly the potential benefits of relaxation intervention, and enlist the client's cooperation. Explore the client's lived experience of relaxation and stress.
- Explain to the client that relaxation may be easier if practiced with the eyes closed. The client may drift off to sleep, but this position allows the client to focus attention inward while remaining awake. This may take practice to accomplish, and many times clients fall asleep as a result of exhaustion or lack of sleep. In such a case, the restorative dimension of relaxation is at work, and the nurse has still introduced therapeutic suggestions.
- Explain that one purpose of breathing and relaxation exercises is to experience inward relaxation and become aware of the body-mind-spirit connections associated with relaxation.

- Emphasize that you are merely a guide, and that any therapeutic results obtained from the session are from the client's natural healing ability, involvement, interest, and practice.
- Let go of outcomes. There is an ebb and flow to the learning experience. Encourage the client to practice for comfort and awareness, noting shifts in breathing, anxiety, and sensations.
- Arrive at mutually agreeable goals for the session, such as reduction of pain, decreased time to sleep onset, reduction of anxiety, or enhanced well-being.
- Have the client quantify the level of the parameter to be changed; for example, "My pain or anxiety level right now is 7 on a scale of 0 (none) to 10 (extreme pain)." Record the level before and after the session.
- Record baseline vital signs. If biofeedback equipment is used, record baseline readings.
- Assure the client that sensations of heaviness, warmth, floating, or lightness are naturally occurring indications of deep relaxation; explain that the client can end the experience at any moment she or he desires by opening the eyes, tightening the fists, or stretching; this will orient the client and enable the exercise to continue.
- Begin soft background music that is pleasing to the client.
- Guide the client through a basic breathing relaxation exercise. Breathing exercises may be repeated slowly for several minutes as an introduction to deeper relaxation.
- Start the session with short breathing or relaxation exercises (5 minutes); lengthen the exercises to 10 to 20 minutes as the client becomes better able to relax and attend to inner thoughts and feelings.

During the session:

- Phrase all therapeutic suggestions and self-statements in a positive form. For example, say, "I am aware of comfort moving down my arm and into my hand," rather than "I am not in pain." These therapeutic suggestions enhance the process and reframe the experience.
- Speak in a relaxed manner. Ask the client for feedback concerning the appropriateness of the practice and his or her ability to hear the background music and instructions. Have the client respond with a finger movement (using signals established before the session) or nod of the head, and make adjustments as necessary.
- Pace your instructions according to the following visual cues from the client. Each indicates a deepening of relaxation.
  - Change in breathing pattern: slower, deeper breaths progressing to slow, somewhat shallower breathing as relaxation deepens
  - More audible breathing
  - Fluttering of eyelids
  - Blanching of the skin around the nose and mouth
  - Easing of jaw tightness, sometimes to the extent that the lips part and the jaw drops slightly
  - If the client is supine, pointing of toes outward rather than straight up
  - Complete lack of muscle holding (ask the client's permission to lift an arm gently by the wrist; no resistance should be felt and the arm should move as easily as any other object of similar weight)
- Modify your instructions and strategies to fit the situation. Encourage an intubated and ventilated patient who cannot control respiratory rate or volume to drop the jaw and allow the rhythm of the ventilator to soothe tight muscles, for example. Gently placing your hand over the clavicle or holding the person's hand as you speak enhances the therapeutic relationship and supports relaxation.
- Intersperse your instructions with therapeutic suggestions of encouragement that the client can use after the session as cues to recapture aspects of the relaxation experience. Examples of such phrases are:
  - Perhaps you are noticing a softening of your muscles.
  - As you take your next breath, become aware of how the warmth is flowing down your arm.

- Deep breathing helps to replenish the oxygen and energy of the body and helps the body heal, relax, restore, and renew.

- As the client relaxes, she or he may experience a release of emotional life issues, which can surface in the conscious mind. Be alert for signs of emotional discomfort or letting go, such as tears or a change in breathing to deeper, faster breaths. If such a sign occurs, ask gentle questions (e.g., "Can you put those feelings into words and express them safely?"), and allow time for the client to express and deal with the material before continuing with or concluding the session. (See the earlier sections relating to cryptotrauma and trauma for more information on helping clients stay grounded if they tap into emotion-laden material.) Often, clients in a deeply relaxed state gain insight into how to resolve problems or which direction to take in their lives.

At the end of the session:

- Bring the client gradually into a wakeful state by suggesting that she or he take deep, energizing breaths, begin to move hands and feet, and stretch; orient the client to the room, talking with the client about the comfort she or he created.

- Have the client reevaluate, on the scale of 0 to 10 used earlier, the level of comfort or severity of the parameter previously selected to be changed. Record the level. Take vital signs again and readings on any biofeedback equipment and record postrelaxation practice readings to monitor any psychophysiologic changes pre- and postpractice.

- Allow time for discussion of the experience, including the techniques that seemed especially effective and the client's physical, emotional, and energy awareness. Invite the client to express his or her experience by writing, making a journal entry, or drawing. Different clients will prefer different methods, such as creating an abstract drawing, offering a story, or writing poetry, to express their experience.

- Ensure that medication changes, if indicated, are appropriately monitored.

- Engage the client in continuing practice on an individually assigned basis until the next session.

- Help the client choose supportive measures for practicing his or her relaxation skill.

- Review a log or journal in which the client records relaxation practice, symptoms, medications, time, and results.

Case Study (Implementation)

Case Study 1

Setting: Outpatient; multidisciplinary holistic healthcare center

Client: S. D., a 47-year-old African American man with family history of stroke

Medical diagnosis: Progressive essential hypertension, unresponsive to any antihypertensive therapy

Current medications: Catapres (clonidine), Lasix (furosemide), Valium (diazepam), Minipress (prazosin), potassium chloride

Patterns/Challenges/Needs:

1. Altered physical regulation (essential hypertension)
2. Anxiety
3. Fear
4. Powerlessness
5. Ineffective coping related to anxiety, job stress, and parenting of five children
6. Self-esteem disturbance, situational

S. D. had been diagnosed with severe uncontrollable essential hypertension. He scrupulously took his antihypertensive medications and had an extensive clinical workup to rule out any secondary causes. S. D. was very frustrated because his father had died of a stroke, and S. D. did not want to have a stroke or "die young." He and his wife cared for their five children. He worked at a job that required him to perform physical labor and walk up and down three flights of stairs.

His physician sent him to learn biofeedback-assisted relaxation as an adjunctive therapy. His blood pressure at rest while on medication ranged from 160/100 to 200/120 mm Hg. To reduce S. D.'s fear and feeling of powerlessness, the nurse explored his lived experience of his condition and used healthcare teaching and stress management counseling to reframe his understanding of what was happening in his body.

The nurse explained to S. D. that his body knew very well how to respond to stress, but that he needed the opportunity and the time to recover from stress and learn less physically distressing ways to respond. S. D. was shown how to use the temperature trainer and a small galvanic skin response unit that indicated sympathetic outflow by measuring sweat gland response. He was taught simple breathing exercises and autogenic phrases while he learned to monitor his body-mind-spirit response on the biofeedback displays.

Because of the urgency and critical nature of his situation, he was invited to participate in three practice sessions a week for 1 month instead of the usual one session per week. He was asked to practice the relaxation two times a day. Within the first 2 weeks, he had brought his blood pressure down to 140/100 mm Hg. He continued sessions each week during the second month and then continued practice on his own. After 3 months, his blood pressure was 140/80 mm Hg while he continued on the same level of medication.

After 1 year, his medication level was reduced, and blood pressure was maintained at 140/80 mm Hg. The nurse scheduled a meeting with S. D., his wife, and all of their children to explore their needs, fears, and concerns about S. D.'s health. The family agreed to help support S. D. in his healthcare practice by ensuring that he was not disturbed during his practice time. The opportunity to share their love and support, and to understand how their loved one was working to help himself, offered them a new understanding of their father and husband, his healthcare issues, and how they could be active in his wellness plan.

Case Study 2

Setting: Home care and outpatient clinic
Client: P. H., a 50-year-old European American teacher with a recurrence of breast cancer discovered in the lymph nodes, which was surgically removed and followed with a course of chemotherapy and radiation
Patterns/Challenges/Needs:

1. Altered physical regulation (chemotherapy and radiation therapy/breast cancer)

2. Anxiety
3. Fear
4. Ineffective coping related to recurrence of breast cancer
5. Powerlessness

P. H. is a 50-year-old teacher who had been diagnosed with breast cancer 5 years ago. At that time, she had a lumpectomy of her right breast, which was followed by a course of chemotherapy, radiation, and hormone therapy. No lymphatic involvement was found. Five years later during her regular checkup with her oncologist, a recurrence was discovered in the lymph nodes, which was treated by surgical removal followed by chemotherapy and radiation. Getting the news, she said she "went into shock" but also became determined to do what was necessary to care for her bodymindspirit. Even with this determination, she still found it difficult to rest or sleep as her fear at times was overwhelming her and was not only running her mind but also exhausting her body. The fact that there had been a recurrence was still hard at times to grasp.

P. H.'s decision to become an active part of her own self-care during the chemotherapy and radiation treatments resulted in her putting together a team of complementary practitioners, including supportive friends and a holistic nurse, to support her healing process.

To nourish and protect her body during the chemotherapy and radiation treatment, she began to work with a nutritionist to guide her diet, help her learn healthier habits, and support her body's well-being during treatment so that food was medicine for her. She also attended weekly yoga classes and began receiving Reiki treatments both in person and through distance Reiki from a local Reiki Master.

P. H. had a longstanding meditation practice that included both centering prayer and mindfulness meditation, but she found it difficult to concentrate and practice her meditation under the current circumstances. This was not unusual, but P. H. found it very discouraging at times. She also suffered from a great deal of pain around the radiation site, which made it even more difficult to rest.

The holistic nurse offered sessions that included guided meditations and conversational therapeutic suggestions to support the healing ability of her body and the healing energy of the treatment. The holistic nurse encouraged P. H.'s trust and confidence in herself, her self-care practices, and her healing team. She also supported P. H.'s connection to her own meditation practice and her meditation practice body. Drawing on the understanding P. H. had shared from her mindfulness meditation wisdom and yoga philosophy, the holistic nurse acknowledged that mindfulness was not just something P. H. did; it was something "she was"—that is, that the energy of her mindfulness practice was alive in every cell of her body, supporting her even if it was difficult at times to concentrate or to trust the support that is present in her meditation and yoga practice and in her bodymindspirit's ability to heal and be at peace no matter what the outcome.

She also offered P. H. deep relaxation practice during sessions both at the clinic, while she was receiving chemotherapy, and during home visits, after her radiation therapy sessions, as a way to reduce fatigue and anxiety, enhance rest, and induce sleep. This was supplemented by P. H.'s use of an MP3 version of recorded guided meditations or relaxation practice. The live deep relaxation practices offered by the holistic nurse lasted 15 to 30 minutes and helped P. H. to rest and fall asleep. Though the holistic nurse would check both pre- and postresponses, there were times when she told P. H. that if she fell asleep during the relaxation (whether live session or MP3) to just allow her body to do what it needed to do. This would mean that there were times that the holistic nurse would check in with her the next day rather than wake her up to check her response. Her falling asleep itself was considered an affirmation of benefits and postevaluation because she had been unable to fall asleep herself at times.

P. H. has completed her treatment and has been gradually regaining her strength, energy, and ease in her bodymindspirit. She is returning to and feeling more at ease with her meditation practice and has attended several weekend meditation and yoga retreats. She continues to work with her healing team, especially for nutrition and yoga, and receives periodic Reiki while

---

EXHIBIT 11-6   Evaluation of the Client's Subjective Experience of Relaxation

1. Was this a new experience for you? Can you describe it?
2. Did you have any physical or emotional responses to the relaxation exercises? If so, can you describe them?
3. Do you feel different after this experience? How?
4. How does your body–mind communicate with you when your stress level is at an uncomfortable point?
5. Would you like to do this again?
6. Were there any distractions to your relaxation?
7. What would make this a more pleasant experience for you?
8. How do you see yourself integrating relaxation skills into your daily life?

---

checking in regularly with the holistic nurse as she continues her healing journey.

Evaluation

With the client, the nurse determines whether the client outcomes for relaxation interventions were successfully achieved (see **Exhibit 11-6**). To evaluate the session further, the nurse may again explore the subjective effects of the experience with the client (see Exhibit 11-6). Because the accomplishment of these interventions may take place over a period of days or weeks, they must be reviewed and reevaluated periodically. Continuing support and encouragement are necessary.

Conclusion

Relaxation exercises can be taught to clients under almost any circumstances. They not only reduce the fear and anxiety associated with many medical and nursing interventions but, once learned, may be used in all aspects of a client's life. They increase the overall movement-toward wholeness and balance for both client and nurse, and they facilitate other interventions by allowing the client to move toward learning and participating more fully in his or her own health promotion.

Directions for Future Research

1. Correlate the changes in psychophysiology with the specific relaxation interventions used to determine the most effective interventions and their presentation.
2. Conduct tightly structured studies to evaluate specific relaxation techniques, using control groups to validate changes brought about by specific forms of relaxation exercises.
3. Monitor and validate the effect of "therapeutic presence" in the relaxation process.
4. Compare effects of live guided relaxation to audio- or video-guided relaxation on specific client populations, conditions, and healthcare environments, using control groups to validate changes brought about by live or recorded forms of relaxation exercises.
5. Conduct qualitative studies to explore how an optimal healing environment is influenced by holistic nurses practicing self-compassionate and relaxation self-care on hospital units.
6. Monitor and validate the effect of conversational suggestion and sustained centering for enhancing comfort and calm in crisis situations.

Nurse Healer Reflections

After reading this chapter, the nurse healer will be able to answer or to begin the process of answering the following questions:

- How does my inner experience of tension or anxiety shift when I release my muscle tightness?
- How do I model relaxation to my family, friends, colleagues, and clients?
- What is my kinesthetic experience of letting go of tension, concerns, and physical and emotional stresses?
- Which cues about my inner experience of tension or relaxation do I receive from my breathing pattern?

- How do I cultivate peace of mind as I move through my potentially stressful job activities?
- Am I aware that my attitudes toward my tasks are contagious to my clients?
- Which ways can I integrate relaxation practice for myself and my colleagues into my workplace culture?
- Which dimensions of resiliency are found or needed in my workplace and community?

NOTES

1. F. Nightingale, *Notes on Nursing: What It Is, and What It Is Not*, Commemorative ed. (Philadelphia: Lippincott, 1992): 28.
2. J. Kabat-Zinn, *Full Catastrophe Living: Using the Wisdom of Your Body and Mind to Face Stress, Pain, and Illness* (New York: Bantam Dell, 1990).
3. D. Ornish, *Dr. Dean Ornish's Program for Reversing Heart Disease* (New York: Ivy Books, 1990).
4. D. Krieger, *Accepting Your Power to Heal: The Personal Practice of Therapeutic Touch* (Rochester, VT: Bear and Co., 1993): 17–20.
5. D. Krieger, "Characteristics of Integration During the Healing Moment" (keynote address at the 5th Annual Holism and Nursing Conference, Zeta Omega Chapter-at-Large of Sigma Theta Tau International, Rye, NY, May 16, 2003).
6. J. Levey and M. Levey, *The Fine Arts of Relaxation, Concentration, and Meditation: Ancient Skills for Modern Minds* (Somerville, MA: Wisdom, 2003): 11.
7. R. Schneider, C. E. Grim, M. Rainforth, T. Kotchen, S. I. Nidich, C. Gaylord-King, J. W. Salerno, et al., "Stress Reduction in the Secondary Prevention of Cardiovascular Disease: Randomized, Controlled Trial of Transcendental Meditation and Health Education in Blacks," *Cardiovascular Quality and Outcomes* 5, no. 6 (2012): 750–758.
8. H. Benson, S. Alexander, and C. L. Feldman, "Decreased Premature Ventricular Contractions Through Use of the Relaxation Response in Patients with Stable Ischaemic Heart-Disease," *The Lancet* 2, no. 7931 (1975): 380–382.
9. J. Kabat-Zinn, L. Lipworth, R. Burncy, and W. Sellers, "Four-Year Follow-Up of a Meditation-Based Program for the Self-Regulation of Chronic Pain: Treatment Outcomes and Compliance," *Clinical Journal of Pain* 2, no. 3 (1986): 159–173.

10. S. Rosenzweig, J. M. Greeson, D. K. Reibel, J. S. Green, S. A. Jasser, and D. Beasley, "Mindfulness-Based Stress Reduction for Chronic Pain Conditions: Variation in Treatment Outcomes and Role of Home Meditation Practice," *Journal of Psychosomatic Research* 68, no. 1 (2010): 29–36.

11. C. Moriconi and S. Stabler-Haas, "Mindfulness-Based Stress Reduction and Its Effect on Test Anxiety and Focused Attention with Baccalaureate Nursing Students: A Pilot Study" (presentation at the Mindfulness in Education Conference, American University, Washington, DC, March 19, 2011).

12. J. J. Arch, K. W. Brown, D. J. Dean, L. N. Landy, K. D. Brown, and M. L. Laudenslager, "Self-Compassion Training Modulates Alpha-Amylase, Heart Rate Variability, and Subjective Responses to Social Evaluative Threat in Women," *Psychoneuroendocrinology* 42 (2014): 49–58.

13. B. L. Fredrickson, M. A. Cohn, K. A. Coffey, J. Pek, and S. M. Finkel, "Open Hearts Build Lives: Positive Emotions, Induced Through Loving-Kindness Meditation, Build Consequential Personal Resources," *Journal of Personality and Social Psychology* 95, no. 5 (2008): 1045–1062.

14. H. E. Tilbrook, H. Cox, C. E. Hewitt, A. R. Kang'ombe, L-H. Chuang, S. Jayakody, J. D. Aplin, et al., "Yoga for Chronic Low Back Pain: A Randomized Trial," *Annals of Internal Medicine* 155, no. 9 (2011): 569–578.

15. J. F. Coleman, "Spring Forest Qigong and Chronic Pain: Making a Difference," *Journal of Holistic Nursing* 29, no. 2 (2011): 118–128.

16. Contemplative Outreach, "Centering Prayer" (n.d.). www.contemplativeoutreach.org/category /category/centering-prayer.

17. The Center for Contemplative Mind in Society, "The Tree of Contemplative Practices" (2014). www.contemplativemind.org/practices/tree.

18. J. B. Bartels, "The Pause," *Critical Care Nurse* 34, no. 1 (2014): 74–75.

19. T. N. Hanh, *The Blooming of a Lotus: Guided Meditation Exercises for Healing and Transformation* (Boston: Beacon Press, 1993): 17.

20. T. N. Hanh, *The Long Road Turns to Joy: A Guide to Walking Meditation* (Berkeley, CA: Parallax Press, 1996).

21. T. N. Hanh, *Teachings on Love* (Berkeley, CA: Parallax Press, 2007): 21.

22. K. Neff, "Guided Self-Compassion Meditations" (2009). www.self-compassion.org/guided-self -compassion-meditations-mp3.html.

23. H. Benson, *Beyond the Relaxation Response* (New York: Times Books, 1984).

24. J. K. Keicolt-Glaser, R. Glaser, D. Williger, J. Stout, G. Messick, S. Sheppard, D. Ricker, et al., "Psychosocial Enhancement of Immunocompetence in a Geriatric Population," *Health Psychology* 4, no. 1 (1985): 25–41.

25. P. Pathak, R. Mahal, A. Kohli, and V. Nimbran, "Progressive Muscle Relaxation: An Adjuvant Therapy for Reducing Pain and Fatigue Among Hospitalized Cancer Patients Receiving Radiotherapy," *International Journal of Advanced Nursing Studies* 2 (2013): 58–65.

26. G. Feldman, J. Greeson, and J. Senville, "Differential Effects of Mindful Breathing, Progressive Muscle Relaxation, and Loving-Kindness Meditation on Decentering and Negative Reactions to Repetitive Thoughts," Behaviour Research and Therapy 48, no. 10 (2010): 1002–1011.

27. G. E. Knowlton and K. T. Larkin, "The Influence of Voice Volume, Pitch, and Speech Rate on Progressive Relaxation Training: Application of Methods from Speech Pathology and Audiology," *Applied Psychophysiology and Biofeedback* 31, no. 2 (2006): 173–185.

28. J. H. Schultz and W. Luthe, *Autogenic Training: A Psychophysiologic Approach in Psychotherapy* (New York: Grune & Stratton, 1959).

29. M. Shinozaki, M. Kanazawa, M. Kano, Y. Endo, N. Nakaya, M. Hongo, and S. Fukudo, "Effect of Autogenic Training on General Improvement in Patients with Irritable Bowel Syndrome: A Randomized Controlled Trial," *Applied Psychophysiology Biofeedback* 35, no. 3 (2010): 189–198.

30. S. L. Fahrion, "Hypertension and Biofeedback," *Primary Care* 18, no. 3 (1991): 663–682.

31. G. Tan, T. K. Dao, L. Farmer, R. J. Sutherland, and R. Gevirtz, "Heart Rate Variability (HRV) and Posttraumatic Stress Disorder (PTSD): A Pilot Study," *Applied Psychophysiology Biofeedback* 36, no. 1 (2011): 27–35.

32. O. M. Giggins, U. M. Persson, and B. Caulfield, "Biofeedback in Rehabilitation," *Journal of NeuroEngineering and Rehabilitation* 10, no. 1 (2013): 60–71.

33. K. McKenna and K. Gallagher, "Ready, Set, Relax: Biofeedback-Assisted Relaxation Training (BART) in a Pediatric Psychiatry Consultation Service," Psychosomatics (June 2014). doi:10.1016/j.psym.2014.06.003.

34. C. A. Prato and C. B. Yucha, "Biofeedback-Assisted Relaxation Training to Decrease Test Anxiety in Nursing Students," *Nursing Education Perspectives* 34, no. 2 (2013): 76–81.

35. R. J. Davidson and G. E. Schwartz, "The Psychobiology of Relaxation and Related States: A Multi-Process Theory," in *Behavioral Control and the Modification of Physiological Activity*, ed. D. I. Mostofsky (Englewood Cliffs, NJ: Prentice Hall, 1976): 399–442.

36. W. Linden, "The Autogenic Training Method of J. H. Schultz," in *Principles and Practice of Stress Management*, 2nd ed., eds. P. M. Lehrer and R. L. Woolfolk (New York: Guilford Press, 1993): 205–230.

37. P. M. Lehrer, J. M. Atthowe, and P. Weber, "Effects of Progressive Relaxation and Autogenic Training on Anxiety and Physiological Measures, with Some Data on Hypnotizability," in *Stress and Tension Control*, eds. F. J. McGuigan, W. E. Sime, and J. M. Wallace (New York: Springer, 1980): 171–184.

38. S. Shapiro and P. M. Lehrer, "Psychophysiological Effects of Autogenic Training and Progressive Relaxation," *Biofeedback and Self-Regulation* 5, no. 2 (1980): 249–255.

39. H. Benson, *The Relaxation Response* (New York: William Morrow, 1975).

40. Personal communication. Dorothy Larkin, assistant professor, College of New Rochelle School of Nursing, June 16, 2003.

41. D. Cheeks, "Hypnosis," in *Health for the Whole Person: The Complete Guide to Holistic Medicine*, eds. A. Hastings, J. Fadiman, and J. S. Gordon (Boulder, CO: Westview Press, 1980): 141–156.

42. B. Rogers, "Therapeutic Conversation and Posthypnotic Suggestion," *American Journal of Nursing* 72 (1972): 714–717.

43. D. Larkin, "Principles of Therapeutic Suggestion (Part I) and Clinical Applications of Therapeutic Suggestions (Part II)," *Explore: The Journal of Science and Healing* 10, no. 6 (2014): 380–388.

44. E. Jacobs and E. Pelier, "Ericksonian Hypnosis and Approaches with Pediatric Hematology Oncology Patients," *American Journal of Clinical Hypnosis* 41, no. 2 (1998): 139–153.

45. S. R. O'Brien, "Staff Wellness Program Promotes Quality Care," *American Journal of Nursing* 98, no. 6 (1998): 16B, 16D.

46. S. E. Taylor, L. C. Klein, B. P. Lewis, T. L. Gruenewald, R. A. R. Gurung, and J. A. Updegraff, "BehavioralResponses to Stress in Females: Tend and Befriend, Not Fight or Flight," *Psychological Review* 107, no. 3 (2000): 411–429.

47. J. V. Domino and J. D. Haber, "Prior Physical and Sexual Abuse in Women with Chronic Headache: Clinical Correlates," *Headache* 27, no. 6 (1987): 310–314.

48. Personal communication. John Draper, director of Public Education and the LifeNet Hotline Network, July 9, 2003.

49. J. Sareen, B. J. Cox, M. B. Stein, T. O. Afifi, C. Fleet, and G. J. Asmundson, "Physical and Mental Comorbidity, Disability, and Suicidal Behavior Associated with Posttraumatic Stress Disorder in a Large Community Sample," *Psychosomatic Medicine* 69, no. 3 (2007): 242–248.

50. E. A. M. Barrett, "The Theoretical Matrix for a Rogerian Nursing Practice," *Theoria: Journal of Nursing Theory* 9, no. 4 (2000): 3–7.

51. J. H. Lasater, *Relax and Renew: Restful Yoga for Stressful Living* (Berkeley, CA: Rodmell Press, 1995).

52. S. C. F. Tolse, "A Case Report of the Design and Implementation of a Hospital Based Therapeutic Yoga Rehabilitation Program" (presentation at the International Association of Yoga Therapists, Los Angeles, CA, January 2007).

53. TRE California, "Neurogenic Yoga" (2014). http://trecalifornia.com/neurogenic-yoga.

54. D. Berceli and M. Napoli, "A Proposal for a Mindfulness-Based Trauma-Prevention Program for Social Work Professionals," *Journal of Evidence-Based Complementary and Alternative Medicine* 11, no. 3 (2006): 153–165.

55. N. Gerlach-Spriggs, R. E. Kaufman, and S. B. Warner, Jr., *Restorative Gardens: The HealingLandscape* (New Haven, CT: Yale University Press, 1998).

56. T. Zborowsky and M. J. Kreitzer, "Creating Optimal Healing Environments" in *Integrative Nursing*, eds. M. J. Kreitzer and M. Koithan (New York: Oxford University Press, 2014): 84–100.

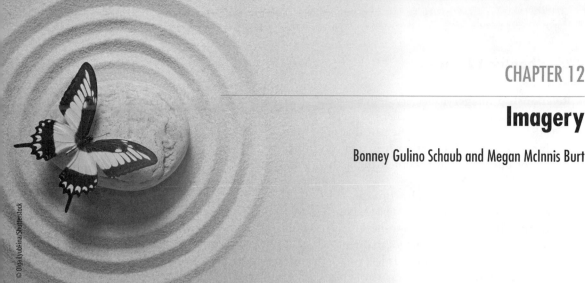

CHAPTER 12

Imagery

Bonney Gulino Schaub and Megan McInnis Burt

Nurse Healer Objectives

Theoretical

- Define and contrast the different types of imagery.
- Discuss the imagery process and the different theories of imagery.
- Explain different imagery interventions.

Clinical

- Incorporate imagery interventions into your clinical practice.
- Appreciate the spectrum and variety of clinical responses to imagery.
- Learn techniques to empower your spoken words.
- Train your voice so that your tone of voice and the pacing of selected words and phrases convey the qualities of calmness, reassurance, openness, and trust.

Personal

- Bring awareness of your own imagery process into your daily life.
- Choose a special healing image to focus on throughout the day.
- Learn to trust and be curious about the meaning of your images.

Definitions

Body–mind imagery: The conscious formation of an image that is directed to a body area or activity that requires attention or increased energy.

Clinical imagery: The conscious use of the power of the imagination with the intention of activating physiologic, psychological, or spiritual healing.

Correct biologic imagery: Biologically accurate images that are visualized to send messages to physiologic processes.

End-state imagery: Images that contain specified imagined hopes and goals (e.g., a healed wound).

Guided imagery: A highly structured imagery technique.

Imagery process: Internal experiences of memories, dreams, fantasies, inner perceptions, and visions, sometimes involving one, several, or all of the senses, serving as the bridge for connecting body, mind, and spirit.

Imagery rehearsal: An imagery technique designed to rehearse behaviors or prepare for activities or procedures.

Impromptu imagery: The nurse's introduction of his or her spontaneous, intuitive images or perceptions into the therapeutic intervention.

Packaged imagery: Commercial tapes that have general images.

Relationship imagery: Imagery designed to explore relationships with other people or with a part of oneself (e.g., the part that is always judgmental) or with a symptom or part of one's body (e.g., connecting with the heart).

Spontaneous imagery: The unexpected reception of an image, as if it "bubbled up," entering the stream of consciousness.

Symbolic imagery: Inner images that represent a person's deeper knowledge, occurring in the form of metaphors or symbols, that may be immediately translatable to rational verbal thought, or their meaning may emerge slowly over time.

Transpersonal imagery: Images that connect one to expanded (i.e., beyond personality) levels of consciousness, such as imagining one's body as a mountain and beginning to feel an inner quality of immovable strength and solidity.

Visualization: The use of external images (e.g., religious paintings, written words, nature photography) to evoke internal imagery experiences that energize desired emotions, qualities, outcomes, or goals.

Theory and Research

Imagery is an essential aspect of holistic nursing practice because it brings the natural powers of the mind into the process of health and healing. Distinct from thinking, imagery as a technique interacts with the image-making function of the brain, which, in turn, acts on the entire physiology. Imagery can be used on its own or in conjunction with therapeutic touch, meditation, biofeedback, Reiki, reflexology, massage, and other holistic practices.

The clinical value of imagery has been well documented in the treatment of a wide variety of conditions such as cancer;[1-3] migraine headaches; irritable bowel syndrome;[4-6] hypertension, anxiety, and depression;[7] fibromyalgia;[8-10] posttraumatic stress disorder;[11-13] immune system disorders;[14, 15] asthma;[16] and Parkinson's disease.[17] Health insurance companies now offer reimbursements for utilization of guided imagery, including Blue Shield of California, which offers its members audiotapes of guided imagery to assist in preparing for and recovering from surgery. In addition, hospitals are now incorporating imagery into the therapeutic services they offer.[18]

The research center at the Institute of HeartMath (www.heartmath.org) is dedicated to the study of the heart and the physiology of emotions. The Institute has conducted extensive research that explores the practice of imagining the experiences of appreciation, gratitude, and compassion. When subjects engaged the imagination in the heartfelt experience of appreciation, studies reflect the outcome of physiologic coherence. The emotional experience of appreciation was found to create a more coherent heart rhythm. This coherent state has been correlated with feelings of emotional well-being and improvements in cognitive, emotional, and physiologic performance.[19, 20]

The research definition of imagery is a perception of a stimulus in the absence of that stimulus. For example, if a person imagines a lemon and begins to taste lemon juice, he or she is having a perception (tasting the juice) of a stimulus (lemon) that is not present. Commonly, in addition to tasting the lemon, the person begins to salivate as well, demonstrating a rapid physiologic alteration in response to the imagery suggestion. Research has shown that our physiology reacts to imagined stimuli. For example, research has shown that imagining an odor results in physical changes as if an actual odor has been experienced.[21] Magnetic resonance imaging (MRI) investigations of the brain's recording of tactile information shows that imaged tactile stimulation and actual tactile stimulation are registered in partially overlapping areas of the brain.[22] Researchers also used functional MRI to examine brain activity in healthy volunteers who mentally imagined walking along a curved path. The outcomes suggest that there is a very close neurophysiologic relationship between locomotion and its mental imagery.[23] In other words, the brain processes our images as if they were real.

This "absence of stimuli" definition is relevant to the crucial issue of the placebo effect, a phenomenon in which the patient thinks (imagines) he or she is receiving a potent medication and experiences the anticipated effects, both positive (placebo) and negative (nocebo), of that medication, when in fact a neutral substance was administered.

A practitioner's suggestions regarding expected outcome influences the effect of a placebo. In a study where subjects were instructed to place their hands in ice water, one group was informed of the beneficial effect of this practice, one group was told of the possible hazards, and the control group was given a neutral suggestion. The pain threshold, tolerance, and endurance of the three groups were compared. The tolerance of participants given the positive suggestion was significantly greater than that of the other two groups. In contrast, the group given the negative suggestion had significantly decreased tolerance and endurance of the test condition.[24]

A study compared the effect of language considered compassionate or instructive with words that offered the imagination something it could directly work with, such as imagining being in a safe and comfortable place or imagining coolness or warmth. Words that may have been thought of as instructive or even compassionate, for example, "it's only going to be a small sting," or "don't worry," registered more distress than when the practitioner offered the patient's mind something positive and therapeutic to work with. Soothing, positive imagery suggestions provided more anxiety reduction and decreased distress.[25, 26]

This information challenges the holistic nurse to understand and work with the power of a patient's imagination when providing care. Clinical imagery is the conscious use of the power of the imagination with the intention of activating physiologic, psychological, or spiritual healing. The key word in this definition is *conscious*. The power of the imagination, for good or bad, is always affecting people. People imagine negative futures and employ their intelligence to worry about that negative future. Their life becomes focused around a negative future that they imagine to be true. Imagery's clinical focus is to use the imagination to promote life-affirming behaviors and goals. In addition to its contribution in promoting physical healing, imagery has great value in wellness education. It has shown value in improving quality of life through decreasing stress, increasing positive mood, and improving general health status.

The effectiveness of imagery in healing has been recognized and used cross-culturally for thousands of years.[27, 28] Imagery, in addition to improving physical symptoms, can be used for promoting psychological and spiritual development. It has the potential for promoting personal transformation through an enhanced sense of the interconnectedness of body, mind, and soul. When bringing imagery into clinical practice, nurses are introducing proven ancient methods of healing into modern health care.

Research on States of Consciousness and Mental Imagery

Several important psychology research findings about the ongoing imagery process, or "stream of consciousness," have implications for the nursing care of patients and clients. Sensory deprivation research in the early 1960s spurred the study of the ongoing imagery process. Initially, the purpose of this research was to examine the functioning of the brain in the absence of sensory input. Much of this research resulted from the space program's need to understand the effect on astronauts of the sensory deprivation, isolation, and confinement of space travel.[29] These studies indicated that an ongoing imagery process is a vital element in human mental experience, particularly when perceptual stimulation is reduced as it is in those who have a sensory impairment, those who are dealing with the monotony of hospitalization—particularly those in intensive care units—and those who work in monotonous environments.

Working with imagery has the potential to tap into memory at extremely deep levels. Wilder Penfield, a Canadian neurosurgeon working in the middle of the 20th century, did extensive experimentation with direct electrical stimulation and mapping of the brain during surgery. In his research on locally anesthetized, conscious subjects, he identified an area of the brain he labeled the "interpretive cortex." Upon electrostimulation of this region, he discovered that there is a brain mechanism

> capable of bringing back a strip of past experience in complete detail without any of the fanciful elaborations that occur in a man's dreaming . . . a record that has not faded but seems to remain as vivid as when the record was made.[30]

Penfield went on to indicate that, although the memories recalled in this manner were predominantly visual or auditory, the memory record included all of the sensory information that had entered consciousness (e.g., smells, tastes, sounds, tactile sensations). In addition, there was a sense of familiarity about the event. Simultaneous with the experience of these memory records, Penfield's subjects retained an awareness of their present situation; namely, that they were on an operating table having their brain probed by a surgeon.

Penfield's studies illustrate the capacity of consciousness to be absorbed in multiple activities at the same time. Penfield's patients were conscious of complete sensory recall of memories, were conscious of being on an operating room table, and were able to verbalize their experiences to Penfield and his staff. Appreciating the potentials of human consciousness is a key element in imagery work.

Clinical Effectiveness of Imagery

A comprehensive survey of the research on the physiologic effects of imagery cites the following results on a wide range of systems and symptoms:[31]

- Increased internal blood flow, demonstrated by increased temperature in specific skin areas
- Increased heart rate resulting from imaging sexually or emotionally arousing situations
- Alterations in body chemistry, such as gastric secretions and salivary pH
- Muscle stimulation, as shown in electromyography
- Immune system responses
- Wound healing

- Heart rate control in response to either relaxing or anxiety-producing images
- Systolic and diastolic blood pressure changes in response to images of fear and anger

Jacobson demonstrated imagery's effect on motor responses in 1929, when he showed that subtle tensions of small muscles or sense organs result from imagining movement.[32] This aspect of imagery was applied in working with patients affected with parkinsonism. Mental images of movement have been demonstrated to help in freeing movement in unmoving body parts, particularly following stroke.[33-35] Patients with chronic hemiparesis worked with imagined wrist movements and imagined movements of reaching and manipulating objects, resulting in significant improvement that remained stable for 3 months.

Simonton and colleagues explored the effect of imagery on immune function and the application of this information in the treatment of cancer,[36] as did Achterberg and Lawlis.[37]

Hall studied the effect of hypnosis and imagery on immune modulation, noting increases in the number of lymphocytes and general increased immune system responsiveness.[1, 38] Schneider and colleagues demonstrated enhanced immune responsiveness in subjects working with imagery of white blood cells attacking germs. They also successfully used imagery to increase adherence, or "stickiness," of neutrophils.[39] Two factors affected the successful use of imagery in these studies. First, the biologic accuracy of the imagery appeared to be significant. Second, the ability to work with the imagery without straining at it played a part in significant outcomes.

One of the clearest reflections of the complex body-mind-spirit-environment interaction is in the chronic pain syndromes.[40-42] A study compared the effectiveness of two different types of imagery in the reduction of daily fibromyalgia pain. In the study, women were assigned to one of three groups. Group 1 received relaxation training and guided instruction in "pleasant imagery" to distract from the pain experience; group 2 received relaxation training and "attention imagery" instruction, encouraging the "active workings of the internal pain control systems"; group 3, the control group, received treatment as usual without any imagery. All of the patients in the study were also randomly assigned to treatment with either 50 mg/day of amitriptyline or a placebo pill. The results showed a significant difference in the reduction of pain in the group receiving the pleasant imagery, but not in the attention imagery group when compared with the control group. In addition, it was found that amitriptyline had no significant advantage over the placebo in reducing fibromyalgia pain during the course of the study.[43]

This information also reflects the fact that if an imagery intervention does not prove to be helpful for a particular patient, the practitioner should not be discouraged but instead should use creativity and try other imagery approaches. The attention imagery may have worked for some, just as the pleasant imagery was not effective with everyone. Statistical significance is helpful and points to a general understanding of effects, but it does not give us the final word on what works for an individual. This information may even suggest what works for an individual under one set of conditions, but it may not apply in other circumstances.

The richness of imagery as an intervention in working with children has been described in many clinical settings. Children's receptivity to imaginative play and interactions is an opening for the nurse's creative use of imagery. The effectiveness of imagery in the decrease of recurrent abdominal pain, in the reduction of postoperative pain, and in pediatric hospice pain management are all areas for additional nursing research.[44-48]

Our access to our imagination, our inner wisdom, and our inner healing resources are all elements of imagery work. Because anyone's experience of imagery is deeply subjective, imagery is a challenge to quantify and objectify through a process of quantitative research. Although research is a vital element in gaining recognition of the clinical value of this exciting and effective tool, research necessitates, by its nature, reducing the questions asked into dichotomous frameworks. Do we even know if it is the image, per se, that is effecting the change?

Or is it the focus, intentionality, and empowerment that we elicit in our patients when we provide them with education about inner skills and potentials that are ultimately creating the therapeutic effect? Imagery researcher Braud states, "Perhaps images are simply clothed intentions—specific intentions or focused intentions that have been dramatized or personified in imagery forms?"[49, p. 466]

Clinical Imagery and States of Consciousness

One of the pioneers and influential innovators in the clinical application of imagery into body-mind-spirit medicine was Dr. Roberto Assagioli, an Italian psychiatrist who introduced these techniques beginning in 1909.[50, 51] His concept of the wholeness of human consciousness, called *psychosynthesis*, has been extensively applied in the helping professions since 1965. He was personally most interested in developing a science of the higher self, a term that he used to describe the aspect of each person that holds inner wisdom and connection with life purpose. He saw the higher self as a developmental step latent inside each person.

Assagioli used imagery in three forms:[52]

1. Inner images, to explore the various levels of human experience, including biologic, social, and transpersonal experience.
2. Inner images, to represent the intentions and goals of the patient.
3. External images—the actual paintings and statues of his city, Florence, Italy—to help encourage transpersonal feelings in his patients. He often suggested that his patients go to a particular museum or church to meditate on a specific work of art because of the spiritual insights and feelings that the artist expressed in the work.

Within his body-mind-spirit context, Assagioli developed a set of principles he referred to as "psychological laws," which describe the interactive effects among images, ideas, emotions, physical responses, behaviors, attitudes, and impulses. According to one such law, "images or mental pictures tend to produce the physical conditions and the external acts that correspond to them." According to a second law, "attitudes, movements, and actions tend to evoke corresponding images and ideas; these, in turn, evoke or intensify corresponding emotions."[51, pp. 51-52] In these and other laws, Assagioli was seeking to outline the ability of the mind through imagery and intention to interact with, and positively affect, the body–mind for healing and psychospiritual growth.

Clinical Techniques in Imagery

It is clear that imagery affects our general physical state and our sense of emotional well-being. Patients with negative imagery will go into physical states of fear and nervous vigilance. If, instead, they choose to focus their minds on specific positive imagery, all of their physical systems will move toward states of ease and harmony. Imagery interacts with physiologic processes, sending messages and information from the right brain to the central nervous system.

Nurses may use specific, highly structured, guided body–mind, correct biological, and end-state imagery techniques. The use of symbolic drawing can also be introduced in the exploration process. Perhaps the most available use of imagery is the nurse's own impromptu imagery. Impromptu imagery is the nurse's unplanned use of an image that arises in her or his own imagery process during a clinical interaction. For example, an emergency room nurse, caring for a woman who had badly injured arms as a result of a car accident, was unable to establish an intravenous (IV) line because the woman's veins were collapsing. The situation was urgent, and there was discussion about the possible need to amputate an arm. The nurse, who had recently started studying clinical imagery, suddenly had an image of this woman holding a baby. She immediately suggested that the woman take a few moments and embrace her injured arm as if it were a tiny baby. She said, "Hold your arm, and send it loving energy." Within moments, the woman was calm, and the nurse was able to start the IV infusion.

Another nurse became aware of a patient's anxiety as she was preparing to administer a transfusion of packed cells. The woman had recently experienced several transfusion reactions and was fearful about the procedure. The nurse, who was meeting the patient for the first time, noticed that the cells had come from a source in Florida. She had an image of the blood donor basking on a warm Florida beach. The nurse told the woman where the blood supply had originated and suggested that she imagine these cells bringing the healing energy of the Florida sun and the gentle breeze of the beach to soothe and calm her. The patient immediately responded favorably to this suggestion, happy to have a calming image with which to engage her mind. The transfusion was a success.

Imagery in Holistic Health Coaching

Imagery clearly taps a deep level of self-knowledge in the patient. One example of this occurs in relationship imagery. In one instance, when a patient was asked to describe his relationship with his father, he offered a few familiar comments. But when he was asked to get an image of his father, the patient suddenly got in touch with the feelings of sadness and hopelessness that his father stimulated in him. This deeper level of self-knowledge allowed the patient to appreciate why he struggled with hopelessness in himself.[52]

Nurses are often working with patients and family members who are grieving past or imminent losses (see Chapter 17). Imagery is a valuable resource at this time because the connection with the loved one is alive in the imagination. People often feel strongly that they have communicated at an extremely deep, meaningful, and comforting way with internal imagery processes.[53, 54] These experiences may be helpful in making decisions, rehearsing new behaviors, understanding relationships, making life choices, and experiencing equanimity in the face of painful challenges.

Values and Spirituality

Nurses often are caring for patients at a stage in their lives when values and spirituality have become a central concern. Illness, divorce, ethical dilemmas, deaths, or other life crises often cause people to slow down and ask basic questions about how they are going to conduct their lives. Changes in physical capacities, the need to find different employment, decisions about education and lifestyle, and retirement all call on people to reassess their deepest values and their sense of spiritual purpose in life.

At these times, rational thought processes are not enough because they do not reveal the big picture. Imagery allows someone to imagine the actual results of a decision. For example, a nurse counseling a 59-year-old elementary school teacher struggling with a decision about retirement suggested that she close her eyes, focus on her breath, and imagine herself retired. After a few moments, the woman experienced an image of herself at home, looking bored and unhappy. She was frustrated with this image. She then tried to imagine her retirement as a time of new growth. She went back into the imagery, trying to imagine herself retiring and going back to school to study something new—she was unable to do so. Her imagination literally refused to see it. She then imagined herself doing service work in the community. Suddenly, during this imagery, she felt a peace and an ease settle into her experience.

Imagining pictures of the future helps a person to make specific behavioral and emotional changes. This information is invaluable for decision making because it provides a holistic level of information that is not available at the purely verbal level.

Transpersonal Use of Imagery

The transpersonal (beyond personality) level of human nature is a fact. Cultures throughout the world have used prayer, meditation, imagery, diet, physical training, contemplation and study, ritual, art, and many other methods to experience transpersonal states of consciousness. People seek these states because they tend to provide a subtler understanding of the universal patterns of reality and a more peaceful perspective on the "little self" living in the immensity of creation. Holistic nurses frequently cite their own transpersonal experiences as one of the reasons they became interested in introducing holistic methods into their work.

Motivated by their own development through such experiences, they desire to pass the potential of transpersonal experiences on to others.

The role of imagery in transpersonal experience is a crucial one. Holistic nurses can use transpersonal imagery to introduce patients safely to the transpersonal level of consciousness.[55-57] This imagery is referred to as transpersonal because it links and identifies the individual experience with universal processes. Transpersonal imagery taps into an expanded experience of the self, an experience that draws on human beings' capacity to connect deeply with the flow of life energy and creation. This connection, and the imagery that emerges from it, can be interpreted as a connection with God, with all of humanity, with a higher power, with the wonder of the universe and nature, or with the mysterious, nonverbal communication that occurs between people at the level of intuitive knowing and caring (see Chapters 4 and 7).

Visualization practice can be helpful for energizing and eliciting transpersonal experiences. Art images, photographs, and picture postcards are all sources for images that can be used in work with transpersonal symbols. The nurse can begin to collect art cards and other images that can be used to help patients. For example, one elderly woman hospitalized with advanced heart disease was feeling lonely, depressed, and fearful. She expressed fear that she was going to die. In sharing this with the nurse, she said she was confused by spirituality and did not know what she believed. The nurse asked if she would like to explore these feelings with imagery, and the woman agreed. The nurse led her in a brief relaxation and then suggested that she experience herself in a place that she felt was sacred. The woman was silent for a long time. The nurse sat silently with her. After a while, the woman opened her eyes. She was surprised by her imagery. She felt herself in Florence, Italy, a place she had never visited. She imagined walking the streets, looking at the beauty of the churches, and feeling deeply connected to the sacredness of the art. She said she always imagined Florence as a sacred place. She deeply loved Renaissance art and imagined the magic of a place where so much beauty had been created. She realized that her love of art was the closest thing she could identify as a spiritual feeling. Recognizing the importance of this imagery for the patient, the nurse said she would bring her a postcard of Florence. This pleased the woman, and the nurse told her that it would be important to honor this inner experience by keeping a reminder of it where she could connect with it over the course of the day.

Working with metaphors and symbols of transcendent experiences is an effective way to help a patient who is experiencing spiritual distress, hopelessness, and helplessness. Bringing a client into deep relaxation and then introducing one of these metaphors in an open-ended, exploratory way can be deeply meaningful. The patient can choose the symbol that he or she wants to explore, or the nurse can create the journey based on information from the patient. In times of illness and crisis, people may have spontaneous spiritual experiences and images. It is advisable to learn about these images so that patients can be supported and derive benefit from their experience (see **Table 12-1**).

Imagery with Disease and Illness

Much emphasis is placed on treating disease, the pathologic changes in organic form either observed or validated by laboratory tests. There is also a great need to address the individual's personal experience of his or her illness, general state of being, anxiety level, state of hopefulness or despair, and the meaning attributed to the situation. The nurse, using imagery, can promote a sense of well-being in clients and help them change their perceptions about their disease, treatment, and inner resources and innate healing ability. The use of an interactive approach to guided imagery with medical patients, which was designed to promote relaxation and cultivate healing intentions, has been significantly helpful in increasing patients' insights into their health problems.[58]

TABLE 12-1 Symbols and Metaphors of Transformation	
Symbol or Metaphor	**Transformative Experience**
Introversion	Exploration of the true self; self-knowledge; inner journey to the soul, to Beingness
Deepening/descent	Journey to the underworld of the psyche; confronting the difficult aspects of the self, the shadow; entering a cave; the heroic journey of facing fears
Ascent/elevation	Climbing a mountain to reach a higher plane of awareness
Expansion/broadening	Enlarging perspective; taking in the wholeness and seeing beyond one's small, individual perspective
Awakening	Awakening from the dream or from illusions; opening to the truth or reality of what really matters
Illumination	Bringing in the light of the human soul; spiritual light to transform or "enlighten" a situation; moving from darkness to light; bringing in life energy
Fire	Purification; spiritual alchemy; candles, lanterns, and bonfires; ceremonies of transformation
Development	Growth, blossoming; potentials waiting to become real
Love	Opening the heart; compassion and generosity; forgiveness
Path/pilgrimage	"Mystic way"; the journey of outward exploration; seeking to be changed by new experience or knowledge
Rebirth/regeneration	Birth of the new being; resurrection
Freedom/liberation	Liberation of psychic, physical, and spiritual energy to align with creation and creativity

Source: Reprinted by permission of SLL/Sterling Lord Literistic, Inc. Copyright © 1965 by Robert Assagioli.

Fear and negative imagery are not unusual in an individual with an undiagnosed or even a known illness. For example, a woman who discovers a palpable breast lump may conjure up frightening images before any tests or diagnoses. These images may include cancer, mastectomy, chemotherapy, radiation, hair loss, nausea and vomiting, severe pain, metastatic disease, the dying process, funeral, and the actual moment of dying. This process may be conscious or pre-verbal. It may be noticed in dreams, daydreams, spontaneous images, and kinesthetic sensings.

Concrete Objective Information

Over the last 30 years, nursing research has been conducted on the use of imagery in preparing patients for difficult procedures. Using concrete objective information and descriptions of a procedure is a form of imagery rehearsal. Its effectiveness lies in the importance of the prepared mind. People are fearful of the unknown and of feeling out of control. This technique addresses both of these fears.

Clients who receive information about both subjective and objective components of tests, procedures, and surgery recover more quickly. They are able to plan and use more effective coping strategies than clients who receive only one of the components. To prepare a patient for surgery, the nurse would describe what the person will experience at each stage of the procedure, including what will be felt, heard, seen, smelled, or tasted before, during, and after the operation. In addition, the imagery includes the sensory experiences of the postsurgical healing incision (e.g., pressure, smarting, tingling), as well as sensations over time (e.g., fleeting sharp sensations from the incision area when turning in bed or when coughing). **Table 12-2** lists sensations evoked by selected procedures.

Objective experiences are observable and verifiable by someone other than the person going through the procedure. Thus, for the surgical patient, an objective experience may include the time and place of the presurgery nurse's visit, the matters to be discussed during the visit, the preoperative preparation of the skin, placement on the stretcher to go to surgery, awakening in the recovery room, and expected sensations. This process reduces the likelihood that the patient will interpret normal sensations or events as signs that "something's wrong." It also allows the nurse and patient to plan specific strategies for the patient to handle difficult parts of the event.

The following procedural points related to the use of concrete, objective information originate in science-based nursing practice:

- Identify the sensory features of the procedure to be used.
- Determine the individual's perception of the procedure, treatment, or test to be experienced.
- Choose words that have meaning for the person.
- Use synonyms that have less emotional weight, such as *discomfort* instead of *pain*.
- Select specific experiences when giving examples, rather than abstract experiences (see Table 12-2).
- Help individuals reframe any negative imagery. For example, patients often fear chemotherapy and think of it as a poison because of all the precautions and side effects associated with it. It is important to have a way of framing the experience that is positive and focuses on healing. For example, the nurse may say, "Chemotherapy is powerful and effective in fighting the most vulnerable cells, the confused and incomplete cancer cells. The healthy cells—most of the cells in your body—are strong and protected."
- Plan specific strategies to be used at different stages of the procedure, such as using a breathing technique while waiting for the procedure to begin, and using imagery of a safe place during the procedure as a distraction from uncomfortable sensations.

Fears in Imagery Work

There are three predictable and understandable fears encountered in imagery work.

1. *Nothing will happen.* Patients fear that they will not be able to imagine anything in response to the nurse's imagery suggestion. Coincidentally, the nurse may share the

TABLE 12-2	Documented Subjective Experience Descriptors by Stressful Healthcare Event

Stressful Event	Descriptors
Gastroendoscopic examination	Intravenous medication; feel needlestick, drowsiness
	As air is pumped into stomach, feeling of fullness like after eating a large meal
	Feel physician's finger in mouth to guide tube insertion
Nasogastric tube insertion	Feeling passage of tube
	Tearing
	Gagging
	Discomfort in nose, throat, mouth
	Limited mobility
Cast removal	Hear buzz of saw
	Feel vibrations or tingling
	See chalky dust
	Feel warmth on arm or leg as saw cuts cast; will not hurt or burn
	Skin under padding looks and feels scaly and dirty
	Arm or leg may feel a little stiff when first trying to move it
	Arm or leg may feel light because cast was heavy
Barium enema	Lying on hard table
	Table feels hard
	Feel fullness
	Feel pressure
	Feel bloating
	Feel uncomfortable
	Feel as if might have a bowel movement
Abdominal surgery	Preoperative medications: feel sleepy, lightheaded, relaxed, free from worry, not bothered by most things, dryness of mouth
	Feel incision: tenderness, sensitivity, pressure, smarting, burning, aching, soreness
	Sensations might become sharp and feel like they are traveling along incision when moving
	Arm with intravenous tube feels awkward and restricted but not painful
	Feel tired after physical effort
	Bloating in abdomen
	Cramping due to gas pains
	Pulling and pinching when stitches are removed

TABLE 12-2	Documented Subjective Experience Descriptors by Stressful Healthcare Event (*continued*)
Stressful Event	**Descriptors**
Tracheostomy	When moving about, swallowing, or during suctioning: feel hurting, pressure, choking
Mastectomy — mean of 5.5 years postoperative	Arm or chest wall pain, "pins and needles," numbness, weakness, increased skin sensitivity, heaviness
	Phantom breast sensations, such as twinges, itching
4-vessel arteriography	Before contrast medium: table is hard, head taping is uncomfortable, cleansing solution is cold
	After contrast medium: hot, burning sensation in face, neck, chest, or shoulders

Source: This article was published in *Nursing Interventions: Essential Nursing Treatments,* 2nd ed., by G. Bulechek and J. McCloskey, p. 145, Copyright WB Saunders 1992.

same fear. The nurse may be afraid that the imagery method will produce nothing of worth for the patient.

The answer to this fear is to be curious about any experience that occurs during the course of the imagery. If, for example, the patient reports that her breathing became faster as soon as she heard the nurse's suggestion to relax, the nurse should be curious about why the patient believes her breathing became faster. The patient may respond that she was afraid of relaxing. On the surface, this may seem a strange statement. How can anyone be afraid of relaxing? In fact, relaxation can be frightening. For example, it can be frightening for someone who has experienced trauma in childhood and feels the importance of maintaining vigilance. Such information can be invaluable in actually helping the patient to enter states of relaxation safely and to engage in imagery work.

2. *Too much will happen.* Patients fear that the imagery will evoke difficult or even overwhelming thoughts and feelings. Coincidentally, the nurse may share the same fear. The nurse may fear that the imagery method will be too evocative and will have negative consequences for the patient.

The answer to this concern is that imagery does not take away a person's defenses. If the imagery suggestion is too evocative, the patient will simply fail to hear it, ignore it, change it into a suggestion that is easier

to work with, or open his or her eyes and stop the process. If a patient does have difficult thoughts and feelings in response to the imagery suggestion, these thoughts and feelings will develop because the patient is ready to receive them.

These statements presuppose that the nurse is skilled in imagery and is not imposing a manipulative imagery practice. Each patient has the potential for important new knowledge and new feeling. The nurse is not using imagery to make something happen. Rather, the nurse is using imagery to evoke what is already present in the patient. Carried out in this spirit, the nurse will not evoke any experiences for which the patient is not ready. The imagery suggestion will instead open the patient to the interior world of latent intuition, knowledge, and creative problem solving already present in the patient's imagination.

3. *It will be done wrong.* Anxious to please the nurse, patients fear that they cannot do imagery the "right way." Coincidentally, the nurse may also harbor the fear that there is a "right way" to do imagery and that his or her personal skills are inadequate for the "right way."

The answer to this fear is to realize that there is no right way. The processes of the imagination are unique to each person; thus, each imagery experience is unique. Furthermore, a nurse may use the same imagery suggestion twice, and the same patient may experience two totally different responses to the imagery. It is important to realize that the patient's experience is the center of all imagery work. The nurse may suggest imaging a walk in an open field, and the patient may respond by imaging the atmosphere in a dark room. The dark room becomes of importance. The original suggestion of an open field is no longer significant. The meaning of the dark room for the patient becomes the source of interest and new learning. The nurse's imagery suggestion is simply that— a suggestion—to evoke the latent powers and intelligence of the imagination in the service of the patient. Imagery techniques can be studied for many years, imagery skills can be honed, and yet it remains the unique response of the patient that is central to the work.

Holistic Caring Process

Holistic Assessment

In preparing to use imagery as a nursing intervention, the nurse assesses the following parameters:

- The client's potential for organic brain syndrome or psychosis to determine if general relaxation techniques should be used instead of imagery techniques.
- The client's anxiety/tension levels to determine which types of relaxation inductions will be most effective.
- The client's hopes in regard to the session and reason for seeking help.
- The client's wants, needs, desires, or recurrent and dominant themes.
- The client's understanding that it is not necessary to literally hear, see, feel, touch, or taste when working with imagery; that it is best to trust the inner experience in whatever form the information comes.
- The client's primary sensory modalities when he or she experiences the imagination— visual, auditory, kinesthetic, and so forth.

- The client's understanding that imagery is basically a way in which we communicate with ourselves at a deep level.
- The client's understanding that imagery can bring us into contact with our body and find out what it needs.
- The client's previous experiences with the imagery process.
- The client's emotional comfort level with closing eyes, bringing attention inside, and opening to states of internal awareness; if the client is not comfortable with closing the eyes, the nurse can suggest just lowering the eyes and gazing at a point on the floor approximately 1 or 2 feet in front of him or her. This will cause the client's peripheral vision to blur, eyelids will usually get heavy, and then the eyes will close effortlessly. Some clients need to learn to trust that it is safe to relax, that they are experiencing a natural phenomenon.
- The client's knowledge of relaxation skills; if not skilled in relaxation, the client may need an explanation of what the normal sensations will be and time to shift to the "letting go" state. Once the client becomes skilled at entering a relaxed state, a selected word, phrase, or hand posture can become a signal to relax.
- The client's ability to maintain attention and not drowse off in the session.

Identification of Patterns/Challenges/Needs

The following are the patterns/challenges/ needs (see Chapter 8) compatible with imagery interventions:

- Social isolation
- Role performance
- Caregiver role strain
- Parental role strain
- Spiritual well-being
- Spiritual distress
- Altered effective coping
- Impaired adjustment
- Ineffective denial
- Potential for growth
- Decision conflict
- Health-seeking behaviors

- Sleep pattern disturbance
- Relocation stress syndrome
- Altered self-concept
- Disturbance in body image
- Disturbance in self-image
- Potential hopelessness
- Potential powerlessness
- Pain
- Anxiety
- Fear
- Post trauma response
- Grief

Outcome Identification

Exhibit 12-1 guides the nurse in client outcomes, nursing prescriptions, and evaluations for the use of imagery as a nursing intervention.

Therapeutic Care Plan and Interventions

Facilitation and Interpretation of the Imagery Process

It is essential for nurses to become aware of their own imagery process and familiarize themselves with the rich variety and individuality of imagery experiences. When nurses come together in a group to listen and share personal and professional stories, they hear many perspectives. They can train themselves to listen to the use of metaphors and images and learn from the different types of experiences.

To facilitate the imagery process, the nurse serves as a guide. There is no way to predict what will surface in a client's imagination. Every experience is different, even when the same script is used.

EXHIBIT 12-1   Nursing Interventions: Imagery

Nursing Prescriptions

Following an assessment, guide the client in an imagery exercise.

Assess the client's levels of anxiety with this new process.

After the imagery process experience, assess its effectiveness through client dialogue.

Encourage the client to recognize daily self-talk and the images that lead to balance and inner peace.

Help the client to create images of desired health habits, feelings, and desires for daily living.

Teach the client coping, power over daily events, and the ability to move toward a healthy lifestyle.

Teach the client to recognize images leading to self-defeating lifestyle habits.

Encourage the client to draw images and symbols as a communication process with self.

Evaluation

The client participated in imagery exercise by choice.

The client demonstrated no signs of anxiety with the imagery process.

The client stated that the imagery experience was helpful.

The client reported using self-dialogue with imagery.

The client reported creating images of desired health habits, feelings, and desires for daily living.

The client reported increased coping with daily stressors.

The client reported recognition of negative images leading to self-defeating behavior; the client created positive images.

The client used drawing as a communication process with self.

Client Outcomes

The client will demonstrate skills in imagery.

Nurses who are unfamiliar with imagery and guiding should learn a few basic relaxation and imagery scripts and practice on themselves by making tapes of their own voice and following their own guiding. This will help build confidence with the intervention. It is helpful to learn a variety of scripts pertaining to common problems in clinical practice, such as preoperative anxiety, recovery from surgery, postoperative coughing, effective wound healing, fear, anxiety, pain, and relationship problems. For scripts not frequently used, some nurses keep a notebook or reference book handy. In studying clinical imagery, the nurse needs to be willing to open up and learn it from the inside out, using imagery for personal change and development.

Each individual is the best interpreter of his or her own imagery process. Symbolic information that surfaces in the imagination is rich with personal meaning. Many people have been closed off from or afraid of their imagination. Nurses should encourage clients to record their images in a diary or journal for further exploration. It is easy to lose symbolic imagery in the conscious thoughts that dominate one's attention during a busy day.

When teaching imagery, the nurse listens to the way that a client tells his or her story to get a sense of the client's outlook and orientation to the world. Does the client have a materialistic, concrete outlook on problem solving and life in general, or a more intuitive, spontaneous perspective? For the logical, concrete thinker, written information is useful. For example, if using imagery for hand warming, the nurse may prepare an imagery teaching sheet that includes specific physiologic information and instructions such as the following:

- An explanation of normal blood flow physiology
- A drawing of blood flow to the hands via radial and ulnar arteries that branch into intricate blood vessel networks of the hands and the fingers
- Examples of images that warm the hands

Less structure is necessary for the more intuitive patient. The nurse can go directly to working with imagery and use the teaching sheets to support what the vivid imager has learned.

There is no need to follow teaching sheets explicitly. Suggested images are adapted to fit what feels right to the client. Teaching sheets refresh and reinforce the teaching–learning session and provide additional information to be mastered. Clients can add their own notes about specific images and personalize their practice. The nurse can help clients rework weak or erroneous imagery so that it more accurately reflects healthy outcomes (e.g., images focusing on weak, confused, cancer cells and a strong immune system instead of vice versa).

Guided Imagery Scripts

The guidelines that follow help the nurse in the effective implementation of imagery scripts as nursing interventions:

- Start the session with an induction, a general relaxation—focusing on breath, shortened passive progressive relaxation, or body awareness, for example. (Also see Chapter 11.)
- Reaffirm that there is no right or wrong way for the client to do imagery, that whatever occurs is useful information, and that the client has complete control over the process (e.g., deciding whether to continue or to stop).
- Follow the induction instructions for yourself so that you communicate a calming presence.
- Personalize the imagery by using the client's name or other specific references several times during the process.
- Speak slowly and smoothly, allowing for pauses and silence after each suggestion.
- Observe the client's body language and breathing rhythm to assess responses to suggestions.
- If there are signs of tension, such as shallow breathing, tightness of muscles, or tense facial muscles in response to an imagery suggestion, ask, "What are you experiencing now?"
- If the client appears to be struggling to get into the imagery, pause in the script and

suggest that the client reconnect with the breath and go more deeply into relaxation.

- Avoid saying "yes" or "right" or other words that communicate evaluative reactions to the client's experience. A more supportive comment such as "stay with your experience" can be made.
- Provide encouragement and guidance for those with less vivid imagery. Vivid imagers, on the other hand, prefer more silence: words may be distracting or intrusive to them. Extremely vivid imagers may prefer to keep their eyes partially open to prevent feeling overwhelmed.
- End the session by bringing the person's awareness back to the room. You can do this by encouraging the person to begin to transition back to the room by becoming aware of his or her body in the chair or the bed, by bringing awareness to his or her breath, and then slowly opening his or her eyes. An example of another classic reintegration method is: "At the count of five, you will be fully awake and alert . . . one . . . two . . . three . . . four . . . five."

Induction for Imagery A simple breathing technique or other relaxation technique may be useful to focus the client's mind inward and induce imagery. This allows awareness of subtler aspects of experience to become available to the person. This inward focus can be thought of as reducing external stimuli so that the inner awareness is enhanced.

The following induction script can be used as a preparation for most imagery interventions. It is especially appropriate for a person who needs assistance quieting the body. Resting the hands on the lower abdomen and breathing into the belly (diaphragmatic breathing) is an effective calming posture. In this position, the palms of the hands are resting on the body's energy center. By noting the slowing of breathing, relaxation of facial muscles, and changes in skin color, the nurse can assess the effectiveness of the relaxation technique. The induction for imagery can take 5 to 10 minutes. The most common mistake that new imagery practitioners make is to move too quickly through the suggestions. Go slowly. Allow your client time to connect with a subtler awareness. Learn to become comfortable with silent pauses.

> **Script:** Make yourself comfortable and close your eyes. . . . Put your hands gently on your lower abdomen, just below your navel. . . . Bring all of your attention to the sensations in your hands. . . . Notice the slight rise and fall of your hands as they move with your breathing. . . . Notice the tactile sensations of the surfaces of your hands and fingers. . . . Bring all of your awareness into these sensations. . . . [pause] Now notice the temperature of your hands. . . . [pause] Notice their weight. . . . [pause] Now notice any sensations inside the skin, perhaps tingling or pulsing. . . . [pause] Now bring your attention to the center of your chest and be aware of the sensations. . . . Notice the movement of your chest with each breath . . . the passage of breath into your lungs . . . the tactile sensations of your skin . . . perhaps an awareness of your heartbeat. . . . [pause] Now bring your awareness to your nose and be aware of breath passing through your nostrils. . . . Notice the slight cool sensations of the air touching the inside of your nose.

Connecting with Life Energy Imagery This imagery, which draws on a person's sense of his or her inner energy, focuses on the fact that the body is not just sick. The life force is operating without any conscious effort. This awareness can reframe a person's attitude, bringing a connection with inner healing mechanisms and with what is functioning healthfully, as opposed to focusing on the disease process.

> **Script:** Bring your awareness to your imagination and take a moment to reflect on all of the systems that are functioning in your body–mind at this moment . . . your heart and your circulatory system . . . [pause] your immune system   [pause] your respiratory system . . . [pause] your senses. . . . [pause] Be aware of all of these. . . . [pause] Realize

that you don't need to do anything to make these systems function. . . . They are part of your body's wisdom. . . . [pause] And now be aware that deep within you is a source of life energy . . . a vital spark that has been a part of you since the moment of your conception. . . . It has always been a part of you . . . guiding and energizing your body and mind. . . . Use your imagination to get in touch with this source of life energy. . . . Trust whatever information your imagination gives you. . . . Locate this source in your body. . . . Feel its strength and energy. . . . [pause] Allow your intuition to give you an image or symbol for this source and when you have the image, spend some time with it. . . . [pause] If it feels right, communicate with it. . . . What does it need from you? . . . [pause] If there is anything else that needs to happen in relation to this image, let it happen. . . . Take your time. . . . When you feel ready, bring your awareness back to the room.[59]

B. G. Schaub, "Imagery in Health Care: Connecting with Life Energy," Alternative Health Practitioner 1, no. 2 (1995): 113–115.

Special or Safe Place Imagery Clients need to identify a special place that is a safe retreat. This is an easy place for novices to start. It takes 10 to 20 minutes. Several different approaches can be useful. The first script is more open ended and less specific. The ones that follow are more descriptive. People have different preferences as to what is most helpful.

Script: Let your imagination choose a place that is safe and comfortable . . . a place where you can retreat at any time. This is a healthy technique for you to learn. . . . This place will help you with your daily stressors. [If the client is in the hospital] This safe and special place is very important, particularly while you are in the hospital. . . . Any time that there are interruptions, just let yourself go to this place in your mind.

Form a clear image of a pleasant outdoor scene, using all of your senses. . . . Breathe . . . smell the fragrances around you. Feel . . . feel the texture of the surface under your feet. Hear . . . hear all of the sounds in nature, birds singing, wind blowing. See . . . see all of the different sights around

as you let yourself turn in a slow circle to get a full view of this special space. [Include taste, if appropriate.]

Let a beam of light, such as the rays of the sun, shine on you for comfort and healing. Allow yourself to experience the warmth and relaxation. Form an image of a meadow. Imagine that you are in the meadow. . . . The meadow is full of beautiful grass and flowers. In the meadow, see yourself sitting by a stream . . . watching the water . . . flowing by . . . slowly and gently.

Imagine a mountain scene. See yourself walking on a path toward the mountain. You hear the sound of your shoes on the path . . . smell the pine trees and feel the cool breeze as you approach your campsite. You have now reached the foothills of the mountain. You are now higher up the mountain . . . resting in your campsite. Look around at the beauty of this place.

Imagine yourself in a bamboo forest. . . . You are walking in a large bamboo forest. The bamboo is very tall. . . . You lean against a strong cluster of bamboo . . . hear the swaying . . . and hear the rustling of the bamboo leaves, gently moving in the wind. . . . Look into the sky of your mind. . . . See the fluffy clouds. A cloud gently comes your way. . . . The cloud surrounds your body. You climb up on the cloud and lie down. Feel yourself begin to float off gently in a gentle breeze.

Worry and Fear Imagery Some images can help clients change the internal experience of worry and fear. Clients should set aside 10 to 20 minutes a day to worry, preferably in the morning before they start their daily routines. This approach reassures the subconscious that it has worried, and the person has greater success at stopping the habitual worry during the rest of the day.

Script: Let worries come one by one. . . . Just watch as one replaces the other. As you do this for a short period of time, feel the experience that occurs with each of those worries and fears. Notice how just having a worry or fear changes your state right now.

Stop the images. Focus on your breathing . . . in . . . and out. . . . Allow yourself to have three complete cycles of breathing before continuing. . . . In your relaxed state, become aware of these feelings of relaxed body–mind. This time, take your relaxed state with you into your imagination. Let one worry come to your mind right now. See and feel it. . . . See yourself in that situation relaxed and at ease.

Right now, just say to yourself, "I can stop this worry." Imagine yourself functioning without that worry or fear. See yourself waving goodbye to that worry and fear. See yourself completely free of that worry and fear. Look at the decisions that you can make for your life that will lead you in new directions. Feel your energy as you breathe in. As you exhale, let go of all of the worry, fear, tension, and tightness.

Experience your comfortable body–mind. Know that you can work with many of your worries and fears that surface daily. Whenever they come, let the dominant worry surface. . . . Then feel what it is like as you gradually give up portions of the worry . . . until it is completely gone. If that seems impossible right now, decide which part of that worry and fear you need to keep and which part you can let go. And now, see yourself waving goodbye to the part that you can let go.

Now, feel what it is like in your mind with part of that worry or fear gone. Experience that and feel the changes within the body. Assess the part of the worry or fear that remains. Again, allow a portion of that worry or fear to move away. See yourself waving goodbye. Feel the change inside as more is released.

Let yourself now be in a place where the worry and fear are diminished. Assess what part remains and see if you can now begin to give up that part. Pay attention to the experiences inside your body as you do this.

This script has many variations: writing worries and fears on a seashell and watching a seagull pick up the shell and drop it into the sea; running along a road, dropping the worries and fears by the road, and watching the wind blow them away; letting a picture of worries and fears flow forward in a moving stream. This basic script can also be individualized by putting into words what the client revealed before the session.

Inner Guide Imagery The nurse can assist the client in creating purposeful self-dialogue that gains access to the inner wisdom and personal truth that naturally reside within each of us. It is advisable to allow 10 to 20 minutes for this exercise.

> **Script:** As you begin to feel even more relaxed now . . . going to a deeper place within . . . feeling deeply relaxed . . . peaceful and safe . . . let yourself become aware of a sense of not being alone. With you right now is a guide . . . who is wise and concerned with your well-being. Let yourself begin to see this wise being with whom you can share your fears or your joys. You have a trust in this wise being.
>
> If you do not see anyone, let yourself be aware of hearing or feeling this wise being, noticing the presence of care and concern. In whatever way seems best for you, proceed to make contact with this wise inner guide. Let yourself establish contact with your guide now . . . in any way that comes. Your guide may appear to you in any form, such as a person, an animal, an inner presence or peace . . . or as an image of the very wisest part of you.
>
> Notice the love and wisdom with which you are surrounded. This wisdom and love are present for you now. . . . Let yourself ask for advice . . . about anything that is important for you just now. Be receptive to what emerges. . . . Let yourself receive some new information. This inner guide may have a special message to share with you. . . . Listen with openness and pure intention to receive.
>
> Allow yourself to look at any issue in your life. It may be a symptom, a choice, or a decision. . . . Tell your wise guide anything that you wish. . . . Listen to the answers that emerge. Imagine yourself acting on the answers and directions that you received. . . . Imagine yourself calling on the wisdom and love of this wise guide to help you in the days to come. Now in whatever way is best for you . . . bring closure to the visit with this inner guide. You can come back here any time that you wish. All you have to do is take the time.

This script helps clients gain an awareness of their own inner wisdom. It is best to introduce this exercise after a client has done several imagery sessions. Word choices should take into account the client's dominant sense. If a client prefers the visual, for example, the nurse uses the word *see*; if the client prefers the auditory, the word *hear*; if the client prefers the kinesthetic, the word *feel*.

Seeking an inner guide can be done over many sessions. The client should be aware that many different guides or advisors will surface over time. The guide may also appear as a traditional religious figure such as a shaman, the Virgin Mary, a saint, Moses, or Buddha. It can be interesting and surprising when someone meets a spiritual figure not from his or her own religious tradition. The guide may also emerge as an admired historical or living person such as a favorite author or artist, a philosopher, or a heroic leader such as Martin Luther King, Jr.

There are many versions of this script, so the nurse can add, invent, and explore. Much detail can be added to this imagery script to lengthen the session. When time is extended, a wealth of insight can emerge for the client. The nurse should pause frequently and let a few moments pass in silence during the guiding, as indicated by his or her intuition.

Pain Reduction Imagery   The red ball of pain. To decrease psychophysiologic pain, clients can learn to use distraction. This kind of imagery is good for both acute and chronic pain, as well as for the discomfort or pain of procedures. It takes 10 to 20 minutes.

> **Script:** Scan your body. . . . Gather any pains, aches, or other symptoms up into a ball. Begin to change its size. . . . Allow it to get bigger. . . . Just imagine how big you can make it. Now make it smaller. . . . See how small you can make it. . . . Is it possible to make it the size of a grain of sand? Now allow it to move slowly out of your body, moving farther away each time you exhale. . . . Notice the experience with each exhale . . . as the pain moves away.

Give suggestions to the client to change the size of the ball several times in both directions. This serves as a distraction and an exercise in manipulating the pain experience rather than being trapped or overwhelmed by it. This imagery provides a tremendous sense of control as well as pain relief for the client. The person's body cues indicate how many times to go in each of the opposite directions.

Pain Assessment Imagery   Imagery helps access and control both acute and chronic psychophysiologic pain. The following exercise can be done in 10 to 20 minutes.

> **Script:** Close your eyes and let yourself relax. . . . Begin to describe the pain in silence to yourself. Be present with the pain. . . . Know that the pain may be either physical sensations . . . or worries and fears. Let the pain take on a shape . . . any shape that comes to your mind. Become aware of the dimensions of the pain. . . . What is the height of the pain? . . . The width of the pain? . . . And the depth of the pain? Where in the body is it located? . . . Give it color . . . a shape. . . . Feel the texture. Does it make any sound?
>
> And now with your eyes still closed, let your hands come together with palms turned upward as if forming a cup. Put your pain object in your hands. [Once again, the nurse asks these questions about the pain, preceding each question with this phrase, "How would you change the size, etc.?"]
>
> Let yourself decide what you would like to do with the pain. There is no right way to finish the experience. . . . Just accept what feels right to you. You can throw the pain away . . . or place it back where you found it . . . or move it somewhere else. Let yourself become aware . . . of how pain can be changed. . . . By your focusing with intention, the pain changes.

It is not unusual for the pain to go completely away, or at least lessen after this exercise. The client also learns to manipulate the pain so that it is not the controlling factor of his or her life. The exercise is also effective with severe pain. After giving pain medication, the nurse can have the client relax during the imagery process.

Correct Biologic Imagery Teaching Sheets and Scripts

The nurse elicits from a client or patient images and symbols that have special healing meaning and value, and then makes an audio recording for the client or patient that includes correct biologic images, specific concrete objective information, specific symbols, and specific types of imagery.

It may seem that the following scripts are suitable only for well-educated, sophisticated individuals, but this is not the case. However, it is necessary for the nurse to assess the individual's education level and adapt these scripts to fit the person's needs and cultural beliefs. Imagery is an important tool, particularly for those clients who do not read.

Bone Healing Imagery   An imagery exercise for bone healing may be done in 20 to 30 minutes.[56] Prior to imagery, to teach basic biologic imagery of bone healing, the nurse should explain the following concepts:

- *Reaction (cellular proliferation).* Within the hematoma surrounding the fracture, cells and tissues proliferate and develop into a random structure.
- *Regeneration (callus formation).* At 10 to 14 days after the fracture, the cells within the hematoma become organized in a fibrous lattice. With sufficient organization, the callus becomes clinically stable. The callus obliterates the medullary canal and surrounds the two ends of bone by irregularly surrounding the fracture defect.
- *Remodeling (new bone formation).* Approximately 25 to 40 days after the fracture, calcium is laid down within the bone that has spicules perpendicular to the cortical surface. Osteonal bone gradually replaces and remodels fiber bone. The fracture has been bridged over by new bone. Conversion and remodeling continue up to 3 years following an acute fracture.

Immune System Odyssey Imagery   Patients can be taught correct biologic images of the normal process of the immune system.[60, pp. 317-328] The nurse should explain the following concepts prior to the imagery exercise:

- *Neutrophils.* The most numerous cells, billions of neutrophils swim in the bloodstream; when they sense unhealthy tissue, they pass through the blood vessel, move to the unhealthy tissue or cells, surround it, shoot caustic chemicals, and destroy the unhealthy tissue or cells.
- *Macrophages.* Moving throughout the body, always ready to eat, macrophages travel in hordes; each one swells up, consuming the enemy (e.g., bacteria, viruses, yeast, cancer cells).
- *T cells.* Born in the bone marrow, millions of T cells go from infancy to adolescence each minute. They go to the thymus gland, where they get a special imprint; some are designated killer cells, while others become helpers or suppressors. All of these specialized cells keep a watchful vigil in the lymph nodes and tissue until needed.
- *B cells.* For years, B cells wait and mature in the bone marrow until needed. They can change like caterpillars to butterflies, becoming plasma cells that manufacture magic bullets—the protein called *antibodies*. Operating like a guided missile, they can shoot the target, paralyze the enemy, shoot caustic chemicals, and explode the bad cells and tissue. B cells can clone themselves and create whatever number it takes to win the battle.

In 20 to 30 minutes, the nurse can guide the client through an intervention, modifying the script as needed.

Script: You are about to embark on the most incredible journey imaginable, a journey through your own immune system, touching your body's healing forces with your mind; you will sense, feel, and envision a miracle. A miracle of defense and protection, a miracle of the billions of honorable, persistent warriors within you that have but one mission: to guard you from disease, injury, and invasion.

To fully appreciate this odyssey, which is as complex as it is magnificent, it is important to clear and focus your mind, which will help you relax your body. The bridge between your mind and body is easily crossed when your mental distractions are released, when a sense of peace and calm spreads warmly from the top of your head to your toes. As you let go of stress, your immune system is activated. Relax, now, as you participate in and observe your own healing process.

As your mind becomes clearer and clearer, feel it becoming more and more alert. Somewhere deep inside of you, a brilliant light begins to glow. Sense this happening. . . . The light grows brighter and brighter and more intense. . . . This is your body–mind communication center. Breathe into it. . . . Energize it with your breath. The light is powerful and penetrating, and a beam begins to grow from it. The beam shines through your body into any area you wish. It is your searchlight, your bridge into the glorious mysteries about to unfold. Practice shining it into your body. Sometimes this is easier to do than other times. Just allow it to happen.

The immune journey begins inside your bones. So, take this most intelligent beam of light and shine it into a long bone . . . a leg bone perhaps. Penetrate deeply into the marrow. This is the birthing center for all of your blood cells. Just imagine if you can, . . . feel if you can, . . . billions . . . of young cells being born . . . many kinds, each with a task to nurture and protect you. As we go through this exercise, we will focus on a few types of cells that are vital to defending you. They have names: neutrophils, macrophages, T cells, B cells, natural killer cells. One by one, we will shine the light on them, watching them work to guard, protect, and remove cells that no longer serve you.

The most numerous cells are called *neutrophils*. They eat and engulf the invaders in a most ingenious way. Imagine them maturing, moving into your bloodstream, floating, ever alert for a call to work in your defense. As a call warns them of an invader, they become exceedingly alert. No longer swimming freely, millions, billions of them sense the danger and move methodically and directly, preparing for attack. The blood vessels become sticky, attracting the neutrophils to their surface. The small opening in the blood vessel walls dilates in the vicinity of the attack.

Imagine the neutrophils being attracted to the walls. They move quickly along the vessel walls until they know with absolute certainty that the invader is near. Now, they extend a small foot, a pseudopod, into the walls, and changing shape, they slither through, entering your tissues. Moving forward now, as they approach the invader, they send another small foot out, surrounding the enemy, shooting caustic chemicals into it, wearing it thin. The enemy is halted, destroyed, may even explode into harmless bits. Imagine this happening, constantly, protecting you from the dangers of living in a hostile world. Billions and billions of neutrophils are born every day.

Now, shining the beam of light back into the bone marrow, imagine the macrophages, or the giant eaters . . . fewer of them, but with long lives and many talents. As they mature, watch them move into tissues and organs and blood. They line the walls of the lungs and liver . . . waiting, surveying, watching, constantly ready to move. Bacteria, viruses, yeast cells, even cancer cells trigger the alarm. As the warning of an invader sounds, the macrophages swell up, becoming large and powerful. They may even mesh together with the other macrophages, moving rapidly in a powerful, connecting flank. They reach out for the enemy, lasso it with their arm-like extensions, and bring the invader into their bodies, injecting it with potent enzymes. With lightning speed, they consume an enemy. What they can't destroy, they encircle and preserve, protecting you from its dangerous acts. The macrophages are also your scavengers. They can and will digest anything and everything in your body that you no longer have use for. Imagine this happening for a moment.

The macrophages and neutrophils are nonspecific, nondiscriminating in their attack and cleanup activities. Other cells, the lymphocytes, or the T cells and the B cells, have an assigned function, a target that they spend their entire lives stalking. It might be a special virus, or bacteria, or cancer cell, or other foreign tissue. Let's look at these cells in action.

Shining the beam, again, into the bone marrow, observe the T cells being born. Millions . . . more than you could possibly count . . . move from infancy to adolescence each minute. The T cells will each be given a special task as they are processed in the thymus gland. Shine your imagery light into the middle of your chest; here is the thymus gland. Feel it pulsating with energy. Watch, now, as the adolescent T cells flow in rapidly, each touched with a spark of wisdom, each challenged with a mission. Some will be killers, assassins with a single target. Others will be helpers for your B cells. Still others will be suppressors, signaling that the battle is over, protecting your body from excessive immune activity. Imagine these—the killers, the helpers, and the suppressors—maturing quickly and with glorious specificity in your thymus. When each has been imprinted, they leave the thymus to go about their tasks. The T cells keep a wakeful vigil in your lymph nodes, your spleen, and other lymph tissue. Think of this for a time. . . .

Back in the bone marrow once again, the B cells are highlighted by the beam. They mature and move into the lymph tissues and blood, waiting for the encounter. Each has a specific enemy to protect you from, and they can wait patiently for years, patrolling, waiting, and watching. When the encounter finally takes place, the B cells change, like cocoons into butterflies, becoming a plasma cell. The plasma cells manufacture magic bullets, which are proteins called *antibodies*. Each antibody is like a guided missile. . . . It moves directly for its target and hooks on to it, like a key in a lock. The enemy is paralyzed and its surface damaged. Other chemicals are liberated in the blood by this action, and they burn holes in the wall of the enemy, causing an explosion. The B cells also clone themselves, creating whatever number is needed to do pure and perfect battle in your defense.

One last time, peering into the birthing center of the immune system, the light shines onto natural killer cells. The natural killers are wondrous defenses against cancer. Like viruses and bacteria, cancer cells are not especially unusual in the human body. The body simply recognizes them as invaders and sends out the forces of defense. Only in the most unusual circumstances (e.g., when cancer cells wear a disguise) does the immune system fail to find them. Watch now, as the natural killer cells are born and move into the bloodstream. Take the light and shine it on one cell, and watch its action. Ever alert, it senses a cancer cell in the vicinity. Moving at lightning speed, it collides with the cancer cell. Its mere touch paralyzes the cell. Fingers of the natural killer cell reach into the cancer cell, oozing in its power and might. Then, a small cannon-like structure within the natural killer cell tilts, aims, and fires deadly chemicals into the cancer cell. Already paralyzed, the cancer cell develops blisters, peels like an orange. Its cellular matter dissolves, leaving only harmless skeletal remains. The natural killer cell, alive and well, continues its alert patrol of your body.

Before you end this exercise, go over the immune process once more, sensing all of the immune cells working in a superbly coordinated team of defense. In the bone marrow, billions of cells are being born each minute, in exactly the number and combinations that you need to stay healthy. As the white blood cells mature, each develops a remarkable intelligence. Each has a dedicated task. Witness these cells moving out of the bone marrow, into blood tissue, watching and waiting for the opportunity to protect and cleanse you. Feel the presence of these magnificent guardians, and sense their power. These dedicated warriors, this system of defense has a universe of its own. That universe is you. By relaxing, as you have just done, and concentrating on this process, you have actively participated in keeping yourself healthy.[32]

Imagery and Drawing

In the imagery process, drawing is an effective way to open up communication with the self and others. It externalizes previously internal mental images and emotions. The emphasis in this intervention is not on how well the client can draw but on the client's ability to get in touch with feelings and healing potential through drawing. Drawing, as a way of externalizing inner images and deepening understanding of inner processes, may be a safer way to talk about difficult feelings. When clients are overwhelmed with emotions, drawing images of the feelings can be therapeutic. Drawing is especially helpful with children who are not verbally sophisticated.

Drawing after being guided through an imagery exercise can bring further insights. The creativity that is evoked is different from the logical mode of explaining the experiences in words. This creative process can also evoke transcendent experiences and healing energy. Drawing works well when a client is crying and is unable to talk easily but wants to express what he or she is experiencing. When introducing drawing, the nurse can make some of the following suggestions:

- Express yourself with a few images. There is no one correct way to draw. Drawings can be either realistic or symbolic. The most important thing is that you express yourself in a nonlogical way. This can bring new awareness and understanding into your life.
- If you find that you are too focused on the result of the drawing exercise, use your nondominant hand. With your eyes closed, allow yourself to get into the expressive quality of drawing.
- Do not judge your drawing. Allow your body, mind, and spirit to connect as you begin simply to be with the paper and crayons in the present moment.
- Notice the energy flow from you. Let your body energy resonate with your imagery and spirit energy. Let the energies slowly begin to resonate together. Do not try to control the process because this inner quality comes from being immersed in the imagery and drawing experience.
- On the blank piece of paper, allow an image to begin to form that represents your feelings and thoughts in this moment. Choose colors that speak to you. If you wish to change the color that you started working with, feel free to do so.
- After you have drawn, you might want to write some details of your images. Often, what you felt or heard during the imagery drawing may surface into conscious awareness and provide new insights about your important images.

When working with drawing for a client's specific disease or symptoms, it is helpful for the nurse to educate the client about the body processes that are being affected. It is therapeutic for the client to have an understanding of, and an image for, the healthful state; the disease or symptoms and the medication, treatments, and associated procedures; and his or her personal belief systems. Asking the client to draw the disease or symptoms in a way that has self-meaning often reveals a client's constricted view of healing possibilities or misunderstanding of the disease or symptoms, either of which may impair recovery. The drawing process helps the client recognize that the disease need not control his or her life. Insight from drawing helps the client reframe experiences of illness, let go of the inner judgments and struggles, and mobilize his or her creativity for achieving desired outcomes.

Some of the challenges for nurses are to develop innovative teaching worksheets, booklets, and verbal descriptions of body–mind healing; to integrate imagery as part of each nursing interaction and intervention; and to develop assessment tools.[60] The nurse and client should identify the following elements for the best outcome:

- *Disease or disability.* The vividness of the client's view of the disease, illness, or disability and, if the process is ongoing, the strength of the disease or illness to decrease health or the client's focus on the reverse—the vividness and the strength of the client's ability to stabilize the disease or illness or stop the process.
- *Internal healing resources.* The vividness of the client's perception of his or her healing ability and the effectiveness of this ability to combat the disease.
- *External healing resources.* The vividness of the treatment description and the effectiveness of the positive mechanism of action.

Case Study (Implementation)

Case Study

Setting: Coronary care unit (CCU), followed by outpatient cardiac rehabilitation program
Client: J. D., a 48-year-old man with acute myocardial infarction complicated by congestive heart failure and pericarditis secondary to the infarction

Patterns/Challenges/Needs:

1. Decreased cardiac output related to mechanical factors (congestive heart failure)
2. Altered comfort related to inflammation (pericarditis)
3. Anxiety related to acute illness and fear of death

The nurse asked J. D. several questions to explore with him his psychospiritual state. Following the interaction, the nurse felt that further exploration of the negative images that he conveyed and the meaning behind them was essential to his recovery. She asked him if he wanted to pursue some new ideas that might help him access his inner healing resources and strengths. He said that he would.

Nurse: In your recovery now with your heart healing, how do you experience your healing?

J. D.: There is this sac around my heart, and every time I take a deep breath, my breath is cut off by the pain [pericarditis]. My heart is like a broken vase. I don't think it is healing.

Nurse: I can understand why you are discouraged. However, some important things that are present right now show that you are better than when you first came to the CCU. Your persistent chest pain is gone, and your heartbeats are now regular. If you focus on what is going right, you can help your heart and lift your spirits. Let me help you learn how to think of some positive things.

J. D.: I don't know if I can.

Nurse: I would like to show you how to breathe more comfortably. Place your right hand on your upper chest and your left hand on your belly. I want to show you how to do relaxed abdominal breathing. With your next breath in, through your nose, let the breath fill your belly with air. And as you exhale through your mouth, let your stomach fall back to your spine. As you focus on this way of breathing, notice how still your chest is.

J. D.: [After three complete breaths] This is the easiest breathing I've done today.

Nurse: As you focused on breathing with your belly, you let go of fearing the discomfort with your breathing. Can you tell me more about the image you have of your heart as a broken vase?

J. D.: I saw this crack down the front of my heart right after the doctor told me about my big artery that is blocked, that runs down the front of my heart, which caused my heart attack.

Nurse: [Taking a small plastic bag full of crayons out of her pocket and picking up a piece of paper] Is it possible for you to choose a few crayons and draw your broken heart using those images you just talked about?

J. D.: I can't draw.

Nurse: This exercise has nothing to do with drawing, but something usually happens when you draw an image of your words.

J. D.: Do you mean the image of a broken vase? [When halfway through with the drawing] I know this sounds crazy, but my father had a heart attack when he was 55. I was visiting my parents. Dad hadn't been feeling well, even complained of his stomach hurting that morning. He was in the living room, and as he fell, he knocked over a large Chinese porcelain vase that broke in two pieces. I can remember so clearly running to his side. I can see that vase now, cracked in a jagged edge down the front. He made it to the hospital but died 2 days later. You know, I think that might be where that image of a broken heart came from (see **Figure 12-1a**).

Nurse: Your story contains a lot of meaning. Remembering this event can be very helpful to you in your healing. What are some of the things that you are most worried about just now?

J. D.: [Tears in his eyes] Dying young. I have this funny feeling in my stomach just now. I don't want to die. I'm too young. I have so much to contribute to life. I've been driving myself to excess as far as work. I need to learn to relax and manage my stress, even drop some weight, start exercising, and change my life.

Nurse: J., each day you are getting stronger. You might even consider that this time of rest after your heart attack can be a time for you to reflect on what are the most important things in life for you. Whenever you feel discouraged, let images come to you of a beautiful vase that has a healed crack in it. This is exactly what your heart is doing right now. Even as we are talking, the area that has been damaged is healing. As it heals, there will be a solid scar that will be very strong, just in the same way that a vase can be mended and become strong again. New blood supplies also come into the surrounding area of your heart to help it heal. Positive images can help you heal because you send a different message from your mind to your body when you are relaxed and thinking about becoming strong and well. You help your body, mind, and spirit function at their highest level. Let yourself once again draw an image of your heart as a healed vase, and notice any difference in your feelings when you do this.

With a smile, he picked up several crayons and began to draw a healing image to encourage hope and healing (see **Figure 12-1b**).

When J. D. entered the outpatient cardiac rehabilitation program following his acute myocardial infarction, he was motivated to lower his cholesterol, lose weight, learn stress management skills, and express his emotions. Two weeks into the program, J. D. did not appear to be his usual extroverted self. The cardiac rehabilitation nurse engaged him in conversation, and before long, he had tears in his eyes. He stated that he was very discouraged about having heart disease. He said, "It just has a grip on me." The nurse took him into her office, and they continued the dialogue. After listening to his story, she asked J. D. if he would like to explore his feelings further. He shyly nodded yes.

To facilitate the healing process, she thought it might be helpful to have J. D. get in touch with his images and their locations in his body. She began by saying, "If it seems right to you, close your eyes and begin to focus on your breathing just now." She guided him in a general exercise of head-to-toe relaxation, accompanied by an audio recording of sounds in nature. As his breathing patterns became deeper, indicating relaxation, she began to guide him in exploring "the grip" in his imagination.

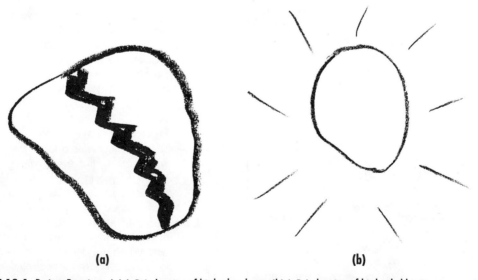

(a)　　　　　　　　　　　　**(b)**

FIGURE 12-1 Patient Drawings. (a) J. D.'s drawing of his broken heart. (b) J. D.'s drawing of his healed heart.

Nurse: Focus on where you experience the grip. Give it a size, . . . a shape, . . . a sound, . . . a texture, . . . a width, . . . and a depth.

J. D.: It's in my chest, but not like chest pain. It's dull, deep, and blocks my knowing what I need to think or feel about living. I can't believe that I'm using these words. Well, it's bigger than I thought. It's very rough, like heavy jute rope tied in a knot across my chest. It has a sound like a rope that keeps a sailboat tied to a boat dock. I'm now rocking back and forth. I don't know why this is happening.

Nurse: Stay with the feeling, and let it fill you as much as it can. If you need to change the experience, all you have to do is take several deep breaths.

J. D.: It's filling me up. Where are these sounds, feelings, and sensations coming from?

Nurse: From your wise, inner self, your inner healing resources. Just let yourself stay with the experience. Continue to use as many of your senses as you can to describe and feel these experiences.

J. D.: Nothing is happening. I've gone blank.

Nurse: Focus again on your breath in . . . and feel the breath as you let it go. . . . Can you allow an image of your heart to come to you under that tight grip?

J. D.: It is so small I can hardly see it. It's all wrapped up.

Nurse: In your imagination, can you introduce yourself to your heart as if you were introducing yourself to a person for the first time? Ask your heart if it has a name?

J. D.: It said hello, but it was with a gesture of hello, no words.

Nurse: That is fine. Just say, "Nice to meet you," and see what the response might be.

J. D.: My heart seems like an old soul, very wise. This feels very comfortable.

Nurse: Ask your heart a question for which you would like an answer. Stay with this and listen for what comes.

J. D.: (After long pause) It said practice patience, that I was on the right track, that my heart disease has a message, I don't know what it is.

Nurse: Just stay with your calmness and inner quiet. Notice how the grip changed for you. There are many more answers to come for you. This is your wise self who has much to offer you. Whenever you want, you can get back to this special kind of knowing. All you have to do is take the time. When you set aside time to be quiet with your rich images, you will get more information. You might also find special music to assist you in this process. . . . Your skills with this way of knowing will increase each time you use this process . . . now that whatever is right for you in this moment is unfolding, just as it should. In a few moments, I will invite you back into a wakeful state. On five, be ready to come back into the room, wide awake and relaxed. One . . . two . . . three . . . four . . . eyelids lighter, taking a deep breath . . . and five, back into the room, awake and alert, ready to go about your day.

J. D.: Where did all that come from? I've never done that before.

Nurse: These are your inner healing resources that you possess to help you recognize quality and purpose in living each day. In our future sessions, we will teach and share more of these skills.

Evaluation

With the client, the nurse determines whether the client outcomes for imagery were successful (see **Exhibit 12-2**). To evaluate the session further, the nurse may again explore the subjective effects of the experience with the client (see Exhibit 12-1).

> **EXHIBIT 12-2   Evaluating the Client's Subjective Experience with Imagery**
>
> 1. Was this a new kind of imagery experience for you? Can you describe it?
> 2. Did you have a visual experience? Of people, places, or objects? Can you describe them?
> 3. Did you see colors while being guided? Did the colors change as the guided imagery continued?
> 4. Were you aware of your surroundings? Were you able to let the imagery flow?
> 5. Did you like the imagery?
> 6. Did the imagery produce any feelings or emotions?
> 7. Did you notice any textures, smells, movements, or tastes while experiencing the imagery?
> 8. Was the experience pleasant?
> 9. Did you feel relaxed and refreshed after the experience?
> 10. Would you like to try this again?
> 11. What would make this a better experience for you?
> 12. What is your next step (or your plan) to integrate this on a daily basis?

Conclusion

Imagery is a tool for connecting with the unlimited capabilities of the body–mind. The client can experience more self-awareness, self-acceptance, self-love, and self-worth. Clients learn a skill for self-care and self-knowledge that will be useful throughout their life. The best way for nurses to develop confidence and skill in using clinical imagery is for them to use it in their own life as a part of self-care and enrichment.

Directions for Future Research

1. Determine whether a client's specific images increase the client's psychophysiologic healing.
2. Develop valid and reliable tools that measure imagery.
3. Compare the stress level, attitudes, and work spirit of nurses who routinely use imagery as a nursing intervention to those of nurses who do not use imagery.
4. Evaluate the relationship between imagery scripts, physiologic responses, and healing in different clinical settings.
5. Determine whether subjects can learn through manipulation of both imagery scripts and their verbal reports to eliminate or modify negative psychophysiologic responses.

6. Examine cultural diversity through specific types of imagery and symbols.

Nurse Healer Reflections

After reading this chapter, the nurse healer will be able to answer or to begin a process of answering the following questions:

- How do I feel about my imagination?
- When I work with imagery, what inner resources can assist me in my life processes?
- How am I able to remove the barriers to my imagery process?
- In what way do I recognize the nonrational part of myself?
- Can I allow my clients to interpret their own imagery to facilitate their own healing?

NOTES

1. H. Hall, "Imagery and Cancer," in *Healing Images: The Role of Imagination in Health*, ed. A. A. Sheikh (Amityville, NY: Baywood, 2003): 408–426.
2. D. Serra, C. R. Parris, E. Carper, P. Homel, S. B. Fleishman, L. B. Harrison, and M. Chadha, "Outcomes of Guided Imagery in Patients Receiving Radiation Therapy for Breast Cancer," *Clinical Journal of Oncology Nursing* 16, no. 6 (2012): 617–623.
3. K. King, "A Review of the Effects of Guided Imagery on Cancer Patients with Pain,"

Complementary Health Practice Review 15, no. 2 (2010): 98–107.

4. V. Miller and P. J. Whorwell, "Hypnotherapy for Functional Gastrointestinal Disorders: A Review," *International Journal of Clinical and Experimental Hypnosis* 57, no. 3 (2009): 279–292.

5. M. Shinozaki, M. Kanazawa, M. Kano, Y. Endo, N. Nakaya, M. Hongo, and S. Fukudo, "Effect of Autogenic Training on General Improvement in Patients with Irritable Bowel Syndrome: A Randomized Controlled Trial," *Applied Psychophysiology and Biofeedback* 35, no. 3 (2010): 189–198.

6. M. C. Mizrahi, R. Reicher-Atir, S. Levy, S. Haramati, D. Wengrower, E. Israeli, and E. Goldin, "Effects of Guided Imagery with Relaxation Training on Anxiety and Quality of Life Among Patients with Inflammatory Bowel Disease," *Psychology and Health* 27, no. 12 (2012): 1463–1479.

7. J. L. Apóstolo and K. Kolcaba, "The Effects of Guided Imagery on Comfort, Depression, Anxiety, and Stress of Psychiatric Inpatients with Depressive Disorders," *Archives of Psychiatric Nursing* 23, no. 6 (2009): 403–411.

8. S. L. Riedel, "Effects of Guided Imagery in Persons with Fibromyalgia" (doctoral dissertation, University of Virginia, Charlottesville, 2012).

9. R. Verkaik, M. Busch, T. Koeneman, R. van den Berg, P. Spreeuwenberg, and A. L. Francke, "Guided Imagery in People with Fibromyalgia: A Randomized Controlled Trial of Effects on Pain, Functional Status and Self-Efficacy," *Journal of Health Psychology* 19, no. 5 (2014): 678–688.

10. V. Menzies, D. E. Lyon, R. K. Elswick, N. L. McCain, and D. P. Gray, "Effects of Guided Imagery on Biobehavioral Factors in Women with Fibromyalgia," *Journal of Behavioral Medicine* 37, no. 1 (2014): 70–80.

11. J. S. Gordon, J. K. Staples, A. Blyta, M. Bytyqi, and A. T. Wilson, "Treatment of Posttraumatic Stress Disorder in Postwar Kosovar Adolescents Using Mind–Body Skills Groups: A Randomized Controlled Trial," *Journal of Clinical Psychiatry* 69, no. 9 (2008): 1469–1476.

12. S. Jain, G. F. McMahon, P. Hasen, M. P. Kozub, V. Porter, R. King, and E. M. Guarneri, "Healing Touch with Guided Imagery for PTSD in Returning Active Duty Military: A Randomized Controlled Trial," *Military Medicine* 177, no. 9 (2012): 1015–1021.

13. D. J. Libby, C. E. Pilver, and R. Desai, "Complementary and Alternative Medicine in VA Specialized PTSD Treatment Programs," *Psychiatric Services* 63, no. 11 (2012): 1134–1136.

14. E. C. Trakhtenberg, "The Effects of Guided Imagery on the Immune System: A Critical Review," *International Journal of Neuroscience* 118, no. 6 (2008): 839–855.

15. O. Eremin, M. B. Walker, E. Simpson, S. D. Heys, A. K. Ah-See, A. W. Hutcheon, K. N. Ogston, et al., "Immuno-modulatory Effects of Relaxation Training and Guided Imagery in Women with Locally Advanced Breast Cancer Undergoing Multimodality Therapy: A Randomised Controlled Trial," *Breast* 18, no. 1 (2009): 17–25.

16. C. Lahmann, P. Henningsen, C. Schulz, T. Schuster, N. Sauer, M. Noll-Hussong, J. Ronel, et al., "Effects of Functional Relaxation and Guided Imagery on IgE in Dust-Mite Allergic Adult Asthmatics: A Randomized, Controlled Clinical Trial," *Journal of Nervous and Mental Disorders* 198, no. 2 (2010): 125–130.

17. I. Schlesinger, O. Benyakov, I. Erikh, and M. Nassar, "Relaxation Guided Imagery Reduces Motor Fluctuations in Parkinson's Disease," *Journal of Parkinson's Disease* 4, no. 3 (2014): 431–436.

18. D. Wood and G. E. Patricolo, "Using Guided Imagery in a Hospital Setting," *Alternative and Complementary Therapies* 19, no. 6 (2013): 301–305.

19. R. McCraty and D. Tomasino, "Emotional Stress, Positive Emotions, and Psychophysiological Coherence," in *Stress in Health and Disease*, eds. B. B. Arnetz and R. Ekman (Weinheim, Germany: Wiley-VCH, 2006): 342–365.

20. G. Rein, M. Atkinson, and R. McCraty, "The Physiological and Psychological Effects of Compassion and Anger," *Journal of Advancement in Medicine* 8, no. 2 (1995): 87–105.

21. M. Bensafi, J. Porter, S. Pouliot, J. Mainland, B. Johnson, C. Zelano, N. Young, et al., "Olfactomotor Activity During Imagery Mimics That During Perception," *Nature Neuroscience* 6, no. 11 (2003): 1142–1144.

22. S. S. Yoo, D. K. Freeman, J. J. McCarthy III, and F. A. Jolesz, "Neural Substrates of Tactile Imagery: A Functional MRI Study," *Neuroreport* 14, no. 4 (2003): 581–585.

23. J. Wagner, T. Stephan, R. Kalla, H. Brückmann, M. Strupp, T. Brandt, and K. Jahn, "Mind the Bend: Cerebral Activations Associated with Mental Imagery of Walking Along a Curved Path," *Experimental Brain Research* 191, no. 2 (2008): 247–255.

24. P. Staats, H. Hekmat, and A. Staats, "Suggestion/Placebo Effects on Pain: Negative as Well as Positive," *Journal of Pain Symptom Management* 15, no. 4 (1998): 235–243.

25. P. Burhenn, J. Olausson, G. Villegas, and K. Kravits, "Guided Imagery for Pain Control," *Clinical Journal of Oncology Nursing* 18, no. 5 (2014): 501–503.

26. E. V. Lang, O. Hatsiopoulou, T. Koch, K. Berbaum, S. Lutgendorf, E. Kettenmann, H. Logan, et al., "Can Words Hurt? Patient-Provider

Interactions During Invasive Procedures," *Pain* 114, nos. 1–2 (2005): 303–309.

27. J. Achterberg, *Imagery in Healing: Shamanism and Modern Medicine* (Boston: Shambhala, 1985).

28. A. A. Sheikh, R. G. Kunzendorf, and K. S. Sheikh, "Healing Images: Historical Perspective," in *Healing Images: The Role of Imagination in Health*, ed. A. A. Sheikh (Amityville, NY: Baywood, 2003): 3–26.

29. J. L. Singer, *Imagery and Daydream Methods in Psychotherapy and Behavior Modification* (New York: Academic Press, 1974).

30. W. Penfield, *The Mystery of the Mind* (Princeton, NJ: Princeton University Press, 1975): 35.

31. A. A. Sheikh, R. G. Kunzendorf, K. S. Sheikh, and S. M. Baer, "Physiological Consequences of Imagery and Related Approaches," in *Healing Images: The Role of Imagination in Health*, ed. A. A. Sheikh (Amityville, NY: Baywood, 2003): 27–52.

32. E. Jacobson, "Electrical Measurements of Neuromuscular States During Mental Activities: Imagination of Movement Involving Skeletal Muscle," *American Journal of Physiology* 91 (1930): 567–608.

33. A. Y. Kho, K. P. Liu, and R. C. Chung, "Meta-Analysis on the Effect of Mental Imagery on Motor Recovery of the Hemiplegic Upper Extremity Function," *Australian Occupational Therapy Journal* 61, no. 2 (2014): 38–48.

34. M. Ietswaart, M. Johnston, H. C. Dijkerman, S. Joice, C. L. Scott, R. S. MacWalter, and S. J. Hamilton, "Mental Practice with Motor Imagery in Stroke Recovery: Randomized Controlled Trial of Efficacy," *Brain* 134, Pt 5 (2011): 1373–1386.

35. S. M. Braun, D. T. Wade, and A. J. Beurskens, "Use of Movement Imagery in Neurorehabilitation: Researching Effects of a Complex Intervention," *International Journal of Rehabilitation Research* 34, no. 3 (2011): 203–208.

36. O. C. Simonton, S. Matthews-Simonton, and T. F. Sparks, "Psychological Intervention in the Treatment of Cancer," *Psychosomatics* 21, no. 3 (1980): 226–227.

37. J. Achterberg and G. F. Lawlis, *Imagery and Disease* (Champaign, IL: Institute for Personality and Ability Testing, 1978).

38. H. Hall, "Imagery, PNI and the Psychology of Healing," in *The Psychophysiology of Mental Imagery: Theory, Research, and Application*, eds. R. G. Kunzendorf and A. A. Sheikh (Amityville, NY: Baywood, 1990).

39. J. Schneider, W. Smith, C. Minning, S. Whitcher, and J. Hermanson, "Guided Imagery and Immune System Function in Normal Subjects: A Summary of Research Findings," in *Mental Imagery*, ed. R. G. Kunzendorf (New York: Plenum Press, 1991): 179–191.

40. W. Lewandowski and A. Jacobson, "Bridging the Gap Between Mind and Body: A Biobehavioral Model of the Effects of Guided Imagery on Pain, Pain Disability, and Depression," *Pain Management Nursing* 14, no. 4 (2013): 368–378.

41. C. L. Baird, M. M. Murawski, and J. Wu, "Efficacy of Guided Imagery with Relaxation for Osteoarthritis Symptoms and Medication Intake," *Pain Management Nursing* 11, no. 1 (2010): 56–65.

42. F. Büyükyýlmaz, "Non-Pharmacological Intervention in Orthopedic Pain: A Systematic Review," *International Journal of Caring Sciences* 7, no. 3 (2014): 718–726.

43. E. A. Fors, H. Sexton, and K. G. Götestam, "The Effect of Guided Imagery and Amitriptyline on Daily Fibromyalgia Pain: A Prospective, Randomized, Controlled Trial," *Journal of Psychiatric Research* 36, no. 3 (2002): 179–187.

44. M. M. Huth, D. M. Van Kuiken, and M. E. Broome, "Playing in the Park: What School-Age Children Tell Us About Imagery," *Journal of Pediatric Nursing* 21, no. 2 (2006): 115–125.

45. F. Hartmann and A. M. Vlieger, "Effects of Mind–Body Therapies in Children," *Focus on Alternative and Complementary Therapies* 17, no. 2 (2012): 91–96.

46. J. A. Weydert, D. E. Shapiro, S. A. Acra, C. J. Monheim, A. S. Chambers, and T. M. Ball, "Evaluation of Guided Imagery as a Treatment for Recurrent Abdominal Pain in Children: A Randomized Controlled Trial," *BMC Pediatrics* 6 (2006): 29.

47. W. H. Kline, A. Turnbull, V. E. Labruna, L. Haufler, S. DeVivio, and P. Ciminera, "Enhancing Pain Management in the PICU by Teaching Guided Mental Imagery: A Quality-Improvement Project," *Journal of Pediatric Psychology* 35, no. 1 (2010): 25–31.

48. C. Russell and S. Smart, "Guided Imagery and Distraction Therapy in Paediatric Hospice Care," *Paediatric Nursing* 19, no. 2 (2007): 24–25.

49. W. Braud, "Transpersonal Images: Implications for Health," in *Healing Images: The Role of Imagination in Health*, ed. A. A. Sheikh (Amityville, NY: Baywood, 2003): 448–470.

50. R. Assagioli, *Psychosynthesis: A Manual of Principles and Techniques* (New York: Hobbs, Dorman, 1965).

51. R. Assagioli, *The Act of Will* (New York: Viking Press, 1973).

52. R. Schaub and B. G. Schaub, *Dante's Path: A Practical Approach to Achieving Inner Wisdom* (New York: Gotham Books, 2003).

53. J. K. Morrison, "The Dynamic, Clinical Use of Imagery to Promote Psychotherapeutic Grieving," in *Healing with Death Imagery*, eds. A. A.

Sheikh and K. S. Sheikh (Amityville, NY: Bay-wood, 2007): 139–164.

54. R. G. Kunzendorf, "Confronting Death Through Mental and Artistic Imagery," in *Healing with Death Imagery*, eds. A. A. Sheikh and K. S. Sheikh (Amityville, NY: Baywood, 2007): 47–65.

55. R. Schaub and B. G. Schaub, *Transpersonal Development: Cultivating the Human Resources of Peace, Wisdom, Purpose and Oneness* (Huntington, NY: Florence Press, 2013).

56. B. G. Schaub and R. Schaub, "Imagery and Spiritual Development," in *Healing Images: The Role of Imagination in Health*, ed. A. A. Sheikh (Amityville, NY: Baywood, 2003): 489–498.

57. B. G. Schaub and R. Schaub, "Spirituality and Clinical Practice," *Alternative Health Practitioner* 5, no. 2 (1999): 145–150.

58. L. W. Scherwitz, P. McHenry, and R. Herrero, "Interactive Guided Imagery Therapy with Medical Patients: Predictors of Health Outcomes," *Journal of Alternative and Complementary Medicine* 11, no. 1 (2005): 69–83.

59. B. G. Schaub, "Imagery in Health Care: Connecting with Life Energy," *Alternative Health Practitioner* 1, no. 2 (1995): 113–115.

60. J. Achterberg, B. Dossey, and L. Kolkmeier, *Rituals of Healing: Using Imagery for Health and Wellness* (New York: Bantam Books, 1994).

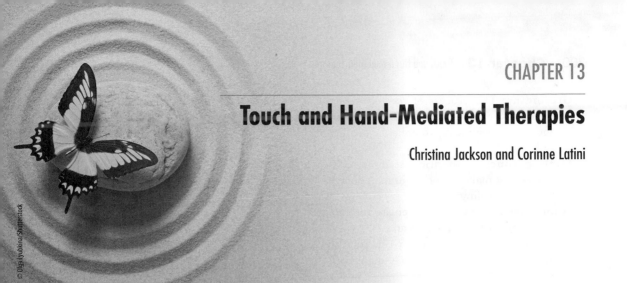

CHAPTER 13

Touch and Hand-Mediated Therapies

Christina Jackson and Corinne Latini

Nurse Healer Objectives

Theoretical

- Describe various types of touch therapies.
- Compare and contrast the various touch therapies.
- Articulate physiologic changes that can result from touch therapies.
- Describe psychoemotional changes that can result from touch therapies.

Clinical

- Develop your abilities to become calm and focused before you use touch therapies in your practice.
- Experiment with soothing music, guided imagery, and aromatherapy as adjuncts to the touch session.
- Observe subjective and objective changes in the client experiencing a touch therapy session.

Personal

- Examine the significance of touch in your personal and professional relationships.
- Create opportunities to practice touch therapies in your clinical practice.

Definitions

Acupressure (Shiatsu): The application of finger and/or thumb pressure to specific sites along the body's energy meridians for the purpose of relieving tension, reestablishing the flow of energy along the meridian lines, and restoring balance to the human energy system.

Body therapy and/or touch therapy: The broad range of techniques that a practitioner uses in which the hands are on or near the body to assist the recipient toward optimal function.

Centering: A calm and focused sense of mindful presence, a place of quietude within oneself where one feels integrated and focused.

Chakra or energy center: Specific center of consciousness in the human energy system that allows for the inflow and directing of energy from outside, as well as for outflow from the individual's energy field. There are seven major energy centers in relation to the spine and many minor centers at bone articulations in the palms of the hands and the soles of the feet.

Energy meridian: An energy circuit or line of force. Eastern theories describe meridian lines flowing vertically through the body, culminating at points on the feet, hands, and ears.

Grounding: The process of connecting to the Earth's energy field, to calm the mind and focus as a means to enhance healing endeavors.

Healing Touch: A specific system of techniques that make use of the human energy system for healing.

Human energy system: The entire interactive, dynamic system of human subtle energies, consisting of the energy centers, the multidimensional field, the meridians, and acupuncture points.

Intention: The motivation or reason for touching; the direction of one's inner awareness and focus for healing.

'M' Technique: A registered method of gentle, structured touch suitable for the very fragile or actively dying, or when the giver is not trained in massage. Simple to learn, the 'M' Technique is profoundly relaxing to both the giver and the receiver. Essential oils are used in specific ways with this technique.

Procedural touch: Touch performed to diagnose, monitor, or treat an illness; touch that focuses on the end result of curing the illness or preventing further complications.

Reflexology: The application of pressure to points on the feet, hands, and ears thought to correspond to other structures and organs throughout the body. Access to the entire nervous system is accomplished through the network in these distal structures.

Reiki: A form of energy healing in which the practitioner uses light touch through a series of hand positions over chakras to channel energy. *Reiki* means "universal life force energy" and is composed of two Japanese words, *rei*, meaning universal, and *ki*, meaning life force.

Therapeutic massage: The use of the hands to apply pressure and motion to the recipient's skin and underlying muscle to promote physical and psychological relaxation, improve circulation, relieve sore muscles, and accomplish other therapeutic effects.

Therapeutic touch: A specific technique of centering intention while the practitioner moves the hands through a recipient's energy field for the purpose of assessing and treating energy field imbalance.

Theory and Research

Touch is unique among all of the senses in that although we can see or hear without being seen or heard ourselves, we cannot touch another without being touched ourselves. A profound exchange occurs whenever we touch, and the power of this exchange cannot be underestimated. By respecting this potential, we can better learn to use touch to promote healing in others and ourselves.

Touch in Ancient Times

Healing through touch is as old as civilization itself. Practiced extensively in all cultures, this ancient treatment is instinctive—it feels natural to rub or hold any part of one's body that hurts and to do so for others. The ancient Egyptians used bandages, poultices, touch, and manipulation. Inside the Pyramids, illustrations thousands of years old show representations of one person holding hands near another, with waves of energy depicted moving from the hands of the healer to the body nearby. The oldest written documentation of the use of body touch to enhance healing comes from Asia. The *Huang Ti Nei Ching* is a classic work of internal medicine that was written 5,000 years ago. The *Nei Ching*, a 3,000- to 4,000-year-old Chinese book of health and medicine, records a system of touch based on acupuncture points and energy circuits. The ancient Indian Vedas also described healing massage, as did the Polynesian Lomi practice and the traditions of Native Americans.

During the height of classical Greek civilization, Hippocrates wrote of the therapeutic effects of massage and manipulation; he also gave instructions for carrying out these practices. He wrote during the time of the great Aesculapian healing centers, at which many whole-body therapies included touch. Touch therapies were also employed at healing centers to assist individuals who wished to make the transition to a higher level of functioning. Massage was used as a mode of preparation for dream work, which was a significant part of therapy in the healing rites. The Roman historian Plutarch wrote that Julius Caesar was treated for epilepsy by being pinched over his entire body every day.

Biblical accounts of the healings performed by Jesus of Nazareth frequently include the use of touch in the form of laying hands on the body. In two New Testament passages (using the new revised standard version), the human energy field is described. In Mark 5:25–34, a woman who had been bleeding for 12 years touched the back hem of Jesus's garment with an inner sense of knowing that this would heal her. Jesus felt that "power had gone forth from him" and turned around quickly, asking who had touched his clothing. Luke 6:18–19 tells of a crowd that had come to be healed of their diseases and demons through Jesus's touch, for "power came out from him and healed all of them."

Both shamans and traditional practitioners used touch widely until the rise of the Puritan culture during the 1600s, including the shift from primitive healing practices to modern scientific medicine. Puritan culture equated touch with sex, which was associated with original sin. During the late 19th and early 20th centuries, health care moved away from anything associated with superstition and primitive healing and was directed toward scientific medicine. All unnecessary touch was discouraged because of the association of touch with primitive healing and because of the prevailing Puritan ethic. Consequently, touch as a therapeutic intervention remained undeveloped in U.S. health care until research into its benefits began in the 1950s.

Cultural Variations

The fact that many cultures, both ancient and modern, have developed some form of touch therapy indicates that rubbing, pressing, massaging, and holding are natural manifestations of the desire to heal and care for one another. However, attitudes toward touch vary among cultures. One society may view touch as necessary, whereas another may view it as forbidden. The nurse must be aware of personal and cultural views and reactions to touch in addition to particular gender prohibitions within cultures.

Philosophic and cultural differences have influenced the development of touch in various areas of the world. The Eastern worldview is founded on energy, whereas the Western worldview is based on reductionism of matter. This basic cultural difference has led to the evolution of widely differing approaches to touch. The Eastern worldview holds that qi (or chi), also described as energy or vital force, is the center of body function. A meridian is an energy circuit or line of force that runs vertically through the body. Magnetic or bioelectrical patterns flow through the microcosm of the body in the same way that magnetic patterns flow through the planet and the universe. Meridian lines and zones are influenced by pressure placed on points along those lines.

Expert practitioners in acupuncture and acupressure purport to send healing energy to the recipient via an energy flow that moves through the body and out through their hands. In contrast, the Western worldview holds that it is the physical effect of cellular changes occurring during touch that influences healing. For example, massage stimulates the cells and aids in waste discharge, promotes the dilation of the vascular system, and encourages lymphatic drainage.[1] Swedish and therapeutic massage techniques were developed to produce these physical changes.

A blending of Eastern and Western techniques has resulted in an explosion of new and widely practiced modalities. The modern-day renaissance in body therapies is likely a healthy response to the fast-paced technologic revolution that has swept Western culture, bringing back a sense of balance and caring.

Modern Concepts of Touch

Evidence is mounting that supports what healers have intuitively known—touch is a vital aspect of human health and well-being. Some of the first studies documenting the significance of touch involved infant monkeys and surrogate mothers.[2] In the 1950s, Harlow caged one group of infant monkeys with a monkey-shaped wire form that served as a surrogate mother and a second group with a soft cloth mother surrogate. When frightened, the monkeys housed with the wire form reacted by running and cowering in a corner. The other group reacted to the same stimuli by running and clinging to the soft cloth surrogate for protection. These infant monkeys even preferred clinging to an unheated cloth surrogate mother to sitting on a warm heating pad. Although the cloth surrogate was unresponsive, the offspring raised with it developed basically normal behavior. This and other classic studies conclusively documented the significance of touch in normal animal growth and development.

Studies of human development soon followed. A study examining abandoned infants and infants whose mothers were in prison found that infants whom the nurses held and cuddled thrived, whereas those who were left alone became ill and died.[3] These studies led to the development of the concept of touch deprivation.

These early studies in the 1950s and 1960s awakened scientific interest in the phenomenon of Healing Touch. Bernard Grad, a biochemist at McGill University, was one of the first to investigate healing by the laying on of hands. He conducted a series of double-blind experiments with the renowned healer Oskar Estebany.[4] In these studies, wounded mice and damaged barley seeds were separated into control and experimental groups. After Estebany used therapeutic touch to manipulate the energy fields of the mice and seeds in the experimental groups, these groups demonstrated a significantly accelerated healing rate in comparison to the control groups. In a subsequent study, an enzymologist worked with Grad using the enzyme trypsin in double-blind studies.[5] After the trypsin was exposed to Estebany's treatments, its activity was significantly increased.

Within the past two decades, there has been a renaissance in the use of touch as a therapeutic practice. A proliferation of research publications, books, continuing education offerings, and Web resources document the effectiveness of these practices. Both the American Nurses Association and the National League for Nursing endorse the use of biofield and touch therapies. The North American Nursing Diagnosis Association includes the diagnosis *Disturbed Energy Field*, defined as a disruption of energy flow surrounding a person that disrupts harmony of body, mind, and/or spirit. Many healers who use biofield therapies claim that they either direct or channel energy to the recipient. Others say that energy will go where it is needed. Nurses are using hand-mediated therapies with increasing frequency as they seek ways to help or heal those for whom they care.

Touching Styles

Data collected through in-depth interviews with eight experienced intensive care nurses reveal two substantive processes—the touching process itself and the acquisition of a touching style—neither of which had been previously reported in the literature. The touching process is more than skin-to-skin contact; it involves entering the patient's space, connecting, talking, following nonverbal cues, and eventually touching. Nurses learn about touch from their culture, family, street knowledge, personal experience, and nursing school. The phenomenon of the healer's touch has been researched, and there are distinct characteristics that emerged. Touch is gestural, effective, and reciprocal. This is inclusive of the fact that the practitioner will also experience these three responses. Emotions, past experiences, and receptivity to healing can emerge from the touch experience. As the practitioner touches the client, relaxation of the muscles may be felt and a change in the breathing pattern may be observed. An openness for the healing power of touch is necessary between the patient and the client, which constitutes the "I–Thou relationship."[6]

There is power demonstrated through the use of touch, and it is important for nurses to be mindful of this when using touch techniques. In Guéguen and Vion's study, touch was used to emphasize and anchor a particular message regarding the taking of antibiotics. Those clients who were touched by the general practitioners while instructions were given had significantly higher compliance rates. This underscores the risk for touch to become coercive or to facilitate hierarchical relationships. Our intention as practitioners should always be examined, and touch should be offered with the best of intention for our patients/clients.[7]

Body–Mind Communication

Touch is perhaps one of the most frequently used and yet least acknowledged of the five recognized senses. It is the first sense to develop in the human embryo and the one most vital to survival. Figurative references to touch in our daily language such as "That speech really touched me" or "This conversation helped me get in touch with my feelings" attest to its deep importance and value to us. As the largest and most ancient sense organ of the body, the skin enables us to experience and learn about the environment. We use touch to help us perceive the external world.

A piece of skin the size of a quarter contains more than 3 million cells, 12 feet of nerves, 100 sweat glands, 50 nerve endings, and 3 feet of blood vessels. There are estimated to be approximately 50 receptors per 100 square centimeters—a total of 900,000 sensory receptors over the human body.[8] Viewed from this perspective, the skin is a giant communication system that, through the sense of touch, brings messages from the external environment to the attention of the internal body-mind-spirit.

Because health care is increasingly delivered in complicated technologic settings, nurses are concerned with ensuring that the human, spiritual, and social needs of patients are not overlooked. This is particularly valuable when working with the geriatric population, an often touch-deprived group. Yet nurses must take into account social contexts and cultural differences before engaging in efforts to provide touch therapy. In addition, it is important to remember that for many an experience of unwanted touch in the form of physical and/or sexual abuse may have occurred, leaving lasting fears related to receiving and giving touch. Nurses must respect and be vigilant about their own boundaries as well as their clients' as related to touch. A nurse should never assume that a client will find touch comforting and should always ask before touching. If the suggestion evokes no response or a wary expression, the nurse may try a tentative touch and observe the client's response carefully. To be truly effective, touch must be given authentically by a warm, genuine, caring individual to another who is willing to receive it. Unwelcome, uncaring, or boundary-violating touch is likely more upsetting than none at all.

Like any other nursing intervention, hugging and touching demand careful assessment. Nurses need to recognize their own feelings, as well as consider the client's age, sex, and ethnic background. A few key questions (e.g., "Would a back massage help you relax?" or "Would it help if I held your hand?") can help the client clarify his or her own beliefs, values, and desires regarding different types, locations, and intensities of touch.

The nurse's perception of touch and the patient's body also need to be considered. As with all aspects of nursing, there is a complexity surrounding how nurses view the patient's body and their desire to provide care. The intimacy of touch and nurses' ability to overcome possible affective and emotional issues can influence how they approach using touch in their practice. Bathing a patient, giving a backrub, and performing invasive procedures all have profound ramifications on the nurse–patient relationship. A qualitative study of "nurses' ambiguous experiences in clinical practice" yielded the following themes: (1) approaching the patient's body, (2) caring for the body, (3) touching a diseased body, (4) difficulties in caring for the body, and (5) staying away from the body. Nurses view the caring aspect of their practice in many different ways. For some, standing or sitting quietly with the patient provides needed patient support. For others, touch is what connects the nurse to the patient for a caring, healing experience. The findings also identified that, while there is respect and privilege associated with caring for the patient's body, other more negative feelings can be experienced.[9]

There are many variations in and names for the touch therapies available for use as nursing interventions. Some are basic human contacts, such as hand holding and hugging. Holding hands with patients who have dementia has been noted as a form of communication by volunteers in a nursing home. This form of touch can be more profound than words for clients with moderate to advanced stages of Alzheimer's disease.[10] However, some clients react strongly to touch, especially if they have been exposed to inappropriate or uncomfortable touch at other times. The touch therapies described here are used by holistic practitioners who often advocate and teach healthy lifestyle behavior patterns to their clients to augment well-being during the course of the touch therapy treatments. The addition of guided imagery and/or music before and during treatment may heighten the relaxation response elicited during touch therapies. The type of setting—acute care, long-term care, home care, rehabilitation center, or wellness center—also affects the focus and length of the treatment.

Overview of Selected Touch Interventions and Techniques

Although touch therapy is as old as civilization, documentation of how and why it works is relatively new in the nursing, medical, and allied health literature. In addition, many special approaches to working with the body and energy field are emerging. The following overview addresses the techniques most frequently encountered and practiced by nurses, including current research findings when available. Touch therapies can be classified into several categories: somatic and musculoskeletal therapies; Eastern, meridian-based, and point therapies; energy-based therapies; emotional bodywork; manipulative therapies; and other holistic touch therapies.

Except for therapeutic touch, Healing Touch, and Reiki, most body therapies involve actual physical contact. The contact usually consists of the practitioner's touching, pushing, kneading, or rubbing the recipient's skin and the underlying fascia. Each of the therapies has an explanatory theory, body of knowledge, history, and techniques. Some techniques are derived from other methods and represent a synthesis of these approaches. Some methods require special licensure or certification, and others can be incorporated into a nurse's practice after minimal instruction via audiovisual media, conference, or classroom presentation.

Somatic and Musculoskeletal Therapies

The category of somatic and musculoskeletal therapies encompasses the generic work known as therapeutic massage. As a nursing intervention, therapeutic massage is effective in stimulating circulation of blood and lymph, dispersing nutrients, removing metabolic wastes, and enhancing relaxation. Several basic strokes are involved, including long smooth strokes (i.e., effleurage), kneading motions (i.e., pétrissage), vibration, compression, and tapping (i.e., tapotement). Although they may be called by different names (e.g., Swedish massage, medical massage), many of the techniques of therapeutic massage are similar. Varying degrees of pressure and various types of oils or creams can be used, depending on client preference and the intention for the treatment. Therapeutic massage has also been referred to as soft massage and has been associated with helping the recipient reestablish balance and as a means to draw attention away from suffering. Offering soft tissue massage to relatives of family members who died while in palliative cancer care has been found to help them through a very emotional time in their lives and gave them the sense of being "valued as a person."[11]

Nurses have routinely performed therapeutic massage primarily on the backs and sometimes on the hands and feet of their clients. Back care is not new; for decades, it has been incorporated into the standard bathing and evening care routine of most hospitals. Because of time constraints and traditional neglect of the body therapies in institutions, these patients receive only a portion of the complete range of touch therapies.

Learning full-body massage greatly augments and expands the nurse's basic knowledge of massage techniques. Most practitioners learn these techniques in continuing education classes, but books on massage that illustrate the techniques are also available. Myriad styles of bodywork literally offer something for everyone. To use these particular techniques, the nurse must take special courses, which often grant a certificate of completion. Massage licensure laws vary from state to state; some states require that even registered nurses take an additional course to become certified prior to practicing massage therapy.

Because no two clients, either within or outside the institutional setting, have the same needs, the nurse must become skilled at adapting the therapy to the setting and the time available. Massage techniques that can be performed quickly, such as massage for the hands, feet, or neck and shoulders, may have beneficial results in short periods of time. One such intervention is hand massage to help alleviate and decrease preoperative anxiety. In one study, hand massage involved a 5-minute massage on each hand that included several purposeful movements. The study took place in a rural community hospital's ambulatory surgery center, and all of the patients were day-surgery candidates. There were two groups: one who had the hand massage and the control group who did not. Both groups completed a Visual Analog Scale (VAS) before either the massage or their preparation for surgery. Just before transport to the operating room, another VAS was completed. Patients who received hand massage experienced lower levels of anxiety than the control group. A serendipitous finding in the hand-massage group was the fact that their preoperative intravenous insertions were facilitated as a result. The increased warmth and vasodilation as well as tactile stimulation may be the causative factors.[12]

Long-term care staff who worked with people with dementia took part in a pilot study that utilized foot massage (N = 9) and a silent resting control group (N = 10). In this study, the caregivers were the recipients of the massage or silent rest time. There were significant decreases in diastolic blood pressure and anxiety levels in the foot-massage group immediately after the session. Interestingly, although not statistically significant, the systolic blood pressure decreased in the silent rest group. The study indicates that it is feasible to provide 10-minute foot-massage sessions during a working shift.[13]

Evidence supports the use of somatic and musculoskeletal therapies to enhance mood, cardiac health, immune function, pain relief, and treatment of clients with cancer. Recent studies support the use of massage therapies to relieve chronic lower back pain, cancer pain, and migraine headache; enhance natural killer cell function; and help relieve depression and anxiety.[14]

In a study involving integrating massage therapy with palliative care, veterans reported significant clinical changes. One hundred and fifty-three patients received massage and 115 were able to provide data on symptom improvement. Participants had advanced illnesses that were both cancer and noncancer related. Pain, anxiety, dyspnea, relaxation, and inner peace were evaluated pre- and postmassage. Short-term changes during the 4-month study included a decrease in pain and anxiety, an increased sense of relaxation, and improved inner peace. One veteran, suffering from end-stage heart failure and chronic back pain, described being able to get his "happy breath" following a massage.[15]

Lymphedema, a complication of mastectomy with lymph node removal, can be relieved through massage. In addition, the massage can benefit the patient with breast cancer who also has skin metastasis with a fungating wound. A patient, who had a brief remission from inflammatory breast cancer, developed a fungating wound that disfigured her chest and neck and left her with a foul-smelling draining wound. Because of the spreading wound and increased lymphedema, the massage regimen was modified but the patient still had the benefits of the light massage on her left hand and arm. This patient reported that the massage gave her a time of peacefulness and that the touch provided a time of relaxation and a feeling of wholeness. Emotional pain was eased through the massage experience.[16]

Even in palliative care situations, patients may actually have a greater sense of well-being when receiving touch therapy. However, if well-being is not measured, a modality can be dismissed as having no significant, measurable, therapeutic benefit. Whenever pain reduction is desired, all of the factors that influence resistance to pain are important in the overall subjective experience for the client. Thus, improvement in well-being is a significant part of pain reduction because the overall degree of suffering is lessened.

Preterm infants have been shown to benefit from the effects of massage on heart rate variability (HRV). In this study, there were two groups: 17 in the massage group and 20 in the control group. Massage was performed twice daily for 20 minutes behind a privacy screen in the NICU. In the control group, the massage therapists stayed behind the screen with the infant for 20 minutes but did not do any massage. There was a positive effect on HRV in the massaged males compared with males in the control group and females in both groups. The physiological effects of stress on preterm infants, especially male infants, who are more vulnerable to the body's stress response, can have important implications for improving survival rates. Massage could play a vital role in alleviating stress in the preterm infant.[17]

Children with asthma ages 9 to 15 were given massage therapy for a 5-week period. Their parents were taught how to perform a 20-minute massage (n = 30). The control group (n = 30) continued with standard asthma treatment. Spirometry was performed and the results recorded on the first and last days of the study using forced expiratory flow in the first second (FEV1), forced vital capacity (FVC), and peak expiratory flow (PEF). The results yielded the following: The FEV1 of the massage group was significantly higher than the control group. The FEV1/FVC ratio was also improved, even though there was no significant difference in FVC or PEF. Further studies are needed, but using massage therapy on children with asthma can have positive benefits.[18] In addition, performing massage on their children can benefit the parents by giving them a therapeutic role and reducing their anxiety. When offering the reciprocal act of touch to their child, they, too, feel the effects of being touched. This facilitates a shift in the direction of healing for all concerned.

Eastern, Meridian-Based, and Point Therapies

The category of Eastern, meridian-based, and point therapies includes modalities that are derived from an Eastern medical approach that is very different from that in our Western training and education. Interested nurses must study these methods in a program that teaches about fields that emanate from our bodies, meridians, pressure points, reflex points, imbalances in the energy system, and Eastern healing philosophy. New programs and modalities are being created regularly in this rapidly growing field of energy-based interventions. Several instruments have been used to measure the human energy field, including Kirlian photography and the superconducting quantum interference device. Some of the better-known and well-studied healing methods used by nurses include therapeutic touch, Healing Touch, Reiki, acupressure, and reflexology.

The nurse's knowledge of biofield therapies is vital as there are concerns raised in some of the literature that equate these therapies with religion and religious ideation. These therapies are not to be construed as belonging to a specific religion or to take the place of religious beliefs and practices or to be thought of as such. They are strictly meant to offer a means of help and a relief of pain and suffering that would be found in any intervention that is being used to treat an illness or disease, or to promote wellness and well-being.

Energetic touch therapies typically involve four phases.

1. Centering oneself physically and psychologically; that is, finding within oneself an inner reference of calm focus
2. Exercising the natural sensitivity of the hand to assess the energy field and/or chakras of the client for clues to understand the quality and balance of energy flow
3. Using the hands and intention to mobilize areas in the client's energy field that appear to be nonflowing (e.g., sluggish, congested, or static), smooth and harmonize areas that seem perturbed, or work with balance and flow within chakras and along meridians
4. Allowing energy flow and exchange to assist the client to repattern and balance his or her energies; some modalities

emphasize directing energy, others view the practitioner as a conduit to channel energy, and many practitioners state that energy will move and go where it is needed

The energetic healing process should be halted when there are no longer any differences in body symmetry relative to density or temperature variation, or when balance is perceived. Four commonly observed responses are (1) flushed skin, (2) deep sighs, (3) physical relaxation, and (4) verbalized relaxation. A caution when using these therapies is to limit the amount of time and/or energy spent in working with the very young, the old, and the infirm. When the client's energy field is full, the energy pushes the nurse away. Nurses can monitor clients for physical and emotional responses throughout the session and be supportive of the client.

Healing modalities that involve touching with the conscious intent to help or heal, therapeutic touch, Healing Touch, and Reiki decrease anxiety, relieve pain, and facilitate the healing process. Most of the energy-based touch therapies have certain common tenets, although the methods for applying them can vary. Nurses are becoming increasingly involved in the use of energy-based modalities for reducing anxiety and pain, inspiring balance, and bringing the body–mind connection into focus. They can be used in any type of environment, and interest in using these low-tech interventions in high-tech environments such as critical care is growing.[6] Over the past three decades, Krieger, Hover-Kramer, Quinn, and others have documented the importance of therapeutic touch.[19-22]

Therapeutic Touch

Therapeutic touch (TT) can be learned by anyone; however, there is a credentialing process with requirements to become a qualified therapeutic touch practitioner and teacher. In an effort to give credibility to the practice, the credentialing process is important, but the founders of TT hoped that everyone would learn and practice this modality. It is taught at beginning, intermediate, and advanced levels in continuing education programs.

A study of postoperative patients on the vascular surgical unit at Massachusetts General Hospital recovering from vascular surgery who received therapeutic touch as an intervention for pain yielded positive results. Those who received therapeutic touch had significantly lower levels of pain, lower cortisol levels, and higher levels of natural killer cells when compared to those who received usual postoperative care. The VAS was used by the patients to assess their pain, with participants having their blood drawn immediately before the TT or usual care and 1 hour after. The VAS was completed before and after treatment as well. One of the outcomes of the study identified that, even if patients wanted to participate in the study, the frequent blood draws made them hesitant to do so.[23]

A review of the literature showed that TT can help with providing relief for those suffering bone pain. Interventions such as TT offer another means of support and comfort for oncology patients. However, even when positive results are noted, more studies with larger sample sizes are needed to support sustained relief and symptom management.[24]

Healing Touch

Healing Touch (HT) involves working with the energy fields (auras) as well as with energy centers (chakras). Janet Mentgen, founder of the Healing Touch Program, believed that anyone can learn to facilitate healing if they have a compassionate heart and a desire to help others. During an HT session, the practitioner moves his or her hands over the client to assess for disturbances in the energy field. Treatment can be done by holding the hands just above the body or by applying gentle touch to parts of the body to clear and balance the energy. The premise is that by restoring balance, the human energy system will promote healing for the mind, body, and spirit.[25]

Healing Touch is also taught in levels and offers a certificate of completion at each stage, with eventual certification upon completing Level 5. Level 6 is the instructor level for those who would like to teach HT. Formal training and certification are available through the Healing Touch Program. The Healing Touch Program curriculum is endorsed by the American Nurses Credentialing Center and the American

Holistic Nurses Association for continuing education credits.

A feasibility study with HT as an intervention for persistent pain in older adults used the Verbal Descriptor Scale (VDS), Pain Assessment Tool in Cognitively Impaired Elders (PATCHIE), and Katz Index of Independence in Activities of Daily Living (ADL) for assessing the HT group and the Presence Care Group. Although comparisons and outcome data were not statistically significant, the study demonstrated that HT is a feasible intervention for older adults. The ADLs improved over time for the HT group, and pain decreased in both groups, though the change was not statistically significant. With nurses caring for an aging population, this study illustrates the importance of interventions that can improve quality of life and decrease pain without the serious side effects of some pain medications.[26]

The complexity of Alzheimer's disease (AD) and the need for early interventions to slow the progression of cognitive decline and memory loss was the focus of an innovative study at the University of Iowa using HT and body talk cortices (BTC). The BTC technique is thought to help reestablish brain function through a noninvasive, nonmanipulative tapping of different parts of the head and sternum to help balance the brain. The technique is easily taught to patients and their families. The control group did not have an intervention, and both groups continued their usual medical regimens. Over a 6-month period, the HT-BTC group received HT once a week, and the patient was to practice BTC technique daily. There was a 76% adherence to the BTC due to memory issues associated with AD. Assessments were done at baseline, 3 months, and 6 months. Positive outcomes of this pilot study showed significant improvement in cognitive function, mood, and depression from baseline to 6 months. Practitioners and healthcare providers must be open to combining interventions as a means to provide improved care and outcomes for our patients.[27]

Healing Touch has also been implemented as a complementary modality for pediatric patients and their families at Nemours/Alfred I. duPont Hospital for Children in Wilmington, Delaware. The facility supports and encourages the use of some complementary therapies and has a special room where Healing Touch practitioners can offer patients HT therapy. Families are also taught how to perform Healing Touch on their loved ones. The hospital is sensitive to the needs of its staff as well and offers a Day of Caring during Nurses Week to minister to the mind, body, and spirit. Healing Touch sessions, chair massages, healthy snacks, and peaceful music give attendees an opportunity for self-care during break times. Recognizing the need for self-care is an important part of practice.

Reiki

Reiki, another energy–biofield modality, also involves training and levels of certification (visit www.reiki.org and www.reikialliance.com for more information). The term *Reiki* (universal life force energy) is derived from the Japanese words *rei*, meaning universal, and *ki*, meaning life force. Originating more than 3,000 years ago and practiced in Tibet, Reiki was rediscovered in the late 1900s in Japan by Dr. Mikao Usui. The practitioner uses various hand positions to facilitate the flow of life force energy. The hands can be place directly on the client or held just above the body. The nurse should always inform the patient that Reiki is being performed.

Healing can be at any level, and the premise is for the practitioner to come into intention with the client and have the energy flow to the client's greatest area of need. Reiki may be used alone or in conjunction with nursing and medical interventions. Research has been conducted on the results of using Reiki, and it has been reported to produce a decrease in pain, alleviation of anxiety, and a reduction in depression. Improved well-being in the mind, body, and spirit has been reported by many who have experienced Reiki therapy. Reiki gives power and control for healing to the receiver. The intention for healing is set by the practitioner and the client, and through the relaxation response, healing is encouraged at all levels within the body.[28]

In an experimental study of 25 community-dwelling older adults, Reiki was found to provide relaxation, with the effects lasting longer after the second session. Sessions were given one day a week for 45 minutes, which included 30-minute Reiki treatments, over a period of 8 weeks.

Participants reported decreased back spasms, decreased shoulder and neck pain, and improved sleep patterns. The authors of the study also found that there was potential for Reiki to be used as a coping resource for older adults.[29]

The use of Reiki in providing improved health-related quality-of-life outcomes in patients with cancer has yielded significant reduction in reported pain and pain assessment findings in a review of studies of biofield therapies. While pain medication was still needed, the significant decrease in pain the day following Reiki treatments prompted the inclusion of Reiki in the comprehensive pain control regimens for these patients.[30]

Magnet hospitals are incorporating biofield therapies for patients as part of integrated care. Practitioners work with healthcare providers to plan the sessions, and the term *Clinical Reiki* has been used to describe how the Reiki session is tailored to meet the needs of the in-patient recipients. Families and friends of the patient recipients also have the opportunity to receive a Reiki treatment. The University Medical Center in Tucson, Arizona, is an example of a highly successful Reiki program that started with two practitioners and now has 16 volunteers. According to the program coordinator, Mega A. Mease, 4,000 people have been touched since the program started in 2006. Many benefits have been noted by patients and their healthcare providers, including the need for less pain medication, improved sleep and appetite, and a decrease in side effects from chemotherapy drugs and radiation.[31]

Patients are not the only ones who can benefit from a Reiki session. Nurses can experience a decrease in work-related stress by learning Level-1 Reiki and practicing self-Reiki. A study of 26 nurses at a large urban medical center used the Perceived Stress Scale (PSS) to do a baseline and follow-up evaluation of their stress. The follow-up evaluation was done at 21 days. During that time, the nurses were to perform self-Reiki on at least 15 out of the 21 days for 10 minutes a day. A journal was kept by each participant, and 17 nurses completed the 3-week pilot study. The PSS follow up by the 17 nurses showed an 82% decrease in PSS. The diary comments supported the PSS data, with improvements in sleep, relaxation, and overall calm being noted as outcomes for the participants.[32]

A best-evidence synthesis from the literature evaluated 66 clinical studies that used various types of biofield therapies and patient populations. The results yielded strong evidence that pain is reduced, negative behaviors in dementia patients decrease, improved quality of life for cancer patients is experienced, and anxiety is decreased in cardiovascular patients. The need for interprofessional collaboration when performing clinical studies is important to provide the data that will encourage the use of biofield therapies as a means of reducing suffering and promoting wellness in various patient populations.[33]

Energy Field Disturbance

In the 1995–1996 *Nursing Diagnoses: Definitions and Classification*, by the North American Nursing Diagnosis Association, the definition of energy field disturbance made its entry into the world of professional nursing. Now referred to as Disturbed Energy Field, the definition given is as follows:

> Disruption of the flow of energy surrounding a person's being [which] results in a disharmony of the body, mind, and/or spirit. [Defining characteristics include] perceptions of changes in patterns of energy flow, such as movement (wave, spike, tingling, density, flowing); sounds (tones, words); temperature changes (warmth, coolness); visual changes (image, color); disruption of the field (deficit, hole, spike, bulge, obstruction, congestion, diminished flow in energy field).[34]

Nursing Interventions Classification

The Nursing Interventions Classification, which lists therapeutic touch, also specifies Healing Touch and Reiki. The use of these modalities calls for a focus on inner self, intention, and healing at all levels of consciousness.[34]

Acupressure and Shiatzu (Shiatsu)

The Eastern energy system of meridian lines and points is the foundation of acupressure and Shiatzu. The word *Shiatzu* comes from the Japanese words *shi* (finger) and *atzu* (pressure). The technique is a product of 4,000 years of Eastern medicine and philosophy. Although widely known and practiced in Japan, Shiatzu was virtually unknown in Western culture until acupuncture began receiving widespread public attention. Shiatzu is based on the same 657 energy points running along 12 pathways or meridians that are used in acupuncture. Instead of inserting needles, however, the practitioner applies pressure on these points with the thumbs, fingers, and heel of the hand. According to the theory underlying these practices, the application of pressure releases congestion and allows energy to flow. Another difference between acupuncture and Shiatzu is that the main function of Shiatzu is to maintain health and well-being (prevention), rather than to treat imbalance, as often occurs in acupuncture.[35]

Reflexology

In the early 1900s, William FitzGerald noted that application of pressure to certain points on the hands caused anesthesia in other parts of the body. Another physician, Edwin Bowers, learned of FitzGerald's work and joined him in the exploration and development of this zone therapy. The technique became more specific as it evolved into reflexology, which encompasses many more pressure points.

Reflexology is based on the theory that 10 equal longitudinal zones run the length of the body from the top of the head to the tips of the toes. This number corresponds to the number of fingers and toes. Each big toe matches to a line that runs up the medial aspect of the body, through the center of the face, and culminates at the top of the head. The reflex points pass all the way through the body within the same zones. Congestion or tension in any part of a zone affects the entire zone running laterally throughout the body. More than 72,000 nerves in the body terminate in the feet. A problem or disease in the body often manifests itself through formation of deposits of calcium and acids on the corresponding part of the foot. It is thought that hand and ear reflexology work in the same way, with points corresponding to

distant structures.[12] The purpose of reflexology is twofold. First, relaxation itself is an important goal. Good health is dependent on one's ability to return to homeostasis after injury, disease, or stress. From this perspective, reflexology is effective in helping the body–mind restore and maintain its natural state of health because foot manipulation triggers deep relaxation. The second goal of this therapy is to stimulate the proprioceptive reflexes in the feet, thereby triggering a corresponding release that affects the endocrine, immune, and neuropeptide systems. Manuals with specific diagrams are used to instruct the therapist. An example of a foot reflexology chart is shown in **Figure 13-1**.

The evidence base supporting the effectiveness of reflexology for physical and psychological symptoms is growing rapidly. In a large, longitudinal, randomized clinical trial examining health-related quality-of-life outcomes in patients with advanced-stage breast cancer, significant improvements in physical functioning and reduction in dyspnea were found in the reflexology group. No adverse effects were noted.[36]

A controlled study of 80 participants in two different institutions compared level of fatigue, pain, and cramps in hemodialysis patients receiving foot reflexology versus those not receiving reflexology. The intervention group received three 30-minute reflexology sessions following dialysis over the course of a week. Results revealed significant reduction in fatigue, pain, and cramps in those receiving reflexology.[37]

The effects of foot reflexology massage on patients' anxiety levels following coronary artery bypass graft surgery was examined in a randomized controlled clinical study. After surgery, the experimental group received reflexology on their left foot 20 minutes a day for 4 days, while the control group received a gentle foot rub. Measurement using two different anxiety tools (state-trait inventory and VAS) confirmed a significant decrease in anxiety following reflexology.[38]

In a blinded, randomized controlled investigation of reflexology's effects on anxiety and level of sedation required in intensive care patients on mechanical ventilators, researchers used the American Association of Critical Care Nurses Sedation Assessment Scale to collect

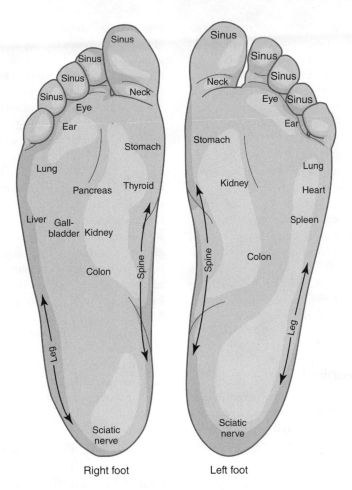

Right foot   Left foot

FIGURE 13-1 Foot Reflexology Chart

data. The intervention group (n = 30) received 30 minutes of reflexology on their feet, hands, and ears for 5 days. Those receiving reflexology had significantly lower heart rate, systolic and diastolic blood pressure, and respiratory rate than those in the control group. Patients receiving reflexology also required less sedation and had better patient–ventilator synchrony than control group participants.[39]

Deep Tissue Techniques

This approach to bodywork aims to affect structure by releasing chronic patterns of muscle tension and held trauma or restriction in connective tissue. This work is done with great intention, and deep finger pressure is used to penetrate through layers of muscle, fascia, and tendons. This work can involve crossing or following the direction of muscle fibers. Sports massage, myofascial release, somatic neuromuscular integration (i.e., soma), Aston-Patterning, Zen therapy, Rolfing, and Hellerwork are examples of this type of massage.

Emotional Bodywork

The category of emotional bodywork includes numerous techniques developed by individuals operating in the various fields that combine psychotherapy and bodywork. Some of the specific techniques include Lomilomi, Rosen Method, somatic experiencing, Trager, and psychoenergetic balancing. Some of these methods derive from ancient traditions, others from established health fields, such as chiropractic care. In general, it is important to remember that all touch therapies can trigger memories, physical and emotional release, and catharsis. This can be unexpected and frightening to clients, and they should be reassured that this is a common occurrence. This release can be related to the assumption of a body position that triggers state-dependent memory or to cellular memory stimulation.[1]

Occasionally, individuals who have experienced abuse or trauma will release long-held emotional or physical tension during a touch session. This can manifest as laughter, tears, uncontrollable twitching, shaking, deep sighs, anger, or a variety of other expressions. Displaying calm acceptance, touching a neutral area of the body (determine this ahead of time with the client), and allowing the client time to release emotion are all therapeutic responses to this type of occurrence. Appropriate referral for counseling is important.

Manipulative Therapies

Manipulative therapies often involve more invasive bodywork and demand a complete program of education often considered separate from nursing. Some nurses study these techniques to augment their nursing endeavors. Manipulative therapies include chiropractic and osteopathy (which involve manipulation of bones, ligaments, and soft tissue areas, including work on the head and dura). A similar, related field of practice is physical therapy.

Other Holistic Therapies and Programs Related to Touch

The number of bodywork, somatic therapies, and touch-related programs is too extensive to cover completely in this chapter. Instead, a sampling is included here to awaken nurses to the magnitude and scope of what is available. Additional touch therapies not discussed in this chapter are noted in **Table 13-1**.

Various types of massage and therapies have been developed for those with specific needs. Chair massage, geriatric massage, prenatal and perinatal massage, and infant massage are but a few examples. Healing Touch International has a program called "Bosom Buddies" for those with breast cancer. Manual lymphatic drainage is available for postmastectomy patients who have lost lymph nodes. Craniosacral therapy is available for infants who have experienced birth trauma. With the proliferation of approaches, a style of touch is available for anyone who may benefit.

The Namaste Care program was developed to provide patients with advanced dementia soothing and calming touch, along with the use of sound, smell, and taste. The main premise, though, is the importance of touch in a person's life and its ability to help them recall a better time in their lives. Joyce Simard, a social worker and dementia specialist, started the program in Florida in 2003 and it is being used internationally to aid patients in end-of-life and advanced dementia care. In England, nurses in Park Avenue Care Center reported that, since implementing the program, use of antipsychotic medications has decreased, urinary tract infections have declined, and sleep schedules have improved. Nurses can play an integral role in supporting a program such as Namaste Care in their area of practice.[40]

Holistic Caring Process

Holistic Assessment

In preparing to use touch interventions, the nurse assesses the following parameters:

- The client's perception of his or her body–mind situation
- The client's potential physical problems that may require referral to a physician for evaluation
- The client's history of emotional and psychiatric disorders (The nurse must modify the approach with clients who have present or past psychiatric disorders. Touch itself may present a problem, and the deeply relaxed, semihypnotic state that a balanced person finds enjoyable may actually frighten or alarm an unbalanced individual.)
- The client's values and cultural beliefs about touch and energy therapies
- The client's past experience with body therapies

TABLE 13-1   Additional Touch Therapies

Therapy	Originator	Primary Purpose and Function
Applied kinesiology	George Goodheart	Focuses on the relationship of muscle strength and energy flow. The theory is that, if muscles are strong, then circulation and other vital functions are also strong.
Chiropractic	D. D. Palmer	Based on alignment of spinal vertebrae. This therapy involves manipulations to restore natural alignment.
Feldenkrais method	Moshe Feldenkrais	Gives the client gentle manipulations to heighten awareness of the body. As awareness increases, clients can make more informed choices about how to move the body in daily situations.
Jin Shin Jyutsu	Master Jiro Murai of Japan in early 1900s	A milder form of acupressure that involves pressure along eight extra energy meridians.
Kofutu touch healing	Frank Homan	Developed in the early 1970s when a series of symbols for use in touch came to the originator during meditation. It is called "Kofutu" for the symbols and "touch" healing because the auras of the healer and recipient must touch. This therapy uses higher consciousness energy symbols to promote self-development and spiritual healing.
Lomilomi	Ancient Hawaii	Practitioners knead, rub, and press with intention—and often prayer. Holistic attention is given to the client's nutrition, and meditation and herbs can be recommended.
Polarity therapy	Randolph Stone	Repatterns energy flow in the individual by rebalancing positive and negative charges. The practitioner places a finger or the whole hand on parts of the client's body of opposite charge to facilitate energy balancing where it is needed. Through these contacts, with the help of pressure and rocking movements, energy can reorganize and reorder itself.
MaríEL	Ethel Lombardi	A 1980s variation of Reiki.
Neuromuscular release		Involves movement of the limbs toward and away from the body by the practitioner to assist the client in learning to let go for the purpose of enhanced circulation and emotional release.
Rolfing	Ida P. Rolf	A form of bodywork that reorganizes the fascia (connective tissues) that permeate the entire body, thus enabling the body to regain the natural integrity of its form. Rolfing enhances structural alignment, postural efficiency, comfort, and freedom of movement.
Trager work	Milton Trager	Involves rhythmically rocking the limbs and often the whole body to aid relaxation of the muscles and promote optimal flow of blood, lymph, nerve impulses, and energy.

The knowledge level of clients varies widely. The approach will differ markedly depending on the client's previous experience. Assisting a client in transferring prior learning such as from childbirth preparation classes to a new situation is helpful.

Identification of Patterns/ Challenges/Needs

The following patterns/challenges/needs are compatible with the interventions for touch:

- Altered circulation
- Impairment in skin integrity
- Social isolation
- Altered spiritual state
- Impaired physical mobility
- Altered meaningfulness
- Altered comfort
- Anxiety
- Grieving
- Fear
- Energy field disturbance

Outcome Identification

Table 13-2 guides the nurse in client outcomes, nursing prescriptions, and evaluation for the use of touch as a nursing intervention.

Therapeutic Care Plan and Interventions

Before the session:

- Wash your hands.
- Have the client empty his or her bladder to reduce muscle tension.
- Prepare the hospital bed, therapy table, or surface on which you will be working. If you will be using a therapy table, drape it with a cotton blanket and place a sheet over the top. Lay out a blanket or sheet for the client to use as a cover when he or she lies on the table. Adjust the height of the table or bed to protect your back.

- Have small pillows, bolsters, or towel rolls available for supporting the head, back, or lower legs.
- Control the environment so that the room is warm, dimly lit, and quiet. If you are in a client's hospital room, draw the curtain and turn off the television set.
- Use relaxation and breathing techniques, imagery, or music to elicit the relaxation response.
- After you have talked with the client, spend a few moments to quiet and center yourself, focus on your healing intention, and then begin.

At the beginning of the session:

- Explain to the client the steps in the touch process to be used. Ask permission to proceed.

TABLE 13-2 Nursing Interventions: Touch		
Client Outcomes	**Nursing Prescriptions**	**Evaluation**
The client is relaxed following a touch therapy session.	Encourage the client to receive touch therapy to evoke the relaxation response. During the touch therapy session, help the client: ▪ Decrease anxiety and fear ▪ Decrease pulse and respiratory rate ▪ Recognize a feeling of body–mind relaxation ▪ Develop a sense of general well-being ▪ Increase effectiveness in individual coping skills ▪ Increase a sense of belonging and lessened loneliness ▪ Feel less alone and express that feeling	The client received benefits from touch therapy. The client: ▪ Exhibited decreased anxiety and fear ▪ Demonstrated a decrease in pulse and respiratory rate ▪ Reported muscle relaxation ▪ Exhibited satisfied facial expression and expressed inner calmness ▪ Reported greater satisfaction in individual coping patterns
The client has improved circulation.	Provide the client with information about how touch therapies improve circulation and tissue perfusion.	Clients with white skin had a reddened color in the area where the nurse had used effleurage and pétrissage massage strokes. Skin in the massaged area is warmer than before the therapy.
The client receives touch therapy to maintain and enhance health.	Encourage the client to ask for touch therapy, suggest that the client seek out the nurse, and recommend that the client accept touch when offered by the nurse.	The client asked for touch therapy.

- As you progress through the intervention, explain what you are about to do before you actually begin. Encourage the client to address concerns or discomfort at any time.
- Position the head comfortably. If the client has long hair, pull it up and away from the neckline.
- If you are using massage techniques, have the client disrobe to his or her level of comfort. The client lies on a padded therapy table or hospital bed that is covered with a cotton blanket and sheet. The sides of the sheet and blanket are then wrapped over the client so that he or she feels protected and warm. (This procedure is used for physical touch therapies and is not needed for TT, HT, Reiki, or other energy-based interventions, which may be done with the client fully clothed. However, remember that when the client experiences the relaxation response, the body may undergo cooling, so a blanket may be necessary.)
- Uncover only the body area that is being massaged or pressed as the therapy proceeds. You may leave the client covered during energetic treatments.
- In most cases, begin with the client lying on his or her back.
- Encourage the client to take slow, deep, releasing breaths.
- During the turning process, slide the sheet or towel around the client's body to ensure that the client will not be exposed.

During the session:

- Be attuned to the client's responses to therapy. This will help the client build trust and achieve optimal relaxation. Be prepared for an emotional or physical release, and calmly remain with the client should this happen.
- In initial sessions, continue to explain what the client can expect to happen so that he or she feels comfortable with the continued direction of the touch sessions. After trust has been established and the relaxation response is learned, the client will relax more quickly and move to deeper levels in subsequent sessions.

At the end of the session:

- When you have finished the touch therapy session, verbally let the client know that it is time to return gradually to the here and now, to begin to move around slowly, and to awaken fully.
- Anticipate that the client will take a few minutes to reorient to time and place after being in a deep state of relaxation.
- Allow a period of silence for the client to appreciate fully the experience and benefits of his or her relaxed body–mind.
- Stay in the room while the client rouses and sits up. Give necessary assistance to ensure a safe transfer to an ambulatory position.
- Allow time to receive the client's verbal feedback about the meaning of the session if the client feels the need to talk. If this does not occur spontaneously, ask for feedback. The insight gained provides guidelines for further sessions or specific ideas that the client can follow up on in daily life.
- When the touch therapy is used for relaxation or sleep induction for hospitalized patients, close the session by softly pulling the bedcovers up over the patient's back and quietly turning off the light as the patient moves into sleep. Let the client know in advance that you will leave quietly at the end.
- Use the client outcomes that were established before the session (see Table 13-2) and the client's subjective experience (**Exhibit 13-1**) to evaluate the session.

Case Study (Implementation)

Case Study 1

Setting: Medical/surgical unit of a general hospital
Patient: E. S., a 68-year-old single man with chronic obstructive pulmonary disease
Patterns/Challenges/Needs:

1. Anxiety
2. Altered comfort
3. Social isolation (related to chronic obstructive pulmonary disease and pneumonia)

EXHIBIT 13-1   Evaluation of the Client's Subjective Experience of Touch Therapies

1. Was this a new kind of experience for you? Can you describe it?
2. Did this feel like a comforting or stimulating tactile sensation or both?
3. Was it pleasurable on all planes—physical, mental, emotional, and spiritual—or more focused in one area than another?
4. Were you aware of your surroundings during the experience, or did you sink into a sense of timelessness?
5. Did emotions surface during the experience? If so, what were they? Can you focus on them now?
6. Did you experience any imagery during the touch session?
7. Did you feel comfortable with the therapist? Is there anything that you want to do to increase your comfort level with the touch therapist?
8. Did you feel relaxed and refreshed after the experience?
9. Would you like to try this again?
10. What would be helpful to make this a better experience for you?
11. Can you develop a plan or strategy to integrate more of the touch therapies into your life on a regular basis?

E. S. was oxygen dependent and no longer ambulatory. After a history of heavy smoking for 40 years, his lungs continued to deteriorate in spite of quitting smoking at age 60. His stomach frequently felt upset, and it was difficult for him to eat much. He could not tolerate liquid nutritional supplements, he worked very hard to breathe, and his weight had dropped from 160 to 100 pounds over a 2-year period. He had become very weak. Because E. S. had become sedentary and very bony, he was uncomfortable most of the time, with stiffness and body aches. E. S. had grown up in the city in which he now found himself hospitalized. He had never married and had no remaining living family.

E. S. declined massage because he was afraid it would hurt him. He felt very fragile and very much alone. He became especially anxious and fearful at nighttime. One of the nurses caring for him had attended a local course and learned the basics of therapeutic touch. She knew that TT would not cause any physical pain for E. S. because it did not involve actually touching him. She also knew that it might be very relaxing for him, perhaps even easing his respiratory effort. She offered E. S. a "trial" session for 10 minutes to see if this might be a helpful modality for him. Pulling the curtain around his bed, she encouraged him to relax and breathe slowly and fully. She calmed herself and took a few deep, slow breaths to increase her sense of

focus. Working about 7 to 10 inches away from his body, she began to move her hands through his field from head to toes with the intention of moving energy and balancing his field. After only 5 minutes, she saw E. S. relax as his shoulders released and his facial expression softened.

E. S. reported that he slept better that night than he had for a long while. It was decided that he would receive a TT session each evening for the remainder of his hospitalization. The nurse who had performed the first session taught several of the other nurses how to do the basic techniques she had used. As they saw the positive effects of their interventions with E. S., they became interested in learning more and sought their own formal training in energetic healing.

Case Study 2

Setting: Long-term care facility
Client: J. S., a 76-year-old widow
Patterns/Challenges/Needs:

1. Anxiety related to painful arthritis in hands
2. Altered self-image related to deformity of hands

J. S. is a delightful woman who has lived in the long-term care facility for 2 years. She is generally healthy and has loving family who visit her regularly. The pain in her hands from arthritis has grown, and she has become increasingly intolerant of the medications used to ease her pain and inflammation. Nurses who care for J. S. have decided to incorporate hand massage twice daily into her routine care. Although they are very busy, they plan to spend at least 5 minutes per hand, using gentle stroking and kneading motions along with lotion. J. S. likes the smell of lavender, and essential oil of lavender is mixed into the lotion that is kept in her room because it is thought to enhance relaxation and pain relief.

Sometimes, when the nurses are very busy, they massage one of her hands and then come back later to do the other hand. J. S. loves this time and says that it is giving her noticeable pain relief and a feeling of greater relaxation. The nurses enjoy this time as well and report that it gives them a chance to get more information from J. S. as to how she is doing in general. Over time, J. S.'s daughter and granddaughter start to massage her hands when they come to visit. Other residents request hand massage, and those clients who are able begin to offer this to one another as well.

Case Study 3

Setting: Patient's home
Client: J. H., a 45-year-old single female minister
Patterns/Challenges/Needs:

1. Anxiety related to pain
2. Ineffective breathing pattern
3. Altered spiritual state
4. Energy field disturbance

J. H., who was suffering from end-stage pancreatic cancer, gently closed her eyes. The practitioner explained the Reiki treatment that the patient was about to experience. J. H.'s breathing began to slow and her body relaxed. She had been short of breath and unable to get comfortable for most of the morning. The music played softly, the lavender candle flickered gently, and the light touch of the Reiki practitioner began to have an immediate effect on the client. As the hour-long treatment ended, the client opened her eyes and said she had been able to breathe more deeply and to experience a sense of well-being and comfort that had not been present for several months. The calmness in her expression and the deep, rhythmic breathing pattern lasted for several hours after the session. J. H. died a few

weeks later. Her experience and testimony demonstrate how comfort can be brought into the lives of others through the use of energetic touch therapies and the practitioner's healing presence.

Evaluation

With the client, the nurse determines whether the client outcomes for touch therapies were successfully achieved (see Table 13-2). To evaluate the session further, the nurse may again explore the subjective effects of the experience with the client using the evaluation questions in Exhibit 13-1.

Directions for Future Research

1. Develop valid and reliable tools to measure the effects of touch and hand-mediated therapies.
2. Investigate hand-mediated techniques practiced in conjunction with other modalities to mirror real-world usage of these modalities.
3. Continue to strengthen the evidence base for practicing touch and hand-mediated therapies.
4. Discern which therapies are best suited for various health concerns and populations.
5. Examine the use of touch and hand-mediated therapies in ambulatory and community settings.
6. Examine the long-term cost effectiveness of touch and hand-mediated techniques.
7. Investigate whether periodic hand-mediated therapy sessions can increase work performance or productivity.
8. Evaluate length of stay, complications, and well-being as related to the use of touch techniques.
9. Examine the responses to touch and hand-mediated therapies related to developmental stage.
10. Investigate how touch can be taught effectively in nursing schools and which methods are best suited to accomplish this.
11. Explore ways in which nursing students' cultural learning pertaining to touch affects performance of clinical care.

12. Measure parental and caregiver satisfaction when taught to offer touch and hand-mediated therapies to loved ones.

Nurse Healer Reflections

After reading this chapter, the nurse healer will be able to answer or to begin the process of answering the following questions:

- How do I feel about using touch and hand-mediated therapies as healing interventions?
- What does the process of centering myself feel like?
- How does the use of my intention alter my experience of offering touch?
- How astute am I at observing my client's response to touch interventions?
- How can I increase my skill pertaining to the use of touch and hand-mediated therapies?
- Who might be a good mentor for me as I increase my repertoire of healing modalities?
- What other modalities can I learn and include to enhance the effectiveness of touch?

NOTES

1. K. Fontaine, *Complementary and Alternative Therapies for Nursing Practice*, 3rd ed. (Upper Saddle River, NJ: Prentice Hall, 2010).
2. H. Harlow, "Love in Infant Monkeys," *Scientific American* 200 (1958): 68–74.
3. R. Spitz, *The First Year of Life* (New York: International Universities Press, 1965).
4. B. Grad, "Some Biological Effects of the Laying on of Hands: A Review of Experiments with Animals and Plants," *Journal of the American Society for Psychical Research* 59 (1965): 95–127.
5. M. J. Smith, "Enzymes Are Activated by the Laying on of Hands," *Human Dimensions* 1 (1973): 46–48.
6. E. D. Papathanassoglou and M. D. Mpouzika, "Interpersonal Touch: Physiological Effects in Critical Care," *Biological Research for Nursing* 14, no. 4 (2012): 431–443.
7. N. Guéguen, S. Meineri, and V. Charles-Sire, "Improving Medication Adherence by Using Practitioner Nonverbal Techniques: A Field Experiment on the Effect of Touch," *Journal of Behavioral Medicine* 33, no. 6 (2010): 466–473.
8. A. Montagu and F. Matson, *The Human Connection* (New York: McGraw-Hill, 1979): 89.
9. E. Picco, R. Santoro, and L. Garrino, "Dealing with the Patient's Body in Nursing: Nurses' Ambiguous Experience in Clinical Practice," *Nursing Inquiry* 17, no. 1 (2010): 38–45.
10. J. Ellis, "The Touch That Means So Much," *Nursing Older People* 22, no. 8 (2010): 10.
11. B. S. Cronfalk, B. M. Ternestedt, and P. Strang, "Soft Tissue Massage: Early Intervention for Relatives Whose Families Members Died in Palliative Cancer Care," *Journal of Clinical Nursing* 19, nos. 7–8 (2010): 1040–1048.
12. L. R. Brand, D. J. Munroe, and J. Gavin, "The Effect of Hand Massage on Preoperative Anxiety in Ambulatory Surgery Patients," *AORN Journal* 76, no. 6 (2013): 708–717.
13. W. Moyle, M. Cooke, S. T. O'Dwyer, J. Murfield, A. Johnston, and B. Sung, "The Effect of Foot Massage on Long-Term Care Staff Working with Older People with Dementia: A Pilot, Parallel Group, Randomized Controlled Trial," *BMC Nursing* 12, no. 5 (2013): 1–9.
14. R. Lindquist, M. Snyder, and M. F. Tracy, *Complementary and Alternative Therapies in Nursing*, 7th ed. (New York, Springer, 2014).
15. A. Mitchinson, C. E. Fletcher, H. M. Kim, M. Montagnini, and D. B. Hinshaw, "Integrating Massage Therapy Within the Palliative Care of Veterans with Advanced Illnesses: An Outcome Study," *American Journal of Hospice and Palliative Medicine* 31, no. 1 (2014): 6–12.
16. S. Fenton, "Reflections on Lymphedema, Fungating Wounds and the Power of Touch in the Last Weeks of Life," *International Journal of Palliative Nursing* 17, no. 2 (2011): 60–66.
17. S. L. Smith, R. Lux, S. Haley, H. Slater, J. Beechy, and L. J. Moyer-Mileur, "The Effect of Massage on Heart Rate Variability in Preterm Infants," *Journal of Perinatology* 33, no. 1 (2013): 59–64.
18. M. A. Fattach and B. Hamdy, "Pulmonary Functions of Children with Asthma Improve Following Massage Therapy," *Journal of Alternative and Complementary Medicine* 17, no. 11 (2011): 1065–1068.
19. D. Hover-Kramer, *Healing Touch: A Guidebook for Practitioners*, 2nd ed. (Albany, NY: Thomson Delmar Learning, 2001).
20. D. F. Bruce and D. Krieger, *Miracle Touch: A Complete Guide to Hands-On Therapies That Have the Amazing Ability to Heal* (New York: Three Rivers Press, 2003).
21. D. Krieger, *Accepting Your Power to Heal: The Personal Practice of Therapeutic Touch* (Santa Fe, NM: Bear & Company, 1993).

22. J. F. Quinn and A. J. Strelkauskas, "Psychoimmu-nologic Effects of Therapeutic Touch on Practitioners and Recently Bereaved Recipients: A Pilot Study," *Advances in Nursing Science* 15, no. 4 (1993): 13–26.

23. A. B. Coakley and M. E. Duffy, "The Effect of Therapeutic Touch on Postoperative Patients," *Journal of Holistic Nursing* 28, no. 3 (2010): 193–200.

24. A. Running and E. Turnbeaugh, "Oncology Pain and Complementary Therapy: A Review of the Literature," *Clinical Journal of Oncology Nursing* 15, no. 4 (2011): 374–379.

25. L. Gordon, C. Hutchinson, N. Lockwood, L. Pointer, and M. Tovey, eds., *Healing Touch Level 2 Notebook*, 7th ed. (San Antonio, TX: Healing Touch Program, 2011).

26. S. Decker, D. W. Wardell, and S. G. Cron, "Using a Healing Touch Intervention in Older Adults with Persistent Pain: A Feasibility Study," *Journal of Holistic Nursing* 30, no. 3 (2012): 205–213.

27. D. Lu, L. K. Hart, S. K. Lutgendorf, H. Oh, and M. Schilling, "Slowing Progression of Early Stages of AD with Alternative Therapies: A Feasibility Study," *Geriatric Nursing* 34, no. 6 (2013): 457–464.

28. R. Keyes, *The Healing Power of Reiki* (Woodbury, MN: Llewellyn, 2012).

29. N. E. Richeson, J. A. Spross, K. Lutz, and C. Peng, "Effects of Reiki on Anxiety, Depression, Pain, and Physiological Factors in Community-Dwelling Older Adults," *Research in Gerontological Nursing* 3, no. 3 (2010): 187–199.

30. J. G. Anderson and A. G. Taylor, "Biofield Therapies and Cancer Pain," *Clinical Journal of Oncology Nursing* 16, no. 1 (2012): 43–48.

31. W. L. Rand, "Reiki at University Medical Center, Tucson, Arizona, a Magnet Hospital: Mega R. Mease Is Interviewed by William Lee Rand," *Holistic Nursing Practice* 25, no. 5 (2011): 233–237.

32. C. L. Cuneo, M. R. C. Cooper, C. S. Drew, C. Naoum-Heffernan, T. Sherman, K. Walz, and J. Weinburg, "The Effect of Reiki on Work-Related Stress of the Registered Nurse," *Journal of Holistic Nursing* 29, no. 1 (2011): 33–43.

33. S. Jain and P. J. Mills, "Biofield Therapies: Helpful or Full of Hype? A Best Evidence Synthesis," *International Journal of Behavioral Medicine* 17, no. 1 (2010): 1–16.

34. B. J. Ackley and G. B. Ladwig, *Nursing Diagnosis Handbook: An Evidence-Based Guide to Planning Care*, 9th ed. (St. Louis, MO: Mosby Elsevier, 2011): 345.

35. M. Micozzi, *Fundamentals of Complementary and Integrative Medicine*, 4th ed. (St. Louis, MO: Saunders Elsevier, 2010).

36. G. Wyatt, A. Sikorskii, M. H. Rahbar, D. Victorson, and M. You, "Health-Related Quality-of-Life Outcomes: A Reflexology Trial with Patients with Advanced-Stage Breast Cancer," *Oncology Nursing Forum* 39, no. 6 (2012): 568–577.

37. G. Ozdemir, N. Ovayolu, and O. Ovayolu, "The Effect of Reflexology Applied on Hemodialysis Patients with Fatigue, Pain and Cramps," *International Journal of Nursing Practice* 19, no. 3 (2013): 265–273.

38. M. Bagheri-Nesami, S. A. Shorofi, N. Zargar, M. Sohrabi, A. Gholipour-Baradari, and A. Khalilian, "The Effects of Foot Reflexology Massage on Anxiety in Patients Following Coronary Artery Bypass Graft Surgery: A Randomized Controlled Trial," *Complementary Therapies in Clinical Practice* 20, no. 1 (2014): 42–47.

39. E. A. Korhan, L. Khorshid, and M. Uyar, "Reflexology: Its Effects on Physiological Anxiety Signs and Sedation Needs," *Holistic Nursing Practice* 28, no. 1 (2014): 6–23.

40. C. Duffin, "How Namaste Principles Improve Residents' Lives," *Nursing Older People* 24, no. 6 (2012): 14–17.

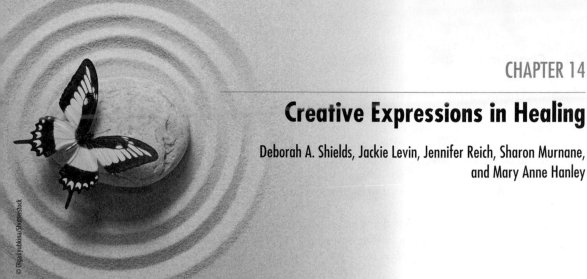

CHAPTER 14

Creative Expressions in Healing

Deborah A. Shields, Jackie Levin, Jennifer Reich, Sharon Murnane, and Mary Anne Hanley

Nurse Healer Objectives

Theoretical

- Describe creative expressions in healing.
- Outline underlying concepts central to the use of various creative expressions.
- Discuss theories integral to creative expressions.
- Explore the concept of time in nature.
- Appreciate the interdisciplinary foundation of creative expressions.

Clinical

- Identify specific ways that creative expression strategies affect healing and clinical practice.
- Explore the relationship between creativity and holism.
- Examine evidence that supports the healing power of creativity.
- Describe approaches to facilitate the integration of creative expression strategies with clients.
- Relate associated creative expression strategies to specific health and wellness needs of clients.

Personal

- Explore one or more creative expression strategies that are unfamiliar to you as a nurse healer.

- Identify one or more creative expression strategies to use as part of your holistic self-care practice.
- Develop a self-development plan that includes the integration of creative expression strategies.

Definitions

Aesthetics: Commonly thought of as the art of nursing; a complex, beautiful pattern of knowing and being that integrates ethical, empiric, intuitive, and personal knowing. Aesthetics invites the exploration of the meaning of experiences (e.g., life, health, well-being, illness, death) with self and/or another.[1]

Healing-healing: The emergence of right relationship at one or more levels of the bodymindspirit system.[2]

Improvisation: The capacity to transform knowledge, imagination, and aesthetics creatively through actions that address the anticipated and actual needs of another.[3]

Reflection: Inner awareness of our thoughts, feelings, judgments, beliefs, and perceptions.[4]

Self-care: Tending to (or attention to) the mind, body, and spirit through activities such as creative expression, physical exercise, time in nature, mindfulness, and healthy eating.

Self-development (holistic self-care): The lifelong commitment to and process of actualizing one's potential for well-being. The core of self-development is developing the Beingness of the nurse through the intentional development of self-awareness, self-reflection, and commitment to higher purpose.[5]

Stillpoint: A core essence to our Being experienced as a point of stillness that connects us directly to expanded levels of consciousness.[5]

Unknowing: A state of being that is open to not knowing.

Background

> Purplecluster Healing*
> *Stepping*
> *dawn of the new*
> *dewdrop fields twinkle*
> *soft magenta horizon*
> *breath of discovery*
> *greets the walker*
> *beginning . . .*

The art of nursing requires creative expression innovatively designed in concert with conventional healing approaches. In this chapter we purposefully use the labyrinth as a model for inner reflection and outer expression of aesthetics in holistic nursing. Aesthetics in holistic nursing require us to have a solid foundation in the fundamentals of holism as well as in the research and evidence that support artistic expression. Frequently, art leads us to new healthcare and self-care practices before theory or evidence does. Art allows us to find ways to express our world and our relationship with our world through nonverbal means. Having made that journey, we are able to begin to express meaning and create new patterns of being.

Creative has been described as inventive, imaginative, innovative, experimental, original, expressive, inspired, visionary, enterprising,

and resourceful.[6] Does this not describe most of the nurses you know, including yourself? Adapting a piece of equipment for a home-bound patient, sneaking in a pet for comfort, taking a hospice patient outside to feel the sun, organizing a spontaneous chorus of staff to sing to hospitalized children—these are all creative actions nurses do in the service of healing in our patients. It may be difficult to think how you might be creative within the context of your nursing work. Creativity needs to have some spaciousness with which to flow. So does healing.

Creative acts require acceptance of uncertainty. In working through the nonlinear process of creativity we develop resilience and promote healing.[7] We propose an arts-based model of interprofessional health care. As holistic nurses we tend to the whole person, mind-bodyspirit; however, our time may be limited due to factors such as patient assignment, complexity of care, and/or staffing levels. Through our relationship and intent to help others, we draw on knowledge, skills, arts, science, and evidence to demonstrate the standards of holistic nursing.

Improvisation, frequently associated with performing arts, offers a framework for integrating nursing expertise and the creative arts within a given patient or caring situation to create innovative solutions to caring. The foundations of a holistic philosophy and knowledge of holistic practices serve as the base for integrating creative expressions within holistic nursing. The transformation of knowledge, skills, and science into the art of holistic nursing requires mastery and creativity. Improvisation becomes evident as the holistic nurse elaborates on the known and creatively brings together the fundamental care patterns with aesthetics and an appreciation of the uncertain and unknown to facilitate new healing patterns. In such instances, the master or virtuoso holistic nurse improviser often acts in ways that appear to be spontaneous to the onlooker.

Although aesthetics offer us new ways of connecting the inner and the outer worlds of healing, improvisation serves as the bridge for that connection. Prior to integrating aesthetics, the holistic nurse needs to have gained the

---

*Reader's Note: This poem, *Purplecluster Healing* by D. Shields (Bremen, OH, 2014), continues throughout the chapter, identified by an asterisk.

discipline of her or his practice, confidence in skills and knowledge, and imagination to consider alternative ways of being and relating. Integrating aesthetics into holistic nursing often requires us to challenge established standards as well as to move forward to evaluate new practices and create innovative approaches where standards do not exist.[7] This continuum is reflected in how we each choose to integrate aesthetic practices. If the holistic nurse fails to adhere to foundations and standards of care while using an aesthetic practice, he or she fails to responsibly care for another and such action would be considered careless and negligent. Along the continuum, the holistic nurse thoughtfully considers and appreciates the role of a specific creative practice in benefiting a person's well-being, clearly within standards of practice. This might include, for example, adding an aesthetic practice to other practices, such as using imagery at the same time as teaching a person breathing patterns to relax, or it might be using the aesthetic practice alone. At the other end of the caring continuum, holistic nurses are faced with situations that do not have standards, new illnesses, or new behavior patterns; it is in these situations that the virtuoso holistic nurse introduces imaginative aesthetics or practices, founded in philosophy, theory, and science, to extend creative approaches to care beyond the known to address the unknown.

Creativity is an act of movement that requires self-reflection, vulnerability, and the courage to take off our masks and invite our authentic selves to emerge. The late Gabrielle Roth, creator of the 5Rhythms movement practice, stated, "The spirit in motion heals, expands, circles in and out of the body, moving through the layers of consciousness from inertia to ecstasy. Open to the spirit, and you will be transformed."[8, p. 207]

Self-reflection allows us this opening of spirit, to knowing self. There are many approaches to create the space for this self-exploration, and many of the emergent tools such as metaphors, symbols, silence, acceptance, and listening to the deeper meanings repeat themselves throughout the journey to healing. Nurses must be gentle and respectful of their inner guidance with the arising sensations, thoughts, and emotions as they engage and immerse themselves. As

you explore the self-reflection strategies offered throughout this chapter, tune in to what resonates with your spirit. As nurse healers, it is helpful to become familiar with a self-reflection strategy through personal experience before introducing it to a patient or client.

As holistic nurses, we purposefully engage in partnership with patients or clients, colleagues, and self to bring new solutions, practices, and patterns to life. Within holistic nursing we have been challenged to use evidence to support caring relationships, to make decisions regarding the interventions we use, and to demonstrate the *rightness* of care. Conversely or simultaneously, as holistic nurses we are often at the leading edge of knowledge and theory development. We are not satisfied with established standards, the status quo. We address the uncertainties of our practices and continuously search for new ways of being and doing.

The Labyrinth

In this chapter, following the path of the labyrinth as a metaphor for an inward and outward journey of healing, we explore creative expressions in holistic nursing (**Figure 14-1**). Through our description and application of selected creative expressions, we will demonstrate how the creative use of self and aesthetics serve to elaborate on existing standards as well as acknowledge improvisation as a way of creating imaginative new patterns and relationships that will inform future standards and foundations for evaluation and inquiry.

The labyrinth holds a particular vibration based on its shape and form. Artress proposed the labyrinth as an archetype of wholeness that helps us rediscover our soul.[9] It speaks to us from a place of unpredictability, tapping our wild and primordial inner nature. Walking in the labyrinth fosters letting go of control and the need to predict or direct the journey. Instead, we open to a more free-form experience, a guided journey from an Unknown Source. The labyrinth creates a path to the inner realms. Time in the labyrinth holds the possibility of tapping into deeper aspects of ourselves that may have been denied, hidden, or even berated. Our walk can create spaciousness and heart

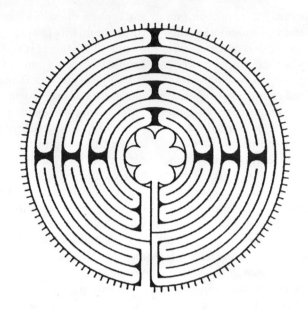

FIGURE 14-1 Labryinth

expansiveness as well as moments of deep self-reflection and inner dialogue.

Entering a walk into a labyrinth is a metaphor as much as it is a literal/physical experience. It is a spiritual experience of quieting the mind, opening the heart, and becoming grounded. The walk is a journey into a creative dimension of the self. With its one winding path into the center and the same path guiding us out, the labyrinth allows us to let go of the need to direct ourselves anywhere. We trust the path; while it does not control us, it does provide a structure for the journey of self-discovery. Creativity, healing, and the holistic nursing process are expressed in this journey through our being present, paying attention mindfully, and letting go of the outcome.

While each labyrinth includes turns and path-changing patterns, the classic Chartres Cathedral labyrinth includes a unique design element—*labyrs*—the turns or the butterfly shape in the path that illustrate the creation of moments of change. Such a change may represent a change in ideas, direction, or pattern. We often think of the labyrinth as the flowing path; however, without the labyrs we would not come face to face with shifts in the pattern of the labyrinth or the shifts in our own patterns of health

and being. The labrys give us a place to pause and ponder.

As we walk the labyrinth, we might move fast, slow, skip, hop on one foot, walk backward, or use a walker, wheelchair, or unicycle; we might even use a finger or hand in a modified labyrinth or our imaginations, whichever is the best means of making the journey. Whatever our mode of travel, we usually end up in the center. There might be a time when we step off of or skip over the path and turn around to retrace our earlier steps; this is a journey in and of itself—yet another way of self-discovery that we can appreciate with loving gentleness. The labyrinth invites us to let go of what we think we know and rest in unknowing. Unknowing allows us the freedom to explore old territory in new ways and unchartered territory without vigilance.[10]

We invite you to take a moment to gaze upon the labyrinth and, then, enter the journey when it feels right. Enter with love, knowing that this self-exploration will be just what you need it to be. It is an opportunity to be with what is in your life. Trust your intuitive knowing—there are no rules, no expectations. This is just for you.

As you travel along the labyrinth, you might be called to open your being, moving more and more inward. Stop along the way to breathe and be, trusting your heartfeet to know when to continue. Throughout the various sections of this chapter, as labrys along the path, you will meet a variety of self-reflection expressions to consider for use in your personal life and in your holistic nursing practice. Take time to pause and ponder.

You will likely reach the center, a place to pause and listen. You may be called to be still, to dance, to laugh, to cry, to write; whatever it is, trust that you are in the right place and that your inner self is expressing your deep wisdom. Perhaps you are becoming more conscious of what you know as your truth. Stay in the center as long as it feels right, and, when you are ready, begin to journey outward.

On your return journey outward, do you notice anything? Are your steps the same? Lighter? More integrated? There are no right answers—you are within your own journey. You continue to meet self-reflection expressions, to pause and ponder as you wish. Glimpses of your connection with a healing community may appear. How is your heart? Are you beginning to envision the integration of creative expressions into your personal life and your holistic nursing practice?

This chapter is designed to be read in snippets; there are no rules and regulations. Be spontaneous and trust. Allow the labyrinth to nourish you—to be a source of creative expression in healing. Welcome.

Entering, Embodiment, and Embeingment

*Stillness
morning larks
soar with ease and grace
she breathes
seeking the quiet
of rumbling mind-monkeys
breathe . . . be
breathe . . . be
larksongs
felt in the depths
breathe
accept
the walker enters . . .*

*This is a continuation of *Purplecluster Healing*.

Movement

Movement is expansive and includes a variety of practices that promote whole person well-being. As part of the fabric of cultures worldwide, movement and dance have historically been a part of ritual (e.g., worship, successful hunts, fertile fields) and healing traditions and practices engaged in by individuals and communities. This is true today. A broad range of Eastern and Western approaches to movement exist. Eastern movement (e.g., tai chi, qi gong, yoga) began as spiritual and even self-defense practices. Many Western movements arose from dance, physical therapy, forms of bodywork, and ways to recover from an injury or even approach death. The whole-person benefits of movement practices are plentiful and include physical (e.g., increased flexibility, muscle tone, cardiovascular stimulation, pain relief, resiliency, endurance), mental–emotional stillness and clarity, and spiritual connection. Movement practices can also promote a sense of belonging and community as one participates in shared activities.[11] Reflect for a moment on movement and consider the following thoughts.

Exercise can be a pathway to self-reflection. Individuals who regularly engage in physical activity often speak of the insights they receive during a walk, run, swim, or other form of exercise. In addition to the numerous physiologic benefits of physical activity, exercise has positive mental health benefits, such as reduced incidence of depression.[11] Some practices, such as yoga, tai chi, and qi gong, combine breath work, meditation, and physical movement to deepen awareness of the present moment. Some individuals keep exercise logs, noting not only their activity and time/distance but also insights and feelings that arise during the session.

You might consider other movements that awaken the rhythm of your inner being. Dancing may do this and can be delightful fun. You might move slowly and gracefully or engage in the rapid, sweat-producing steps of fast dances. The dancer entrains with the sound and rhythm of the music and the instruments and becomes one with them. It can be solo or with a partner(s). Consider: Dancers do not sweat, they glisten and glow!

Importantly, there may be situations that prevent physical movement. Whether a temporary or more permanent reality, you can still reap the benefits of movement. You might work with your body, moving selected parts with other parts and noting at your deepest level the sensations you are experiencing. It might be helpful to have a trusted person help you with these movements. There are also those who mentally rehearse movements in their mind's eye, enjoying the swim, the dance, the walk—enjoying the mental clarity and liberation that manifests with movement.

Pause to Ponder: Movement

Explore exercise as a self-reflective practice. Keep a reflective journal of your experience with a familiar or new form of activity. Reflect on how your body felt before, during, and after the session. How did you feel mentally? Was it hard *to get out the door*? Did you experience any *aha* moments? Note any changes in mood during these time periods. Did you enjoy this activity? Is it feasible to incorporate the activity into your self-development plan? What other forms of physical activity might you try to enhance your self-development practice?

Nature

Climb the mountains and get their good tidings. Nature's peace will flow into you as sunshine flows into trees. The winds will blow their own freshness into you, and the storms their energy, while cares will drop off like autumn leaves.

—Muir[12]

Time in nature as a creative expression in healing is a practice that can soothe a weary heart, calm a stressed body, and clear a cluttered or confused mind. Human beings need nature. Urban dwellers bring plants into their homes, workers place plants on their desks, preschool educational programs encourage outdoor time, gardeners plant flowers for no other reason than their beauty, and vacationers go to the wilderness and experience greater well-being. Nature is defined broadly here; it might be sitting with a favorite plant or pet, lying in the grass cloud watching, visiting a neighborhood park or

venturing further into forests or mountains, or taking a walk at the ocean shore.

Even as you read this chapter, most likely there is something from nature within view. Take a moment and look around. Maybe you see a seashell or a stone on a desk or a shelf, a tree outside your window or a photograph from a vacation. Take a moment and behold this; let your whole being rest with what you see. Notice any sensations, thoughts, and feelings that arise. What is this impulse to bring what is wild into our domesticated lives?

Edward Wilson called this impulse *biophilia*, described as "the urge to affiliate with other forms of life."[13] Louv's description of Wilson's theory is that "humans have an innate affinity for the natural world, probably a biologically based need integral to our development as individuals."[13] Later, Louv defined the field of "ecopsychology," emerging in the early 1990s and bridging the divide the modern world and sciences created between our natural inner life with the life outside our self.

Nature, Wholeness, and Healing

There is not a "fragment" in all nature, for every relative fragment of one thing is a full harmonious unit in itself.

—Muir[14]

Healing, like nature, is the vibration of unity and wholeness. And it is this wholeness that we seek even amidst the busyness of daily life. Modern life is often spent comparing, sorting, and separating—in other words, extracting parts and creating fragments. But within that stone or seashell, the woodpecker or the earthworm, is a relationship to an Oneness that gives us a sense of place within the whole. Contrary to our human endeavors to simplify life by reducing things to its parts, it is within wholeness that we find healing.

Does time in Nature actually heal? A growing body of research shows, as seen in the following examples, that time in nature or environments that bring the natural world inside benefits health and well-being. The Center for Health Design (www.healthdesign.org/chd), a nonprofit research organization, promotes the transformation of our current healthcare environments into places of healing and well-being, benefitting patients as well as healthcare staff. Research on nature as a therapeutic healing practice demonstrated the healing power of garden walking and journaling for depression;[15] time spent in woodlands increased perceived restorativeness;[16] exposure to Nature during the workday decreased generalized health complaints and stress;[17] and plants in hospital rooms enhanced patient recovery from surgery.[18] Seventeen participants in the McCaffrey, Hanson, and McCaffrey study journaled about their time in a walking garden, describing a feeling of unity and its connection to healing.[15]

One participant shared that the garden walks gave her a greater peace and awareness of beauty. Another person felt life had more meaning and that he knew his sense of place. Yet another described an experience of joy, clearing "out negative and confusing thoughts" and focusing on the positive aspects of her life.

Louv coined the phrase *nature-deficit disorder*, referring to the amount of time we spend devoid of nature substituted with time in front of a computer or television screen.[13] Emerging research suggests that the amount of time spent in front of our electronic media screens (handheld devices, computers, tablets, televisions) relates to increases in childhood obesity and poses a greater risk for reducing children's sense of well-being.[19]

If scientific research does not shed sufficient light on the benefits of being in Nature, poets, writers, and artists expand on this theme for us.

Lost*

Stand still.
The trees ahead and bushes beside you
Are not lost.
Wherever you are is called Here,
And you must treat it as a powerful stranger,
Must ask permission to know it and be known.
The forest breathes. Listen. It answers,
I have made this place around you.
If you leave it, you may come back again, saying Here.
No two trees are the same to Raven.
No two branches are the same to Wren.

*David Wagoner, "Lost," Collected Poems 1956–1976, Indiana University Press, http://writersalmanac.publicradio.org/?date=2006/01/11

If what a tree or a bush does is lost on you,
You are surely lost. Stand still. The forest knows
Where you are. You must let it find you.

—Wagoner[20]

When we try to pick out anything by itself, we find it hitched to everything else in the Universe.
—Muir[21]

Intention, Healing, and Time in Nature

Deliberately creating an intention for your time in nature can serve as a mirror for inner awareness and insight and therefore can be healing. Taking a medicine walk, similar to that of walking a labyrinth, is an example of time in Nature as mirror, guide, and healer.

The medicine walk is an indigenous practice of going into nature with a question or intention for insight into a problem or personal dynamic. Indigenous peoples teach that the natural world is both teacher and mirror, reflecting clearly one's unique gifts, strengths, and limiting patterns; it is a doorway to greater insight and transformation through the metaphorical and symbolic messages.[4]

The word *medicine* is used to imply the healing aspect of this practice. Domestic and wild animals, insects, birds, and reptiles cross our paths in both the natural and human-made worlds. Most often these beings are not thought of as bringing messages for self-reflection. However, Sams and Carson in *Medicine Cards* and Andrews in *Animal-Speak* describe how these creatures can teach us about aspects of our own natures that may need greater attention or activation.[4] Deeper meanings and patterns emerge from other messages from nature, such as sounds, smells, rocks, trees, vegetation, and bodies of water, when our contact with these aspects of nature are reflected on.

The medicine walk involves three phases: (1) preparation, (2) solo time, and (3) returning to community. Preparation readies the individual for the coming journey within the context of a supportive community. The individual sits with a trusted friend or group or uses a journal to practice reflective listening to his or her issues and concerns. Emerging from this reflection is the intention for the walk. The intention, set as a question, may be general, as in, "What can I learn about myself today?" Or a health question, such as, "What do I need to know about my illness?" Or even as specific as, "Should I take this job?" Setting an intention calls on the unseen forces to co-create in expanding the individual's conscious awareness of what is needed for healing and insight.

Solo time involves going out on the medicine walk. The individual creates a threshold demarcating a separation from the ordinary material world and the luminous and mysterious world. The threshold may be a doorway, an entrance to a park, or simply a stick placed on the ground to be stepped over to represent moving into the nonordinary world of nature. Before stepping over the threshold, the individual calls up his or her intention and can ask for spiritual guidance in the mini *quest* of discovery. This practice can be done in the wilderness, one's own home or backyard, a neighborhood park, the busy streets of a city, or the hallways of a clinical practice setting.

Pause to Ponder: Medicine Walk

- Reflect on a conflict or question.
- Frame the issue in your mind in an open manner. For example, "I'd like to gain insight into my conflict, illness, relationship, or work choices." Let go of preconceived ideas of any outcome.
- Create a "threshold" separating your ordinary time into sacred reflective time. Use a doorway, gate, stick, or imaginary line.
- Step through this threshold into timeless time and begin your walk, allowing an inner freedom to be your guide. Notice what path you take, who or what crosses your path, and any thoughts and feelings you experience. Allow your senses to guide you; let your rational and critical mind rest. For example, instead of thinking that you see a flower, shift your experience to sensing the flower seeing you. This shift in awareness integrates you into the wholeness of the unfolding universe instead of keeping you separate and in *control*.
- When you complete your walk, step back over the same threshold if possible; if not, create a new threshold.

- Write down the story of your medicine walk in the first or third person. Reflect on and self-mirror this story, noticing metaphors and symbols. Glean any new insights and understandings.

Returning to community is done through sharing the story of the walk. The story, witnessed by trusted others or through journaling, can be told in first or third person: "I/she started out by heading down the street. It was crowded and colorful. I/she then noticed a person looking confused and asked if she needed help. . . ."

When the story is complete, the individual and the trusted other reflect on and mirror it. Mirroring is an advanced level of listening and reflecting back, not simply repeating what was said. To continue with the preceding example, the one acting as mirror might suggest to the walker, "I hear the story of a woman who notices the vibrancy of her surroundings (life?) and who knows how to help people find their way." Upon hearing his or her story mirrored (reflected back), the walker can consciously integrate the deeper meanings and new insights into nursing practice and/or self-directed care. The process of reflection and mirroring can help develop and refine the advanced skills of reflective listening.

Nature, Nursing, and Creative Expressions in Healing

> Since the human body is the world, every individual in this world, regardless of background or race, has an indigenous soul struggling to survive in an increasingly hostile environment created by that individual's mind, which subscribes to the mores of the machine age. Because of this, a modern person's body has become the battleground between the rationalist mind and the native soul.[22]

How can you bring the creative healing aspect of Nature to your nursing practice and your patients? In environments where a patient may stay for a few hours or days, invite him or her or family members to bring in pictures of nature scenes that are particularly meaningful. As the holistic nurse, you can also have on

Here is an example of journaling about my own medicine walk in the woods behind my home in the Northwest United States. I create a threshold and set my intention. I'm feeling the need to shake things up a bit but don't know in what way. I simply ask, "Please show me something that will illuminate my understanding of myself." I'm feeling I need to stand at the red gate and spontaneously twirl three times to the right. Why? I want to enter my nature time a bit off balance. I want less control. I open the gate and turn to the right. I see the path down to the Pond Hut. I'm drawn to a spot near the edge of the shingled roof that's filled with sunlight coming in through the treetops. I follow the sun's dappled light in places and look up. I'm searching for the heron nest in hopes I might find another feather. Ugh, still an agenda.

Then I notice all of the places the sun comes through and where it is blocked by the forest canopy. All day long, the sun arcs across the sky, its light nondirected; it simply exists. It has huge power, and yet it is the forest canopy that creates the places where the light gets in.

As I cross back through my threshold, I reflect on this. Can I be more like the sun and the forest floor below, the dynamic dance between shadow and light?

hand posters or cards of nature scenes to hang on the wall or give to the patient to hold and look at. When using guided imagery, ask the patient if there is a place in nature that he or she finds relaxing and soothing. When a relaxing place in nature is identified, bring it into the guided imagery. In the home setting, remind the patient to spend time when possible outside, on the porch, in the yard or garden, or in a local park or woods.

Nature can bring the patient *back home*, a deep sense of being connected to the universal, to themselves, to the cycles of life, and to healing.

> **She spins*
> *a whirling deva*
> *amidst the white pines*
> *the walker's heart*
> *alive with laughter*
> *she notices*
> *slowing rumbles*
> *as beats quicken*
> *stillness*
> *a blanket of being . . .*

Sound, Rhythm, and Voice

Primordial sound is that sound heard and felt below the perception of hearing, associated with spiritual traditions and scientific discoveries.[23] Many consider *Om* as the primordial sound made, manifest through our experience and awareness. Through a variety of spiritual traditions *Om*, from Hinduism (pronounced Aum), was translated by other traditions. The Tibetan sacred word *Hum*, Muslim *Amin*, and Egyptian, Greek, Roman, and Christian *Amen* are all considered to be primordial sounds.[24] In Hebrew, Amen means sure or faithful. Whittle, an astronomer at the University of Virginia, connected primordial sound with the Big Bang, tracing vibrations to our earliest known source.

> As is often the case with Nature, things are not so simple, and a more accurate description would be something like this: a descending scream, building into a deep rasping roar, and ending in a deafening hiss. As if this were not impressive enough, the entire acoustic show is itself the prelude to a wonderful transformation: the highest pitch sounds ultimately spawn the first generation of stars, while the deep bass notes slowly dissolve to become the tapestry of galaxies which now fills all of space. The birth of the Universe, it turns out, had its own primal scream.[25, p. 1]

Whittle's assertion reinforces our understanding that we are birthed from vibrations of energy that are transformed into sound and light. Ultimately, sound and light become more dense and physical. Hence, our physical bodies became manifested through an evolving energetic transformation. Native Americans often refer to the *star people*—those souls who have left their physical bodies and have returned to the energies of the Universe from whence they came.

**This is a continuation of *Purplecluster Healing.*

Thanks to the intense work of French scientist Alfred Tomatis (described as the "Einstein of sound and Sherlock Holmes of sonic detection"), we understand that the voice can only reproduce what the ear can hear.[26] He examined more than 100,000 clients in listening centers throughout the world for listening disabilities as well as learning disorders. Curiosity led him to his work in the field of embryology and to the discovery that "the mother's voice serves as a sonic umbilical cord for her developing baby and a primal source of nurturing."[26, pp. 16-17] We begin hearing low-frequency sounds close to 4.5 months of fetal life; we hear the sound of the breath moving in and out, our mother's heartbeat, and her stomach rumbling (in hunger and satisfaction). The fetal environment is a constant cacophony of interactive sound.

Awakening through awareness to sound and vibration, remembering, and being present to sound and vibration around us affects us in multidimensional realms. Generally speaking, our worlds are abundant with sound and stimulation. We experience both as a welcome and constant aspects of our environments. Is it no wonder that we often seek a place and space of less sound, peaceful nurturing sounds, and even silence. We yearn for silence from the chatter, both internal and external, and a relief from the background noise that is a constant in our lives for better or for worse. Are we aware of how these and all sounds affect us?

Pause to Ponder: Sound

Take yourself through "a day in your life": Observe the first/earliest sounds or sounds that begin your day and, hour by hour, remember what you typically hear and listen to. How do these sounds affect you physically, mentally, emotionally, spiritually? Perhaps you might journal your thoughts.

The Deep Listening*
What is the deep listening?
Sama is a greeting from the secret ones inside . . .

*"Listening," from THE GLANCE: RUMI'S SONGS OF SOUL-MEETING by Rumi, translated by Coleman Barks, translation copyright ©1999 by Coleman Barks. Used by permission of Viking Penguin, a division of Penguin Group (USA) LLC.

I should sell my tongue and buy a thousand ears
when that one steps near and begins to speak.
—Rumi[27]

Sound may be both positive and negative; it requires both consciousness and management. Koch suggested, "One day man will have to combat noise as he once combated cholera and the plague."[26, p. 35] As people and as holistic nurses it is important to be mindful of the presence of noise stimulation and its effects on healing. In *Timeshifting: Creating More Time to Enjoy Your Life*, Rechtschaffen discussed how living beings become entrained or synchronized with the rhythms around them.[28] If the environment is frenetic, our inner rhythms may become ones of pressure and stress. Without awareness, we may become chronically stressed. When we are not feeling well, we may say that we feel *out of synch*. Sounds that ground us have a calming effect. For instance, Friedman noted that Andrew Neher "focused on the effects on the central nervous system with rhythmic drumming." He found drumming could entrain his subjects' brain waves into "alpha and theta states, states commonly associated with relaxation, a sense of well-being, and deep drowsiness."[29, p. 44] Raising our awareness can help us to intervene and intercept the neural pathway messages we are receiving. When we find ourselves in the midst of rhythms that do not serve us, Rechtschaffen suggested that we create a "pause button" to help us stop our frenetic pace, breathe, and come into a rhythm that is comfortable and good for us, our patients, and our colleagues.[28]

Sound and rhythm are energetic pulsations that are universal. We are one song, however in or out of tune or synchronicity we may be. Rhythm is a given; if you have a heartbeat, you have rhythm. It is inherently this "rhythm from within" where we may find a connectedness with self. Too many people are told that "they have no rhythm" or they say, "I have no rhythm." These are erroneous statements and beliefs. If you are breathing you have rhythmic breath, your heart beats rhythmically; energetically, the soul's heartbeat is a constant. The energy center or chakra of the heart holds the vibrational quality for each individual's own unique rhythm—as unique as a fingerprint or the iris.

Our heart–mind is in constant flux, but the rhythm exists within a complex constellation of multidimensional influences. Rather than viewing the heart in a healthy or unhealthy rhythm, think of every heart with the potential to create and/or be in synchrony with its environment. Some hearts benefit or need support from a variety of sources; for example, a sad heart needs more love, patience, and caring, or perhaps an antidepressant herb or medication to survive. On the other hand, one may require less medication if the ancient practices of rhythm and music as medicine are recognized, researched, and incorporated into healing practices today as they have been used by indigenous healers since ancient times.

Shamans and communities, where song and dance are important aspects of healing create a sense of connection, feelings of well-being, and ways of communicating. Healing is a naturally occurring phenomenon revealed through the sounds and rhythms that create internal synchrony with one's environment. Friedman noted that "everything we perceive is based on rhythm."[29, p. 26] Slower rhythms represent the changing of the seasons, the rotation of the sun and moon in perfect order, and the constellations of stars as they shift position through the sky and with the seasons. Close your eyes and recall hearing the rhythm of the waves lapping on the shore. In Native American traditions, the oceans, rivers, and lakes are known as the blood of the Mother Earth. The winds that circumnavigate the globe, constantly and rhythmically, are all life-giving elements moving in a rhythm that creates the miraculous planet we inhabit. Again, we are One Song, in concert together. The more we listen to our own rhythms and learn how to synchronize with our environment, the healthier we become.

This brings us to the art of listening. Campbell noted that, compared to hearing, which is the ability to receive auditory information through the ears, skin, and bones, listening is the ability to filter, selectively focus on, remember, and respond to sound; while we may hear, we do not always listen.[26, p. 44] All too often we and our patients may experience the phenomenon of truly not being heard due to lack of authentic, active listening skills. Before we can authentically listen to others, we must be able to listen to our own heart song as part of our holistic self-development practice.

We may deny or simply neglect our potential for healing with sound and song. Since ancient times, mantras, chanting, toning, and, more commonly in our culture, humming (a quiet form of toning) are ways to enliven the vocal cords that actually create a healing vibration throughout our bodymindspirit. In the beginning, the birthing mother often cries out in one form or another; the next most significant sound is the first cry of the just-born infant, signifying first breath, first sound, and life itself. It is a powerful sound to parent and child alike. Producing and listening to sound vibrations are empowering approaches to self-reflection. By cultivating our appreciation of sound, we deepen our ability to listen to our inner wisdom.

Pause to Ponder: Listening

You may begin with a simple exercise in your home. Set a timer for 15 to 30 minutes and blindfold your eyes (depending on your ability to sit quietly without stimulation or movement) and listen to any and all sounds that you hear. In this way, you are practicing active listening and setting your intention to pay attention to the full spectrum of sounds in the world around you. You are now in and experiencing the present moment. If your mind begins to chatter, just as in meditation, bring your attention back to your intention: Take a breath and refocus on listening (rather than hearing mind chatter). What are you noticing?

Take a moment, if it is comfortable, to ponder your labyrinth walk thus far. What is your sense of what will nourish you in this moment? Continuing? Stopping for a time? Listen. Know.

Voice

Continuing our exploration of sound, we consider the power of our voice, which is the throat or fifth chakra and a major energy center. The sounds we can generate are freeing, releasing, and healing. The sense of freedom is commonly evidenced by how wonderful we feel when we sing loudly and privately in the shower or in our vehicles when no one else can hear our sometimes out-of-tune voices.

The throat is a physical and symbolic bridge between the head and the heart. Singing connects the mind with the emotions. Gaynor noted, "To the Sufis, singing is (prana), the breath of life itself, and the most potent of all the musical healing modalities."[30] Yet singing is often not enjoyed by adults (except for a fortunate few) because as children they may have received messages, directly or implied, such as they could not and should not sing as indicated by the frown from a parent/elder/teacher or anyone in a position of authority, or they were ridiculed by siblings and/or classmates, which shut them down. How might we alter these messages and create a new experience? Let's consider the wisdom of indigenous practices.

In Native American traditions, drumming circles are also singing circles. Individuals gathered around the circle are asked to lead the group in a song. The group will drum and sing because every song is considered a prayer, whether reverent or playful. A collective deep breath, silence, and pause at the end of a drumming song allows the vibrations and energy to be deeply felt and permits oneself to be in a conscious act of gratitude. The emphasis is on connection and the shared experience, not the voice.

Drumming

Ancient instruments like the drum, in all of its forms, along with the flute, didgeridoo (Australian Aboriginal culture), Tibetan 7-metal singing bowls, gongs, and other lesser known instruments from a wide variety of ancient and indigenous cultures are known to be powerful healing tools. Weaving awareness of percussion and the beat–rhythm into our personal and professional practice can be transformative. In contemporary culture, this transformation is often facilitated with the drum.

Of all of the instruments in the world, the drum stands firmly in the place of universality. Its prominence in numerous cultural traditions is depicted in historical images and narrative. Women from many cultures are portrayed in carvings, cave drawings, and symbols as they were drumming and serving as the eternal connection to rhythm, particularly to the moon. Women honored the "Mother Goddess, and the five phases of the moon cycle mirror the natural cycle of birth, growth, fruition, desolation and death which is always followed by a new cycle, initiated with birth."[31] The frame drum has long been an essential tool and voice of shamans, the ancient medicine people, and healers and professional interworld travelers. The shrine painting of dancers holding the frame drum and rattle (both percussion instruments) at Catal Huyuk is believed to have been created circa 5800 BC.[31]

Today, we are culturally reconnecting with the essence of our innate rhythms through drumming. Drumming is done as meditation, alone or in concert with others. The cadence can be drumming a singular beat (as often used in Native American cultures) or a repeated rhythm pattern. Regardless of how simple or complex the practice, drumming alters our state of consciousness. It has the potential to support our connection to self, our breath, and our heartbeat. Our "inner space" connects to the universal world of which we are wholly a part, rhythmically, vibrationally, and spiritually. Through the drum the soulful part of our being connects to the Earth and to one another. We take a deep, cleansing breath, which signals a shift in consciousness; we become aware of our physical bodies vibrating. It is a vibration of peacefulness, openness, and wholeheartedness.

When we drum as a practice, we deepen our connections to self-healing. In this way, we can drum (and sing) as nurse healers with our patients. Drumming mindfully, we can release stress and negative emotions (fear, anger, sadness, loneliness) into a safe, grounded space. We can drum intuitively because we trust that the rhythm is occurring within us with every breath and heartbeat. "When we let go of our words, we are left with our emotions; when we release our emotions, we are left only with sounds. When we release our sounds, we are left only with the drum."[29]

Stevens described four drum circle principles:[32]

1. There is no audience; everyone is part of the musical experience.
2. There is no rehearsal; the drum circle is a safe, permissive, explorational environment, regardless of size.

3. There is no teacher; the drum circle may be led by a facilitator who builds a sense of community and connection.
4. It is inclusive; everyone is welcome.

Drumming can be helpful to people with varied health challenges. Oncology patients may drum to reconnect with their wholeness. People living with Parkinson's disease may be able to walk with improved balance, stride, and arm swing when specific rhythms are played, suggesting that the drumming improves neural pathway reconnections. Seniors living with Parkinson's, with and without cognitive deficits, can drum to reconnect with vital life-giving neural pathways. Drumming allows them to experience a sense of reconnection and the ability to create sounds and rhythms, often from times and memories of long ago. They are empowered to connect and create and have a sense of being more alive in the present moment. Often, severely disabled patients in nursing homes will experience the joy and amazement of *playing* once again. The power of the drumming experience is expansive and deeply healing.

Pause to Ponder: Drumming

Take your drum and sit with it. When you are ready, walk, play, listen, feel your experience. What is your felt sense? How are the rhythms? Are you comfortable? Uncomfortable? What might this mean to you? Is there room for both comfort and discomfort in healing? Can you envision that you are healing yourself? Then, when you are ready to share, bring the healing dream of drumming to others.

Music

Music therapy can be defined as the controlled use of music and its influence on the human being to aid in physiologic, psychological, and emotional integration of the individual during the treatment of an illness or disease.[33] When in good health, our body is in tune and more in synchrony with all parts—harmony prevails. In illness or disease, one or more of the body's instruments is out of tune—flat, sharp, deficient—creating symptoms of disharmony. To heal with music means to become present but also to transform into a state of *holos*,

becoming whole, as in harmony and balance. "Defining wholeness in musical terms means we must go beyond the contemporary model of the body and think of it as an orchestra receiving and producing a symphony of sounds, chemicals, electrical charges, colors and images."[26, p. 62] Music therapy helps the body rebalance, allowing the music of one's own heart song to strengthen and regain a sense of peace, healing, and wholeness, whether into life or death.

Music is a social behavior in people from before birth to transition. Rhythm, a dominant feature of the universe—indeed, ubiquitous in nature—emanates from all musical genres. Exploring the relationship between rhythm and vibration deepens our understanding of the scientific foundation of music as energy and its effect on us.

Seward posited, "Quantum physics established the theory that everything is energy, hence, the effect of vibrations on anything can be powerful."[34, p. 171] Every cell is vibrating at a particular resonance; each organ and tissue is pulsing in continuous motion. Energy (qi/chi) pulses throughout us along meridian lines. Vibrating atoms create our energy field, which extends outward from our body to interact with all in our environment. This is the mystery and magnificence of the orchestra within. Vibrations are powerful and can be healing—and possibly harmful. Thus, musical vibrations can be wonderful—or not. Let's consider music as a creative expression. As holistic nurses, we are mindful that sound and music are subjective. Music's power needs to be felt as a healing therapy rather than as something that activates negative or extremely distressing emotions of any kind (anger, depression, even violence). As co-partners in healing, through the use of music as gentle medicine, we connect with ourselves and support our patients through our collective interaction with sound, rhythms, and music in whichever form is healing and therapeutic for each individual. As co-partners in healing, holistic nurses support the whole person—body-mindspirit—to a place and space of self-healing.

Pause to Ponder: Inner Rhythms

Listening to your own rhythms offers you the opportunity to embark on a self-reflective journey as you prepare for the music of your heart and soul to reveal itself to you in an awakened state of awareness.

Go to your soundless center. Take a moment to again listen deeply from a place of silence. What do notice?

> *Silence, you are the diamond in me,*
> *the Jewel of my real wealth!*
> *From your self earth grows thousands of rose gardens*
> *whose perfumes drown me in my heart.*
>
> —Rumi[35]

> *Coming to center*
> *the walker pauses*
> *skies brightening*
> *into the blue of the morning day*
> *she breathes . . .*

The Center

Centering, Celebrating, Contemplating: Take some moments here, as many moments as you wish, to sink gently into your contemplative space, connected to that deeper place of your inner wisdom and grace. Honor and celebrate yourself in an open and allowing state of being, fully present and feeling deeply connected, inspired, and grateful. You trust that all is as it is. What are you noticing? What messages are you receiving from your stillpoint, your inner self? The center is not a place of pushing or forcing. It is a space of openness and receiving. And you remember—silence is a message. From this place/space, you are more fully prepared as a holistic nurse to bring the gifts and wisdom of creative expression to those you serve.

> *The walker*
> *enfolded in light*
> *listens to the sounds*
> *of stillness . . .*
> *blue skies*
> *blankets of peace*
> *stir within her*
> *wonderment*
> *what will the center*
> *reveal?*
> *She trusts . . .*

*This is a continuation of *Purplecluster Healing.*

Reflective Writing

Writing for self-reflection takes many forms. Some individuals feel drawn to creative forms of writing, such as poetry and story writing, to reflect on their conscious experiences. Others use a daily journal for ongoing thoughts, brainstorming creative ideas, and recording insights. Journaling has also been cited in the literature as a tool to help nursing students reflect on their clinical experiences and understand the links between theory and practice.[36] With advances in technology over the past decade, blogging has become an alternative to traditional journaling for self-reflection. Whether traditional or high-tech, journal writing reveals to us our unique inner world while also connecting us to the shared experience of being human.

Pause to Ponder: Journaling

Gather a notebook and pen, or have your computer nearby. Set a timer for 10 to 20 minutes. Sit in quiet meditation for a few moments, paying attention to the breath flowing in and out of your body. Then, begin to write. Allow whatever wants to be expressed to take form on the page. Write until the buzzer goes off, or beyond, *without* editing. The writing may take any number of forms: a poem, narrative, lists, pictures, and doodles. Use this writing as a guide for reflection throughout the day.

Storytelling

Sturm explained that listening to stories can lead to changes in the experience of reality. He called this the *storytelling trance*, describing how listeners transcend normal waking consciousness as the story takes on new dimensions. Listeners experience the story with "remarkable immediacy," becoming part of the characters and plot of the story.[37, p. 2] In listening to stories, we are drawn to archetypes. Smith noted that human beings have always used stories as a means to receive information as well as to create structure around it. We are meaning seekers and makers, and we create symbolic stories that exemplify the universality of our experiences.[38]

Pause to Ponder: Storytelling and Story Sharing

1. Take yourself to a professional storytelling performance. As you listen, notice where you find yourself in the story. Did you find yourself entering the storytelling trance?

2. Invite a group of colleagues to participate in a story circle. Allow space and time for everyone in the circle to be heard and witnessed.

Listening, Metaphors, and Images

Listening occurs on multiple depths simultaneously. The first depth of listening is listening to a person's words and interpreting the meaning through your own lens of life experiences and beliefs. The second depth of listening is listening deeply to the words without judgment, allowing a fuller understanding of a person's experience. The third depth of listening includes listening to the greater environmental field of language and messages beyond the words. At this depth the listener is tuning into body language, tone, pace, and the metaphoric and symbolic language, as well as to synchronistic events occurring in the environment.[39]

A metaphor is the use of an image, word, or phrase to represent something else. For example, when describing a neck pain, the patient explains, "It feels like a tight knot." When exploring the knot, the nurse asks the patient to describe the knot in detail. "It's a thick, coarse rope and very heavy." Metaphors enrich our understanding and take us deeper into the underlying patterns. The nurse might venture further, asking, "Does anything else in your life right now feel like it's tied up in a knot?"

Smith wrote, "Metaphor is the product of an intuitive grasp of a unity of meaning; in it a familiar image used in an unfamiliar context fosters a holistic insight in a moment."[38, p. 48] This insight can become a source of information (expanding consciousness) for the person, who, with the use of imagery, can begin to "untie the knot."[38]

This deeper level of listening requires the holistic nurse to entrain herself or himself to the unity of experience in the mutual process of pattern appreciation and recognition.

Listening Beneath the Words

When entering into pattern appreciation with the patient or client, take three breaths and set your intention to listen to his or her story uninterrupted. To begin the connection, ask the patient one of the following or another open-ended question:

- Can you tell me what is most distressing for you right now?
- Can you describe to me what is most important to you right now?
- What has occurred over the last few days, weeks, or months that has led up to this [event or situation]?

Listen to the meaning beneath the words, listen to the messages hidden in metaphors and symbolic language, and notice if events occur in the environmental field that would give greater significance or understanding to the patient's situation (e.g., a bird flies at the window, rain starts to fall, a car honks when a significant insight occurs). Engage in unknowing and allow the unfolding to occur.

Pause to Ponder: Poetry as Creative Expression

Find a quiet space to sit. Close your eyes and take three slow breaths, expanding the belly as you breathe in and fully emptying the belly before your next breath. Gently open your eyes and come back to the room. Now, try writing a poem about a personal experience.

Pause to Ponder: Synchronicity

Take a moment to reflect on experiences of synchronicity. For example, knowing who is on the other end of the phone before you answer, or perhaps thinking about someone and then running into that person at the same time or shortly after. Are there instances when you received the very sign you needed to move forward on your journey? For the next 7 days, keep a journal of these types of experiences, even if

---

Exemplar: Paying Attention

What does it mean to "pay attention"? Reflect on the following story. How does life show us our connection through people we do not know? What do we miss when we move through life without paying attention?

Trip the Light Fantastic

I met Henry at the coffee shop. He sat down across from me, and I smiled and said hello. As he was leaving, I wished him a good day, and he said he appreciated that I was smiling and enjoying what I was doing. I told him I was a nurse poet and writing poetry and he said he was a poet also. He explained that he had been a banker before he had a bad car accident about 10 years ago. He said he almost died in the accident and had a near-death experience. He had a scar across his head and told me he was in the hospital for more than a year after his accident. Not long after he woke up, he started getting poetry in "downloads." He asked me to read him a poem, and then he recited an amazing poem for me. This poem had personal meaning, and I was overcome with emotion. Then he said, "I have one more for you." This poem had a message for me, and I started to cry. He ended with the line "trip the light fantastic," which has special significance for me. At that point, I knew I was experiencing a connection with my spirit guidance.

---

they seem insignificant. Reflect on how "paying attention" may have shifted your worldview.

Art

Little as we know about the way in which we are affected
by form, by colour, and by light, we do know this,
that they have an actual physical effect . . .
People say the effect is only on the mind.
It is no such thing.
The effect is on the body, too . . .
Variety of form
and brilliancy
of color in the objects presented to patients
are actual means of recovery.

—Nightingale[40]

Art has been a part of culture since ancient times; archaeological evidence includes a variety of art forms that reveal insight into people's daily lives, ceremonies, rituals, and transitions.[41, 42] From paintings on cave walls to archaeological excavations where beautiful pieces of sculptures are discovered, we understand the significance of art throughout our evolution.

Art can be active (creating art) and/or passive/receiving (gazing upon it).[41] Both of these art forms are valuable and engage our inner being. Creating art may take many forms: drawing, painting, writing, sculpting, fabric work,

photography, singing, and dancing. We are able to appreciate receiving art from many sources, such as through galleries, concerts, street fairs, reading, theaters, and special items that we use in our personal and professional lives. Holistic nurses are mindful of environments within which practice unfolds, considering light, color, air quality, scents, sounds, and general ambience. We strive to create caring spaces designed to support healing-healing of self and others.

According to Kovalesky, we are increasingly aware of the mind–body effects of art. The pleasure associated with creating or gazing upon aesthetically pleasing art can stimulate endorphin release. A stress response may be modulated, as engaging in art seems to increase natural killer cells and T cells. Art helps with whole-brain integration, bringing together the emotional, intuitive, nonverbal right side with the logical, problem-solving left side of the brain. Indeed, through art, the brain reveals its plasticity.[41]

Art can be a powerful expression of self-reflection, moving us to depths not yet discovered but alive with wisdom. We are often reluctant to undertake art projects because we believe that we are not artistic or that we lack in some way the abilities needed to create art. As a self-reflective expression, we are invited to consider that the healing journey is about process, not outcome. Who are we when we gaze upon a work that we find beautiful, or when we create a piece that represents something deep within our hearts? There are no rules, no requirements, as we pick up the paintbrush or sing the song. It is our chance to express, to feel the joy of liberation!

Mandala Art

The deepest and most profound aspects of any art form, traditional or spontaneous, will be felt and recognized as universal; a mandala is one of these. Rooted in Sanskrit, the word *mandala* is translated to mean circle.[43] The circle represents a sacred container that most traditions have used as a meditative and/or spiritual symbol for thousands of years. Crafting a mandala is an ancient form of creative expression used for insight, healing, self-reflection, and self-expression. The mandala is said to be the bridge between the higher and lower realms. Nature is the most fertile and abundant source of mandalas.

Mandalas are thought to support our connection with our Self. Jung believed,

> The mandala is an archetypal image whose occurrence is attested throughout the ages. It signifies the wholeness of Self. This circular image represents the wholeness of the psychic ground, or, to put it in mythic terms, the divinity incarnate in man.[44]

Fincher noted,

> The Self generates *patterns* within your inner life. Your mandalas reveal the dynamic of the Self as it creates a matrix where your unique identity unfolds. The mandala circle mirrors the Self as the container for the psyche's striving toward self-realization or wholeness. Within the mandala motifs from the shared past of all human beings, symbols of individual experience find expression.[45, p. 20]

Consider Susanne's mandala journey:

Susanne's knowledge and deep connection to the mandala came directly from her personal life experience and dark night of the soul as she sought healing while deeply grieving the death of a child and a painful divorce.

She intuitively began drawing circles that made her feel better. Eventually discovering art as therapy, she pursued training to become a highly accomplished art therapist and author.

How then, might we create our own mandala journey and, as holistic nurses, support one another?

> *Though we seem to be sleeping,*
> *there is an inner wakefulness that directs the dream*
> *and that will eventually startle us back*
> *to the truth of who we are.*
> —Rumi, An Inner Wakefulness, translated by Coleman Barks, http://www.poetry -chaikhana.com/blog/2013/12/18 /mevlana-jelaluddin-rumi -inner-wakefulness-2[46]

Mandala creation establishes a deeper connection to the innermost self and to subconscious thoughts and feelings otherwise unable or unwilling to reveal themselves. These sacred circles are used as a form of creative expression and meditative contemplation leading to the center, that mysterious core of our being where inner wisdom resides and beckons to be revealed. Revealing and releasing insights of our innermost selves supports harmony and healing from the multidimensionality of the physical, mental–emotional, and spiritual aspects of the self. Cornell asserted, "Deep within our psyches, the *universal light of consciousness* awaits our remembering and expressing who we really are."[47]

The center within oneself, the *Hara* or center point, represents the original spark of one's pure, clear light. You enter into the world with this light at birth. Intuition and inner wisdom develop at an early age; then, over time, the inner knowingness may (or may not) become gradually less accessible for any number of reasons (family, environment, workplace, attitudes, values, and beliefs of those surrounding us). The mandala process reconnects us to that original spark of light and inner wisdom.

What is the mandala process? It is a merging of art, science, and ancient wisdom for reconnection to meaning and purpose within the sacred circle as an opportunity for the authentic self to be revealed through the quiet, introspective space of self-reflection. The mandala process may serve several purposes or needs: (1) a reflective process (anywhere from 20 to 60 minutes); (2) a self-care practice of awareness and healing; (3) a potential healing tool for anyone wishing to experience a nonverbal expression of thoughts or feelings with a release of emotions related to relationships, transitions, or challenges; (4) an opportunity for gaining insight, stress management, and personal/professional and/or spiritual growth along the continuum of holism in self-health care; and (5) a nonverbal expression of inner wisdom, light, love, and peace. In other words, it is a remembering of our authentic self and/or a letting go of what no longer serves us. We might, for example, create a mandala of what it would be like if we were *not* carrying the burden of fear, hurt, resentment, or similar feelings. Regardless of the intention, the mandala helps us move energy and/or build and replenish energy.

The goal of the mandala process is to create an instance where one can experience or reexperience a sense of well-being, gratitude, self-awareness, inner peace, and healing into wholeness. This shift toward deeper meaning occurs through the process of grounding and embracing the experiential and creative expression that needs no artistic ability (only the intention to heal). The basic tools required include an unlined sheet of white or black paper with a circle; black, white, or colored pencils; a simple pencil sharpener; pictures and symbols; and scissors and paste.

Mandalas can be brought to patients to use in their healing journey. Within a "healing presence moment," share your experience with this creative expression and ask your client or patient if he or she would be willing to quietly work with this simple and enjoyable process. As you create the space, inquire as to the patient's preferred healing or calming music and assist him or her to set an intention (e.g., sense of calm and trust, letting go of tightness, fear, anxiety, and pain to increase comfort, peace, and relaxation) for the mandala creation. It is important for us to be mindful and to be individually creative—making adjustments as we discover how patients relate to others, to the idea of this experience, and to how they reveal their wants and needs. The first time you work

with the mandala process, you may invite the patient to close his or her eyes and go to a special place that is safe, comfortable, and healing, whether real or imagined. Even if addressing pain or a negative emotion, always ask for a healing symbol to dissipate any negative energy. The essence and nature of the mandala as a creative expression is to allow energy to move and shift consciousness. Ideally, a quiet, uninterrupted time of 30 to 45 minutes or longer is helpful. In this created space one does the work and receives the gift of self-healing. Sharing a few examples of simple mandalas can be helpful, such as geometric designs or examples from nature such as flowers, snowflakes, and webs; free templates are available on several websites. Trust the process and allow the pencil to move inside the circle until the design feels complete (at least for now). The possibilities are limitless. As the nurse you might stay and hold the sacred space; you might, however, determine that it is best to offer the patient privacy, checking back at a predetermined time. It is wonderful to sit with the patient in order that he or she might share the experience. It is critical to not judge or to make a conjecture about what an image may mean to you; this is the patient's process. Instead, allow the patient to share the meaning of the mandala to him or her. If the patient does not really know or seems perplexed, encourage him or her to simply sit and/or meditate with it. Often, insights will be revealed in time.

We are all part of the great mandala, the sacred hoop of life, rich with sound, vibration, light, color, feelings, thoughts, and actions— a mandala in the making continually being recreated.

*The walker experiences
soothing swirls of color
vibrancy
softness
creating a tapestry
of possibilities
she is the painter
she is the singer
she is . . .*

This is a continuation of Purplecluster Healing.

Pause to Ponder: Art

Take a moment to sit and be. Allow beautiful breaths to move inward and outward with ease. So much unfolding on this labyrinth journey. You continue to move out from center. How are you feeling? Who is the artist within you?

You might enjoy taking a few moments to doodle or paint or color in your favorite coloring book. Perhaps this playful idea brings a smile to your heart.

You may want to take a moment and visit the creative expressions used in healing in two communities:

Mirror Mirror Project: Creating Connections Between Artists and Homeless Youth in L.A., where approximately 40% of the homeless population are 21 and under. The Mirror Mirror Art Project is a simple program of creating art and creating relationships. Visit the website (http://www.themirrormirrorproject.com /about/).

Starving Artists Project: The New York homeless community presents a new initiative, which strives to give voice to the homeless population and display their creativity, often manifested in signs. Read about the project online (http://www.huffingtonpost .com/2013/03/06/starving-artists-project -homeless-community-photos_n_2821633 .html).

There are many others. . . . What is calling your heart?

Dreams

Dreams are filled with symbols, metaphors, premonitions, and insights delivered each night from the realms of our unconscious as well as the metaphysical world.[48, 49] These nightly visitations come as bizarre, strange, or scary tales. They involve those we know and those we do not, places we have never been or a familiar home, and are speckled with animals, insects, parties, weddings, birth, and death. These images are to inform, serve, and expand our consciousness. Often, dreams represent parts of ourselves that are still hidden and their messages cryptic. Jung called this unknown or repressed aspect "the shadow."[50, 51] The way one makes heads or tails of the stories created while we sleep is to develop an understanding of one's personal iconography. Thus, to make sense of the messages from one's dreams, we can view the images, the literal words, and the symbolic language all as parts of a puzzle. Jung also stated that dreams make more sense when we connect them to personal events and issues in the dreamer's life.[50, 51]

Each dream is specific to the dreamer, as if sent by a mysterious source hoping to illuminate the person's intuitive mind. Over time and with the practice of writing and reflecting on dreams, the dreamer develops skill in interpreting his or her own metaphorical dream language. In addition, archetypal patterns and generalities can be utilized, but these are related to the individual dreamer and his or her life particulars. Dream work helps to bring our inner world (dream world) and outer world (awake world) into alignment.

For example, a client dreamed the following: "I was meeting an elderly man at a nuclear reactor. We got onto the elevator and he took me down to the core." One might connect literally to recent events regarding the Japanese nuclear power plant meltdowns of 2011.

Metaphorically, however, one might wonder about *nuclear* as an energy source; or *nucleus* as meaning center, heart, basis; and *core* as the core of oneself. The older man may represent the higher self–teacher. Reflecting on current events in his life, the client is contemplating changing careers and has yet to get to the core of what this will look like. We considered phrasing the dream events this way: "My higher self wants me to get to the core of an issue or what are the particulars for the core of my work?"

Pause to Ponder: Dream Exploration

Keep a journal or notebook by your bed. Upon awaking, remain in the same position to remember your dream. This engages your "body memory." Then, write down the dream or parts of the dream that you remember. Circle specific words, phrases, and numbers that stick out, as well as images, animals, location, cast of characters, and the overall feeling you get from the dream. See how these images may relate to your current life, issues at hand, or events from your past. Notice in the days to come whether the events in the dream coincide with events in your physical life or the pandimensional environment. Move the pieces of the puzzle around; play with the different meanings that emerge. In this way, the dream itself becomes a guide and a bridge from the metaphysical to the physical. Ask yourself, "Why was this dream sent to me?" "What does it want me to reflect on?"

Reflections on the Walk

And so we are coming to the place where we entered; this labyrinth walk is coming to a close. As you near the entrance, consider slowing your pace or even stopping a moment to reflect on your journey. What have you discovered? Are there creative expressions that call to you in your personal self-development practice? How about as a nurse?

As holistic nurses, we can shape healing experiences as we integrate creative expressions into our lives and those of our patients and clients. In this way, our holistic nursing philosophy more fully manifests into thoughts, words, and actions as we walk our talk as a way of being and becoming. We live more consciously, which prepares us to effectively co-create and co-partner with our patients, colleagues, friends, and family in so many meaningful ways.

Standing at the entry, we look back upon the labyrinth—gratitude fills our being. All is . . .

*She gazes upon
the labyrinth of grass
and flowers and brush
sacred collection
transfixed
surrounded within
unitary unity
hawks soar
on the breadth of the winds
the walker
so still
her eyes drawn
to a cluster
purple panorama
she beholds
the flower so named
self-healing
pausing
ah what a journey
she smiles
as tears trickle down
lighter in being
peaceful in heart
and she walks*

*This is a continuation of *Purplecluster Healing*.

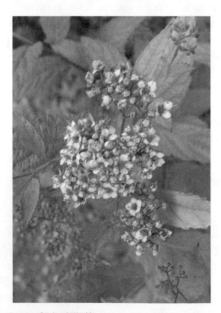

Source: Courtesy of Deborah Shields.

Directions for Future Research

As we have explored the integration of creative expressions of aesthetics in holistic nursing practice, several ideas for future areas of inquiry emerged. These areas of interest draw upon traditional quantitative and qualitative modes of inquiry as well as emerging modes, such as appreciative inquiry and quality improvement science. Consider additional topics for holistic nursing discovery, including:

1. Explore the sense of empowerment and/or insight experienced when using art forms as self-development practices.
2. Does a nurse taking time in Nature enhance the quality of patient care?

3. How do nurses bring creative expressions into their clinical practice?

4. Explore the lived experience of nurses and clients who incorporate creative expression strategies into health and wellness programs.

5. Examine the effect of creative expression programs in healthcare settings (nursing homes, hospitals, community agencies).

6. Determine how healing is supported using nonlinear modalities of music and art.

Nurse Healer Reflections

Through our labyrinthian journey, we have taken time out of time to explore the interface of our experiences and the meaning these have for our personal lives and holistic nursing practice. Our ongoing personal and professional development flourish as we purposefully and intentionally ponder and invite ourselves to imagine the unknown through reflection. Consider these as initial guides for future journeys.

- The journey of holistic care can be felt when nurses and patients are engaged in creative expressions that allow mindful self-reflection.

- Which creative expression strategies do you currently practice and which new strategy might you try in the future for your own inner growth?

- Bring yourself into attunement with your client and the environment simultaneously; which creative strategy can you draw on to enhance your client's healing relationship with the environment and with you?

NOTES

1. B. M. Dossey, "Nursing: Integral, Integrative, and Holistic—Local to Global," in *Holistic Nursing: A Handbook for Practice*, 6th ed., eds. B. M. Dossey and L. Keegan (Burlington, MA: Jones & Bartlett Learning, 2013): 3–58.

2. J. F. Quinn, "Transpersonal Human Caring and Healing," in *Holistic Nursing: A Handbook for Practice*, 6th ed., eds. B. M. Dossey and L. Keegan (Burlington, MA: Jones & Bartlett Learning, 2013): 107–116.

3. M. A. Hanley and M. V. Fenton, "Improvisation and the Art of Holistic Nursing," *Beginnings* 33, no. 5 (2013): 4–5, 20–22.

4. J. D. Levin and J. L. Reich, "Self-Reflection," in *Holistic Nursing: A Handbook for Practice*, 6th ed., eds. B. M. Dossey and L. Keegan (Burlington, MA: Jones & Bartlett Learning, 2013): 247–260.

5. D. Shields and S. Stout-Shaffer, "Self-Development: The Foundation of Holistic Self-Care," in *Holistic Nursing: A Handbook for Practice*, 7th ed., eds. B. M. Dossey and L. Keegan (Burlington, MA: Jones & Bartlett Learning, 2015).

6. Oxford Dictionaries, "Creative" (2014). www.oxforddictionaries.com/definition/american_english-thesaurus/creative.

7. R. Ettun, M. Schultz, and G. Bar-Sela, "Transforming Pain into Beauty: On Art, Healing, and Care for the Spirit," *Evidence-Based Complementary and Alternative Medicine* 2014 (2014). doi:10.1155/2014/789852.

8. G. Roth, *Maps to Ecstasy: A Healing Journey for the Untamed Spirit* (Novato, CA: World Library, 1998): 207.

9. L. Artress, *Walking a Sacred Path* (New York: Riverhead Books, 1995).

10. P. Munhall, "Unknowing: Toward Another Pattern of Knowing," *Nursing Outlook* 41, no. 3 (1993): 125–128.

11. U.S. Department of Health and Human Services, *Healthy People 2020* (Washington, DC: U.S. Department of Health and Human Services, 2010).

12. J. Muir, *Our National Parks* (Boston: Houghton Mifflin, 1901): 56.

13. R. Louv, *Last Child in the Woods: Saving Our Children from Nature-Deficit Disorder* (Chapel Hill, NC: Algonquin Books, 2008): 43.

14. J. Muir, *A Thousand Mile Walk to the Gulf* (Boston: Houghton Mifflin, 1916): 164.

15. R. McCaffrey, C. Hanson, and W. McCaffrey, "Garden Walking for Depression," *Holistic Nursing Practice* 24, no. 5 (2010): 252–259.

16. L. Tyrväinen, A. Ojala, K. Korpela, T. Lanki, Y. Tsunetsugu, and T. Kagawa, "The Influence of Urban Green Environments on Stress Relief Measures: A Field Experiment," *Journal of Environmental Psychology* 38 (2014): 1–9.

17. E. Largo-Wight, W. W. Chen, V. Dodd, and R. Weiler, "Healthy People in a Healthy Environment," *Public Health Reports* 126, Suppl 1 (2011): 124–130.

18. S. Park and R. Mattson, "Ornamental Indoor Plants in Hospital Rooms Enhanced Health Outcomes of Patients Recovering from Surgery,"

Journal of Alternative and Complementary Medicine 15, no. 9 (2009): 975–980.

19. S. S. Tiberio, D. C. Kerr, D. M. Capaldi, K. C. Pears, H. K. Kim, and P. Nowicka, "Parental Monitoring of Children's Media Consumption: The Long-Term Influences on Body Mass Index in Children," *Pediatrics* 168, no. 5 (2014): 414–421.

20. D. Wagoner, *Collected Poems (1956–1976)* (Bloomington: Indiana University Press, 1976).

21. J. Muir, *My First Summer* (New York: Dover, 1911): 110.

22. M. Prechtel, *Secrets of the Talking Jaguar: Memoirs from the Living Heart of a Mayan Village* (New York: Putnam, 1998): 281.

23. Pop Tech, "Milton Garcés: Primordial Sounds" (2011). http://poptech.org/popcasts /milton_garc%C3%A9s_primordial_sounds.

24. "(Om)—The Primordial Sound, The Eternal Syllable," *Akhandjyoti Magazine* (September–October 2005). www.akhandjyoti.org/?Akhand-Jyoti/2005 /Sep-Oct/OmEternalSyllable.

25. M. Whittle, "Primordial Sounds: Big Bang Acoustics" (June 1, 2004). www.astro.virginia .edu/~dmw8f/sounds/aas/press_release.pdf.

26. D. Campbell, *The Mozart Effect* (New York: Avon Books, 1997).

27. J. Rumi, "The Deep Listening," in *The Glance: Songs of Soul-Meeting*, trans. C. Barks (New York: Viking Penguin, 1999): 90.

28. S. Rechtschaffen, *Timeshifting: Creating More Time to Enjoy Your Life* (New York: Doubleday, 1996).

29. L. Friedman, *The Healing Power of the Drum* (Reno, NV: White Cliffs Media, 2000): 39.

30. M. Gaynor, *Sounds of Healing* (New York: Broadway Books, 1999): 101–102.

31. L. Redmond, *When the Drummers Were Women* (New York: Three Rivers Press, 1997): 9.

32. C. Stevens, *The Art and Heart of Drum Circles* (Milwaukee, WI: Hal Leonard, 2003).

33. L. Freeman and F. Lawlis, *Mosby's Complementary and Alternative Medicine: A Researched Based Approach*, 3rd ed. (St Louis, MO: Mosby, 2009).

34. L. Seward, *Achieving the Mind-Body-Spirit Connection* (Sudbury, MA: Jones and Bartlett, 2005): 171.

35. J. Rumi, *A Year of Rumi*, trans. A. Harvey (Boston: Shambhala, 1998).

36. R. Van Horn and S. Freed, "Journaling and Dialogue Pairs to Promote Reflection in Clinical Nursing Education," *Nursing Education Research* 29, no. 4 (2008): 220–225.

37. B. W. Sturm, "The Enchanted Imagination: Storytelling's Power to Entrance Listeners," *School Library Media Research* 2 (July 1999). www.ala.org/aasl/sites/ala.org.aasl /files/content/aaslpubsandjournals/slr/vol2 /SLMR_EnchantedImagination_V2.pdf.

38. C. Smith, "Metaphor in Nursing Theory," *Nursing Science Quarterly* 5, no. 2 (1992): 48–49.

39. J. Levin and S. Maida, "Four Shields of Leadership" (self-published course material, 2008).

40. F. Nightingale, *Notes on Nursing: What It Is, and What It Is Not* (New York: Dover, 1969): 59.

41. A. Kovaleski, "Increasing the Use of Arts in My Personal and Professional Life" (presentation at the American Holistic Nurses Association Annual Conference, Portland, OR, June 2014).

42. M. Samuels and M. R. Lane, "Creative Healing with Visual Arts, Words, Music, and Dance" (Healing with the Arts Series, Session 5, August 19, 2013).

43. The Mandala Project, "What Is a Mandala?" (2010). www.mandalaproject.org/What/Index .html.

44. C. Jung, *Memories, Dreams and Reflections* (New York: Random House, 1965): 334–335.

45. S. Fincher, *Creating Mandalas* (Boston: Shambhala, 1991): 20.

46. Daily Celebrations, "Favorite Quotations: Life and Living" (2014). www.dailycelebrations.com /living.htm.

47. J. Cornell, *Mandala* (Wheaton, IL: Theosophical, 1994): 18.

48. R. Kamenetz, *The History of Last Night's Dreams: Discovering the Hidden Path to the Seat of the Soul* (New York: HarperCollins, 2007).

49. S. Krippner, F. Bogzaran, and A. P. DeCarvalho, *Extraordinary Dreams and How to Work with Them* (Albany, NY: State University of New York Press, 2002).

50. C. Jung, *On the Nature of Dreams*, eds., R. Soulard, Jr. and K. Kramer (Seattle, WA: Scriptor Press, 1945).

51. C. Jung, *Dreams*, trans. R. F. C. Hull, eds. W. McGuire, H. Read, M. Fordham, and G. Adler (Princeton, NJ: Princeton University Press, 1974).

Additional Resources

1. L. Schwartzberg, "Nature. Beauty. Gratitude." *TED Talk* (June 2011). www.ted.com/talks/louie_schwartzberg_nature_beauty_gratitude.
2. University of Minnesota, "Taking Charge of Your Health and Wellbeing" (2014). www.takingcharge.csh.umn.edu/enhance-your-wellbeing/environment/nature-and-us/how-does-nature-impact-our-wellbeing.
3. B. W. Sturm, "The Enchanted Imagination: Storytelling's Power to Entrance Listeners," *School Library Media Research* 2 (1999). www.ala.org/ala/mgrps/divs/aasl/aaslpubsandjournals/slmrb/slmrcontents/volume21999/vol2sturm.cfm.

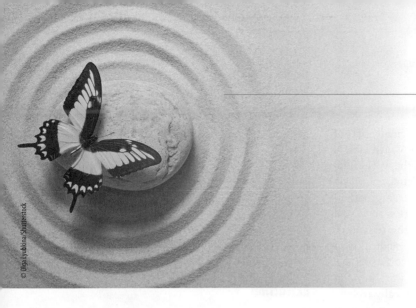

CHAPTER 15

Aromatherapy

Jane Buckle

Nurse Healer Objectives

Theoretical

- Describe the historical path of aromatherapy, from ancient times to the present renaissance.
- Describe the relevance of learned memory in the choice of essential oil.
- Compare the different methods of using essential oils.
- Discuss the safety issues of using essential oils.

Clinical

- Describe the use of aromatherapy for insomnia.
- Describe the use of aromatherapy for chronic pain.
- Describe the use of aromatherapy for infection.
- List three uses for essential oil of *Lavandula angustifolia*.
- List three uses for essential oil of *Eucalyptus globulus*.
- List three uses for essential oil of *Mentha piperita*.
- List three uses for essential oil of *Melaleuca alternifolia*.
- List three uses for essential oil of *Boswellia carteri*.

Personal

- Integrate aromatherapy into your daily life to enhance your well-being.
- Experience each of the five essential oils mentioned previously, both inhaled and topically.

Definitions

Aromatherapy: The use of essential oils for therapeutic purposes.

Chemotype: A cloned variety of a plant that always has the same chemistry.

Clinical aromatherapy: The use of essential oils for specific, measurable outcomes.

Essential oil: The distillate from an aromatic plant, or the oil expressed from the peel of a citrus fruit.

Learned memory: The ability of the mind to condition the response to an aroma based on previous experience.

Limbic system: The oldest part of the brain; it contains the amygdala, hippocampus, thalamus, and hypothalamus.

'M' Technique: A registered form of gentle, structured touch suitable when the receiver is very fragile or actively dying, or when the giver is not trained in massage. Recognized as part of holistic nursing care.

History

The use of aromatic plants was originally part of herbal medicine. According to the World Health Organization, more than 85% of the world population still relies on herbal medicine, and many of the herbs are aromatic. However, aromatherapy only began in France just prior to World War II, at about the same time the first antibiotics were being introduced. A medical doctor, Jean Valnet, a chemist, Maurice Gattefosse, and a nurse, Marguerite Maury, were key figures. They used aromatherapy clinically to help wounds heal, fight infections, and reduce skin problems, and they used essential oils topically.

This more clinical approach to aromatherapy has survived in France and Germany, where aromatherapy is seen as an extension of orthodox medicine.[1] German doctors and nurses are tested in the use of essential oils to become licensed. The clinical use of aromatherapy is easy to understand, as many of today's drugs originally came from plants—for example, aspirin from willow bark and digoxin from foxglove. Even the contraceptive pill originally came from a plant—the humble yam—and the yew tree produces a cytotoxic drug to fight cancer.

Theory and Research

Aromatherapy uses essential oils to improve physical, psychological, and spiritual health. Essential oils are powerful; they can be up to 100 times more concentrated than the herb itself. Many essential oils have familiar smells, such as lavender, rose, and rosemary. Essential oils are highly volatile droplets created by the plant to prevent (or treat) infection, regulate growth, and mend damaged tissue. These tiny droplets are stored in veins, glands, or sacs by the plant, and when they are crushed or rubbed, the essential oil and its aroma are released. Some plants store large amounts of essential oil; some store very little. This, along with the difficulty of harvesting the essential oil, dictates the price of each type of oil. More than 220 pounds (100 kilograms) of fresh rose petals are needed to produce a little more than 2 ounces (60 grams) of essential oil, making

rose one of the most expensive essential oils and, therefore, one of the most frequently adulterated.

There are some important things to know about essential oils before they can be used safely: extraction, the botanical name (for clear identification), method of application, safety, storage, and contraindications. These topics are discussed in the following subsections as well as in Exhibit 15-2 later in this chapter.

Extraction

Only steam-distilled or expressed extracts produce essential oils. These two methods give a product with no additional solvent or impurity. However, many "essential oils" on the market are extracted with solvent that can produce allergic or sensitivity reactions in the user. A bottle of essential oil should state that the contents are pure essential oils: steam distilled or expressed. (Only the peel from citrus plants, such as mandarin, lime, or lemon, produces an *expressed* oil.)

Identification by Botanical Name

It is important to know the botanical name of a plant. The common name can often include different species that may have very different chemistry and therefore very different actions. For example, there are three species of lavender (and many hybrid clones) and 400 species of eucalyptus. Only the full botanical name (the genus, species, and, where relevant, the chemotype) can identify the plant. The genus of lavender is *Lavandula*, thus all lavender names start with *Lavandula*. The species is the second part of the botanical name. The chemotype, if there is one, comes last. See **Table 15-1** for a list of botanical and common names of the essential oils mentioned in this chapter.

Do not buy just anything that is labeled "lavender oil" because there is no way of knowing which lavender is in the bottle. One lavender (*Lavandula angustifolia*) is soothing, calming, and exceptional for burns, but another lavender is a stimulant and expectorant (*Lavandula latifolia*). This second lavender will not promote sleep or soothe burns.

TABLE 15-1 Essential Oils Mentioned in This Chapter	
Common Name	**Botanical Name**
Aniseed	*Pimpinella anisum*
Basil	*Ocimum basilicum*
Chamomile, German	*Matricaria recutita*
Chamomile, Roman	*Chamaemelum nobile*
Clary sage	*Salvia sclarea*
Coriander seed	*Coriandrum sativum*
Eucalyptus	*Eucalyptus globulus*
Fennel	*Foeniculum vulgare var. dulce*
Geranium	*Pelargonium graveolens*
Ginger	*Zingiber officinale*
Hyssop	*Hyssopus officinalis*
Lavender, true	*Lavandula angustifolia*
Lemongrass	*Cymbopogon citratus*
Neroli	*Citrus aurantium var. amara*
Palmarosa	*Cymbopogon martinii*
Parsley	*Petroselinum sativum*
Pennyroyal	*Mentha pulegium*
Peppermint	*Mentha piperita*
Rose	*Rosa damascena*
Rosewood	*Aniba rosaeodora*
Sage	*Salvia officinalis*
Sandalwood	*Santalum album*
Tarragon	*Artemisia dracunculus*
Wintergreen	*Gaultheria procumbens*

EXHIBIT 15-1   Methods of Application

1. Inhalation: usually 1 to 5 drops undiluted
2. Topical:
   - In baths: 1 to 8 drops
   - Compresses: 1% to 8%
   - 'M' Technique or massage: 1% to 10%
   - Wounds: 12% to 40% (depending on chemistry of essential oil)
   - Burns, bites, and stings (first aid): 100%
   - Radiation burns: 3% to 10%
3. Vaginal: Useful for yeast infection or cystitis. Use 1% to 5% diluted on tampon.
4. Ingestion: This is not accepted as part of holistic nursing care.

Methods of Application

Essential oils can be absorbed by the body in three ways: through ingestion, olfaction, and topical application (using internal and external skin). For methods of using essential oils that are congruent with holistic nursing practice, see **Exhibit 15-1**.

Touch in Aromatherapy

Aromatherapy often is used with massage or the 'M' Technique.[1] This registered method of simple structured touch is suitable when massage is inappropriate, either because the receiver is too fragile or the giver is not trained in massage.[2] The 'M' Technique is used in hospitals, hospices, and long-term care facilities in the United States, the United Kingdom, the Netherlands, Japan, and South Africa.[3] It is simple to learn and produces a profound relaxation response in just a few minutes. It can be useful for treating dementia,[4] special needs,[5] chronic pain, and end-of-life issues.[6] Research has shown that the 'M' Technique has a more relaxing effect than conventional massage as well as an accumulative effect.[7] Gentle stroking enhances absorption of essential oils through the skin into the bloodstream. (For more details on 'M' Technique, including training programs and DVDs, see www.rjbuckle.com.)

Olfaction

The fastest effect from aromatherapy is through olfaction.[6] Essential oils are composed of many different chemical components that travel via the nose to the olfactory bulb. There is debate as to whether the components are recognized by shape or vibration;[7] either way, they trigger responses in the limbic system of the brain—the oldest part of the brain—where the aroma is processed. The limbic part of the brain contains the amygdala, where fear and anger are analyzed; the thalamus, where pain is analyzed; and the hippocampus, which is involved in the formation and retrieval of explicit memories. This is why an aroma can trigger memories that have lain dormant for years. Smell is very important, beginning with the newborn baby's identification of its mother and continuing into old age, where studies show that the depression of residential older adults can be reduced with the aromas of familiar fruits and flowers.

The effect of odors on the brain was "mapped" using computer-generated graphics.[8] Brain Electrical Activity Mapping indicates how a subject, linked to an electroencephalogram, rates different odors even when the subject is asleep.[9] These maps indicate that aromas can have a psychological effect even when the aroma is subliminal (i.e., below the level of human awareness), and that, provided the olfactory nerve is intact, the aroma still has a measurable effect on the brain.

Topical Applications

Components within essential oils are absorbed into, and through, the skin via diffusion. The two layers of the skin, the dermis and fat layer, together act as a reservoir before the components within the essential oils reach the bloodstream. There is some evidence that massage or hot water enhances absorption. Essential oils, because they are lipophyllic (dissolve in fat), can be stored in the fatty areas of the body and can pass through the blood–brain barrier and into the brain itself.

Negative Reactions

Essential oils are commonly used in the pharmaceutical, perfume, and food industries.[10] Pure essential oils rarely produce an allergic effect. However, as synthetic aromatic components are becoming more common in everyday products, cross-sensitization will increase.

Nursing Theory

Aromatherapy links into many of the most recognized nursing theories, including Watson's Theory of Human Caring, because aromatherapy allows nurses a method of showing their care at a deep level.[11] It resonates with Barrett's Theory of Power because it allows the patient to participate knowingly in change and offers a model for change through empowerment.[12] Nightingale put forward the first theory of nursing—putting the patient in the best condition for Nature to act—and thus aromatherapy clearly fits here because it allows the patient to relax sufficiently for the healing process to occur from within.[13] Nightingale also suggested creating an environmental space conducive to healing—aromatherapy fits very well here as well because essential oils create a safe environment at many levels. Erickson's work led to Modeling Theory,[14] which requires building trust, encouraging positive orientation, promoting strength, and setting mutual health-directed goals—these requirements also fit exceptionally well with aromatherapy. Rogers's theory suggests that human beings are more than just physical entities and have specific energy fields. Aromas clearly affect both the psyche and the human energy field.

How Aromatherapy Works

The term *aromatherapy* refers to the therapeutic use of essential oils—the volatile organic constituents of plants. Essential oils are thought to work at psychological, physiologic, and cellular levels. This means that they can affect our body, our mind, and all of the delicate links in between. The effects of aroma can be rapid, and sometimes just thinking about a smell can be as powerful as the actual smell itself. Take a moment to think of your favorite flower. Then, think about a smell that makes you feel nauseated. The effects of an aroma can be relaxing or stimulating depending on the individual's previous experience (called the *learned memory*), as well as the actual chemical makeup of the essential oil used.

Who Uses Aromatherapy?

Aromatherapy is used by nurses in many countries, including the United Kingdom, France, Germany, Switzerland, Sweden, South Africa,

---

EXHIBIT 15-2   Warnings, Contraindications, and Precautions When Using Essential Oils

1. Use caution with patients with severe asthma or multiple allergies.
2. Do not take by mouth (unless guided by a person trained in aromatic medicine).
3. Do not use essential oils near the eyes. If essential oils get into eyes, rinse out with milk or carrier oil (essential oils do not dissolve in water), and then water.
4. Store away from fire or naked flame. Essential oils are volatile and flammable.
5. Store in a cool place out of sunlight, in colored glass—amber or blue. Store expensive essential oils in a refrigerator.
6. Ensure that you have accountability by being properly trained. For a clinical home study course see www.rjbuckle.com.
7. Do not use phenol-rich essential oils undiluted on the skin (e.g., *Thymus vulgaris*).
8. Keep away from children and pets.
9. Only use essential oils from a reputable supplier who can supply the correct botanical name, place of origin, part of plant used, method of extraction, and batch number when possible. See **Table 15-2** for recommended suppliers.
10. Always close the container immediately.
11. Use care during pregnancy.
12. Be aware of which essential oils are photosensitive, such as bergamot (*Citrus bergamia*).

Australia, New Zealand, Korea, and Japan. In France and Germany, medical doctors and pharmacists use aromatherapy as part of conventional medicine, often for the control of infection. Aromatherapy is the fastest growing therapy among nurses in the United States.[6]

Although essential oils are very safe to use, there are some guidelines that must be followed. Reference-backed, patient-centered clinical training is strongly recommended (see www.rjbuckle.com for classroom or home study courses). **Exhibit 15-2** provides relevant warnings, contraindications, and precautions. Possible drug interactions are listed in **Exhibit 15-3**.

EXHIBIT 15-3   Drug Interactions When Using Essential Oils

1. Avoid strong aromas such as peppermint and eucalyptus with patients receiving homeopathy.
2. People who are allergic to ragweed may be allergic to chamomile.
3. The effect of tranquilizers, anticonvulsants, and antihistamines may be slightly enhanced by some sedative essential oils.

Adverse Reactions

There is some evidence of adverse skin reactions caused by sensitivity in rare instances. The majority of cases were from extracts rather than pure essential oils. Topically applied bergamot (*Citrus bergamia*), used in conjunction with sunshine or tanning beds, can result in skin damage ranging from redness to full-thickness burns.[15] It is recommended that essential oils be used with caution during pregnancy, although the risk is extremely small when the essential oils are used only topically or inhaled; however, sage, pennyroyal, camphor, parsley, tarragon, wintergreen, juniper, hyssop, and basil should be avoided.[16] Tisserand and Young state that there is no evidence that essential oils are abortificient in the amounts used in aromatherapy.[17]

Administration

Essential oils can be used topically or inhaled. A typical topical application for relaxation uses a 1% to 5% mixture: 1 to 5 drops of essential oils diluted in 5 cc (a teaspoon) of cold-pressed vegetable oil such as sweet almond oil. Wound infections, contusions, and inflammation may require higher concentrations—up to 20%. Certain essential oils, such as lavender (*Lavandula angustifolia*) and tea tree (*Melaleuca alternifolia*), can be topically applied undiluted for stings or bites. Others, like clove and thyme, should never be used undiluted on the skin because their high phenol content would cause burning. For insomnia, nausea, or depression, the patient can inhale the correct oil for 5 to 10 minutes as necessary, using a cotton ball, personal inhaler (aromastix), aromapatch, or personal packet. The nurse can also use massage or the 'M' Technique where appropriate. Simple stress management can be incorporated into an everyday regime with the use of aromatic baths and foot soaks, vaporizers, and sprays. Oral intake of essential oils, while extremely effective for acute infection or gastrointestinal problems, is not recognized as part of holistic nursing care at this time.

Self-Help

Aromatherapy can be very helpful when self-applied for stress management, insomnia, or depression because the oils are portable and can be used anywhere at any time. A drop of peppermint can help clear your mind at the end of a busy day, or a drop of ylang ylang can help soothe nerves.

Credentialing

There is currently no recognized national certification for clinical aromatherapy. The closest is the exam set by the Aromatherapy Registration Council, a nonprofit entity that provides a national exam for lay people (see www.aromatherapy council.org for exam details). The exam is open to anyone who has studied aromatherapy for 200 hours and meets the criteria. There is little, if any, clinical content in the exam. There are two professional bodies: the National Association for Holistic Aromatherapy and the Alliance of International Aromatherapists, with the latter taking a more clinical approach. Aromatherapy training can range from 1 day to several years. However, because nurses are accountable, if a nurse wants to use aromatherapy as part of nursing care, it is strongly recommended that he or she is able to show documented evidence of clinical training, preferably one that is nurse taught and patient centered. See the American Holistic Nurses Association website (www.ahna.org) for endorsed and approved aromatherapy courses for nurses.

Aromatherapy for Dementia

A Chinese systematic review of 11 randomized controlled trials shortlisted from electronic databases between 1995 and 2011 found that aromatherapy reduced the behavioral and psychological symptoms of dementia.[18] It also improved cognitive functions, increased quality of life, and enhanced independence of daily living activities. The authors conclude that aromatherapy is safe and effective to use in dementia.

A British study explored the effect of weekly aromatherapy massage on the stress and well-being of 12 caregivers of patients with Alzheimer's disease over a period of 8 weeks.[19] Outcome measures were taken at 1, 4, and 8 weeks; measures included MYMOP2 (Measure Your Medical Outcome Profile), HADS (Hospital Anxiety and Depression Scale), and VAS (Visual Analogue Scale). Results showed that aromatherapy reduced stress levels across all measures. Another British study found that Melissa (*Melissa officinalis*) was as effective as donepezil in a double-blind parallel-group placebo-controlled randomized trial across three specialist old-age psychiatry centers over 12 weeks.[20]

R. J. Buckle Associates students conducted six small pilot studies on dementia between 1999 and 2005.[1] The most common essential oil used was lavender (*Lavandula angustifolia*), but there were also pleasing results from mandarin (*Citrus reticulata*) and frankincense (*Boswellia carteri*). Room diffusers, nebulizers, and personal patches can be useful in situations where patients with dementia are confined to bed or dislike any form of touch.

Aromatherapy for Pain

Published studies on aromatherapy for pain suggest that both inhaled and topically applied essential oils can affect the perception of pain. More recent research indicates that some essential oils have intrinsic analgesic properties. When essential oils are combined with the 'M' Technique, this can increase the effectiveness in chronic pain.

Ko and colleagues conducted a placebo-controlled study on 153 patients with fibromyalgia using a mixture of essential oils (camphor, eucalyptus, peppermint, rosemary, lemon, and orange in aloe).[21] The mixture was applied topically. Results from the VAS found reduced night pain (p = .018), increased Jamar grip strength (p < .001), and reduced number of Trigeminal-evoked potentials (p < .001).

Ayan and coauthors explored the use of inhaled rose oil (*Rosa damascena*) on a group of 80 patients with renal colic.[22] Half of the group received conventional analgesic (diclofenac sodium, 75 mg intramuscularly) plus a placebo smell of saline. The other group received the same intramuscular injection plus inhaled rose essential oil. Pain was measured using the VAS (worst pain = 10; no pain = 0). The perception of pain was measured after 10 and 30 minutes. After 30 minutes, the difference in the two groups was 3.75 +/– 2.08 for the conventional therapy plus placebo group versus 1.08 +/– 1.07 for the conventional therapy plus rose group.

Kim and colleagues explored the effect of inhaled lavender (*Lavandula angustifolia*) via a face mask in a randomized controlled study.[23] Participants were healthy volunteers who rated stress and pain during needle insertion. The results showed the pain intensity of needle insertion was significantly decreased after aromatherapy compared with the control (p < .001).

R. J. Buckle Associates students conducted 13 pilot studies on pain between 1997 and 2011.[1]

Aromatherapy for Infection

There is considerable published research on the in vitro antibacterial, antifungal, and antiviral effects of many essential oils. Methicillin-resistant *Staphylococcus aureus* (MRSA) has become endemic.[24] Even vancomycin, used to treat MRSA, has shown disappointing cure rates: 44% failure in treating bacteria and 40% failure in treating lower respiratory tract infections.[25] Some antifungal drugs are no longer working,[26] and some antivirals are no longer effective.[27]

Warnke and colleagues tested tea tree against MRSA, four *Streptococcus* strains, and three *Candida* strains including *Candida krusei*.[28] Tea tree showed considerable efficacy. Bowler and coauthors used tea tree in conjunction with conventional antibiotics to control MRSA spread in residents of five nursing homes in Wisconsin.[29] After intervention and follow up for 12 months

or more, the prevalence of MRSA carriage at the nursing homes decreased by 67% (p < .001), and 120 of 147 (82%) nursing home residents and 111 of 125 (89%) clinic patients remained culture negative for MRSA. Tea tree was one of the essential oils originally tested by Edwards-Jones and colleagues in a wound-dressing pack.[30] They looked at both the vapor and topical effects of essential oils and found that geranium and tea tree were the most effective against MRSA in a dressing. Chin and coauthors conducted an in vivo study based on Edwards-Jones's in vitro study.[31] Ten participants who had wounds infected with MRSA volunteered for the study. Four of the 10 were used as matched subjects to compare standard treatment to treatment with tea tree oil. The differences were striking and, it is hoped, will lead the way to a larger study.

Sherry and Warnke broke new ground when they applied essential oils directly into the bones of patients suffering from osteomyelitis (MRSA) and presented their findings at the American Academy of Orthopedic Surgeons.[32] Twenty-five patients with MRSA infections were treated: 16 involved bone, 6 a joint, and 3 soft tissue. Ten patients were diabetic. Following debridement, diluted essential oils were applied to the infected sites. In the case of bone, calcium (Osteoset) beads soaked in essential oils were used. In 22 cases, the infection was completely resolved either without antibiotics (19) or with antibiotics (3). In Australia, 90% of hospital-acquired infections are MRSA. In vitro studies on tea tree and eucalyptus show that both were effective within 1 minute against 90% of the five multiple-resistant tuberculosis (TB) organisms tested. The paper concludes that essential oils could be a possible mass treatment for TB.

Finally, the following three studies may also be useful in nursing care:

1. An essential oil mixture of diluted tea tree, peppermint, and lemon reduced malodor and volatile sulfur compounds in intensive care unit patients.[33]
2. Inhaling black pepper (*Piper nigrum*) for 1 minute stimulated swallowing reflex in people with swallowing dysfunction following stroke compared to lavender oil or distilled water (p < .03) (n = 105).[34]

3. Diffused essential oils can reduce the incidence of hospital-acquired and ventilator-associated pneumonia.[35]

Several exhibits follow that contain descriptions of the therapeutic value of five of the most useful and commonly available essential oils suitable for holistic nursing care:

Lavender	*Lavandula angustifolia*	**Exhibit 15-4**
Peppermint	*Mentha piperita*	**Exhibit 15-5**
Tea tree oil	*Melaleuca alternifolia*	**Exhibit 15-6**
Blue gum	*Eucalyptus globulus*	**Exhibit 15-7**
Frankincense	*Boswellia carteri*	**Exhibit 15-8**

The method of application depends on whether you are targeting a psychological or physiologic response. Nurses must ensure that they have adequate training first before asking their patients if they like the aroma. Essential oil companies used by the author are listed in **Table 15-2**.

EXHIBIT 15-4   Properties of Lavender (*Lavandula angustifolia*)

1. Skin regenerative: for burns, wound healing, insect bites, mild eczema[36] (applied topically)
2. Calming,[21, 37] good for insomnia and depression,[38] good for stress[39, 40] (inhaled)
3. Reduces agitation in dementia[19] (inhaled or applied topically)
4. Enhances sense of well-being[41] (inhaled)
5. Effective against ticks[42]
6. Fungistatic, not fungicidal[43]

EXHIBIT 15-5   Properties of Peppermint (*Mentha piperita*)

1. Analgesic,[44] migraine,[45] postherpetic neuralgia[46] (when applied topically)
2. Antinausea,[47–49] opiate detoxification[50] (when inhaled)
3. Useful for irritable bowel syndrome (antispasmodic)[51] (enteric coated capsules taken orally)
4. Antibacterial,[52–54] useful in sinusitis[55]
5. Virucidal[56]

EXHIBIT 15-6   Properties of Tea Tree (*Melaleuca alternifolia*)

1. Bacterial infections,[57] acne.[58]
2. Fungal infections including athlete's foot, tinea.
3. Most skin infections, including impetigo, cold sores, herpes,[59] and warts.[60]
4. Mouth infections.[61]
5. Effective against MRSA.[29–31, 62]
6. Antiviral, including influenza.[63, 64]
7. Antitumoral.[65, 66]
8. Vaginal infections, especially *Candida albicans*.[67] Tea tree can be diluted and used as a vaginal douche for infections, or it can be diluted in carrier oil and used on a tampon: Put 2 to 3 drops of tea tree oil in 1 teaspoonful of carrier oil, roll tampon in mixture, and insert into vagina. Repeat with fresh tampon every 4 hours and leave in overnight. Relief should occur within 48 hours. Vaginal thrush should not reoccur.

EXHIBIT 15-7   Properties of Blue Gum (*Eucalyptus globulus*)

1. Respiratory complaints, including TB[54, 68–70]
2. Effective against pneumonia in ventilated patients[36, 71]
3. Antibacterial;[72] effective against MRSA[54]
4. Effective against head lice[73]

EXHIBIT 15-8   Properties of Frankincense (*Boswellia carteri*)

1. Good for relaxation, meditation, and spiritual renewal
2. Very useful in terminal agitation[74]
3. Good for scars[75]
4. Anti-inflammatory[76, 77]
5. Useful in asthma[78]
6. Antiparasitic[79]
7. Anticancer[80, 81]

TABLE 15-2   Essential Oils Distributors Used by the Author
Nature's Gift 316 Old Hickory Boulevard East Madison, TN 37115 615-612-4270 www.naturesgift.com
SunRose Aromatics, LLC 1120 Dean Avenue Bronx, NY 10465 718-794-0391 www.SunRoseAromatics.com
Florihana Les Grands Prés 06460 Caussols, France +33 (0) 493 09 06 09 www.florihana.com
Recommended Diffusers
Plant Extracts International, Inc. 600 11th Avenue South Hopkins, MN 55343 952-935-9903 www.plantextractsinc.com
Aromapatches (for individual use, either plain or with integral essential oils)
Bioesse Technologies, LLC PO Box 1182 Minnetonka, MN 55345 sales@bioessetech.com www.bioessetech.com
Aromapackets (for individual use; comes with essential oil blends)
Aeroscena, LLC Cleveland Clinic GCIC 10000 Cedar Road Cleveland, OH 44106 800-671-1890 www.aeroscena.com

Holistic Caring Process

There is tremendous emphasis on "doing" in the Western world, where we are judged (and tend to judge others) on what we "do" rather than on our ability "to be." But illness takes away a patient's ability "to do" and forces attention on "being." This can be intimidating. Aromatherapy enables the nurse to share at a deep level, thus demonstrating care for the soul, mind, and body—a true holistic therapy. And it smells good!

Holistic Assessment

In preparing to use essential oils clinically, the nurse assesses the following parameters:

- The patient's like or dislike of particular aromas because this affects the choice of essential oils
- The patient's like or dislike of touch because this affects which method is chosen
- The patient's perception of the problem because this indicates the targeted outcome
- The patient's level of stress because this directly affects the oils chosen
- The patient's understanding of aromatherapy—this indicates whether the patient is expecting cure or care
- The patient's skin integrity because certain essential oils are inappropriate with poor skin integrity
- The patient's age—very young or elderly patients need low percentages of essential oils
- The patient's medical history because previous illness could be related to the current problem
- The patient's current medical status because this indicates which essential oils are safest to use
- The patient's sleep pattern because this indicates whether this is for a targeted outcome
- The patient's weight and height because these indicate the amount of essential oil required
- The patient's blood pressure because this indicates hypotensive or hypertensive essential oils
- The patient's medication because certain medications could be affected by essential oils
- The patient's respiratory pattern because this indicates whether there is chronic obstructive pulmonary disease or asthma
- The patient's reproductive status because this indicates whether the patient is pregnant, reducing the choice of essential oils

- The patient's allergy status, particularly to ragweed, because some essential oils would then be inappropriate
- The patient's close proximity to others who may be affected by the aromas because this will affect which essential oils are chosen

Identification of Patterns/ Challenges/Needs

The following patterns/challenges/needs (see Chapter 8) compatible with aromatherapy are:

- Altered circulation
- Risk of infection
- Constipation: real, perceived, or risk of
- Altered tissue perfusion (peripheral)
- Ineffective breathing pattern
- Dysfunctional ventilatory weaning response
- Impaired tissue integrity or risk of
- Energy field disturbance
- Impaired verbal communication
- Social isolation
- Risk for loneliness
- Sexual dysfunction
- Caregiver role strain
- Ineffectual individual/family coping
- Defensive coping
- Family coping with potential for growth
- Decisional conflict
- Impaired physical/bed mobility
- Activity intolerance
- Fatigue
- Sleep pattern disturbance
- Delayed surgical recovery
- Adult failure to thrive
- Ineffective breastfeeding
- Bathing or hygiene self-care deficit
- Relocation stress syndrome
- Body image disturbance
- Chronic low self-esteem
- Sensory or perception alterations, such as olfactory or tactile
- Hopelessness
- Powerlessness
- Chronic confusion
- Impaired memory
- Chronic pain
- Nausea
- Dysfunctional grieving

- Chronic sorrow
- Post-trauma response
- Anxiety
- Fear

Outcome Identification

Table 15-3 guides the nurse in patient outcomes, nursing prescriptions, and evaluations for the use of aromatherapy as a nursing intervention.

Setting Goals

It is important to establish mutually acceptable goals prior to beginning aromatherapy and 'M' Technique sessions. These outcomes may be immediate or long term but should be relevant to aromatherapy and the role of holistic nursing care. Patients are more likely to be content with the outcomes if they are perceived to be achievable within a specified time frame and are deemed successful with recognizable tools such as a visual analog. It is recommended that such goals are judged by using the VAS (0–10), where 0 is lack of the symptom (such as pain) and 10 is the worst imaginable symptom. Informed consent (with written consent where possible) is required before using essential oils.

Therapeutic Care Plan and Interventions

Before the session:

- If in a clinical area, inform other people that aromatherapy will be used and assess whether they are comfortable with the aromas that will be used.
- Request no interruptions for the period required. This could be 5 minutes for a hand 'M' Technique using essential oils, or 15 minutes for hand, face, and feet. Allow 5 to 15 minutes for inhalation, 5 minutes for wound application, 5 to 10 minutes for sitz or hand bath, and 10 to 15 minutes for compress. Individual patches, aromastix, or aromapackets will not affect other people in the room.
- Discuss the length of the session, the required outcome, and the method to be used.

TABLE 15-3   Nursing Interventions: Aromatherapy

Patient Outcomes	Nursing Prescriptions	Evaluations
The patient will choose aromas from a selection offered by the nurse.	Provide the patient with various aromas to choose from that are suitable for the patient's condition.	The patient chose aromas from a selection offered by the nurse.
The patient will demonstrate positive physiologic outcomes in response to the aromatherapy and the 'M' Technique sessions, such as the following: • Decreased respiratory rate • Decreased heart rate • Decreased blood pressure • Decreased muscle tension • Decreased fatigue • Decreased pain • Improved physical mobility • Improved bed mobility • Improved activity tolerance • Improved sleep pattern • Improved surgical recovery • Improved ability to thrive • Improved breastfeeding • Improved self-care • Reduced nausea • Reduced constipation • Reduced risk of infection	Assess the patient's physiologic outcomes in response to the aromatherapy and the 'M' Technique before and immediately after each session. Evaluate the patient for the following: • Decreased respiratory rate • Decreased heart rate • Decreased blood pressure • Decreased muscle tension • Decreased fatigue • Decreased pain • Improved physical mobility • Improved bed mobility • Improved activity tolerance • Improved sleep pattern • Improved surgical recovery • Improved ability to thrive • Improved breastfeeding • Improved self-care • Reduced nausea • Reduced constipation • Reduced risk of infection	The patient demonstrated the following: • Decreased respiratory rate • Decreased heart rate • Decreased blood pressure • Decreased muscle tension • Decreased fatigue • Decreased pain • Improved physical mobility • Improved bed mobility • Improved activity tolerance • Improved sleep pattern • Improved surgical recovery • Improved ability to thrive • Improved breastfeeding • Improved self-care • Reduced nausea • Reduced constipation • Reduced risk of infection
The patient will demonstrate positive psychological outcomes in response to the aromatherapy and the 'M' Technique sessions, such as the following: • Improved body image • Improved self-esteem • Improved olfactory ability • Improved tactile ability • Reduced hopelessness • Reduced powerlessness • Reduced confusion • Improved memory	Assess the patient's psychological outcomes in response to the aromatherapy and the 'M' Technique before and immediately after each session. Evaluate the patient for the following: • Improved body image • Improved self-esteem • Improved olfactory ability • Improved tactile ability • Reduced hopelessness • Reduced powerlessness • Reduced confusion	The patient demonstrated the following: • Improved body image • Improved self-esteem • Improved olfactory ability • Improved tactile ability • Reduced hopelessness • Reduced powerlessness • Reduced confusion • Improved memory • More functional grieving • Reduced sorrow

(continues)

TABLE 15-3   Nursing Interventions: Aromatherapy (*continued*)

Patient Outcomes	Nursing Prescriptions	Evaluations
▪ More functional grieving	▪ Improved memory	▪ Improved trauma response
▪ Reduced sorrow	▪ More functional grieving	▪ Reduced anxiety
▪ Improved trauma response	▪ Reduced sorrow	▪ Reduced fear
▪ Reduced anxiety	▪ Improved trauma response	▪ More effective coping
▪ Reduced fear	▪ Reduced anxiety	▪ Less decisional conflict
▪ More effective coping	▪ Reduced fear	▪ Better family coping
▪ Less decisional conflict	▪ More effective coping	
▪ Better family coping	▪ Less decisional conflict	
	▪ Better family coping	

- Ask the patient to empty the bladder for comfort.
- Prepare the hospital bed or surface on which you will be working. Adjust the bed height for your convenience.
- Ensure that the temperature of the room is appropriate.
- Ask the patient to remove eyeglasses if using direct inhalation as a method.
- Prepare the environment for optimal relaxation if this is the purpose of the session.
- Place a clean towel under the hand or foot for 'M' Technique.
- Wash your hands.
- Prepare mixture of essential oils in carrier oil/aloe vera gel if being applied topically.
- Prepare diffuser with mixture of undiluted essential oils if inhalation is being used.
- Prepare compress with either water or carrier oil for wound care.
- Prepare bath for immersion of limb or body.
- Prepare basin with very hot water for steam inhalation.
- Prepare basin with warm water and essential oils for body wash.
- Select individual aromapatch or aromapacket, or make up aromastix as per instructions.
- Focus on your healing intention, and then begin.

At the beginning of the session:

- Tell the patient what you are going to do before you do it.
- Tell the patient which part of the body you are going to touch before you touch it.
- Make sure that the limb is supported.
- Ask the patient to tell you what the pressure feels like to him or her (on a scale of 0–10) if you are using the 'M' Technique. It should be a 3.
- Warm your hands by rubbing them together.
- Apply a small amount of diluted essential oil into one hand if using the 'M' Technique.
- Put required number of drops of essential oil in basin for steam inhalation.
- Put required number of drops of essential oil in diffuser.
- Begin slowly and rhythmically if using the 'M' Technique.
- Help position the patient above steaming bowl for inhalation, and place towel over head and shoulders.
- Begin applying diluted essential oils to wound or burn.
- Apply aromapatch to patient's chest area, or give aromastix or aromapacket to patient and ask patient to hold the aromatherapy personal device and breathe in several times.

During the session:

- Maintain constant pressure, rhythm, and speed if using the 'M' Technique.
- Discourage conversation.
- Encourage the patient to focus on the treatment.
- If the patient is using inhalation method, encourage him or her to breathe deeply.
- Have tissues available for expectoration if steam inhalation is used.
- Have empty basin available if essential oil is being used for nausea.
- Stay with a confused, elderly, infirm, or very young patient if inhalation or bath is being used.
- Reassess the patient as you move through the session.

At the end of the session:

- Remove any apparatus used for aromatherapy (basin, bath, diffuser).
- If the patient has gone to sleep, gently wake him or her after a few moments.
- Tell the patient that you have finished the session.
- Dry skin if bath has been used.
- Wash your hands.
- Leave individual aromapatch in situ so the aroma can gently diffuse up toward the patient's nose.
- Leave the individual aromastix or aromapacket with the patient for him or her to use when needed for symptoms such as nausea, headache, or depression.

Specific Interventions

- Have the patient discuss any changes or experiences that occurred during the session.
- The nurse may reassess physical parameters such as blood pressure, pulse, and respiration.
- The nurse may suggest that the treatment be self-applied at regular intervals.
- The nurse may make up a series of treatments in a bottle for such self-application.
- The nurse may schedule a follow-up treatment.

Case Study (Implementation)

Case Study 1

Setting: Outpatient unit
Patient: G. D., a 54-year-old Caucasian woman with mild asthma
Patterns/Challenges/Needs:

1. Altered physical regulation
2. Anxiety
3. Fear
4. Powerlessness
5. Ineffective coping related to anxiety around asthma attacks

G. D. is a 54-year-old woman who has had asthma with frequent wheezing and coughing problems for the last 10 years and fears each attack when she feels she "just cannot get enough air." The attacks are triggered by very cold weather, exercise, and stress. She has tried relaxation techniques, but none has really worked. G. D. developed asthma as a child, but during her teenage years her symptoms resolved and only reappeared about 10 years ago. She has been wheezing on a daily basis for the last 9 months, and currently the wheezing is controlled with fluticasone propionate and salmeterol (Advair).

Prior to commencing Advair, G. D. required emergency department treatment as a result of an asthma flare-up. At the time, she was prescribed a course of oral corticosteroids and antibiotics, albuterol and amoxicillin. This resolved the asthma completely, and she was much better for a month. But after a month, she felt the albuterol did not really help, so her physician switched her to Advair. This seems to be controlling the asthma; however, when she exercises, her chest tightens and she coughs. She particularly resents that the asthma prevents her from exercising because she is trying to lose weight. She has allergies to mold and some animals, she does not smoke, and there are no pets in the house. Her father has eczema.

The nurse outlined the use of inhaling essential oils and their effect on opening up the respiratory tract. She invited G. D. to smell the aromas of *E. globulus*, *E. smithii*, *E. citriadora*, *Ravansara aromatica*, *L. latifolia*, and *Boswellia carteri*. The patient liked *E. globulus* and *B. carteri* best. The nurse prepared an aromastix with six drops of *E. globulus* and six drops of *B. carteri*. The nurse asked the patient to hold the aromastix close to one nostril and inhale the aroma, then to the other nostril, and to repeat this several times until the patient felt symptoms abating. The patient did so. The nurse reassured her that she (the nurse) would stay with her initially. The patient was asked if she could feel the essential oils deep within her chest, and the patient said yes. The session was concluded after 8 minutes when the patient felt that she had received enough.

The patient stated that the effect of inhaling the essential oils appeared to open up her airway almost immediately. She felt the aromas were familiar and calming—and it was a simple treatment to receive. The nurse told G. D. she could keep the aromastix to use when necessary and to return in a week. G. D. continued to use the aromastix four times a day. She found the aromastix calmed her asthma and the effect lasted for about 3 hours. She was surprised that something so simple was so effective, and she felt empowered and no longer helpless. She was particularly pleased that she did not need to see her physician, and her supply of Advair lasted a long time. She reduced her use of Advair to once a day and sometimes would go for several days without needing to use it at all.

The nurse showed G. D. how to make up a personal inhaler and where she could purchase essential oils.

Evaluation

The nurse determined with G. D. whether the desired outcomes had been achieved. Both the nurse and G. D. felt that the inhaled essential oils had proved effective on all five outcomes:

1. Altered physical regulation (asthma) went from a 7 to a 3.
2. Anxiety went from an 8 to a 2.
3. Fear went from a 7 to a 2.
4. Powerlessness went from an 8 to a 2.
5. Ineffective coping related to anxiety around asthma attacks went from a 7 to a 3.

Case Study 2

Setting: Hospital inpatient

Patient: B. S., an 82-year-old Caucasian woman with unresolved chronic pain resulting from severe spinal degeneration

Patterns/Challenges/Needs:

1. Chronic pain
2. Anxiety
3. Fear
4. Powerlessness
5. Ineffective coping related to chronic pain

B. S. is an 82-year-old woman who had been experiencing severe back pain. X-rays revealed spondylolisthesis of L4 and L5 secondary to severe degenerative changes, a central spinal stenosis of L1 through L4, and a mild compression fracture of L2. B. S. had a caudal epidural block without relief. For the following 10 days, she had been on bed rest with bathroom privileges only. She was on 6-hour medication for pain control, but the medication (morphine derived) left her nauseated and confused. The pain remained at a 5 to 6 on a scale of 0 to 10. Prior to the aromatherapy session, she was lying rigid in bed with her eyes closed, her respirations were shallow, and her skin was very pale. When she was called by name, her eyes seemed glazed and her lips stuck to her teeth when she tried to reply. She said that she had been given pain medication about 3 hours previously, but it "hadn't helped much." She had been unable to eat because she felt so nauseated. Her oxygen saturation was 94%, her heart rate was 89 beats per minute, and her breathing was shallow (24 breaths per minute).

The nurse asked B. S. if she had any likes or dislikes when it came to aromas. She said she liked flowery smells and disliked the smell of food at the present time. She was open to being touched and said she would prefer her hands and face to be touched rather than her feet and legs. The nurse chose specific essential oils to alter perception of pain (*Rosa damascena* and *L. angustifolia*), relieve nausea (*Zingiber officinalis*), and give comfort and relaxation (*Salvia sclarea* and *Chamaemelum nobile*). She made a 5% solution of the essential oils in jojoba oil.

The nurse centered herself before making her touch known so that B. S. would know the texture and temperature of her touch. Then, the nurse carried out a 5-minute 'M' Technique with 5% solution of *L. angustifolia*, *Z. officinalis*, *C. nobile*,

S. sclarea, and *R. damascena* (one drop each essential oil in 5 cc of grapeseed carrier oil) on each of her hands. She worked slowly and rhythmically, keeping her pressure light. She checked with B. S. that the pressure was a 3 (on a scale of 0–10). B. S. nodded but did not say anything. The nurse wrapped each hand in a hand towel at completion. Then, the nurse completed an 'M' Technique of B. S.'s face; this took an additional 5 minutes. B. S.'s face began to soften a little toward the end of the technique and her breathing became less shallow. She sighed several times. At the end of the treatment, B. S. was nearly asleep. The nurse checked B. S.'s oxygen saturation (97%) and her heart rate (74 beats per minute). Her respirations were down by 14 breaths a minute.

B. S. slept for 2 hours and later stated it was the first time she had been without pain since the accident. The nurse continued to return to give the aromatherapy treatment using the 'M' Technique each day. Each time, B. S. experienced profound pain relief that was unobtainable through medication. Immediately following the 'M' Technique, her pain was rated as a 1. This effect lasted for 3 hours. The relaxing effect of the 'M' Technique coupled with the analgesic effect of the essential oils seemed to enable B. S. to relax into her pain and thus achieve relief.

Evaluation

The nurse determined with B. S. whether the desired outcomes had been achieved. Both the nurse and B. S. felt that the 15 minutes of 'M' Technique with diluted essential oils had proved effective on all five outcomes:

1. Chronic pain went from a 5 to a 1.
2. Anxiety went from a 7 to a 1.
3. Fear went from a 7 to a 2.
4. Powerlessness went from a 9 to a 2.
5. Ineffective coping related to chronic pain went from a 7 to a 2.

Directions for Future Research

1. Evaluate the outcome of diffused essential oils to reduce airborne infection in intensive care units.
2. Evaluate the outcome of inhaled aromas on posttraumatic stress disorder.

3. Evaluate the effect of topically applied diluted essential oils on postradiation burns.
4. Evaluate the effect of topically applied essential oils and the 'M' Technique on chronic pain.
5. Evaluate the effect of inhaled essential oils on nicotine withdrawal.

Nurse Healer Reflections

After reading this chapter, the nurse healer will be able to answer or to begin the process of answering the following questions:

- What is important for me to know before I begin using essential oils?
- How do I know whether to apply an essential oil topically or ask the patient to inhale it?
- What is my experience of inhaling the five essential oils discussed in this chapter?
- How do I feel about using aromatherapy with the 'M' Technique for chronic pain?
- How do I feel about using essential oils for infection?
- How do I feel about using aromatherapy as part of holistic nursing care?

NOTES

1. J. Buckle, *Clinical Aromatherapy: Essential Oils in Healthcare*, 3rd ed. (St. Louis, MO: Elsevier, 2015).
2. J. Buckle, "Take Five and Relax," *Nursing Spectrum* 18A, no. 11 (2006): 23.
3. J. Buckle, "The 'M' Technique for Dementia," *Working with Older People* 13, no. 3 (2009): 22–24.
4. J. Buckle, "The 'M' Technique: Touch for the Critically Ill or Actively Dying," *Positive Health* 152, no. 1 (2008). www.positivehealth.com/article/bodywork/the-m-technique-touch-for-the-critically-ill-or-actively-dying.
5. J. Buckle, A. Newberg, N. Wintering, E. Hutton, C. Lido, and J. T. Farrar, "Measurement of Regional Cerebral Blood Flow Associated with the 'M' Technique—Light Massage Therapy: A Case Series and Longitudinal Study Using SPECT," *Journal of Alternative and Complementary Medicine* 14, no. 8 (2008): 903–910.
6. J. Buckle, "Should Nursing Take Aromatherapy More Seriously?" *British Journal of Nursing* 16, no. 2 (2006): 116–120.

7. C. Burr, *The Emperor of Scent* (New York: Random House, 2003).

8. C. Brownlee, "Mapping Aroma: Smells Light Up Distinct Brain Parts," *Science News* 167, no. 22 (2005): 340–341.

9. N. Goel, H. Kim, and R. Lao, "The Olfactory Stimulus Modifies Nighttime Sleep in Young Men and Women," *Chronobiology International* 22, no. 5 (2005): 889–904.

10. Y. Fu, Y. Zu, L. Chen, X. Shi, Z. Wang, S. Sun, and T. Efferth, "Antimicrobial Activity of Clove and Rosemary Essential Oils Alone and in Combination," *Phytotherapy Research* 21, no. 10 (2007): 989–994.

11. J. Watson, *Caring Science as Sacred Science* (Philadelphia: F. A. Davis, 2005).

12. E. Barrett, "The Theoretical Matrix for a Rogerian Nursing Practice," *Theoria: Journal of Nursing Theory* 9, no. 4 (2000): 3–7.

13. B. Dossey, *Florence Nightingale: Mystic, Visionary, Healer* (Philadelphia: F. A. Davis, 2009).

14. H. L. Erickson, "Philosophy and Theory of Holism," *Nursing Clinics of North America* 42, no. 2 (2007): 139–163.

15. K. Kejlovia, D. Jirova, H. Bendova, P. Gajdos, and H. Kolarava, "Phototoxicity of Essential Oils Intended for Cosmetic Use," *Toxicology in Vitro* 24, no. 8 (2010): 2084–2089.

16. J. Bastard and D. Tiran, "Aromatherapy and Massage for Antenatal Anxiety: Its Effect on the Fetus," *Complementary Therapies in Clinical Practice* 12, no. 1 (2006): 48–54.

17. R. Tisserand and R. Young, *Essential Oil Safety*, 2nd ed. (New York: Churchill Livingstone, 2014).

18. J. K. Fung, H. W. Tsang, and R. C. Chung, "A Systematic Review of the Use of Aromatherapy in Treatment of Behavioral Problems in Dementia," *Geriatrics and Gerontology International* 12, no. 3 (2012): 372–382.

19. R. C. Atkins, "The Use of Aromatherapy Massage with Carers of Dementia Patients: A Preliminary Evaluation," *International Journal of Clinical Aromatherapy* 6, no. 2 (2009): 9–14.

20. A. Burns, E. Perry, C. Holmes, P. Francis, J. Morris, M.-J. R. Howes, and P. Chazot, "A Double-Blind Placebo-Controlled Randomized Trial of *Melissa officinalis* Oil and Donepezil for the Treatment of Agitation in Alzheimer's Disease," *Dementia and Geriatric Cognitive Disorders* 31, no. 2 (2011): 158–164.

21. G. D. Ko, A. Hum, G. Traitses, and D. Berbrayer, "Effects of Topical O24 Essential Oils on Patients with Fibromyalgia Syndrome: A Randomized, Placebo Controlled Pilot Study," *Journal of Musculoskeletal Pain* 15, no. 1 (2007): 11–19.

22. M. Ayan, U. Tas, E. Sogut, M. Suren, L. Gurbuzler, and F. Koyuncu, "Investigating the Effect of Aromatherapy in Patients with Renal Colic," *Journal of Alternative and Complementary Medicine* 19, no. 4 (2013): 329–333.

23. S. Kim, H-J. Kim, J-S. Yeo, S-J. Hong, J-M. Lee, and Y. Jeon, "The Effect of Lavender Oil on Stress, Bispectral Index Values, and Needle Insertion Pain in Volunteers," *Journal of Alternative and Complementary Medicine* 17, no. 9 (2011): 823–826.

24. C. A. Arias and B. E. Murray, "Antibiotic-Resistant Bugs in the 21st Century: A Clinical Super Challenge," *New England Journal of Medicine* 360, no. 5 (2009): 439–443.

25. D. L. Wegner, "No Mercy for MRSA: Treatment Alternatives to Vancomycin and Linezolid," *Medical Laboratory Observer* 37, no. 1 (2005): 26–29.

26. A. Espnel-Ingroff, "Mechanisms of Resistance to Antifungal Agents: Yeasts and Filamentous Fungi," *Revista Iberoamericana de Micologia* 25, no. 2 (2008): 101–106.

27. C. Gilbert and G. Bolvin, "Human Cytomegalovirus Resistance to Antiviral Drugs," *Antimicrobial Agents and Chemotherapy* 49, no. 3 (2005): 873–883.

28. P. H. Warnke, S. T. Becker, R. Podschun, S. Sivananthan, I. N. Springer, P. A. J. Russo, J. Wiltfang, H. Fickenscher, and E. Sherry, "The Battle Against Multi-Resistant Strains: Renaissance of Antimicrobial Essential Oils as a Promising Force to Fight Hospital-Acquired Infections," *Journal of Craniomaxillofacial Surgery* 37, no. 7 (2009): 392–397.

29. W. Bowler, J. Bresnahan, A. Bradfish, and C. Fernandez, "An Integrated Approach to Methicillin-Resistant *Staphylococcus aureus* Control in a Rural, Regional-Referral Healthcare Setting," *Infection Control and Hospital Epidemiology* 31, no. 3 (2010): 269–275.

30. V. Edwards-Jones, R. Buck, S. Shawcross, M. Dawson, and K. Dunn, "The Effect of Essential Oils on Methicillin-Resistant *Staphylococcus aureus* Using a Dressing Model," *Burns* 30, no. 8 (2004): 772–777.

31. K. B. Chin and B. Cordell, "The Effect of Tea Tree Oil (*Melaleuca alternifolia*) on Wound Healing Using a Dressing Model," *Journal of Alternative and Complementary Medicine* 9, no. 12 (2013): 942–945.

32. E. Sherry and P. Warnke, *Alternative for MRSA and Tuberculosis (TB): Eucalyptus and Tea Tree Oils as New Topical Antibacterials* (paper presented at the Orthopedic Surgery Conference, February 13–17, 2002, Dallas, TX).

33. M. Hur, J. Park, W. Maddock-Jennings, D. Kim, and M. Lee, "Reduction of Mouth Malodor and Volatile Sulphur Compounds in Intensive Care Patients Using Essential Oil Mouthwash," *Phytotherapy Research* 21, no. 7 (2007): 641–643.

34. T. Ebihara, S. Ebihara, M. Maruyama, M. Kobayashi, A. Itou, H. Arai, and H. Sasaki, "A Randomized Trial of Olfactory Stimulation Using Black Pepper Oil in Older People with Swallowing Dysfunction," *Journal of the American Geriatric Society* 54, no. 9 (2006): 1410–1416.

35. E. Lesho, "Role of Inhaled Antibacterials in Hospital-Acquired and Ventilator-Associated Pneumonia," *Expert Review of Anti-Infective Therapy* 3, no. 3 (2005): 445–451.

36. J. Valnet, *The Practice of Aromatherapy* (Rochester, VT: Healing Arts, 1990).

37. F. Xu, K. Uebaba, H. Ogawa, T. Tatsuse, B. H. Wang, T. Hisajima, and S. Venkatraman, "Pharmaco-Physio-Psychologic Effect of Ayurvedic Oil-Dripping Treatment Using an Essential Oil from *Lavandula angustifolia*," *Journal of Alternative and Complementary Medicine* 14, no. 8 (2008): 947–956.

38. I. Lee and G. Lee, "Effects of Lavender Aromatherapy on Insomnia and Depression in Women College Students," *Taehan Kanho, Hakhoe Chi* 36, no. 1 (2006): 136–143.

39. E. Pemberton and P. Turpin, "The Effect of Essential Oils on Work-Related Stress in Intensive Care Unit Nurses," *Holistic Nursing Practice* 22, no. 2 (2008): 97–102.

40. B. Bradley, N. Starkey, S. Brown, and R. Lea, "Anxiolytic Effects of *Lavandula angustifolia* Odour on the Mongolian Gerbil Elevated Plus Maze," *Journal of Ethnopharmacology* 111, no. 3 (2007): 517–525.

41. J. Lehrner, G. Marwinski, S. Lehr, P. Johren, and L. Deecke, "Ambient Odors of Orange and Lavender Reduce Anxiety and Improve Mood in a Dental Office," *Physiology and Behavior* 86, nos. 1–2 (2005): 92–95.

42. K. Pirali-Kheirabadi and J. Teixeira da Silva, "*Lavandula angustifolia* Essential Oil as a Novel and Promising Natural Candidate for Tick (*Rhipicephalus (Boophilus) annulatus*) Control," *Experimental Parasitology* 126, no. 2 (2010): 184–186.

43. F. D. D'Auria, M. Tecca, V. Strippoli, G. Salvatore, L. Battinelli, and G. Mazzanti, "Antifungal Activity of *Lavandula angustifolia* Essential Oil Against *Candida albicans* Yeast and Mycelial Form," *Medical Mycology* 43, no. 5 (2005): 391–396.

44. H. Gobel, "Mint Oil Solution in Tension Headache Is Comparatively as Effective as Paracetamol or Acetylsalicylic Acid," *Notfall Medizin* 27 (2001): 12.

45. A. Borhani Haghighi, S. Motazedian, R. Rezali, F. Mohammadi, L. Salarian, M. Pourmokhtari, S. Khodaei, M. Vossoughi, and R. Miri, "Cutaneous Application of Menthol 10% Solution as an Abortive Treatment of Migraine Without Aura: A Randomised, Double-Blind, Placebo-Controlled, Crossed-Over Study," *International Journal of Clinical Practice* 64, no. 4 (2010): 451–456.

46. S. Davies, L. Harding, and A. Baranowski, "A Novel Treatment for Postherpetic Neuralgia Using Peppermint Oil," *Clinical Journal of Pain* 18, no. 3 (2002): 200–202.

47. A. Piotrowski, "Inhale Peppermint to Relieve Postoperative Nausea" (R. J. Buckle Associates certification no. 293, 2005).

48. S. Irby, "Peppermint for Chemo-Induced Nausea" (R. J. Buckle Associates certification no. 322, 2005).

49. G. Lowdermilk, "Peppermint and Ginger for Chemo-Induced Nausea" (R. J. Buckle Associates certification no. 348, 2007).

50. M. Chalifour, "Peppermint as Anti-Emetic in Opiate Detox" (R. J. Buckle Associates certification no. 270, 2005).

51. R. M. Kline, J. J. Kline, J. Di Palma, and G. J. Barbero, "Enteric-Coated, pH-Dependent Peppermint Oil Capsules for the Treatment of Irritable Bowel Syndrome in Children," *Journal of Pediatrics* 138, no. 1 (2001): 125–128.

52. H. Salari, G. Amine, M. Shirazi, R. Hafezi, and M. Mohammadypour, "Antibacterial Effects of *Eucalyptus globulus* Leaf Extract on Pathogenic Bacteria Isolated from Specimens of Patients," *Clinical Microbiology Infection* 12, no. 2 (2006): 194–196.

53. A. Tyagi and A. Malik, "Antimicrobial Action of Essential Oil Vapors and Negative Air Ions Against *Pseudomonas fluorescens*," *International Journal of Food Microbiology* 143, no. 3 (2010): 205–210.

54. A. Tohidpour, M. Sattari, R. Omidbaigi, A. Yadegar, and J. Nazemi, "Antibacterial Effect of Essential Oils from Two Medicinal Plants Against Methicillin-Resistant *Staphylococcus aureus* (MRSA)," *Phytomedicine* 17, no. 2 (2010): 142–145.

55. L. Pitcher, "*Mentha piperita* to Reduce Sinus Pain and Congestion" (R. J. Buckle Associates certification no. 153, 2000).

56. A. Schumacher, J. Reichling, and P. Schnitzler, "Virucidal Effect of Peppermint Oil on the Enveloped Viruses Herpes Simplex Virus Type 1 and Type 2 In Vitro," *Phytomedicine* 19, no. 607 (2003): 504S–510S.

57. J. Kwiecinski, S. Eick, and K. Wojcik, "Effects of Tea Tree (*Melaleuca alternifolia*) Oil on *Staphylococcus aureus* in Biofilms and Stationary Growth Phase," *International Journal of Antimicrobial Agents* 33, no. 4 (2009): 343–347.

58. S. Enshaieh, A. Jooya, A. Siadat, and F. Iraji, "The Efficacy of 5% Topical Tea Tree Oil Gel in Mild to Moderate Acne Vulgaris: A Randomized, Double-Blind Placebo-Controlled Study," *Indian Journal of Dermatology, Venereology, and Leprology* 73, no. 1 (2007): 22–25.

59. A. Astani, J. Reichling, and P. Schnitzler, "Comparative Study on the Antiviral Activity of Selected Monoterpenes Derived from Essential Oils," *Phytotherapy Research* 24, no. 5 (2010): 673–679.

60. B. C. Millar and J. E. Moore, "Successful Topical Treatment of Hand Warts in a Paediatric Patient with Tea Tree Oil (*Melaleuca alternifolia*)," *Complementary Therapies in Clinical Practice* 14, no. 4 (2008): 225–227.

61. J. Bagg, M. S. Jackson, M. P. Sweeney, G. Ramage, and A. N. Davies, "Susceptibility to *Melaleuca alternifolia* (Tea Tree) Oil of Yeasts Isolated from the Mouths of Patients with Advanced Cancer," *Oral Oncology* 42, no. 5 (2006): 487–492.

62. A. Brady, T. Farnan, J. Toner, D. Gilpin, and M. Tunney, "Treatment of a Cochlear Implant Biofilm Infection: A Potential Role for Alternative Antimicrobial Agents," *Journal of Laryngology and Otology* 124, no. 7 (2010): 729–738.

63. A. Garozzo, R. Timpanaro, B. Bisignano, P. M. Furneri, G. Bisignano, and A. Castro, "In Vitro Antiviral Activity of *Melaleuca alternifolia* Essential Oil," *Letters in Applied Microbiology* 49, no. 6 (2009): 806–808.

64. F. Mondello, A. Girolamo, M. Scaturro, and M. L. Ricci, "Determination of *Legionella pneumophila* Susceptibility to *Melaleuca alternifolia* Cheel (Tea Tree) Oil by an Improved Broth Micro-Dilution Method Under Vapor Controlled Conditions," *Journal of Microbiology Methods* 77, no. 2 (2009): 243–248.

65. S. J. Greay, D. J. Ireland, H. T. Kissick, P. J. Heenan, C. F. Carson, T. V. Riley, and M. W. Beilharz, "Inhibition of Established Subcutaneous Murine Tumour Growth with Topical *Melaleuca alternifolia* (Tea Tree) Oil," *Cancer Chemotherapy and Pharmacology* 66, no. 6 (2010): 1095–1102.

66. G. Bozzuto, M. Colone, L. Toccacieli, A. Stringaro, and A. Molinari, "Tea Tree Oil Might Combat Melanoma," *Planta Medica* 77, no. 1 (2011): 54–56.

67. A. Catalán, J. Pacheco, A. Martínez, and M. Mondaca, "In Vitro and In Vivo Activity of *Melaleuca alternifolia* Mixed with Tissue Conditioner on *Candida albicans*," *Oral Surgery, Oral Medicine, Oral Pathology, Oral Radiology, and Endodontology* 105, no. 3 (2008): 327–332.

68. E. Sherry, M. Reynolds, S. Sivananthan, S. Mainawalala, and P. H. Warnke, "Inhalational Phytochemicals as Possible Treatment for Pulmonary Tuberculosis: Two Case Reports," *American Journal of Infection Control* 32, no. 6 (2004): 369–370.

69. A. Sadlon and D. Lamson, "Immune-Modifying and Antimicrobial Effects of Eucalyptus Oil and Simple Inhalation Devices," *Alternative Medicine Review* 15, no. 1 (2010): 33–47.

70. E. Ben-Ayre, N. Dudai, A. Eini, M. Torem, E. Schiff, and Y. Rakover, "Treatment of Upper Respiratory Tract Infections in Primary Care: A Randomized Study Using Aromatic Herbs," *Evidence-Based Complementary and Alternative Medicine* (2011). doi:10.1155/2011/690346.

71. C. Cermelli, A. Fabio, G. Fabio, and P. Quaglio, "Effect of Eucalyptus Essential Oil on Respiratory Bacteria and Viruses," *Current Microbiology* 56, no. 1 (2008): 89–92.

72. H. Daroui-Mokaddem, A. Kabouche, M. Bouacha, B. Soumati, A. El-Azzouny, C. Bruneau, and Z. Kabouche, "GC/MS Analysis and Antimicrobial Activity of Essential Oil of Fresh Leaves of *Eucalyptus globulus* and Leaves and Stems of *Smyrnium olusatrum* from Constantine (Algeria)," *Natural Products Communication* 5, no. 10 (2010): 1669–1672.

73. A. Toloza, A. Lucia, E. Zerba, H. Masuh, and M. Picollo, "Eucalyptus Essential Oil Toxicity Against Permethrin-Resistant *Pediculus humanus capitis*," *Parasitology Research* 106, no. 2 (2010): 409–414.

74. K. Eaton-Kelley, "Frankincense and the Terminally Ill Patient" (R. J. Buckle Associates certification no. 303, 2006).

75. P. Calzavara-Pinton, C. Zane, E. Facchinetti, R. Capezzera, and A. Pedretti, "Topical Boswellic Acids for Treatment of Photoaged Skin," *Dermatology Therapy* 23, Supplement 1 (2010): S28–S32.

76. E. Blain, A. Ali, and V. Duance, "*Boswellia frereana* (Frankincense) Suppresses Cytokine-Induced Matric Metalloproteinase Expression and Production of Pro-Inflammatory Molecules in Articular Cartilage," *Phytotherapy Research* 24, no. 6 (2010): 905–912.

77. S. Singh, A. Khajuria, S. C. Taneja, R. K. Johri, J. Singh, and G. N. Qazi, "Boswellic Acids: A Leukotriene Inhibitor Also Effective Through

Topical Application in Inflammatory Disorders," *Phytomedicine* 15, nos. 6–7 (2008): 400–407.

78. M. E. Houssen, A. Ragab, A. Mesbah, A. Z. El-Samanoudy, G. Othman, A. F. Moustafa, and F. A. Badria, "Natural Anti-Inflammatory Products and Leukotriene Inhibitors as Complementary Therapy for Bronchial Asthma," *Clinical Biochemistry* 43, nos. 10–11 (2010): 887–890.

79. A. Amer and H. Mehlhorn, "Larvicidal Effects of Various Essential Oils Against *Aedes*, *Anopheles*, and *Culex* Larvae (*Diptera, Culicidae*)," *Parasitology Research* 99, no. 4 (2006): 466–472.

80. M. B. Frank, Q. Yang, J. Osban, J. T. Azzarello, M. R. Saban, R. Saban, R. A. Ashley, J. C. Welter, K-M. Fung, and H-K. Lin, "Frankincense Oil Derived from *Boswellia carteri* Induces Tumor Cell Specific Cytotoxicity," *BMC Complementary and Alternative Medicine* 18, no. 9 (2009): 6.

81. X. Pang, Z. Yi, X. Zhang, B. Sung, W. Qu, X. Lian, B. B. Aggarwal, and M. Liu, "Acetyl-11-Keto-Beta-Boswellic Acid Inhibits Prostate Tumor Growth by Suppressing Vascular Endothelial Growth Factor Receptor 2–Mediated Angiogenesis," *Cancer Research* 69, no. 14 (2009): 5893–5900.

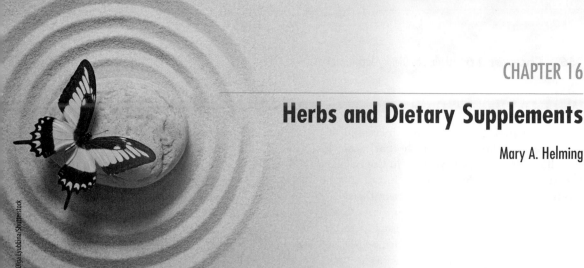

CHAPTER 16

Herbs and Dietary Supplements

Mary A. Helming

Nurse Healer Objectives

Theoretical

- Identify the historical perspective of herbal medicines.
- Define ways in which herbal medicines and supplements are now monitored for safety and efficacy.
- Describe the difference between dietary supplements and herbal supplements or botanicals.

Clinical

- Gain insight into a wide variety of herbs and dietary supplements that may augment allopathic disease treatment.
- Understand safety issues and contraindications of dietary and herb supplements.
- Identify several health conditions that have herbal or dietary supplement recommendations.

Personal

- Increase your knowledge of herbs and supplements to answer patient/client questions effectively and safely.
- Consider the potential use of appropriate herbs or dietary supplements for self-care.

Definitions

Botanical: Plant or plant part valued for its medicinal or therapeutic properties, flavor, and/or scent.

Dietary supplements: Products that supplement the diet and are typically vitamins, minerals, and amino acids. Sometimes herbal products are added to this definition.

Extract: Created by a botanical soaking in a liquid that removes some chemicals. The resultant liquid may be used by itself or evaporated in order to create a dry extract to place into tablets or capsules.

Good manufacturing practices: Statement for herbal products that sets the standard for purity, potency, and strength of substances to be truthful to statements on the label.

Herbs: Subset of botanicals. Products made from botanicals that are used to maintain or improve health may be called *herbal products*, *botanical products*, or *phytomedicines*.

Tea: (*infusion*) Adds boiling water to dried or fresh botanicals and steeps them.

Tincture: Created by soaking a botanical in a water and alcohol solution and sold as liquid concentrates in different strengths

© Olga Lyubkina/Shutterstock

Historical Perspectives

The use of herbal medicine has increased in recent years, although it is likely that most, if not all, of these herbs have been in use by our ancestors all over the globe for hundreds or thousands of years. Due to more scientific investigation into the components, properties, beneficial actions, and contraindications of these herbal remedies, there has been an upsurge of interest in herbs and supplements as well as use by the population in general. The German E Commission first began scientific studies of these preparations from 1983 to 1995,[1] and now the National Center for Complementary and Integrative Health (NCCIH), formerly known as the National Center for Complementary and Alternative Medicine (NCCAM), a federal government agency, is pooling and examining the information available on these herbal medicines.

Supplements refer to products that supplement the diet and are typically vitamins, minerals, and amino acids. While most of our supplements are based in nature, many of them are now made synthetically in the United States. Some herbal preparations, based on natural products, are being created synthetically as well. Some herbs and supplements may treat diseases and conditions, while others can be used as preventive measures to maintain health. It is vital for holistic nurses to be knowledgeable about these preparations, know where to find more information on them, and be ready to answer patients' questions about their use.

Introduction to the Tables

A general description of herbs by category of use and supplements by category of use is presented in **Table 16-1** and **Table 16-2**. Detailed information includes:

- Common and/or biological names
- Desirable medicinal actions of the herb or supplement
- Contraindications and risks/adverse drug reactions of the herb or supplement
- Usual dosing of the herb or supplement

While selected common herbs and supplements have been included, these tables are not all inclusive; thus, the reader is directed to the resources in the Notes list, especially the Natural Standard database (https://naturalmedicines .therapeuticresearch.com), which keeps current information. There the reader may find additional herbs and supplements that have not been included, as well as further details on each. Please refer to Chapter 31 for a more in-depth discussion of vitamin and mineral supplements.

Prevalence of Use and Safety Issues

Safety of herbs and supplements is sometimes questioned, but Adams noted that statistics from the National Poison Safety Data in 2009 showed that no one in the United States died from use of amino acids, vitamins, minerals, or herbs, in comparison to the more than 100,000 U.S. citizens per year who die from issues related to prescription pharmaceuticals.[2] The NCCIH reports that approximately 38% of the adult U.S. population and 12% of the pediatric-aged population currently use complementary and alternative medicine, and the highest percentage of use is for nonvitamin, nonmineral natural products.[3] Women and others who suffer from recurrent or chronic illness and who also receive allopathic or conventional medical care are among the highest users of herbal or botanical medicine.[4] Farina, Austin, and Lieberman reported that approximately one-third of the U.S. population concomitantly used dietary supplements with prescribed medications, according to survey data.[5] Multivitamins with other ingredients, followed by antacids, and then by multivitamins with botanical ingredients were the top three categories of dietary supplements noted. There are no universally accepted guidelines for managing herbal medicines used concomitantly with prescription medicines, but the Joint Commission mandates that dietary supplements (minerals, vitamins, and herbs) conform to the identical hospital standards as prescription medicines.[4]

Because of the potential for risks and adverse effects of herbs (botanicals) and other dietary supplements, it is essential for healthcare providers, including holistic nurses and holistic nurse practitioners, to directly question patients on their use of over-the-counter (OTC), herbal, and supplementary products. It is useful to ask patients to bring the associated bottles to the nurse or provider. Some patients do not consider these as "medicines" and may not feel it is important to report them. Some patients are disinclined to report them for fear of disapproval by healthcare providers. It is also important to recall that, globally, many people use botanical products, especially in other cultures; they may be prescribed routinely by healthcare providers, or they may be part of indigenous folk medicine practices. When global citizens immigrate to the United States, they usually bring their medicinal traditions with them. At times, the herbs are in combination products, which may not be easily identifiable.

The Dietary Supplement and Health Education Act was enacted into law in 1994, and there are many provisions that have changed the way herbals are sold in the United States. This law permits dietary supplements (vitamins, minerals, and herbs) to be marketed without approval of their safety and efficacy by the Food and Drug Administration (FDA). Manufacturers of herbal products must have evidence of the veracity of claims made on the product labels, but they are allowed to claim the product affects particular functions or structures of the body provided that there is no claim of effectiveness made for prevention or treatment of a certain disease and that a disclaimer that the FDA has not evaluated the product appears on the product container. However, the FDA has created a Good Manufacturing Practices statement for herbal products that sets the standard for purity, potency, and strength of substances to be truthful to statements on the label.[4] The Dietary Supplement and Nonprescription Drug Consumer Protection Act was passed into law in 2006. Features of this law include that the healthcare provider is encouraged to submit drug–herb interactions or adverse effects to MedWatch, an FDA-sponsored drug safety program. Adverse effects of herbs may be reported to the local poison control center, and the herb manufacturer is then required to send information on serious adverse effects to the FDA within 15 days. Important label logos identify dietary supplements and herbals that have been tested. These include the National Products Association seal certification process for ingredient quality and contaminants; the United States Pharmacopeia seal certification, a process that tests for pharmacologic properties,

contamination, adulteration, and proper manufacturing; the Consumer Lab seal certification, a process of testing for composition, purity, potency, bioavailability, and consistency of products; and the NSF International (National Sanitation Foundation) seal, a certification of Good Manufacturing Practices and persistent monitoring.[4] These seals are useful to identify quality natural products due to ongoing concerns about contamination of natural products through pesticides, microorganisms, heavy metals, misidentification of products, and adulteration of products with prescription medicines. In addition, quality of plant materials varies depending on where the product is grown or harvested, how it is dried, and even the quality of the soil and climate. As NCCIH reports:

> There have been reports of Chinese herbal products being contaminated with drugs, toxins, or heavy metals or not containing the listed ingredients. Some of the herbs used in Chinese medicine can interact with drugs, have serious side effects, or be unsafe for people with certain medical conditions.[6]

Therefore, the reader is cautioned about Chinese herbal products from China. Potentially, these products may instead be available from a U.S. company and should ideally be dispensed from a medical provider.

Reputable Resource and Research Organizations

The NCCIH is committed to the study of natural products, which it lists as being produced from plants, bacteria, fungi, and marine organisms. The NCCIH researchers also study vitamins, minerals, and probiotics, or any other natural product that can be linked to traditional medicine or other integrative or complementary health practices. Funding opportunities are available through the Natural Products Research division.[7] The NCCIH has therefore provided, to the public and to health professionals, a sizable list of herbs with associated information titled "Herbs at a Glance."[8] This list includes the herbs' common names, information on traditional or folk use, scientific evidence, potential adverse effects and cautions, and resources for additional information. Each fact sheet may be printed individually, or the entire packet of information may be downloaded as an ebook, if desired.

The FDA evaluates the safety of natural products on the market through research and through tracking reports of adverse or side effects. If the FDA feels that a product is not safe, it may issue a warning or require that the product be removed from the market. The FDA also monitors package inserts and label claims, and the Federal Trade Commission may become involved if information is not truthful or is misleading. The federal government has acted legally in cases of deceptive or false marketing of supplements, including on websites, and in cases of product safety concerns.

Evidence-based resources of dietary supplement information include the following national websites:[4]

- NCCIH: https://nccih.nih.gov/
- MedlinePlus: www.nlm.nih.gov/medlineplus/druginfo/herb_All.html
- Office of Dietary Supplements: http://ods.od.nih.gov/

Other trustworthy websites include:

- American Botanical Council: http://abc.herbalgram.org
- Cochrane Complementary Medicine Field: http://cam.cochrane.org/
- HerbMed (part of American Botanical Council): www.herbmed.org/
- The Natural Standard, available for purchase

In addition, AltMedDex's website features World-Cat (www.worldcat.org/), an international catalog that provides an extensive list of hard copy and electronic books and other resources on herbs.

Botanicals and Preparations

A botanical is a plant or plant part valued for its medicinal or therapeutic properties, flavor, and/or scent. Herbs are a subset of botanicals. Products made from botanicals that are used to maintain or improve health may be called *herbal products*, *botanical products*, or *phytomedicines*.[9] Botanical preparations can be made in several forms:[9]

- *Tea*. Also called an *infusion*, adds boiling water to dried or fresh botanicals and steeps them.
- *Decoction*. This is for some barks, berries, and roots that require longer periods of simmering in boiling water than teas in order to extract their beneficial ingredients.
- *Tincture*. This is created by soaking a botanical in a water and alcohol solution. The tinctures, sold as liquid concentrates, are made in different strengths according to botanical-to-extract ratios by volume or weight.
- *Extract*. This is created by the botanical soaking in a liquid that removes some chemicals. The resultant liquid may be used by itself or evaporated in order to create a dry extract to place into tablets or capsules.

Examples of Herbs and Supplements Used for Selected Common Conditions

Dermatologic

Eczema. This condition, also known as atopic dermatitis, is characterized by chronically pruritic and inflamed skin that can be exacerbated at times. It is known to be allergy and stress related and to have genetic and food allergy links. In addition to, or in place of allopathic medicine treatments, there are natural supplements and herbal treatments.

Natural supplements for eczema include high-potency multivitamin and mineral supplements; vitamin E 400 IU daily; fish oil (eicosapentaenoic acid [EPA] and docosahexaenoic acid [DHA]) 1000 to 3000 mg daily; probiotics *lactobacillus* and *bifidobacteria*; and colloidal oatmeal topical preparations.

Herbal remedies include grape seed or pine bark extract, 50 to 100 mg before meals; chamomile and oatmeal preparations for topical use.[10]

Seborrheic dermatitis. This skin issue is characterized by erythematous papules and/or scaling skin, especially on the cheeks, scalp, neck, and skin folds. It has been associated with genetic predisposition, diet, stress, food allergies, yeast organisms, and acquired immune deficiency syndrome (AIDS). In the scalp, its common term is *dandruff*, or *cradle cap* in infants. Vitamin B deficiency has also been linked to the disorder. In addition to, or in place of allopathic medicine treatments, there are natural supplements and herbal treatments of value.

Natural supplements include vitamins B_6 and B_{12} combined with folic acid.

Herbal remedies include aloe vera gel topically applied and tea tree oil for its antifungal effect, including 5% tea tree oil for the scalp or 1 tablespoon tea tree oil for 8 ounces of shampoo.[10]

Migraine headache. This subtype of headache is thought to be associated with strong vasodilators, such as substance P, released by cranial nerve V. This affects blood vessels in the scalp and meninges, causing edema and inflammation. Nitric oxide and the neurotransmitters glutamate and serotonin are also involved. Migraine headaches have a familial influence and can be prompted by stress, certain foods, menses, weather changes, fatigue, and sunlight.

Botanical supplements that have proven useful for migraine headache include feverfew (*Tanacetum parthenium* leaf), which may work by inhibiting inflammatory promoters, serotonin, and prostaglandin, in addition to inhibiting platelet aggregation. Studies are difficult to replicate due to variations in standardization of the dried leaf, and there have been no long-term studies on safety. Oral dosage of up to 125 mg/day of the dried leaf standardized to a minimum of 0.2% parthenolide has been recommended, but the effect may take weeks to develop. Sudden cessation of feverfew can cause increased headache and agitation. Adverse effects are gastrointestinal irritation and apthous ulcers. It is not recommended in pregnancy as it prolongs bleeding times. Another botanical is butterbur (*Petasites hybridus* root), which showed in studies that migraine frequency was reduced about 50% over a 4-month period. The extract of butterbur is commonly standardized at 15% of petasins, and carcinogens are removed. The starting dose is 50 mg three times per day for a month, then 50 mg twice a day. Pregnancy risks are unknown, and the main adverse effect is belching. Melatonin or valerian root have also been used for sleep management if that is an issue causing migraines.[4]

Upper respiratory. Most of these infections, known as URIs or "common colds," occur from viruses. Sometimes there are secondary bacterial infections that occur subsequently. There is a seasonal pattern to the various causative viruses. Botanical supplements include echinacea, which has three subtypes: angustifolia, purpurea (used most widely), and pallida. From the coneflower plant, this herb has even been incorporated into many OTC products. Due to a paucity of studies, in general it is not recommended for children or pregnant women. Most, but not all, studies of the effectiveness of echinacea have tended toward positive results by decreasing the duration and symptoms of URI because it is thought that this herb has immunologic activity, including cytokine and macrophage activation. It seems to be most beneficial in the first few days of URI symptoms.[4] Dosing may range from 500 to 1000 mg up to three times a day for the period of illness.[11] According to the Natural Standard, some authorities discourage the use of echinacea, due to concern about exacerbating conditions in such illnesses as autoimmune diseases, cancer, and tuberculosis.[11]

In Traditional Chinese Medicine, Astralgus extracts have been used for the prevention and treatment of the common cold, but there is a lack of research studies. Theoretically, it can have antiviral or immunomodulation activity. Chamomile has been used for a variety of conditions, including URI, most often in a tea. Elderberry (*Sambucus nigra*) studies show some antiviral, anti-influenza, and anti-inflammatory activity. Garlic, ginseng, and peppermint are other herbs that are under study as supportive for URI.

Nutritional supplements for URI include vitamin C, for prevention and treatment, after the studies of Dr. Linus Pauling. A Cochrane Systematic Review reveals that vitamin C plays some role in respiratory defense mechanisms, but not all studies have been positive. The average dosing recommended for prevention is 200 to 500 mg daily, and vitamin C-rich foods are also recommended. Large doses may cause gastrointestinal distress. Zinc preparations in studies reveal positive benefits about half of the time. The recommendation is for frequent dosing of oral preparations, dependent on type, but often every 2 to 3 hours in lozenge form. Taste has been bitter, but newer preparations are more palatable; food cannot be consumed for a period of time after a lozenge is consumed. Nasal zinc preparations are not recommended because they have caused a loss of smell in some users.[4]

Asthma. This disease is characterized by inflammation and spasm of the bronchial airways, plus production of excessive, viscous mucous that all contribute to respiratory distress. Many people with asthma wheeze, while others have only the cough-variant form of asthma, and it is graded into mild, moderate, and severe categories. The etiologies of asthma are potentially as follows: allergic, respiratory infection exacerbations, exercise induced, chemical induced, and stress related.

Depending on the etiology, several botanical herbs have shown efficacy in treating asthma. *Boswellia serrata* is an Ayurvedic Indian herb with both anti-inflammatory and antiallergy effects; one study showed improvement in symptoms and a decrease in the number of asthma attacks. Aloe vera extract may help to improve the immune system in asthma. Ginkgo biloba extract contains ginkolides, terpene molecules that oppose platelet-activating factor, a key mediator of asthma. Licorice root is known to have anti-allergy and anti-inflammatory actions, as well as being an expectorant; unless licorice is taken in the deglycyrrhizinated form, it can elevate blood pressure and cause electrolyte imbalance. Interestingly, capsaicin, the active ingredient in cayenne pepper, desensitizes airway mucosal response to mechanical and chemical irritants, and the mechanism is thought to be decreasing substance P in the respiratory tract.

Nutritional supplementation may be even more useful in asthma. Studies have revealed that supplementation with vitamin C, vitamin E, and antioxidants have proven beneficial. Vitamin C is a major antioxidant in the fluid lining airway surfaces, and low levels of vitamin C are associated with a risk for asthma. Vitamin C may also lower histamine levels, important in allergic asthma. Flavonoids are antioxidants, which act to prevent release of allergic mediators. Quercetin is a key flavonoid, but others include grape seed and pine bark extracts, green tea, passion fruit peel, and ginkgo. Carotenoids (e.g., beta-carotene) are strong antioxidants that

potentially improve the lining of the respiratory tract and decrease inflammatory leukotriene formation. Lycopene may be the most significant carotenoid, and supplementation has been experimented with, as has tomato juice and extract, which are high in lycopene. Vitamin B_{12} by injection has shown some efficacy in trials, as has vitamin D supplementation, which acts to block the inflammatory-causing protein cascade in asthma. Magnesium has often been found deficient in asthmatics, and treatments have included intravenous (IV), nebulized, and oral magnesium supplementation for asthma improvement. Finally, omega-3 fatty acid supplementation has shown improvement in respiratory function, likely related to decreasing arachidonic acid, which can lead to production of inflammatory leukotrienes. Some children with asthma have improved with vitamin B_6 supplementation, likely linked to a metabolic defect involving tryptophan.[10]

Cardiac

Dyslipidemia. This general term may refer to abnormalities in lipids, including total cholesterol, low-density lipoprotein (LDL-C) cholesterol, high-density lipoprotein (HDL-C) cholesterol, and triglyceride (TG) levels, in addition to others. Dyslipidemias are very common in the United States and are especially associated with aging, obesity, and diabetes mellitus. The risk for coronary artery disease increases with dyslipidemias, and there are dietary-induced, genetically induced, and secondary disease-associated causes of dyslipidemias. There are no botanical products recommended for dyslipidemia.

Dietary supplements for dyslipidemia include fiber, which may be in the form of natural fiber supplements (e.g., Metamucil, psyllium) or flaxseed. Fiber intake primarily acts to decrease LDL-C. Soy foods are also considered beneficial to reduce total cholesterol alone, but there are contraindications to the use of soy, such as history of some breast and cervical cancers. Fish oil provides omega-3 fatty acids that act to reduce TG and increase HDL-C (which is favorable, as it is protective). Omega-3 fatty acid content can vary with DHA and EPA content, but on average, a 1-gram capsule contains 120 mg of DHA and 180 mg of EPA. For general lipid benefit, 1 to

4 g/day is recommended, but higher doses, up to 3 to 4 g/day, are needed for hypertriglyceridemia. A prescription medication, Lovaza, is available for high-dose TG supplementation, as some people experience gastrointestinal side effects from fish oil. Plant stanols and sterols are mixtures usually extracted from soybean oil or pine tree wood pulp. These increase fecal elimination of cholesterol, both dietary and biliary. Stanols and sterols are most commonly added to foods such as margarines, rice milk, soy milk, and juices. Plant sterols can elevate dangerously in a rare condition with the inability to clear sterols, but stanols have no such risk and so may be safer. Gastrointestinal adverse effects are possible. Finally, red yeast rice is a fermented product of rice that has been used as a preservative and spice in China for centuries. It has been shown effective in U.S. studies at decreasing cholesterol up to 30% and TG up to 12% to 19%. It contains monaclins and sometimes lovastatin, which is a prescription statin or HMG Co-A reductase inhibitor. Red yeast rice has the same potential to cause side effects as prescription statins, although it is known to cause less risk of myopathy. Liver enzymes must be periodically monitored because they can elevate just as with prescription statins, and the drug would be discontinued. Standard dosing is 1200 mg twice daily, but doses range from 600 to 3600 mg per day. The FDA has sought to regulate red yeast rice supplements because standardized dosing and manufacturing reliability are not available, and because it can contain lovastatin; in fact, inappropriate fermentation processes can cause a nephrotoxic contaminant to arise, so caution must be observed with the use of this preparation.[4] An important supplement to take with statins is Coenzyme Q10 (see the next section), so it would be recommended with red yeast rice as well.

Coronary artery disease (CAD). This disease genetic and environmental etiologies, and the essential issue is atherosclerotic plaque deposition in coronary arteries, leading to risk of angina and myocardial infarction, or death. The earlier discussion regarding dyslipidemia factors into environmental and genetic causes of CAD; thus, all of the earlier-mentioned supplements can be useful for CAD. However, additional dietary and other supplements have been proposed as useful in the treatment of CAD. Niacin, a B vitamin, has been helpful in

decreasing LDL-C by 15% to 20%. However, its most bothersome adverse effect, systemic flushing, is common in up to 50% of those taking niacin. "No flush" niacin preparations remove the active ingredient that decreases LDL-C. The best manner of taking niacin is with food, especially with dinner, and often with applesauce after dinner (possibly due to the quercetin component in applesauce). An aspirin tablet or nonsteroidal anti-inflammatory drug (e.g., ibuprofen) taken just before the niacin also seems to decrease flushing incidence. Vitamin D has been found in heart muscle cells and arterial walls; a deficiency in vitamin D has been linked to cardiovascular risk. Development of myalgias from statins also appears to be more commonly seen in vitamin D deficiency. Vitamin D levels should be over 30 ng/mL; mild deficiencies for cardiac health can be treated with OTC vitamin D_3 in doses of 1000 to 5000 units per day, depending on the level of deficiency. Excess vitamin D can cause hypercalcemia. Folic acid and other B vitamins had been considered useful supplements in CAD because of their ability to decrease homocysteine levels, which have, if elevated, increased CAD and stroke risk. However, studies have shown no actual benefit to folic acid supplementation in CAD, but dietary supplementation of foods high in folate, especially dark green leafy vegetables, has shown benefit in CAD.[4]

Coenzyme Q10, known as CoQ10, is considered a worthy supplement both for avoidance or treatment of statin-related myalgias and for systolic function improvement in congestive heart failure. CoQ10 is a mitochondrial compound that acts in electron transport and energy production. Any patient on a statin drug develops lower levels of CoQ10, potentially lower energy levels, and higher risk for myalgias. Supplementation with CoQ10 at a 100-mg/day dose appears to be adequate.[4]

Diabetes Mellitus Type 2

Diabetes mellitus type 2. This condition increasingly prevalent in today's society. Factors that cause risk for type 2 diabetes include genetics, obesity, insulin resistance, the metabolic syndrome, a diet high in refined carbohydrates and low in fiber, a sedentary lifestyle, a low intake of antioxidants, and a higher presence of free radicals, which damage tissues, activate inflammation, and cause insulin resistance. It is clear that diet, exercise, and lifestyle changes play a large role in managing type 2 diabetes, but dietary supplements and some botanicals have also proven effective in improving disease management.

Dietary supplements studied in type 2 diabetes include chromium, a mineral that is essential to glucose tolerance factor, a molecule that facilitates insulin effectiveness. Chromium helps insulin take up glucose into cells. Chromium deficiency is now thought to be common in the United States, and it may factor into the increased prevalence of diabetes. Studies have shown both efficacy and no change when chromium supplementation was used in diabetes type 2; it appears most useful if there is a chromium deficiency. There is no recommended daily intake for chromium, but it is estimated that at least 200 mg/day is required. Patients with type 2 diabetes should supplement with chromium polynicotinate or picolinate at 400 to 600 mg/day. Chromium with 2 mg biotin showed efficacy as well, dropping HgbA1C levels by 0.54%. Vitamin C transport into cells is enhanced by insulin; therefore, it is known that many diabetics have vitamin C deficiency and should take supplementation. Due to other functions of vitamin C, deficiency in diabetics can lead to elevated cholesterol, impaired wound healing, and depressed immunity. Vitamin C also causes some reduction in HgbA1C levels and in blood pressure (improves elasticity of blood vessels). Vitamin E is an antioxidant that protects cell membranes; nerve cells are especially vulnerable to damage in diabetes, and vitamin E appears to prevent this. Further, vitamin E improves insulin action, prevents free radical damage to LDL-C and vascular lining, increases magnesium intracellularly, decreases C-reactive protein (inflammatory marker), improves electrical conduction through the nervous system, improves blood flow to the eye to decrease diabetic retinopathy, and improves kidney function and creatinine clearance. Vitamin E dosing at 400 to 800 IU/day appeared most useful, with precautions for bleeding risk and, in some cases, for systolic blood pressure elevation.

Other dietary supplements that may have use in type 2 diabetes include the B vitamins niacin

and B_6. A study showed that niacin given as niacinimide 500 mg three times daily improved C-peptide release (reflects how much insulin is being manufactured by the pancreas) and blood glucose control. Vitamin B_6, especially at a dose of 25 mg/day, assists in protection against diabetic neuropathy. Biotin, another B vitamin, is important in sugar metabolism and it enhances insulin sensitivity. Minerals that may be useful in diabetes include magnesium, zinc, and manganese. Greater than 50% of all diabetics show evidence of magnesium deficiency, and this can worsen diabetic retinopathy and neuropathy. Magnesium supplemented at 300 to 500 mg/day is suggested, especially because diabetics may lose magnesium through the kidneys. Adequate B_6 is necessary for moving magnesium intracellularly. Zinc is an enzyme cofactor in greater than 200 enzyme reactions. Diabetics and the elderly tend to have lower levels of zinc, and this affects wound healing, sense of taste and smell, and skin disease. Zinc is protective against beta cell destruction; the recommended supplementation for diabetics is at least 30 mg/day. Manganese is involved in energy production and blood glucose control, as well as in thyroid function. Animal studies reveal that a deficiency in manganese produces diabetes. Average supplemental dosing of manganese is 3 to 5 mg/day. Finally, omega-3 fatty acids promote insulin sensitivity and are anti-inflammatory, so 1 g/day is recommended for diabetics.

Botanical and other supplements for diabetes include fenugreek seeds, which have shown antidiabetic effects as well as reductions in LDL-C and TG. Taken as 1 g/day as fenugreek seed extract, fasting blood glucose levels dropped and insulin sensitivity increased. Alpha-lipoic acid is vitamin-like but also an antioxidant. It functions to stop free radicals intracellularly. In Germany, it has been used successfully for diabetes for the past 30 years. Part of its effect is improving diabetic neuropathy, probably because of the free radical scavenging. A dosage of 400 to 600 mg/day has been used in studies, which have also shown improved glucose metabolism, improved peripheral nerve circulation, and regeneration of nerve fibers. Flavonoids show promise in diabetes treatment; quercetin, for example, improves insulin secretion. Bilberry extract is a type of flavonoid that seems to have benefit for preserving the eye in early diabetic retinopathy and cataracts. Dosing is 160 to 320 mg/day for bilberry. Other flavonoids that show promise in diabetes include ginkgo biloba extract, at a dose of 120 to 240 mg/day, especially for patients over age 50. It has benefit for improved extremity circulation and is brain- and vascular-lining protective. Grape seed or pine bark extract are systemic antioxidants and are considered the best choice for diabetics under age 50, particularly if there is diabetic retinopathy, hypertension, or CAD. Hawthorne extract is a flavonoid to be considered if there is accompanying CAD or hypertension, at a dose of 450 to 600 mg/day. Bitter melon has been used in folk medicine for diabetes and has shown blood glucose-lowering effectiveness. It can be found in Asian grocery stores because the fresh juice, although it is bitter, is the best supplement. American ginseng has properties that show a reduction in postprandial blood glucose, whereas *Panax* ginseng extract has also shown improved HgbA1C levels. Finally, onions and garlic appear to lower blood glucose. Garlic seems to be the more potent of the two, and it also lowers cholesterol and blood pressure in diabetes.[10]

Nutraceuticals

Nutraceuticals are foods that promote medical or health benefits. Dietary supplements such as plant stanols and sterols, cereals fortified with omega-3 fatty acids, sports drinks with ginseng, orange juice with calcium added, soy products in energy bars, iron supplements in food, and dairy products with probiotics added all are examples of nutraceuticals.[12] While there is overlap between dietary supplements and herbs, a discussion of greater depth on nutraceuticals and food as medicine is beyond the scope of this chapter.

Examples of Herbs That May Have Preoperative Contraindications Due to Bleeding and Other Risks

A review of Tables 16-1 and 16-2 will demonstrate that numerous medicinal herbs and some dietary supplements may cause risk of bleeding, sometimes by themselves or sometimes in combination with other anticoagulants such as warfarin. This may especially be a risk during surgery and/or anesthesia. In 2011, the American Association of Nurse Anesthetists produced a list of herbs and supplements that are potentially hazardous for surgery and anesthesia.[13] They recommend that all products be stopped 1 to 2 weeks prior to surgery and that the surgeon and anesthetist or anesthesiologist be made aware of all of the patient's OTC medications and supplements. It may be the role of the nurse or advanced practice nurse, when seeing a patient for preoperative examination, to determine if there are any risks with herbs and supplements. If this is unknown, the registered nurse or advanced practice nurse should contact the surgeon and anesthesia providers to discuss whether such medications and supplements need to be stopped ahead of time, and if so, how long preoperatively. Some surgical offices provide patients with information sheets describing which herbs or supplements may need to be stopped, but many patients are unaware of these risks and are not notified by surgeons. Some examples follow.

Black cohosh can increase bleeding and decrease blood pressure. Echinacea can suppress the immune system and inflame the liver. Feverfew can increase the risk of prolonged bleeding. Garlic can alter blood pressure and cause prolonged bleeding. Ginger can be sedating and can risk increased bleeding, especially if combined with aspirin and ginkgo. Ginkgo biloba may increase bleeding. Ginseng may cause insomnia and risk cardiac effects. Hoodia may cause blood sugar imbalance and, potentially, arrhythmias. Kava kava has sedative properties, which can be an additive to some medications, and it has a potential for severe liver toxicity (this can occur in general use, so it is not recommended). St. John's wort can alter blood pressure, cause sedation, and create a risk of interacting with other medications that may prolong the effects of anesthesia. Valerian (root) has increased sedative effects that could combine dangerously with anesthetics or pain medications.[13] Saw palmetto has been known to cause excess bleeding. Dietary supplements such as vitamin E and fish oil, which also can have anticoagulant properties, are normally stopped as well.

TABLE 16-1 Selected Common Herbs, Alphabetical

Common/Biological Name	Desirable Medicinal Actions	Contraindications and Risks (Adverse Drug Reactions [ADRs])	Typical Dosing
Acai (ah-sigh-EE) ■ Berry from South and Central America	**Uses:** anticancer, antioxidant, anti-inflammatory **Studies:** no scientific studies conducted on use for medical conditions	■ Allergic to acai or plants in palm family ■ May affect magnetic resonance imaging (MRI) results **ADRs** ■ Hypertension ■ Gastrointestinal (GI) bleeding ■ Ulcers	**Form:** juice, capsules, powder, tablets **Dose:** widely used, no specific dosing
Aloe Vera "burn plant," "lily of the desert" Leaves contain a clear gel that can be used topically ■ Green part of leaf that surrounds gel produces juice or dried substance (latex) that can be taken orally ■ Used as far back as 6,000 years ago in Egyptian times	**Uses:** laxative effect taken orally, inactivates herpes simplex virus 2, bacteriostatic properties, contains sterols with anti-inflammatory properties **Studies:** show benefit for the topical gel to heal burns and abrasions; however, may not work for deep surgical wounds or radiation wounds	■ Toxicology study of oral whole leaf extract found risk of carcinogenicity in lab animals ■ Topical aloe has no known side effects **ADRs with oral aloe** ■ Lowers blood sugar by stimulating insulin ■ Diarrhea/abdominal cramps ■ Arrhythmia from hypokalemia ■ Contact dermatitis, stinging, soreness ■ Acute hepatitis, renal failure, nephritis ■ Abortifacient, may increase uterine bleeding ■ Avoid in pregnancy/lactation ■ Avoid perioperatively: has caused bleeding	

Ashwaganda

"*withania somnifera*"

Uses: adaptogen, antiarthritis, antiaging, type 2 diabetes mellitus, hyperlipidemia, Parkinson's disease

- Do not use in pregnancy: has been used as abortifacient

ADRs

- Decreases blood pressure
- Decreases blood sugar
- Increases white blood count
- Increases platelets
- Lowers testosterone/FSH levels

Drug Interactions

- Alcohol, sedatives, anxiolytics: increases sedation
- Avoid with diuretics: increases effect
- Anticoagulants: increases bleeding
- Antidiabetic agents: increases hypoglycemia
- Antihypertensives: increases hypotension
- Thyroid hormones: alters effect

Form: capsules, tablets, tea; tablets are standardized

Dose: 1 to 6 g in capsule, tea daily, or 3 to 12 g in combination with other herbs

Pediatric dose (8 to 12 years only): 2 g daily for no >60 days

---

Asian Ginseng

"Korean ginseng," "Chinese ginseng"

- Note: Siberian ginseng is not ginseng at all

Uses: adaptogen, stamina, mental and physical performance, hepatitis C, menopause, erectile dysfunction, hypertension, diabetes mellitus

Studies: may lower blood glucose; may help immune function; NCCIH research currently in cancer and Alzheimer's disease

Other: increases T cell and lymphocyte activity; may inhibit RNA-type viruses; may have antioxidant properties

- Risk of allergic reactions
- Not recommended in pregnancy/lactation due to hormonal and toxic effects, teratogen
- Increases risk of breast cancer, stimulates breast cancer cells
- Avoid in asthma, arrhythmia, hypertension, psychiatric disorder
- Stop preoperatively due to bleeding effect

ADRs

- Headache
- GI disturbance, appetite changes
- Sleep disturbance
- Arrhythmia
- Anemia

Form: root is dried for tablets, capsules, extracts, teas; tablets and capsules standardized to 4% ginsenosides (active ingredient)

Short-term use: up to 2 g/day *Panax* ginseng

Long-term use: 1 g/day *Panax* ginseng

Note: ginseng is added to many commercial beverages

(continues)

TABLE 16-1 Selected Common Herbs, Alphabetical (*continued*)			
Common/Biological Name	**Desirable Medicinal Actions**	**Contraindications and Risks (Adverse Drug Reactions [ADRs])**	**Typical Dosing**
Asian Ginseng (*continued*)		▪ Stevens-Johnson syndrome	
		▪ Increases estrogenic effect	
		▪ Menstrual changes: increases bleeding	
		▪ Mastalgia, breast growth	
		▪ Mania in bipolar disorder	
		Drug Interactions	
		▪ Anticoagulants: increases bleeding	
		▪ Antidiabetic agents: increases or decreases blood sugar	
		▪ Antihypertensives: alters effect	
		▪ Antipsychotics: increases sedation, increases effect	
		▪ Estrogen: increases effect	
		▪ Sedatives: increases sedation	
Astraglus "milk vetch" ▪ Traditional Chinese Medicine for immunity, cancers, and hepatitis ▪ In legume family ▪ 300 species grow in North America; some toxic to livestock	***Uses:*** antioxidant effects, CAD, diabetes mellitus, hepatitis, HIV, hepatoprotection, chemotherapy side effects, mental performance, smoking cessation, URI, burns ***Studies:*** potential benefits for immune system, liver, heart, and adjunctive cancer therapy; 2005 Cochrane study found some immune stimulation and decreased nausea and vomiting in colorectal cancer	▪ Some astragalus species, mostly not found in dietary supplements used, might be toxic; some species contain toxic levels of selenium and some contain neurotoxin swainsonine, which has caused "locoweed" poisoning in animals ▪ Dietary supplement astralgus is generally considered safe for most adults	***Form:*** root used in teas, soups, capsules, extracts, tinctures, intramuscularly (IM), and IV ***Dose:*** no specific dosing recommendations; mostly used as dried root, considered nontoxic

Astralgus (continued)

ADRs

- Decreases blood sugar and heart rate
- Diarrhea
- Bleeding: interacts with anticoagulants
- Avoid in pregnancy/lactation
- Avoid in immune disorders, transplants, bleeding disorders

Drug Interactions

- May interact with immune suppressants, such as the cancer drug cyclophosphamide and organ transplant drugs

Bilberry
"huckleberry," "European blueberry"

- Related to blueberry
- Berries or dried leaves are medicinal
- Used for 1,000 years in European folk medicines; especially for scurvy and diarrhea

Contains: anthocyanosides (type of flavonoid): increases microcirculation

Uses: antioxidant, platelet inhibitor, anti-inflammatory (decreases capillary fragility and preserves endothelium), atherosclerosis, peripheral vascular disease, diabetes mellitus, peptic ulcer disease, diarrhea, cataracts and glaucoma, retinopathy

Studies: four studies showed no benefit for night vision; one study showed possible antiproliferative effects on colon cancer cells; not enough scientific evidence for other indications

- Avoid in allergy to blueberries or same family of berries
- Avoid in pregnancy/lactation

ADRs

- Decreases blood pressure
- Increases or decreases blood sugar
- Diarrhea, nausea
- Hepatotoxicity
- Bleeding

Drug Interactions

- Anticoagulants: increases bleeding
- Antidiabetic agents: increases or decreases blood sugar
- Antihypertensives: decreases blood pleasure
- Estrogen: may decrease absorption

Form: dried leaves, berries, extracts, tinctures, capsules, tablets

Dose: No specific dosing recommendations

(continues)

TABLE 16-1 Selected Common Herbs, Alphabetical (*continued*)

Common/Biological Name	Desirable Medicinal Actions	Contraindications and Risks (Adverse Drug Reactions [ADRs])	Typical Dosing
Black Cohosh "black snakeroot," "bugbane," "bugwort" ▪ Not the same as blue cohosh ▪ Contains salicylic acid ▪ Member of the buttercup family ▪ Used in Native American and American folk medicine for menopausal symptoms, induction of labor, rheumatism	***Uses:*** menopausal symptoms most traditional ***Studies:*** mixed results: NCCIH study found that black cohosh failed to relieve night sweats and hot flashes; 2008 National Institutes of Health study discovered inadequate support for use; German Commission approved for menopausal symptoms, not > 6 months; 2004 North American Menopause Society states use of the product should be from a reputable source and for the shortest time possible (2012). Insufficient studies for safety > 6 months or for rheumatism	▪ United States Pharmacopeia: women should discontinue use of black cohosh and consult a healthcare practitioner if they have a liver disorder or develop symptoms of liver trouble, such as abdominal pain, dark urine, or jaundice ▪ Several case reports of hepatitis and liver failure; not known if black cohosh was cause ▪ Avoid in pregnancy/lactation: can induce labor **ADRs** ▪ Stomach pain, constipation ▪ Headache, rash, dizziness ▪ Bleeding, bruising ▪ Increased risk of cerebrovascular accident ▪ Mastalgia, uterine bleeding ▪ Increased risk of hormone-associated female cancers ▪ Hepatotoxicity **Drug Interactions** ▪ CYP450 2D6 drugs ▪ Anticoagulant drugs: increases bleeding from salicylate ingredient ▪ Antihypertensives: decreases blood pressure ▪ Hepatotoxic drugs: liver failure ▪ Chemotherapeutic drugs ▪ Tamoxifen, antiestrogens, hypertension, oral contraceptive pill: estrogenic effect ▪ Thyroid: causes hyperthyroidism	***Form:*** extract from dried rhizome and root; caplets, capsules, powdered root, dried rhizome, tea, tinctures ***OTC:*** black cohosh as Remifemin 20 mg twice daily ***Other brands:*** Menopause Support Estroven (includes other ingredients)

Butterbur
"Petadolex" patented name

■ Perennial shrub

■ Leaf, root, and rhizome used for extract

Uses: asthma, allergic rhinitis, migraine prophylaxis, smooth muscle relaxant, leukotriene and COX-2 inhibitor, anticholinergic effects possible

Studies: show as much effectiveness as antihistamine for allergies; some studies show effectiveness for migraine treatment; conflicting results on asthma

Danger: natural product contains pyrrolizidine alkaloid (PA), which can cause liver damage and increased risk of carcinogenicity

■ Only butterbur products that have been processed to remove PAs and are labeled or certified as PA-free should be used

■ Avoid if allergic to *Asteraceae* family: ragweed, marigold, daisies, chrysanthemums

■ Avoid in pregnancy/lactation

ADRs

■ Belching, abdominal pain, nausea, vomiting, diarrhea

■ Depression

■ Urinary retention

■ Rash, pruritus

■ Pruritus eyes, asthma

■ Drowsiness

Drug Interactions

■ Calcium channel blockers

■ Anticholinergics: increases symptoms

■ Vasodilators (vasodilates)

■ Testosterone: decreases levels

■ Chronotropes and isotropes: negative activity

Form: softgels, powder, tinctures, extracts, capsules; extract is standardized

Allergic rhinitis: Petasin (Tesalin) 8 mg up to four times daily

Asthma: Petaforce 50 to 150 mg 2 to 3 ×/day or as needed

Migraine prevention: Petadolex 50 to 75 mg twice daily up to 4 months

Cat's Claw

■ Central and South America

■ Dates to use by Incas

Uses: immunostimulant, anti-inflammatory effects, enhances DNA repair, increases phagocytosis, free radical scavenger

Studies: show possible benefit in rheumatoid arthritis and osteoarthritis; in vitro study found possible use as antiviral, antitumor agent; possible research on Alzheimer's disease benefit

■ Some preparations from Peru may be contaminated with fungus, other herbs, and aerobes, and be toxic

ADRs

■ Sedation

■ Decreases blood pressure

■ Decreases estradiol and progesterone

■ One report of renal failure in systemic lupus erythematosus patient

Form: capsules, tablets, tinctures, tea, bark/leaves/roots in dried, cut, or powdered forms

General use: 250 to 1000 mg 1 to 3 ×/day

Freeze-dried extract: 100 mg/day

Note: other forms available

(continues)

TABLE 16-1　Selected Common Herbs, Alphabetical (*continued*)

Common/Biological Name	Desirable Medicinal Actions	Contraindications and Risks (Adverse Drug Reactions [ADRs])	Typical Dosing
Cat's Claw (*continued*)		▪ Avoid in pregnancy/lactation: traditional use as abortifacient ▪ Avoid with history of autoimmune disease, hypotension, renal transplant, renal disease, immunosuppression, bleeding disorders **Drug Interactions** ▪ CYP3A4: increases levels ▪ Antihypertensives: decreases blood pressure ▪ Antiarrhythmics: increases arrhythmias ▪ Anticoagulants: increases bleeding risk ▪ Calcium channel blockers: increases effect ▪ Immunosuppressants: decreases levels ▪ Nephrotoxic drugs: causes renal failure ▪ Iron: decreases absorption	
Chamomile ▪ German chamomile is more common for supplements	***Uses:*** radiation skin issues, wound healing, anxiety ***Studies:*** indicate some benefit for generalized anxiety disorder; infant colic, children's diarrhea, and GI upset; and mouth ulcers in radiation or chemotherapy ***Other:*** anti-inflammatory and antispasmodic effects, sedative effects may be from binding to benzodiazepine receptors	▪ Avoid in allergies to daisy family: ragweed, chrysanthemums, marigolds, daisies: risk of anaphylaxis or other allergic reaction ▪ Avoid with allergies to onions, garlic, and artemesia ▪ Avoid taking with alcohol **ADRs** ▪ Sedation ▪ Decreases blood pressure and blood sugar, increases heart rate ▪ Vomiting ▪ Asthma ▪ Alters menses ▪ Increases bleeding risk	***Form:*** flowers used to make tablets, extracts, tea, creams, mouth rinse, bath additives ***Tea:*** up to 8 g dried flowers ***Capsules:*** up to 1600 mg/day ***Cream:*** 2% to 10% chamomile extract

Dandelion

- Used in Native American and Arabic medicine

Uses: liver or kidney tonics, diuretics, GI disturbances, high vitamin A content and high potassium content in dried herb

Studies: no scientific evidence for medical conditions

Other: May have diuretic and immune-modulating effects, antioxidant effects

Drug Interactions

- CYP450 interactions
- Central nervous system depressants: increases sedation
- Warfarin: increases international normalized ratio
- Antidiabetic agents: decreases blood sugar
- Anticoagulants: increases bleeding risk
- Antiarrhythmics: increases heart rate
- Some allergies/anaphylaxis to dandelions
- Some reports of GI upset with use
- Do not use with gallbladder disease as it increases bile secretion

ADRs

- Exacerbates asthma
- Decreases platelets
- Increases potassium
- Ventricular tachycardia, ventricular fibrillation
- Decreases blood sugar
- Alters estrogen, progesterone, FSH

Form: leaves and roots or whole plant, used fresh or dried in teas, capsules, or extracts; dandelion leaves used in salads or as cooked greens; flowers used for wine

Dong Quai

- From *Angelica sinensis* plant

Uses: dysmenorrheal, menopausal symptoms, menstrual headache

Other: possible anti-inflammatory, antioxidant effects; antispasmodic, GI stimulant effects; antiplatelet effects (coumarin derivative); antiarrhythmic effects

Drug Interactions

- Antidiabetic agents
- Estrogens: increases effect
- Diuretics: increases effect
- Niacin: increases effect
- Antiarrhythmics: increases arrhythmia
- Avoid in pregnancy/lactation: can cause uterine contractions and congenital malformations
- Avoid in bleeding disorders, do not use with anticoagulants
- Possible carcinogenic potential

Form: root used as capsules or tablets

Dose: Medicinal use, safety is unclear

(continues)

TABLE 16-1 Selected Common Herbs, Alphabetical (*continued*)

Common/Biological Name	Desirable Medicinal Actions	Contraindications and Risks (Adverse Drug Reactions [ADRs])	Typical Dosing
Dong Quai (*continued*)		**ADRs** ■ Sedation ■ Increases blood pressure ■ GI symptoms ■ Bleeding **Drug Interactions** ■ Anticoagulants ■ Hormonal medications ■ Antihypertensives	
Echinacea "purple coneflower"	**Uses:** immune stimulant; URIs and other infections, including wounds; genital herpes **Studies:** conflicting studies on usefulness for treating URIs, some positive; NCCIH studies on usefulness for immunity; German Commission-approved for treatment of colds, chronic respiratory, and GI tract infections A Cochrane review (2014) revealed the overall evidence for clinically relevant treatment effects is weak, though preventive care points to a small positive effect. **Other:** may have anti-inflammatory, antifungal, and free radical scavenger effects	Potential anaphylactic or allergic reactions, asthma, especially with allergy to daisy family: marigolds, chrysanthemums, daisies, ragweed Allergies more common in those who are atopic, with eczema or asthma Avoid in people needing immunosuppression Avoid in pregnancy/lactation Discontinue before surgery or may affect wound healing and infection rate Avoid in autoimmune disease, collagen vascular disease, HIV, liver disease, multiple sclerosis, tuberculosis **ADRs** ■ Rashes ■ GI side effects ■ Dizziness, nervousness, headache ■ Atrial fibrillation, palpitations	**Form:** plant and roots used to make juice (expressed), teas, extracts, other forms **Dose:** URI 500 to 1000 mg three times daily **Pediatric dose:** usually weight based, see other sources

Ephedra **"ma huang"** Evergreen shrub that has been used for 5,000 years in India and China - Powerful stimulant of nervous system and heart used to treat respiratory conditions, flu, asthma, fever	**Uses:** weight loss, energy supplement, athletic performance, amphetamine-like; primary component is ephedrine **Studies:** higher rate of calls to poison control centers about severe side effects; increases risk of stroke, hypertension, cardiac problems, GI side effects **Risks:** benefit for short-term weight loss is outweighed by risks	- Hypertension - Asthma exacerbation - May aggravate autoimmune disease or increase immune response **Drug Interactions** - Amoxicillin: rhabdomyolysis, death - Anticoagulants: increases bleeding - Corticosteroids: decreases immunosuppressive effect - Statins, acetaminophen: increases risk for hepatotoxicity	- United States banned sale of dietary supplements with ephedra in 2004 - Reports of stroke, myocardial infarction, sudden death - Can worsen diabetes, cardiovascular disease, renal disease - Can cause seizures - Do not use in pregnancy/lactation **ADRs** - Anxiety, psychosis, tremors - Dry mouth, GI irritation, nausea - Hypertension, arrhythmia, heart damage - Urinary obstruction - Sleep problems **Drug Interactions** - Anesthetics: alters effect, increases blood pressure - Ethanol: psychosis with caffeine - Caffeine: increases toxicity - Antidiabetic agents: decreases effect - Anticonvulsants: decreases effect - Ergot alkaloids: increases hypertensive crisis - Phenothiazines: increases arrhythmia, death	**Form:** dried stems and leaves make tablets, tinctures, capsules, teas **Note:** Ephedra still allowed in Chinese herbal remedies and teas

(continues)

TABLE 16-1　Selected Common Herbs, Alphabetical (*continued*)

Common/Biological Name	Desirable Medicinal Actions	Contraindications and Risks (Adverse Drug Reactions [ADRs])	Typical Dosing
Evening Primrose Oil ■ Yellow flower: contains gamma-linolenic acid (GLA), essential fatty acid, required by the body and obtained from the diet	**Uses:** eczema, inflammation, mastalgia, premenstrual syndrome, menopause symptoms, cancer, diabetes mellitus **Studies:** show some benefit for rheumatoid arthritis, eczema, premenstrual syndrome, mastalgia **Other:** May have anti-inflammatory, vasodilatory, and antiplatelet effects	■ Not for pregnancy/lactation: increases risk complications, rupture of membranes **ADRs** ■ GI upset ■ Headache ■ Rash ■ Depression ■ Seizures in patients without seizure risk **Drug Interactions** ■ Anesthesia: decreases seizure threshold ■ Anticoagulants: increases bleeding risk ■ Antihypertensives: decreases blood pressure ■ Tricyclic antidepressant: decreases seizure threshold ■ Anti-seizure agents: increases seizure risk	**Form:** oil extracted from seeds and put in capsules **Dose:** products standardized for 8% GLA and 72% linoleic acid
Fenugreek ■ Used back to Egyptian times ■ Used to induce childbirth ■ Used to help digestion and menopause symptoms	**Uses:** in cooking, for diabetes mellitus, hyperlipidemia, loss of appetite **Other:** Stimulates milk production	■ Avoid in pregnancy **ADRs** ■ Bloating, flatulence, diarrhea ■ Hypoglycemia ■ Hypokalemia ■ Miscarriage **Drug Interactions** ■ Alcohol: decreases hepatotoxicity ■ Analgesics: additive effect ■ Anticoagulants: increases bleeding risk ■ Antidiabetic agents: increases hypoglycemia	**Form:** seeds are ground and taken orally or put in paste for skin **Dose:** 25 g seed powder daily in divided doses

Feverfew

"bachelor's buttons," "wild chamomile"

- Used as antipyretic by ancient Greeks

Uses: migraine headaches, psoriasis, asthma, tinnitus, nausea, vomiting

Studies: may help prevent (not acutely treat) migraine headaches and rheumatoid arthritis pain

- Allergic risk with ragweed, chrysanthemum allergies
- Not for use in pregnancy/lactation: can cause miscarriage, premature birth
- Avoid in children
- Avoid prior to surgery or dental procedures

ADRs

- Canker sores, sore tongue
- Loss of appetite
- Nausea/GI symptoms
- Risk of worsened depression
- Dizziness, fatigue, anxiety
- Palpitations, increased heart rate

Drug Interactions

- Anticoagulants: increases bleeding risk
- Vasodilators: increases vasodilitation

Form: dried leaves primarily used; stems and roots sometimes used; extracts, tablets, capsules

Standardized dose: up to 250 mg daily; take with food

Garlic

- Edible herb from the lily family

Uses: hyperlipidemia, CAD, hypertension, colon and gastric cancer, URI prevention, peripheral vascular disease

Studies: varying benefit on lowering cholesterol; positive for decreasing blood pressure and atherosclerosis; shows that it affects dilation and constriction of blood vessels

- Safe for most adults
- Does have blood-thinning effect; stop preoperatively
- Mild risk of allergy, mostly raw form; cross-allergies with onions, leeks, chives

ADRs

- Raw: halitosis, GI upset, body odor
- Contact dermatitis, blisters
- Bleeding
- Asthma, rhinitis

Drug Interactions

- Anticoagulants: increases bleeding

Form: raw, cooked, dried, powdered

Dose: 600 to 900 mg garlic powder (in standardized 1.3% allicin active ingredient) daily in divided doses or 3 to 5 mg allicin daily (equivalent to 2 to 5 g fresh garlic)

(continues)

TABLE 16-1 Selected Common Herbs, Alphabetical (*continued*)

Common/Biological Name	Desirable Medicinal Actions	Contraindications and Risks (Adverse Drug Reactions [ADRs])	Typical Dosing
Garlic (*continued*)		■ Antihypertensives: decreases blood pressure	
		■ Antidiabetic agents: increases or decreases blood sugar	
		■ Anesthetics: prolongs effect	
		■ Acetaminophen: alters effect	
		■ Protease inhibitors: decreases effect	
		■ Oral contraceptive pill with estrogen: decreases effect	
Ginger ■ Tropical plant often used in Asian medicine	***Uses:*** postsurgical and motion nausea, GI upset, chemotherapy nausea, pregnancy nausea (hyperemesis gravidarum), arthritis pain, muscle pain ***Studies:*** short-term effectiveness in pregnancy nausea, variable effectiveness in other forms of nausea; ongoing studies on inflammation ***Other:*** may inhibit serotonin $5\text{-}HT_3$ receptors in GI tract and platelet aggregation; may have lipid-lowering, antihypertensive effects	■ Avoid in lactation: safety not established ■ Avoid perioperatively due to bleeding risk ■ Avoid in CAD, arrhythmia history **ADRs** ■ Mostly with powdered ginger: bloating, gas, heartburn, nausea ■ Depression ■ Arrhythmias ■ Increases bleeding risk **Drug Interactions** ■ Calcium channel blockers: decreases blood pressure ■ Antidiabetic agents: decreases blood sugar ■ Cardiac agents: may alter effect ■ Anticoagulants: increases bleeding risk ■ Antiarrhythmics: increases risk	***Form:*** fresh, powder, tablets ***Dose:*** up to 4 g/day in divided doses

Ginkgo

"Japanese silver apricot," "fossil tree"

- Seeds of ginkgo tree used for thousands of years in Traditional Chinese Medicine

Uses: memory enhancement, prevention of Alzheimer's disease and dementia, ischemic stroke, decreases intermittent claudication, multiple sclerosis, tinnitus, sexual dysfunction

Studies: most show no improvement for memory or prevention of dementia or decreasing blood pressure; minimal benefit possible for intermittent claudication and tinnitus (variable); being studied for electric shock memory loss

- Possible severe allergic reactions
- Avoid preoperatively or before dental procedures: increased bleeding risk
- Avoid raw ginkgo seeds: contain toxin that can cause seizures and death

ADRs

- Headache, dizziness
- GI symptoms
- Increases bleeding risk

Drug Interactions

- Antidiabetic agents: increases blood sugar
- Anticoagulants: increases bleeding
- Anticonvulsants: decreases effect
- Antihypertensives: decreases blood pressure
- Antipsychotics can cause priapism
- Estrogens may have estrogenic effect
- Nifedipine: increases concentrations
- Prilosec: decreases levels
- SSRIs: increases serotonin syndrome
- Trazadone: risk of coma

Form: ginkgo leaf abstracts used in tablets, capsules, teas, and skin preparations; also in nutrition bars, sublingual spray; standardized extracts

Dose: 80 to 240 mg/day divided 2 to 3 ×/day

Goldenseal

"yellow root"

- Native American remedy
- Now grown commercially due to short supplies

Uses: URIs, digestive disorders, diarrhea, some cancers, vaginitis, wounds, canker sores, chloroquine resistant malaria, hyperlipidemia, stimulates immune system

Studies: some antibacterial effects and lipid-lowering effects; possible benefit for diarrhea and eye infections

- Avoid in pregnancy/lactation: contains berberine, which can cause jaundice
- Not for infants or young children

ADRs

- Arrhythmias, bradycardia
- Headache
- Decreases blood pressure

Form: stems and roots dried for extracts and teas; mouth rinses; sometimes combined with echinacea for URIs

Tablets/capsules: 0.5 to 1 g orally three times daily

Extract: 0.3 ml to 1 ml

Note: also IV and ophthalmic forms

(continues)

TABLE 16-1   Selected Common Herbs, Alphabetical *(continued)*

Common/Biological Name	Desirable Medicinal Actions	Contraindications and Risks (Adverse Drug Reactions [ADRs])	Typical Dosing
Goldenseal *(continued)*		▪ Decreases blood sugar ▪ GI irritation, nausea ▪ Dry mucous membranes ▪ Seizures **Drug Interactions** ▪ Antiplatelet agents ▪ Antilipemic agents: increases effect ▪ Antimalarials: additive effect ▪ Beta blockers: changes effect ▪ Phenylephrine: increases effect ▪ Warfarin: decreases effect	
Hoodia "Kalahari cactus" ▪ Kalahari bushmen ate this to suppress hunger and thirst while hunting	**Uses:** appetite suppressant (weight loss) while elevating energy No reliable scientific evidence published and no studies in people	▪ Drug risks, interactions, adverse effects have not been studied ▪ Avoid in pregnancy	**Form:** often combined with green tea or chromium; dried extracts from stems and roots make capsules, extracts, powders, teas, chewable tablets **Dose:** dried extract up to 800 mg/day
Horse Chestnut "buckeye" ▪ Only seed extract is safe ▪ Do not use any other parts of plant, which may be toxic	**Uses:** chronic venous insufficiency, ankle edema, night leg cramps **Studies:** as effective for venous insufficiency as supportive compression stockings	▪ Contraindicated in hepatic and renal impairment; inflammatory bowel disease; latex allergy ▪ Avoid in pregnancy/lactation **ADRs** ▪ Calf spasm ▪ GI upset	**Form:** standardized for 15% to 20% **Dose:** 300 mg extract twice daily **Topical gel:** 3 to 4 ×/day **Note:** short-term use only

Kava

"Kava kava"

- Member of the pepper family
- Ceremonial beverage in the South Pacific

- Bleeding
- Renal/liver damage

Drug Interactions

- Anticoagulants: increases bleeding
- Antidiabetic agents: increases hypoglycemia
- Antihypertensive: increases hypotension

Uses: anxiety, insomnia, menopausal symptoms

Studies: NCCIH studies halted due to risk of severe liver damage; earlier studies showed some benefit with anxiety, but dangers outweigh risks

Other: may affect cerebellar and GABA functions

- Risk of severe liver damage, including liver failure and hepatitis, and dystonia (abnormal muscle movements)

ADRs

- Drowsiness
- Ataxia
- Dizziness, dyskinesia
- Headache
- Tachycardia
- Contact dermatitis, kava dermopathy (long-term rash with yellow discoloration)
- GI upset: increases transaminases
- Parkinsonism

Drug Interactions

- Acetaminophen: increases liver toxicity
- Psychotropics: altered mental status
- Ethanol: increases toxicity
- Anxiolytics: increases effect
- Sedatives: increases effect
- Opioids: increases sedation, central nervous system depression

Form: root and rhizome make beverages, capsules, tablets, extracts, topical solutions

(continues)

TABLE 16-1 Selected Common Herbs, Alphabetical (*continued*)

Common/Biological Name	Desirable Medicinal Actions	Contraindications and Risks (Adverse Drug Reactions [ADRs])	Typical Dosing
Lavender "English lavender"	**Uses:** anxiety, depression, insomnia, GI upset, alopecia, topical antiseptic aromatherapy **Studies:** do not confirm any benefits for certain except for alopecia used topically	■ Avoid in pregnancy/lactation **ADRs** ■ Headache, photosensitivity ■ GI symptoms ■ Skin pigment changes **Drug Interactions** ■ Anxiolytics: increases side effects ■ Sedatives: increases side effects ■ Antidepressants: increases side effects	**Form:** dried lavender teas or extracts can be taken orally; essential oils can be made from flowers and used topically and in aromatherapy **Note:** poisonous if taken internally
Licorice Root ■ Glycyrrhizin is the most dangerous compound ■ Deglycyrrhizinated form "DGL" is safer	**Uses:** stomach ulcer, hepatitis, sore throat, bronchitis **Studies:** none show significant effectiveness except IV form for hepatitis C; not available in the United States	■ Glycyrrhizin can cause low potassium, high blood pressure, salt and water retention, all risks for cardiovascular disease ■ Avoid high levels of licorice: affects cortisone ■ Not for pregnancy: can cause preterm labor ■ Not for hypertension or CAD **Drug Interactions** ■ Avoid with medications that affect potassium, diuretics, prednisone ■ Antiarrhythmics: increases risk ■ Anticoagulants: increases bleeding ■ Immunosuppressants: decreases effect ■ Antidiabetics: alters effect ■ Antihypertensives: decreases effect	**Form:** use safer DGL form

Herb	Uses / Studies / Risks	ADRs / Drug Interactions	Form / Dose / Note
Milk Thistle "holy thistle," "silymarin" ▪ Used for thousands of years for liver assistance	**Uses:** chronic hepatitis, cirrhosis, liver damage from drugs and toxins, alcoholic liver disease, hyperlipidemia **Studies:** prior studies showed benefit of protecting and promoting growth of liver cells; later studies show conflicting results; benefit in hepatitis C showed fewer, milder liver disease symptoms but no effect on amount of viral load **Risks:** can decrease insulin resistance in patients with diabetes mellitus and cirrhosis, breast, cervical, and prostate cancers	▪ Avoid in allergies in daisy family: ragweed, chrysanthemums, daisies, marigold ▪ Not recommended in pregnancy/lactation **ADRs** ▪ Decreases blood sugar ▪ GI side effects ▪ Headache, insomnia ▪ Exacerbates hemochromatosis ▪ Arthralgia **Drug Interactions** ▪ Alcohol: decreases alcohol-induced hepatoxicity ▪ Statins: inhibits effect ▪ Antineoplastic drugs: increases effect ▪ Antidiabetic agents: decreases blood sugar	***Form:*** silymarin (active ingredient) from seeds used to make tinctures, capsules, extracts ***Dose:*** 230 to 800 mg/day divided in 2 to 3 doses ***Note:*** generally considered safe
Noni "Indian mu berry" ▪ History of topical use for joint pain and dermatological issues	**Uses:** juice as health tonic, chronic conditions (e.g., diabetes, cardiovascular disease), cancer, hearing loss **Studies:** early studies show anticancer effects, antioxidant, and immune-stimulating effects; NCCIH study on prostate cancer; National Cancer Institute study on breast cancer prevention	▪ Risk of liver toxicity ▪ High in potassium: avoid in renal disease ▪ Not for use in pregnancy (traditional abortifacient) **ADRs** ▪ Decreases blood pressure **Drug Interactions** ▪ Anticoagulants: contains vitamin K in some, not all, preparations ▪ ACE inhibitors: increases potassium ▪ Numerous others that affect potassium	***Form:*** fruit used in fruit juices, mostly with grape; fruit and leaves can make tablets, capsules, teas ***Dose:*** up to 2 ounces twice daily for 3 months
Panax Ginseng "American ginseng"	*See Asian Ginseng* **Uses:** attention deficit hyperactivity disorder (ADHD), chronic hepatitis B, congestive heart failure, dementia, CAD, hyperlipidemia, menopausal symptoms, idiopathic thrombocytopenic purpurea methicillin-resistant *Staphylococcus aureus* (MRSA), diabetic renal disease	*See Asian Ginseng ADRs*	*See Asian Ginseng Dosage*

(continues)

TABLE 16-1   Selected Common Herbs, Alphabetical (*continued*)

Common/Biological Name	Desirable Medicinal Actions	Contraindications and Risks (Adverse Drug Reactions [ADRs])	Typical Dosing
Peppermint Oil ■ Cross between spearmint and watermint	***Uses:*** seasoning and medicinal, nausea, GI upset, indigestion, irritable bowel syndrome, URI, headache, asthma, muscular, antispasmodic, nerve pain, halitosis, nasal congestion ***Studies:*** peppermint may help irritable bowel syndrome; peppermint with caraway may help indigestion	■ Oil is safe in small doses ■ Not for pregnancy/lactation **ADRs** ■ Heartburn ■ Abdominal pain ■ Acute renal failure ■ Contact dermatitis ■ Burning mouth syndrome **Drug Interactions** ■ Antacids, H2 blockers, PPIs: may prematurely dissolve enteric coating ■ CYP450 interactions possible	***Form:*** essential oil of peppermint; in small doses in capsules or liquids; in teas; mixed with other ingredients in topical preparations ***Dose:*** by-mouth digestive: 0.2 to 0.4 ml twice daily (average one a day, 6 to 12 gtts) ***Capsules:*** 1 to 2 capsules by mouth twice daily every half hour as needed ***Other:*** teas with dried leaves; topical preparations
Red Clover "meadow clover" ■ Legume family ■ Contains phytoestrogens that act like estrogen ■ Past use for pertussis, asthma, bronchitis, cancer	***Uses:*** menopausal symptoms, mastalgia, osteoporosis, benign prostatic hypertrophy, hyperlipidemia ***Studies:*** not enough evidence for effectiveness or safety in menopause; NCCIH studying how it affects prostate cells; study to determine if it causes endometrial cancer risk	■ Avoid in pregnancy/lactation: unsafe in medicinal amounts ■ May increase risk of breast cancer or other hormone-sensitive cancers **ADRs** ■ Mastalgia ■ Menstrual changes ■ Vaginal spotting ■ Headache, rash **Drug Interactions** ■ Anticoagulants: increases bleeding ■ Tamoxifen: alters effect ■ Estrogens: alters effect	***Form:*** flowers used in tablets, capsules, teas, extracts ***Dose:*** 40 to 80 mg red clover isoflavones/day

Rhodiola

- Considered adaptogen

Uses: energy and exercise enhancement, fatigue, generalized anxiety disorder, bladder cancer, hypoxia

- Avoid in pregnancy/lactation

ADRs

- Insomnia
- Increases blood pressure
- Dermatitis
- Irritability
- Dry mouth
- Leukocytosis

Drug Interactions

- Antidepressants: additive effect
- Anxiolytics: additive effect
- Central nervous system depressants: additive effect
- Opioids: additive effect
- Antihypertensives: additive effect

Capsules: 100 to 400 g daily

Sage

- Fertility drug in ancient Egypt
- Cleansed and stopped bleeding in ulcers/wounds in ancient Greece

Uses: spice and seasoning, mouth inflammation and sore throat, indigestion, menopausal symptoms, improve mood and boost memory/performance

Studies: show mental and mood improvements; memory boosting in older adults; thinking/learning improvement in Alzheimer's disease; essential oil has antimicrobial properties

- Safe, but some varieties contain thujone, which can affect the nervous system, causing restlessness, tremor, seizures, renal toxicity
- Ingesting sage powder can cause asthma
- Inflammation with skin contact
- Avoid in pregnancy: risk of abortifacient and hormonal effects
- Contraindicated in seizure disorders

ADRs

- Seizures
- Contact dermatitis
- Hypertension
- Sedation

Form: dried leaves, essential oils, sprays, extracts

Menopausal symptoms: 120 mg every day

Pharyngitis: 15% spray

Mood enhancement: dried leaf 300 to 600 mg every day

Alzheimer's disease: essential oils

(continues)

TABLE 16-1　Selected Common Herbs, Alphabetical (*continued*)

Common/Biological Name	Desirable Medicinal Actions	Contraindications and Risks (Adverse Drug Reactions [ADRs])	Typical Dosing
Sage (*continued*)		**Drug Interaction** ■ Antidiabetic drugs: increases hypoglycemia ■ Anticonvulsants: alters effect ■ Thyroid hormones: alters effect	
Saw Palmetto "dwarf palm" native to United States, "cabbage palm" ■ Seminole Native Americans used for urinary symptoms	***Uses:*** prostate (BPH) problems, prostatitis, pelvic pain, bladder problems, prostate cancer, libido issues, alopecia, increase testosterone ***Studies:*** conflicting reports of benefits on BPH symptoms; does not affect PSA; being studied for affect on prostate cancer; German-Commission approved for BPH early stages I and II ***Other:*** May be an anti-inflammatory and immune stimulant	■ Mild GI symptoms can be decreased by taking with food ■ Do not use in pregnancy/lactation due to hormonal effect **ADRs** ■ Abdominal pain ■ Diarrhea ■ Nausea, vomiting ■ Fatigue ■ Sexual dysfunction **Drug Interactions** ■ Antibiotics (ciprofloxacin azithromycin especially): additive effect ■ Androgens: decreases effect ■ Anticoagulants: increases bleeding ■ Anti-inflammatories: additive effect	***Form:*** whole or ground berries or dried fruit; in liquid extracts, tablets, capsules, as infusion or tea, topical for alopecia ***Capsule:*** 320 mg every day ***Ground, whole, or dried berries:*** 1 or 2 every day

St. John's Wort

"hypericum," "goat's weed"

- Flower blooms around feast time of St. John the Baptist in late June
- Used for centuries to treat mental disease, nervousness, as sedative
- Used to treat malaria, was balm for wounds, burns, and insect bites

Uses: depression, anxiety, sleep disorders, premenstrual syndrome, seasonal affective disorder, somatoform disorders, ADHD, burning mouth syndrome, obsessive-compulsive disorder

Studies: may not be any more effective than placebo for major depression of moderate severity: NCCIH and National Institute of Mental Health studies showed neither antidepressant nor St. John's wort treated mild depression any more effectively than placebo; 2008 Cochrane review showed better than placebo and similar to standard antidepressants with fewer side effects; hyperforin component inhibits neuronal uptake of dopamine, serotonin, norepinephrine, GABA, and L-glutamate

- Avoid use with other antidepressants: can lead to serotonin syndrome
- Do not use with MAOIs
- Stop 5 to 14 days preoperatively
- Do not use with suicidal ideation
- Do not use in pregnancy/lactation

ADRs

- Drowsiness
- GI symptoms
- Hypertension/hypertensive crisis (could act like MAOI)
- Mania
- Serotonin syndrome
- Delirium
- Confusion
- Psychosis
- Myocardial infarction
- Palpitations
- Increases thyroid-stimulating hormone
- Increases adrenocorticotropic hormone
- Photosensitivity
- Dry mouth
- Dizziness

Drug Interactions

- Anesthetics
- SSRI antidepressants: serotonin syndrome
- Anticancer drugs

Form: flowering tops used for teas, tablets, capsules, extracts, liquids, topical agents

Standardized extract dose: 300 mg by mouth three times daily for 4 to 6 weeks

Note: sudden discontinuation may cause adverse reaction

(continues)

TABLE 16-1 Selected Common Herbs, Alphabetical (*continued*)

Common/Biological Name	Desirable Medicinal Actions	Contraindications and Risks (Adverse Drug Reactions [ADRs])	Typical Dosing
St. John's Wort (*continued*)		▪ Anticoagulants: decreases effect ▪ Antihypertensives: increases blood pressure ▪ Alcohol: increases sedation ▪ Oral contraceptives: decreases contraception, possible breakthrough bleeding ▪ Cyclosporin and transplant drugs: decreases digoxin, decreases serum level ▪ Statins: decreases level ▪ HIV drugs: may affect ▪ Seizure drug: may affect ▪ OTC cold/flu meds: may increase MAO inhibition	
Tea Tree Oil ▪ Used by Australian aborigines for centuries ▪ From tea tree	***Uses:*** athlete's foot (tinea pedis), nail fungus (onychomycosis), wounds, infections, acne, dandruff, lice, oral candidiasis, skin lesions, antibacterial, antifungal, anti-MRSA ***Studies:*** show benefit for treatment of MRSA wounds; some positive benefit for acne, onychomycosis, tinea pedis, and dandruff	▪ Do not take orally: poisonous, can lead to coma, especially in children ▪ Can be a topical irritant or cause contact dermatitis ▪ Can be used topically in pregnancy according to Ulbright **ADRs** ▪ Contact dermatitis ▪ Skin dryness ▪ Ototoxicity if instilled in ear **Drug Interactions** ▪ Topical drying agents: increases dryness ▪ Tretinoin: increases dryness	***Topical:*** 5% to 100% oil, safer in adults; topical use of styling gel and shampoo caused breast growth in young boy ***Note:*** is in some mouthwashes but, based on the concerns with oral use, do not recommend

Thunder God Vine

- Found in China
- Used in Traditional Chinese Medicine for overactivity of immune system or inflammation

Uses: multiple sclerosis, systemic lupus erythematous, rheumatoid arthritis, excessive menses, HIV/AIDS, hyperlipidemia, osteoarthritis

Studies: show anticancer and anti-inflammatory effects; suppression of immune system; benefits for rheumatoid arthritis pain as good as sulfasalazine

Other: may have immune stimulant effects

- Highly poisonous leaves, flowers, and skin of root
- Avoid in pregnancy/lactation

ADRs

- GI symptoms
- URI symptoms
- Loss of bone mineral density
- Decrease male fertility
- Alopecia, rash, headache

Drug Interactions

- Antihypertensives: alters effect
- DMARDs (anti-inflammatories): increases effect
- Immunosuppressants: increases effect

Form: extracts made from skinned root

Note: no consistent, high-quality products are made in the United States yet; Chinese products may not be reliable

Turmeric

"Indian saffron"

- Related to ginger, bitter taste, gold color
- Used for spice and color
- Used in Traditional Chinese Medicine and Ayurvedic medicine for liver function, digestion, menstrual regulation, and arthritis pain

Topical uses: wound healing and eczema

Oral uses: ulcers, cancer, GI problems, inflammation, gallstones

Studies: curcumin chemical in turmeric has anti-inflammatory, anticancer, and antioxidant properties in early studies; NCCIH funding studies on acute respiratory distress syndrome, osteoporosis, and liver cancer

- High doses or long-term use have caused GI problems and liver issues
- Do not use with gallbladder disease: can worsen
- Considered safe as a spice in pregnancy but can stimulate uterus in high doses

ADRs

- GI problems
- Hypotension
- Alopecia
- Contact dermatitis

Drug Interactions

- Anticoagulants: increases bleeding
- Antidiabetic agents: increases hypoglycemia
- Antihypertensives: excessive decrease in blood pressure

Form: rhizomes (underground stems) dried and used as oral powder and in capsules, teas, or liquid extracts; turmeric paste used on skin

Dose: root 1.5 to 7 g in divided daily doses

Tea: 1 to 1.5 g dried root steeped 15 minutes in 150 ml water twice daily

(continues)

TABLE 16-1 Selected Common Herbs, Alphabetical (*continued*)

Common/Biological Name	Desirable Medicinal Actions	Contraindications and Risks (Adverse Drug Reactions [ADRs])	Typical Dosing
Valerian "all heal," "garden heliotrope" ▪ Used back to ancient Greece and Rome ▪ Described by Hippocrates and Galen (for insomnia)	***Uses:*** sleep disorders, anxiety, depression, headache, arrhythmia ***Studies:*** NCCIH researching effect on sleep in older adults and Parkinson's patients; suggest helpful with insomnia, not enough research on anxiety and depression; German-Commission approved to treat sleep disorders from nervous conditions and restlessness ***Other:*** may be adenosine agonist, GABA receptor modulator; may have central nervous system neuroprotective effects	▪ Studies show safe for short periods: up to 4 to 6 weeks ▪ Not for use in pregnancy: possible teratogenic effects **ADRs** ▪ Morning fatigue ▪ GI upset ▪ Dizziness ▪ Headache ▪ Hallucinations ▪ Ataxia ▪ Decreased heart rate, blood pressure ▪ Dry mouth ▪ Muscle relaxation ▪ One report of withdrawal symptoms **Drug Interactions** ▪ Alcohol: increases effect ▪ Antidepressants: increases effect ▪ Benzodiazepines: increases effect ▪ Central nervous system depressants: increases effect ▪ Antihypertensives: decreases blood pressure	***Form:*** roots and rhizomes (underground stems) make tablets, teas, capsules, liquid extracts ***Dose:*** use 30 minutes to 2 hours before bed if for sleep ***Anxiety:*** 80 to 300 mg by mouth every day ***Insomnia:*** 400 to 900 mg 30 to 60 minutes before bedtime ***Note:*** monitor liver function tests

Yohimbe

"yohimbe bark"

- From bark of African evergreen tree

Uses: female libido, SSRI-induced libido issues, sexual dysfunction, aphrodisiac, athletic performance

Studies: no adequate studies conducted; yohimbe hydrochloride form has been studied for erectile dysfunction

Other: contains alpha-2 blocker: increases norepinephrine cholinergic and sympathetic tone

- Avoid in pregnancy: fetal toxicity, uterine relaxation
- Do not use in lactation
- Do not use with MAOIs, caution with other antidepressants and phenothiazines
- Do not use with psychiatric or renal disorders: can exacerbate
- One report of hypertensive crisis
- Overdose: severe effects, possibly fatal

ADRs

- Insomnia
- Increases or decreases blood pressure
- Irritability, psychosis
- Nausea, vomiting
- Anxiety
- Headache
- Renal failure
- Lupus-like syndrome

Drug Interactions

- Antidiabetic: decreases blood sugar
- Benzodiazepines: increases sedation
- Ethanol: increases intoxication
- Naloxone/naltrexone: increases yohimbine toxicity, alters opioid withdrawal symptoms
- Central nervous system stimulants: increases effect
- Anticoagulants: increases bleeding
- Central sympathomimetics: increases yohimbine toxicity

Form: some products contain very little yohimbe; bark used in capsules, tablets, tea; standardized yohimbe available by prescription

Dose: 5 to 50 mg in divided doses for erectile dysfunction

Note: monitor blood pressure, heart rate

Source: Data from National Center for Complementary and Integrative Health, "Herbs at a Glance" (2012). https://nccih.nih.gov/health/herbsataglance.htm; M. Iannuzzi-Sucich and C. A. Sanoski, *Herbal Notes: A Complementary and Alternative Medicine Pocket Guide* (Philadelphia: F. A. Davis, 2011); *Natural Standard*, from Quinnipiac University; MedlinePlus, "Herbs and Supplements" (2014). www.nlm.nih.gov/medlineplus/druginfo/herb_All.html; C. Ulbright, *Davis' Pocket Guide to Herbs and Supplements* (Philadelphia: F. A. Davis, 2011).

TABLE 16-2   Selected Common Dietary Supplements, Alphabetical

Common/Biological Name	Desirable Medicinal Actions	Contraindications and Risks (Adverse Drug Reactions [ADRs])	Typical Dosing
Acidophilus ■ Main types: *lactobacillus* species (*acidophilus, casei, plantarum, delbrueckii*) ■ *Bifidobacterium* species (*brevis, infantis, longum*)	***Uses:*** maintain or restore microbial balance in GI and GU tracts ***Other:*** may produce bacteriocins and lactic acid, which impair growth of pathogens	■ May cause morbidity or mortality if patients are immunocompromised or debilitated ■ Avoid in pregnancy: risk of amnionitis, sepsis, endometritis ■ Avoid with artificial heart valves, radiation therapy, oral surgery, GI surgery, chronic diarrhea, and with immunocompromised, debilitated patients	***Form:*** liquids, capsules, powders, tablets, milk, vaginal and anal suppositories; some yogurts with live cultures; some are kept refrigerated ***Dose:*** varies depending on number of living organisms in product; take 2 hours after antibiotics; do not take with immunosuppressants
Alpha Lipoic Acid ■ Found especially in potatoes, spinach, liver, and broccoli	***Uses:*** diabetes mellitus, cataracts, retinopathy, peripheral neuropathy, nephropathy from diabetes mellitus, HIV, cirrhosis, glaucoma, lead toxicity, burning mouth syndrome, ischemic injury to liver, brain, or heart ***Actions:*** improves microcirculation in peripheral neuropathy in diabetes mellitus; antioxidant; increases insulin-stimulated glucose in diabetes mellitus; increases CD4 and CD8 levels in HIV	■ Avoid in thiamine deficiency (alcoholism especially) ■ Avoid in pregnancy/lactation ■ Caution with bleeding disorders ■ Interactions with anticoagulants, antiplatelets, NSAIDs/ASA: may increase bleeding risk ■ May decrease effectiveness of chemotherapy ■ May decrease blood sugar and worsen hypoglycemia ■ Vertigo, headache, nausea, vomiting, rash	***Dose:*** oral; for most indications average dosing is 300 to 600 mg every day; IV
Arginine ■ Semi-essential amino acid ■ Especially in corn, dairy, oats, meat, grains, brown rice, nuts, chocolate, raisins	***Uses:*** CAD, congestive heart failure, hypertension, peripheral vascular disease, hyperlipidemia, breast cancer, asthma ***Actions:*** precursor of nitric oxide, a vasodilator; increases relaxation of smooth muscle; decreases white blood cell adhesion, platelet aggregation, fibrin formation; immune stimulant	■ Anaphylaxis to IV arginine in children ■ Atrioventricular block ■ Headache, dizziness, atypical chest pain ■ Increases bleeding risk ■ Increases or decreases blood sugar ■ Decreases blood pressure ■ Avoid in pregnancy/lactation ■ Avoid after acute myocardial infarction ■ Avoid IV forms in acidosis or hypotension	***Form:*** sufficient amounts made in body; if supplemented, cream, capsule, IV, nutrient bar; no established standards

Bee Pollen

- Flower pollen collected on bodies of worker bees mixed with nectar and bee saliva

- Commercial bee pollen may just be pollen harvested from plants

- Not the same as honey or royal jelly

- Contains essential amino acids, essential fatty acids, hormones, minerals, vitamins B and C coenzymes, sterols, lipids, carbohydrates, and more

Uses: athletic performance, memory booster, multiple sclerosis, menopause, premenstrual syndrome

Actions: reduces cancer chemotherapy side effects, antioxidant, immune stimulant, antifungal

- Allergic reactions: anaphylaxis, edema, shortness of breath, pruritus, eosinophilia, risk of asthma exacerbation

- Avoid in pregnancy/lactation

- Contraindicated in allergy to pollens

ADRs

- Nausea, vomiting, diarrhea, abdominal pain

- Hepatitis

- Headache, malaise

- Photosensitivity

- Vertigo

- Hayfever

- Decreased memory

Form: capsules, tablets, liquid, granules, extracts, food supplements; no standardized products; often in combination products

Note: pollen content varies depending on plant and geographic location

Capsicum

"cayenne," "chili pepper," "paprika," "capsaicin"

- Possible that capsaicin releases substance P from neurons, which decreases pain sensation

Uses: clotting disorders, GI disorders, cluster headaches, musculoskeletal pain, neuropathic pain, postoperative nausea and vomiting, perennial rhinitis

Other: may be immunosuppressant, anti-inflammatory, antimicrobial

- Risk of allergic reactions

ADRs

- Increases heart rate

- Increases blood pressure transiently

- Topical burning on skin, contact dermatitis

- Pharyngitis, rhinorrhea (nasal)

- Eye burning and tearing

- Sweating, flushing

Drug Interactions

- ACE inhibitors: increases cough

- Antiarrhythmics: increases heart rate

- Anticoagulants: increases bleeding

- Antidiabetic agents: decreases blood sugar, increases insulin

- Antiulcer agents: increases stomach acid

Form: powder, topical creams, intranasal spray; Zostrix cream contains 0.025% capsaicin; law enforcement uses in pepper spray

(continues)

TABLE 16-2 Selected Common Dietary Supplements, Alphabetical (*continued*)

Common/Biological Name	Desirable Medicinal Actions	Contraindications and Risks (Adverse Drug Reactions [ADRs])	Typical Dosing
Chasteberry "vitex" ■ Used by monks to decrease sexual desire, thought to promote chastity ■ Inhibits prolactin by binding to dopamine receptors	**Uses:** menopause symptoms, breast milk production, infertility, acne **Studies:** show positive evidence for hyperprolactinemia and premenstrual syndrome; possible benefit for breast pain and infertility, more studies needed	■ Do not take in pregnancy/lactation: secondary to hormonal effect ■ Do not take with dopamine medications (some antipsychotics, Parkinson's drugs): affects dopamine ■ Do not take with oral contraceptives or hormone-related cancer (e.g., breast cancer) ■ Contraindicated with bromocriptine, also used for hyperprolactinemia **ADRs** ■ Acne ■ GI symptoms ■ Dizziness ■ Depression, fatigue	**Form:** dry commercial extract, aqueous alcohol extract **Dose:** varies; up to 600 mg/day for dried fruit extract **Note:** not on the FDA Generally Recognized as Safe (GRAS) list
Chondroitin Sulfate ■ Glucuronic acid and galactosamine molecule ■ Found in mammalian cartilage, supplement derived from bovine, shark, or synthetic material	**Uses:** Osteoarthritis, especially of hip and knee; psoriasis **Studies:** show positive evidence for osteoarthritis, with or without glucosamine, and in urinary incontinence **Other:** may be anti-inflammatory, protective of joints	■ Avoid in bleeding disorder, preoperatively ■ Avoid in persons with psychiatric disorders: possible euphoric effect ■ Caution with bovine type: risk of bovine spongiform encephalopathy (mad cow disease) ■ Although found naturally in breast milk, it has not been studied sufficiently for safety in pregnancy/lactation ■ Some concern for shellfish allergies but in combination with glucosamine	**Form:** capsules or combined with glucosamine **Dose:** may be able to dose intermittently; 200 to 400 mg two or three times daily for osteoarthritis; used intravesically for urinary incontinence and interstitial cystitis **Note:** not on the FDA GRAS list

	Uses/Studies	ADRs/Drug Interactions	Form/Dose/Note
		ADRs ▪ Increases or decreases blood pressure ▪ Euphoria, headache ▪ Asthma exacerbation ▪ Bleeding risk, decreased hemoglobin **Drug Interactions** ▪ Anticoagulants: increases bleeding ▪ Iron: increases absorption	
Cinnamon ▪ From bark of cinnamon tree ▪ Many varieties: Ceylon and Chinese (cassia) cinnamon most common	**Uses:** most promising for diabetes mellitus, bronchitis, GI symptoms, loss of appetite, angina, CAD	▪ Avoid consuming large amounts of cassia cinnamon: contains coumarin of the anticoagulant family ▪ Has been used unsafely to get "high" in youth by inhaling powder or ingesting oil; unsafe to swallow in quantity, can cause burning, coughing, respiratory irritation ▪ Allergic/hypersensitivity reaction ▪ Not tested for safety in children **ADRs** ▪ Asthma ▪ Glossitis, gingivitis, stomatitis **Drug Interactions** ▪ Antidiabetic agents: decreases blood sugar	**Form:** powders, extracts, capsules, teas **Dose:** 1 to 6 g/day in divided doses up to 16 weeks, or 333 mg capsules up to twice daily for up to 8 weeks, for type 2 diabetes mellitus; two 250-mg capsules twice daily with water-soluble Cinnulin PF for metabolic syndrome **Note:** on the FDA GRAD list
CoQ10 or Coenzyme Q-10 "ubiquinone" ▪ Tends to decline with age ▪ Organ meats have highest levels so less often ingested in the United States, creating lower overall CoQ10 levels	**Uses:** prevention of statin-induced myopathy (statins may deplete CoQ10); conditions associated with deficits: diabetes mellitus, Parkinson's disease, muscular dystrophies, cancer, HIV/AIDS, cardiovascular disease; congestive heart failure **Studies:** show positive evidence for CoQ10 improving heart function in heart failure	▪ Low toxicity ▪ Potential for interactions with numerous drugs and supplements ▪ Has been used in children for specific conditions ▪ Can be toxic in high doses ▪ FDA approved as orphan drug for certain mitochondrial disorders ▪ ADRs lacking: possibly allergy, nausea, GI symptoms, rash in fewer circumstances	**Form:** variation of bioavailability depending on product **Dose:** ranges from 22 to 400 mg per day, depending on condition and product

(continues)

TABLE 16-2　Selected Common Dietary Supplements, Alphabetical (*continued*)

Common/Biological Name	Desirable Medicinal Actions	Contraindications and Risks (Adverse Drug Reactions [ADRs])	Typical Dosing
Cranberry ■ No longer thought to acidify urine ■ Instead, contains proanthocyanidins, which prevent bacterial adhesion in bladder	**Uses:** urinary tract infections, *H. pylori* stomach infections that cause ulcers, antioxidant anticancer, prevention of dental plaque **Studies:** dispute that cranberries can treat urinary tract infections, but they may help prevent them; may prevent *E. coli* organisms from adhering in urinary tract walls and may prevent *H. pylori* organisms from surviving in stomach; possible antioxidant properties; possibly prevents dental plaque	■ Excess cranberry juice can cause GI upset ■ Use cautiously if taking with anticoagulants, aspirin, or medications that affect the liver ■ Insufficient evidence for use in children medicinally **ADRs** ■ Increases risk of bleeding **Drug Interactions** ■ Antibiotics: additive ■ Anticoagulants: increases bleeding ■ Aspirin: increases bleeding	**Form:** juices, sauces, jellies, tablets, capsules **Capsules:** 200 to 500 mg daily in divided doses, or 6 Azo-cranberry capsules every day up to 3 months **Juice cocktail:** 300 ml/day, or 10 ounces each day
Creatine ■ Produced in body from amino acids ■ Stored in muscles ■ Found especially in meat and fish	**Uses:** enhancing muscle mass, hyperlipidemia **Studies:** show positive evidence for athletic performance enhancement, congestive heart failure; conflicting reports about possible renal dysfunction; effects only in short duration of physical activity	■ Avoid in bipolar, arrhythmia, diabetes mellitus ■ Allergy has been reported, causing asthma ■ Avoid with caffeine products **ADRs** ■ Headache, sedation, seizures ■ Arrhythmia, edema ■ GI symptoms ■ Muscle cramping ■ Aggression, irritability, mania in bipolar, depression, anxiety **Drug Interactions** ■ Antiarrhythmics: increases arrhythmia ■ Antidiabetic agents: alters blood sugar ■ Diuretics: increases effect ■ NSAIDs: increases nephrotoxicity	**Form:** made in many combination products for sports drinks, risk of overuse by teens and athletes **Dose:** varies depending on products **Note:** FDA recommends consultation with healthcare provider before using

DHEA

- Produced by adrenals, liver, testes, neurons, and brain
- Precursor of estrogens and androgens
- Steroids, oral contraceptives, and antipsychotics are among the drugs that lower DHEA
- Alzheimer's disease, HIV/AIDs, diabetes mellitus, depression, osteoporosis, and adrenal insufficiency are among the disorders associated with low DHEA

Uses: increase strength

Studies: show positive evidence for improving bone density, obesity, depression, adrenal insufficiency, systemic lupus erythematosus, and sexual dysfunction/erectile dysfunction

Note: Banned substance by the National Collegiate Athletic Association

- Avoid in pregnancy/lactation

ADRs

- Deepening voice
- Arrhythmia, hypertension
- GI symptoms
- Agitation, confusion, depression, psychosis
- Insulin resistance

Drug Interactions

- Antihypertensives: increases blood pressure
- Antipsychotics: increases mania
- Lithium: increases mania
- Antidiabetic agents: increases insulin resistance

Form: tablets, capsules, creams, IV/IM

Dose: dependent on condition, ranges from about 5 to 200 mg

Note: Plasma levels of DHEA should be taken prior to beginning treatment and should be reexamined periodically during treatment; not on the FDA GRAS list

Fish Oil

"omega 3 oils"

- From oily fish
- Contains DHA omega 3 fatty acid and EPA

Uses: hypertriglyceridemia, prevention of CAD, mild decrease in blood pressure, decrease atherosclerotic plaque, decrease triglyceridemia

Studies: show positive evidence for hyperlipidemia (specifically triglycerides), CAD, hypertension, prevention of CAD, and rheumatoid arthritis

Other: may be antiarrhythmic, antithrombogenic

- Avoid in fish allergy
- Avoid perioperatively: bleeding risk
- Avoid in pregnancy/lactation: risk of mercury contamination
- Avoid in bleeding disorders
- Fish oil has been used in children, but mercury, dioxin, and PCB contaminants in fish are concerning for children

ADRs

- Decreases blood pressure
- Increases LDL cholesterol
- Increases ALT level in cystic fibrosis
- Increases risk of mania
- Fishy taste, belching

Drug Interactions

- Anticoagulants: increases bleeding
- Antihypertensives: decreases blood pressure
- Vitamins A and D: may cause toxicity with cod liver oil
- Vitamin E: increases bleeding

Form: fish liver oil supplements (potential toxicity of vitamins A and D), fat-soluble vitamins

Dose: 2 to 4 g EPA+DHA daily to lower triglycerides per American Heart Association; other doses vary according to condition treated

Note: FDA approved; DHA/EPA are safe and lawful provided not more than 3 g/day in both food and supplementary sources

(continues)

TABLE 16-2   Selected Common Dietary Supplements, Alphabetical (*continued*)

Common/Biological Name	Desirable Medicinal Actions	Contraindications and Risks (Adverse Drug Reactions [ADRs])	Typical Dosing
Flaxseed oil/seed "linseed oil" ■ Flaxseed contains lignans, or phytoestrogens ■ Flaxseed oil does not contain lignans ■ Source of fatty acid alpha linolenic acid, which is a precursor to omega 3s	***Uses:*** menopause symptoms, arthritis, hyperlipidemia, cancer ***Studies:*** show positive evidence for constipation; German Commission-approved for chronic constipation, irritable bowel syndrome, diverticulitis, enteritis, gastritis; suggest helps lower elevated lipids; suggest alpha-linoleic acid (type of omega 3 fatty acid) helps heart disease; mixed results on hot flashes; may reduce some cancers' risks, unclear	■ Not for pregnancy: risk of spontaneous delivery ■ Risk of allergy, type I hypersensitivity **ADRs** ■ Severe diarrhea ■ Abdominal pain, bowel obstruction ■ Decreases platelet aggregation ■ Increases triglycerides ■ May affect sex hormones **Drug Interactions** ■ Acetaminophen: decreases absorption ■ Anticoagulants: increases bleeding ■ Antidiabetic agents: increases or decreases blood sugar ■ Antihypertensives: decreases blood pressure ■ Furosemide: decreases absorption	***Form:*** flaxseed oil in liquid or capsule form; flaxseed whole or crushed can be mixed with water or used with food; also in powder form ***Dose:*** Take both seed and oil with sufficient water to avoid intestinal obstruction and constipation; do not take together as may decrease absorption ***Oil:*** up to 2 g/daily ***Powder/flour:*** up to 60 g/daily, divided doses with liquid up to 4 weeks
Glucosamine ■ An amino monosaccharide that is produced normally in the body and is part of cartilage	***Uses:*** rheumatoid arthritis, TMJ, diabetes mellitus, chronic venous insufficiency ***Studies:*** show positive evidence for arthritis, especially of the knee; most studies use glucosamine sulfate, some with chondroitin	■ Avoid in pregnancy/lactation ■ Avoid with history of shellfish or iodine allergy: some preparations are from marine exoskeletons ■ Caution in diabetes mellitus: may increase blood sugar **ADRs** ■ Dizziness, headache, somnolence ■ Increases blood pleasure, heart rate, palpitations ■ GI side effects ■ Asthma exacerbation	***Dose:*** 500 mg twice daily for up to 6 months, but varies depending on product and condition; takes average 2 to 4 weeks for benefit ***Note:*** on the FDA GRAS list

Grape Seed Extract

- Leaves and fruit of grapes have been used medicinally since ancient Greece
- Extract made from grape seeds left over from winemaking

Uses: atherosclerosis, CAD, hyperlipidemia, hypertension, circulatory issues from diabetes, in eyes (macular degeneration and vascular disease), peripheral vessels, cancers, edema, antioxidant effects

Studies: show positive evidence for edema, chronic venous insufficiency, diabetic retinopathy, and vascular fragility; studies in process are examining breast, prostate, and colon cancer prevention, and Alzheimer's treatment

Drug Interactions

- Antihypertensives: decreases effect
- Anticoagulants: increases bleeding
- Antidiabetic agents: decreases insulin production or increases insulin resistance
- Stop 2 weeks perioperatively and before dental procedures due to risk of bleeding
- Avoid in pregnancy/lactation
- Avoid with bleeding disorders, iron deficiency

ADRs

- Headache, dizziness
- Hypertension
- Itchy scalp
- GI symptoms

Form: capsules, tables, juices, also available in a powder that can be mixed with water

Capsules or tablets: up to 300 mg/day by mouth

Juice: Concord grape juice has been used at a dose of 480 ml daily for 12 weeks with similar efficacy

Green Tea

"Chinese Tea," "Japanese Tea," *Camellia seniisis*

- Active ingredient is EGCG
- High in polyphenols and antioxidants
- Contains 50 mg caffeine per average cup, compared to 65 to 175 mg caffeine per cup of coffee
- Decaffeinating green tea does not seem to reduce polyphenols

Uses: mental alertness, weight loss, hyperlipidemia, cancer treatments (gastric, breast, skin)

Studies: show positive evidence for genital warts and hypercholesterolemia; mixed results on prevention or slowing of some cancers; improves mental alertness, likely from caffeine

Drug Interactions

- Anticoagulants: increases bleeding
- Antihypertensives: increases effect
- Antidiabetic agents: decreases blood sugar
- Iron: decreases amount
- Avoid if on anticoagulants: contains vitamin K
- Avoid if caffeine sensitive
- Avoid using concentrated green tea extracts if have or develop liver issues; some risk of liver toxicity

ADRs

- Caffeine related: insomnia, irritability, palpitations, GI upset, urinary frequency, increases psychiatric symptoms

Form: primarily used as a beverage by steaming green tea leaves; can be made into capsules or put with other products; some topical products

Dose: 250 to 950 ml tea by mouth daily up to 4 weeks for CAD benefits; 400 ml twice daily for mental alertness; green tea extracts in varying amounts of 100 to 750 mg per capsule, but liver toxicity is a risk; topical ointments may be used for genital warts, acne, and skin aging

(continues)

TABLE 16-2   Selected Common Dietary Supplements, Alphabetical (*continued*)

Common/Biological Name	Desirable Medicinal Actions	Contraindications and Risks (Adverse Drug Reactions [ADRs])	Typical Dosing
Guarana ■ Has among highest caffeine content of all plants ■ Guarana = 2.5% to 7% caffeine ■ Coffee = 1% to 2% caffeine	***Uses:*** cognitive and mood enhancement, obesity, athletic performance, fatigue reduction	■ Not to be used in pregnancy/lactation: high percentage of caffeine and associated risks of miscarriage and intrauterine growth restriction ■ Not to be used with anticoagulants: decreases platelet aggregation ■ Avoid in anxiety, panic, and bipolar disorders ■ Not to be used in children **ADRs** ■ Related to caffeine content: agitation, anxiety, insomnia, arrhythmia, hypertension, headache, GI symptoms, tachycardia, psychosis ■ Decreases platelet aggregation **Drug Interactions** ■ Alcohol: increases effect ■ Analgesics: increases effect ■ Anticoagulants: increases bleeding ■ Antihypertensives: decreases effect ■ Antibiotics: alters effect ■ Central nervous system depressants: antagonistic ■ Ephedrine: additive ■ Dopaminergic: additive ■ Beta-blockers: antagonistic	***Form:*** dry extract doses, tablets, capsules, teas; found in Brazilian sodas and increasingly in U.S. energy products and energy drinks; usually standardized by the amount of caffeine contained

Kelp

"seaweed"

- Brown seaweed has been used for food and medicine
- Contains sodium alginate
- Multicellular, brown or green seaweed

Uses: anticoagulant, antiviral, wound repair, goiter, weight loss, cancer

Studies: evidence of antioxidant and antibacterial actions; anticoagulant effects in lab

- Iodine may cause hypersensitivity, rash, including angioedema, thrombotic thrombocytopenic purpura, death
- Not for pregnancy/lactation: abortifacient effect
- Iodine content is beginning to be included; toxicities can be from iodine or other contaminants
- Insufficient evidence for use in children

ADRs

- Decreases blood pressure in some species
- Increases or decreases thyroid
- Laxative effect
- Bleeding
- Peripheral neuropathy from arsenic content
- Nephrotoxicity

Drug Interactions

- Laxatives: increases effect
- Antidiabetic agents: decreases blood sugar
- Anticoagulants: increases bleeding
- Antihypertensives: decreases blood pressure in some
- Estrogens: antiestrogenic effect

Form: aqueous extract, powder, granules, capsules, tablets; no standardization of iodine content

Dose: 200 to 600 mg in soft capsules used daily

Melatonin

- Neurohormone secreted by pineal gland due to darkness
- Produced from tryptophan
- Influences circadian rhythm and sleep initiation

Uses: ADHD, Alzheimer's disease, immune stimulant, antioxidant

Studies: show positive evidence for insomnia in children and elderly, jet lag, sleep disorders, and sleep enhancement

Other: may affect brain sleep center

- Do not use in pregnancy/lactation

ADRs

- Confusion
- Depression (transient)
- Dizziness
- Dream disturbance
- Drowsiness
- Irritability
- Neurobehavioral alteration

Dose: 0.3 to 5 mg up to 2 hours before bedtime in elderly; doses of 0.1 to 0.3 mg may be adequate

Jet lag: 0.1 to 0.5 mg taken on day of travel and every 24 hours

Note: not approved for safety over 3 months of use; safety not established for children's use

(*continues*)

TABLE 16-2 Selected Common Dietary Supplements, Alphabetical (*continued*)

Common/Biological Name	Desirable Medicinal Actions	Contraindications and Risks (Adverse Drug Reactions [ADRs])	Typical Dosing
Melatonin (*continued*)		**Drug Interactions** ■ Anticoagulants: decreases effectiveness ■ Antihyperlipidemics: increases atherosclerosis ■ Anti-seizure drugs: increases seizure risk ■ Sedatives: increases sedation	
Policosanol ■ Alcohols from sugar cane wax	**Uses:** hypercholesterolemia, cholesterol lowering (even as effectively as some statin drugs), inhibits cholesterol synthesis in liver, LDL degradation, antioxidant **Studies:** show positive evidence for platelet aggregation inhibition, coronary heart disease, and intermittent claudication; many studies from Cuba, source of sugar cane, some conflicting data from non-Cuban studies	■ Not recommended in pregnancy/lactation **ADRs** ■ Antiplatelet effect ■ Headache, dizziness, decreased blood pressure **Drug Interactions** ■ Antidiabetic agents: decreases blood sugar ■ Antihypertensives: decreases blood pressure ■ Antiparkinsonians: increases dyskinesias ■ Anticoagulants: increases bleeding ■ Nitrates: decreases blood pressure	**Form:** capsules, tablets **Dose:** 5 to 40 mg daily for coronary heart disease; 5 to 10 mg daily for hypertension; 10 to 20 mg daily for intermittent claudication
Red Yeast Rice ■ Extract from fermenting rice with yeast ■ FDA warns not to buy on Internet due to lovastatin component in some products ■ Contain sterols, fatty acids, isoflavones	**Studies:** show positive evidence for hyperlipidemia, anti-inflammatory potential	■ Avoid in pregnancy/lactation **ADRs** ■ Rash, anaphylaxis ■ Dizziness, headache ■ Decreases blood pressure ■ Decreases blood sugar ■ GI symptoms ■ Decreases Hgb, BUN	**Form:** gel capsules **Dose:** 1200 mg capsules of red yeast rice powder twice daily with food; do not take with grapefruit juice or alcohol **Note:** Cholestin, containing red yeast rice, is no longer available to purchase in the United States; several other varieties are available; not on the FDA GRAS list

		Drug Interactions	Form / Dose / Note
		■ Alcohol: increases liver toxicity ■ CoQ10: decreases, needs supplement ■ Antidiabetic: increases or decreases blood sugar ■ Antihyperlipidemics: increases risk of adverse effects ■ Statins: increases risk of adverse effects ■ Increases risk of rhabdomyolysis with azalides, cyclosporine, nefazodone, others	**Form:** tablet only in the United States; poor bioavailability due to first pass effect **Dose:** 400 mg/day in 2 to 3 divided doses for 4 weeks for ADHD; 800 to 1600 mg/day for up to 6 weeks for depression **Note:** monitor glucose, liver function tests
SAMe *S-adenosylmethionine* ■ Methionine is converted to SAMe with enzyme methionine adenosyl transferase	**Studies:** show positive evidence for osteoarthritis, alcoholic liver disease (liver disease has decreased hepatic SAMe, which decreases glutathione needed for hepatic detoxification and prevention of oxidative liver damage), depression, osteoarthritis, ADHD, fibromyalgia, analgesic, anti-inflammatory; SAMe transmethylation necessary to synthesize and metabolize neurotransmitters, proteins, hormones, and membrane phospholipids; production of SAMe associated with adequate B$_{12}$ and folate levels; SAMe converted to *S-adenosylhomocysteine*, which increases glutathione liver antioxidant; can increase dopamine and norepinephrine; 2006 Cochrane study found no evidence for or against use in alcoholic liver disease; 2008 Cochrane review on osteoarthritis use pending	**Drug Interactions** ■ Avoid in pregnancy/lactation ■ Avoid in bipolar disease: increases mania or hypomania ■ Avoid in CAD: thromboembolism risk ■ May worsen Parkinson's symptoms **ADRs** ■ Dizziness, headache, palpitations ■ Diaphoresis, rash, itchy or hot ear ■ Anxiety, insomnia, fatigue ■ Anorexia, constipation, nausea, vomiting, diarrhea, dry mouth **Drug Interactions** ■ Serotoninergic/SSRI: causes serotonin syndrome ■ St. John's wort: causes serotonin syndrome ■ Tricyclic antidepressants: causes serotonin syndrome ■ Tramadol: causes serotonin syndrome ■ MAOI: causes serotonin syndrome, hypertensive crisis ■ Dextromethorphan: causes serotonin syndrome ■ Meperidine: causes serotonin syndrome ■ Levodopa: decreases effect	

(continues)

TABLE 16-2   Selected Common Dietary Supplements, Alphabetical (continued)

Common/Biological Name	Desirable Medicinal Actions	Contraindications and Risks (Adverse Drug Reactions [ADRs])	Typical Dosing
Soy ■ Soybeans contain isoflavones similar to estrogen	**Uses:** menopausal symptoms, osteoporosis, breast and prostate cancer (may be contraindicated in breast cancer due to estrogenic effect) **Studies:** show positive evidence for hyperlipidemia (cholesterol and triglycerides), pediatric diarrhea, menopause symptoms, and hypertension; reduces LDL cholesterol and hot flashes	■ Rare allergies ■ Avoid soy in hormone-related cancers or risk of cancers (breast, endometrial, ovarian) **ADRs** ■ Mild GI symptoms ■ Headache **Drug Interactions** ■ Anticoagulants: increases bleeding ■ Antihypertensives: decreases blood pressure ■ Tamoxifen: alters effect ■ Estrogen: alters effect	**Form:** soybeans, tofu, soy milk, powders, capsules, supplements, nutrition bars **Dose:** 25 g soy daily for CAD risk and other conditions **Note:** on the FDA Everything Added to Food list
Spirulina "blue-green algae"	**Uses:** diabetes, allergic rhinitis, weight loss **Studies:** show positive evidence for hypercholesterolemia use	■ Avoid in pregnancy/lactation **ADRs** ■ Headache, nausea, vomiting ■ Hepatotoxicity	**Dose:** 1 g by mouth twice daily with meals for diabetes mellitus; 1000 to 2000 mg once daily for 12 weeks for allergic rhinitis; up to 1 g spirulina twice daily for type 2 diabetes mellitus
Wild Yam ■ Considered natural source of estrogen, progresterone, and/or DHEA	**Uses:** hyperlipidemia, menopausal symptoms	■ Avoid in pregnancy/lactation **ADRs** ■ GI upset ■ Contact dermatitis **Drug Interactions** ■ Antidiabetic agents: decreases blood sugar ■ Hormones: alters effect	**Forms:** capsules, tinctures, dried root, vaginal creams **Dose:** 250 mg 1 to 3 ×/day

Source: Data from National Center for Complementary and Integrative Health, "Herbs at a Glance" (2012). https://nccih.nih.gov/health/herbsataglance.htm; M. Iannuzzi-Sucich and C. A. Sanoski, *Herbal Notes: A Complementary and Alternative Medicine Pocket Guide* (Philadelphia: F. A. Davis, 2011); *Natural Standard,* from Quinnipiac University; MedlinePlus, "Herbs and Supplements" (2014). www.nlm.nih.gov/medlineplus/druginfo/herb_All.html; C. Ulbright, *Davis' Pocket Guide to Herbs and Supplements* (Philadelphia: F. A. Davis, 2011).

Directions for Future Research

1. Should detailed information about herbs and dietary supplements be a required part of undergraduate and graduate nursing programs?
2. Should questions on herbal medications and dietary supplements be included in the board certification exams?
3. Because so many people are now using herbs and supplements, which are the most important ones for nurses to thoroughly understand, in view of drug interactions and preoperative risks?

Nurse Healer Reflections

- What websites are essential for me to familiarize myself with in order to better understand herbs and dietary supplements and their benefits, risks, and contraindications?
- What is most important for me to know about herbs and supplements to provide quality, holistic nursing care?
- How do I feel about using herbal medication or dietary supplements for myself?

NOTES

1. Zentrum Publishing, "German Commission E Monographs Validate Herbs" (2014). www.herbal-software.com/german_commission_e_monographs.htm.
2. M. Adams, "Zero Deaths Caused by Vitamins, Minerals, Amino Acids or Herbs," *Natural News* (January 21, 2010). www.naturalnews.com/027993_vitamins_nutritional_supplements.html.
3. National Center for Complementary and Integrative Health, "The Use of Complementary and Alternative Medicine in the United States" (December 2008). https://nccih.nih.gov/news/camstats/2007/camsurvey_fs1.htm.
4. D. Rakel, *Integrative Medicine*, 3rd ed. (Philadelphia: Saunders, 2012).
5. E. K. Farina, K. G. Austin, and H. R. Lieberman, "Concomitant Dietary Supplement and Prescription Medication Use Is Prevalent Among US Adults with Doctor-Informed Medical Conditions," *Journal of the Academy of Nutrition and Dietetics* 114, no. 11 (2014): 1784–1790.
6. National Center for Complementary and Integrative Health, "Traditional Chinese Medicine: An Introduction" (2009). https://nccih.nih.gov/health/whatiscam/chinesemed.htm.
7. National Center for Complementary and Integrative Health, "Natural Products Research—Information for Researchers" (2014). https://nccih.nih.gov/grants/naturalproducts.
8. National Center for Complementary and Integrative Health, "Herbs at a Glance" (2012). https://nccih.nih.gov/health/herbsataglance.htm.
9. National Institutes of Health, "Botanical Dietary Supplements: Background Information" (June 24, 2011). http://ods.od.nih.gov/factsheets/BotanicalBackground-HealthProfessional/.
10. M. T. Murray and J. Pizzorno, *The Encyclopedia of Natural Medicine*, 3rd ed. (New York: Atria, 2012).
11. *Natural Standard* (professional electronic database, Quinnipiac University, Hamden, CT, 2014).
12. M. H. Frisvold, "Functional Foods and Nutraceuticals," in *Complementary and Alternative Therapies in Nursing*, 7th ed., eds. R. Lindquist, M. Synder, and M. F. Tracy (New York: Springer, 2014): 365–373.
13. American Association of Nurse Anesthetists, *Herbal Products and Your Anesthesia* (Parkridge, IL: American Association of Nurse Anesthetists, 2011).

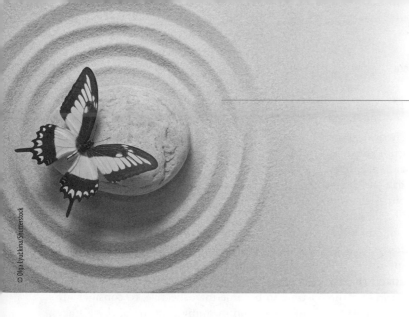

CHAPTER 17

Dying in Peace

Lynn Keegan and Carole Ann Drick

Nurse Healer Objectives

Theoretical

- Apply theories of grief, self-transcendence, and culture to assist the dying in peaceful and meaningful death.
- Discuss with colleagues difficult issues surrounding the care of the dying.
- Interview patients who have experienced nearing death awareness.

Clinical

- Contribute to the dying person's peace of mind through comeditation practices.
- Promote the dying person's sense of integration through life process review.

Personal

- Explore personal myths and beliefs about death with colleagues.
- Plan your own ideal death.
- Experience "letting go" through self-recording of imagery scripts and periodically experiencing them.

Death: A moment in time.

Dying: The final stage of physical life that fits into a broader awareness, giving meaning to both death and life.

Grief: A response to loss, characterized as dynamic, pervasive, individual, yet normative.

Loss: The absence (or anticipated absence) of someone or something of real or symbolic meaning.

Mourning: The expression of a sadness or sorrow resulting from a loss.

Myth: Story lines created by individuals and cultures about meaning and journeying in life.

Nearing death awareness: The dying person's knowledge of death and attempts to describe this experience to healthcare providers, family, and friends.

Perideath: The last hours of life, the actual death, and the care of the body after death.

Self-transcendence: A spiritual concept referring to moving one's self into a wider sense of consciousness and understanding.[2]

Spirituality: "The essence of our being." (See also Chapter 7)

Definitions

Culture: Socially transmitted ways of life including but not limited to language, arts and sciences, thought, spirituality, social activity, and interaction.[1]

Theory and Research

To die well is to die peacefully, with the knowledge that life has had meaning and that one is connected through time and space to others, to God, and to the universe. Assisting people to die well requires knowledge and skill, as well as a willingness to be intensely involved in the most intimate phases of another's life. Physical, spiritual, psychological, and social distress must be addressed with concern and compassion. Nurses being present "in the moment" with the dying and their family inevitably confront their own mortality. Care for the caregiver, both professional and personal, is a necessity and an often overlooked part of caring for the dying. The dying and their family are the unit of care.

One holistic overarching approach to easing the burden for those who are caring for the terminally ill is based on Watson's Theory of Human Caring, which focuses on the relationship between the whole person of the caregiver (nurse) and the whole self of the client/family as it protects and preserves the humanity and dignity of the client.[3] In this partnership or relationship between caregiver and client and family, the burden becomes shared; each can ease the other's burden.

Developing theories to guide end-of-life care are based on standards of care, like those identified by professional associations, state laws, and culture. Theories related to grief and loss, self-transcendence, myths and beliefs (two components of culture), and nearing death awareness are particularly useful in formulating effective plans for care for the dying.

Grief and Loss

Grief theory links concepts of loss, bereavement, and mourning into a fabric of ideas that assist in deciding actions on the part of caregivers, family members, and the dying. Grief is not only normative but also dynamic, pervasive, and individual. Each person moves through bereavement at a different pace and copes in a different manner, depending on inner resources, support, and relationships. Society may think that the period of mourning has been long enough (a normative statement), but the individual may need more (or less) time before beginning to take charge of a changed life.[4]

Grief is a necessary process for both the dying person and his or her significant others. The more bonded and intimate two people have been, the more intense grief can be. Grief

is pervasive, affecting every area of life. Therefore, it affects relationships, physical symptoms, schedules of care, feelings, spirituality, and one's sense of meaning in life. The person who is dying integrates care (e.g., regular laboratory tests, visits to healthcare providers, various therapies) into an already full schedule. That gradually changes in content from outer activities to inner, more personal, physical, emotional, and mental activities. As death grows closer, visits by family and friends may be welcome. But there comes a point when the one who is dying needs time to become introspective, to consider life's messages and meanings. At any of these stages, caregivers may feel excluded from the dying one's life, wanting to be present yet having difficulty "reaching" the loved one. Once caregivers understand this increasing need for introspection by the dying person, they are better able to realize that this is a normal part of the dying process that the dying person must enter more and more on his or her own. Nurses can respond with gentle touch and loving words.

Hope increases as death approaches, but the nature of hope changes. Hope for less pain, for example, is common, when hope for a cure has been abandoned. Hope is a basic construct of spirituality and has been recognized as having both physiologic and psychological value. Families and staff caregivers share in hope as it relates to spirituality and the end of life. The whole team grieves, and the whole team helps one another through the process.[5] The nurse can spiritually support the family during this time by creating space to allow for the expression of emotions and spiritual beliefs and to encourage meaning-based coping behaviors.[6]

Spiritual development is related to the phases of grief originally identified by Kübler-Ross.[7] Nursing care during each of the phases takes into account the spiritual maturity of the griever, whether it is the dying person or those who love that person. A person who is in the early stages of spiritual maturity, whether a child or an adult, needs much external help, information, communication, and the ability to develop trust. This person may not achieve acceptance (and transcendence) without moving to a higher level of spiritual development. Persons who have a more formal spiritual practice may use rituals, rites, symbols, and activities that incorporate them; thus, they may find comfort in planning their own funeral.

It is becoming increasingly acceptable to plan one's own funeral. Just the act of planning can create a peace of mind not only for oneself but also for loved ones after you are gone. Preplanning is seen by many as a selfless act and a last and lasting gift to loved ones that extends beyond actual death.[8]

Nursing care requires a careful assessment of a dying person's spiritual resources to assist with peaceful death. In one survey of registered nurses caring for the actively dying in an academic medical center, it was found that nurses' self-perceived professional capability and comfort levels in caring for dying patients is positively influenced by older age, greater clinical experience, and extensive continuing education. This suggests that it is important to recruit experienced nurses to care for the dying and their families and to mentor inexperienced nurses to increase their comfort in working with the dying.[9]

The nurse's own developing spiritual maturity can be a useful support, as when one accompanies an acquaintance for a while along a road. The nurse maintains an attitude of being open, listening, and assessing the client's path, even when his or her own journey changes directions. Successfully dealing with grief allows the dying client to achieve peace and allows the family and significant others to move on with a changed life, cherishing memories while creating new ones.

Self-Transcendence

Many people have studied self-transcendence, the sense of a temporal integration of self, the feeling that past and future enhance the present. In studying survivors of concentration camps, Frankl discovered that those who survived seemed to transcend (beyond self) either toward other people or toward meaning.[10]

One study tested whether nurse–patient interaction affects cognitively intact nursing home patients' interpersonal and intrapersonal self-transcendence. In this instance, self-transcendence was considered a spiritual developmental process of maturity in adulthood and a vital resource of well-being at the end of life.[11]

Those with a sense of transcendence have a greater sense of well-being and a greater ability to cope with grief. These people live in the present and usually see death as a normal part of life. Encouraging people to seek meaning and connections, either in the present or through the ages, helps people move toward self-transcendence to achieve peace.

In recent years, personal and clinical dilemmas relating to terminally ill patient care medical decisions have increased significantly. It is important to understand the patient's medical, nursing, and social background. In order to garner this information, a comprehensive appraisal essential for treating the "whole patient" includes a spirituality assessment.[12]

Much of this information can be derived directly from the person using the process of reminiscence and life review. Life review is the story of this life, of living in this space on this Earth in this time. Studies show that systematic life review helps reduce depression and anxiety, and it promotes a feeling of "This was my life, no one else would have done it this way, and I have a unique place in this universe."[13]

Myths and Beliefs

Myths are our story lines, values, beliefs, and images; they are our personal manual about the meaning and the journeys of the human spirit.[14] Myths help us seek the unfolding mystery in life. In seeking life's meaning and purpose, personal myths help us manifest hope, learn to accept daily struggles and challenges, and deal with ambiguity and uncertainty. Myths help us recognize strengths, choices, goals, and faith. They also help us to assess our perception of our world, recognize our capacity to pursue personal interests, and demonstrate love of self and self-forgiveness. Myths provide a sense of connection and of oneness with all of life and nature.

Throughout life, we create many myths; some serve us well while others hinder our healing journey. More than 30 years ago, the Senior Actualization and Growth Exploration study began to question society's beliefs about older people and their potential.[15] The researchers taught seniors deep relaxation, biofeedback, breathing exercises, meditation, yoga, and ways to expand creativity through movement, music, art, education, and group discussion. This project not only helped the participants reshape their declining years to an understanding of healthy aging and lifestyles that promote the goal of healthy aging, but it also gave them new, practical ways to cope with personal problems and a more confident self-image. With healthier lifestyles, most people can add a vital 30 or more years to their life span. There is also more time to practice a new way of living so that dying in peace is a clear choice for each person.

Nearing Death Awareness

When people become aware that they are approaching death, they often talk about two things. They may attempt to describe what they are experiencing while dying, and they may request something that they need for a peaceful death. This awareness is not to be confused with near-death experiences that happen as a result of cardiac arrest, drowning, or trauma in which a person feels the self suddenly leave this life but quickly return. In a state of nearing death awareness, a person's dying is slower, often because of a progressive illness such as acquired immune deficiency syndrome (AIDS), cancer, or heart or lung disease. The person becomes aware of a dimension that lies beyond, a drifting between this world and another, perhaps a space of transcendence, yet not one that touches "an Ultimate." The slower dying process allows the dying person to have more time to assess his or her life and to determine what remains to be finished before death. Some dying patients try to describe being in two places at once or somewhere in between. It is a time for a caregiver to respond to the dying person's wishes and needs and to listen to what dying is like for that person. It is at this time that the patient's wishes for cardiopulmonary resuscitation should be heard if this topic has not been previously discussed.[16] This can be a period of challenge for many caregivers, and yet it can help each of us to prepare for what may happen in our dying. Those individuals who are tired of living but who do not believe that it is time to die describe the dying process differently from those who are truly ready to depart. The statements of those

who are truly ready are different in the clarity with which the words are spoken, the look in their eyes, or their touch. Their statements, looks, or touches are like no others that have been made before or during the dying process.

Holistic Caring Process

Holistic Assessment

In preparing to use interventions for promoting peaceful dying, the nurse assesses both the dying person and the family or significant others in the following areas:

- The different emotions that can surface during the process include:
  - *Guilt:* Blame of self and others over management of the dying person; distress over inability to decrease pain
  - *Anger:* Toward God, disease, family or significant others, doctors, or survivors; over inability to fix things physically, emotionally, and spiritually
  - *Ability to laugh:* The shortest distance between two people; the relationship between comedy and tragedy as joy and sadness pathways cannot operate simultaneously
  - *Love:* An essential element in living and in dying; a state of self-giving and presence of being a person, where openness and willingness exist for self or another; the network that brings and weaves families and significant others together to work through the dying process and move into total acceptance of death
  - *Fear:* Often evocation of separateness and aloneness, but it can become a path leading deeper into the present moment; useful in that it reveals areas of resistance; return to unconditional love and a sense of equanimity after release of fear
  - *Forgiveness:* Essential element for inner peace; an exercise in compassion that is both a process and an attitude; not necessarily reconciliation
  - *Faith:* The larger vision of existence, which is different for each person; helps

to harness energy to evoke healing resources and power
- *Hope:* Support of patient or family and significant others during death's darkness; an inner moment that perceives lightness when in the midst of darkness and has the potential for leading to deeper love; hope for decreased pain and increased physical and spiritual comfort, for a miracle, for peace of mind, for a remission, for peaceful death transition, and for acceptance of a shorter life than expected or the death of a loved one
- The patient's interactions with others and the effect of the patient's emotions on these interactions
- The need for education about what will happen and what can be done to help, for the family and the patient
- Comfort needs, assessed according to the patient's culture and wishes for:
  - Pain control and symptom management
  - Hydration
  - Nutrition
  - Respiratory assistance
  - Movement
  - Touch
- Signs of psychiatric illness, under- or overmedication that may interfere with a patient's ability to cope with dying:
  - Hallucinations
  - Delusions
  - Depression
  - Denial that interferes with the ability to move toward comfort and peace
  - Excessive anxiety
  - Confusion, agitation, or memory loss, especially in older adults
  - Advanced dementia

Identification of Patterns/ Challenges/Needs

The following are the patterns/challenges/needs compatible with dying in peace interventions (see also Chapter 8):

- Altered circulation
- Altered oxygenation
- Altered body systems

- Altered communication
- Effective communication (see the section on Nearing Death Awareness earlier in this chapter)
- Spiritual distress
- Spiritual well-being (see the section on Nearing Death Awareness earlier in this chapter)
- Ineffective individual or family coping
- Self-care deficit
- Body image disturbance
- Powerlessness
- Hopelessness
- Pain
- Anxiety
- Death anxiety
- Grieving
- Fear

Outcome Identification

Table 17-1 guides the nurse in identifying patient outcomes, nursing prescriptions, and evaluation for assisting patients and their families and significant others during the dying process.

Therapeutic Care Plan and Interventions

The following guidelines are appropriate both for the dying person and the caregiver, whether family, friends, or nurse. They are helpful in all settings. The guidelines are beneficial from the first awareness of a coming interaction with a patient and family who are moving through the dying process, through dying, and afterward.

Before the interaction:

- Spend a few moments centering yourself to recognize and honor your presence there.
- Become a healing presence, be in the present moment with the client/family, believing in and affirming their dignity and wholeness.
- Begin the session with intention to facilitate healing and peaceful dying. This may be a prayer.

At the beginning of the interaction:

- Encourage the patient and the family and significant others as the caregiver(s) to do the following:
  - Set realistic goals.

TABLE 17-1　Nursing Interventions: Dying in Peace

Client Outcomes	Nursing Prescriptions	Evaluation
The patient will demonstrate an understanding of the reasons for ongoing assessment and management of anxiety, including: ■ Quiet environment ■ Explanations of all personnel, procedures, and equipment ■ Touch and reassurance by nurse ■ Relaxation skills	Continue to reassess states of anxiety and provide ways to decrease anxiety: ■ Provide a quiet environment. ■ Explain all interventions. ■ Offer reassurance. ■ Teach relaxation and imagery skills.	The patient demonstrated an understanding of the reasons for assessment and management of anxiety.
The patient will verbalize feelings of anxiety and will talk spontaneously about fears. (If the patient is intubated, the patient and the nurse use specific communication codes.)	Provide high-quality time for the patient to share worries and fears. Use common symbols for communication if the patient is intubated.	The patient verbalized anxiety and fears.
The patient will use effective coping mechanisms during the course of illness.	Focus on the patient's strengths.	The patient used effective coping mechanisms during the course of illness. (List specific examples.)
The family will communicate stressors associated with the patient's illness to staff.	Allow time for the family to express worries and fears.	The family or significant others communicated stressors to staff.
The patient will verbalize fears of death.	Be present with the patient, and allow time for the patient to talk about fears of dying.	The patient talked of death.
The family and significant others will verbalize fears that the patient may die and what this means to them.	If death seems imminent, be with the patient and family to assist them through the death.	The family or significant others acknowledged the impending death and shared feelings about death.
The family and significant others will receive support from nurses and clergy.	Provide spiritual support for the patient through presence, life review, prayer, talking, and handholding. Allow the family to be with the patient. Call clergy for assistance, if requested.	The family or significant others received spiritual support and talked to nurses and clergy.
The patient, family, and significant others will express fears and other feelings associated with dying and death.	Assist the patient and the family to focus on what has been accomplished in life. Provide as much privacy as possible.	The patient and the family focused on life accomplishments.
The patient will experience closure on matters of daily living.	Provide the opportunity to complete "unfinished business." Fulfill the patient's requests to see a family member, lawyer, clergy member, or physician.	The patient and the family completed unfinished business.
The patient will be comfortable and participative until death occurs.	Evaluate the procedures and treatments that can be discontinued to make the patient more comfortable. Make provisions for someone to remain with the patient all the time if so desired by the patient.	Procedures and treatments were used for comfort only.

- Identify different behaviors that have surfaced in their interactions with one another during this period.
- Gather a healing team and honor the patient's personal needs and feelings to avoid more suffering.
- Accept current circumstances, and release things that are beyond their control. Accept the fact that release may not be possible at this time, but they can work toward it.
- Take frequent breaks, at least 20 minutes daily, to evoke high-quality quiet time with relaxation, imagery, music, meditation, prayer, journal keeping, or dream work to assist in the process of letting go.
- Exercise, take long hot baths or showers, eat nutritious foods, eliminate excess caffeine or junk food, and ask other people for relief.
- Encourage the patient and caregivers to tell themselves over and over what a good job they are doing and that it is the best job that they can do. Repeating it helps in releasing guilt, anger, and frustration.

During the dying process:

- Recognize the one who is dying as the person who is usually the best teacher about what is right. The place of death is not as important as the care, trust, compassion, acceptance, and love that was provided and shared in the perideath interactions.
- Determine the care needed. The whole family should consider the following questions and issues:
  - Will the dying person receive better care in a hospital, in a hospice, or at home?
  - Which kinds of medical treatment, technology, and equipment are needed?
  - What information is needed to make decisions about care choices (e.g., providing hydration, withholding nutrition)?
  - Can a hospice nurse or healthcare professional assist with treatments and medication?
  - Is a parish nurse or congregational nurse available for liaison with the congregation involved?
  - What expenses will be involved? What expenses will be covered by insurance? Is the patient eligible for state or federal disability payments, veterans or Social Security benefits, or Medicaid or Medicare?
  - Who will assume the care 24 hours a day? Who will provide respite care? Are there children at home who also need continuous care? Can the care of the dying person and young children both be managed?
  - Will some or all of the organs be donated?
- Explore the advantages and disadvantages of dying at home (or alternative sites). Advantages for staying in the home include the freedom of the patient and the family to do anything they wish because they can change or alter routines and schedules at will. In addition, staying in the home makes the continuous support of family, friends, and even pets available. It allows meals to be prepared fresh and served with attention to details; it eliminates the stress of traveling to and from the hospital or hospice; it provides the unique beauty of familiar surroundings; it makes high-quality time available to focus on inner work for the moment of death; and it permits the patient and family to experience feelings and emotions in a different way because their closeness is subject to fewer interruptions. Finally, the patient and family can make most of the decisions regarding care, medication, and treatments and can ask advice from professionals when needed. Disadvantages to staying at home may include inadequate support for coping with care needs or competing needs for care by small children, older adults, and other sick or disabled family members. When available, inpatient hospice units may help blend some of the advantages of care in the home with the additional support an individual may need that significant others cannot provide.
- Integrate therapies.
  - Does the dying person believe that medical and nonmedical modalities are complementary?

- How motivated is he or she to try non-medical resources (e.g., acupuncture, aromatherapy, touch therapies, music)?
- Which nonmedical resources are available?
- Does the dying person really want to try different modalities, or is he or she receiving so much advice about therapies that the response is passive rather than active?
- Is the dying person choosing to try therapies to please caregivers? A patient should feel free to choose not to include complementary therapies if they are not wanted.

- Incorporate the senses in rituals.
  - *Touching.* Lovingly, freely, and joyfully convey through your hands what your heart is feeling. Touching is a powerful way to break the illusion of separateness, loneliness, and fear; it may evoke laughter, calmness, or tears. Create times to give and get hugs. Hold a hand now and then. Avoid touching if it is not welcome.
  - *Smelling.* Use lotions and colognes with mild fragrances, remembering that illness will likely change the types of fragrances that can be tolerated. Use caution because some odors cause nausea and unpleasant feelings. Try light, natural scents such as rosemary or vanilla, perhaps as a plant growing in the room or a candle in the bathroom (remembering safety considerations with an open flame).
  - *Tasting.* Remember that taste varies with degrees of illness but stays with us until the end of life. Tasting and eating have social and symbolic meaning to patients and family. Explain what will happen if the patient stops eating within the progression of terminal illness, that it may be normal and may not cause undue suffering. Provide tastes and foods that are desired.
  - *Seeing.* Arrange in a pleasing manner healing objects and different touch-stones that have special meaning and symbolize people, places, and events in the patient's life. A room that receives soft, subdued rays from the sun can bring balance to surroundings. Sitting out on the patio in good weather allows the patient to feel the sun as well as see the sunlight. Light colors are usually more soothing than dark colors.
  - *Hearing.* Remember that the sense of hearing is often sharp to the end of life, so special words at death can be heard. Be present in silence also, sitting or holding one another. Music can be nice, but not all the time.

- Practice sitting quietly with relaxation, meditation, or prayer. Gentle sounds from wind chimes or environmental recordings of ocean waves, wind, rain, birds, and music (e.g., harp, flute, stringed instruments) can offer a sense of peace. Music thanatology, referred to as sung prayer, uses the human voice when chanting or singing to bring balance to the dying, dissolving fears and lessening the burden, sorrows, and wounds.[17] Use words ending in *ing*, such as *releasing, letting, floating, softening,* or words ending in *ness,* such as *openness, beingness, awareness, vastness,* to help the patient to relax.
- Recognize the patient's going in and out of awareness. The moment of death itself has no pain but is a reflex last breath. It opens up very special exchanges of intention, intimacy, and bonding where the patient may share between the dying spaces. The patient's eyes can take on a staring, glazing, or spaciness so different that the patient appears to be going to another realm of knowing or to be focusing on something that the caregiver cannot see; the dying person can return with a smile and possibly share that he or she was in a space of peace.
- Learn about the normal natural changes in the body and how it functions during the dying process. Knowing what body changes to expect as death approaches helps the family anticipate personal healing rituals and removes the fear, shock, and mystery from the moment of death.
- Understand and accept the body's shutting down. The conscious dying person knows

that it is time to leave the physical body and can choose to shut physical life down. The caregiver and family journey with the dying person as far as possible, and then tell the person it is all right to leave; this can evoke the purest, most special moments for all involved. For those people who wish to experience every morsel of life, even if that morsel is physical agony, respect the choice. For them, it may be inappropriate to suggest that they leave. Tell them that you love them and will stay with them as long as they need you (or a significant other).

At the moment of death:

- Prepare rituals for the moment of death. The dying person usually has serenity and inner calm, particularly if healing rituals have been carried out prior to death. Before the dying moment, the eyes begin to stare and blinking ceases, tight brow muscles may become relaxed; the peace in the face or within the room is often palpable. Trust your inner wisdom for how to touch, hold, talk, and be with the dying one in ways that deepen hope and faith for a peaceful crossing into death and beyond.

- Surround yourself and the dying person with the peace and light of love, taking the energy of love and light in with each breath; imagine and experience literally going inside the breath, flowing inside the breath with comeditation (see the scripts in the following section on Specific Interventions) into the death of each moment.

- Continue to communicate with family caregivers and to those there to support the dying patient. Talk to the dying loved one as restlessness or agitation moves to unresponsiveness; give gentle love squeezes, touches, and hugs; play favorite music; read poems; or say mantras and prayers. Shut the half-closed eyes, stroke and hug the physical body, and adjust the loved one's head on the pillow for the last time. Give permission for this special person to be free, to soar, to meet God and others who have died before, if this is appropriate. Say all you need to say, and share your own kind of blessings for the smooth transition.

- If appropriate, when the person has taken a last breath, carry out additional rituals that may be helpful to those present. Holding hands around the bed, saying a blessing or prayer, or anointing with healing oil, for example, may be planned ahead of time for this moment.

- Schedule a follow-up session or visit with family and significant others, if appropriate. If grief support groups are available, a referral may be helpful.

- Take care of yourself. Adequate rest, relaxation, exercise, and nutrition are always important; the person who cares for dying people needs to "go apart for a little while." Center, meditate, celebrate, or plan your own self-renewal times. There are retreat centers and sanctuaries for those who wish to use them. Simply sharing your experience with others, either verbally or in writing (e.g., journaling, writing poetry or narratives), is helpful. Be glad for the opportunity to share such a sacred moment with others, and use those special times for your own growth.

Specific Interventions

Planning an Ideal Death   To help patients and families experience peace in the dying process, it is important to engage them in planning. To be of maximum assistance to someone else on the journey toward his or her own death, it is helpful for the nurse to explore this journey as well. The following reflective questions provide enormous insight into death myths, beliefs, problem solving, loving, and forgiving:

- What would an ideal death be like?
- When are you going to die?
- Where are you going to die?
- Who do you want to be with you, or do you want to be alone?
- What legal matters, relationships, or other personal business must be finished?
- What have been and what are the most precious events in your life?
- Who are the important people in your life?
- Have you told them why they are important?
- Are there family or friends who need to be told special things that you have never shared?

- Do you need to forgive or be forgiven?
- Have you written your obituary or your epitaph?
- Have you completed advance directives, in writing, and shared them with those involved?
- Who do you want to care for your pets?
- What are your assets?
- Which treasures do you wish to leave to specific family members or friends?
- Who have you appointed to be in charge of your medical decisions? Does this person know what you want done?
- Have you planned rituals for your burial, or a funeral, memorial service, or cremation? Are they recorded and available to those who will perform them, whether family, religious institution, or funeral home?
- If you are to be buried, what do you want to be buried in?
- What kind of a coffin or container do you want for your body?
- Who will perform your burial ceremony?
- Which kind of a ceremony do you want?
- Do you prefer a wake or another form of ceremony?
- Which prayers, passages, poems, or music do you want to have used?
- Who will direct the ceremony? Or do you want a death day celebration for people to celebrate your life during or in place of a funeral and to be celebrated in subsequent years?

Part of confronting death is deciding how to use medical care and technology. As part of their right to die, individuals can decide whether they want medical treatment; which kind of treatment; and under which circumstances to start, continue, or stop treatment. A power of attorney for health care records the appointment of someone to make medical decisions for the individual should that become necessary. An individual can record his or her wishes as a living will for four different life situations: (1) mental incompetence, (2) terminal illness, (3) irreversible coma, or (4) persistent vegetative state. Recording information about the individual's wishes regarding organ donation is also important. Most hospital and hospice organizations have documents called *advance*

directives available. These documents can be changed by the dying person as long as he or she is competent.

States vary in the legislative details of such documents. Specific information about the details to include in such a document can be found in the office of the state attorney general or by consulting an attorney. Furthermore, because these wishes often reflect philosophic, personal, religious, and spiritual desires, individuals should discuss these matters with the family and friends who will function on their behalf should they become incompetent. It is important for those who will be asked to make decisions to understand fully the nature of the request. Withholding of nutrition and fluids is often thought to be a cruel decision and a cause of suffering, yet history suggests that artificially feeding and hydrating a person who is clearly dying is an anomaly and reflects society's denial of death. Some research indicates that patients who stop taking food and fluids slowly sink into unconsciousness and coma over a period of 5 to 8 days and die several days later. Any discomfort that they experience, such as dry mouth, can be addressed with routine care. Those who make these kinds of decisions need to be fully informed, both about the patient's desires and about the effects of their wishes. Those who cannot do what the patient asks of them should have the choice of withdrawing from the decision-making role.

Learning Forgiveness   Forgiveness is important because it helps us get on with life. Many people are "stuck" in feeling guilt or assigning blame. Self-guilt leads to depression, and blaming others leads to anger. Both of these conditions steal energy and focus, reduce coping ability, and rob a person of precious time that could be used to establish a positive relationship and attend to end-of-life goals. Forgiveness, central to various religions, appears to ease the releasing of anger that may impair our relationships and healing.[18]

Many authors have described steps to forgiving self and others. They include (1) taking responsibility for what we have done; (2) confessing the nature of the wrongs to ourselves, another human being, or God; (3) atonement, or being willing to make amends where possible, as long as we can do this without harm to ourselves or other people; (4) asking for forgiveness, if that is possible; (5) looking to God for help; and (6) receiving or accepting forgiveness. Steps to forgiving others are (1) acknowledging that a wrong has occurred; (2) recognizing that we are responsible for what we are holding onto; (3) confessing our story to ourselves, another person, and God; (4) receiving atonement, or considering whether any specific action needs to be taken; (5) looking to God for help; and (6) offering forgiveness.[19, 20]

These steps take time to complete. As the awareness of forgiving self and others is developed, we recognize unconditional love. Because it helps us connect more with our source of joy, not focusing on loss, sadness, or pain, unconditional love helps release us from fear.

Becoming Peaceful   Use relaxation and imagery scripts. To learn how to let go of attachments, what is right and wrong, and what is good and bad, requires commitment and practice. Nurses encourage patients to hear their inner voice of judging and to release the judging. Nurses encourage patients just to listen, to be ready for the next moment of listening, and to be in the present moment. Centering, meditation, and contemplative prayer are helpful in learning to listen to the inner self. The skill of opening and releasing ordinary fears allows a person to emerge with awareness in the healing moment and to be fully present when assisting another during death.

Patients who are dying and their caregivers may set aside 20 minutes or more several times a day to practice opening to the moment. It may be helpful to create a special relaxation and imagery tape as part of a personal ritual to practice releasing and letting go. The breathing, relaxation, imagery, and music scripts that follow are important experiential exercises to help you and others learn the letting-go experience of calming the mind and creating a sense of spaciousness within the body (see also Chapters 11, 12, 13, and 14). Recording one or several of these scripts, after a 5- to 10-minute relaxation exercise, allows the dying patient and caregivers to use them repeatedly, even when professionals are not present. It is important to be sensitive about which scripts are likely to be useful for particular individuals. A person who has suffered from a respiratory disorder such

as emphysema for many years may not do well with a script focused primarily on breathing, for example. The following scripts are adapted from the work of Stephen Levine in the late 1970s and 1980s and from Julie Burnett in 2012.[21-23]

Script: Introduction. Close your eyes and focus your attention on your breath. Allow your brain to rest. Simply note your breathing pattern; no need to fix or change it. Allow yourself to go deep within your breath, to a place of rest and peace. Feel its warmth and safety. Feel the soft glow of an inner light becoming stronger and more powerful with each breath. Feel this inner core of your being and gently rest in it.

Script: Letting go. From this inner core, gently observe your breathing . . . no effort here . . . simply becoming aware of your breath . . . nice and easy . . . watch the breath . . . in . . . out . . . how easy . . . how effortless. . . . If any thoughts enter your awareness, allow them to pass through like gentle music floating through the air . . . keep going deeper. . . . Begin to notice a slight change as your breath begins to breathe you . . . so gentle . . . so easy . . . so natural. . . . Allow yourself to dissolve into this Universal Breath of Life . . .

Script: Opening the heart. Rest in your breath . . . the breath of life . . . allowing it to breathe you. . . . Notice your heart center and allow the breath to breathe through the heart . . . nice and easy. . . . You have lots of time . . . no effort. . . . Notice that there are some rough edges to your heart where old fearful thoughts or images are hanging on and wanting attention. Place your attention on them now. . . . Remain in the gentle Universal Breath. . . . Allow them to come forward . . . to the center of your heart . . . no longer at the sides. . . . There is plenty of room in your heart for them. . . . Allow the fears to rest in the openness of your heart. . . . Simply watch them begin to open and soften . . . accepting and acknowledging them . . . allowing them to float away.

Script: *Releasing grief and pain.* Rest in your breath, allowing it to breathe you. Feel the gentle rate and rhythm as you turn your attention to thoughts of sadness, grief, and loss. Notice any areas of your body that respond to these thoughts with tension, aches, or pains. Allow yourself to be drawn to the strongest area that demands the most attention. You may return to others later. Focus on this area with your breath, allowing the thought or feeling to become clear; it might be about a personal loss, grief over a loved one, or pain of an unresolved concern.

Rest in your breath as it surrounds and enfolds this heaviness of your sadness, grief, or pain. Gently breathe into the heaviness. Allow the waves of sensation to arise and float back into the nothingness from which they came. Be aware of sensations and emotions, feeling them but not becoming them. . . . Be the watcher. . . . Breathe life into the sensations as they arrive . . .

Gently, gently . . . there is plenty of time. Allow the sensations to arise and be acknowledged. . . . No hurry here. . . . You have all the time you need. Allow whatever needs to be expressed to arise from deep within. It has been there a long time and has many layers to come through. Allow it to slowly come up and open . . . like a lotus flower gently opening. Allow the process to unfold in a kind, gentle way. Remain with your breath. . . . The breath will guide you through . . . allowing, simply allowing, the fears of loss, of losing loved ones and yourself . . . your death, your end . . . all to gently arise, be recognized and released. . . . Allow them from the safety of your breath.

Script: *Forgiving self and others.* Rest in your breath, noting its rate and rhythm as it morphs just slightly and gently begins to breathe you. . . . It feels so natural, so easy. . . . Turn your attention to forgiving . . . forgiving yourself and others. . . . Gently observe the feelings that arise and the person or situation that needs attention. Breathe this in and feel the feelings of resentment, anger, bitterness, or dislike. Stay with your breathing and surround the feelings with this Universal Breath of love and light. . . . Place your hands on your heart and gently say, "I forgive you. I forgive you for any and all. I forgive you. I forgive myself." Repeat this three times while breathing deeply between repetitions.

Stay with your breathing and simply be the breath surrounding the feelings, the person, the situation. . . . Allow the feelings to gradually expand into the breath around them. . . . See them surrounded and enfolded in the breath. . . . No hurry here. . . . Allow this natural healing process to run its full course . . . gently . . . easily. . . . As they expand, observe how they respond to the breath . . . how they respond to your words . . . forgiving others . . . forgiving yourself.

Notice how light you feel . . . how spacious you are becoming . . . how alive. . . . Notice the increasing depth and fullness of your breath. . . . Feel your inhale so clear, so smooth, so deep . . . like you could inhale forever. . . . Notice your exhale so full and complete. It keeps going out farther and farther . . . like you could exhale forever.

While consciously living, it is possible to experience conscious dying. It is helpful to use a relaxation or imagery technique to become grounded before the exercise. After the exercise, this same technique can facilitate the return to full alertness and readiness to proceed with daily activities. These scripts are intended to be a rehearsal, not an actual shutting down and leaving of the physical body.

Learning to confront our own death helps us be more present to assist others in facing their death. It reaffirms that we really need to do nothing but be present with another and speak from our hearts in dying time. The nurse may begin with an extended head-to-toe general relaxation or other breathing exercise (see the previous scripts). Because the experience of dying can be described as melting or dissolving away at the moment of death, the words *dissolving* and *melting* are used in the script. To continue this script, the four elements of the body described by the ancients—earth, water, fire, and air—are used to represent decomposition as the body dissolves.

Script: Conscious dying. Relax into this moment and become aware of the breath. Let the breath just continue to breathe you. As you focus on the breath, . . . begin to notice how the breath lets you move from heavy sensations in the body to the lighter . . . subtle body of awareness . . . all awareness on the breath . . . the breath in . . . and the breath out. . . . Let yourself be in the heavy body . . . and now all awareness on being in the light body. . . . The breath is all that there is . . . just breathing. . . . Let each thought dissolve into the breath . . . melting into the breath . . . awareness of the light body . . . and now letting the breath go. . . . This is the final breath. . . . Let the breath in . . . and the breath out . . . dissolving . . . opening to death . . . and allow yourself to die.

Script: Earth. The body . . . solid . . . heavy . . . mass . . . compact . . . all changing as death comes . . . the vital body losing its form . . . weakening and dissolving . . . becoming thinner like the elements of Earth . . . changing . . . dissolving . . . all parts dissolving . . . organs . . . extremities . . . muscles . . . all senses dissolving . . . fading away . . . melting away . . .

Script: Water. All feelings becoming one . . . dissolving . . . all sensations dissolving . . . body fluids that flow through you . . . drying up . . . all body organs closing down . . . dissolving . . . .

Script: Fire. The fire of life within you . . . going out . . . all body warmth and heat leaving . . . all organs ceasing to function . . . your body becoming cooler and cooler . . . your sense of boundaries slowly dissolving . . . all senses dissolving . . . breath is dissolving . . .

Script: Air. Your body is without function. . . . The air is the element of consciousness . . . dissolving . . . all sensation . . . all feeling. . . . All senses have gone. . . . Body boundaries have disappeared and are no more . . . light . . . melting . . . dissolving . . . no separate body . . . no separate mind . . . all separateness dissolving . . . all in the vastness of oneness . . .

Take a few slow, energizing breaths and, as you come back to this awareness, know that whatever is right for you at this point in time is unfolding just as it should . . . that there is a perfect time and place for your death and that you rest in the peace that passes understanding.

Adapted from Levine's work, the following script is useful for someone who is preparing for the death moment or for a family member or friend whose loved one has just died.[24] It can be expanded as needed. The four-elements part of the imagery script may also be used to assist one whose death is imminent.

Script: Moving into the light. Fill yourself with an awareness or brilliance of clear light . . . a pure light within you and surrounding you. . . . Go forward . . . releasing anything that keeps you separate . . . pushing away nothing . . . spaciousness . . . releasing . . . dissolving . . . all body . . . dissolving into consciousness itself. . . . Let go of all distractions. . . . Listen and be with the transition. . . . What is called death has arrived. . . . You are not alone. . . . Many have gone before you. . . . Let yourself go . . . into the clear light.

The dying person may move in and out of sleep or comatose states after this script or the conscious dying script. The nurse or family member sits with the person as long as necessary to bring closure to this time. If the person lingers a while longer, the nurse or family member may close with the following phrases.

Script: Closure. Take a few slow, energizing breaths and, as you come back to this awareness, know that whatever is right for you at this point in time is unfolding just as it should, that there is a perfect time and place for your death and that you rest in the peace that passes understanding.

The Pain Process   In 90% to 99% of cases, pain can be managed. Pain medication response patterns should be evaluated at least every 72 hours, as well as after each administration. When giving the medication, the nurse reminds the patient that the pain medication is in the body and working. Nurses should understand and use the most current pain management strategies and treatments. These include new medications, methods of administration, physical treatments (e.g., massage, ice, and movement), combinations of treatments, documentation, and evaluation techniques. The administration of medication should precede activity (e.g., positioning).

Although the physical body can experience pain, the mind's fear of the pain is often more intense. Acute pain has qualities of suddenness and surprise that can evoke anxiety and fear. The best thing to do with this suddenness is to encourage the dying person to breathe rhythmically and soften into the pain to decrease the resistance to the experience. Relaxation, imagery, or acupressure may be combined with pain medication. Even the worst of pain can be shifted in many ways. For example, shifting the pain experience by calling it sensations rather than pain often reduces discomfort. It also helps to encourage the person to make decisions over which he or she has control, such as decisions about medications, treatments, and daily routines.

When guiding the person in pain, the nurse may suggest allowing pain images and the different felt experiences to emerge. Each person enters pain in a way that opens in the moment, and each person will know how far to go in exploring the pain. Common expressions an individual may have about the pain (e.g., pain attacks, it has a grip on me and takes my breath away, it has a loud and deafening pulsation, it is violent and unrelenting) create negative images that may interfere with the emergence of healing images. These negative images may become positive if the person focuses on the grip of pain being released, a deep belly breath coming forth evenly and effortlessly, or the pulsating sound becoming like the falling of gentle raindrops or snowflakes. Different relaxation and imagery exercises help the person practice letting go of the perception of the physical body. This letting go helps ease both physical pain, such as

difficult procedures, and emotional pain, such as conflicts, and allows the person to experience death with peace and dignity.

With continued gentle exploration of opening and releasing into the pain, the person may begin to experience the pain as floating and diminishing. This is also a way of expanding one's sense of time. Another suggestion is to have the patient step aside in the mind and watch the pain to see how it might be changed to release some of the pressure, resistance, and holding on to the pain. Such guidance and presence over time will help the person to stay with a focused attention, opening and softening and expanding into the pain.

Blending Breaths and Comeditation   The simple release of the breath and the ah-h-h-h sound is an ancient ritual for dying into peace. Comeditation is based on the principle that respiration evokes a particular state of mind and serves as a direct link to the nervous system. There is a direct correlation between breathing and thinking. At first, the ah-h-h-h sound may be like an echoing of words, but staying with the sound allows the release of tension, fears, and pain.

The following are the steps for comeditation:

1. Position yourself comfortably close to the patient. A session may last 20 to 30 minutes or longer. Obtain whatever is necessary to make you and the person comfortable, such as pillows or a light blanket.

2. Suggest to the person that watching the breath is an ancient method of calming the body and the mind. Let the person first begin noticing the rise and fall of his or her abdomen with each breath in and each breath out.

3. Sitting at the person's midsection, focus on the rise and fall of the abdomen with each inhalation and each exhalation. Focus your attention on the person's lower chest area, and observe closely for the natural flow of the exhalation from the person. With this focused attention, you can begin breathing in unison with the person. At the beginning of the exhalation, begin softly and out loud to make the sound *ah-h-h-h*, matching the respiration of the person.

4. Occasionally, say simple, powerful phrases, such as *peaceful heart* or *releasing into the breath*. The fewer words spoken, however, the more powerful the breath work. If the person should fall asleep, you may wish to sit with the person for a while or until he or she awakes.

Mantras and Prayers   A mantra is the repetition of a word or sound, either aloud or silently. The word may be given by another or discovered. It has meaning to the individual. Repetition moves one toward peace.

A prayer may be special phrases or repeated words, or it may be a unique and spontaneous communication with God. There is considerable evidence for the effectiveness of at least two forms of prayer, the directed and the nondirected. In direct prayer, the individual has a specific goal or outcome in mind. In the nondirected form, the individual takes an open-ended, nonspecific, non-goal-oriented approach. In one form of contemplative prayer, *Rosaries of Divine Union*, one listens in silence for the word of the Divine following a few words of scripture.[25]

In centering prayer, individuals seek a place deep inside themselves, where they live in rich harmony and connection with other people and with God and in the place of wisdom.[26] Every faith group has prayers of the faithful that provide comfort and joy in the last moments.

Saying mantras and prayers can decrease the number of lonely hours at home, as well as in the hospital, although this is not the main reason for the practice. Mantras and prayers serve as an affirmation of a deeper faith. In asking the dying person about wishes for prayers or repeated phrases, we may encourage him or her to select phrases that are short, easy to remember, and rhythmic. The personal selection of focus words enhances the faith factor. It may be helpful to pray for the highest good for the dying one or ourselves rather than for what we want. If we are praying for another, we need to hold the person for whom we are praying in our conscious thought, not ourselves. If we are totally focused on the patient, we cause ourselves less grief, frustration, and fear, recognizing that we are not responsible for outcomes. The nurse and the patient should agree on what

to pray for before the prayer begins, and the nurse must be sensitive to the individual's formal system of belief.

Reminiscing and Life Review   A process basic to human existence is reminiscing and recounting past events, either alone or with friends. We spend much of our time talking, thinking, or writing about plans, goals, resources, successes, disappointments, and failures. This is especially true when facing death. Life review is a more formal process that involves reviewing present and past experiences. A life review experiencing form is useful in ordering questions related to each stage of life from earliest memories to old age.

One way to do life review is through storytelling. The purpose of one exploratory study was to implement a storytelling approach to examine the experience of living with terminal cancer. Storytelling allowed the seven study participants to share personal experiences and achieve a sense of connectedness and intimacy. Holistic nurses can use this intervention as a way to facilitate physical, emotional, and spiritual healing and provide holistic end-of-life care.[27]

Where We Die   The environment in which people die, by choice or not, affects the ability of the person to achieve peace. Hospice and palliative care have evolved and helped to change the way and places where people die. Nurses continue to seek ways to help people die with dignity without needless suffering. As a culture, we are still debating when to stop life-prolonging interventions when one has reached the definitive time to die. However, even as these discussions continue, when it is time to die, where we die becomes a most important consideration.

Many people are alone at their time of death. Countless hundreds come to their end in the nursing homes that permeate every state in the nation. And of these hundreds, many are alone without living or able-bodied family members present. Still others face death at home, many, it is hoped, with hospice care nearby. Unfortunately, many more are surrounded by machines and invaded with tubes in the busy ICU.[28] Those interventions to help them last a few more hours or day are still enforced, and thus they die wrapped in technology and seldom in the arms of caring people.[29]

The literature appears to be consistent in the view that terminally ill patients are best cared for in specialized care settings, such as palliative care units and hospices. In the United Kingdom, approximately 90% of the population spends time in the hospital in the final year of life, with more than half dying in the hospital. Due to the changing demographics of older persons, greater numbers of dying patients are being admitted to the acute hospital setting.[30]

Hospital length of stay may be used to assess end-of-life care aggressiveness and health-care delivery efficiency. One study found that patients admitted to an inpatient palliative care unit had a shorter length of stay than those who only had palliative care consultation.[31]

Another study assessed the effect of a palliative medicine consultation on a medical intensive care unit (MICU) and length of hospital stay, Do Not Resuscitate (DNR) designation, and location of death for MICU patients who died during hospitalization. It found that palliative medicine consultation is associated with an increased rate of DNR designation and reduced time until death. Patients in the intervention group were also more likely to die outside the MICU as compared to controls in the usual care group.[32]

It is encouraging to know that there are alternatives. One of the newest options is a place called the *Golden Room*. This concept is a place that offers a new and expanded way to provide care for the terminally ill. The concept of the *Golden Room* removes the dying patient from the acute care setting into either a cluster of rooms separated from the regular patients in the general hospital and/or the nursing home. Another place for *Golden Rooms* is a free-standing building entirely dedicated to caring for the dying. These rooms are similar to contemporary hospice care but offer expanded facilities and personnel.

The purpose of the *Golden Room* is to facilitate and honor the dying process both for the patients and their loved ones. To create that place all elements of the design are taken into consideration. The physical room reflects calm and inclusion for all members present in the environment. Certain features designed into the space augment the sense of peace and security. A sense of spirit is reflected from the center-piece ceiling mural. Scenes depicting the cosmos with ethereal themes draw the supine patient below upward into a dimension of cosmic design. Some patients may sense a feeling of being drawn upward into their personal conception of spirit. Others may not consciously relate to a star-studded mural or painting of angels bursting from clouds, but subconsciously they will likely be relating to something much greater than themselves.[29]

These *Golden Rooms* will be designed with color schemes, furniture, technology, and comfort features to put the dying person and his or her caregivers in the best possible place for a comfortable, dignified, and peaceful death. Caregivers who render care in this setting will have special skills and, for example, be knowledgeable of the scripts and methods detailed in this chapter.

When these places for end of life are developed, we reason that pending death will not seem so formidable and frightening. Compassionately educated caregivers will be able to ease the transition from life into a peaceful death.

Death Bed Ritual (Basic)   Easing the transition from life to a peaceful death can be helped by the integration of a planned ritual into the process. This may occur at the moment of death or immediately after. If anointing has not already been done and is desired, it may be conducted at this time. Family, special friends, care staff, and clergy may choose to hold hands, surround the bed of the deceased, and share a moment of silence, a prayer, a song, or hugs. They may choose to touch the body, prepare the body according to rituals within the faith community involved, and say goodbye. It is important to allow as much time as needed.

Leave-Taking Rituals (Basic)   A nurse who works with survivors must remember that their grief period is unique for them. Furthermore, grief has no timetable. Healing grief requires a commitment to imagine a fulfilling life without a loved one. Action steps toward continued self-discovery after the death of a loved one may include dream work, meditation, movement, drawing, journal keeping, crying, sighing, drumming, chanting, singing, and music, as well as the following rituals:[24]

- *Celebrating holidays.* Special holidays, birthdays, anniversaries, and other important dates can be a time for creating rituals to ease the pain of loss and acknowledge feelings. For example, a widow fixed a place at the Christmas dinner table for her deceased husband. She and her six children gave him a farewell toast and shared special memories of him before they ate. A young couple who had a stillborn child asked several of the nurses and the attending physician to a memorial service in the hospital chapel before the baby was taken to the funeral home. After her mother died, a woman chose to have her healing team of eight friends with her at a memorial service by the sea. The family of a teenaged girl who died in an automobile accident had a gathering for her class and gave each person an opportunity to say special things about the girl. Her favorite music was played while dancing and singing began in her honor.

- *Rearranging and giving away.* If a loved one has died at home, the family member who shared the bedroom must decide what is best to do. Some wish to rearrange the room and remove hospital beds and other equipment quickly after death. Giving away a loved one's possessions, such as special mementos of jewelry, clothes, shoes, makeup, shaving equipment, and other personal possessions, is healing. Some people need a shrine or memorial for a period of time, however.

- *Letting grief be present.* There are periods after death when a person appears brave, in control, or strong to others. Grief will come, however. It is important to share with the grieving person that there is no special way to grieve. When pain, fear, and anger can dissipate, the bodymindspirit knows the best way to grieve. Grieving allows love to heal the loss one feels for self and the person who has died.

- *Sustaining faith and hope.* There are many ways to sustain faith and awareness toward life, meaning, and purpose during grieving time. For example, survivors sometimes have a sense of talking to deceased loved ones,

being enveloped in their love, and feeling their presence. People have described experiences such as having a faith in oneness, feeling an energy, vaguely sensing the presence of the deceased person, hearing the voice of the deceased giving guidance, or working on the same problem at different energy levels. One woman said, "My [deceased] husband told me how to finish this business deal." Another woman created a healing ritual after the death of her husband. When the weather permitted, she would get in her truck in the evening and drive to her husband's favorite hill on their big Texas ranch. As she looked out over the prairie and gazed into the Milky Way, she would choose a bright star and carry on a dialogue with the star, experiencing a sense of unity with her deceased husband somewhere in infinity. This provided her with calmness, wisdom, and clarity of thought.

- *Releasing anger and tears.* The release of anger, sadness, and tears is a cleansing process of the human spirit that makes a person more open to experience living in the moment. Holding grief in increases the suffering, fear, and separation.

- *Healing memories.* It is not necessary to stop thinking about the person who has died. Often, a grieving person who feels that the grief process is over finds that a memory, a song, or a meal suddenly evokes a sense of loss so deep that it seems as though it will never heal. The person needs to stay with the pain, sadness, guilt, anger, fear, or loneliness. Love and joy will begin to fill the heart again. The wisdom is to let the pain in and to stay open to it, to let the pain penetrate every cell in your body, to trust the pain, to know that what emerges from the pain is a new level of healing awareness.

- *Getting unstuck.* Grieving can bring on suffering; therefore, it may be helpful for survivors to ask for assistance from friends, family, or a healthcare professional to help them move past the blocks. Some people think, "It's been 6 months since my mother died [or a year since my husband, son, or wife died]. Why do I still feel so depressed and cry so frequently?"

Case Study (Implementation)

Case Study 1

Setting: Critical care unit where visiting schedule was one visitor every 2 hours
Patient: S. R., a 30-year-old mother of three children
Patterns/Challenges/Needs:

1. Decreased cardiac output related to end-stage heart failure
2. Grieving related to imminent death
3. Spiritual strength related to dynamic belief systems and family and friend support

S. R. said to the nurse, "I feel death over my right shoulder. Call my husband. I need him to come and bring my children, my parents, and my three friends. Tell them to come as soon as possible." The nurse also had an inner felt sense of the presence of death and began calling S. R.'s family. Four hours before her death, all of her family was present. Her friends sang her favorite songs as one played a guitar.

Case Study 2

Setting: Writing thoughts about healthy grief in a letter, 4 years after son's death
Client: V. D. J., a 45-year-old professional and mother
Patterns/Challenges/Needs: Spiritual strength related to the ability to deliberate the meaning of life, death, grief, and suffering

There is a holy purpose in grief and nothing should stand in its path. Grief begins with so few words. Sounds take shape traveling from a great distance. Within, a reserve is sensed. Something sacred that holds a luminous darkness that stills the mind even as the heart shudders with waves of deep sorrow. The natural quality of grief is ancient and bone bare. It tolerates nothing false. Grief is unrestrained; conscious effort is not required.

A mother who has lost a child learns what true freedom is. It is being cut free from the knot of habit, customs, rules. It is not being bound by considerations or even fear, for the worst has happened. Your child is dead, and you live. A mother's lament begins.

Your heartbeat creates a tone for your body to hear. It drums and moves you slowly forward with your family even as you weep and prepare to say your last goodbye. Now is not the time to be a bystander. It is crucial that you support and include your other children and family in the vigil, the wake, the funeral, and the burial or cremation ceremonies. They, too, are in shock and disbelief. And it does not end there.

Let nothing be left undone, unsaid, unwritten, or unsung in this farewell. This is not the place to lose courage or even your humor, for you will need both to sustain the intense suffering you have yet to bear. Nature provides the exact dosage for dealing with the constant strikes of pain experienced. Usually there is no real need for outside medication. Your body in its perfect wisdom gauges your requirements and numbs you accordingly. You will feel cold, but your mind–body will not allow more pain than you can tolerate. To disrupt the natural safeguards may only postpone the initial pain in your mourning process.

During the vigil and the wake your only thought is to do everything you can do to console your children and other family members. You realize they have the same concern for you. Plan the funeral ceremonies together. In the process, some small consolation may be experienced. The path of grief leads inward when you watch and listen. Did you not bring this spirit child into the world, flesh of your flesh? This last goodbye may enable you to complete the circle; keeping a vigil through the night allows you to be closer to your child.

The vigil with your child provides a place to begin to say goodbye, the goodbye you were both denied by sudden, unexpected death. You hear yourself talking and reassuring your son. You must now help your child to take the first steps into the great mystery, by talking aloud and guiding, much as you did when he was very young. Empty your mind and your heart, and give him all of your love and spiritual strength for his journey.

The week following the funeral I moved everything from my bedroom except basic essentials. I felt driven to sleep on a mat and to make a low altar that I filled with family photographs, mementos, childhood treasures belonging to Sean and my children, family poetry, drawings, vigil candles, prayer fans, fresh flowers, and ceremonial sage.

Prayers became conversations and chants and death songs for the son who had no time to create them for himself. Forty-nine days of talking-prayer, asking the angelic beings to guide my son on his journey. Each member of the immediate family scattered Sean's ashes in places special to him. A spirit bundle was placed and kept before the altar for him. Always the moving between worlds; letting go of the loneliness through weeping, sound, and moving prayer to returning to repose, listening, and sitting. A year goes by.

You find it difficult to speak. Your breathing habits are changing. You become aware of differences in your breath. You sense your heart breathing, your brain breathing. You notice that when you breathe out, you see thought. Some days you do not remember breathing at all.

You keep a journal as an ongoing discussion with your child, seeking solace. You somehow deal with daily life, guilt, illness, helplessness, and the grief of your other children.

Four more years go by; 4 years of dreams, voices, and mourning. I begin to understand the innate usefulness of creative work and humor as an antidote to loneliness and pain. My children need me and continually pull me onto the more solid ground where they stand. Dream walks, drumming, chanting, and round dancing lead me to my tribal traditions. My children personify the creative weaving of compassion, intelligence, and courage and remind me of how precious each individual life is and the miracle of being together with Sean and with each other in this life and in this time and in this place.

My son Sean has taught me that the true object of death is life. I have learned that a dream can be shaped by the dreamer; that in the act of sacrifice, the sacred is manifested through surrender of all that is.

Case Study 3

Setting: Bedroom at home of daughter (M. L.), who recently brought her ill mother (L. Y.) home to care for her

Patient: L. Y., a 90-year-old mother of two middle-aged adults, grandmother of two, who has been ill for 4 months; she had lived alone for the last 40 years

Patterns/Challenges/Needs:

1. Moderate pain related to diagnosis of cancer

2. Decreased cardiac output (including altered oxygenation) related to multisystem organ shutdown
3. Family grieving related to imminent death
4. Spiritual well-being and effective individual coping related to patient desire to care for her grieving family

M. L. checked with her mother to see that she was not in pain or distress prior to going out of the house on a short errand. L. Y. told her daughter to go, adding that she was quite comfortable and would be fine. M. L. noticed her mother's skin was mottled and cool, but her breathing was unlabored and she seemed peaceful. M. L.'s husband remained in the home. When M. L. returned, she found that her mother had stopped breathing. The bedclothes were unruffled, and her mother's face was peaceful. Her husband had heard nothing to indicate when the passing occurred. M. L. called the hospice nurse, the nun who was her neighbor and belonged to the same church, and other family members, and they carried out the ritual that they had planned for this moment. They held hands around the bed, prayed together in the ways of their tradition, and played a hymn that had been taped. After this, they informed the doctor, called the funeral director, and took care of legal obligations. A woman who had lived alone for 40 years had chosen to die alone, but cared for, to the end. The family grieving needs were also addressed.

Evaluation

With the patient (family and significant others), the nurse evaluates whether the patient outcomes for planning and implementing a peaceful death (see Exhibit 17-1) were successfully achieved. To evaluate the interventions further, the nurse may explore the subjective effects of the experience with the patient (family and significant others), using questions such as those shown in **Exhibit 17-1**.

Like peaceful living and dying, the care of a dying person and the family and significant others is an art. Preparing for death can be a series of conscious, spirit-filled, light-filled moments that lead to the ultimate peaceful moment of death. It is different for each person. True

EXHIBIT 17-1   Evaluating the Patient's (Family's and Significant Others') Subjective Experience with Perideath Nursing Interventions

1. How do you continue to recognize your anxiety, fear, and grief at this time?
2. Which of your strengths can best serve you as you move through this difficult time?
3. What are the things that you will do to take care of yourself at this time?
4. What are some questions and concerns that I can help you with now?
5. Will you call on others to help you?
6. Whom can you ask for help?
7. Were the imagery exercises helpful to you? Is prayer helpful to you?
8. Are there images, feelings, or emotions that surfaced during the imagery exercises that I can help you with?
9. Are there rituals that you can begin to create to help you deal with your grief?

Note: These subjective experiences may be used in helping a patient, family members, and significant others during the dying process or with the family or significant others during the grieving process.

healing and dying in peace come from integrating the creative process and the art of healing into our daily lives. The paradox is that, although this healing awareness may appear at first to be rare, it is a very ordinary and natural event that is available to each of us at all times. As each of us seeks to understand and integrate our spirit-filled lives as meaningful and connected with others throughout the ages, we learn about living and dying. The more we integrate solitude, inward-focused practice, and conscious awareness into daily life, the more peaceful is dying and the moment of death.

Directions for Future Research

1. Evaluate the attitudes and stress levels of nurses who work with death; determine whether rituals for nurses to use following death of patients might be useful in decreasing stress and helping grief.

2. Determine effective responses and nursing interventions for the increasing vulnerability of the dying person.
3. Develop empirically based therapeutic interventions to preserve dignity at the end of life.
4. Evaluate the use of life review in assisting patients with a sense of integration of life at the end of that life.
5. Determine the special needs of nurses who work with dying people who are friends and relatives or who have special experiences while dying (such as negative near-death experiences).
6. Explore and evaluate the use and effectiveness of *Golden Rooms* as superior and more satisfactory places to make the final transition.

Nurse Healer Reflections

After reading this chapter, the nurse healer will be able to answer or to begin a process of answering the following questions:

- Do I feel a greater sense of healing intention when I include relaxation, imagery, or music in my life every day?
- What are the effects on me when I guide others in healing modalities to facilitate peace in dying?
- How do I know that I am actively listening?
- Which new death mythologies and skills can assist me in releasing attachment to my physical body, possessions, and people?

NOTES

1. Roshan Cultural Heritage Institute, "Definition of Culture" (2011). www.roshan-institute.org/474552.
2. L. Keegan and C. A. Drick, "Theoretical Frameworks," in *End of Life: Nursing Solutions for Death with Dignity*, eds. L. Keegan & C. A. Drick (New York: Springer, 2011): 118.
3. J. Watson, *The Philosophy and Science of Caring*, rev. ed. (Boulder: University Press of Colorado, 2011).
4. B. Davies and R. Steele, "Supporting Families in Palliative Care," in *Textbook of Palliative Care*

Nursing, eds. B. F. Ferrell and N. Coyle (New York: Oxford University Press, 2011): 613–629.

5. M. Erseck and V. T. Cotter, "The Meaning of Hope in the Dying," in *Textbook of Palliative Care Nursing*, eds. B. F. Ferrell and N. Coyle (New York: Oxford University Press, 2011): 579–597.

6. M. Reblin, S. Otis-Green, L. Ellington, and M. F. Clayton, "Strategies to Support Spirituality in Health Care Communication: A Home Hospice Cancer Caregiver Case Study," *Journal of Holistic Nursing* 32, no. 4 (2014): 269–277.

7. E. Kübler-Ross, *On Death and Dying* (New York: Macmillan, 1969).

8. L. Keegan and C. A. Drick, *The Golden Room: A Practical Guide for Death with Dignity* (North Charleston, SC: CreateSpace Independent Publishing Platform, 2013).

9. R. Powazki, D. Walsh, B. Cothren, L. Rybicki, S. Thomas, G. Morgan, D. Karius, M. P. Davis, and S. Shrotriya, "The Care of the Actively Dying in an Academic Medical Center: A Survey of Registered Nurses' Professional Capability and Comfort," *American Journal of Hospice and Palliative Care* 31, no. 6 (2014): 619–627.

10. V. Frankl, *Man's Search for Meaning*, 3rd ed. (New York: Simon & Schuster, 1963).

11. G. Haugan, T. Rannestad, B. Hanssen, and G. A. Espnes, "Self-Transcendence and Nurse-Patient Interaction in Cognitively Intact Nursing Home Patients," *Journal of Clinical Nursing* 21, nos. 23–24 (2012): 3429–3441.

12. E. Jaul, Y. Zabari, and J. Brodsky, "Spiritual Background and Its Association with the Medical Decision of DNR at Terminal Life Stages," *Archives of Gerontology and Geriatrics* 58, no. 1 (2014): 25–29.

13. Growth House, *Life Review and Reminiscence Therapy* (San Francisco: Growth House, 2011).

14. P. R. Burns, "Myth and Legend from Ancient Times to the Space Age" (January 20, 2011). www.pibburns.com/myth.htm.

15. G. Luce, *Your Second Life: The SAGE Experience* (New York: Delacorte Press, 1979).

16. End-of-Life Nursing Education Consortium, *Graduate Curriculum: Faculty Guide* (Washington, DC: City of Hope and American Association of Colleges of Nursing, 2010).

17. J. L. Hollis, *Music at the End of Life: Easing the Pain and Preparing the Passage* (Santa Barbara, CA: Praeger, 2010).

18. L. J. Lutjen, N. R. Silton, and K. J. Flannelly, "Religion, Forgiveness, Hostility and Health: A Structural Equation Analysis," *Journal of Religion and Health* 51, no. 2 (2012): 468–478.

19. B. M. Reik, "Transgressions, Guilt and Forgiveness: A Model of Seeking Forgiveness," *Journal of Psychology and Theology* 38, no. 4 (2010): 246–254.

20. R. Fehr, M. J. Gelfand, and M. Nag, "The Road to Forgiveness: A Meta-Analytic Synthesis of Its Situational and Dispositional Correlates," *Psychological Bulletin* 136, no. 5 (2010): 894–914.

21. S. Levine, *A Gradual Awakening* (New York: Anchor Press, 1979).

22. S. Levine, *Healing into Life and Death* (New York: Doubleday, 1989).

23. J. Burnett, "Guided Imagery as an Adjunct to Pharmacologic Pain Control at End of Life" (October 2012). www.nacsw.org/Publications /Proceedings2012/BurnettJGuidedImagery.pdf.

24. C. Hammerschlag, *Healing Ceremonies*, Kindle ed. (Amazon Digital Services, 2011).

25. I. N. Oliver, *Investigating Prayer: Impact on Health and Quality of Life* (New York: Springer Science+Business Media, 2013).

26. J. J. Knabb, "Centering Prayer as an Alternative to Mindfulness-Based Cognitive Therapy for Depression Relapse Prevention," *Journal of Religion and Health* 51, no. 3 (2012): 908–924.

27. I. Tuck, S. C. Johnson, M. I. Kuznetsova, C. McCrocklin, M. Baxter, and L. K. Bennington, "Sacred Healing Stories Told at the End of Life," *Journal of Holistic Nursing* 30, no. 2 (2012): 69–80.

28. S. O'Mahony, J. McHenry, A. E. Blank, D. Snow, S. E. Karakas, G. Santoro, P. Selwyn, and V. Kvetan, "Preliminary Report of the Integration of a Palliative Care Team into an Intensive Care Unit," *Palliative Medicine* 24, no. 2 (2009): 154–165.

29. L. Keegan and C. A. Drick, *End of Life: Nursing Solutions for Death with Dignity* (New York: Springer, 2011): 40–41.

30. R. McCourt, J. J. Power, and M. Glackin, "General Nurses' Experiences of End-of-Life Care in the Acute Hospital Setting: A Literature Review," *International Journal of Palliative Nursing* 19 no. 10 (2013): 510–516.

31. S. A. Alsirafy, A. M. Abou-Alia, and H. M. Ghanem, "Palliative Care Consultation Versus Palliative Care Unit: Which Is Associated with Shorter Terminal Hospitalization Length of Stay Among Patients with Cancer?" *American Journal of Hospice and Palliative Care* (December 2, 2013). doi:10.1177/1049909113514476.

32. D. Lustbader, R. Pekmezaris, M. Frankenthaler, R. Walia, F. Smith, E. Hussain, B. Napolitano, and M. Lesser, "Palliative Medicine Consultation Impacts DNR Designation and Length of Stay for Terminal Medical MICU Patients," *Palliative Support Care* 9, no. 4 (2011): 401–406.

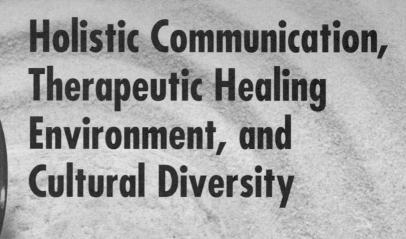

Holistic Communication, Therapeutic Healing Environment, and Cultural Diversity

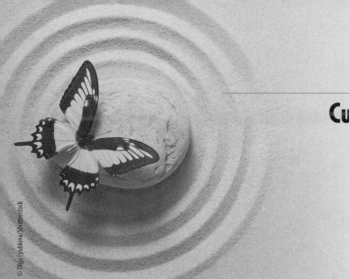

CHAPTER 18

Cultural Diversity and Care

Joan C. Engebretson

Nurse Healer Objectives

Theoretical

- Compare common value orientations associated with culture.
- Describe the influence of technology on cultural development and communication systems.
- Analyze components of cultural diversity.
- Describe the components and principles of cultural competence.
- Discuss cultural influences on beliefs and explanatory systems related to health and illness.

Clinical

- Discuss the role of culture in interactions with clients.
- Use components of transcultural assessment in caring for clients.
- Identify appropriate patterns, challenges, and needs of clients in the cultural domain.
- Explore interventions that reflect cultural competence.
- Discuss ways in which nursing interventions may be evaluated in relation to cultural competence.

Personal

- Clarify your own values, beliefs, and ideas related to your cultural heritage.
- Identify barriers in your own life to acceptance of cultural diversity.
- Explore activities that will increase your awareness and acceptance of cultural differences.

Definitions

Acculturation: The process of the adaptation or accommodation of an individual immigrant or immigrant group to a new culture.

Culturally competent health care: Health care delivered with knowledge of and sensitivity to cultural factors that influence the health and illness behaviors of an individual client, family, or community.

Culture: The values, beliefs, customs, social structures, and patterns of human activity and the symbolic structures that provide meaning and significance to human behavior.

Ethnicity: Designation of a population subgroup sharing a common social and cultural heritage.

Ethnocentrism: A worldview that is based to a great degree on the socialization of individuals within their own culture, to the extent that such individuals believe that all others see the world as they do.

Race: A social classification that denotes a biological or genetically transmitted set of distinguishable physical characteristics.

Stereotyping: Consigning cultural attributes to a group of people based on assumptions, opinions, or attitudes.

Xenophobia: An inherent fear or hatred of cultural differences.

Theory and Research

Culture is the combination of ideas, customs, skills, arts, and other capabilities of a people or group, although as a whole, it is more complex than any one of these elements. Culture is learned from birth through language acquisition and socialization and is the process by which an individual adapts to the group's organized way of life. This process also provides for the transmission of culture from one generation to another. Members of the cultural group share cultural values, beliefs, and patterns of behavior that create and reflect a group identity. This has a powerful influence on behavior, usually on a subconscious level. Culture is largely tacit, meaning it is not generally expressed or discussed at a conscious level. Most culturally derived actions are based on implicit cues rather than on written or spoken sets of rules.

Although many of the underlying beliefs and value systems of a culture are stable, all cultures are inherently dynamic and changing; therefore, it is difficult to generalize from one person, situation, or time to another. Cultural practices are continually adapting to the environment, historical context, technology, and availability of resources. As a result, the context in which people live influences, and is influenced by, cultural practices.

Anthropology, the study of cultures, and nursing are both based on a holistic perspective that incorporates the issues of context. Culture has a significant effect on health and illness behaviors, as well as patterns of response to illness or medical care. It directly influences health behaviors such as diet and exercise. Cultural beliefs and practices also affect the types of health problems that are attended to and the actions taken to deal with them. Activities taken to promote, maintain, or restore health are all performed in a cultural context. Therefore, an understanding of the client's perceptions and the context in which he or she lives is necessary for optimal client care.

Culture also determines much of the relationship and type of communication between a client and a healthcare provider. Given that the United States is a culturally diverse nation, nurses and other healthcare providers encounter individuals and groups whose habits of health maintenance, reactions to illness or disease, and use of healthcare services may differ from their own. An awareness of and accommodation to the cultural aspects of health and illness behaviors enables one to promote health by skillfully blending professional knowledge with knowledge of the individual's or group's beliefs. Culturally appropriate care is the delivery of health care with skill, knowledge, and sensitivity to cultural factors. With the increase of cultural pluralism in North America, it is essential that nurses develop cultural competency to deliver holistic care.

Cultural Competency

With increasing diversity in the population, and the recognition that health disparities exist across ethnic groups, healthcare regulatory agencies recommend that cultural competency become a goal in the provision of health care. In 2000, the Office of Minority Health developed the National Standards for Culturally and Linguistically Appropriate Services (CLAS) in Health and Health Care that included recommendations that applied to the institutional level as well as to the individual provider. These standards were enhanced in 2013 to provide a guide for national leadership to promote CLAS and health equity, support language assistance in institutions providing health care, and outline processes of quality improvement, community engagement, and evaluation.[1]

The idea of developing cultural competence has been increasingly discussed in the literature, and more recently the term *competency* has been challenged; however, it must be remembered that it is a process, not a destination.[2] Other concerns in the development of cultural sensitivity have focused on "cultural humility."[3] The National Center for Cultural Competency at Georgetown University developed an often-cited conceptual framework that describes a continuum from cultural destructiveness to cultural competency.[4] This continuum positions cultural destructiveness at the lowest level, with four intermediary steps to cultural proficiency at the top. This continuum can be viewed as corresponding to well-established values in medicine. **Figure 18-1** illustrates this continuum, along with parallel values in biomedicine and a recent value of evidence-based practice superimposed on the model.[5]

Cultural destructiveness, the lowest level of the continuum, corresponds to maleficence in medicine and this is countered through laws such as the Civil Rights Act of 1964 (Title VI), which mandates that healthcare providers do not discriminate according to race, ethnicity, or creed. The ethic of nonmaleficence, or "do no harm," also addresses this basic level. The second level of the continuum, cultural incapacity, corresponding to incompetence, refers to nonintentional practices that may be harmful to clients through ignorance, insensitive attitudes, or improper allocation of resources. Cultural blindness, the third level that corresponds to standardization, is exemplified by treating all patients alike without accommodating or recognizing cultural differences. Precompetence,

corresponding to outcomes-focused care, is the next step toward cultural competence and proficiency. Providing translators, developing health education aimed at specific cultural groups, and creating programs that address diverse groups' access to care are good examples of cultural precompetence, which is the fourth level. Cultural competence, the fifth level, is best described as an ongoing learning process for the provider, who can integrate cultural knowledge into individualized client-centered care. This eventually leads to the highest level of the continuum, cultural proficiency. These two levels correspond to the movement to patient-centered care, or to what holistic nurses would identify as individually focused holistic care.

Evidence-based practice has been an important issue in healthcare delivery. It grew out of the outcomes-focused value, as an effort to incorporate the best research evidence in healthcare delivery. In the focus on applying these findings, many revert back to standardized care or cultural blindness. According to some of the leaders in the evidence-based practice field, practicing in a culturally competent manner incorporates three aspects of evidence-based practice:

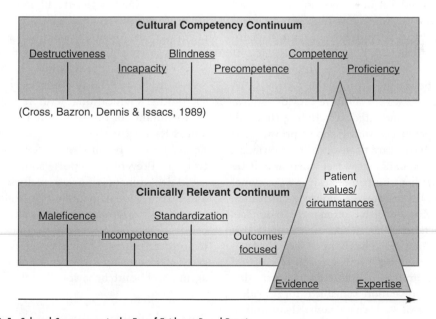

FIGURE 18-1 Cultural Competence in the Era of Evidence-Based Practice

Source: Reprinted from Journal of Professional Nursing 24, no. 3, J. Engebretson, J. Mahoney, and E. Carlson, "Cultural Competence in the Era of Evidence-Based Practice," pages 172–178, Copyright 2008 with permission from Elsevier.

best evidence from valid and clinically relevant research, the provider's clinical expertise, and the client's values, unique preferences, and situation.[6] The emphasis on the client's values, preferences, and situation moves evidence-based practice into cultural competence and proficiency. Much of the literature in cultural competency also tends to focus only on the evidence or the studies or the literature that describe particular ethnic groups. It is important for holistic nurses to recognize that applying that information to clients of a specific ethnic group is only at the precompetence level at best. However, at the individual patient–provider encounter, it must be individually based and patient centered.

Culturally competent health care must be provided within the context of a client's cultural background, beliefs, and values related to health and illness to attain optimal client outcomes. To enhance one's understanding of cultural issues, it is therefore important for nurses to continue their understanding of cultural diversity. In addition to the Transcultural Nursing Society, there is a corpus of literature in nursing about cultural competence.[7-12]

A plethora of sensitivity training and educational programs has been implemented, and curricula have been developed in nursing and other healthcare professions. Lipson and Desantis reviewed several approaches to nursing education and concluded that there is a lack of consensus on what should be taught and how it should be integrated into the curricula.[13] A systematic review of healthcare provider education was also conducted, concluding that cultural competence training shows promise for improving healthcare professionals' knowledge, attitudes, and skills. However, there was little evidence of client outcomes.[14] Most educational approaches have addressed knowledge, attitudes, and skills. Knowledge has often focused on facts and characteristics about specific cultures. This "cookbook" approach has been criticized as leading to stereotyping. The approach of cultural sensitivity training attempts to address attitudes. What seems to be more valuable is for providers to learn a set of skills that enables them to provide high-quality client care to everyone.

In a literature review of cultural competence and the clinical encounter, Betancourt concludes that healthcare providers develop the skills for a client-centered approach that does the following: (1) assesses core cross-cultural issues, (2) explores the meaning of the illness to the patient, (3) determines the social context in which the patient lives, and (4) engages in a negotiation process with the patient.[15] Cultural competence represents an important element of clinical care and skills that are central to professionalism across disciplines. The relationship between cultural competency and improvement in health outcomes is not yet firmly established and more research is warranted.[16] Although there is much emphasis now on developing cultural competency, there is also an increasing awareness that competency is always a growth process, which means that it requires more than an accumulation of facts about different cultures.[17] The clinical encounter, in which cultural competency is most demanding, requires individual- or family-centered care.[18]

Cultural Diversity and Health Disparities

Despite the fact that human beings are 99.9% identical at the DNA level, there are differences in prevalence of illness between groups. This may be explained by genetic differences; dietary, cultural, environmental, and socioeconomic factors; or combinations thereof.[19] Health disparities in the United States exist for multiple health outcomes. For example, in the United States, infant mortality is inversely related to the mother's educational level. It is also highest for infants of non-Hispanic black mothers and is lowest for those of Chinese mothers.[20] According to a recent Centers for Disease Control and Prevention report, some of the key social determinants of health include education and income, inadequate and unhealthy housing, unhealthy air quality, and health insurance coverage.[21] Socioeconomic status underlies three major determinants of health: access to health care, environmental exposure to health-related agents, and health behaviors.[22]

Race and Ethnicity

Ethnicity refers to values, perceptions, feelings, assumptions, and physical characteristics associated with ethnic group affiliation. Often, *ethnicity* refers to nationality—a group sharing a common social and cultural heritage. In contrast, *race* typically refers to a biological, genetically transmitted set of distinguishable physical characteristics. In some literature, however, *race* has often been misused to describe differences in people that have no basis in biology or science. Demographic data are commonly gathered with no differentiation of ethnicity or definitions of race. Both skin color and country of origin have been used to classify race. For example, many natives of India (considered racially Caucasian) have darker skin than do many natives of Africa.

Race and culture have significant relationships to illness states because biological differences can make certain groups of people vulnerable to specific diseases. For example, genetic predisposition for sickle cell disease affects people of African and Mediterranean descent; predisposition for Tay-Sachs disease affects Ashkenazi Jews. Also, certain diseases that may be attributable to a combination of genetic predisposition and lifestyle, including nutritional patterns, are more prevalent in some groups. One example is the disproportionately high prevalence of diabetes in Native Americans and Hispanics. Some diseases are connected to lifestyle risks, such as substance abuse and human immunodeficiency virus (HIV) infection, which are related to particular social behaviors. An emerging body of information on the differences in response to pharmaceuticals by ethnic and racial groups has led to a new field of pharmacogenomics.[23, 24] Cultural subgroups can be identified by virtue of shared experiences or circumstances that may influence values, beliefs, and behaviors. Ethnicity is the most common cultural demarcation, but intraethnic variations may be more pronounced than interethnic variations, especially in a culturally pluralistic society. Other variables that have been proposed as influencing cultural groupings are religion, socioeconomic status, geographic region, age, common beliefs, and professional orientation, such as nursing and medicine.

Factors Related to Culture

Along with ethnicity, religion is an important factor in determining the values and beliefs of a culture.[25] Religion, an organized system of beliefs that binds people together, is differentiated from spirituality, which is born out of each individual's personal experience in finding meaning and significance in life. Religious faith and the institutions derived from that faith have a powerful influence over human behavior. All religions have experiential, ritualistic, ideological, intellectual, and consequential dimensions. Religious views have historically served as a unifying force for groups of people with a set of core values and beliefs.

Socioeconomic status refers to an individual's social status, occupation, education, economic status, or a combination of these. Socioeconomic explanations are often discounted when determining the relationships between ethnicity or race and health status or health. It is necessary to distinguish between cultural identification and the common experience of being poor in our society. By illustration, the experience of being poor in our society is different from that of being Hispanic and also must be further distinguished from being both poor and Hispanic. The effect of socioeconomic status on both morbidity and mortality measures of specific groups is highly significant and is related to health disparities; lower socioeconomic status groups have higher morbidity and mortality rates for various diseases.[26]

The local or regional manifestations of the larger culture bring up such distinctions as rural, urban, southern, or Midwestern. For example, African Americans living in the southern region of the United States may have beliefs and behaviors different from those in the northern region, based somewhat on their heritage of slavery and exposure to the civil rights movement.

Age of the individuals within a cultural group has a profound influence on their beliefs and behaviors as well. Value systems are tied to historically shared events that occur in childhood; therefore, each generation develops a unique value system. For example, there is much in the popular literature about the differences among generations: baby boomers (people born from 1945–1965), Generation X (1966–1980), and Generation Y (1981–2000). As a society, we have moved from the Industrial Age to the

Information Age—and this new age affects everyone through its influence on cultural values, beliefs, and the sharing of information.

Common beliefs or ideologies may unite a cultural group or subculture, as well as differentiate that group from the larger culture. These value systems may be related to religion (e.g., the Amish), lifestyle (e.g., communal groups), sexual orientation (e.g., gay and lesbian groups), or political ideologies (e.g., feminist separatist groups). Social or professional orientations often constitute a type of cultural grouping. Medical anthropologists have described the biomedical system as a cultural system.[27] The biomedical culture of many hospitals constitutes an unfamiliar culture for many laypeople. Healthcare professionals use unique and esoteric language, as well as rituals, roles, expectations, patterns of behavior, and symbolic communication that are often alien to the layperson.

Common Myths and Errors

Errors of stereotyping are common among those who define the world by strict categories of ethnicity or race. It is also problematic to presume that all members of another culture conform to a common pattern without regard to individual characteristics or the variety found within one cultural grouping. For example, some people assume that all African Americans eat soul food or that all Hispanics are Catholic. Failure to recognize that values from a particular cultural group can vary across time and location leads to stereotyping cultures with values that no longer guide the group's or the individual's thinking or behavior. Stereotyping is less obvious in some cases, such as a nurse manager assigning all Hispanic clients to the Mexican American nurse. Such action does not take into account the differences within the Hispanic group, presumes that all Hispanics are alike, and disregards the individual.

The heterogeneity of ethnic groups is often underestimated, but as mentioned earlier, the variations within ethnic groups may be as great or greater than those between ethnic groups. For example, the Hispanic culture includes persons of Puerto Rican, Cuban, Spanish, and South and Central American origins. These people are from many different socioeconomic backgrounds and represent the Caucasian, Mongoloid, and Negroid racial groups. Sometimes Asians from different countries and backgrounds are grouped together and treated as generic Asians, an attitude that totally ignores the historical differences among Asians. Kipnis relates a clinical incident that occurred in Hawaii in which a Korean client with a serious medical condition refused a treatment that promised a better than 50% recovery with minimal risks.[28] Clinical staff were puzzled by his refusal of treatment coupled with his request for life support if he experienced cardiopulmonary arrest. On further investigation, he mentioned that all of his physicians were Japanese. In the early 1900s, Japan had ruthlessly tyrannized Korea, much as the Nazis in Germany tyrannized Poland prior to and during World War II. Thus, the Korean gentleman very much wanted to live, but his cultural history caused him to refuse treatment directed by the Japanese physicians.

Ethnocentrism is the tendency, usually unconscious, for individuals to take for granted their own values as the only objective reality and to look at everyone else through the lens of their own cultural norms and customs. Ethnocentric views often result from a lack of knowledge of other cultures and the presumption that one's own behavior is not influenced by culture. Many people of the dominant culture falsely assume that they have no cultural practices and beliefs. This restrictive view of the world often perceives people and cultures with different beliefs and behaviors as culturally inferior. An extreme and more conscious form of ethnocentrism is xenophobia, an inherent fear of cultural differences, which often leads people to bolster their security in their own values by demeaning the beliefs and traditions of others. This attitude often takes the form of prejudice or racism.

Cultural imposition is the perception that successful cultural adaptation involves a change to the cultural views of the dominant group, regardless of an individual's cultural heritage. This posits an inherent view that the dominant culture is superior, and its values are imposed on others.

Often disguised as equal treatment for everyone, cultural blindness ignores cultural differences as if they did not exist. This view overlooks real diversity and the importance of other perspectives. The concept of the "melting pot" assumes that, in the process of acculturation and assimilation, everyone takes on significant aspects of the dominant culture such that the original culture is largely lost. This assimilation or melting pot view is challenged by concepts of heritage consistency, which is the degree to which one maintains practices and beliefs that reflect one's own heritage. A more appropriate metaphor is a stew where each component retains original characteristics but takes on the overall flavor of the stew.

Development of Cultural Patterns and Behaviors

Anthropologists have studied practices among cultures in relation to the universal experience of being human. Their major focus has been on the variation of ways that humans organize and structure their social world. Some of the factors that contribute to the development of cultural patterns and behavior are geography and migration, gender-specific roles, value orientations and cultural beliefs, and technological development.

Geography and Migration

Social groups evolve through interaction with the climate, as well as in conjunction with the availability of food and resources. The persistence of dietary patterns reflects the types of food available in a particular region. For example, fish constitutes a large portion of the traditional diet of people from Norway and the Philippines, whereas dairy products and meats are dominant in the food patterns of Finland and Germany.

Social organization falls in line with these geographic patterns. For example, the social structure of a fishing village differs from that of a nomadic group that hunts for food, and from that of a settled agrarian culture. Urbanization and industrialization are also important for the way society organizes and social roles develop. Social roles become patterned and often institutionalized into hierarchical structures that reflect social, economic, and political power. These social structures and roles greatly alter

people's daily lives and the economics of providing for families.

Climate, environmental conditions, and political and economic factors are very important in migration patterns. Climate change, famine, political upheaval, and overpopulation have all been responsible for migration. For example, a large wave of Irish immigrants came to the United States in the late 1840s following a potato famine that was causing starvation, disease, and death in Ireland. Many immigrants came to the United States to flee political unrest in El Salvador in the 1980s. Many Vietnamese and Southeast Asians sought political refuge and opportunities in the United States following the Vietnam War. A large number of nurses seeking professional and economic opportunities moved to the mainland United States from the Philippines in the 1980s. Even in the 1990s and the early 21st century, a large number of immigrants have steadily come to the United States seeking economic opportunities or fleeing political oppression.

Cultural patterns change through the sharing of ideas, beliefs, and practices that follow trade or migration. Immigrants bring cultural patterns, values, and beliefs with them. Along with their adaptation to the new host culture, they expose the host culture to a different set of cultural beliefs and practices. Both cultures assimilate aspects of the other.

The historical context of immigration is important and varies among groups. Many African Americans arrived involuntarily and endured a lengthy history of slavery. Hispanics may be immigrants seeking economic opportunity, refugees from political upheavals, or descendants of people living in the Southwest before it became a part of the United States. The fact that many Asian immigrants find it necessary to take a job with lower status than they had in their country of origin creates cultural and economic hardship for the family. In many Hispanic families, the father immigrates alone to establish a better economic future for the family. Estranged from the family, he may be vulnerable to such behavioral health risks as acquired immune deficiency syndrome (AIDS) and alcohol abuse. Health issues may also arise because of low income and low self-esteem.

Acculturation is an important process in the adaptation, assimilation, or accommodation of immigrant groups to a new culture. This is sometimes referred to as hybridization. This is because in the process of adapting to a new culture, immigrants integrate the new culture into their beliefs and lifestyle and yet retain heritage consistency, maintaining pride in and adhering to their parent culture. According to the Theory of Orthogonal Cultural Identification, this process does not take place along a single continuum but rather has numerous dimensions that operate independently from one another.[29] Intergenerational gaps frequently develop because the youth become more quickly acculturated to the dominant society, and they may challenge the more traditional values, beliefs, and customs of their parents. This, in turn, may threaten the integrity and lines of respect in the family and roles within the family and society, particularly the role of women. Conflicts that arise from intergenerational gaps can lead to the alienation of young people and families from both the ethnic culture and the general dominant culture.

Gender Roles

All cultures develop socially sanctioned roles for respective genders. Over the past century, the social role for women in the United States has undergone many changes. The role of women has expanded from its traditional focus on childbearing and child rearing to include participation in the workplace and marketplace. The feminist movement has championed this expanded role and has heightened consciousness about opportunities consistent with the American values of individualism, equality, and political freedom. Furthermore, the feminist movement has challenged the values and structures developed by elite, masculine power, such as competition, a strong focus on objectives and goals, the harnessing and control of nature, principle-based ethics, and productive activities. Feminists often have promoted cultural practices and organizations that espouse more feminine values such as teamwork, focus on social process, working in harmony with nature, relationship-based ethics, and social connections. As people from other cultures move into

the United States, these differing values and expanded roles for women may challenge the traditional family roles. In some cases where women's roles take a more traditional position, a woman may need to get her husband's or father's permission prior to receiving medical care for herself or her children.

Women have played significant roles in the healing arts as well. Historically and cross-culturally, women have discovered and preserved information about healing herbs and plants. In the Middle Ages, women were often persecuted for their knowledge of plants and other healing arts, which were deemed mysterious and suspicious. As medicine became more scientific and moved into a professional and scientific status, women became disengaged from the official healing roles.[30] Women were associated with nature and men with developing technology to tame and control nature. Women's roles in the healing arts reflected this dichotomy. With the establishment of medical professions, women's roles even in midwifery—a traditional role for women—were reduced, and physicians took over the practice and moved childbirth into hospitals. Women who worked in medical professions were often in nonphysician roles or positions of lower power and social status, such as nurses, social workers, and physical therapists. However, women are increasingly moving into leadership positions and have had a strong presence among complementary healers and users of complementary therapies.[31]

Basic Value Orientations and Beliefs

All cultures hold certain value orientations that are central to their cultural patterns of behavior. These values can be both implicit and explicit. They influence an individual's perception of others, direct that individual's responses to others, and reflect his or her identity. These values are the basis for understanding oneself and one's social relationships, political and economic structures, and direct and motivated behavior. These values are generally quite stable and do not change quickly. In a classic work on cultural orientations, Kluckhohn identified five categories by which cultures address universal concerns of human nature.[32]

1. Innate human nature as being good, evil, or mixed
2. Human beings' relationship to nature as being subjugated to the forces of nature, harmonious coexistence with nature, or using human abilities to master nature
3. Relationship to time as past oriented, present oriented, or future oriented
4. Purpose of being seen as focused on self-realization or a more action-orientation focus on doing
5. Relationship to other persons as expressed in individual, familial, or communal orientations

In Western culture and in particular the United States, these value orientations are reflected in a strong emphasis on individualism, mastery over nature, future-focused time orientation, and an action orientation to being. This can be seen in health care when we view the individual as the client and often ignore the family. Our mastery over nature is illustrated in our efforts to understand and cure disease and control health issues. Future orientation is reflected in our goal orientation and an emphasis on the effect our actions may have on the future. Both healthcare providers and clients expect some type of action or treatment from the clinical encounter. This reflects the shared value of an action-oriented culture. The healthcare system both influences and is influenced by the general cultural orientations. Cultural conflicts may occur when we fail to recognize that our clients hold differing value orientations.

Worldviews and cosmologies essential to Western Judeo-Christian-Islam beliefs differ from those of other world religions. Three dominant cosmology assumptions foundational to Western Judeo-Christian-Islam beliefs are monotheism, transcendence, and dualism.[33] Monotheism, the belief in one God or Creator who is separate from humans, contrasts with the beliefs common in many agrarian societies, whose members believe in polytheism (i.e., multiple gods with different attributes) or pantheism (i.e., the locus of the sacred in all living things). The Western view of transcendence, or relating to God as separate from humans and knowing God through prayer, supplication,

and rituals, can be contrasted with the Eastern view of immanence, or finding God by looking inward and doing other spiritual exercises to discover the sacred. Finally, Western dualism, the separation of material from nonmaterial aspects of being, is in contrast to monism, or the essential unity found in both the pantheistic and Eastern belief systems. Many "new age" perspectives are exploring these issues as they are exposed to different cultural beliefs.

Technology and Culture

In contemporary Western culture, as well as in much of the world, technology is widely expanding as we move into the Information Age. The development of technology affects values, religion, politics, economics, and the arts and sciences. Medical technology in particular has progressed in its development of intricate instruments that allow for more complex procedures, such as computer-based imaging, microsurgery, gene mapping, targeted therapies, and pharmacogenomics. The development of these technologies poses new ethical and cultural questions related to the human and social effects this technology may have. Often the use of these technologies challenges existing cultural values. Once the technology is available for use, it often becomes the fuel for ethical debates related to such issues as allocation of resources, fetal tissue transplantation and right to life, and genetic testing and right to privacy.

Technology has also held a powerful influence on culture through its use in communication, which affects not only how information is conveyed, but also what type of knowledge is valued.[34] Traditionally, knowledge was passed on by oral means in stories, parables, and poetry. Essential knowledge (i.e., cultural wisdom associated with oral tradition) was preserved through memory, often aided by rhythm and rhyme. Many cultures today have their roots in oral traditions.

With the advent of written communication, the Western world became a different culture based on the type of knowledge that was conveyed and developed. Printed materials recorded information with detail, precision, and accuracy in a way that oral speech could not. The ability to read this information also facilitated discussions and formation of complex thoughts. Thus, scientific and factual information gained value, giving rise to the development of modern scholarship.

Today's electronic culture, dependent on cell phones, radio, television, tablets, and computers to communicate information, has an enormous influence on the beliefs, values, and behaviors of contemporary society. In relation to health care, clients have access to a plethora of health-related information from multiple sources. This has presented new challenges for healthcare providers to help clients interpret information and make appropriate choices.

Changing Beliefs and Values

Recently, people in the developed and industrialized world have been exposed to several different cultures as a result of both immigration and electronic technology. Electronic media, allowing for fast and more universal dispersal of information, has promoted intercultural communication throughout the world as never before. Such communication has led to unprecedented exposure to different cultures, with results ranging from attempts to integrate diverse ideas to overt conflict and violence. Scientific and technologic advances, as well as global, political, social, and economic changes, have challenged existing cultural systems and increased the velocity of cultural change.

A large marketing survey indicated that the U.S. population could be divided into three groups according to values. Ray identified one of these groups, cultural creatives, as those who were on the leading edge of change, comprising nearly one-quarter of the population.[35] This group held a holistic philosophy of health; valued ecologic preservation, spirituality, relationships, and self-actualization; and expressed interest in other cultures and new ideas. The largest group identified (47%), the moderns, placed a high value on success, consumerism, materialism, and technologic rationality. The third group (29%), the traditionalists or heartlanders, believed in the nostalgic images of small towns and strong churches that defined the "good old American way."

In a survey of more than 1,000 adults, Astin found that those who use alternative and complementary therapies generally have a higher education level, have a more holistic orientation to health, and often have been through a transformational experience that changed their worldview. They also were more likely to have had a chronic health problem or other recent illness.[36] This group expressed a set of values, beliefs, and philosophic orientations that included commitment to environmentalism and feminism and an interest in spirituality and personal growth. Other studies have described these consumers as generally well educated and affluent members of the middle class.[37] The use of complementary therapies and the search for holistic approaches to health care are often associated with the middle class; however, it should be noted that most survey instruments generally do not include ethnic healing practices.

Ethnic Groups in North America

Culturally diverse groups in the United States have grown to substantial proportions of the population. In their practice, nurses are likely to encounter representatives of different ethnicities and cultures. General descriptions of these various ethnic groups may provide helpful orientations to the groups. It is important to remember that there is much diversity within ethnicities and that in the processes of globalization and exposure to other cultures, these cultural beliefs are dynamic. Therefore, it is extremely important for nurses to avoid stereotyping. Reading about and engaging in discussions and activities with members of these cultural groups can help to avoid stereotypic interpretations of these groups and aid in developing cultural competency. The compiled U.S. Census data provide estimates for 2013.[38]

American Indians and Alaska Natives

According to the census data, American Indians and Alaska Natives (AIAN) are classified as AIAN alone or AIAN mixed with another race. The combined group represents 1.7% of the total population.[38] They have a higher rate of poverty than does the population as a whole.

They often cluster in tribal groups, with the largest concentrations located in the Pacific and western mountain regions of the United States. There is considerable variation among the tribes regarding language, beliefs, customs, health practices, and rituals. Tribes or clans constitute a social unit in which members may or may not be blood relatives, and both family and clan are powerful sources of the Native American's identity and support. Largely because of the respect for the wisdom accrued with aging, elders are typically the community leaders. Value orientations center on harmony with nature, a present-time orientation, and an integration of rituals and religion into everyday life. Many Native Americans still adhere to folk healing practices, seeking out local healers before going to a healthcare clinic. Folk healing practices may fall into the shamanic category or often are understood in a supranormal paradigm. Common health problems include diabetes, obesity, infectious disease, alcohol abuse, and diseases associated with poverty. Years of racism, dehumanization, and oppression have left a legacy in which many Native Americans may mistrust Caucasian healthcare providers.

European Americans

The largest ethnic group in North America is made up of European Americans or whites. According to the Census Bureau, they constitute the dominant culture and comprise approximately 76.2% of the population of the United States. However, that percentage is declining. White persons, not Hispanic, constitute 62.4% of the population.[38] The largest emigrations from various regions in Europe occurred in the late 1700s, all through the 1800s, and into the first half of the 20th century. Many immigrants to the United States carried the European ideas of the Age of Reason, dominance over nature, and the belief in progress and technologic advancement. Their quest for freedom enhanced an abiding value of individualism. They are generally action oriented, future directed, and focused on progress and productivity. Families are an important social unit among European Americans, but the value of individualism is pervasive. Although this group is diverse, the values are usually consistent with dominant values of the culture. Therefore, members of this group may not be as aware of the role that culture plays in their lives as the members of other cultural groups are.

African Americans

The 2013 Census estimates the number of African Americans (AA), also classified as AA alone or combined with another group, in the United States to be 13.8% of the population.[38] This number and proportion have grown since the 2000 census. The highest concentrations of African Americans are in the South and on the East Coast. One-third of this population was younger than age 18 in 2000. This group is very heterogeneous and varies in economic status, religion, education, and regional background. Many African Americans are descendants of slaves who were brought to the United States; others are recent immigrants from Africa and the Caribbean Islands. Within the social structure of slavery, families were dispersed and individuals were not allowed to read. Thus, a tradition of strong matriarchal family units with a rich oral tradition developed. Social organization centers on the family, kinship bonds, and the church. Some of the health disparities among African Americans may be related to the disproportional rate of poverty. Many African Americans have absorbed much of the dominant culture, but some adhere to ancestral beliefs of illness as disharmony with nature and supranormal healing rituals or folk healing. The history of slavery and the Tuskegee atrocities have made some African Americans mistrustful of receiving professional health care or participating in clinical research studies.

Asian Americans

Constituting 6.0% of the total U.S. population, Asian Americans are expected to represent 9% of the population by 2050.[38] Approximately two-thirds reside in the western part of the United States. This group is composed of immigrants and refugees from the Pacific Rim countries, such as China, Japan, Korea, Thailand, Laos, Vietnam, Cambodia, the Philippines, and other

Asian countries. People from India are often included in this group as well. There is wide diversity in language, customs, and beliefs in this group. Traditional Asian families tend to be patriarchal, revere their elders, and value achievement and honor. Certain infectious diseases, such as tuberculosis and hepatitis, are common among Asian Americans, depending on the country from which they emigrated. Stress-related diseases and suicides are high, as many do not seek mental health care because of an associated stigma and a threat to honor. Asians' traditional health practices often are oriented around the balance paradigm in which health is equated with balance and unimpeded flow of energy or *chi*. Traditional healing includes the use of herbal preparations, and many families practice traditional dermabrasion procedures such as coining, pinching, or rubbing.

Pacific Islanders and Native Hawaiians

The Native Hawaiian and Other Pacific Islander (NHPI) population constituted 0.4% of the U.S. population in the 2013 estimates.[38] Native Hawaiians are the largest subgroup, although the majority of this group reported one or more other races as well. Nearly three-fourths of this population lives in the West, with more than half living in California and Hawaii combined. There is great diversity in beliefs and customs. As an aggregate group, NHPIs are socioeconomically disadvantaged and underserved in terms of access to social and health services. Pacific Islanders have high rates of health-related risk behaviors, such as smoking, heavy alcohol consumption, and high fat and caloric intake, which leads to obesity.

Hispanics

The Hispanic population in the United States constituted 17.1% of the U.S. population in the 2013 estimates and is rapidly growing.[38] The majority of these immigrants come from Mexico, with others from Puerto Rico, Cuba, and Central and South America. This is the fastest growing group in the United States. Although the Spanish language is a common factor, there is much diversity in dialects and cultural practices. This group comprises indigenous peoples of the Americas, Spanish and other European settlers, and some African-Caribbean groups. Predominant religions are Catholicism and Pentecostalism. The family and extended family are important, and the family unit is traditionally patriarchal. Many believe that illness may be punishment for sins or the result of witchcraft or *brujería*, meaning the "evil eye." Traditional health beliefs regarding hot and cold remedies for various maladies reflect humeral balance beliefs. Healing also incorporates many spiritual elements, such as worship of saints and use of talismans.

Effect of Culture on Health Care

Concepts of health and healing are rooted in culture. The concept of disease generally refers to the diagnostic label or categorization of a disorder that medicine treats, whereas the concept of illness incorporates the personal, social, and cultural aspects of the experience. Cultural practices influence an individual's behavior to promote, maintain, and restore health and how, when, and with whom the individual seeks help or treatment. Cultural beliefs, values, and practices are also extremely important in birth and death.

Cultural understandings of health and illness reflect larger philosophic worldviews, or paradigms, that provide a way of understanding the body and the forces that influence health and illness. According to Andrews and Boyle, there are three major types of cross-cultural paradigms: magicoreligious, holistic, and scientific.[39] Although aspects of all three are found in most cultures, one usually predominates.

In the magicoreligious health paradigm, the fate of the world depends on God, gods, or supernatural forces. Events such as sorcery, breach of taboo, intrusion of a disease-causing spirit, or loss of soul are considered responsible for illness. This paradigm relates to a psychic or metaphysical need of humanity for integration and harmony. For example, people from some African-Caribbean cultures believe that parts of a person such as hair, fingernails, or blood represent the person and can be used in healing.

Also, they may believe that lack of protection for these body parts can make the person vulnerable to illness.

In the holistic health paradigm, the forces of nature must be kept in harmony according to natural laws and the larger universe. These systems often have a strong emphasis on health rather than on the treatment of disease. In ayurvedic medicine from India, for example, health results from being in harmony with oneself, others, and the environment. Diet and activity are adapted according to the individual's *doshas* (i.e., forces of the human body whose composition varies among individuals) and the seasonal variations in the environment. In Western culture, this idea appears in humoral theories, such as the concepts of balancing hot and cold held by Hispanic, Arab, African, Caribbean, and other societies. Holistic health care is regaining some popularity in developed countries, which are currently the bastions of the scientific paradigm, as the focus begins to shift to promoting health.

The scientific or biomedical paradigm is characterized by four main concepts.

1. *Determinism.* A cause-and-effect relationship exists for all natural phenomena.
2. *Mechanism.* The relationship of life to the structure and function of machines suggests the possibility of control through mechanical or engineered interventions.
3. *Reductionism.* The division of all life into isolated smaller parts, such as the dualism of mind and body, facilitates the study of the whole.
4. *Objective materialism.* That which is real can be observed and measured.

This paradigm is the basis for healthcare systems in Western society, where disease is viewed as the "enemy," the body is the "battlefield," and the physician is the "general." Great effort, expense, and technology are invested in determining the underlying cause of disease. The "system at fault" is isolated, and the most medical attention is directed toward measuring the functions of, and repairing, this faulty part. Persons are often placed in foreign environments (e.g., hospitals) in which limited attention is given to individual needs and cultural

beliefs. Anthropologists have also described the healthcare system as a culture with its historical underpinnings in the scientific approach, mind–body dualism, and reflecting American or Western capitalism.[40]

Kleinman, a much referenced medical anthropologist, has described three sectors of health care that are common in all healthcare systems: professional, popular, and folk.[41] Cultures vary widely in the way that they combine these three systems. Usually, one is dominant, although simultaneous use is common. In the United States, the *professional*, or orthodox biomedical, sector of health care has held a legal, political, and ideological monopoly for most of the 20th century. This sector corresponds to the scientific paradigm described earlier. Nurses and other healthcare professionals are part of this sector.

The *popular* sector includes all of the personal and social networks that laypeople use to understand their health and plan their health care. Individuals, family, and social networks determine whom to consult, when to seek a consultation, whether to adhere to suggested treatments, when to switch treatments, and how to evaluate the usefulness of treatments. Nearly all persons are active in their own healthcare decisions and practice some form of private or self-prescribed health care. This is the area where the majority of health decisions are made and the one that is the least studied or understood. All secular and sacred healers who are generally outside the professional sector make up the *folk* sector. This sector also includes healing practices used to promote health and treat illness. Many of the currently popular complementary healing practices are in this sector.

Explanatory Models of Health and Illness

Kleinman describes explanatory models as notions that individuals or groups have about understanding the causes, symptoms, and treatments of illness.[41] Culturally specific explanatory models are interpretations of the culture's worldview as it pertains to health and healing and generally provide an understanding of disease and direct treatment. Explanatory models of health and healing are used to recognize, interpret, respond to, cope with, and make sense of an illness experience. For example, a client who believes that the cause of his or her illness is related to committing a sin or breaking a taboo may not accept biomedical treatment as a cure. Some form of catharsis, forgiveness, or ritual may be necessary. Some of these explanatory models are associated with the three sectors of health care. For example, the professional sector has a particular explanatory mode that may differ from various models in the folk or popular sectors.

Kleinman recommends that clinicians explore the explanatory models of their clients in an effort to promote better communication. These questions elicit a framework that allows the clinician to compare the client's explanatory model of etiology, pathology, course of the disease, treatment, and possible outcomes with those of the medical model. Kleinman recommends specific questions to explore what the client calls the disorder and what caused it, as well as what he or she thinks is happening, will happen, and might make it better or worse.

Giger and Davidhizar and many anthropologists describe explanatory models of folk medicine as classifying diseases or illnesses as natural or unnatural.[42] Natural events arise from the way that a higher power made the world and intended it to be. The basic principle is that everything in nature is connected and events can be explained in terms of this relationship. In some folk sectors, disease represents a disturbance in that relationship with nature. A natural disease or illness results from a disturbance in the person's relationship or balance with nature, and recovery requires the restoration of this relationship. This view is common among Native Americans, whose concept of medicine embraces the forces of nature. Because death is seen as part of the life cycle and a component of natural harmony, a cure for illness is not necessarily sought. Unnatural illnesses are often attributed to punishment from a higher power for one's sins or improper behavior. The origin of unnatural illnesses in folk medicine is based on the continuous battle between good and evil forces. Witchcraft and breaking of a taboo are sometimes considered the origin for unnatural illnesses.

Multiparadigm Model of Healing

As Western culture is becoming increasingly culturally pluralistic, several alternative and complementary healing practices and beliefs are surfacing. The word *holistic* is related to the word *health*, which stems from the root word *hale*, the same root as "to make whole." This definition would necessarily incorporate multiple approaches to support health. One effort to place diverse modalities, including biomedicine, into a unified model is illustrated in **Exhibit 18-1**.[43] Paradigms of health and healing are based in underlying philosophy, cultural beliefs, and explanatory models of health and illness. Hence, there is resonance between the biomedical model and the technologic development of modern society. In this unified model, modalities or healing activities are suggested based on the explanation that healers have given for their use.

The unified model illustrated in Exhibit 18-1 uses four paradigms across the horizontal axis: mechanical, purification, balance, and supranormal. The mechanical paradigm best describes the biomedical model, or the professional sector, in which the prevailing views are that the body is a system of structure and function, disease is a disruption of its mechanism of action, and the purpose of treatment is to restore or replace that function. The mechanical paradigm is self-correcting and produces increasingly sophisticated understandings of the mechanics of the function of the human body.

The purification paradigm underlies many healing and religious healing practices. The general intention is to cleanse and rid the body of polluting influences. This approach to healing is evident as far back as the early Egyptians, who understood and used some of the concepts of purification in the process of mummification. This paradigm was dominant in European medicine as late as the 19th century and was the rationale behind purges, bloodletting, and other cathartic treatments.

Evident in many cultures, the balance paradigm was part of Hippocratic medicine in the form of balancing the humors and still is evident in Mexican dietary patterns used to balance disorders with cold or hot foods. Balance is epitomized in many of the Oriental healing

EXHIBIT 18-1   Multiparadigm Model of Healing

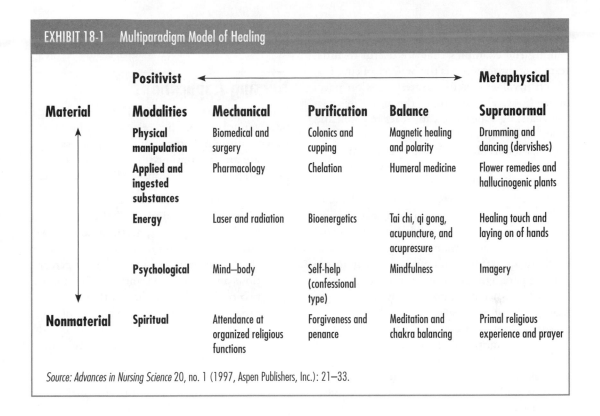

	Positivist ⟷				Metaphysical
Material	**Modalities**	**Mechanical**	**Purification**	**Balance**	**Supranormal**
	Physical manipulation	Biomedical and surgery	Colonics and cupping	Magnetic healing and polarity	Drumming and dancing (dervishes)
	Applied and ingested substances	Pharmacology	Chelation	Humeral medicine	Flower remedies and hallucinogenic plants
	Energy	Laser and radiation	Bioenergetics	Tai chi, qi gong, acupuncture, and acupressure	Healing touch and laying on of hands
	Psychological	Mind–body	Self-help (confessional type)	Mindfulness	Imagery
Nonmaterial	Spiritual	Attendance at organized religious functions	Forgiveness and penance	Meditation and chakra balancing	Primal religious experience and prayer

Source: Advances in Nursing Science 20, no. 1 (1997, Aspen Publishers, Inc.): 21–33.

practices that balance yin and yang and the harmonious flow of chi. There is no English equivalent to the word *chi*, but it is commonly translated as energy. This may be misleading because, according to Kaptchuk, *chi* implies matter at the verge of energy or energy at the point of materializing.[44]

The final paradigm, supranormal, corresponds to some of the magicoreligious healing practices and has been used cross-culturally to address phenomena that physical laws cannot explain. Many paradoxical healings that defy a scientific understanding of physiology may be more clearly understood from this paradigm. Many of the more mystical spiritual practices of ritual, pilgrimage, prayer, and other activities of religious discipline related to healing the mind, body, and spirit stem from this paradigm. Spontaneous healing that has no medical explanation may be attributed to divine intervention, miraculous synergy, vital energies, or capabilities of living organisms beyond the current

understanding of medicine. Many of the explanations refer to abilities acquired in an altered state of consciousness by the healer, healee, or both. Several complementary modalities of healing, such as visual imagery, Healing Touch, or prayer, are best understood through this paradigm. This paradigm is the most distant from the mechanical paradigm, an opposition that may explain some resistance to these types of healing activities.

In the multiparadigm model, the healing activities on the vertical axis are classified as physical manipulation, applied or ingested substances, use of energy, psychological modalities, and spiritual modalities. Each of the paradigms contains all types of healing activities. However, as one moves to the right in the model (see Exhibit 18-1), all healing is conceptualized as more holistic; all activities affect the entire human. For example, a physical manipulation in the supranormal paradigm is assumed to have spiritual effects and vice versa.

Healing activities are inserted in the model as examples; other modalities can be added. Among the examples that are useful to illustrate healing activities is the practice of cupping, which involves placing heated cups on parts of the body. The cooling of the air creates suction, causing superficial capillaries to break and blood to collect in the cup. Cupping exemplifies physical manipulation in the purification paradigm, a healing modality that removes toxins or impurities from the body. Bach flower remedies are viewed as an ingested or applied substance in the supranormal paradigm because their action is understood through a more spiritual or essential manner than a biochemical mechanism. Acupuncture is an energy activity in the balance paradigm because it is the energy or chi that is being acted on, not the physical manipulation of the needles on the physical body.

Mindfulness is a mental discipline based on Eastern thought. This practice is a process of becoming detached and observing thoughts, feelings, and perceptions while remaining fully attentive and in the present. This is a psychological activity in the balance paradigm. Spiritual practices extend through all paradigms. Attendance at organized religious functions is an example of spiritual activities in the mechanical paradigm. Epidemiologic research indicates that attendance at religious events or membership in religious organizations has a salutary effect on health.[45] Some proposed explanatory mechanisms are that these individuals have healthier lifestyles, benefit from social support, or have better stress-coping abilities. This example illustrates the link of mental and spiritual activities to physical outcomes. This understanding has promoted the legitimacy of many of the psychological and spiritual activities that holistic nurses use in encouraging physical health within the mechanical paradigm.

In many cultures, systems of healing combine many levels of activities. For example, shamanism includes physical manipulation, applied and ingested substances, use of vital energy, psychological aspects of belief, and spiritual practices that cluster in the supranormal paradigm. Contemporary complementary healers may use modalities from several paradigms. An understanding of the paradigm from which the modality was developed is important for appropriate use in conducting research.

Nursing Applications

Six phenomena found in all cultural groups have variations that are relevant to the provision of culturally competent nursing assessment and care and are outlined here.[42] It is useful to understand these variations in clinical practice.

1. *Communication.* There are cultural variations in expression of feelings, use of touch, body contact, gestures, and verbal and nonverbal communication. Language shapes experiences and influences perceptions and actions. Warmth and humor are two communication factors that are interpreted differently through various cultures. For example, many Asians may not overtly express their emotions because they may fear "losing face."

2. *Personal space.* Spatial behavior refers to the comfort level related to personal space, meaning the area that surrounds a person's body. Spatial territoriality is the need to have and to control personal space. Cultures vary in the level of proximity to others that is acceptable. For example, Western culture has three zones: the intimate zone (less than 18 inches), the personal zone (18 inches to 3 feet), and the social zone (3 feet to 6 feet). Cultural background also influences aspects of objects within space, such as orderliness, cleanliness, and structural boundaries of furniture and architecture.

3. *Time.* Cultures vary in their orientation toward time, both social time and clock time. *Social time* refers to patterns and orientations related to the ordering of social life, whereas *clock time* represents an objective, ordered approach to viewing time in a linear fashion that implies causality. Some cultures orient around cyclic approaches that attach time to natural events that repeat, such as seasons or migration patterns. For example, in mystical thought, magic or ritual may negate the temporal order of causality and reverse a bad event. All cultures contain the three orientations

of future, present, and past, with one being dominant.

4. *Social organization.* Families, religious groups, kinship groups, workplace groups, and special interest groups are social organizations. Families vary in structure, dynamics, roles, and organizational patterns. Kinship structures and the relative geographic location of family members have cultural implications. Religious organizations provide not only social connections but also a context in which to understand one's relationship to the world, the cosmos, and the meaning in life.

5. *Environmental control.* Different cultures have different perceptions of the ability of an individual to control nature, the environment, and personal relationships. The locus of control may be external (i.e., an event contingent on luck or fate), internal (i.e., an event contingent on one's own behavior or characteristic), or outside (i.e., an event in harmony with nature, as in some Asian cultures). In folk medicine, for example, events are perceived as natural and unnatural. Natural events have to do with the world as God intended and the laws of nature. Unnatural events upset the harmony of nature and are outside the world of nature.

6. *Biological variations.* In a pluralistic culture, it is important to distinguish among factors that are strictly biological (i.e., genetic) and those that are ethnic adaptations related to living in a particular environment (e.g., availability of certain types of food) or in certain social conditions (e.g., socioeconomic status, lifestyle). Biological factors to be considered are body size and structure, including variations in teeth, facial features, and skin color; variations in metabolism and enzyme production that result in drug reactions, interactions, and sensitivities; and susceptibility to disease (e.g., hypertension, diabetes, sickle cell anemia). Nutritional issues, including food preferences, habits, and patterns, as well as deficiencies such as lactose intolerance, all have medical implications.

This information is a helpful guide to thinking about cultural variations. However, no amount of factual knowledge about cultural variation can replace careful individual assessment because there is more intracultural variation than intercultural variation.

Cross-Cultural Communication

Members of minority groups may distrust and fear the Western biomedical healthcare system. Because the element of trust is essential to the formation of a therapeutic nurse–client relationship, clients need to know that nurses are receptive and nonjudgmental regarding their differences. Nurses must approach cultural competency through knowledge of self and knowledge of other cultures. To develop the ability to interact with clients appropriately, nurses should clarify their personal values, recognize the healthcare system as a culture, learn about the specific culture of each client, interact and intervene in a culturally congruent manner, and elicit feedback regularly from the client and family. Skills such as listening, explaining, acknowledging, recommending, and negotiating facilitate a nonjudgmental perspective toward the client's cultural beliefs. Nurses and clients should validate their perceptions and discuss similarities and differences in their perceptions to formulate health-related goals and interventions.

Cultural competency is a dynamic, challenging process faced by all healthcare providers regardless of their cultural background or association. Providers who are members of minority groups also encounter situations in which their cultural competency is desirable. Various principles are important in developing cultural competency. The process of sharing information in a straightforward manner demystifies other cultures and, for example, makes it possible for the nurse and client to find common ground and understand the context of differences. To find common ground, it is necessary to consider terminology. Many individuals may consider some terms such as *Negro, black,* or *foreigner* inappropriate and possibly offensive. The terms *Hispanic, Latino,* and *Chicano* are used to describe people from Spanish-speaking cultures. The terms may be used by the individuals themselves in some cases or, in other cases, may be considered insulting. Individuals working together in provider–client interactions must ensure that the terminology used is mutually understood and acceptable. Researchers and scholars must strive for consensual cultural terminology so that research findings can be appropriately applied and compared.

Professional Recommendations

Many healthcare organizations and regulatory bodies have developed standards and recommendations. The Office of Minority Health issued the CLAS standards in an attempt to synthesize cultural competency definitions and requirements into a single set of standards.[1] The CLAS standards contain several regulations and recommendations for organizations regarding the use of translations and providing culturally appropriate health care. Cultural and linguistic competence has been incorporated into the curricula of medicine, nursing, and other healthcare professions and endorsed by many professional organizations. It is reflected in the standards and guidelines from several health regulatory agencies. Some promising studies support positive results on health and mental health outcomes from culturally and linguistically based programs for specific populations.

Other major governmental agencies have also emphasized the importance of cultural competency in the delivery of health care. The Agency for Healthcare Research and Quality has a focus on health literacy and cultural competency and reducing health disparities.[46] The Health Resources and Service Administration also focuses on culture, language, and health literacy.[47]

The Joint Commission has also put forth cultural competency standards that include patient- and family-centered care.[48] It is noteworthy that several national sources are now linking cultural competency with patient-centered care. The American Academy of Nursing established a Nursing Expert Panel that made the following recommendations for the development of cultural competence and reduction of health disparities:[49]

- *Education.* The integration of knowledge, skills, and basic competencies to develop sensitivity and competence in curricula.

- *Practice.* Healthcare organizations provide a supportive climate for culturally competent care. This includes appreciation of complementary alternative therapies.
- *Research.* Research on diversity, disparities, and culture is necessary. Inclusion of women and minorities for representative samples and adequate funding is needed.
- *Policy.* Education of policymakers is needed to ensure funds and care in areas that can change outcomes.
- *Advocacy.* Advocacy is needed for vulnerable populations.

Communication

All healthcare providers of the professional sector in the United States have acculturated to the biomedical model and accompanying technology by virtue of their education and the sociology of the healthcare institution where they practice. Each institution has its own culture that defines the norms, protocols, and hierarchy, both formal and informal. Most healthcare institutions are based on the biomedical model and accept clients into the system because of a perceived physical or mental disease or illness. In contrast, healers in the folk sector are more likely to approach health from a holistic perspective, with a focus on the emotional and spiritual domains, as well as on the physical domain. Such healers have become acculturated to the holistic model through education, which is often based on an apprenticeship with a more experienced practitioner.

The purposes of communication in the healthcare environment are to create an interpersonal relationship, exchange information, and allow for decision making. Specific barriers may impede the achievement of these goals. First, communication between the provider and client generally involves individuals of unequal positions, with the provider assuming a higher rank to some extent simply by virtue of greater medical knowledge. Second, communication related to health care is often not planned, involves vitally important issues, and is emotionally laden. Finally, differences in language, both verbal and nonverbal, may isolate the client and the family. Nonverbal aspects of oral communication, such as voice tone, eye contact, and body positioning, are often as significant as verbal communication. If the cultural backgrounds of the provider and the client are significantly different, these communication factors may make it difficult to obtain and provide health care without misunderstandings.

Roles in the relationship between the provider and client are frequently derived from cultural norms and can enhance or impede communication. Such roles can be seen as a spectrum of control, ranging from paternalistic to mutualistic.[50] In a paternalistic (i.e., provider-centered) relationship, the provider has the control, directs care, makes decisions about treatment, and is authoritative. A mutual, client-centered relationship involves shared decision making and is more egalitarian. Problems can arise in communication and the therapeutic relationship if the client's expectations do not match those of the provider with respect to control and decision making. Problems can also arise if communication styles, both nonverbal and verbal, differ. Such expectations are often culturally related, and nurses can avoid some problems by developing sensitivity to various communication styles.

Use of Translators

The increasing number of languages and dialects in the United States means that nurses, even those who are bilingual, often rely on translators or interpreters to communicate with clients. Translators play powerful roles in the exchange of valuable information between nurses and their clients. The California Endowment published National Standards of Practice for Interpreters in Health Care.[51] These standards are aligned with the National Code of Ethics and address the ethical issues of accuracy, confidentiality, impartiality, respect, cultural awareness, role boundaries, professionalism, professional development, and advocacy.

Bilingual staff or trained on-site interpreters are preferred over family members. If interpretation is needed immediately or the language is infrequently encountered, then telephone interpreter systems should be used. Untrained interpreters may provide misinformation to the client and also may use words, tones, or gestures that emphasize the translator's own personal preferences, omit portions of a message deemed irrelevant, or diminish the importance of the intended message. Indeed, translators may dominate the conversation. It is best to avoid using family members as translators whenever possible because they are likely to filter information based on what they want the client to hear. Also, it might be culturally inappropriate for the client to discuss some health matters with certain family members. In addition, not all interpreters fully understand issues of confidentiality. Regardless of the source or skill of the translator, nurses should attempt to do the following when using a translator:[52]

1. Orient the client to the process and the purpose of using a translator.
2. Orient the translator to the topics to be covered, the client's situation, and the degree of accuracy required.
3. Avoid standing; sit so that the client can observe the nurse and make eye contact; avoid placing the translator between the nurse and the client.
4. Observe the client for nonverbal communication that does not match the message intended and request clarification.
5. Slow down the communication process.
6. Encourage the translator to let the nurse know when something is difficult to translate so that it may be reworded.
7. Limit the use of medical jargon, slang, and metaphors to reduce the chance for error.
8. Consider the effect of differences in gender, educational level, and socioeconomic status between the client and translator. This is particularly important when topics of a sensitive or personal nature are to be discussed.
9. Ask translators to translate in the client's own words and ask clients to repeat the information communicated to increase accuracy.

Holistic Caring Process

Interactions between the healthcare provider and the client are based on the communication between the two and reflect their respective cultures. Both the provider and the client bring their personal beliefs, values, and cultural backgrounds to the interaction. These factors then affect the transfer of information, decision making, adherence to treatment, and healing outcomes. The professional nature of the encounter brings the culture of the healthcare system into the exchange, even if the meeting occurs in the client's home or a community setting. An understanding of the cultural world of the client and the cultural world of the healthcare system enables the provider to deliver culturally appropriate care. Nurses often act as cultural brokers between the client and the biomedical culture.

A midrange theory of cultural negotiation for clinical nursing was proposed, which links the holistic perspective of nursing theories to the pragmatic elements of the nursing process[53] (see **Figure 18-2**). This situates the clinical encounter between the patient and the clinician within the culture of the biomedical healthcare system, which is located within an ecological hierarchy of cultures reflecting the social world (e.g., Western culture). Both the nurse and the patient bring expert knowledge to this encounter. This expert knowledge includes cultural heritage, personal experiences, formal and informal knowledge, and personal knowing. Both also bring aspects of their cultural heritage, and it is important that the nurse engage in some of the previously mentioned practices to become aware of these influences to better understand that of the patient. Both have a history of experiences. Patients have often had previous experiences with the healthcare system. Nurses have their professional/personal experiences as well. For example, a nurse may have experienced caring for patients from a specific culture or had personal experience as a patient, which influences his or her encounter with a patient. Nurses have formal knowledge that they bring to the encounter and they are responsible for applying this knowledge competently. Nurses are also exposed to a lot of informal knowledge.

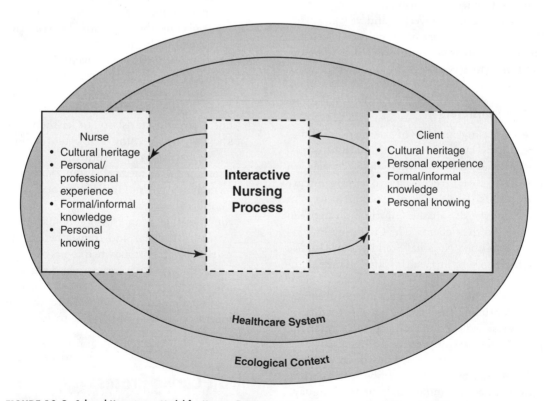

FIGURE 18-2 Cultural Negotiation Model for Nursing Practice

Source: Reprinted from *Nursing Outlook* 49, no. 5, J. Engebretson and L.Y. Littleton, Cultural Negotiation: A Constructivist-Based Model of Nursing Practice," pages 223–230, Copyright 2001, with permission from Elsevier.

Currently, there is an abundance of health information available through the media. Patients also are exposed to various media and have varying levels of formal knowledge. Both nurse and patient have personal or intuitive knowledge that each brings to the encounter.

Central to this encounter is the nursing process. The nursing process is the basic problem-solving approach. Holistic nurses have long advocated that the process reflects an active engagement between the patient and the clinician. This positions the patient to have more agency, or power, in the relationship than the classic nursing process in which the clinician has the agency and the patient complies. In this model the agency is fluid. For example, in a case in which the patient is too ill to exert much agency, the nurse and medical team assume more agency. In contrast, in health promotion or management of chronic conditions, the patient must assume greater agency. Consistent with this perspective, the steps in the nursing process are refigured (see **Exhibit 18-2**).

Holistic Assessment

In this model, nursing assessment becomes the exchange of expert knowledge. This focuses on the sharing of knowledge. The patient is the expert in knowledge about symptoms, history, perceptions, fears, concerns, and expectations. Nurses are experts in using technical skills, professional knowledge, and experience in the examination of the patient and incorporating information from laboratory reports and other medical data. In addition to uncovering

explanatory models, the nurse could ask where the patient gets information about health issues and how the patient integrates that information into health practices.

Data from a brief assessment, including questions about ethnic background and religion, can be used to determine the need for a more in-depth assessment that focuses on specific parameters, such as nutritional patterns, social support networks, and beliefs about treatments and coping. See **Exhibit 18-3** for some suggested areas to question patients to get a better understanding of their cultural orientations.

Nursing Diagnosis, or Analysis and Interpretation of the Information

The nurse begins to interpret and analyze the information and, at this point, brings in the use of both formal and informal knowledge and professional experience concerning problems, risks, patterns, challenges, and needs. Ideally, information is shared in this process so that the nurse can explain to and interpret medical matters for the client, begin the process of consolidating explanatory models, establish a foundation for further communication, and incorporate salient concerns of the patient.

Identification of Patterns/ Challenges/Needs

In addition to the influence of culture on the process of developing a mutual interpretation of needs and establishing common goals and plans for action, there may be specific concerns in the cultural domain. For example, a client's needs

EXHIBIT 18-2 Nursing Process	
Traditional Nursing Process Model	**Negotiated Holistic Model of Nursing Process**
Nursing assessment	Exchange of expert knowledge.
Nursing diagnosis	Analysis and interpretation of information from both client and nurse.
Planning	Joint decision making between client and nurse.
Intervention	Implementation of mutually derived plans for action with specific agreed-upon actions for nurse and client.
Evaluation	Outcomes appraisal of goals and processes. This is also a mutual undertaking.

Everyday health practices

- Nutritional patterns
- Exercise and physical activities
- Health and healing practices
- Sources of information about health

Family organization, structure, and role differentiation and child care practices

- Decision making: how made, who is involved, and why
- Health seeking: who, when, and how to consult about health issues
- Communication style and relationship toward authority
- Social support networks and relationships

Demographics, socioeconomic status, and employment patterns

- Spiritual beliefs, rituals, and practices
- Immigration and cultural history

Explanatory models of illness

typically involve biophysical and psychological disturbances, alterations, impairments, and distresses. These patterns, challenges, and needs are largely derived from the conceptual areas of normalcy based on North American culture and heavily influenced by biomedicine. The patterns/challenges/needs directly related to cultural interventions are as follows (see also Chapter 8):

- Altered or impaired communication related to language differences or communication style: Even with the aid of translators, language and dialect differences may exist based on the region in which the client was born (e.g., China and Mexico have multiple dialects).
- Altered or impaired social interaction related to sociocultural dissonance: Difficulties in relating with members of the healthcare team may occur when there are gender, socioeconomic, or educational gaps.
- Lack of adherence related to incongruent value systems between provider and client:

Clients may be considered noncompliant with follow-up appointments when differences in the perception of time are at the root of missed or late appointments.

- Anxiety related to culturally unusual expectations for behavior and treatment; fear related to unknown environment or customs: The biomedical healthcare system may be particularly anxiety provoking for clients whose custom is to be cared for in the home during an illness.

Outcome Identification

Culturally appropriate outcomes are developed with the client. This incorporates the client's values and explanatory model expectations and allows for accommodations of other outcomes beyond the disease treatment.

Therapeutic Care Plan and Interventions

The nurse and patient conjointly develop an approach to address the mutually identified concerns and the agreed-upon goals. The patient discusses assets, barriers, and priorities, and the nurse shares expert knowledge and may suggest other resources. Based on the mutual decision making, alternative solutions and modalities may be incorporated into the care plan. Explanatory models are often reflected in the care plan.

Cultural healing practices, unless there are clear counterindications, may be incorporated into the care plan. Nurses should convey respect for the practice and make every effort to acquire appropriate foods, people, artifacts, and so on, as well as to secure space and time for such practices. During this clinical process, Leininger's three modes of incorporating cultural practices may be evident.[54]

1. *Cultural preservation and maintenance* refers to professional actions that retain relevant care values to support aspects of the client's culture that positively influence his or her health care.
2. *Cultural accommodation and negotiation* refers to professional actions to bridge the gap between the client's culture and

biomedicine for beneficial health outcomes, by recognizing the cultural relevance of a practice and integrating it into the treatment plan, even though the cultural practice has no scientific basis.

3. *Cultural repatterning and restructuring* refers to professional actions that assist the client in making changes in, but not discarding, practices that may be harmful to his or her well-being.

Therefore, a variety of healing modalities may be used, depending on the illness and cultural preferences. Two aspects of healing, touch and spiritual practices, have deep cultural meaning. Touch, even as an element of communication, has culturally specific meanings. In some Arab and Hispanic cultures, male providers may be prohibited from examining or touching parts of the female body. Some Asians believe that the center of strength lies in the head, and touching the head is a sign of disrespect or threat. Thus, the process of shaving the head preoperatively may be viewed very negatively. Gentle touch may be seen as a caring gesture. Specific healing modalities using human touch are often viewed from an energetic or spiritual framework. Many cultures have traditions of "laying on of hands." Some patients may be suspicious if a nurse uses a touch therapy that is not consonant with or connected to their specific religious beliefs. Spiritual rituals or practices are associated with healing in many cultures. Rituals and practices to protect one from evil, disease, or danger include the use of amulets, talismans, ritualistic behavior, the avoidance of taboos, exorcism, and purification or cleansing rituals. Prayer and other spiritual practices are widely associated with healing. Rituals may be positive in nature, including those related to spiritual growth, redemption, and life transitions, such as birth or initiations into adulthood.[55] Often viewed as having divine gifts, healers or spiritual leaders are believed to be able to negotiate with the spiritual world through prayer, meditation, blessings, chants, and other primal religious experiences, many of which incorporate altered states of consciousness. Individuals also may seek healing forces by sacrifice, penance, and pilgrimages.

Evaluation

Together, the nurse, the client, and any member of the extended family or social group who the client feels is significant should evaluate desired client outcomes. Evaluation must be woven throughout the entire holistic caring process because it is essential to obtain validation through mutual understanding, especially when there are differences between the cultural backgrounds of nurse and client. It is important to note the purpose of the activity in evaluating its effectiveness. A massage that is given for the purpose of comfort must be evaluated on the basis of comfort, for example, not its medical effect on the disease process. A healing activity that is understood by the client as having multiple effects (e.g., spiritual benefits, psychological benefits, better health) should be evaluated on many levels and should not be discounted if the physical benefits are not comparable to those of a pharmaceutical product. Each component of the healthcare plan and each nursing intervention should be carefully examined to ensure that it is understandable and acceptable to the client, effective for achievement of short- and long-term goals, and appropriately revised as necessary during the evaluation process. Cultural modifications can be made upon careful evaluation.

Directions for Future Research

1. Survey patterns of usage of healing modalities from various paradigms and cultural backgrounds.
2. Develop efficient and effective ways of assessing the degree of acculturation in clients with various cultural backgrounds.
3. Analyze effective models for interaction between biomedical and traditional healthcare systems.
4. Evaluate the degree to which healthcare goals are achieved when nurses deliver culturally competent care.
5. Analyze various methods for teaching nursing students or staff how to provide culturally competent care.

Nurse Healer Reflections

After reading this chapter, the nurse healer will be able to answer or to begin a process of answering the following questions:

- What are my values and beliefs regarding health and illness in relationship to models of healing?
- How do I feel when caring for clients whose cultural backgrounds differ from my own?
- What are my biases and attitudes toward clients with various cultural backgrounds?
- How can I determine whether I am offering culturally competent care in a holistic manner?

NOTES

1. Office of Minority Health, "National Standards for Culturally and Linguistically Appropriate Services in Health and Health Care (The National CLAS Standards)" (2013). http://minorityhealth.hhs.gov/omh/browse.aspx?lvl=2&lvlid=53.

2. S. M. Montenery, A. D. Jones, N. Perry, D. Ross, and R. Zoucha, "Cultural Competence in Nursing Faculty: A Journey, Not a Destination," *Journal of Professional Nursing* 29, no. 6 (2013): 51–57.

3. M. Isaacson, "Clarifying Concepts: Cultural Humility or Competency," *Journal of Professional Nursing* 30, no. 3 (2014): 251–258.

4. T. Cross, B. J. Bazron, K. W. Dennis, and M. R. Isaacs, *Towards a Culturally Competent System of Care* (Washington, DC: CASSP Technical Assistance Center, Georgetown University Child Development Center, 1989).

5. J. Engebretson, J. Mahoney, and E. D. Carlson, "Cultural Competence in the Era of Evidence-Based Practice," *Journal of Professional Nursing* 24, no. 3 (2008): 172–178.

6. D. L. Sackett, S. E. Strauss, W. S. Richardson, W. Rosenberg, and R. B. Haynes, *Evidence-Based Medicine: How to Practice and Teach EBM*, 2nd ed. (New York: Churchill Livingstone, 2005).

7. J. Campinha-Bacote, "A Model and Instrument for Addressing Cultural Competence in Health Care," *Journal of Nursing Education* 38, no. 5 (1999): 203–207.

8. M. Douglas, "Developing Frameworks for Providing Culturally Competent Health Care," *Journal of Transcultural Nursing* 13, no. 3 (2002): 177.

9. L. Purnell and B. Paulanka, *Transcultural Health Care: A Culturally Competent Approach* (Philadelphia: F. A. Davis, 1998).

10. J. Giger and R. Davidhizar, *Transcultural Nursing: Assessment and Intervention*, 5th ed. (St. Louis, MO: Mosby Elsevier, 2007).

11. R. E. Spector, *Cultural Diversity in Health and Illness*, 5th ed. (Upper Saddle River, NJ: Prentice Hall, 2000).

12. M. Leininger, *Culture Care Diversity and Universality: A Theory of Nursing* (Sudbury, MA: Jones and Bartlett, 2001).

13. J. G. Lipson and L. A. Desantis, "Current Approaches to Integrating Elements of Cultural Competence in Nursing Education," *Journal of Transcultural Nursing* 18, no. 1 (2007): 10S–20S.

14. M. C. Beach, E. G. Price, T. L. Gary, K. A. Robinson, A. Gozu, A. Palacio, C. Smarth, M. W. Jenckes, C. Feuerstein, E. B. Bass, N. R. Powe, and L. A. Cooper, "Cultural Competence: A Systematic Review of Health Care Provider Educational Interventions," *Medical Care* 43, no. 4 (2005): 356–373.

15. J. R. Betancourt, "Cultural Competency: Providing Quality Care to Diverse Populations," *Consultant Pharmacist* 21, no. 12 (2006): 988–995.

16. J. R. Betancourt and A. R. Green, "Commentary: Linking Cultural Competence Training to Improved Health Outcomes: Perspectives from the Field," *Academic Medicine* 85, no. 4 (2010): 583–585.

17. G. R. Gregg and S. Saha, "Losing Culture on the Way to Competence: The Use and Misuse of Culture in Medical Education," *Academic Medicine* 81, no. 6 (2006): 542–547.

18. M. Dreher and N. MacNaughton, "Cultural Competence in Nursing: Foundation or Fallacy?" *Nursing Outlook* 50, no. 5 (2002): 181–186.

19. F. Collins, "Genomics and Health Disparities," in *Disparities in Health in America: Working Toward Social Justice* (summer workshop, Houston, TX, 2003).

20. M. F. MacDorman and T. J. Mathews, "Infant Deaths—United States 2000–2007," *Morbidity and Mortality Weekly Report* 60, no. 1 (2011): 49–51.

21. Centers for Disease Control and Prevention, "CDC Health Disparities and Inequalities Report—United States, 2011," *Morbidity and Mortality Weekly Report* 60, Supplement 1–2 (2011): 1–114.

22. N. E. Adler and K. Newman, "Socioeconomic Disparities in Health: Pathways and Policies," *Health Affairs* 21, no. 2 (2002): 60–76.

23. V. J. Burroughs, R. W. Maxey, and R. A. Levy, "Racial and Ethnic Differences in Response to

Medicines: Towards Individualized Pharmaceutical Treatment," *Journal of the National Medical Association* 94, no. 10 (2002): S1–S25.

24. American Society of Health-System Pharmacists, "ASHP Statement on Racial and Ethnic Disparities in Health Care" (2008). www.ashp.org /DocLibrary/BestPractices/SpecificStDisparities .aspx.

25. A. Rundle, M. Carvalho, and M. Robinson, eds., *Cultural Competence in Health Care: A Practice Guide* (San Francisco: Jossey-Bass, 1999).

26. T. R. Marmor, M. L. Barer, and R. G. Evans, *Why Are Some People Healthy and Others Not? The Determinants of Healthy Populations* (New York: Aldine de Gruyter, 1994).

27. M. Lock and D. Gordon, *Biomedicine Examined* (Dordrecht, Netherlands: Kluwer, 1988).

28. K. Kipnis, "Quality Care and the Wounds of Diversity" (paper presented at the meeting of the American Society for Bioethics and Humanities, Houston, TX, November 18, 1998).

29. E. R. Oetting and F. Beauvais, "Orthogonal Cultural Identification Theory: The Cultural Identification of Minority Adolescents," *International Journal of Addiction* 25, nos. s5–s6 (1991): 655–685.

30. J. Achterberg, *Woman as Healer* (Boston: Shambhala, 1990).

31. J. Engebretson, "Comparison of Nurses and Alternative Healers," *Journal of Nursing Scholarship* 28, no. 2 (1996): 95–99.

32. F. R. Kluckhohn, "Dominant and Variant Value Orientations," in *Transcultural Nursing: A Book of Readings*, ed. P. J. Brink (Englewood Cliffs, NJ: Prentice Hall, 1976): 63–81.

33. J. Engebretson, "Considerations in Diagnosing in the Spiritual Domain," *International Journal of Nursing Terminologies and Classifications* 7, no. 3 (1996): 100–107.

34. N. Postman, *Technopoly* (New York: Vintage Books, 1993).

35. P. H. Ray, "The Emerging Culture," *American Demographics* 19, no. 2 (1997): 28–34.

36. J. A. Astin, "Why Patients Use Alternative Medicine: Results of a National Study," *Journal of the American Medical Association* 279, no. 19 (1998): 1548–1553.

37. D. M. Eisenberg, R. B. Davis, S. L. Ettner, S. Appel, S. Wilkey, M. Van Rompay, and R. C. Kessler, "Trends in Alternative Medicine Use in the United States, 1990–1997: Results of a Follow-Up National Survey," *Journal of the American Medicine Association* 280, no. 18 (1998): 1569–1575.

38. U.S. Census Bureau, "Schedule of New Estimates" (July 1, 2013). www.census.gov/popest /schedule.html.

39. M. M. Andrews and J. S. Boyle, eds., *Transcultural Concepts in Nursing Care*, 4th ed. (Philadelphia: J. B. Lippincott, 2002).

40. M. O. Loustaunau and E. J. Sobo, *The Cultural Context of Health, Illness, and Medicine* (Westport, CT: Bergin & Garvey Press, 1997).

41. A. Kleinman, *Patients and Healers in the Context of Culture: An Exploration of the Borderland Between Anthropology, Medicine and Psychiatry* (Berkeley: University of California Press, 1980).

42. J. Giger and R. Davidhizar, *Transcultural Nursing: Assessment and Intervention*, 3rd ed. (St. Louis, MO: Mosby Elsevier, 1999).

43. J. Engebretson, "A Multiparadigm Approach to Nursing," *Advances in Nursing Science* 20, no. 1 (1997): 22–33.

44. T. J. Kaptchuk, *The Web That Has No Weaver: Understanding Chinese Medicine* (New York: Congdon & Weed, 1983).

45. J. S. Levin, "Religion and Health: Is There an Association, Is It Valid, and Is It Causal?" *Social Science in Medicine* 38, no. 11 (1994): 1475–1482.

46. Agency for Healthcare Research and Quality, "Cultural and Linguistic Competence" (2013). www.ahrq.gov/health-care-information/topics /external/Cultural-and-Linguistic-Competence .html.

47. U. S. Department of Health and Human Services, "Health Resources and Services Administration" (n.d.). www.hrsa.gov.

48. The Joint Commission, "Advancing Effective Communication, Cultural Competence, and Patient- and Family-Centered Care" (July 28, 2014). www.jointcommission.org /Advancing_Effective_Communication/.

49. J. Giger, R. E. Davidhizar, L. Purnell, J. T. Harden, J. Phillips, and O. Strickland "American Academy of Nursing Expert Panel Report: Developing Cultural Competence to Eliminate Health Disparities in Ethnic Minorities and Other Vulnerable Populations," *Journal of Transcultural Nursing* 18, no. 95 (2007): 95–102.

50. D. W. Sue and D. Sue, *Counseling the Culturally Different: Theory and Practice*, 4th ed. (New York: Wiley, 2003).

51. National Council on Interpreting in Health Care, *National Standards of Practice for Interpreters in Health Care* (Washington, DC: National Council on Interpreting in Health Care, 2005).

52. C. Degazon, "Cultural Diversity and Community Health Nursing Practice," in *Community Health Nursing: Promoting Health of Aggregates, Families and Individuals*, 4th ed., eds. M. Stanhope and J. Lancaster (St. Louis, MO: Mosby Elsevier, 1996): 117–134.

53. J. Engebretson and L. Littleton, "Cultural Negotiation: A Constructivist-Based Model for Nursing Practice," *Nursing Outlook* 49, no. 5 (2001): 223–230.

54. M. M. Leininger and M. R. McFarland, *Transcultural Nursing: Concepts, Theories, Research and Practices*, 3rd ed. (New York: McGraw-Hill, 2002).

55. D. Kinsley, *Health, Healing, and Religion: A Cross-Cultural Perspective* (Upper Saddle River, NJ: Prentice Hall, 1996).

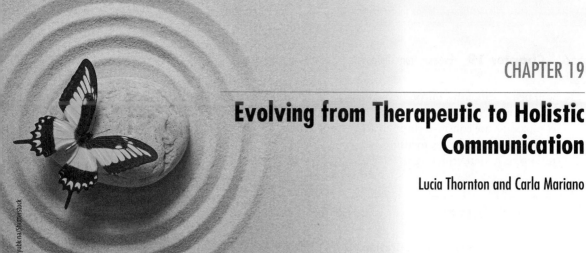

CHAPTER 19

Evolving from Therapeutic to Holistic Communication

Lucia Thornton and Carla Mariano

Nurse Healer Objectives

Theoretical

- Identify foundational theories and concepts in the development of therapeutic communication.
- Describe contemporary nursing theories and concepts foundational to the development of holistic communication.
- Identify and describe the concepts that distinguish holistic communication.

Clinical

- Integrate foundational holistic communication processes into clinical practice.
- Integrate and utilize intention, centering, grounding, caring, healing, transcendent presence, and intuition in establishing a caring, healing field of communication.

Personal

- Engage in reflective practices to increase self-awareness and personal growth.
- Integrate and utilize intention, centering, presence, caring, and intuition in creating and maintaining a healing field of communication in daily life.

Definitions

Energy field: The fundamental unit of the living and nonliving. *Field* is a unifying concept. *Energy* signifies the dynamic nature of the field; a field is in continuous motion and is infinite.[1, p. 7]

Holistic communication: A caring, healing process that calls forth the full use of self in interacting with another. It incorporates the constructs and processes of therapeutic communication within a framework that acknowledges the infinite, spiritual, and energetic nature of Being, the centrality of being heart centered, and the importance of intention, self-knowledge, transcendent presence, and intuition in our interactions.[2, p. 619]

Person: An energy field that is infinite and spiritual in essence and is in continual, mutual process with the environment. Each person manifests unique physical, mental, emotional, and social or relational patterns that are interrelated, inseparable, and continually evolving.[3, p. 42]

Therapeutic communication: A goal-directed form of communication used to achieve goals that promote client health and well-being. Empathy, unconditional regard, genuineness, respect, concern, caring, and compassion are conveyed through active listening, active observing, focusing, restating, reflecting, and interpreting.[2, pp. 619–620]

Theory and Research

Pioneers in Therapeutic Communication

Therapeutic communication is a field of study that has been influenced by theorists, researchers, and clinicians from a multitude of professions including nursing, psychology, sociology, and physics. These early pioneers created a rich foundation of ideas and constructs, many of which were holistic in nature. It is important to understand these perspectives to gain a greater understanding of how this work has evolved and its usefulness in holistic practice. Some of the significant contributions of nurse theorist Hildegard Peplau and those of Martin Buber, Carl Jung, Harry Stack Sullivan, and Carl Rogers are presented.

Peplau: A Visionary in Relationship-Based Caring

Peplau, the "mother of psychiatric nursing," was the first to emphasize the nurse–client relationship as being the foundation of nursing practice.

The concept of partnership between nurse and client originated in Peplau's interpersonal model. The idea that the nurse helps guide the patient and the patient takes an active role in the treatment plan was indeed revolutionary in 1952 and was in opposition to mainstream thinking, which promoted a role in which the client was dependent on the nurse.

The essence of Peplau's work revolved around the concept of the shared experience. She shifted the focus of nursing practice from one that was based on medical intervention to an interpersonal model in which the nurse became the therapeutic agent. Peplau identified nursing roles during the course of the nurse–client relationship. The roles include *Stranger*, providing acceptance and trust; *Resource*, answering questions and giving information; *Teacher*, giving instruction and analyzing the learner

experience; *Counselor*, helping the client derive meaning from the current experience; *Surrogate*, advocating for the client and clarifying dependence, independence, and interdependence; and *Leader*, assisting the client to assume maximum responsibility for meeting goals that are mutually established.[4, p. 89]

Peplau's concepts provided a bridge between the old paradigm, in which the client was dependent on the healthcare system, to one in which the client was an active participant in treatment and care. Her ideas paved the way for communication that involved the whole person.

Cogent Concepts from Other Disciplines

In the field of therapeutic communication, many rich ideas and constructs originated with psychotherapists. Concepts and ideas from Buber, Sullivan, Rogers, and Jung are similar to concepts that are foundational to holistic communication.

Martin Buber introduced the idea that the therapeutic process involves mutual discovery and emphasized the importance of mutual respect in the client–therapist interaction. He coined the term *I-Thou relationship*, which reflects a reverence in the client–therapist relationship. In this orientation, the therapist consciously creates a transcendent space in the relationship, fostering shared authenticity and compassion.

Harry Stack Sullivan was a contemporary of Peplau and influenced the development of her interpersonal model. Sullivan introduced the idea of the therapeutic relationship and described it as being a human connection that heals. Carl Rogers saw the therapist as an agent of healing. The hallmark characteristics that Rogers identified as being essential to the client-centered relationship were unconditional regard, empathy, and genuineness. Carl Jung examined the complexity of gender roles and our universal heritage as human beings. He described the first half of life as a search for self and the second half of life as a search for soul.[4, pp. 9–13]

All of these therapists, and many others not mentioned, have contributed ideas that have significantly influenced the development of the therapeutic communication process. The concepts of partnership, healing, reverence, unconditional regard, empathy, genuineness, spirituality, and many more first found their place in therapeutic communication before being embraced by holistic nursing.

Nursing Theory Related to Holistic Communication

The nursing theorists whose theories and concepts have facilitated the evolution of therapeutic communication toward holistic communication are Martha Rogers, Margaret Newman, and Jean Watson. Concepts related to holistic communication are explicated and briefly discussed. For an overview of these theories, see Chapter 5, *Nursing Theory*.

Martha Rogers

Rogers uses the term *unitary human being* in place of *person* and defines who we are as "an irreducible, indivisible, pan-dimensional energy field identified by pattern and manifesting characteristics that are specific to the whole and which cannot be predicted from knowledge of the parts." Rogers further defines energy field as "the fundamental unit of the living and non-living. Field is a unifying concept. Energy signifies the dynamic nature of the field; a field is in continuous motion and is infinite."[1, p. 7]

The nature of therapeutic communication changes when Rogers's definitions are applied. How does one communicate with an energy field that is infinite in nature? Also, if we accept Rogers's definitions, then communication shifts from being a linear or circular process to a pan-dimensional energetic process. Accepting Rogers's definition also shifts our thinking to view communication as a *field phenomenon*. And finally, Rogers's definition invites us to entertain the idea that our interactions can extend beyond the realm of this physical universe, beyond the space-time continuum and into dimensions that are infinite.

Rogers's Principle of Integrality also has implications for the nature of holistic communication. Rogers defines integrality as a "continuous mutual human field and environmental field process."[1, p. 8] Rogers describes

person and environment as "open systems" and states that "man and environment are continuously exchanging matter and energy with one another."[5] This implies that *all* that we are—our thoughts, behaviors, emotions, that which is conscious, and that which is unconscious—interacts and affects everything and everyone in our environment. Likewise, everyone and everything that exists in our environment are continuously exchanging matter and energy with us. Integrating this concept into our lives challenges us to transform our lives and our way of being. If we are to act in a way that is therapeutic, in a way that promotes healing, we ourselves must be whole and healed. This concept reinforces the importance of self-awareness and self-knowledge.

Margaret Newman

The task of nursing intervention, according to Newman, "is not to try to change another person's patterns but to recognize it as information that depicts the whole and relate to it as it unfolds."[6] The nurse must first be able to recognize her or his own patterns before entering into this process with a patient. Again, self-knowledge is paramount for the nurse to be effective in a caring, healing relationship.

The responsibility of the nurse is not to make people well or to prevent their getting sick but to assist people in recognizing the power that is within them to move to higher levels of consciousness. The nurse's awareness of *being* rather than *doing* is the primary mechanism for helping. Newman quotes Thomas Moore to emphasize the importance of staying fully present to all that life offers, without trying to fix or intervene:

> By doing less, more is accomplished . . . what is needed is not taking sides when there is a conflict at a deep level. It may be necessary to stretch the heart wide enough to embrace contradiction and paradox.[7]

Newman illuminates the concepts of pattern recognition, being fully present, and the importance of self-awareness and transformation in the holistic communication process.

Jean Watson

Watson defines person as "an embodied spirit; a transpersonal, transcendent, evolving consciousness; unity of mind-body-spirit; person-nature-universe as oneness, connected."[8] Watson is the first nursing theorist to address the concept of soul, as in the following passage:

> My conception of life and personhood is tied to notions that one's soul possesses a body that is not confined by objective space and time. . . . Notions of personhood, then, transcend the here and now, and one has the capacity to coexist with past, present, future, all at once. As a result of this view, there is a great deal of regard, respect, and awe given to the concept of a human soul (spirit, or higher sense of self) that is greater than the physical, mental, and emotional existence of a person at any given point in time.[9, p. 45]

How does one address the soul in the process of therapeutic communication? Watson's answer to this is the transpersonal caring relationship. Engaging with another at the transpersonal level is not a technique that can be learned. Rather, it is the ability of the person to access the higher self and move from that place of higher consciousness in interactions with another. This process calls for the "full use of the self."[9, p. 69] Watson's description of the art of transpersonal caring also serves as a description of the caring, healing process of holistic communication.

> The nurse is able to form a union with the other person on a level that transcends the physical, and that preserves the subjectivity and physicality of persons without reducing them to the moral of objects. . . . The union of feelings can potentiate self-healing and discovery in his or her own existence. That is the great attractive force of the art of transpersonal caring in nursing.[9, p. 68]

Another concept that Watson expanded on and that has significance in the application of holistic communication is that of the phenomenal field.

> The phenomenal field incorporates consciousness along with perceptions of self and others; feelings, thoughts, bodily sensations, spiritual beliefs, desires, goals, expectations, environmental considerations, meanings, and the symbolic nature of one's perceptions—all of this based upon one's life history and the presenting moment as well as the imaged future.[9, pp. 55–56]

From Watson's perspective, "an event or actual caring occasion" occurs when two persons come together with their unique life histories and their phenomenal fields.[9, p. 58] When people come together they share a phenomenal field, which becomes part of the life history of both and alters the dynamics of the present and the future. From this perspective, holistic communication can be viewed as a field experience.

This is consistent with Rogers's Principle of Integrality in relation to the open and infinite nature of energy fields, where person and environment are in continuous mutual interaction. Watson, through the descriptions of her model, shows how Rogers's Principle of Integrality can be applied.

A field perspective adds a richer and more holistic approach to therapeutic communication, wherein the gestalt of one person interacts with another. It challenges us to develop ways of being and ways of interacting that embrace the whole.

Therapeutic Communication Skills: A Prerequisite for Holistic Communication

Traditional models of therapeutic communication do the following: define and prescribe various stages or phases, delineate various roles for the nurse or therapist, identify verbal and nonverbal communication skills, and identify therapist characteristics that are essential to creating a therapeutic milieu.

It is important for nurses to be familiar with the various stages of relationship formation and to develop and refine communication skills. It is also important for nurses to understand and integrate the qualities and attributes that are important in creating a therapeutic exchange. Empathy, unconditional regard, genuineness, respect, concern, caring, and compassion are vital and essential attributes for therapeutic communication. Developing and refining communication skills, including active listening, active observing, focusing, restating, reflecting, and interpreting, are also important in facilitating the therapeutic process. The aforementioned knowledge, skills, techniques, and attributes are foundational to the therapeutic communication process and are prerequisites to engaging in the caring, healing exchange that characterizes holistic communication. Acquiring these skills takes time and is enhanced by experience. Mastering these skills is a lifelong process that is facilitated by reflective practices, guidance, sage mentoring, and a commitment to self-knowledge and awareness.

The next step is to identify how a holistic approach to therapeutic communication would manifest itself. It is important to consider the distinguishing characteristics of holistic communication and how we can integrate these to create a caring, healing environment.

Distinguishing Characteristics of a Holistic Orientation to Communication

Preaccess and Assessment Phase

The holistic communication process acknowledges the importance of being centered and creating an intention before engaging in a caring, healing interaction with another. These two processes, being centered and creating intention, constitute the preaccess phase involved in holistic interactions. This phase lays the foundation for caring, healing communication and occurs before any person-to-person interaction takes place. As the nurse stays present to the moment, to self, and to the person, a healing environment is maintained. Consciously creating a healing

environment, no matter where one is working, nurtures both the client and the self at a deep level.[2, p. 623]

It is useful to note the distinction between *accessing* and *assessment*. The term *accessing* is preferred because it has the connotation of being open to receiving information in a nonjudgmental way. The term *assessment* implies appraising, evaluating, and judging. An essential characteristic of holistic communication is the mutuality inherent in the experience—this means that both the nurse and the client participate equally in the process. Utilizing language that supports the concept of partnership reinforces a commitment to mutuality.

Acknowledgment of the Infinite and Sacred Nature of Being

Holistic nursing acknowledges that people are infinite, sacred, and spiritual beings. Florence Nightingale spoke of human beings as a "reflection of the Divine with physical, metaphysical, and intellectual attributes." Jean Watson teaches that we are "sacred beings," and Martha Rogers speaks of unitary human beings as "energy fields that are infinite in nature." The Model of Whole-Person Caring combines these concepts to define person as "an energy field that is open, infinite, and spiritual in essence and in continual mutual process with the environment. Each person manifests unique physical, mental, emotional, and social or relational patterns that are interrelated, inseparable, and continually evolving."[3, p. 42] Thus, from the perspective of holistic nursing theorists and models, people are infinite and sacred in nature. This orientation makes a difference in how we approach one another. It shifts how we speak, listen, relate, and interact. When we perceive human beings as sacred, our words, actions, and behaviors are significantly affected.

Moreover, when we view ourselves and others as spiritual, infinite beings with finite bodies, our relationship to illness, disease, and death shifts dramatically. Communication may be oriented to the soul's purpose in addition to symptom relief. This orientation creates a potential to explore and derive meaning from life's challenges and create a healing environment even in the face of death and terminal illness. Nurses who care for patients with terminal illnesses often are uncomfortable discussing prognosis, hospice care, advanced care planning, and spirituality.[10]

When one understands that this physical life is a small part of the infinite journey, the stigma of death becomes obsolete and allows the nurse to be fully present to persons with terminal illnesses and facing imminent death.

Heart-Centering, Heart Coherence, and the Intuitive Heart

Heart-centering is one of the first processes the nurse engages in prior to any interaction. This process involves the nurse focusing her or his attention on the heart, setting aside concerns and thoughts, and connecting with feelings of love and compassion.

Maintaining this heart-centeredness throughout interactions has many positive effects for the nurse. Research conducted at the Institute of HeartMath shows that the resultant feelings of caring and appreciation from heart-centering creates coherence in the electromagnetic energy field; balances heart rhythms; increases IgA (immunoglobulin A) levels and natural killer cell levels; increases mental clarity and problem solving; and reduces sleeplessness, body aches, fatigue, anger, sadness, hypertension, and other chronic problems.[11] Heart coherence, also referred to as physiologic coherence, cardiac coherence, or resonance, is a functional mode measured by heart rate variability analysis, wherein a person's heart rhythm pattern becomes ordered.[12]

In addition to the positive mental, psychological, and physiologic effects, coherence may help to connect people with their intuitive inner guidance. Research suggests that the heart's energy field (energetic heart) is coupled to a field of information that is not bound by the classic limits of time and space. This evidence comes from a rigorous experimental study that investigated the proposition that the body receives and processes information about a future event before the event actually happens.[13] McCraty

and Childre explain that the intuitive heart or heart intelligence is coupled to a deeper part of oneself, what some may call their *higher power* or their *higher capacities*. When we are heart-centered and coherent, we have a tighter coupling and closer alignment with our deeper source of intuitive intelligence.[12, pp. 15–16]

Research also shows that the positive mental and physiologic effects experienced by the nurse can be transmitted to the person. When a person maintains a coherent electromagnetic field through the process of centering, that person's energy field positively affects those in the surrounding environment. Morris reports that a coherent energy field can be generated and/or enhanced by the intention of small groups of participants trained to send coherence-facilitating intentions to a target receiver.[14] It is believed that information about a person's emotional state is encoded in the heart's electromagnetic field and is communicated into the external environment.[12, p. 20] When the nurse becomes heart-centered, a caring, healing field is created in which the person feels safe, nurtured, and loved; this is in an optimal environment for healing communication to occur.

Grounding

Grounding is the process of connecting to the Earth and the Earth's energy field to calm the mind and focus one's inner flow of energy as a means to enhance healing endeavors.[15] Centering and grounding may be considered a single continuous process because one flows into the other. As such, grounding can also be viewed as part of the preaccess phase of the holistic communication process.

Often, communication can bring up many feelings and thoughts that are emotionally charged and difficult for the nurse to deal with. Grounding provides the nurse with a steady physical, psychological, and energetic platform on which to anchor the communication process. In physical terms, grounding provides a connection between an electric circuit and the Earth. In psychological terms, grounding helps establish a feeling of self-awareness and provides a connection to the consciousness of one's own self.

Energetically, grounding establishes an awareness of the unity of body, mind, and spirit, as stated by McCartney:

> The practice of grounding connects you with your spiritual intelligence, which opens a cornucopia of wisdom tools for creating health and keeping you in emotional balance and harmony. To heighten this experience, visualize your spiritual intelligence as energy or light. To ground your spiritual intelligence into your body, visualize this light in the center of your head expanding straight down your body and anchoring into the earth. In this way you are affirming [that] "I am a spirit grounded in my body and anchored to the earth."[16]

Creating Intention

Creating an intention ideally precedes interaction with a person and is part of the preaccess phase of the holistic nurse caring process. Intention can be defined as "the direction of one's inner awareness and focus for healing."[15]

Creating an intention is a process that affects not only the mental and emotional realms but also the physical world. Tiller demonstrated that conscious intent can be imprinted in materials that can be shipped to a distant laboratory, where they bring out the intentional effect that is imprinted on them. Recent advances in theoretical physics suggest that the space between atoms and molecules is not inert. Tiller and Dibble speculate that this "vacuum" may be where the intent is imprinted.[17]

Thus, creating an intention is a powerful way for the nurse to establish an optimal environment for a caring, healing interaction. Examine the following intention: "I am here for the greater good of this person. I set aside my own concerns and worries and am fully present to the person here and now." With this intention the nurse is consciously setting aside her or his own concerns and focusing on the patient, thus putting into motion the dynamic that this interaction will be "for the greater good of this person." The nurse is also making a conscious decision to be fully present. Through this intention the nurse creates an environment that promotes and sustains a caring, healing interaction.

Caring, Healing, Transcendent Presence

Presence has been defined as a way of being, a way of relating, a way of being with, and a way of being there. These perspectives each speak to different facets of the quality and characteristics of the attention that one person gives to another in a relationship.

Osterman and Schwartz-Barcott characterize four ways of "being there" as presence, partial presence, full presence, and transcendent presence.[18] McKivergin describes three levels of presence as physical presence, psychological presence, and therapeutic presence.[19]

What distinguishes holistic communication from other types of communication is the depth and profound quality of presence. Watson speaks of the full use of self in the transpersonal caring process. When the nurse becomes heart-centered, she or he has the capacity to resonate with the person at a heart-and-soul level. At this level, the nurse connects with the person at a deep psychosocial, heartfelt, and spiritual level. This is a difficult concept to describe and remains more of a felt experience. The nurse must be able to access and rest in the depth of her or his own Beingness before bringing this caring, healing, transcendent presence into a relationship.

Being able to communicate from more profound levels of presence is the result of experience and engaging in processes of deep reflection and inquiry. However, cultivating this type of presence is something that also can be taught through experiential techniques and role modeling. Various self-reflective practices such as journaling, meditation, relaxation, contemplation, dream analysis, narrative, and storytelling in one's personal daily practice can help cultivate a deeper relationship with the essence of one's existence that can then be brought into a relationship with another. The nurse must be able to connect with her or his own heart, soul, and transcendent nature before establishing that connection with others.

Intuition

Intuition is a useful and foundational element in the holistic communication process. It is defined as "the perceived knowing of things and events without the conscious use of rational processes; using all of the senses to receive information"[20, p. 722] The usefulness of intuition in the nursing process is well researched and documented. Although intuitive knowing is something that occurs more readily with the experienced nurse, it can be consciously cultivated through various practices.

Ways to cultivate intuition are listening to music, engaging in relaxation techniques, and journal writing, which can be useful in increasing one's intuitive and spiritual development. Meditation also increases one's intuitive knowing. Regular meditation practice enables one to enter the intuitional state at will.[2, p. 625]

When the nurse utilizes intuition she or he engages the full use of self, which is essential in accessing and communicating with the whole person. Intuition allows the nurse to access the subtle energies and the conscious and unconscious fields that are not readily perceived. This process allows the nurse to sense into the Being of another and communicate at levels where profound healing occurs.

Tools and Practices to Enhance Holistic Communication

Knowing Self

Awareness and understanding of one's self and one's values, beliefs, motivations, goals, feelings, and actions are imperative to relating in a caring, healing manner. When we are aware of ourselves and understand who we are and the basis for our own attitudes, preconceptions, and reactions, we are in a much better position to empathize, appreciate other people's differences and uniqueness, and encourage their self-revelations. To nurture caring, healing communication and relationships, we need to conduct assessments of ourselves as individuals, as well as our communications, spirituality, and cultural beliefs and traditions. All of these factors influence behavior and, without a thoughtful reflection

and understanding of them, we deny the very people we care for the opportunity to understand themselves.[21]

Meditation

Meditation is a quiet turning inward—the practice of focusing one's attention internally to achieve clearer consciousness and inner stillness. Meditation is both a state of mind and a method. The state is one in which the mind is quiet, open, and receptive. The meditator is relaxed but alert. The method involves the focusing of attention on something such as the breath, an image, a word, or an action such as tai chi or qi gong. There is a sustained concentration, but it should be effortless. Meditation allows a better understanding of the self and increased receptivity to insights arising from one's deeper being. There are numerous methods and schools of meditation. However, all methods believe in emptying the mind and letting go of the mind's chatter that preoccupies us.[22] Various forms of meditative practice can be found in Chapter 11.

According to Benor:

> Meditation is healing in and of itself. Meditation is a gateway into spiritual awareness and healing. By quieting our mind we can access dimensions in which spiritual healing can occur. Meditation allows us to quiet the mind from its chatter and its focus on everyday, outer-world matters. It helps us open into transcendent awareness.[23]

John Kabat-Zinn, a teacher of mindfulness meditation, describes his practice in the following way:

> It has everything to do with waking up and living in harmony with oneself and with the world. It has to do with examining who we are, with questioning our view of the world and our place in it, and with cultivating some appreciation for the fullness of each moment we are alive. Most of all, it has to do with being in touch.[24, p. 3]

Meditation is perhaps the single most useful reflective practice to help gain self-awareness, self-knowledge, increase intuition, and enhance one's spiritual development. Because self-awareness, self-knowledge, and intuition are foundational to creating a caring, healing presence, meditating regularly is an important practice in which to engage.

Like any reflective and contemplative process, it takes discipline and practice to reap the benefits of meditation. When nurses first begin to meditate, they can start with 5-minute sessions, and then increase by 5 more minutes every couple of weeks. Meditating from 30 minutes to an hour daily will help the nurse realize maximum benefits. Setting aside time to meditate in the morning to begin the daily routine is a wonderful way to start the day. Meditating first thing in the morning allows one to access one's spiritual essence and to approach life from a place of peace and equanimity.

Engaging Your Observer

Engaging your Observer is a process that is useful when confronting a situation or communication that is particularly difficult and emotionally charged. It also helps the nurse be present to a person or situation with clarity and without bias. This practice has its roots in Buddhist psychology.

The nonjudgmental aspect of your self is called the *Observer* or *Witness*. Some perceive this aspect as our higher Self. It can be likened to a wise grandparent who looks lovingly on the thoughts and reactions of our childlike minds. The Witness is our ability to observe life without engaging our past patterns of reacting and becoming emotionally charged. The Observer acts as a third party who allows the nurse to separate from difficult emotions and feelings in situations so that communication occurs from a space of clarity and wisdom. Utilizing this technique enhances self-knowledge and self-awareness because it provides constant feedback related to one's responses and reactions to situations. The Observer is able to transcend the ego while embracing the whole of the moment so that one responds with wisdom rather than reacting from conditioned response.[25]

Engaging the Observer involves centering, being aware of internal reactions, gratefully acknowledging these reactions, and responding from the higher Self. This is a technique that allows one to access the higher Self and move from that place of higher consciousness in interactions with another. This is central to the transpersonal caring process and communicating from a holistic perspective.[3, p. 104] (See **Exhibit 19-1**.)

EXHIBIT 19-1   Engaging Your Observer in a Difficult Situation

Situation: You just realized that you gave your patient the wrong medication.

- *Center yourself and create an intention.* Take a breath and bring your consciousness or attention to the area around your heart; connect with a feeling of love and compassion. You might imagine holding a newborn baby, hugging a loved one, or cuddling your pet.

- *Observer relates your internal reactions — emotionally, mentally, and physically.* This makes you feel horrible. You are upset that you made this mistake. You are concerned about your patient, what your supervisor will say, and filling out an incident report. Your stomach is churning and you feel like crying.

- *Acknowledge your reactions.* "Yes, I feel horrible when I make mistakes and I am concerned about my patient, my supervisor's response, and having to fill out an incident report. My stomach hurts and I feel like crying."

- *Respond from a place of wisdom and compassion.* Take another deep breath, bring your attention to the area around your heart, connect with a feeling of love and compassion, and respond silently to yourself with a self-compassionate remark: "Making mistakes is part of being human. Don't be so hard on yourself. This is a valuable opportunity to learn and grow and become a better nurse."

This entire process takes about 5 seconds and allows the nurse to set aside thoughts and feelings that interfere with a caring, healing interaction.

Source: L. Thornton, *Whole Person Caring: An Interprofessional Model for Healing and Wellness* (Indianapolis, IN: Sigma Theta Tau International, 2013): 104.

CLEAR Communication

Sometimes it is useful to use an acronym when acquiring or trying to remember new skills. Nurses use an acronym to help remember some of the processes involved in holistic communication. Being CLEAR in communication stands for Center, Listen, Empathize, Attention, and Respect.[3, p. 190] (See **Exhibit 19-2**.)

Drawing Out the Person's Story

We as humans ascribe unique meanings to our experiences. A person's perception of meaning is related to all factors in health-wellness-disease-illness and can influence his or her response to it. If these are not clearly articulated, either because the person is unable or, more commonly, is not given the opportunity to express comprehension and feelings about the situation—be it the illness, treatment, responses, or reason for his or her actions—meaning is then left up to the interpretation or preconceived ideas of the helper. A cornerstone of holistic communication is assisting individuals to find meaning in their experience, meanings such as the person's concerns regarding health and family economics, as well as deeper meanings related to the person's purpose in life. Nurses should ask clients, patients, and families to share the meaning that something has for them

---

EXHIBIT 19-2   Holistic Communication: Be CLEAR

Center yourself

- Pause for a moment.
- Breathe deeply.
- Connect with a feeling of love and compassion.
- Create a silent intention that your thoughts, words, and actions will be for the greater good.

Listen wholeheartedly

- Set aside your own thoughts, emotions, and feelings.
- Focus on the person's agenda.
- Do not judge or analyze.
- Open your heart to what is being communicated.

Empathize

- Come from a place of genuine concern.
- Ask yourself: How does this person perceive the situation? What does the world look like through this person's eyes? What is he or she feeling?
- Empathy involves an understanding that comes from sensing into the being of another.

Attention: Be Fully Present

- Be aware of what you are feeling and sensing. Stay present to yourself.
- Bring the fullness of yourself to every moment: emotionally, mentally, physically, and spiritually.

Respect

- Respect all that is.
- Respect yourself. Set boundaries if needed.
- Respect person. Honor cultural, social, ontological, and ideological differences.
- Welcome diversity.

Source: L. Thornton, *Whole Person Caring: An Interprofessional Model for Healing and Wellness* (Indianapolis, IN: Sigma Theta Tau International, 2013): 190–191.

(e.g., symptoms, illness, treatment, outlook, fears). Only then will we truly glean an understanding of the individual's experience as he or she sees it and shape our interventions to meet the person's needs.

One of the best ways to understand what the person is most concerned about and the meaning something has for that person is through the use of narrative and story. Client narratives, whether they arise from individuals, families, or communities, provide the context of the experiences and are used as an important focus in understanding the person's situation. The nurse first ascertains what the individual thinks or believes is happening to him or her, and then assists the person to identify what will help the situation. The assessment begins from where the individual is. Space and time are allowed for exploration. Each person's health encounter is truly seen as unique. This requires a perspective that the nurse is not the "expert" regarding another's health/illness experience.[26, p. 66] Simply asking, "What do you think is going on with you (or is happening to you)?" and "What do you think would help?" allows patients time to tell their story and give their perspective. The same principle applies to cultural competence. Asking, "What do I need to know about you culturally (or your culture) to care for you?" provides much more individualized and useful information about various cultures, their health beliefs and practices, and needs. The nurse then discusses options, including the person's choices, across a continuum, including the possible effects and implications of each.[26, p. 70]

Listening to the patient's story provides a holistic perspective and allows the nurse to get an overall sense of what the person is experiencing. This is more than simply using therapeutic techniques such as responding, reflecting, and summarizing. This is deep listening or, as some say, "listening with the heart and not just the ears." It is done with conscious intention and without preconceptions, busyness, distractions, or analysis. Using active listening responses, such as "Uh huh . . . uh huh," "Oh," "I see," and "Can you tell me more?" indicate that the nurse is listening, gives the person permission to continue, and keeps the patient focused on the story. It takes place in the "now" within an atmosphere of shared humanness—that is,

human being to human being. Through presence or "being with in the moment," nurses provide each person with an interpersonal encounter that is experienced as a connection with one who is giving undivided attention to the needs and concerns of the individual. Using unconditional positive regard, nurses convey to the individual receiving care the belief in his or her worth and value as a human being, not solely the recipient of medical and nursing interventions.[26, p. 69]

Caring, Healing Responses to Frequently Asked Questions and Statements

The following are some of the questions clients, patients, and families regularly ask nurses. A brief description of the underlying dynamic of the question or statement, ineffective responses, and caring, healing responses are identified.[27]

1. "Am I dying?"
   - *Dynamic:* Request for information, reassurance.
   - *Ineffective responses:* "I really am not able to discuss that. You should talk with your doctor." or "You always have to keep hope." or "Don't say that. Look how you are improving every day."
   - *Caring, healing response:* In a very gentle voice, "Do you think you are dying? Can you tell me why you think you are dying?" Follow up by asking, "What does death mean to you?"
2. "Why did God (or whomever one believes in) do this to me?" and "I don't want to go on living."
   - *Dynamic:* Spiritual distress.
   - *Ineffective responses:* "Sometimes in life, bad things happen to people who don't deserve them." or "Don't feel that way. God has not abandoned you." or "We can't always understand why things happen, but there is a reason."
   - *Caring, healing response:* Be silent. If acceptable, hold the person's hand and convey by your full attention and presence that you are willing to bear witness to her or his deepest despair and sorrow.

"This seems to be a very difficult time for you on many different levels." Wait for a response. If none, gently ask, "Can you explain that to me so that I can understand?"

3. "Don't tell anyone else what I am telling you."
   - *Dynamic:* Can I trust you?
   - *Ineffective responses:* "You can trust me not to tell anyone else." or "Your request makes me really uncomfortable."
   - *Caring, healing response:* "Is there a particular reason why you do not want me to share this information?" Wait for a response. Depending on the answer, "I understand your wish to keep this between us, but others may need to know this information to provide you with (what you need, or the best care possible, or to help you make a decision, etc.)." or "If it is not imperative for anyone else to know, certainly I will keep it confidential."

4. Repeated requests for the nurse's personal information.
   - *Dynamic:* A need to be connected.
   - *Ineffective responses:* "I don't talk with clients or patients about my personal life," or answering every question that the individual asks.
   - *Caring, healing response:* "Is there a reason why you would like to know about (the topic asked about)?"

5. Silence.
   - *Dynamic:* Individual is thinking, processing, feeling, cannot put thoughts and feelings into words, or is physically or emotionally exhausted. Silence is a form of communication and has a great deal of meaning.
   - *Ineffective responses:* Filling the silence with any words to keep conversation alive, or "I can see that you do not want to talk now. I will come back later."
   - *Caring, healing response:* "You seem quiet." Wait for a response. "Would you like to talk or would you just like me to sit here with you for a while?" Get in touch with your own discomfort if this is an issue for you. Relax into the silence,

understanding that this is what the person needs at this time. Communicate through presence and intent that you are there for this person.

6. "What should I do? What would you do?"
   - *Dynamic:* Insecurity about decision, lack of knowledge, second guessing, too much input.
   - *Ineffective responses:* "Well, I would . . ." or "When this happened to (me, my brother/friend/another patient), I/she/he did . . ." or "I think you should discuss this with your doctor."
   - *Caring, healing response:* "First, tell me what you understand about your illness and treatment." Wait for a response. Then, "Tell me what you think you should do or what you feel would be best or most helpful for you." The nurse is an option giver. Discuss the options, the implications of each option, and the individual's thoughts, feelings, beliefs, and concerns about each option so that the person has sufficient information to make an informed decision with which he or she is comfortable.

7. Anger.
   - *Dynamic:* Powerlessness.
   - *Ineffective responses:* "Don't get angry at me. I am just trying to help you." or "I don't have to take this from (a patient, a colleague, a family, the doctor, etc.)." or "Call security."
   - *Caring, healing response:* Stop and center, and then send peace. Visualize the person as he or she was as an innocent, precious baby. The energy tends to change immediately when we image babies because they connect with our joy. Wait calmly until the angry person completes the attack, and then begin the discussion.

8. Fear.
   - *Dynamic:* Projection, misperception. Fear and worry are the most common forms of imagery.
   - *Ineffective response:* "Don't worry, everything will work out."
   - *Caring, healing response:* "Can you share with me what your understanding is or

what you think is going to happen?" Then, reality test by gently asking, "What do you think is the worst that can happen?" and "What might be a positive that can happen in this circumstance?"

9. Anxiety.
   - *Dynamic:* Projection, unknowing, too much input, inability to stay in the present or listen to and trust one's own inner wisdom.
   - *Ineffective responses:* "Constantly thinking or worrying about this is not going to help. It will only make it worse." or "Try to get your mind off of it."
   - *Caring, healing response:* "It sounds like a lot is going on, so let's see if we can focus on right now and deal with it after that." or "What do you think is best or necessary for you? What are your body, mind, and gut telling you?"

10. "It's all my fault."
   - *Dynamic:* Guilt often rooted in shame.
   - *Ineffective responses:* "Of course you are not to blame." or "Well, it was going to happen some time or another. It's not your fault."
   - *Caring, healing response:* "Can you tell me why you think you are responsible for (or are to blame for) it?"

11. "I am such a burden (e.g., bothering you, having you see me like this, having to clean me up, can't do anything for myself)."

   - *Dynamic:* Guilt as an assault on one's assumptions and beliefs about oneself and what one wants others to believe about him or her, creating vulnerability and exposure.
   - *Ineffective response:* "Oh, I've seen (or dealt with) worse. You're not so bad."
   - *Caring, healing response:* "It is a gift to care for you and share this part of your journey (your experience) with you." or "It is my pleasure."

Conclusion

Holistic communication is a caring, healing process that calls forth the full use of self in interacting with another. The elements that distinguish holistic communication are acknowledgment of the infinite and sacred nature of Being; the use of centering, grounding, intention, and intuition; and caring, healing, transcendent presence. Holistic communication can be viewed as a field experience in which there is constant mutual exchange between the nurse's field and the patient's field. Communication is constantly occurring on physical, mental, emotional, and energetic levels. We are never not communicating.

Self-knowledge and self-awareness are foundational to the process of holistic communication. Tools and practices that help the nurse gain a greater understanding and awareness of self include journaling, dream analysis, relaxation techniques, self-reflective practices, and meditation. Growing in self-knowledge and self-awareness increases the nurse's effectiveness as an instrument in the caring, healing process. Holistic communication invites us to engage our higher Self as we meet another in that transcendent space where profound healing occurs. When this happens, a "healing field of communication" is created in which both the nurse and the person are enriched and nurtured.

Directions for Future Research

1. Explore research findings related to holistic communication.
2. Examine how various aspects of holistic communication are implemented in nursing and healthcare settings.
3. Explore ways in which cultural learning can be incorporated into nurses' practice to influence the effectiveness of holistic interactions.

Nurse Healer Reflections

After reading this chapter, the holistic nurse will be able to answer or to begin a process of answering the following questions:

- How does being centered and creating an intention affect the quality of my communication?

- When I view another as sacred, how does this affect the quality of my interaction?
- What are my attributes as a holistic communicator?

NOTES

1. M. E. Rogers, "Nursing: Science of Unitary, Irreducible, Human Beings: Update 1990," in *Visions of Rogers' Science-Based Nursing*, ed. E. A. M. Barrett (New York: National League for Nursing, 1990): 5–11.

2. L. Thornton and C. Mariano, "Evolving from Therapeutic to Holistic Communication," in *Holistic Nursing: A Handbook for Practice*, 6th ed., eds. B. M. Dossey and L. Keegan (Burlington, MA: Jones & Bartlett Learning, 2013): 619–632.

3. L. Thornton, *Whole Person Caring: An Interprofessional Model for Healing and Wellness* (Indianapolis, IN: Sigma Theta Tau International, 2013).

4. E. Arnold and K. Underman-Boggs, *Interpersonal Relationships: Professional Communication Skills for Nurses*, 6th ed. (St. Louis, MO: Saunders, 2011).

5. M. Rogers, *An Introduction to the Theoretical Basis of Nursing*, 7th ed. (Philadelphia: F. A. Davis, 1977): 54.

6. M. A. Newman, *Health as Expanding Consciousness*, 2nd ed. (Sudbury, MA: Jones and Bartlett, 1999): 13.

7. T. Moore, *Care of the Soul* (New York: HarperCollins, 1992): 10.

8. J. Watson, *Postmodern Nursing and Beyond* (New York: Churchill Livingston, 1999): 129.

9. J. Watson, *Nursing: Human Science and Human Care: A Theory of Nursing* (Sudbury, MA: Jones and Bartlett, 2007).

10. J. Goldsmith, B. Ferrell, E. Wittenberg-Lyles, and S. Ragan, "Palliative Care Communication in Oncology Nursing," *Clinical Journal of Oncology Nursing* 17, no. 2 (2012): 163–167.

11. R. McCraty and R. Reese, *The Central Role of the Heart in Generating and Sustaining Positive Emotions*, Institute of HeartMath, Publication No. 06-022 (Boulder Creek, CA: HeartMath Research Center, 2009).

12. R. McCraty and D. Childre, "Coherence: Bridging Personal, Social, and Global Health," *Alternative Therapies* 16, no. 4 (2010): 10–24.

13. R. McCraty, M. Atkinson, and R. T. Bradley, "Electrophysiological Evidence of Intuition: Part 1. The Surprising Role of the Heart," *Journal of Alternative and Complementary Medicine* 10, no. 1 (2004): 133–143.

14. S. Morris, "Achieving Collective Coherence: Group Effects on Heart Rate Variability Coherence and Heart Rhythm Synchronization," *Alternative Therapies* 16, no. 4 (2010): 62–72.

15. C. Jackson and C. Latini, "Touch and Hand-Mediated Therapies" in *Holistic Nursing: A Handbook for Practice*, 6th ed., eds. B. M. Dossey and L. Keegan (Burlington, MA: Jones & Bartlett Learning, 2013): 418

16. Personal communication. F. McCartney, August 13, 2014.

17. W. Tiller and W. Dibble, *A Brief Introduction to Intention-Host Device Research* (Payson, AZ: William A. Tiller Foundation, 2009): 10.

18. P. Osterman and D. Schwartz-Barcott, "Presence: Four Ways of Being There," *Nursing Forum* 31, no. 2 (1996): 23–30.

19. M. McKivergin, "The Nurse as an Instrument of Healing," in *Holistic Nursing: A Handbook for Practice*, 5th ed., eds. B. M. Dossey and L. Keegan (Sudbury, MA: Jones and Bartlett, 2009): 721–738.

20. P. Potter and N. Frisch, "The Holistic Caring Process," in *Holistic Nursing: A Handbook for Practice*, 6th ed., eds. B. M. Dossey and L. Keegan (Burlington, MA: Jones & Bartlett Learning, 2013): 146

21. C. Mariano, "Holistic Nursing as a Specialty: Scope and Standards of Practice," *Clinics of North America* 42, no. 2 (2007): 165–188.

22. C. Mariano, "Holistic Integrative Therapies in Palliative Care," in *Palliative Care Nursing: Quality Care to the End of Life*, 4th ed., eds. M. Matzo and D. Sherman (New York: Springer, 2015): 235–267.

23. Personal communication. D. Benor, August 13, 2014.

24. J. Kabat-Zinn, *Wherever You Go There You Are: Mindfulness Meditation in Everyday Life* (New York: Hyperion, 1994): 3.

25. L. Thornton, "Self-Compassion: A Prescription for Well-Being," *Imprint* 58, no. 2 (2011): 42–45.

26. C. Mariano, "Holistic Nursing: Scope and Standards of Practice," in *Holistic Nursing: A Handbook for Practice*, 6th ed., eds. B. M. Dossey and L. Keegan (Burlington, MA: Jones & Bartlett Learning, 2013): 59–84.

27. C. Mariano, "Therapeutic Interactions" (adapted course materials, New York University and Pacific College of Oriental Medicine, 2014).

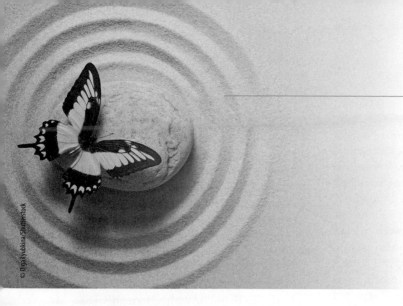

CHAPTER 20

Relationships

Mary A. Helming

© Olga Lyubkina/Shutterstock

Nurse Healer Objectives

Theoretical

- Define three areas in which nurses are required to develop effective relationships.
- List seven issues that either strengthen or interfere with relationships.
- Identify ways in which selected nursing theorists inform therapeutic relationships.
- Identify ways that the humanistic psychologies of Rogers and Maslow, as well as the positive psychology of Seligman, expand holistic thinking.
- Identify four archetypes of human relationships that address physical, emotional, mental, and spiritual domains, using Jung and Arrien.

Clinical

- Identify core elements that lead to establishing and maintaining effective relationships.
- Implement and evaluate effective negotiating styles that address issues while maintaining a sense of relatedness.
- Gain insight into problematic aspects of relationships and how to manage them more effectively.

Personal

- Increase your use of key effective personal relationship characteristics.

- Develop strategies to incorporate effective boundaries in relationships.
- Strengthen your concepts of spiritual relationship.

Definitions

Archetype: Name given by Jung and Arrien to specific patterns of human collective awareness that symbolically represent human potential, such as the Healer, the Warrior, the Mother, or the Wise Person.

Boundaries: Artificial separations between people that define the perimeters of the relationship.

Complementary transaction: An interaction in which the ego states match (e.g., adult-to-adult communication). Complementary transactions support and strengthen relationships.

Defense patterns: Protective mechanisms that justify individual action while detracting from relationship building.

Emotional intelligence: Awareness and attention to personal emotional needs that allow individuals to be in a position of equality with others, rather than seeking power and control or becoming overly passive.

Forgiveness: A willingness to acknowledge one's own mistakes and shortcomings and to allow others room to acknowledge their shortcomings as well.

Theory and Research

Relationship refers to kinship, passionate attachment, or a connection between those having relations or dealings. A relationship refers to two or more persons or things working together, belonging together, or being part of a whole, as in relatives within a family. Throughout history, relationships have existed between human beings, between the divine and human beings, and between the earthly environment and human beings. It is evident that no human being was intended to live alone. This concept is repeated in many world religions. Throughout the ages, the great religions have spoken of the necessity of loving, caring human relationships. Keegan and Drick explain the term *interconnectedness* as implying that people may share the "universal reciprocity of love and responsibility" without regard to their culture, politics, or religion.[1]

Relationship Theories

The Theory of Human Relatedness, according to Hagerty and Patusky, suggests that people are "relational beings who experience some degree of involvement with external referents, including people, objects, groups, and natural environments."[2, pp. 147-148] The theory emphasizes that some human relationships serve to lessen anxiety and improve wellness, and others promote distress and anxiety. The following are the four stages of human relatedness:

1. Connection means there is active involvement with another, associated with enhanced comfort and wellness.
2. Disconnection involves lack of involvement and is associated with lack of wellness and distress.
3. Parallelism implies disengagement, or the lack of involvement with others. This can have a positive effect of creating solitude with associated physical and psychological replenishment.
4. Enmeshment often describes negative, overinvolved relationships, fraught with anxiety, distress, and functional disability.

It is also possible for people to be in relationships in all of these quadrants simultaneously.

Hagerty and Patusky further suggest that there are four social competencies vital for relationships:

1. Sense of belonging means there is an appropriate "fit" with the environment, group, or individual. There is a sense of being valued and needed in the relationship.
2. Reciprocity is a positive aspect of relationship in which there is a perceived equal exchange between parties.
3. Mutuality represents how people tend to join with those they believe share similarities to them, or with whom they share an acceptance of differences.
4. Synchrony is a person's perception of congruent feelings or behaviors with another with whom the individual shares a relationship.

The term *interrelationship* implies the existence of a subtle web of life that connects all human beings, their environment, and spirituality. Each person's actions can directly and indirectly affect others and can create a healing or toxic response or energy. Holistic nurses have identified interrelationship as a key element of their practice. For holistic nurses, relationship transcends patient care and includes patient families and significant others, interactions with coworkers, interdisciplinary associates, and authority figures. Jackson cites 12 essential values to guide relationship-based care, evolving from care theory, holistic concepts, and loving care, as referenced in Koloroutis's classic work, *Relationship-Based Care: A Model for Transforming Practice.*[3] Seven of the 12 values include relationship, and they are as follows:

1. The meaning and essence of care are experienced in the moment when one human being connects with another.
2. Feeling connected to one another creates harmony and healing; feeling isolated destroys spirit.
3. The relationship between patients and their families and members of the clinical team belongs at the heart of care delivery.
4. Care providers' knowledge of self and self-care are fundamental requirements for high-quality care and healthy interpersonal relationships.

5. Healthy relationships among members of the healthcare team lead to the delivery of high-quality care and result in high patient, physician, and staff satisfaction.

6. The value of relationship in patient care must be understood, valued, and agreed to by all members of the healthcare organization.

7. A therapeutic relationship between a patient/family and a professional nurse is essential to high-quality patient care.

Therapeutic Relationships in Holistic Nursing

The *therapeutic relationship* has traditionally been associated with psychological counseling processes, but it is highly adaptable to holistic nursing. A therapeutic relationship is a professional alliance between the nurse and the client or patient, working together for a defined period of time to accomplish specific health-related goals.[4] Further, a therapeutic relationship can occur even if a patient is in the end stages of life or is generally uncooperative with health and wellness initiatives.

The patient must feel supported as well as listened to, and the nurse should feel valued in his or her role. A significant point is that patients may not listen well to their healthcare providers unless they themselves feel listened to. Discontent with healthcare providers can cause patients to avoid treatment, take longer to recover, have more complications, and misunderstand vital information.

The therapeutic relationship is considered to be essential to psychiatric nursing, yet Dziopa and Ahern note that it is not instinctive but requires high-level skills, including advanced practice skills.[5] Nine primary concepts explain the therapeutic relationship, according to their review of the literature: (1) demonstrating respect, (2) being genuine, (3) being there/being available, (4) accepting individuality, (5) having self-awareness, (6) maintaining boundaries, (7) demonstrating understanding and empathy, (8) providing support, and (9) promoting equality. Therapeutic relationships can be utilized in many areas of nursing. In hospice and palliative care nursing, the therapeutic relationship with patients has given nurses "a 'privileged' experience that may lead to existential growth and job satisfaction."[6, p. 75] The therapeutic relationship has been considered the cornerstone of mental health nursing.[7] In critical care, the therapeutic relationship often extends to family members and requires the nurse to use sound emotional intelligence. Advanced practice nurses in primary care may form beneficial therapeutic relationships with their patients. Likewise, many psychotherapists consider the therapeutic relationship vital to therapy. It is well known that the provider–patient relationship plays a potentially large role in healing. In this light, it is important to discuss selected psychological theorists whose work encourages the use of the therapeutic relationship. Many other healthcare workers, such as licensed clinical social workers, marriage and family counselors, psychologists, psychiatrists, peer counselors, occupational therapists, physical therapists, and psychotherapists, utilize the concept of the therapeutic relationship, which promotes a healing relationship. *Being therapeutic* implies using oneself as an agent of healing in the dynamic relationship between provider and patient or client. It is meaningful for holistic nurses to have a basic knowledge of selected psychological modalities that have influenced models of therapeutic relationship, counseling, and therapy. It is vital to comprehend some of the primary psychology theories that influence understanding of human behaviors and relationships. To understand others, it is necessary to understand ourselves and why we do the things we do. Because human lives are built on interrelationships, it is plausible that the sources of our conflicts and troubles are often associated with unhealthy relationships with a Higher Power, with other human beings, with the environment, and with one's self.

Table 20-1 highlights selected influential psychologists and their theories, ranging from traditional theories to humanistic psychology to positive psychology. First, Pavlov described *behavioral psychology*, with the belief that most human actions are conditioned behaviors. This concept was followed by traditional

TABLE 20-1 Relationship Theorists	
Psychologist	**Theories and Applications**
Eric Berne	Transactional Analysis.
	Concept: Three ego states, people move among states; unconscious games played between people may be a substitute for true intimacy. Three ego states are Adult (rational, objective), Parent (authoritative figure), and Child (playful, curious, stubborn). All human beings need social interaction, even if it is negative interaction.
	Book: Games People Play: The Psychology of Human Relationships (1964)
Erik Erikson	Eight psychosocial stages of life; psychoanalytic approach:
	1. Trust versus mistrust (infancy)
	2. Autonomy versus shame (early childhood)
	3. Initiative versus doubt (preschool)
	4. Competence versus incompetence (elementary school)
	5. Identity versus role confusion (middle/high school)
	6. Intimacy versus isolation (college)
	7. Generativity versus stagnation (adult)
	8. Ego integrity versus ego despair (older age)
	Concept: Tasks of each age group must be completed; youth often develop identity crisis in their 20s after completing higher education.
	Book: Identity, Youth, and Crisis (1968)
Carl Jung	Freudian psychoanalytic psychology.
	Concept: Collective unconscious as the inherited human unconscious composed of universal mental images and thoughts, which are archetypes.
	Archetypes: Concepts of personality expressed in myths and fairy tales; people fit into these roles interchangeably.
	Mother archetype: Most important, role of nurse, Mother of God, grandmothers, church, Earth, and Nature.
	Crone archetype: The wise old woman who is a visionary, who at the crossroads of life chooses the path of the soul rather than the ego, and she speaks the truth always.
	Book: Development of Personality (1981)
Angeles Arrien	Transpersonal psychology; views life holistically.
	Concept: Evolved Jungian archetypes, four primary archetypes identified.
	Healer archetype: Holistic nursing professionals manifest this archetype by relating to others compassionately and with love. Other essential characteristics of the Healer include bringing caring to human relationships, viewing others in a positive light, and bringing emotional comfort.
	Teacher archetype: The Teacher represents the mental quality in relationships, helping learners to achieve new knowledge, wisdom, and insight. Teachers are also very open to learning. Holistic nurses often exhibit the teacher quality as well.

TABLE 20-1 Relationship Theorists (*continued*)	
Psychologist	**Theories and Applications**
	Warrior archetype: The Warrior symbolizes physical qualities of relationship building. This archetype uses courage to help improve behaviors of self and others, is firm, and uses knowledge, especially facts, effectively. Holistic nurses are very interested in helping patients improve their health and wellness behaviors and can use facts and their knowledge effectively in this endeavor.
	Visionary archetype: The Visionary archetype symbolizes the spiritual aspect of relationship. The Visionary is nonjudgmental and assists in conflict resolution. This personality model exemplifies sound intuitive knowing to assist others in achieving their highest good. Holistic nurses need to focus on the spiritual aspect of relationship, which, in itself, tends to move others toward their highest potential.
	Book: *The Four-Fold Way* (1993)
Isabel Briggs Myers	***Concept:*** Jungian based. Myers-Briggs Type Indicator (MBTI) test widely used to identify personality types. Basis of much psychometric testing; often used to gauge appropriate career choices for individuals, to describe marriage compatibility, and for personal development.
	The MBTI results are expressed in four-letter codes representing how personalities fall into four different domains. Possible to have a total of 16 combinations of domains. Manner in which a person perceives reality is described as either "sensing" type (relies on the five senses) or "intuiting" type (relies on the unconscious to confirm what is real and what is not). Second area of personality involves the way a person judges, either through "thinking" (using logic in interpersonal relationships) or "feeling" (interpreting what something means to themselves as individuals). The third domain involves being an "extravert" (outgoing, makes quick decisions, attempts to influence situations) or an "introvert" (more interested in the inner world of ideas, needs time to develop ideas and insights, quieter). The final domain involves deciding between dominant and auxiliary processes. Sensing (S), intuition (N), thinking (T), and feeling (F) are placed together in pairs. Of these pairs, one function is "dominant" and the other is "auxiliary" (additional), which helps in ordering the letters. Extraverts (E), introverts (I), judgment (J), and perception (P) round out the personality symbols.
Abraham Maslow	Father of human psychology.
	Concept: Hierarchy of needs. People move from lowest physiologic needs (food, water, oxygen) to safety and security, to love and belonging, to esteem and respect, to the highest level, self-actualization (need to do and be the person one is meant to be).
	Other significant concepts of humanistic psychology:
	▪ Identifying one's own voice as the self, rather than listening to society or the parental figure
	▪ Realization that life is a series of choices, one leading to personal growth and the other to regression
	▪ Being honest and taking responsibility for one's feelings, even if not popular
	▪ Being the best one can be in one's work; think outside the box, creative
	▪ Seeing others at their best, finding the good in others
	▪ Abandoning psychological defense mechanisms
	Book: *Toward a Psychology of Being* (1968)
Carl Rogers	Humanistic psychologist.
	Concept: Patient-centered or client-centered therapy; some people have experienced being in open, trusting dialogue with another, without being judged, and have felt a sense of healing from this relationship. Based on Buber's I–Thou philosophy of treating the other as person, not object.

(*continues*)

TABLE 20-1 Relationship Theorists (*continued*)	
Psychologist	**Theories and Applications**
Carl Rogers (*continued*)	Preferable to listen to what clients are saying, rather than trying to "fix" them. Therapist did not need to remain detached and objective; could respond emotionally to the client. **Book:** *On Becoming a Person: A Therapist's View of Psychotherapy* (1995)
Daniel Goleman	**Concept:** Began new movement looking at significance of emotional versus intellectual intelligence. Qualities such as optimism, empathy toward others, resilience (the ability to recover from adversity), and ability to adapt to change are considered part of emotional intelligence. Also conscientiousness, goal orientation with delayed gratification to achieve goals, awareness of one's own shortcomings, confidence in being able to handle most problems, and ability to interact well with others, be cooperative, and manage close personal relationships. **Book:** *Emotional Intelligence* (1995)
Martin Seligman	Father of Positive Psychology. <ul><li>The study of emotions that are positive.</li><li>The study of traits that are positive, including virtues, intelligence, strength, and athleticism.</li><li>The study of social institutions or concepts that possess positive qualities (e.g., functional family units, freedom of inquiry, and democracy) and support a virtuous life. Virtues include integrity, loyalty, valor, and equity.</li></ul>**Concept:** Positive emotions such as trust, hope, and confidence help us most in times of distress. Optimistic people interpret problems as controllable, transient, and limited to one situation. Pessimistic people believe troubles last forever, are uncontrollable, and undermine them. **Learned helplessness:** Concept that studied human and animal responses to uncontrollable events. Linked to passivity in emotionally stressed and traumatized human beings. Linked to depression and victim abuse because of learned helplessness. **Book:** *Authentic Happiness: Using the New Positive Psychology to Realize Your Potential for Lasting Fulfillment* (2002)

Source: Data from T. Butler-Bowden, *50 Psychology Classics: Who We Are, How We Think, What We Do* (Boston: Nicholas Brealey, 2007).

psychoanalytical psychology, which views the subconscious as the key motivator for human behavior, as exemplified by Freudian psychology. Then, in the 1960s, the *humanistic psychology* movement brought with it the concept that caring, trust, and understanding of human complexity are key. The person is viewed holistically, and human creativity and transcendence are valued.[8] The distinction among humanistic psychologists is their belief that human beings are not just controlled by subconscious forces or their environments but are people of free will who maintain the ability to reach for their highest potential. Key concepts of humanistic psychology include self-actualization, creativity, intrinsic nature, individuality, becoming, and meaningfulness. *Positive psychology* developed on the heels of human psychology.

Holistic nurses may select which theories they find most reasonable to use in their practice settings and in their own sphere of personal relationships.[9] (See **Table 20-2**.)

The Healing Relationship

In addition to pursuing a therapeutic relationship with their patients or clients, holistic nurses have identified that the act of relating to another human being can be accomplished in a healing environment, and this is termed

TABLE 20-2   Case Studies Using Theoretical Models

Using the Rogerian Model	The nurse provides client-centered care in her psychiatric setting. The nurse listens to Shelly, a 16-year-old female who has just lost her mother, and allows her to tell stories of how her mother was her best friend. The nurse nonjudgmentally allows Shelly to describe her guilt over having an argument with her mother the day before she died.
Using the Myers-Briggs Type Indicator	The nurse is providing care to 43-year-old JoEllen who talks excessively about her past. The nurse recognizes that JoEllen may have the Feeler personality type, and talking is her way of expression. Another patient, Ryan, is a 35-year-old executive who has a Thinker personality, consistent with his job as a manager. The nurse recognizes that Thinkers prefer direct information rather than excessive conversation.
Using Seligman's Positive Psychology	The nurse assists 28-year-old Amy, a victim of physical abuse, to avoid the passivity and pessimism that often comes with being abused. The nurse points Amy in the direction of hope, positive change, lack of acceptance of this "learned helplessness," and optimism about a new future.

the *healing relationship*. Nightingale characterized the healing relationship as that which puts the patient in the best position for Nature to act on him or her. Dossey describes Nightingale as a mystic, visionary, and healer.[10] Nightingale, as a visionary, described many aspects of healing with which nurses can empower patients. Promoting a healing relationship is both an art and a relational skill.

Healthcare providers, including holistic nurses, can create healing relationships by becoming more *patient centered*. According to Remaking American Medicine, a return to the ideals of patient-centered care includes the following concepts for all healthcare providers:[11]

- *Dignity and respect.* Healthcare practitioners listen to and honor patient and family perspectives and choices. Patient and family knowledge, values, beliefs, and cultural backgrounds are incorporated into the planning and delivery of care.
- *Information sharing.* Healthcare practitioners communicate and share complete and unbiased information with patients and families in ways that are affirming and useful. Patients and families receive timely, complete, and accurate information in order to effectively participate in care and decision making.
- *Participation.* Patients and families are encouraged and supported in participating in care and decision making at the level they choose.

- *Collaboration.* Patients and families are also included on an institution-wide basis. Healthcare leaders collaborate with patients and families in policy and program development, implementation, and evaluation; in healthcare facility design; and in professional education, as well as in the delivery of care.

Time Urgency in Nursing

Too often, the fast pace of care causes providers only to nod to patients' stories and move on to complete the exam or task at hand. Nurses and other healthcare providers are so busy in this era of managed care that it is difficult to find the time to really listen to patients. Relationships take time to establish rapport and trust. How can healing take place when there is no time to listen to patients?

Jean Watson refers to the importance of *caring moments* between nurses and others.

> A caring moment involves an action and choice by both the nurse and the other. . . . If the caring moment is transpersonal, each feels a connection with the other at the spirit level, thus it transcends time and space, opening up new possibilities for healing and human connection at a deeper level than physical interaction.[12]

These moments of eye contact or touch can be transforming, even though they take only seconds. Amplified by the intention of the nurse, powerful healing can be facilitated even while doing task-oriented nursing activities. Often there is no time to establish trust, yet trust on specific levels occurs all of the time; for example, one trusts a nurse one has only just met at a physician's office to give a safe injection of a correct substance at an appropriate dose. The importance of here-and-now interactions is emphasized. Rather than being discouraged with time restrictions, nurses should see their interactions as caring and healing.

The Nurse–Patient Relationship

Nurses can foster truly mutual healing relationships using patient-centered care. Beyond establishing rapport, holistic nurses utilize authentic relationships, which represent true sharing of self and a willingness to be open and genuine within certain limits that protect patient well-being. Patient-centered care has been represented as a key means to achieve a healing relationship. Analogous to patient-centered care is the concept of the nurse–patient relationship.

Hagerty and Patusky assert that the nurse–patient relationship is foundational to good nursing care.[2] The nurse–patient relationship is traditionally defined as having three distinct phases: a beginning phase involving the development of trust; a middle phase, which is the active working phase; and the ending phase, in which the relationship may be terminated. However, Hagerty and Patusky disagree with this traditional approach because even single encounters or short-term relationships with patients can possess as much value as this three-step nurse–patient relationship. Shorter hospital stays and quick primary care or urgent care visits exemplify this shortened relationship.

Jackson describes Halldorsdottir's classic qualitative research on nurse-patient relationships, which are categorized as uncaring and destructive to caring and healing using four terms: the *biocidic* relationship is considered toxic, the *biostatic* relationship is considered cold, the *biopassive* relationship is considered detached and apathetic, while the ideal relationship is *bioactive*.[3] The bioactive relationship is described as concerned, kind, and life sustaining, as well as being the classic ideal nurse–patient relationship. Bioactive relationships are described as loving, full of compassion, fostering of spiritual growth and freedom, and restoring of dignity and well-being. These high-level interactions are likely the most supportive of healing.

Theories About Relationships

Barbara Dossey's Theory of Integral Nursing, a grand theory, transcends holistic nursing theory and includes multiple dimensions of interrelationships. As mentioned earlier in this text, within the theory are four quadrants demonstrating how human beings experience their world through relationships. The "I" quadrant represents the individual; the "We" quadrant demonstrates relationship to others within the context of culture, values, and vision; the "It" quadrant represents the physical body; and the "Its" quadrant represents relationships to environment and social systems. Further, integral nursing values the patient–practitioner relationship, the community–practitioner relationship, and the practitioner–practitioner relationship. The patient-practitioner relationship is an ideal combination of psychosocial spiritual care along with biotechnological care that favors holistic ideals. The community–practitioner relationship involves working with families, coworkers, companions, community, hospital, and religious organizations within the sphere of the practitioner. The practitioner–practitioner relationship involves collaborative and interdisciplinary work with the goal of improving patient care.[13]

Nurse theorists Paterson and Zderad describe the importance of person-to-person relationships in their humanistic nursing theory.[14] Relationship occurs through presence, inferring, being with, and doing with another. These theorists believe that presence is a gift of self. People grow and improve through relationships. Learning to understand others gives each person the opportunity to appreciate the uniqueness of his or her self. Presence is characterized by spontaneity, availability, and reciprocity in a mutual nurse–patient relationship. Reciprocity is considered a flow between two people in a shared situation. The nurse's goal is to nurture well-being. The nurse–patient relationship is a type of community, implying two or more people moving toward a common goal.

Nurse theorist Jean Watson developed a Caring Science over the past 3 decades, drawing from the work of Florence Nightingale and Martha Rogers, and this science is said to be the hallmark of nursing practice.[12] One of the major concepts of Caring Science is that it is *transpersonal*, defined as a subjective human-to-human relationship in which the nurse affects and is affected by the person of the other. Both are fully present in the moment and feel a union with the other and thus share a phenomenal field that becomes part of the life history of both. Nightingale described this concept of transpersonal caring long ago by advocating that nurses maintain full use of self, connect with humanity, the environment, Nature, the cosmos, and the divine within and without.[15]

Relationships, according to Watson, may develop a spiritual dimension as in the transpersonal human relationship that transcends person-to-person relationship and evolves into spirit-to-spirit relationship within a "caring moment." This segment in time is capable of connecting the spirits of two or more people on a spiritual level. According to Watson, a transpersonal caring relationship, such as that typifying the nurse–patient relationship, involves an energetic communication of intentionality (i.e., desiring the highest good of the other), consciousness, and full presence. Outcomes of transpersonal healing include improved self-knowledge, self-healing, and self-control. The Ten Caritas Processes affiliated with Caring Science, as shown in **Exhibit 20-1**, describe the values in the ideal nurse–patient relationship and transcend to describe other life relationship ideals.[12]

Erickson, Swain, and Tomlin used the work of Maslow, Erikson, Piaget, and Selye (Adaptation Response); Seligman (Positive Psychology); and Bowlby (Attachment Theory) to develop their theory called *Modeling and Role-Modeling*. This theory posits that the nurse–client relationship is the essence of nursing and that it should be interactive and interpersonal. Dr. Erikson's newest book on modeling and role modeling explores additional concepts.[16] Five significant goals of nursing interventions include creating trust, assisting the client to maintain control,

EXHIBIT 20-1   Ten Caritas Processes

1. Embrace altruistic values and practice loving kindness with self and others.
2. Instill faith and hope and honor others.
3. Be sensitive to self and others by nurturing individual beliefs and practices.
4. Develop helping, trusting, caring relationships.
5. Promote and accept positive and negative feelings as you authentically listen to another's story.
6. Use creative scientific problem-solving methods for caring decision making.
7. Share teaching and learning that address the individual needs and comprehension styles.
8. Create a healing environment for the physical and spiritual self that respects human dignity.
9. Assist with basic physical, emotional, and spiritual human needs.
10. Open to mystery and allow miracles to enter.

Source: Caring Science Theory and Research. Watson Caring Science Institute and International Caritas Consortium. (2014).

encouraging a positive orientation, promoting client strength, and assisting the client to set goals as well as promoting needs such as love, belonging, self-esteem, safety, and biophysical wellness. It is evident that modeling and role modeling represent a theoretical framework that promotes a therapeutic healing relationship as well as a patient-centered nurse–client relationship.[16] Key concepts for nurses to consider in using this holistic nursing theory include the following: unconditional acceptance of the patient, no matter his or her background; facilitating the identification of personal strengths; and nurturing the client to utilize his or her affective and cognitive abilities, as well as physical abilities, toward improved health.[17]

Relationship to Other Living Beings

For many people, relationships with animals are as important as relationships with other people. Pets—in particular, dogs and cats—are capable of providing love, affection, companionship, and fidelity in an unconditional manner. Animal-assisted therapy has become very popular, and studies have shown remarkable health benefits. Stewart, Chang, and Rice described the highly developed relationship with a therapy animal and how it is capable of affecting the therapeutic process.[18] Animals, especially dogs, have been used to provide an incredible number of services in such areas as hearing and vision impairment, palliative care, geriatrics, Alzheimer's units, pediatrics, physical therapy, and correctional facilities. More than 60% of U.S. households include pets, and holistic nurses must be aware of the many benefits of animal-assisted therapies, or of just owning or being with a pet.

Relationship to Nature is yet another means to interact with living things. Many people feel at peace being in Nature, hiking on a tree-shaded forest path, sitting by the ocean in the salt air and feeling the sea breezes, or lovingly tending a home garden. All of these, and other activities involving Nature, demonstrate relationship to living plants, living waters, and living ecosystems. McCaffrey studied the benefit of garden walking on older adults with depression and found it efficacious.[19] She notes that gardens have been shown to be a distraction from negative stimuli, relaxation enhancers, and a means to promote positive attitude. Lowe and Benton also describe the positive benefit of a healing garden for nurses.[20]

Spirituality and Relationship to a Higher Power

Physician Herbert Benson, cardiologist and a legendary mind–body researcher, stated years ago that human beings are "wired" for God,[21] and others have agreed. This implies that no human being can achieve true happiness without a relationship with a Higher Power, also variably called the Source, the Divine, God, Christ, Buddha, Yahweh, Spirit, Universal Energy, and more. Maslow's hierarchy of needs suggests that those moving closer to self-actualization also move closer in their search for the Source. Nurses need to acknowledge that people of different religions may view relationship with a Higher Power in myriad ways, and some religions do not worship one God, or they may worship many gods.

How does a human being develop a relationship with the Divine? According to Burkhardt and Nagai-Jacobson, prayer is considered the most fundamental and primordial language human beings use.[22] Through prayer, which can be accomplished at any moment of the day or at a set time, in such modalities as silence, contemplative prayer, meditation, chanting, music, reading of scripture, or simple conversation with God, human beings can form increasingly intimate relationships with the Divine. Helming describes the lived experience of being healed through prayer.[23, 24] Sixteen of 20 participants who attributed most of their healing to prayer, even if they utilized allopathic and integrative modalities, described the essence of this healing as *spiritually transformative.*

In monotheistic religions, such as Christianity, Judaism, and Islam, many feel that God reaches out to people through the Old or New Testament or the Koran. Some religions assist people to find spirituality in themselves; through other inspirational readings; through nature, art, and music; through speaking with God in prayer; and through silent times spent in meditation or contemplative prayer. Other religions, such as Buddhism and Hinduism, place much importance on spirituality and peace. Buddhists do not believe in one God but rather in the potential perfection of man as exemplified by Buddha,[25] while Hindus believe in one Supreme Being, Brahman, represented by multiple gods and goddesses.[26]

Some feel that people never reach their potential without having a right relationship with the Divine. Communicating with and about a Higher Power may take many forms, such as prayer, journaling, inspirational writing about spirituality, sermons, prayer groups, meditation, and contemplation. For some, it is necessary to have periods of solitude away from the noise of daily life, to "hear" the still, small voice of God within. Some people believe that "Higher Power" does not need to be God but may be Nature or a sense of spirituality outside of oneself, a power larger than oneself.

It is indeed possible to develop an enhanced relationship with the Divine, just as one gets to know a friend better by spending time with him or her. This requires daily thought and communication, not only once a week or when in crisis. As with any other healing relationship, this requires complete honesty and trust. It requires time to build, and work to maintain, this relationship. This two-way relationship may be the most significant relationship that any human being needs to develop.

Qualities That Enhance Relationships

Three of the most vital concepts in healthy relationships are trust, forgiveness, and appropriate boundary setting.

Trust

It has been traditionally felt that an ideal nurse–patient relationship requires the development of trust before patients can open up and engage in active problem resolution. Trust is an essential element of the therapeutic healing relationship as well. First, people who believe in a Higher Power tend to develop an intrinsic trust that God is ever present and caring. The popular phrase "Let go and let God" implies a willingness to trust the Higher Power's direction, assistance, and concern. Second, a sense of hope in the essential goodness of humankind assists people to trust rather than distrust on most occasions.

Messina defines trust as "the glue or cement of relationships" and further describes trust as having several beliefs and attitudes implicit in its development.[27] Another vital step in building trust includes the ability to risk being vulnerable, to risk criticism through self-revelation of one's weaknesses and strengths. This self-disclosure is usually necessary for trust to grow. Self-acceptance is a meaningful component of building trust because it implies self-trust and self-love, vital to the development of strong, healthy relationships. According to Messina, the building of trust can be impaired if individuals have:[27]

- Experienced a great deal of emotional and/or physical abuse and/or neglect.
- Been chronically put down for the way they feel or for what they believe.
- Been emotionally hurt in the past and are not willing to risk getting hurt in the future.
- Had problem relationships in the past where they were belittled, misunderstood, or ignored.
- Experienced the loss of a loved one through death. They can get so caught up in unresolved grief that they are unable to open themselves up to others, fearing they will be left alone again due to death or abandonment.
- Experienced a hostile or bitter divorce, separation, or end of a relationship. They may be unable to believe anyone who opens up to them in a new, committed relationship.
- Been reared in or have lived in an environment that is emotionally and/or physically unpredictable and volatile.
- Experienced a great deal of pain at the hands of another. Even if the other finally recognizes and accepts the responsibility to change such behavior, the person fears that by letting his or her guard down, the pain and hurt will begin again.
- Low self-esteem and difficulty believing that they are deserving of the attention, care, and concern of anyone. They have problems even trusting the positive, healthy, and reinforcing behavior of another who is sincere.
- Experienced a great deal of nonprovoked victimization in their lives. They are unwilling to trust people, situations, or institutions for fear of being victimized again.

Forgiveness

A highly significant hallmark of a healing relationship is forgiveness. To be empowered to forgive, it is necessary to release the anger that is part of resentment. This can alter a relationship immeasurably. There are all levels of forgiveness: of self, of spouse or significant other, of children, of parents, of coworkers, of friends or family, and of God.

Dincalci believes that forgiveness is transformative:

> People who have completely forgiven all the people and situations in their

lives have a much more joyful existence. They get sick less often. In fact, some say they don't get sick at all as long as they hold no grudges or resentments toward people. Their interactions with others are much more pleasant and productive than they were before their forgiveness transformations.[28]

Through his work in Forgiveness Therapy, he has found that some clients who learn to forgive are transformed spiritually, emotionally, and physically.

Delaney, Barrere, and Helming completed a research study that included community-dwelling older adults utilizing a Heart Touch meditation technique to help heal and appreciate personal relationships.[29] Forgiveness was a prominent theme, as noted by such statements as:

> I had not spoken to my sister for several years and I realize now that it is time for us to reconnect. I was able to let go and to focus on bringing in joy to my life and spreading it around. I called her last week for the first time in years.

The Heart Touch, used in addition to meditation, encouraged the participants to feel connected to others by imagining a circle of light moving from their heads to their hearts, along with remembering a time of feeling loved or loving. This Heart Touch technique enhanced connection to the Higher Power and the sending of loving energy to the persons being visualized.

Boundaries

Boundaries are artificial separations between people that can be either healthy or unhealthy. They define the perimeter of a relationship. In psychotherapeutic work and in the therapeutic nurse–patient relationship, it is vital to recall that the nurse or therapist should have therapeutic neutrality, that he or she should not give directives about major life decisions to the patient or client. Nurses and others in therapeutic roles are often held in high esteem, and the patient should not assume the "child" role if adhering to major life decisions set forth by the nurse or therapist. The patient–provider relationship assumes the

provider has power because the patient is seeking help from the provider. This is an asymmetrical relationship. The nurse or therapist is not intended to remain totally neutral, and emotion can be expressed, but neither should the nurse nor the therapist reveal significant personal information to the patient. This is a healthy boundary, with attempts to keep the relationship objective and helpful.

Therapeutic relationships between provider and patient are often considered a dyad, but in reality they are a triad because the family is always the third aspect of the relationship triangle, even if family is not physically present. This occurs because many people act within family relationships and are highly influenced by them. Parents may feel they are to blame for their child's emotional disorders, and this is exaggerated by keeping parents out of child counseling. Family members can be extremely useful in counseling because they give the nurse or therapist another perspective on the patient's life, and they can be helpful in the patient's recovery. Family therapy allows the nurse or therapist to view family interactions, but this dynamic can be just as visible in a hospital setting or home care visit where the patient is observed interacting with family members in front of the nurse.

Boundaries can be considered rigid, permeable, or semipermeable. A formal relationship may be seen as more rigid and family relationships as more permeable (i.e., with ease of exchange between parties). An example of a boundary issue occurs when a parent acts as too much of a "friend" or "peer" to his or her adolescent child, and thus the boundary is too permeable to promote executive decisions that the parent must make regarding the adolescent.[30]

Nurses are constantly faced with boundary issues. In hospital and home situations, nurses see very personal sides of their patients and their families. Nurses must maintain professional boundaries, being cautious with personal information, and always keeping safety in mind. However, the nature of nursing and therapeutic relationships is such that we may transcend ordinary conversation and converse with patients and clients on a much deeper level.

Signs of ignored boundaries are presented in **Table 20-3**.

TABLE 20-3   Signs of Ignored Boundaries

Ignored Boundaries	Symptoms
Overenmeshment	This symptom requires everyone to follow the rule that everyone must do everything together and that everyone is to think, feel, and act in the same way. Uniqueness, autonomy, and idiosyncratic behaviors are viewed as deviations from the norm.
Disassociation	This symptom involves blanking out during a stressful emotional event. This blanking out results in your being out of touch with your feelings about what happened. It also may result in your inability to remember what happened.
Excessive detachment	This symptom occurs when neither you nor anyone else in the group or family is able to establish any fusion of emotions or affiliation of feelings. You and they seem to lack a common purpose, goal, identity, or rationale for existing together.
Victimhood or martyrdom	In this symptom, you identify yourself as a violated victim and become overly defensive to ward off further violation. Or it can be that once you accept your victimization you continue to be knowingly victimized and then let others know of your martyrdom.
Chip on the shoulder	Because of your anger over past violation of your emotional and/or physical space and the real or perceived ignoring of your rights by others, you have a "chip on your shoulder" that declares, "I dare you to come too close!"
Invisibility	This symptom involves your pulling in or overcontrolling so that others, even yourself, never know how you are really feeling or what you are really thinking. Your goal is not to be seen or heard so that your boundaries are not violated.
Aloofness or shyness	This symptom is a result of your insecurity from real or perceived experiences of being ignored or rejected in the past. Once rejected you take the defensive posture to reject others before they reject you. This keeps you inward and unwilling or fearful of opening up your space to others.
Cold and distant	This symptom builds walls or barriers to ensure that others do not permeate or invade your emotional or physical space. This, too, can be a defense due to previous pain from being violated, hurt, ignored, or rejected.
Smothering	This symptom results when another is overly solicitous of your needs and interests. It can be so overwhelming that you feel like you are being strangled, held too tightly, and lack freedom to breathe on your own.

Source: Modified from J. J. Messina and C. G. Messina, Chapter 12, "Establishing Healthy Boundaries," in *Growing Down: Tools for Healing the Inner Child.* Retrieved from www.jamesjmessina.com/growingdowninnerchild/healthyboundaries.html.

Disorders in Relationships

Selected psychological issues that create unhealthy relationships are discussed in this section. These include an explanation of psychological defense mechanisms, anger, power and control issues, as well as attachment disorders.

Defense Mechanisms

According to Grohol, defense mechanisms are thought processes that allow people to distance themselves from unpleasant feelings, behaviors, and thoughts.[31] In their daily interactions, nurses frequently encounter these most common defense mechanisms. *Denial* is a defense mechanism that involves ignoring or denying reality. This mechanism can be harmful, as in the case of an addicted person who does not address his or her addiction. *Regression* is reverting to an earlier stage of development because of overwhelming fears. This defense mechanism can be harmful, as in the case of an adult refusing to leave his or her bed and function normally because of overwhelming stress. Children and adolescents may show regression to earlier stages by acting in more juvenile ways or reverting to bedwetting, for example. *Acting out* is a primitive defense mechanism wherein individuals attempt to injure themselves or others instead of verbally confronting the situation. Angrily throwing an object at the person who is the focus of the individual's anger, instead of verbally discussing the situation, is an example of acting out.

Projection is a defense mechanism used when one does not want to take responsibility for one's own thoughts and feelings. With this mechanism one ascribes one's feelings or motives to another person and does not take ownership of those thoughts or feelings. An example is when a person strongly dislikes another person but uses projection to assume that person does not like him or her instead. *Displacement* involves transferring unpleasant emotional pain from the direct source of the pain to another, less threatening person or thing. For example, someone who is angry with his or her boss but who does not feel comfortable confronting the boss instead may become angry with a colleague or a family pet. *Rationalization* is a process of filtering or reframing reality to make that reality more acceptable. For example, a student might blame her poor exam grade on the professor, rationalizing that his teaching was ineffective, rather than taking responsibility for her lack of studying. *Repression* is the unconscious denial of painful thoughts or feelings. However, this unconscious material may affect a person's behaviors, moods, and health in undesirable ways until the content is brought to conscious awareness and healed. An example of repression is when a victim of childhood abuse has trouble forming normal adult relationships.[32]

Defense mechanisms can interfere with healthy relationships. They can create distance from the truth and block honest dialogue. Many of the psychological frameworks discussed in this chapter address why people use defense mechanisms and how to manage them effectively in counseling.

Anger

Anger is a transient but forceful emotion arising out of a threat. It may be expressed openly, or it may be suppressed quietly and persist as chronic resentment. Resentment is the long-term persistence of the pain of anger, long after the initial situation that sparked the anger has subsided. People may suppress their anger because it makes them feel ashamed or is inconsistent with their image of themselves as good people. Anger can serve the following functions:[33]

- It may give a sense of power, strength, and pride.
- It can be a motivator of change, but it generates fear and opposition as well.
- It can control others by manipulating them or making them feel guilty.
- It may keep others away so that the angry person feels less vulnerable and safer.
- It can be used as a defense mechanism to avoid communicating about painful or difficult topics, including the situation that caused the anger.
- It can keep a person in the role of victim, and there is sometimes secondary gain to feeling the victim or the martyr.

Psychologically, some people are passive-aggressive. This implies that they remain passive and quiet externally, but they are repressing anger internally. The anger seeps out in small ways, such as going behind another's back to gossip about him or her in a spiteful way while remaining superficially pleasant to the other. Defensive mechanisms that are commonly used in anger include a penchant to withdraw and isolate oneself, as well as the impulse to express anger openly in out-of-control rage, verbal abuse, and insults. Anger can become extreme and manifest in explosive anger and rage. Holistic nurses frequently have to handle patients and clients who are angry at life, at others, at themselves, and at their illnesses. Helping patients to comprehend their anger, particularly when it is repressed, and assisting them to move toward forgiveness are essential aspects of the therapeutic nurse–patient relationship.

Power and Control Issues

Dominant personality patterns can cause relationship conflicts. Controlling people tend to assert themselves over others and exert power over them. Although there are people who are willing to be subservient to controlling personalities, others reject this and power battles ensue. People with obsessive-compulsive personality disorder tend to be highly controlling, rigid, and perfectionistic. They often fail to allow others to participate in projects or discussions, feeling that their way is the only right way. These people are capable of being highly devoted to their work, which can be seen in a positive or negative light. There is a preoccupation with inflexible rules, details, and lists. The disorder termed *obsessive-compulsive personality disorder* is different from *obsessive-compulsive disorder*, in which the person feels compelled to repeat specific behaviors, such as hand washing and counting.

The nurse seeking to develop and maintain caring relationships understands the inherent inequities of power that exist in most encounters between health providers and patients. Inequities regarding the hierarchical structure of institutions, race, sex, gender, education, occupation, and socioeconomic status must be monitored as the nurse seeks to collaborate with patients and families in promoting health and planning care. The unique language of health care, the schedules and routines within these environments, and the lack of partnership between patients and their care providers all reinforce these power differentials. By offering clients more choices, using language that is free of jargon, and sharing important information relevant to their care, nurses can reduce the power differential between patients and providers, thus increasing the likelihood of a partnership and aiding in the facilitation of healing. Nurses are in an ideal position to maximize the potential benefits of this healing alliance because they are inherently often more approachable than, for example, physicians.

The quality of nursing care is greatly affected by the quality of relationships between nurses and those they care for, as well as by the relationships among caregivers in the professional setting. This web of relationships creates a community complete with its own cultural norms, and this environmental context has a tremendous effect on the delivery of care. Interprofessional education and practice is a current theme that has its focus on preparing healthcare students, including nursing students, how to practice well with other health team members.

Holistic Caring Process

Holistic Assessment

In preparing to use relationship interventions, the nurse should assess the following parameters:

- The client's social support system and social network
- The quality of the client's relationships as perceived by the client, including the client's satisfaction with these relationships
- The client's use of clear communication and patterns of relating
- Predominant relational styles (e.g., shy and withdrawn, outgoing and gregarious, controlling, passive, aggressive, mutual)
- Use of defense mechanisms
- Evidence of boundaries
- Boundary issues (e.g., evidence of codependency in relationship)

Identification of Patterns/ Challenges/Needs

The patterns/challenges/needs (see Chapter 8) compatible with relationship interventions are as follows:

- Withdrawal
- Denial
- Repression
- Rationalization
- Regression
- Changes in parenting and family structure
- Human sexual dysfunction
- Lack of social coherence
- Spiritual disconnectedness and distress
- Altered family process
- Ineffective coping
- Self-care deficits
- Self-care dysfunction
- Anxiety
- Grief
- Fear
- Response to trauma

Outcome Identification

Table 20-4 guides the nurse in client outcomes, nursing prescriptions, and evaluations for effective relationship interventions.

In addition to effective outcomes with clients, it is important to examine possible outcomes for nurses and clients as follows:

- The nurse will recognize family and relationship patterns.
- The nurse will identify healthy boundaries in each interaction, assertively confronting any putdowns or defense patterns.
- The nurse will recognize opportunity for effective negotiations and conflict management, using the characteristics of effective communicators.
- The nurse will work from the dimension of mutual respect, valuing both self and others without discounting either.
- The nurse will increasingly see opportunities for new relational patterns in challenging situations.

Therapeutic Care Plan and Interventions

The holistic nurse's careful planning and preparation enhance the effectiveness of relational interactions. The following are guidelines for planning and implementing effective relational patterns.

Before the session:

- Take a moment to set your intent and focus, allowing yourself to breathe fully, to sense your center, and to align with your sense of purpose.
- Take several deep breaths and relax the body.
- Rehearse a new pattern, such as giving accurate facts, in your mind.
- Imagine the successful outcome.
- Acknowledge your positive intent.
- Be willing to learn from each experience.

During the session:

- Notice the ego states that are in evidence, specifically the feelings that are triggered within yourself.
- Be aware of ways that finding common ground enhances rapport.

- Consider options that can achieve the communication goal.
- Make "I" statements when speaking about your personal point of view or experience; avoid "you" statements, which can be taken defensively and negatively.
- Set limits by determining the time frames, the topics to be discussed, the context, and the environment.
- Be willing to change direction or reconsider a point to come to feasible compromises.
- Above all, keep the intent of the communication positive and maintain a relationship of mutual respect, even though specific content areas may be questioned and differing viewpoints may be expressed.

At the end of the session:

- Use the client outcomes (see Table 20-4) to assess the ways in which you assisted the client in moving toward goals of understanding relationship patterns.
- Consider alternatives and make concrete plans for future action.
- Evaluate your own relational skills, your use of different ego states, your use of the archetypes, your own personality style, your Myers-Briggs pattern, and so forth.
- Honor your learning process by accepting mistakes and thinking about what you might have done differently.
- Consider methods that will make trying new behaviors safe and enjoyable, such as sharing your process with a friend or mentor.

Ways in which holistic nurses can assist in improving their patients' and clients' relationship issues include the following:

- *Facing fears.* People may have difficulty altering relationship patterns because of fear. Holistic nurses can help patients and clients become aware of their nonverbalized fears and rationally evaluate them. People tend to expect the worst, when in fact, that is not usually what happens.
- *Improved communication.* Nurses can assist clients to verbalize their emotions and fears by identifying and labeling them. Nursing knowledge of psychological defense

TABLE 20-4   Nursing Interventions: Relationships

Client Outcomes	Nursing Prescriptions	Evaluation
The client will recognize personal and relationship patterns and how they support or detract from quality of life.	Assist the client in identifying the following: ■ The importance of relationships ■ The patterns that increase comfort and effective communication ■ Family relationship patterns and areas that could be improved ■ Sources of emotional stress in his or her relationships ■ The human needs that are fulfilled by quality relationships ■ The effect of relationships on health and illness	The client verbalized the dynamics within the family relationship patterns. The client stated the importance of his or her relationships to quality of life. The client identified areas in which relationships could be improved. The client recognized factors that create stressors in relationships. The client stated understanding of the interconnection between relationships and health or illness.
The client will recognize and identify harmful defense mechanisms in relationships.	Demonstrate examples of defense mechanisms and help the client to identify such problems in family and caregiver relationships.	The client identified defense mechanisms in use within the relationship.
The client will increase awareness of parent, adult, and child ego states.	Demonstrate examples of the differences among the three ego states.	The client identified his or her personal use of parent, adult, and child ego states.
The client will identify personal response patterns to others' ego states.	Assist the client in identifying personal response patterns to others' ego states, and help the client improve the effective expression of inner feelings. Describe the four archetypes and their applications in communicating physical, emotional, mental, and spiritual perspectives.	The client recognized another person's use of an ego state and his or her personal response.
The client will incorporate new strategies to improve the quality of interpersonal relationships.	Provide the client with techniques to improve relationships, such as making "I" statements (e.g., "This is how I feel. . . . My feeling is . . ."), noting ego states in a transaction, and activating the four archetypes.	The client showed interest in the four archetype patterns and willingness to try new communications from each perspective.
The client will increase awareness of the physical, emotional, mental, and spiritual aspects of relationship interactions.	Teach the client to express awareness of physical needs and take responsibility for practical aspects of his or her care, such as a need for more information and an understanding of optimal outcomes.	The client demonstrated the ability to express personal feelings using "I" statements.
The client will recognize opportunities for effective negotiations with willingness to reconsider ineffective aspects.	Assist the client to identify areas where he or she can negotiate, make choices, or reconsider previous decisions; see the open-ended nature of present relationships, especially with caregivers and family; and view the present disease as an opportunity for learning and change.	The client negotiated effectively after considering options. The client reconsidered relationship interactions that were ineffective. The client expressed interest in the open-ended nature of learning from his or her illness and treatment.

mechanisms, factors that improve or destroy relationships, and psychological theories all play a role in identifying appropriate communication styles that create healthy relationships.

- *Counseling.* Nurses are skilled at interpersonal relationship work and can counsel patients effectively. Nurses are fully capable of counseling patients for wellness interventions, such as smoking cessation, weight control, and proper nutrition. Many nurses without advanced psychiatric skills are still capable of beginning therapeutic counseling and then referring patients to higher-level mental health care. Understanding the basic psychological theories and concepts within this chapter can assist holistic nurses in beginning levels of counseling.

- *Storytelling.* Telling stories about one's experiences and problems can be highly therapeutic. It is common to feel a sense of relief in sharing personal experiences and thoughts with another. This is a very significant nursing role. Nurses can help clients to acknowledge their strengths, as well as weaknesses, through the power of story. Use of story may enhance relationship building by helping the client empathize or understand the life stories of others. If the nurse repeats the story back to the client, there is the potential for the client to see relationships in a new light.

- *Nurses' relationships with others, including coworkers.* First and foremost, nurses accept responsibility for bringing caring and sensitivity into their relationships with their patients or clients. If effectively relating to clients were enough, nursing professionals would have an easy task because most nurses demonstrate deep caring and respect for those for whom they have responsibility. It is also necessary, however, to address intricate interactions with coworkers, who possess a wide variety of backgrounds, skills, and educational levels. Thus, nurses may have ongoing transactions with colleagues ranging from a sophisticated medical specialist who focuses solely on a single domain, to a nursing aide who may have little training in interpersonal skills or understanding of

person-centered values. Bringing these various interactions into harmony with holistic ethics, theory, and philosophy is a challenging task. It also offers a grand opportunity for building teamwork through effective relationship interventions.

Healing the Healer

Wise nurse educators and leaders build in time, as in staff debriefings, that decreases the isolation of the healer, enabling nurses to regularly share feelings and responses to the difficult physical, emotional, and intellectual work that is nursing. A concept exists that all healers (physicians, nurses, etc.) are emotionally "wounded" in some ways in their own lifetimes, and this wounding may enable them to care for their patients in a more sensitive way. However, wounded healers may also react negatively to patients, without being aware of their subconscious motivations, as, for example, when a nurse whose father was an alcoholic cannot tolerate alcoholic patients and displays no empathy toward them. Conti-O'Hare, who has written extensively about wounded healers in nursing, describes two types of wounded healers:[34]

- *Walking wounded:* "An individual who remains physically, emotionally and spiritually bound to past trauma. This wounding can be reflected in the nursing practice of the individual in many ways. The walking wounded have limited consciousness related to how their pain is manifested in their lives."

- *Wounded healer:* "Through self-reflection and spiritual growth, the individual achieves expanded consciousness, through which the trauma is processed, converted and healed."

The ideal situation is for healers to work through their own traumas and woundings so that they can use themselves therapeutically in healing patients.

Conclusion

How, then, can holistic nurses apply these skills to therapeutic relationships with patients or clients? First, the holistic nurse brings a sense of

---

EXHIBIT 20-2   Evaluating the Nurse's Subjective Experience with Relationship Interventions

1. Can you continue to identify and be aware of a relationship that is troublesome to you?
2. Is it possible for you to be clear about your wants and expectations in this relationship?
3. Have you tried out new patterns, such as making a conscious choice of a different ego state? What was the result?
4. Have you considered the transactions in this relationship to make them more complementary? Have you considered how to make the transactions in this relationship more complementary?
5. Is it possible for you to communicate your strengths in this relationship? What are the strengths and intent of the other person that you could also acknowledge?
6. Can you imagine how the Healer in you could approach this relationship? How about the Teacher? The Visionary? The practical, grounded Warrior?
7. What would a healed relationship with this person be? How would you feel?
8. Can you identify the steps you could take to move in this direction?
9. Which interventions would be most helpful in moving toward healing this relationship?
10. Do you have any questions about any of the new strategies that you have learned for healing this relationship?
11. What is your next step?

---

presence to the encounter. He or she can calmly focus on the here and now and be totally present for the other. Mindfulness practices, breath awareness, body scan, and yoga are examples of practices that can enhance self-care, increasing self-awareness and compassionate presence in helping professionals. As previously explained by Watson's caring moment theory, the energy fields of the nurse and patient may overlap. In a momentary glimpse of time, the nurse and patient may become one in relationship.

Right relationship implies a therapeutic and, therefore, helpful relationship. As explained, there are many ways for relationships to become destructive. However, holistic nurses are focused on helping patients achieve healing of the body-mindspirit. Even without extensive psychiatric training, nurses can incorporate tenets of one or more psychological models into their therapeutic and healing relationship skills. We know it is vital for patients to tell their stories. People need to be heard, and in this day of abbreviated nursing encounters, it is difficult to have the time simply to listen to detailed patient stories. Nonetheless, there is a universal human need to be heard, and if nurses bear that in mind, the accuracy and compassion of the nursing care are amplified, enriching the healing relationship for both the client and the nurse. **Exhibit 20-2** lists several questions that help to evaluate a nurse's subjective response to relationship interventions.

Directions for Future Research

1. Which tools can be used to measure the quality of the nurse–patient relationship?
2. How does the quality of the nurse–patient relationship influence patient outcomes?
3. How does the quality of the nurse–patient relationship influence nurse satisfaction?
4. Is it feasible to include the quality of a nurse's therapeutic relationships as part of the nurse's performance evaluation?
5. Does a program of "relationship training" for nurses enhance patients' perceptions of quality of care?

Nurse Healer Reflections

After reading this chapter, the nurse healer will be able to answer or to begin a process of answering the following questions:

- How do I feel at the end of the workday?
  - Can I acknowledge the child within?
  - What gives me pleasure?
  - What bothers me?
  - Which defenses do I use?
  - What do I wish I had done differently?

- Were there any unpleasant interactions?
  - What other options could have been considered?
  - Do I need to forgive anyone?
- Are there repeated patterns in my relationships?
  - Are there anger or control issues?
  - How can I change the pattern?
- Will I be able to practice new responses with a friend or coworker?
  - What will I do differently?
  - Will I have support from trusted friends?
  - Will I honor and acknowledge myself as a growing, learning being, aligned with inner light and truth?

NOTES

1. L. Keegan and C. Drick, *End of Life: Nursing Solutions for Death with Dignity* (New York: Springer, 2011): 108.

2. B. M. Hagerty and K. L. Patusky, "Reconceptualizing the Nurse–Patient Relationship," *Journal of Nursing Scholarship* 35, no. 2 (2003): 145–150.

3. C. Jackson, "Using Loving Relationships to Transform Health Care," *Holistic Nursing Practice* 24, no. 1 (2010): 181–186.

4. E. C. Arnold and K. U. Boggs, *Interpersonal Relationships*, 6th ed. (St. Louis, MO: Saunders, 2011).

5. F. Dziopa and K. Ahern, "What Makes a Quality Therapeutic Relationship in Psychiatric/Mental Health Nursing: A Review of the Research Literature," *Internet Journal of Advanced Nursing Practice* 10, no. 1 (2009): 11–19.

6. R. Dobrina, M. Tenze, and A. Palese, "An Overview of Hospice and Palliative Care Nursing Models and Theories," *International Journal of Palliative Nursing* 20, no. 2 (2014): 75–81.

7. J. Cahill, G. Paley, and G. Hardy, "What Do Patients Find Helpful in Psychotherapy? Implications for the Therapeutic Relationship in Mental Health Nursing," *Journal of Psychiatric and Mental Health Nursing* 20, no. 9 (2013): 782–791.

8. Association for Humanistic Psychology, "Humanistic Psychology Overview" (2014). www.ahpweb.org/about/history/what-is-humanistic-psychology.html.

9. T. Butler-Bowdon, *50 Psychology Classics: Who We Are, How We Think, What We Do* (Boston: Nicholas Brealey, 2007).

10. B. M. Dossey, *Florence Nightingale: Mystic, Visionary, Healer*, Commemorative ed. (Philadelphia: F. A. Davis, 2010).

11. Remaking American Medicine, "Receiving Patient-Centered Care" (2006). www.pbs.org/remakingamericanmedicine/care.html.

12. Watson Caring Science Institute, "Caring Science Theory and Research" (2014). http://watsoncaringscience.org/about-us/caring-science-definitions-processes-theory/.

13. B. M. Dossey, "Nursing: Integral, Integrative, and Holistic—Local to Global," in *Holistic Nursing: A Handbook for Practice*, 6th ed., eds. B. M. Dossey and L. Keegan (Burlington, MA: Jones & Bartlett Learning, 2013): 3–58.

14. N. O'Connor, *Paterson and Zderad: Humanistic Nursing Theory* (Newbury Park, CA: Sage, 1993).

15. J. Watson, "Florence Nightingale and the Enduring Legacy of Transpersonal Human Caring-Healing," *Journal of Holistic Nursing* 28, no. 1 (2010): 107–108.

16. H. Erikson, ed., *Exploring the Interface Between the Philosophy and Discipline of Holistic Nursing: Modeling and Role Modeling at Work* (Cedar Park, TX: Unicorns Unlimited, 2010).

17. Nursing Theory, "Modeling and Role Modeling Theory" (2013). http://nursing-theory.org/theories-and-models/erickson-modeling-and-role-modeling-theory.php.

18. L. A. Stewart, C. Y. Chang, and R. Rice, "Emergent Theory and Model of Practice in Animal Assisted Therapy in Counseling," *Journal of Creativity in Mental Health* 8, no. 4 (2013): 329–348.

19. R. McCaffrey, "The Effect of Healing Gardens and Art Therapy on Older Adults with Mild to Moderate Depression," *Holistic Nursing Practice* 21, no. 2 (2007): 79–84.

20. L. Lowe and B. Benton, "In the Elements," *Nurse.com* (July 11, 2011). http://news.nurse.com/article/20110711/NATIONAL01/107110040#.VG56GouKxtc.

21. H. Benson, *Timeless Healing: The Power and Biology of Belief* (New York: Simon & Schuster, 1996).

22. M. A. Burkhardt and M. G. Nagai-Jacobson, "Spirituality and Health," in *Holistic Nursing: A Handbook for Practice*, 6th ed., eds. B. M. Dossey and L. Keegan (Burlington, MA: Jones & Bartlett Learning, 2013): 721–750.

23. M. A. Helming, "The Lived Experience of Being Healed Through Prayer Among Adults Active in a Christian Church" (doctoral dissertation, Union Institute and University, Cincinnati, OH, 2007).

24. M. Helming, "The Lived Experience of Healing Through Prayer: A Qualitative Study," *Holistic Nursing Practice* 25, no. 1 (2011): 33–44.

25. Buddha Dharma Education Association, "Buddhism and the God Idea" (2014). www.buddhanet.net/e-learning/qanda03.htm.

26. S. Das, "Top Ten Hindu Deities" (2014). http://hinduism.about.com/od/godsgoddesses/tp/deities.htm.

27. J. J. Messina, "Building Trust" (2010). www.jamesjmessina.com/toolsforpersonalgrowth/buildingtrust.html.

28. J. Dincalci, "Forgiveness Transforms!" (n.d.). http://howtoforgivewhenyoucant.com/whyforgive.php.

29. C. Delaney, C. Barrere, and M. Helming, "The Influence of a Spirituality-Based Intervention on Quality of Life, Depression, and Anxiety in Community-Dwelling Adults with Cardiovascular Disease: A Pilot Study," *Journal of Holistic Nursing* 29, no. 1 (2011): 21–32.

30. J. J. Messina and C. G. Messina, "Establishing Healthy Boundaries," in *Growing Down: Tools for Healing the Inner Child* (2010). www.jamesjmessina.com/growingdowninnerchild/healthyboundaries.html.

31. J. M. Grohol, "15 Common Defense Mechanisms" (2014). http://psychcentral.com/lib/15-common-defense-mechanisms/0001251.

32. L. Fritscher, "Defense Mechanisms: The Ego's Coping Skills" (January 1, 2014). http://phobias.about.com/od/causesanddevelopment/qt/Defense-Mechanisms.htm.

33. R. Casarjian, *Forgiveness: A Bold Choice for a Peaceful Heart* (New York: Bantam Books, 1993).

34. M. Conti-O'Hare, "The Theory of the Nurse as Wounded Healer: Finding the Essence of the Therapeutic Self" (n.d.). http://drconti-online.com/theory.html.

CHAPTER 21

Nurse Coaching

Barbara Montgomery Dossey and Susan Luck

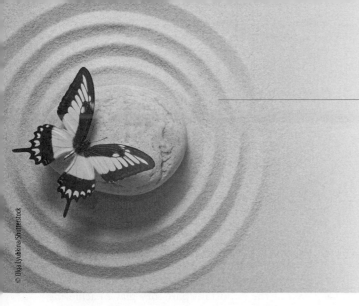

Nurse Healer Objectives

Theoretical

- Define the terms *professional nurse coach* and *nurse coaching*.
- Compare the nursing process and the nurse coach process.
- Examine the Theory of Integrative Nurse Coaching and the five components of the Integrative Nurse Coach Leadership Model.

Clinical

- Explore the nurse coaching process and the nurse coaching core competencies.
- Increase the use of deep listening skills.

Personal

- Engage in one or more reflective practices to deepen presence and intuition.
- Consider finding a nurse coach and entering into a coaching agreement to reach desired health and wellness goals.

Definitions

Middle-range nursing theory: Focused on a specific nursing phenomenon; offers a bridge between grand nursing theories that encompass the fullest range or the most global phenomena in the nursing discipline; broad enough to be useful in complex situations; leads to implications for instrument development, theory testing through research, and nursing practice strategies.

Professional nurse coach: A registered nurse who incorporates coaching skills into her or his or professional nursing practice and integrates a holistic perspective. This perspective, as applied to both self and client in a coaching interaction, emerges from an awareness that effective change evolves from within before it can be manifested and maintained externally. The professional nurse coach works with the whole person to utilize principles and modalities that integrate body-mind-emotion-spirit-environment.[1]

Professional nurse coaching: A skilled, purposeful, results-oriented, and structured relationship-centered interaction with clients provided by registered nurses for the purpose of promoting achievement of client goals.[1]

Theory of Integrative Nurse Coaching (TINC): A middle-range nursing theory that contains healing, the metaparadigm in nursing theory, patterns of knowing, five components—(1) Integrative Nurse Coach Self-Development (Self-Reflection, Self-Assessment, Self-Evaluation, Self-Care); (2) Integral Perspectives and Change; (3) Integrative Lifestyle Health and Well-Being;

(4) Awareness and Choice; and (5) Listening with HEART (*Healing, Energy, Awareness, Resiliency, Transformation*)—energy fields, and internal and external healing environments.[2]

The Evolution of the Field of Health Coaching and Nurse Coaching

Prior to the 1980s, the term *coach* was used to refer to a role in the field of human performance, specifically in athletics. Coaches training athletes for the Olympic games began introducing relaxation, imagery rehearsal, and somatic awareness practices to enhance athletic performance. Winners of the Olympic games popularized these practices.

During the 1960s, with the beginning of the human potential movement, coaching moved outside of sports and into organizational settings. There was an increased demand for greater productivity and enhanced employee performance. This led to programs and coaching designed to promote employee self-development. In addition, there was a desire to be able to measure and document the effectiveness of these initiatives in meaningful ways. New challenges emerged with the increase in technology, globalization, and multicultural teams located in different countries. Professional coaching and executive coaching became important factors in business. Formal coaching programs were still in their infancy.

By the 1990s, formal coaching programs, courses, and certifications emerged outside of the nursing profession. Most recently, many nurses have added coaching skills to their professional nursing practice. The time has arrived for nurse coaching to be recognized as embedded within the nursing profession and to be fully integrated into all nursing curricula. In 2013, the American Holistic Nurses Credentialing Corporation began a nationally and internationally recognized Nurse Coach Certification program.[3]

Nursing, recognizing the importance of the emerging nurse coach role, is stepping forward and claiming its rightful position in this major shift from disease care to disease prevention, improved health, and enhanced well-being. Nurses constitute the largest group of healthcare providers and are uniquely situated for this role. Professional nursing practice is rooted in efforts to assist clients to achieve optimal health. Nurses partner with clients to assess, strategize, and plan. Nurses utilize professional nursing knowledge and skills in their role as nurse coaches.

Professional nurse coaches are emerging as leaders who are informing governments, regulatory agencies, businesses, and organizations about the important part they play in achieving the goal of improving the health of the nation as well as health at a global level.

The Science and Art of Nurse Coaching

Nurse coaches incorporate approaches to nursing practice that are holistic, integrative, and integral and that include the work of numerous nurse scholars. Coaching is a systematic and skilled process grounded in scholarly, evidence-based professional nursing practice. All of the chapters in this text can inform a nurse coaching practice.

At the heart of nurse coaching is support for the client's healing process as it manifests in bodymindspirit. Nurse coaches realize that by being open and curious, and by asking powerful questions, they may guide the client in the healing process while at the same time provide the client choices in determining priorities for change.

The quality of human caring is central to the relationship between the nurse coach and the client. The nurse is fully present in the coaching relationship, honoring the wholeness of the patient/client. This allows clients a safe environment in which to express their goals, hopes, and dreams, as well as a setting where their vulnerability can be spoken of and addressed. Nurse coaches utilize a full spectrum of coaching strategies, as listed in **Exhibit 21-1**, to engage the client in meeting desired goals.

In 2013, *The Art and Science of Nurse Coaching: A Provider's Guide to Scope and Competencies*[1] clarified nursing perspectives concerning the role of the nurse coach in four key ways: (1) It specifies

---

EXHIBIT 21-1   Interventions Frequently Used in Nurse Coaching Practice

Affirmation	Holistic self-assessments	Prayer
Appreciative inquiry	Humor and laughter	Presence
Aromatherapy	Intention	Probing questions
Art	Journaling	Reflection
Celebration	Meditation	Relaxation modalities
Client assessments	Mindfulness practice	Ritual
Cognitive reframing	Motivational interviewing	Self-care interventions
Contracts	Movement	Self-reflection
Deep listening	Music and sound	Silence
Exercise	Observation	Somatic awareness
Goal setting	Play	Stories
Guided imagery	Powerful questions	Visioning

Source: Used with permission by the American Nurses Association. Copyright © 2013. D. R. Hess, et al., *The Art and Science of Nurse Coaching: A Provider's Guide to Scope and Competencies.* Silver Spring, MD: Nursesbooks.org.

---

the philosophy, beliefs, and values of the nurse coach and the nurse coach's scope of practice; (2) it articulates how *The Art and Science of Nurse Coaching* aligns with the American Nurses Association's *Nursing: Scope and Standards of Practice, 2nd Edition;*[4] (3) it provides the basis for continued interprofessional conversations related to professional health and wellness coaches and lay health and wellness coaches; and (4) it provides the foundation for an international certification process in professional nurse coaching.

Nurse coaches are guided in their thinking and decision making by the following four professional resources:

1. *Nursing: Scope and Standards of Practice, 2nd Edition*, outlines the expectations of the professional role of registered nurses and the scope of practice and standards of professional nurse practice and their accompanying competencies.[4]
2. *Code of Ethics for Nurses with Interpretive Statements* lists the nine provisions that establish the ethical framework for registered nurses across all roles, levels, and settings.[5]

3. *Nursing's Social Policy Statement: The Essence of the Profession* conceptualizes nursing practice, describes the social context of nursing, and provides the definition of nursing.[6]
4. *Holistic Nursing: Scope and Standards of Practice, 2nd Edition*, provides the philosophical underpinnings of a holistic nurse coaching practice.[7]

Description of Professional Nurse Coaching Practice

Nurse coaches work with individuals and groups and are found in all areas of nursing practice, serving as staff nurses, ambulatory care nurses, case managers, advanced practice registered nurses, nursing faculty, nurse researchers, educators, administrators, nurse entrepreneurs, and nurse coaches in full-time private practice. For some, nurse coaching is their primary role. The depth and breadth to which registered nurses engage in the total scope of nurse coach practice depend on education, experience, role, and the population they serve.

Professional Nurse Coaching Scope of Practice

Effective nurse coaching interactions involve the development of a coaching partnership, creation of a safe space, and sensitivity to client issues of trust and vulnerability as a basis for further exploration.[1] The nurse coach must be able to structure a coaching session, explore client readiness for coaching, facilitate achievement of the client's desired goals, and co-create a means of determining and evaluating desired outcomes and goals.[1] Nurse coaching is grounded in the principles and core values of professional nursing.

Nurse Coaching Core Values

The following five professional nurse coaching core values are adapted from and congruent with *Holistic Nursing: Scope and Standards of Practice, 2nd Edition:*[7]

1. Nurse Coach Philosophy, Theories, Ethics
2. Nurse Coaching Process
3. Nurse Coach Communication, Coaching Environment
4. Nurse Coach Education, Research, Leadership
5. Nurse Coach Self-Development (self-reflection, self-assessment, self-evaluation, self-care)

Core Value 5 is worded according to a nurse coaching model. These core values and the specific nurse coaching competencies (see the Nurse Coaching Process section later in this chapter) are aligned with *Nursing: Scope and Standards of Practice, 2nd Edition.*[4] Nurse coaches understand that professional nurse coaching practice is defined by these core values and competencies. Professional nurse coaching capabilities enhance foundational professional nursing skills and are acquired by additional training.

Nurse Coaching and Change

Nurse coaches work with people to assist them in improving their overall wellness and gaining an enhanced sense of well-being and balance in their lives. Nurse coaching helps clients to flourish by making healthful choices and adopting healthier behaviors. *Wellness* is integrated and congruent functioning is aimed at reaching one's highest potential. *Human flourishing* is when an individual finds and creates meaning in life and identifies his or her purpose in life, however defined; it includes taking charge of one's own health. Nurse coaches see clients/patients as whole beings, each with the capacity to connect deeply with her or his own inner wisdom and truth.

Self-development (self-reflection, self-assessment, self-evaluation, self-care) promotes the recognition of what is going right in life, allowing for the celebration of little successes each day. Coaching is an opportunity to promote and acknowledge success, however small, and then to build on that to achieve further success.

In coaching sessions, the client may also access vulnerable moments and share pain and suffering. *Pain* is a physical and/or emotional discomfort or experience; *suffering* is the story people create around pain.[8] Signs of suffering may be physical, mental, emotional, social, behavioral, and/or spiritual. This is why it is so important for nurse coaches to develop a reflective practice to strengthen their own capacity to sit with the pain and suffering clients express without trying to fix the discomfort. A useful saying is "soft front and strong back." This relates to the nurse coach's skill and capacity to bear witness and engage in inner stillness, to be with the suffering and the sufferer fully in the moment, bearing witness without judgment.

Clients seek professional coaching for many reasons, including to help them explore possibilities and new directions in life, celebrate successes and identify opportunities for personal and professional development, enhance quality of life, and improve relationships. Clients who come for coaching for such reasons usually are not focused solely on problems to overcome or issues to manage but are seeking opportunities to enrich a current way of being.

Other clients come with specific problems and health challenges, seeking nurse coaching to improve management of acute or chronic conditions. Their challenges may be related to self-esteem and self-image, fear and self-confidence, and general adaptation to actual or perceived changes. Other clients seek coaching to learn to handle personal and workplace challenges and stressors or to learn new behaviors in relation to improving health through nutrition, exercise, weight management, enhanced sleep, or stress management. An important area for nurse coaching is in working with clients who are facing end-of-life issues, either their own or those of loved ones, as well as those clients/patients who are living with loss and grief.

By using a patient-centered, relationship-centered process, the nurse coach accompanies the client through the change and discovery processes during coaching sessions. Held within this safe relationship and environment, the coaching journey can arrive at a successful outcome.

Coaching Conversations

Coaching conversations have a beginning (reasons for seeking coaching, a greeting, quick update), a middle (where the majority of time is spent), and an end (agreeing on the next session date, reviewing action plans and other possibilities, completing coaching session). After the client determines the topic for the coaching session, the nurse coach uses presence, intention, intuition, and deep listening to determine the most powerful questions to ask the client.

Use of silence, often referred to as the "power of the pause," throughout a coaching session allows time for both the client and the nurse coach to reflect on the process of discovery and insight. Further possibilities also emerge in the conversation, and the integrative nurse coach may rephrase what the client shares, leading to an opportunity to go deeper into the client's story.

As the coach listens to the client's responses to questions or insights, it is important for the coach to remember that moments of insight and *aha* moments are often examples of the mind grasping something new.[1] This insight is often transitory and not yet embodied as a lived experience. This is where the coaching agreement and coaching sessions evolve to guide the client to desired skill building and commitments to specific actions.

Not all coaching leads to action. Insights can be very useful in understanding barriers to change. They may result in identifying thoughts that get in the way of achieving goals. In this way, they are extremely beneficial. Assisting a person in the recognition of the need for an adjustment in attitude or in challenging a belief may, in and of itself, be the catalyst for change.

The nurse coach is aware that although clients may be expressive and make many connections, this does not indicate embodiment of insights, goals, and actions. For a change to become embodied, a practice must be repeated over and over again. This leads to the creation of new capacities and competencies. Clients learning how to use self-awareness and self-observation throughout the day become able to understand and recognize thoughts, actions, behaviors, body sensations, and postures in the moment when they occur and how they relate to the desired changes

The Transtheoretical Model of Behavior Change (introduced in Chapter 34 in the discussions on weight management, motivational interviewing, and appreciative inquiry) is important in nurse coaching because it is necessary to determine which stage a client is in regarding readiness to make changes.[9] The challenge of change also includes the client's willingness to sustain new behaviors and ways of being. The five stages of change are (1) precontemplation, (2) contemplation, (3) preparation, (4) action, and (5) maintenance; each stage is predictable and identifiable. Motivational interviewing and appreciative inquiry (see Chapter 23) are essential skills that the nurse coach can use to help clients recognize resistance, ambivalence, and change talk.[10, 11]

The Nursing Process and the Nurse Coaching Process

The nursing process involves six focal areas: assessment, diagnosis, outcomes, plan, implementation, and evaluation. These six areas are conceptualized as bidirectional feedback loops from each component.[12]

The nurse coaching process uses the holistic caring process[1] (see Chapter 8), with a shift in terminology and meaning to understand and incorporate the client's subjective experience:

from *assessment* to establishing the relationship and identifying readiness for change; from *diagnosis* to identifying opportunities, issues, and concerns; from *outcomes* to establishing client-centered goals; from *plan* to creating the structure of the coaching interaction; from *implementation* to empowering clients to reach goals; and from *evaluation* to assisting clients to determine the extent to which goals were achieved. The nurse coach understands that growth and improved health, wholeness, and well-being are the result of an ongoing journey that is ever expanding and transformative.

Establishing Relationship and Identifying Readiness for Change (Assessment)

Professional Nurse Coach Role

In a coaching model, the foundation for coaching is laid during the assessment phase of the coaching interaction and establishes the relationship and identifies readiness for change. The nurse coach begins by becoming fully present with self and client before initiating the coaching interaction. The session proceeds with an assessment, establishing the relationship with the client and listening to the client's subjective experience or story. The nurse coach helps the client assess readiness for change. Assessment is dynamic and ongoing. The nurse coach then determines if the client's concerns are appropriate for coaching or if the client would be better served through a referral to psychotherapy or other services and resources.

Identifying Opportunities, Issues, and Concerns (Diagnosis)

Professional Nurse Coach Role

The nurse coach and the client together explore assessment data to determine areas for change. There is no attempt or need to assign labels or to establish a diagnosis. Instead, the nurse coach is open to multiple and fluid interpretations of an unfolding interaction in partnership with the client. This process identifies opportunities and issues related to growth, overall health, wholeness, and well-being. Opportunities for

celebrating well-being are explored. The nurse coach understands that acknowledgment promotes and reinforces previous successes and serves to enhance further achievements.

Establishing Client-Centered Goals (Outcomes)

Professional Nurse Coach Role

The nurse coach assists the client in identifying goals that will lead to the desired change. The nurse coach values the evolution and process of change as it unfolds. The nurse coach employs an overall approach to each coaching interaction that is designed to facilitate achievement of client goals.

Creating the Structure of the Coaching Interaction (Plan)

Professional Nurse Coach Role

The nurse coach develops a coaching plan with the client that identifies strategies to attain goals. The nurse coach structures the coaching interaction with a coaching agreement that identifies specific parameters of the coaching relationship, including coach and client responsibilities.

Empowering Clients to Reach Goals (Implementation)

Professional Nurse Coach Role

The nurse coach supports the client's coaching plan while simultaneously remaining open to emerging goals based on new insights, learning, and achievements. The nurse coach supports the client in reaching for new and expanded goals using a variety of specific communication skills to facilitate learning and growth.

As key components of the coaching interaction, the nurse coach employs effective communication skills such as motivational interviewing, appreciative inquiry, deep listening, and powerful questioning. In partnership with the client, the nurse coach facilitates learning and results by co-creating awareness, designing actions, setting goals, and planning and addressing progress and accountability. The nurse coach chooses interventions based on the client's statements and actions and interacts with intention and curiosity in a manner that assists the client to achieve his or her goals. The nurse coach effectively utilizes her or his nursing knowledge and a variety of skills acquired with additional coach training.

Assisting Clients to Determine the Extent to Which Goals Were Achieved (Evaluation)

Professional Nurse Coach Role

The nurse coach partners with the client to evaluate progress toward attainment of goals. The nurse coach is aware that the evaluation of coaching (the nursing intervention) is done primarily by the client, not the nurse, and is based on the client's perception of success and the achievement of client-centered goals. In the next section, a brief overview of the Theory of Integrative Nurse Coaching and the Integrative Nurse Coach Leadership Model are discussed to further ground nurse coaching in a nursing theory and a nursing leadership model.

The Theory of Integrative Nurse Coaching and the Integrative Nurse Coach Leadership Model

Health and wellness coaching is a multidimensional concept across the healthcare professions, and it acquires multiple meanings depending on the discipline from which it is viewed. The Theory of Integrative Nurse Coaching (TINC) contains healing, the metaparadigm in nursing theory, patterns of knowing in nursing, and the five components of integrative nurse coaching (see **Exhibit 21-2**), referred to as theoretical niches that acquire the TINC meaning and context within the component in which it resides. The TINC coauthors—Barbara Dossey, Susan Luck, and Bonney Gulino Schaub—believe that the TINC is essential to the continued evolution of the nurse coach role.[2] They also believe that nurse coaches, with their leadership capacities,

> **EXHIBIT 21-2   The Theory of Integrative Nurse Coaching and the Integrative Nurse Coach Leadership Model: Five Components**
>
> Component 1: Integrative Nurse Coach Self-Development (Self-Reflection, Self-Assessment, Self-Evaluation, Self-Care)
> Component 2: Integral Perspectives and Change
> Component 3: Integrative Lifestyle Health and Well-Being
> Component 4: Awareness and Choice
> Component 5: Listening with HEART (Healing, Energy, Awareness, Resiliency, Transformation)
>
> *Source:* Used with permission. Copyright © 2015. B. M. Dossey, S. Luck, & B. G. Schaub, *Nurse Coaching: Integrative Approaches for Health and Wellbeing.* North Miami, Fl: International Nurse Coach Association. www.inursecoach.com.

interactions with clients/patients, and other interprofessional collaborations, are leaders in the evolution of healthy people living in a healthy world. See Chapter 30 and the Integrative Health and Wellness Assessment research tool that supports the TINC.[13] (For a complete discussion of the Theory of Integrative Nurse Coaching, the reader is referred to B. M. Dossey, S. Luck, and B. G. Schaub, *Nurse Coaching: Integrative Approaches for Health and Wellbeing*, North Miami, FL: International Nurse Coach Association, 2015. www.iNurseCoach.com.)

The Integrative Nurse Coach Leadership Model (INCLM) components are the same as in the TINC. The INCLM expands nursing's visibility in how to create a culture of health and well-being.[14] Nurses are challenged to be leaders and the driving force in healthcare reform and in the health and wellness coaching movement. Nurse coaches are uniquely positioned to coach and engage individuals in the process of behavior change in hospitals, clinics, and communities and to advance steps toward healthier people living on a healthy planet—local to global.

Because the details of the TINC and INCLM are beyond the scope of this chapter, the reader is referred to *Nurse Coaching: Integrative Approaches for Health and Wellbeing*. The TINC is the organizational framework for the International Nurse

Coach Association's Integrative Nurse Coach Certificate Program, a 3-semester credit hour (SCH) undergraduate nurse coach course, a 3-SCH graduate-level nurse coach course, a 1-SCH undergraduate nurse coach course, and a 1-day Introduction to Integrative Nurse Coaching workshop (6.5 contact hours). For information on this certificate program, see www .inursecoach.com/programs.

The Nurse Coach Five-Step Process

The Nurse Coach Five-Step Process (see Figure 21-1 later in the chapter) actualizes and integrates the TINC. The five process steps are as follows:[8]

Process 1: Connecting to the story
Process 2: Deep listening and skillful questioning
Process 3: Inviting opportunities, potentials, and change
Process 4: Practicing, integrating, and embodying change
Process 5: Guiding and supporting the transforming self

Process 1: Connecting to the Story

Before the coaching session begins, the nurse coach becomes fully present, centered, and grounded. This allows the nurse coach to be completely attentive to the client's topic and the elements of the story. This includes noticing both the affective and energetic state of the client, as well as the content of what the person presents in the initial meeting.

As a starting point, the client may bring a topic or specific intention or goal to the coaching session. If the client cannot clearly identify a topic on which to work, the nurse coach, through skillful questioning and/or introducing awareness practices, can assist the client to identify what he or she is hoping for. The nurse coach conveys curiosity about what the client brings to the coaching session. The client provides the subject and direction of the coaching conversation. The nurse coach is open and attentive to what the coaching client presents.

Topics for exploration may be generated by the client's responses and reactions to such tools such as the Integrative Health and Wellness Assessment and the action plan (see Chapter 30).

Nurse coaches align their intentions with clients' goals and attend to clients' subjective experiences and internal frames of reference. This builds trust and respect. The nurse coach's belief in the client's capacity to connect with inner resources, wisdom, and potentials supports the client's current self in the journey toward desired changes and goals. Being present with the client's process of discovery helps the nurse coach to step back from the nurse expert role, remembering the wisdom of "less is more" in the coaching conversation.

Process 2: Deep Listening and Skillful Questioning

The nurse coach lets go of trying to fix a client. The session is conducted through deep listening and skillful questioning. If and when the client moves into vulnerable moments, bearing witness to the client's narrative is essential. Bearing witness to a story means being present with patience and respect for things just as they are. This includes learning to be with the client's joys and successes as well as giving full permission for the client to express pain and suffering. Being curious and open is attending to the present moment, allowing whatever emerges to come forth. By bringing awareness to her or his own inner wisdom, wealth of experience, and intuition, the nurse coach draws from inner resources to guide the direction of the questioning.

Cultivating a connection with the client that communicates safety and respect creates the opportunity for the client to explore vulnerability, doubts, and challenges as well as strengths, potentials, and successes. Skillful questions move the client toward goals by identifying attitudes, behaviors, and beliefs that have led to past successes and accomplishments. They also help identify blocks and obstacles, both internal and external, that have created limitations. Skillful questioning supports the client in identifying habits of thought and feeling that are self-defeating. Bringing awareness to these patterns provides the client with the possibility of making different choices.

When issues arise in coaching that are outside the scope of the nurse coach's expertise, the coach can make referrals. It is essential that the nurse coach be knowledgeable about and have information and referral sources for professional colleagues and the spectrum of community resources.

Process 3: Inviting Opportunities, Potentials, and Changes

The nurse coach recognizes and respects the client's subjective experiences, perceptions, learning style, and culture (e.g., beliefs, values, and customs). In addition, the nurse coach continually exhibits authenticity through honesty, sincerity, personal integrity, and maintenance of professional ethics. Nurse coaching includes planning and negotiating clear actions and agreements as part of the coaching conversation. Following up on agreements and reevaluating their effectiveness or appropriateness are parts of the process, as is altering or creating new action plans when appropriate.

Before any coaching occurs, the nurse coach enters into a coaching agreement with the client. In returning sessions, the nurse coach explores with the client which plans have been kept and reexamines the plans that have not been realized. Periodically reviewing the coaching plan with the client stimulates engagement and helps to identify barriers to change. Holding the person accountable for planned actions, results, and related time frames allows progress to continue as a result of the dynamics in the trusting relationship.

A client's new ideas, behaviors, and actions may feel uncomfortable or even risky as old patterns and habits are challenged. Fear of failure is often an issue. The nurse coach offers ongoing support. When unrealistic or unmanageable goals are established, the nurse coach suggests that the client apply the 50% rule, cutting a goal in half to maximize the potential for an initial success.

Process 4: Practicing, Integrating, and Embodying Change

Employing deep listening and powerful questioning, the nurse coach focuses more completely on what the client is communicating. Changing behavior means practicing, integrating, and embodying change and bringing this awareness to day-to-day activities. This awareness opens the opportunity for the client to choose to take new actions and create new ways of thinking and being. This helps in planning ahead, rather than engaging in mindless, habituated behavior. This embodied change brings the possibility of being liberated from self-defeating patterns and thoughts with the spirit of engagement in new health behaviors and choices.

Encouraging and supporting the client in experimenting and applying what has been learned from the coaching interaction leads to new behaviors and sustained change. The nurse coach is an ally and support in this relationship. Being mindful of the power inherent in the coaching relationship, the nurse coach offers encouragement and feedback that is nonjudgmental, respectful, and appropriate. This frees the client to express strong feelings without fear of judgment.

When assessing the client's communication process, the nurse coach attends to the person's breath pattern, facial expressions, body language, vocal quality, and energy. In Skype or phone coaching conversations, the nurse can observe breathing patterns, vocal quality, and energy. When clients acknowledge that change is hard, they can identify their resistance and ambivalence to change. Clients who understand their own patterns of resistance gain an opportunity for self-awareness and growth.

Process 5: Guiding and Supporting the Transforming Self

The integral perspective honors the fact that every individual is always negotiating her or his experience at many levels. People observe their present interaction at the same time they are affected and shaped by past experiences, some remembered and some forgotten. Individuals function in a bio-psycho-social-environmental-spiritual reality. Both challenges and opportunities can present themselves in any of these aspects of being.

Skillfully, the nurse coach assists clients in exploring and navigating the narrative of their life stories. Profound changes can occur in this coaching journey when clients are introduced to the power of their imagination. Introducing clients to meditative and imagery awareness practices may offer them an opportunity to identify metaphors, images, or words that resonate with their story. The intimate, personally meaningful quality of these experiences can help in keeping clients aligned with envisioned hopes and intentions. These images, metaphors, and other creative aspects of the coaching experience become useful resources that may be referred to frequently in coaching sessions. These symbols and stories are not static. They become part of a transformative process that can release or reconcile parts of clients' stories that no longer serve them. This coaching discovery process inspires clients to be open to broader perspectives and new ways of being.

As shown in **Figure 21-1**, the client current self (CS) includes the person's current reality.

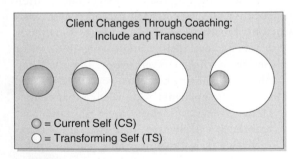

FIGURE 21-1 Client Changes Through Coaching

Legend: Clients bring to coaching their current self (CS) and life story. Through coaching, the client's current self (CS) opens to new opportunities, potentials, and change. The current self (CS) begins to shift and a transforming self (TS) emerges, with the outer circle going from black (CS) to gray. With the widening of awareness, transformation (TS) occurs, allowing desired goals and changes to be realized.

Source: Copyright 2012. Integrative Nurse Coach Certificate Program (INCCP). Used with premission from Dossey, B. M., Luck, S., and Schaub, B. G. Integrative Nurse Coaching For Health and Wellness. Huntington, NY: Florence Press, 2012. www.iNurseCoach.com

As changes are made, the old story remains but also opens into another way of being and transcends into the changing and transforming self (TS). The nurse coach recognizes this new way of being and acknowledges the changed behaviors and new commitments.

This process assists the client in recognizing what worked in moving forward. Clarity in what works provides the client with a strong foundation on which to build in the future when other challenges occur. This recognition also provides more insights and elicits opportunities for new commitments or actions. The client's old worldview and assumptions have been challenged. The transforming self becomes integrated into the broadened sense of self, leading to increased self-efficacy, self-esteem, and confidence.

Case Studies

The reader is referred to the following chapters and case studies in this text that integrate nurse coaching:

Chapter 24: Environment and specific nurse coaching interactions

Chapter 23: Brief case studies and coaching interactions using motivational interviewing and appreciative inquiry

Chapter 31: Nutrition and specific nurse coaching interactions

Chapter 34: Weight management and the five stages of change details

Conclusion

Nurse coaches are uniquely positioned to engage individuals in the process of meaningful and health-promoting behavioral change. With a renewed focus on prevention and wellness in healthcare reform, now is an important time for the nursing profession to expand its visibility in the emerging coaching paradigm. Professional nurse coaching promotes opportunities for nurses to practice to the full extent of their education and experience in a way that leads to healthy people living in a healthy nation on a healthy planet.

Directions for Future Research

1. Develop a qualitative research study to identify themes in nurse coach self-development and in coaching skills mastery.
2. Identify the most effective ways to incorporate nurse coaching into acute care settings.
3. Evaluate the effectiveness of nurse coaching in your institution and analyze themes.
4. Determine whether nurse coaching in the clinical setting increases job satisfaction and nurse retention.
5. Develop nurse coaching worksite wellness programs and evaluate the long-term effects on finances, retention, quality indicators, and patient experiences.

Nurse Healer Reflections

After reading this chapter, the nurse healer will be able to answer or to begin a process of answering the following questions:

- How do I describe the role of nurse coach and nurse coaching to colleagues and others?
- What new understanding and insight do I have about my own capacity to change a behavior(s) considering an integral perspective and the four quadrants?
- In what ways have I become more aware of phrasing questions to clients/patients and others?
- Do I slow down to listen more deeply?

NOTES

1. D. Hess, B. M. Dossey, M. E. Southard, S. Luck, B. G. Schaub, and L. Bark, *The Art and Science of Nurse Coaching: A Provider's Guide to Coaching Scope and Competencies* (Silver Spring, MD: Nursesbooks.org. 2013).
2. B. M. Dossey, "Theory of Integrative Nurse Coaching," in *Nurse Coaching: Integrative Approaches for Health and Wellbeing*, B. M. Dossey, S. Luck, and B. G. Schaub (North Miami, FL: International Nurse Coach Association, 2015): 29–49.
3. American Holistic Nurses Credentialing Corporation, "Holistic Nurses Certification" (n.d.). www.ahncc.org/certificationprocess.html.
4. American Nurses Association, *Nursing: Scope and Standards of Practice*, 2nd ed. (Silver Spring, MD: Nursesbooks.org, 2010).
5. American Nurses Association, *Code of Ethics for Nurses with Interpretive Statements* (Silver Spring, MD: Nursesbooks.org, 2001).
6. American Nurses Association, *Nursing's Social Policy Statement: The Essence of the Profession* (Silver Spring, MD: Nursesbooks.org, 2010).
7. American Holistic Nurses Association and American Nurses Association, *Holistic Nursing: Scope and Standards of Practice*, 2nd ed. (Silver Spring, MD: Nursesbooks.org, 2013).
8. B. M. Dossey, "Stories, Strengths, and the Nurse Coach 5-Step Process," in *Nurse Coaching: Integrative Approaches for Health and Wellbeing*, B. M. Dossey, S. Luck, and B. G. Schaub (North Miami, FL: International Nurse Coach Association, 2015): 85–108.
9. J. Prochaska, J. C. Norcross, and C. C. Di Clemente, *Changing for Good: A Revolutionary Six-Stage Program for Overcoming Bad Habits and Moving Your Life Positively Forward* (New York: HarperCollins, 1995).
10. M. A. Dart, *Motivational Interviewing in Nursing Practice* (Sudbury, MA: Jones and Bartlett, 2011).
11. M. E. Southard, L. Bark, and D. Hess, "Motivational Interviewing and Appreciative Inquiry," in *Holistic Nursing: A Handbook for Practice*, 7th ed., eds. B. M. Dossey and L. Keegan (Burlington, MA: Jones & Bartlett Learning, 2015).
12. P. Potter and N. C. Frisch, "The Holistic Caring Process," in *Holistic Nursing: A Handbook for Practice*, 7th ed., eds. B. M. Dossey and L. Keegan (Burlington, MA: Jones & Bartlett Learning, 2015).
13. B. M. Dossey, "Integrative Health and Wellness Assessment," in *Nurse Coaching: Integrative Approaches for Health and Wellbeing*, B. M. Dossey, S. Luck, and B. G. Schaub (North Miami, FL: International Nurse Coach Association, 2015): 109–122.
14. B. M. Dossey and S. Luck, "Nurse Coaching and Leadership," in *Nurse Coaching: Integrative Approaches for Health and Wellbeing*, B. M. Dossey, S. Luck, and B. G. Schaub (North Miami, FL: International Nurse Coach Association, 2015): 387–402.

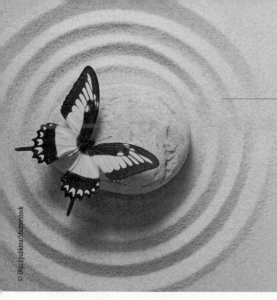
© Olga Lyubkina/Shutterstock

CHAPTER 22

Applying Cognitive Behavioral Therapy in Everyday Nursing

Eileen M. Stuart-Shor, Carol L. Wells-Federman, and Shanna D. Hoffman

Nurse Healer Objectives

Theoretical

- Define cognitive behavioral therapy.
- Identify the three main principles of cognitive behavioral therapy.
- Discuss the connection between cognition(s), health, and illness.
- Identify four major contributors to the development of cognitive behavioral therapy.
- Compare and contrast potential bio-psycho-social-spiritual-behavioral responses to stress and their effects on health and illness.
- Discuss the roles of contracting and goal setting in cognitive restructuring.

Clinical

- Discuss the major diagnoses and health problems that respond favorably to cognitive behavioral therapy.
- Describe ways to facilitate cognitive restructuring.
- Identify stress warning signals.
- Describe and identify automatic thoughts.
- Describe and identify cognitive distortions and irrational beliefs.
- Describe a simple model for cognitive restructuring.
- Outline the guidelines for organizing a cognitive behavioral therapy session.

- Explore different practice settings in which cognitive restructuring can be used.

Personal

- Identify stress warning signals.
- In response to stress, stop, take a breath, reflect on the cause of the stress, and choose a more healthy response.
- Develop a list of meaningful personal rewards.
- Begin a healthy lifestyles and healthy pleasures journal.

Definitions

Cognition: The act or process of knowing.

Cognitive: Of or relating to consciousness, or being conscious; pertaining to intellectual activities (such as thinking, reasoning, imagining).

Cognitive behavioral therapy: A therapeutic approach that addresses the relationships among thoughts, feelings, behaviors, and physiology.

Cognitive distortions: Inaccurate, irrational thoughts that generate stress-producing thoughts and maladaptive behaviors.

Cognitive restructuring: Examining and reframing one's interpretation of the meaning of an event.

Theory and Research

Historically, cognitive behavioral therapy (CBT) is rooted in the treatment of anxiety and depression; however, its application has now broadened greatly. This chapter explores the application of CBT in the context of nursing practice along the wellness–illness continuum and the bio-psycho-social-spiritual domains. The myriad ways in which CBT is integrated into holistic nursing practice and the unique perspective that nurse healers bring to the application of CBT are addressed throughout this chapter.

Cognitive behavioral therapy is based on the premise that stress and suffering are influenced by perception, or the way people think, and that thoughts that create stress are often illogical, negative, and distorted. These distorted, negative thoughts can affect emotions, behaviors, and physiology and can influence the individual's beliefs. By changing negative, illogical thoughts that trigger distress, the individual can change physical and emotional states.

In this chapter, to illustrate the relationship between illogical thoughts that trigger and perpetuate stress and changes in physical and emotional states, we draw from the biopsychosocial model,[1] and we have added spirituality to the biopsychosocial existing model.[2] In this bio-psycho-social-spiritual model, there is an understanding that stress, or the perception of threat, can lead to changes in physical, emotional, behavioral, and spiritual states. Knowing that stress causes changes in physical and emotional states and is influenced by perception, and that perception is influenced by distorted thinking patterns (exaggerated negative thoughts), we can understand the link between CBT, which restructures distorted negative thinking patterns, and mind–body interactions, which influence health and illness. This link has implications for health promotion, symptom reduction, and disease management. Because understanding the dynamic interaction of CBT and the psychophysiology of mind–body connections is fundamental to the application of CBT in nursing, it is explored in greater detail later in this chapter.

Cognitive behavioral therapy was first used for depression and anxiety as a short-term treatment that focused on helping people to recognize and change automatic, distorted thoughts that trigger and perpetuate distress.[3] It is now being applied successfully to reduce health-risking behaviors, physical symptoms, and the emotional sequelae of a variety of illnesses to which stress is an important causative or contributing factor.[4] Cognitive behavioral therapy is also useful in value clarification, which is the first step in establishing meaningful health goals.[4] Interestingly, it has ancient origins. A millennium ago, the Greek philosopher Epictetus described how people most often are disturbed not by the things that happen to them but by the opinions they have about those things. Theorists including Beck, Ellis, Meichenbaum, and Burns have advanced the modern interpretation of cognitive therapy.[5-7] In the late 1960s, Beck conceptualized cognitive theory as a model to treat depression and anxiety and developed effective intervention strategies to restructure cognitive distortions and successfully mitigate the symptoms of depression and anxiety. Ellis developed the approach known as rational emotive therapy to recognize and challenge distorted thinking. He was particularly interested in uncovering those beliefs and assumptions that people hold as absolutes and that provide the lens (or filter of life experience) that causes distortions. Meichenbaum and Burns further enhanced the theory and practice of CBT through research and clinical experience.

Research on CBT continues to provide evidence of its broad application to both psychological and physical health problems. Beck, in a 40-year retrospective review of the current state of CBT, affirmed the utility of CBT (often referred to as cognitive therapy) in treating an array of psychological disorders and medical symptoms.[3, 8] A significant contributor to this extensive review, Butler and colleagues analyzed the current literature on outcomes of CBT.[9] They provided a comprehensive assessment of 16 methodologically rigorous meta-analyses and focused on effect sizes that contrast outcomes for CBT with outcomes for various control groups for each disorder. Large effect sizes were found for unipolar depression, generalized anxiety disorder, panic disorder with or without agoraphobia, social phobia, posttraumatic stress disorder, and childhood depressive and anxiety disorders.[9] Effect sizes for CBT of marital distress, anger, childhood somatic disorders, and chronic pain were in the moderate range. Cognitive behavioral therapy was somewhat superior to antidepressants in the treatment of adult depression and was equally effective as behavior therapy in the treatment of adult depression and obsessive-compulsive disorder.

Recent comparisons of CBT to other forms of psychotherapy showed that CBT was superior to psychodynamic therapy among patients with anxiety or depressive disorders at both treatment and follow up. The results suggest that CBT should be a first line of treatment for patients with anxiety and depressive disorders.[10-13] A review and meta-analysis of five randomized controlled trials of individuals treated within 3 months of trauma indicated that early trauma-focused CBT is more effective than supportive counseling in preventing chronic posttraumatic stress disorder.[14]

Evidence continues to grow in support of the application of CBT to treat a wide variety of physical symptoms. Researchers have reported its effective use in the treatment of chronic low back pain,[15] diabetes,[16] insomnia,[8] irritable bowel syndrome,[17] posttraumatic stress disorder,[1] chronic pain,[18-20] fibromyalgia,[21] tension headache,[22] spinal cord injuries,[23, 24] postconcussion syndrome,[25] seizures,[26] and chronic fatigue syndrome.[27, 28] In addition, it is found to be efficacious in the treatment of congestive heart failure,[29] obesity,[30] alcohol abuse,[31] binge eating,[32] tinnitus,[33] cigarette smoking cessation in teens,[34] and pregnant adolescents.[35]

Effects of Cognition on Health and Illness

Stress (the perception of a threat to one's well-being, and the perception that one cannot cope) can cause physical, psychological, behavioral, and spiritual changes. Both cognition (the way one thinks) and perception (the way one views, interprets, or experiences someone or something) are important to an understanding of cognitive restructuring. If individuals change the way they think (cognition), they may change their perception of the situation. And if they change their perception of a situation so that they no longer view that situation as threatening, they may not experience stress. Thus, changing thoughts and perceptions can influence physiologic, psychological, behavioral, and spiritual processes. The following sections delineate the effects of stress on physical, psychological, social, behavioral, and spiritual pathways.

Physiologic Effects of Stress

In response to a perceived threat (stress), the body gears up to meet the challenge. This perception of threat (stress) stimulates a cascade of biochemical events initiated by the central nervous system (see **Figure 22-1**). Termed the *fight-or-flight response* and later *the stress response*,[36] this heightened state of sympathetic arousal prepares the body for vigorous physical activity.[37] Repeated exposure to daily hassles or prolonged stress activates the musculoskeletal system, increasing muscle tension. Concurrently, the autonomic nervous system, via the sympathetic branch, produces a generalized arousal that includes increased heart rate, blood pressure, and respiratory rate. In addition, there is a heightened awareness of the environment, causing shifting of blood from the visceral organs to the large muscle groups, altered lipid metabolism, and increased platelet aggregability.[38] The neuroendocrine system, in response to stimulation of the hypothalamic-pituitary-adrenal axis and the secretion of corticosteroids and mineralocorticoids, increases glucose levels, influences sodium retention, and increases the anti-inflammatory response in the acute phase.[39] Over time, however, immune function decreases.[40] In addition, there is evidence that levels of other hormones regulated by the neuroendocrine system, such as reproductive and growth hormones, endorphins, and encephalins, can be affected.[40]

When the stress response is activated, the body must then adapt to the situation to mitigate the response. This adjustment is termed *allostasis*.[37] High allostatic load, or repeated stimulation of the stress response, decreases the body's resiliency against stressors and has been known to

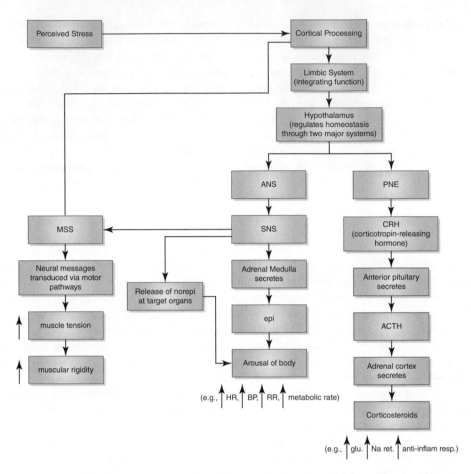

FIGURE 22-1 Stress Response. ACTH = adrenocorticotropic hormone; ANS = autonomic nervous system; BP = blood pressure; epi = epinephrine; glu. = blood glucose level; HR = heart rate; MSS = musculoskeletal system; Na ret. = sodium retention; norepi = norepinephrine; PNE = pituitary-neuroendocrine system; RR = respiratory rate; SNS = sympathetic nervous system.

Source: Reprinted with permission from C. L. Wells-Federman et al., *Clinical Nurse Specialist*, Vol. 9, No. 1, p. 60, © 1995, Williams & Wilkins.

either cause or exacerbate physical and mood-related symptoms.[37, 39, 41] New understanding and imaging of the brain shows that chronic stress activation leads to physiological brain changes, resulting in decreased concentration, problem solving, and memory storage.[37, 39, 41, 42] These effects mean that stress can negatively influence an individual's ability to engage in health promotion and manage existing disease.

In addition, chronic inflammation has been identified as one likely mechanism through which stress affects disease risk.[43] For example, C-reactive protein (CRP), an inflammatory marker, is emerging as a predictor of cardiovascular disease. McDade and colleagues investigated the contribution of behavioral and psychosocial factors to variation in CRP concentrations in a population-based sample of middle-aged and older adults.[44] They found that psychosocial stresses, as well as health behaviors such as smoking, waist circumference, and latency to sleep, were important predictors of an increased concentration of CRP.

Prolonged or repeated exposure to stress has been shown to cause or exacerbate disease or symptoms of diseases such as angina, cardiac dysrhythmias, pain, tension headaches, insomnia, and gastrointestinal complaints. This influence is documented in extensive experimental and clinical literature.[45] Stress has been found to influence the development of coronary artery disease in women[46] and pain perception in older adults.[40]

Psychological Effects of Stress

The psychological effects of stress are manifested by negative mood states such as anxiety, depression, hostility, and anger. These emotions (mood states) can, in turn, negatively influence a person's ability to concentrate and effectively problem solve. In addition, a growing body of research demonstrates the correlation between prolonged negative mood states and increased morbidity and mortality in several diseases.[40, 47–49] Doering and colleagues found that after bypass surgery, depressive symptoms were associated with an increase in infections, impaired wound healing, and poor emotional and physical recovery.[47] In addition, hostility has been found to play a role in a chronic cycle of inflammation among older adults and can dramatically affect their health.[40]

Concurrently, a growing body of research supports the importance of managing stress in the treatment of many diseases. Cancer[50–52] and other diseases of the immune system have been shown to respond to interventions that reduce the stress response, as have arthritis,[53] chronic pain,[54] hypertension and stroke,[55–57] diabetes,[30] asthma,[58] infertility,[59] and the symptoms of chronic diseases.[60–62]

A seminal study found that a pessimistic explanatory style was significantly associated with a self-report of poorer physical and mental functioning 30 years later.[63] It is theorized that a pessimistic explanatory style or attitude, in addition to adversely affecting behavior, may weaken the immune system through a prolonged increase in sympathetic arousal. In addition, pessimists have more health-risking behaviors such as smoking, alcohol misuse, and sedentary lifestyle.

Social and Behavioral Effects of Stress

In response to stress, people often revert to less healthy behaviors.[64] The social and behavioral pathway is best illustrated by appreciating the effect of behavior patterns on the incidence and progression of disease. How and what people eat, drink, and smoke, as well as how they take prescribed or illegal drugs, influence health. For many, stressful events can increase behaviors such as overeating or excessive intake of alcohol.

As stress increases, self-control decreases. Lapsing to behaviors that provide immediate gratification is more likely when stress is high. This inability to control health-risking behaviors as a result of increased stress is called the *stress-disinhibition effect*.[42, 65]

Behaviors such as social isolation, which may be influenced by stress and negative thinking patterns, have been shown to be associated with higher morbidity and mortality in the first year after myocardial infarction.[66] Conversely, social support has been found to have a positive effect on health outcomes in medical settings.

Positive health outcomes in labor and delivery appear to be affected by emotional support as well. The most common surgical procedure performed in the United States is cesarean section (c-section). Delivery by c-section increases the risk of complications for mother and child and extends the length of their hospital stay. The presence of a supportive woman during labor and delivery has been shown to reduce the need for c-section, shorten labor and delivery time, and reduce perinatal problems.[67] Interestingly, greater benefits are realized when the provider is not a member of the hospital staff but rather a lay volunteer such as a female friend or family member taught supportive techniques.[68] This implies obvious cost benefits and continues to underscore the implications of social support to both the patient's health and the healthcare system.

Recent research on programs that influence behavior change have shown positive modification of some of the most widespread diseases. Lifestyle behavior change has been demonstrated to influence regression of coronary artery disease and reduce cardiac risk factors, as well as improve the management of chronic cardiac disease.[69, 70] These are only a few of the hundreds of studies that provide continuing evidence of the multidirectional relationships among thoughts, feelings, beliefs, behaviors, and physiology.

Spiritual Effects of Stress

In response to stress, people can become disconnected from their life's meaning and purpose. In *Man's Search for Meaning*, Frankl draws a parallel between connection with life's meaning and survival.[71] He describes the survivors of the World War II concentration camps as individuals who were able to retain their sense of meaning and purpose and who were able to draw meaning and purpose from their experiences. A feeling of disconnection, however, in addition to being an effect of stress, can also be a precursor to stress. Several studies have examined the effects of spirituality, defined as connection with life's meaning and purpose, on health. Increased scores on measures of spirituality correlated with increased incidence of health-promoting behaviors.[72] Other studies have explored the association between religious affiliation and health and have found a positive correlation.[73-75] This area of study is of considerable interest in the scientific literature today.

The Psychology of Optimism

Through research in the field of positive psychology, it is now known that positive perspectives reduce the ill effects of the stress response and increase resilience.[76, 77] The link between optimism and health was made by researchers tracking the lives of a group of Harvard alumni who graduated in 1945. They found that individuals who were optimistic in college were healthier in later life, whereas those who were pessimistic experienced more health problems by middle age. More recently, research conducted after the September 11, 2001, terrorist attacks found that individuals with positive worldviews have a significantly improved ability to cope with biological and psychological stressors.[78, 79]

Healthier models of living have been learned from the study of individuals who display an optimistic worldview. Positive perspectives are associated with increased health-promotion behaviors, improved relationships, and feelings of well-being in times of adversity.[80] It was found that positive emotional reactivity increases the pleasure one experiences from enjoyable activities.[81] Therefore, even subtle positive shifts in perspectives potentiate health-promoting cycles. In addition, positive emotions are associated with increased observational abilities, flexible attention, and nonreactivity to inner turbulence and empathy.[76, 81, 82] Through CBT, patients can move toward more optimistic perspectives and healthier lifestyle behaviors.

Cognitive Behavioral Therapy

In the preceding pages, a foundation has been established for how cognitions, influenced by perception, can affect physiologic, psychological, social and behavioral, and spiritual processes. Because of this influence, CBT is an important intervention in optimizing positive links between mind, body, and spirit and minimizing the negative consequences of adverse interactions. Cognitive behavioral therapy helps individuals reappraise or reevaluate their thinking and adopt a healthier perspective. It is often referred to as cognitive restructuring because the intent of the intervention is to change or restructure the distortions in thinking patterns that cause stress. The basic principles of CBT are as follows:[7, 83]

- Our thoughts, not external events, create our moods and emotions.
- The thoughts that create stress are usually unrealistic, distorted, and negative.
- Distorted, illogical thoughts and self-defeating beliefs lead to physiologic changes and perpetuation of painful feelings, such as depression, anxiety, and anger.
- By changing maladaptive, unrealistic, distorted thoughts, individuals can change how they feel (physically and emotionally).

The goals of CBT include training patients to do the following:[7]

- Pinpoint the negative, automatic thoughts and silent assumptions that trigger and perpetuate their emotional upsets.
- Identify the distortions, irrational beliefs, or cognitive errors.
- Substitute more realistic, self-enhancing thoughts, which will reduce the stress, symptoms, and painful feelings.
- Replace self-defeating, silent assumptions with more reasonable and flexible belief systems.
- Develop improved social skills, as well as coping, communication, and empathic skills.

The Process of Cognitive Behavioral Therapy

Cognitive behavioral therapy is a short-term intervention used to help modify habits of thinking that may be distorted, negative, or irrational. In the context of CBT, cognitive restructuring is an approach or series of strategies that helps people assess their thoughts, challenge them, and replace them with more rational responses. Importantly, cognitive restructuring does not deny affliction, suffering, misfortune, or negative feelings. There are many experiences in life where it is appropriate to feel angry, sad, depressed, or anxious. The technique of cognitive restructuring is used to help people experience a broader range of emotions and avoid becoming "stuck" in powerful negative mood states, which generate additional stress.

The nurse provider serves as a guide in the process of CBT. Unlike in biomedical interventions, the provider cannot perform this intervention to or for the patient but instead guides the individual to do it for himself or herself. There is no way to predict what will surface during the therapy or what meaning it will have to the individual. The nurse must honor the premise that each individual can best interpret his or her own experience(s), belief(s), and distortion(s).

Step 1: Awareness

Developing awareness is the first step in a systematic approach to guide patients to a restructuring of their cognitive distortions. Patients are asked to bring to their conscious awareness two things. First is an awareness of how habits of distorted, negative thinking and silent assumptions influence them physically, emotionally, behaviorally, and spiritually. Second is awareness that a habit pattern (silent assumptions, irrational beliefs, and cognitive distortions) underlies these automatic, negative thoughts. To facilitate development of this awareness, a four-step approach is used to explore a stressful situation systematically. Patients are asked to stop (break the cycle of "awfulizing," escalating thoughts—become aware that a stress has taken place); take a breath (release physical tension, promote relaxation—become aware of physical changes that have occurred in response to stress); reflect (realize what is going on—become aware of automatic thoughts, distortions, beliefs, assumptions); and

choose (decide how to respond—become aware of choices in responding).[84]

Patients are first asked to identify their warning signals of stress. **Exhibit 22-1** is a sample form for identifying and recording this information. These cues (or signals) can be physical, emotional, behavioral, or spiritual. When asked to monitor responses to a particular event, patients become more consciously aware of these cues. **Exhibit 22-2** is an example of a format for recording this information. Although it may initially increase an individual's perception of physical pain or emotional discomfort, conscious awareness is a necessary first step in recognizing the relationship of thoughts, feelings, behavior, and biology to distorted thinking patterns.

Often, patients have long ignored the cues that their minds or bodies have given them. Consider the patient with disabling headaches who may ignore the shoulder and neck tension that precedes his headaches. Had he attended to his early stress warning signs (neck and shoulder tension), he might have avoided the headache. Becoming aware of these stress warning signs is the first step. Attending to the cues is the next. Once they make this connection, patients can more easily develop skills to reduce negative mood states, unhealthy behaviors, and physical symptoms. To continue with the preceding example, it is easier to prevent a tension headache when the patient notices shoulder tension and then stops, takes a few deep, diaphragmatic breaths, and gently stretches the area than it is to wait for the headache to become incapacitating before acting.

Exercise 22-1

Ask the patient to identify his or her stress warning signals. Then, have the patient identify a stressful experience and the physical or emotional reaction to this particular experience. For example, after being instructed to stop, take a breath, and notice the physical and emotional response to a stressful situation, one patient related the following:

On my way home from work yesterday I sat in traffic. I noticed that my hands were gripping the steering wheel, my neck and shoulders were tight, and my jaw was clenched. I felt angry and frustrated because I wanted to be home.

EXHIBIT 22-1   Stress Warning Signals

Physical Symptoms	Behavioral Symptoms	Emotional Symptoms	Cognitive Symptoms
❑ Headaches	❑ Excess smoking	❑ Crying	❑ Trouble thinking clearly
❑ Indigestion	❑ Bossiness	❑ Nervousness, anxiety	❑ Forgetfulness
❑ Stomachaches	❑ Compulsive gum chewing	❑ Boredom — no meaning to things	❑ Lack of creativity
❑ Sweaty palms	❑ Attitude critical of others	❑ Edginess — ready to explode	❑ Memory loss
❑ Sleep difficulties	❑ Grinding of teeth at night	❑ Feeling powerless to change things	❑ Inability to make decisions
❑ Dizziness	❑ Overuse of alcohol	❑ Overwhelming sense of pressure	❑ Thoughts of running away
❑ Back pain	❑ Compulsive eating	❑ Anger	❑ Constant worry
❑ Tight neck, shoulders	❑ Inability to get things done	❑ Loneliness	❑ Loss of sense of humor
❑ Racing heart		❑ Unhappiness for no reason	
❑ Restlessness		❑ Easily upset	
❑ Tiredness			
❑ Ringing in ears			

Do any seem familiar to you?

Check the ones you experience when under stress. These are your stress warning signs.

Are there any additional stress warning signals that you experience that are not listed? If so, add them here.

_____

_____

_____

_____

Source: Reprinted with permission from H. Benson and E. M. Stuart, *The Wellness Book: The Comprehensive Guide to Maintaining Health and Treating Stress-Related Illness,* p. 182, © 1992, Carol Publishing.

EXHIBIT 22-2   Challenging Stress and Winning with a More Positive Perspective

Describe the situation:

Stop	Breathe	Reflect				Choose	
Break the cycle of escalating, awfulizing thoughts.	Elicit the relaxation response to counteract the stress response.	Physical response: Describe your physical symptoms and behaviors in response to the stressor.	Emotional response: What was your emotional response to the situation?	Automatic thoughts: Write your automatic thoughts to the situation.	Exaggerated beliefs: What distorted beliefs are you hooked to in this situation?	Positive perspectives: What are more optimistic or self-enhancing perspectives of this situation?	Reappraised thoughts: Construct some thoughts that reflect this more positive perspective.

Source: Reproduced from Benson H, Stuart EM. The wellness book: A comprehensive guide to maintaining health and treating stress-related illness. New York: Fireside, Simon & Schuster; 1993[4] and The Benson-Henry Institute for Mind Body Medicine. Stress management and resiliency training: Providers manual. Boston: author; 2014.[85]

Becoming aware of stress warning signals is an important first step. Although this seems very straightforward, the average person is often unaware of the effects of stress on the body–mind. Once the patient is aware of the effects of stress, he or she may be able to release tension more easily. Patients build on this awareness as they proceed through cognitive restructuring.

Step 2: Automatic Thoughts

Once the patient has been able to identify a stress or a stressful situation and the changes in the body–mind that accompany this stress, the next step is to identify the automatic thoughts. These thoughts usually occur automatically in response to a situation. Because these thoughts occur automatically and often are not in the conscious awareness of the individual, they are described as knee-jerk responses. Patients are taught a systematic approach to identifying these self-defeating automatic thoughts.

Automatic thoughts have the following characteristics in common:

- Reflex or knee-jerk responses to a perceived stressor
- Usually negative
- Quick, fleeting, a kind of shorthand (e.g., *should, ought, never, always*)
- Usually not in our conscious awareness
- Frequently unrealistic, illogical, and distorted

Because these thoughts form so quickly, it is often difficult to notice that they have occurred. Typically, people attribute the stress they experience or the feeling they have to the person or situation that is causing the stress. By stopping, taking a breath, and asking the question "What is going on here?" patients gradually become aware that their stress does not always come from an outside event or situation but may come from the way they interpret these events. Automatic thoughts can be viewed as habits of thinking, inner dialogue, or perceptions that, in turn, create the experience and influence the individual's physiology, emotions, and behaviors.

One of the most important and difficult tasks in cognitive restructuring is developing an awareness that these automatic thoughts

---

Example

A popular and successful teacher was reviewing the student evaluations at the end of the semester. He read 20 very positive reviews. Then he read one that contained some criticism of his teaching style. Instantly he felt a tense sensation in his stomach and chest. After stopping and taking a breath, he was able to identify the following automatic thoughts: "There's always one in a crowd ... ought to have done [*whatever*] ... never could teach that concept well ... should have included the new material I saw in the library ... I always come up short."

Notice that the teacher had an instant reaction to this stress (perception of threat) and that his automatic thoughts were quick, fleeting, negative, and probably not in his conscious awareness. (Does he really believe that he always comes up short?) Identifying automatic thoughts is an important step in allowing patients to look realistically at their automatic reaction to a stressor and put it into perspective.

---

occur. One reason that these reflex, knee-jerk responses are so pervasive is that the body does not know the difference between things that are imagined and things that are actually experienced. Another reason is that people are always talking to themselves, and after they say something to themselves often enough, they begin to believe it. A third reason is that people rarely stop to question their thoughts or emotions. For these reasons, patients need to be taught a structured way of exploring stress and uncovering these automatic thoughts.

Here is an exercise to uncover automatic thoughts, feelings, and physical responses (see also Exhibit 22-2):

Exercise 22-2

Stop: Break the cycle of escalating, awfulizing thoughts.
Take a breath: Release physical tension, promote relaxation.
Reflect:

- Physically, how do I feel?
- Emotionally, how do I feel?
- What are my automatic thoughts (e.g., *should, always, ought, never*)?

Step 3: Cognitive Distortions

Once patients have learned to identify stressful situations; their physical, emotional, and behavioral responses to stress; and the automatic thoughts that precipitate the experience, the next step in the process is to teach patients to identify distortions in thinking. Cognitive distortions are illogical ways of thinking that lead to adverse body-mind-spirit states. The problem is not that these thoughts are wrong or bad but that people hold the beliefs so strongly. Cognitive distortions are based on beliefs or underlying assumptions that are generally out of proportion to the situation. These beliefs or assumptions are usually long held, based on life experience, and often not in one's conscious awareness.

Through years of research and clinical experience, Burns identified the following 10 general categories of cognitive distortions that lead to negative emotional states:[86]

- *All-or-nothing thinking.* Viewing things in black or white; considering oneself as a total failure when a performance falls short of perfection. (Think back to the example of the teacher. In the face of 20 excellent evaluations and 1 constructive criticism, the teacher immediately focused all of his attention on the imperfection and felt anxious and upset. "I should have taught the course all differently." "I never get a good review.")
- *Overgeneralization.* Viewing a single negative event as a never-ending pattern. "Fixing my car cost twice what they said it would. All mechanics are dishonest and always will be."
- *Mental filtering.* Picking out a negative detail and dwelling on it exclusively, "catastrophizing," or "awfulizing." "I got a lousy grade on that test. I'll probably have to drop out of school. I won't be able to find a decent job and will have to move back in with my parents."
- *Disqualifying the positive.* Rejecting positive experiences as if they do not count. "It was nothing." Being unable to accept praise. "You're just saying that because you have to."
- *Jumping to conclusions.* Reading the minds of others or predicting negative outcomes without sufficient evidence. "He went off to bed without saying anything. He's angry with me for working late again."
- *Magnification.* Exaggerating the importance of mistakes or inappropriately minimizing the significance of one's own assets. "My performance tonight was horrible—I'll never get the lead part."
- *Emotional reasoning.* Assuming that one's emotions reflect the way things are. "I feel worthless—I must be worthless."
- *"Should" statements.* Trying to motivate oneself with shoulds and shouldn'ts. "Good employees should always get to the office early and be willing to stay late."
- *Labeling.* Name calling; labeling oneself a "loser" if a mistake is made; making an illogical leap from one characteristic to a category. "She's blond. What do you expect? She's an airhead."
- *Personalization.* Blaming oneself inappropriately as the cause of a negative event; seeing events only in relation to oneself. "It's my fault that my child didn't do well in school because I work."

Exaggerated, unrealistic, illogical, and distorted automatic thoughts are a result of deeply held silent assumptions and beliefs that are usually not in one's conscious awareness. A patient is more likely to experience stress in any given situation if he or she holds these beliefs as absolutes. Situations that are encountered are far more likely to precipitate stress if the world is viewed in terms of black or white (e.g., all good or all bad) than if there is room for shades of gray. An important understanding for the clinician is that it is often not the belief that needs to be examined but the degree to which the belief is held. All patients are entitled to their individual sets of beliefs. Assigning any value, right or wrong, to their beliefs is not in the nurse's purview. The nurse is simply inviting patients to examine their beliefs in the context of their stress and to assess whether the degree to which they hold these beliefs serves them well or contributes to stress. Patients can very easily be alienated if they feel the nurse is making value judgments about their beliefs. The core concept here is not to examine beliefs to decide whether they are right or wrong but for the patient to decide whether these beliefs serve him or her well. Some commonly held assumptions and beliefs include the following:[87]

- If I treat others fairly, then I can expect them to treat me fairly.
- I must always have the love and approval of family, friends, and peers to be worthwhile.
- I must be unfailingly competent and perfect in all that I do.
- My worth as a human being depends on my achievements (or intelligence or status or attractiveness).

Everyone has a right to his or her beliefs and opinions. Problems develop when these beliefs are held as absolutes and provide no room for flexibility in an imperfect world.

Example

Reflect back on the previous example of the teacher reading course evaluations who had a strong reaction to criticism. After taking a breath, interrupting his automatic response, and identifying his automatic thoughts, he was able to identify his cognitive distortions and irrational beliefs. They included all-or-nothing thinking (must be perfect all the time), overgeneralization (never will get it right), disqualifying the positive (20 excellent reviews wiped out by 1 negative review), and the belief that "I must be unfailingly competent and perfect in all I do to be loved and respected by family, friends, and peers."

The following is an extension to the exercise to uncover cognitive distortions:

Exercise 22-3

Stop: Break the cycle of escalating, awfulizing thoughts.
Take a breath: Release physical tension, promote relaxation.
Reflect:

- Physically, how do I feel?
- Emotionally, how do I feel?
- What are my automatic thoughts (e.g., *should, always, ought, never*)?
- What is going on here?
- Is it really true?

- Am I jumping to conclusions?
- Am I catastrophizing, awfulizing, getting things out of perspective?
- Is it really a crisis?
- Is it as bad as it seems?
- Is there another way to look at the situation?
- What is the worst that can happen?

Because these strongly held assumptions and beliefs are mostly silent or not in people's conscious awareness, it is a challenge to discover their existence and, consequently, their influence on people's thoughts, emotions, and behaviors. In addition to the systematic approach described here to explore a stressful situation (stop, take a breath, reflect, and choose), another strategy that is helpful in discovering underlying assumptions and beliefs is the vertical arrow technique developed by Burns.[7]

Exercise 22-4: Vertical Arrow

Ask the patient to identify a stressful situation and to challenge the underlying assumptions in this stress. The patient can challenge the assumptions by asking the question, "If that is true, why is it so upsetting?"

For example, a nursing school student had severe panic that kept her from speaking up in class. Class participation was 50% of the grade, so she wanted to change this behavior. When she was asked why it was stressful to ask a question, the following sequence of thoughts emerged.

"If I speak up, I may say something stupid."

↓

If this is true, why is it so upsetting?

↓

"They will think I'm stupid."

↓

If this is true, why is it so upsetting?

↓

"The smart students won't invite me to join their study group."

↓

If this is true, why is it so upsetting?

↓

Exercise 22-4: Vertical Arrow (*continued*)

"I won't pass unless I'm in a good study group."
↓
If this is true, why is it so upsetting?
↓
"I'll flunk out of school."
↓
If this is true, why is it so upsetting?
↓
"My family and friends will be embarrassed."
↓
If this is true, why is it so upsetting?
↓
"They won't love me."
↓
If this is true, why is it so upsetting?
↓
"I'm unlovable."

Using this vertical arrow technique allowed the student to see how out of perspective her automatic thoughts were. She could clearly see that her stress was influenced by the exaggerated belief that to make a mistake would make her less than perfect and to be less than perfect was bad and would make people cease to love her. The awareness of this pattern of thinking allowed her to put the situation in perspective and helped her to get past her fear of asking a question.

Once a fear is recognized, it can be approached like any other stressor. If it is irrational, it can be challenged through cognitive restructuring. If it is rational, then appropriate problem-solving and coping strategies are required.

Identifying Emotions The way people feel emotionally is an important part of health. Feelings of vigor, vitality, and general well-being are important correlates of health; conversely, feelings of anger, hostility, anxiety, or depression can contribute to ill health. Many people find their emotions troubling, either because they are out of touch with them or because they feel overwhelmed by them. Family and cultural influences have a great deal to do with the way emotions are experienced. Many families and cultures do not encourage the expression of emotions, and individuals learn to ignore this aspect of their lives. As individuals become aware of their body-mind-spirit responses to stress by identifying their emotional stress warning signals, they become aware of their feelings and emotions and the connection between these feelings and emotions and stress.

Feelings of depression, anger, fear, and guilt are all part of the human experience; however, individuals may need to be encouraged to acknowledge and honor these emotions. Emotions are genuine, and people are entitled to the way they feel. On the other hand, emotions, particularly exaggerated emotions, can interfere with effective problem solving. Individuals need to be guided through the process of recognizing their emotions and the thoughts that underlie these feelings. For example, anger is often perpetuated by thoughts of unfair treatment. Frustration is often the result of unmet expectations. Thoughts related to loss contribute to the feeling of depression, and perception of a loss of control often causes anxiety. It is important to distinguish healthy fear from neurotic anxiety. Thoughts underlying healthy fear are realistic, keep one alert, and warn one of dangers. Neurotic anxiety is related to thoughts that are distorted and unrealistic and often contain "what ifs": "What if I don't get the job?" "What if I don't find a partner?" A great deal of time and energy are wasted on events that may never take place. The nurse must guide the patient in discovering the thoughts that are behind the emotion. In this way, the nurse can facilitate a process of challenging the thoughts and dealing with the emotions.

When feelings are ignored, denied, or suppressed, they often become intertwined with stress. In this case, patients sometimes have difficulty identifying either the emotion or the automatic thoughts related to the emotion. Cognitive restructuring allows individuals to become aware of the emotions, the automatic thoughts related to a particular emotion, and the connection with stress. Reflecting on these underlying themes often helps individuals to explain why they feel as they do and, in turn, to choose a more effective coping mechanism.

Another danger in denying feelings is that individuals can become trapped in one of these emotional states so that the mind becomes a filter, letting into conscious awareness only material that confirms or reinforces their mood. For example, when people are depressed, they notice and experience only things that depress them more; nothing that would bring joy and pleasure is allowed into their awareness. Through cognitive restructuring, they can learn to reduce the frequency, length, and intensity of these feelings.

This variation of the exercise uncovers the relationship between thoughts and feelings:

Exercise 22-5

Stop: Break the cycle of escalating, awfulizing thoughts.
Take a breath: Release physical tension, promote relaxation.
Reflect: What am I feeling? What am I thinking? Is there a theme that underlies my stress triggers?

Feeling	Thoughts related to
Anger	Being treated unfairly
Frustration	Unmet expectations
Depression	Loss
Anxiety	Loss of control, fear of the unknown

As an example, consider the situation of a person who is laid off from his or her job. An angry person often views situations through the lens of his or her standard of fairness. In response to being laid off, such a person might be angry and think, "Why me? I've worked hard all these years, never complaining, doing more than I was asked, and this is how they reward me?" A depressed individual often responds with distortions such as all-or-nothing thinking, personalization, and overgeneralization. In response to being laid off, such a person might become depressed and think, "This shows what a complete failure I am. I'll never amount to anything." In the same situation, an anxious person might experience an entirely different set of distortions. This person might predict dire consequences (jump to conclusions) and take them as facts. An anxious person who just got laid off might think, "What if I never get a job again. I'll be broke, on the street, and living on welfare in a matter of months."

The nurse helps the patient become aware of the relationship of these emotional themes to stress triggers and cognitive distortions. When the nurse guides the patient through a stress

awareness exercise, if the patient identifies his or her emotional response as anger, the nurse helps the patient to make the connection with automatic thoughts related to being treated unfairly (e.g., "This shouldn't have happened to me." or "Why me? This is so unfair.").

Because patients have often spent so many years ignoring their emotional cues, they sometimes have difficulty recognizing either the thoughts or the emotions that are related to stressful situations. Keeping a diary or journal to reflect on thoughts and feelings about stressful events has been found to be a valuable tool that patients can use to identify automatic thoughts and underlying emotions.[88] This method is explained further in the following section on coping. In addition to understanding stressors and common themes that trigger stress, acknowledging and honoring emotions is important to a healthy sense of self. Healthy self-esteem, in turn, is an important ingredient in stress hardiness or the ability to greet stressful events as challenges to be met rather than as threats to be feared.

Step 4: Choosing Effective Coping

The final step in the process of CBT is to help the patient restructure or reframe distortions and beliefs and choose a more effective way of responding or coping. To accomplish this, one must recognize that stressful situations have two components, which Ellis termed the *practical problem* and the *emotional hook*.[6, 87] The practical problem is the situation at hand, or the problem that needs to be addressed. The emotional hook is the patient's opinion about the problem or the individual(s) who have caused the problem. Quite often people respond to situations as if they can solve the problem by addressing the emotional hook. In the following example, note the difference in these two elements of the stress.

Example

John related that he became very upset when he was late for an appointment and, while he was in line at the grocery store, someone cut in front of him.

Example (*continued*)

To cope effectively with this situation, John needed to separate the practical problem (getting through the line) from the emotional hook (his opinion about people who cut in line and his "right" to be treated fairly). When asked to stop, take a breath, and reflect, he was able to uncover his physical response (tense, tight jaw), his emotional response (anger), his automatic thoughts ("This always happens to me," "People ought not to cut in line," "Late."), and silent assumptions underlying the distorted thinking ("I treat others fairly, and I expect to be treated fairly.").

This example shows that the process of solving the practical problem is different from the process of addressing the emotional hook. If John were to expend his energy in convincing the person who cut in front of him of the error of his ways regarding behavior in line, John would be unlikely to solve his problem (he was late and needed to get through the line efficiently). Moreover, in practical terms, John had no control over this other person. How likely was it that John could influence this person's behavior in future situations? Automatic thoughts—shoulds, nevers, always, musts, and oughts—often interfere with finding practical solutions to the problem. The emotional hook robs individuals of their ability to see the options for responding. This failure can make it impossible for patients to recognize when they have no control over a situation and need to concentrate on the practical problem rather than the emotional hook.

In order to help a patient become "unhooked" from a distorted belief that continues to cause repeated distress, the nurse can help the patient substitute a more positive perspective. In this example, John recognizes how his underlying beliefs and assumptions are influencing his choices. John identifies the exaggerated thinking that is trapping him in the experience of anger, frustration, and anxiety.

- "This always happens to me." = Overgeneralization
- "People ought not to cut in line." = Should statements
- "I'm late for my appointment, which makes me unprofessional." = Magnification

Now John can choose a healthier perspective that will allow him to move through the painful emotions and adapt to the situation.

- "I am not always going to be treated fairly by others."
- "But really, it's not all that bad. I'll just let it go."
- "I can ask the individual to go to the end of the line."
- "Or I can choose to go to a different line."
- "Actually, I am a generally nice, reliable, calm guy and I do not have to be bothered by this unpleasant experience."

This process involves making a decision about how to respond from conscious awareness and without continued emotional arousal. He might see several options. For example, he might choose to change lines or to calmly ask the person who cut in front of him to go to the end of the line (direct action). Or he might choose just to let it go because, although it is important to be treated fairly, in this instance he is in a hurry and does not have the time or desire to deal with this individual; further, because this does not always happen to him, it is not worth getting upset about (acceptance, reframing). Whatever the decision, it can be made with awareness and choice, not in reaction to a deeply held belief about how people ought to behave, and without further escalating emotional distress.

Exercise 22-6: Reframing and Problem Solving

Stop: Build recognition of physical symptoms of stress so that when they occur action can be taken to stop further arousal. Train a patient to stop each time a stress is encountered, before thoughts escalate into the worst possible scenario. The simple act of thinking "Stop" can help break a pattern of automatic response.

Breathe: Teach the patient to breathe deeply and release physical tension. Physically taking a deep, diaphragmatic breath can be important because, during times of stress, most people hold their breath. Taking a deep breath can elicit the physiologic changes of the relaxation response, the opposite of the stress response. This practice facilitates awareness of stress warning signals and the interaction between stress and bodymindspirit changes.

Reflect: Teach patients to ask themselves several questions about their automatic thoughts and underlying beliefs. Is this thought true? Is this thought helpful? (This is the process of developing awareness of automatic thoughts and cognitive distortions and challenging these distorted thoughts, beliefs, and assumptions.)

Choose: Train patients to select the most effective way to cope with or solve the problem. Instruct the patient to ask a series of questions:

- What is the practical problem?
- What is the emotional hook?
- How can I substitute more realistic, self-enhancing thoughts to reduce the painful feelings?
- How can I replace self-defeating silent assumptions (e.g., by substituting "I'm doing the best I can" for "I can't cope with this")?
- What do I need?
- What can I do?
- What do I want?
- What is possible?
- Do I have the time, skills, and personal investment to achieve a practical solution? Is the practical problem within my control to solve?
- Is it possible to deal with the practical problem? Is it within my control?
- Do I need to temper my emotional response before I can act responsibly, practically, and appropriately?
- Am I avoiding the best solution because it will be difficult for me?

Many techniques can be used to help patients effectively problem solve and cope with stressors. Effective coping requires that one attend to both the practical problem and the emotional hook. This sometimes requires two different approaches. Careful thought must be given to each stressful situation to choose the most effective coping strategy. The following list suggests a few ways to cope:[7]

Distraction. Worry about resolving a stress can be put off until the time is right. For example, the patient receives a letter from the manager of the bank asking to speak with the patient as soon as possible, but it is after closing hours. Distraction involves putting this worry aside until the bank opens the next day, at which time the patient can deal directly with the situation. This is different from procrastination or denial because it is a necessary delay as opposed to avoidance.

Direct action. The problem can be dealt with directly to resolve it.

Relaxation. Using relaxation techniques to reduce emotional arousal is a way of coping with a stress that cannot be changed or avoided. Techniques to elicit the relaxation response include meditation, yoga, mindfulness, and tai chi, as well as many others. Relaxation techniques are discussed in Chapter 11.

Reframing. Looking at a situation differently can help individuals cope. A glass filled halfway can be labeled either half full or half empty. This label changes the experience greatly. Illness, for example, can be viewed as catastrophic and life shattering or as an opportunity for reconnection to what is meaningful in one's life.

Affirmations. Positive thoughts can be used to recondition one's thinking. For example, individuals frequently tell themselves they cannot do something, and the statement becomes a self-fulfilling prophecy. Affirmations are a way of countering self-defeating silent assumptions. An affirmation is simply a positive thought, a short phrase, or a saying that has meaning for the individual. Patients can be coached to create an affirmation as a way of reframing or choosing a more helpful, reasonable belief system.

Exercise 22-7: Developing an Affirmation

Ask the patient to choose an aspect of life that is causing stress, such as work, family, or health. Have the patient decide what he or she would want to have happen or how he or she would want to feel in the situation. Formulate the goal as a first-person statement, in the present, and in the positive (e.g., "I am confident in my work," "I can handle it," "I am peaceful," or "I am becoming healthy and strong."). Have the patient repeat the affirmation often during the day, perhaps before or after eliciting the relaxation response or as part of a breathing exercise.

In a short time, affirmations can become second nature and help to enhance self-esteem and reduce stress.

Spirituality. A sense of connection to the universe, God, or a higher power, or connecting with what is important and meaningful in our life, can aid in coping with stress. Connection with life's meaning and purpose is addressed in greater detail in Chapter 7.

Catharsis. Emotional catharsis, either laughing or crying, can be very effective in relieving emotional distress.

Journal writing. Using a journal to write about thoughts, feelings, and experiences is often helpful in processing emotions. Pennebaker and colleagues found that writing to get in touch with one's deepest thoughts and feelings can measurably improve physical and mental health.[88] Suggest to patients that they get a special notebook and colorful pens for their journal. Several other chapters in this text contain more detailed information on journal writing (see, for example, Chapter 14).

Social support. Having supportive family, friends, and coworkers is important to effective coping and has been shown to contribute to stress hardiness. Talking out problems is often helpful to obtain good advice or uncritical support. Social support has been found to reduce the incidence of heart disease as well as other health problems. In the social support literature, it has been noted that both the number of supporters and the quality of the relationships are important.

Assertive communication. Communication is an important skill to help in solving problems and reducing conflicts and stress. Communication (also addressed in Chapter 19) is considered in some detail in the next section because it is an important coping and problem-solving skill that can be adversely affected by deeply held beliefs and silent assumptions. Cognitive restructuring can influence the ability to communicate effectively and, in turn, improve coping.

Empathy. Empathy is the ability to take into consideration the other person's perspective. It is an effective coping technique because it facilitates communication. It helps patients become better listeners. Empathy is described in more detail in the next exercise.

Developing Communication Skills

People who have problems with communication usually experience the following challenges:[54]

- Disparity between what they say (statement) and what they want (intent).
- Confusion about or resistance to stating clearly how they feel, what they want, or what they need (assertiveness); there is a tendency to deny their own feelings (passiveness) or to be indifferent toward the feelings of others (aggressiveness).
- Inability to listen.

The importance of matching the statement with the intention is illustrated by the following example:

Example

After spending a long day at work and stopping to pick up some groceries at the store, Jill arrives home to find her husband Jack at his desk in his office going over some bills. Coming in the door, she remarks, "Wow, busy day. I just picked up some groceries." She begins bringing the bags of groceries into the kitchen, walking past him. Following each trip to the garage, she shuts the door a little more forcefully and sets each bag down a little more loudly as Jack continues to sit at his desk.

When he finally says, "Anything wrong?" Jill answers, "Nothing!" and storms out of the room, feeling that, if he loved her, he would know what she needed and wanted.

The first principle of effective communication is to be clear about what one wants and needs (intent) in statements to others. Although it would be wonderful if spouses, friends, and others were mind readers, assuming that they are does not help with communication. Matching statements with intentions is an art and a skill. It requires that individuals recognize their automatic thoughts, emotions, and cognitive distortions and take responsibility for their part of the conversation.

Consider the preceding example. If Jill's intention was for her husband to help bring the groceries into the house, then her statement should have reflected this. She might have said, "Wow, what a busy day. I just picked up some groceries. Could you help me bring them into the house?" Patients must understand that the other person is not obligated to respond as they would wish. However, what they are asking for will be a lot clearer to others if the statement reflects the intent.

The next principle of effective communication is to be assertive. In most cases, assertive communication is the most effective way to communicate. An assertive statement expresses one's feelings and opinions and reaffirms one's identity and rights. It is not judgmental. The general format of an assertive statement is "I feel [*label the emotion*] when you [*label the behavior*] because [*provide an explanation*]." The formula requires that all three elements be included. Cognitive restructuring facilitates assertive communication because it requires patients to identify their thoughts and feelings. In the example, Jill would:

- **Stop:** Break the cycle of escalating, awfulizing thoughts.
- **Take a breath:** Release physical tension, promote relaxation.
- **Reflect:**
  - Emotionally, how do I feel? (frustrated)
  - What are my automatic thoughts? ("If he loved me, he would get up and help me! He never helps me with the house. He always expects me to do everything around here. He doesn't care about me. He's never going to change.")

Recognizing her thoughts and feelings would help Jill to formulate an assertive statement when her husband asks, "Anything wrong?" She could then say, "I feel frustrated [*emotion*] when you don't help me bring in the groceries [*behavior*] because if you cared for me you would help me more with the chores around the house [*explanation*]." In this way, she would have made her feelings clear and have explained why she felt that way. This, in turn, would have provided a better opportunity to work on problem solving. If patients cannot articulate both their feelings and their needs, they leave it up to others to figure them out. When others fail to do so correctly, the patients feel let down and blame others for not understanding. The nurse can help patients to recognize that they have a right to speak up and a responsibility to do so in an assertive rather than passive or aggressive way. The nurse can guide patients in matching their emotions with the explanation (e.g., frustration = unmet expectation) by reviewing the exercise on matching thoughts and emotions as in the preceding example. Patients should be reminded that this technique will feel awkward and uncomfortable at first. They may have to practice it many times before communications improve. Other people need time to adjust to the changes they are trying to make. Effective communication takes practice as well as patience with oneself and others.

Developing Empathy Skills

Here is an exercise nurses can introduce to patients to help them develop skills in empathy:

Exercise 22-8: Promoting Empathy

Empathy can be facilitated through active listening. This technique requires conscious, nonjudgmental awareness. It helps to clarify the issues involved and can deescalate many emotional exchanges. Consider a situation in which the mother announces, "I can't stand this room anymore. It's a mess." The response to this statement may be critical to resolving the issues without contributing to further miscommunication and escalating the problem. Instead of becoming hooked by a defensive emotional reaction, patients can learn to operate from empathy using the four-step approach.
Stop: Break the cycle of escalating, awfulizing thoughts.
Take a breath: Release physical tension, promote relaxation.
Reflect:

- Emotionally, how do I feel? (hurt, angry)
- What are my automatic thoughts? ("How could she say that? I work hard too. I'm always being blamed for how things are around here. No one understands kids.")

Exercise 22-8: Promoting Empathy (*continued*)

- What are the thoughts and emotions being expressed by the other person? (The simple practice of asking this question provides a very different perspective as the patient begins to formulate a response.)

Choose:

- My feelings are hurt, but I choose not to react defensively.
- I choose to listen actively to the other person's response and will try to understand that person's perspective, using this phrase: "You sound [*emotion*] about [*situation*]."

Rogers suggested using this last phrase as a way to facilitate communication and gain awareness of another person's perspective.[89] In the preceding scenario, the teenage child might say, "You sound upset about the messy house." Possible responses might include: "It's not just the room, everything seems to be in a mess, here and at the office. I can't seem to get anything done." Or the mother might say, "You're right about that. I hate coming home to a messy house after a busy day."

When a patient uses the skill of active listening, the other person often feels heard, which may help to defuse further emotional arousal and defensive behavior. In addition, he or she now has an opportunity to clarify any misunderstanding. Also, active listening allows the patient to buy time to obtain a better perspective on what the other person is thinking and feeling. Patients can then choose how they want to respond. This may be a time to use assertive communication or problem solving, or a time to step away from the interaction until emotions and defenses have settled. Active listening allows reflective, empathic, objective, and nonjudgmental communication. Coaching patients to use cognitive restructuring skills that include active listening techniques facilitates effective communication, in turn reducing conflict and stress.

Acceptance. Acceptance is facing the fact that some situations or people cannot be changed or avoided and letting go of resentment. Forgiveness is often a part of acceptance. Coping successfully means gaining the wisdom to achieve the delicate balance between acceptance and action, between letting go and taking control. It is the art of choosing the right strategy at the right time.

When patients feel that they can cope effectively, the harmful effects of stress are buffered. The situation is perceived not as a threat but as a challenge. This subtle difference has profound physiologic, psychological, behavioral, and spiritual effects. It is what allows people facing great adversity (such as illness) to see the opportunity the situation presents. Above all, as noted earlier, patients need to recognize that coping is the art of finding a balance between acceptance and action, between letting go and taking control. Cognitive restructuring helps patients distinguish these differences by providing a format for observing or objectifying their experiences. In so doing, they gain a sense of control that minimizes or buffers the harmful effects of stress.

Cognitive Behavioral Therapy in Children and Adolescents

Cognitive behavioral therapy is an effective treatment modality for children and adolescents, but it is modified to take into consideration the unique developmental needs of this population. The same basic principles discussed earlier are applied; however, factors such as cognitive, social, and emotional maturity are taken into consideration. Whereas adults can reflect on their thought processes, identify their responses to stressful situations, and develop alternative strategies, children often do not have the capacity for this type of mental activity. An individualized treatment plan can be developed based on assessment of these factors. Families and school personnel should also be included in the treatment plan to promote continuity and support across the environments where children spend most of their time.[90] Involvement of family members in CBT interventions has been demonstrated to show higher response rates than CBT for children alone, both after intervention and at 1-year follow up. By the 6-year follow-up assessment, the two groups showed similar numbers of diagnosis-free individuals.[91] In addition, children and youth are less likely to identify a need for treatment; therefore, a critical factor in implementing CBT is engaging them in treatment. Interventions should be fun and build on specific interests and strengths of the child or youth, rather than following a standardized approach. Research identifies the importance of building positive perspectives as an essential part of cognitive therapy with early adolescents.[92]

A review of CBT for anxiety and phobic disorders in children and adolescents discusses application of this treatment for generalized and separation anxiety disorders, social phobia, specific phobias, and school refusal.[91] For these individuals, therapy might be conducted either individually or in a group. Group intervention has the added value of providing both peer modeling and a built-in opportunity for social exposure. School-based cognitive intervention is also described and has been shown to be successful. A discussion of CBT intervention for children with depression addresses the importance of school-based interventions for reducing depressive symptomatology.[93, 94] This review of 25 studies emphasizes that interventions for children and youth address both cognitions and behavior and include self-instruction retraining, problem-solving training, attribution retraining, and cognitive restructuring approaches. Techniques such as modeling, role playing, and positive role playing are effective techniques for working with young people. The evidence points to a strong role for school mental health practitioners such as school psychologists, nurses, school counselors, and special educators.

Techniques for working with the younger child include the following:[90]

- To help children identify the somatic manifestations of anxiety, have them trace their body shape on a large piece of paper and then color the areas where they might feel different when they are anxious.
- Read children's books that discuss different emotions.
- Create a reward list based on the child's interests and developmental level. These can be tangible or social rewards.
- Actively include family members in the treatment plan so that they can gradually integrate strategies into the family's routine.

Techniques for working with adolescents:

- Make a collage from teen magazines with images that display different emotional states.
- Invite the youth to participate by using examples from the teen's life—for example, an interest in a particular sport or other activity.
- Provide age-appropriate rewards.

Example: School Refusal

An 8-year-old child refuses to go to school every morning and displays symptoms of separation anxiety. Treatment might include phased-in exposure to the school setting, application of social and other reinforcements, and training of parents and teachers about the various aspects of the intervention, such as coping skills training, holding the child responsible for his or her behavior, and fostering self-efficacy.[91]

Reproduced from N. J. King, D. Heyne, and T. H. Ollendick, "Cognitive-Behavioral Treatments for Anxiety and Phobic Disorders in Children and Adolescents: A Review," Behavioral Disorders 30(3) (2005): 241–257.

Application of the General Principles of Cognitive Behavioral Therapy

Cognitive behavioral therapy is most useful for individuals, not for relationship problems or interpersonal conflict.[95] The nurse must be imaginative and tenacious. Cognitive behavioral therapy requires constant shifting between technique and process. The therapy combines problem resolution using cognitive and behavioral techniques with empathic focus on the patient's feelings. The process requires the skills of presence, intention, and communication. Several attempts and several different ways of looking at a situation may be required before a patient recognizes the automatic thoughts and underlying beliefs involved.

Cognitive behavioral therapy can be used in both inpatient and outpatient settings, but the goals and process are different in these settings. The goal of CBT in the outpatient setting is generally to restructure cognitive distortions to enhance a variety of self-management skills and healthy lifestyle behaviors that, in turn, help to promote health, reduce symptoms, or manage illness. Outpatient CBT can be provided either individually or in a group. The majority of this chapter has been written for this application.

The goal of CBT in the inpatient setting is typically confined to assisting the patient to cope more effectively with those stresses that arise during hospitalization for an acute illness. In this context, the nurse must remember that he or she is viewing the patient from a cross-sectional perspective (through one episode in the continuum of the patient's life). Patients bring to this hospital experience a reliance on long-standing coping styles—some adaptive, some maladaptive, and many influenced by cognitive distortions. In view of the short hospital stay and critical needs during this time, long-standing maladaptive coping patterns are best left to be addressed after discharge from the hospital.

In the hospital, CBT can be integrated effectively into the many nurse–patient communications that occur each day. Each interaction can be an occasion to assist patients in identifying the relationship of thoughts, feelings, and behaviors to biology as it applies to their current symptoms and illness. The nurse can utilize the structure of CBT to assist the patient in identifying distorted thinking patterns and realistically appraising the situation as well as in seeing opportunity in adversity. Thus, the patient can often choose a more realistic and less stressful way to view the situation. This, in turn, can decrease physical and emotional symptoms.

Hospitalization can be a time of opportunity despite its difficulties. Because hospitalization usually occurs when individuals are in need or crisis, they often feel vulnerable and may be more open to exploring different ways of thinking. In addition, they may be more open to discussing the role that negative thoughts, pessimism, and stress play in their illness, or the role that enhanced self-management skills would play in promoting wellness. For this reason, the inpatient stay offers multiple opportunities for the nurse to integrate CBT. Such integration can help establish a care plan that is congruent with the patient's core values and beliefs.

Therapeutic Care Plan and Interventions

Together, the holistic nurse and the patient develop a plan to attend to the identified

concerns and mutually established goals. The holistic nurse's careful planning will affect the success of this interaction. The following are guidelines for developing a therapeutic care plan and intervention:

Before the session:

- Establish a therapeutic relationship by creating a space in which both you and the patient feel physically and emotionally safe and comfortable.
- Provide materials for recording cognitive distortions and alternative rational thoughts and statements (e.g., paper and pen, blackboard, preprinted forms).
- Center yourself; clear your mind of personal or professional issues to be fully present.
- Establish the long-term goals (outcome) of therapy with the patient.

At the beginning of the session:

- Assess the patient's level of mood, discomfort, or relaxation.
- Review homework from the previous session, if appropriate. Ask the patient to describe any changes that have occurred since the previous session.

During the session:

- Determine, with the patient, which issues need to be addressed and set short-term goals for the session.
- Listen and guide with focused intention. Provide appropriate feedback, clarification, support, or interpretation.

At the end of the session:

- Have the patient identify and verbalize changes that have occurred during the session. Assess progress toward goals.
- Assign homework to be done for the next session.
- Schedule a follow-up session.

Case Study

The same process that has been discussed throughout this chapter can also be used for inpatients, but the nurse would typically guide the patient through the process at the time of the stress. The following example considers the situation of a patient newly admitted to the coronary care unit who experiences chest pain. As the nurse responds to this potentially urgent clinical situation, he or she can gently guide the patient through the following exercise:

- **Stop:** Break the cycle of escalating, awfulizing, negative, automatic thoughts. "I need you to stop and focus on letting go of the worry cycle. If we work together, we will get the best outcome. We have things under control, and I want you to let me worry about the technical things that need to be done. I want you to . . ."
- **Breathe:** Release physical tensions. "Focus on your breathing and leave the rest to me. Take nice, slow breaths, in and out. Concentrate on letting go of tension in your hands, jaw, and feet. Put all of your effort into feeling your fingers and toes, and let the jaw be relaxed and easy. Do you still feel tension somewhere in your body? If so, begin to relax that area. With each breath in, breathe in relaxation; with each breath out, breathe out tension. Now, begin to think about a favorite place and, as you breathe in, feel the peace of that place fill you; as you breathe out, let the worries and tension of the moment flow out."

The nurse guides the person through this relaxation/distraction exercise as he or she proceeds to treat the patient's chest pain. It is not in the patient's best interest for the nurse to stop what he or she is doing; rather, this skill needs to be such an integral part of the nurse's practice that it can be done while technologic tasks are performed. Empathic communication, presence, and touch enhance the process.

The next steps occur after the acute situation is over. "Tidying up" might be useful as a metaphor for dealing with the feelings that likely emerged in the patient. To continue with the chest pain example, the nurse guides the patient through the remainder of the cognitive restructuring steps.

- **Reflect:** Think back on what happened during the chest pain.
  - "Physically, how did you feel? Were there any areas that you felt were particularly tense? Were you able to release physical tension? What works for you to release tension?" The nurse discusses the effect of relaxation on ischemia and mental stress. The nurse empowers the patient with a specific skill that can be called on to help treat his or her myocardial ischemia.
  - "Emotionally, how did you feel?" The nurse invites the patient to talk about his or her feelings during this episode (e.g., worry, fear, anger, sadness). Using the concepts of awareness, automatic thoughts, and cognitive distortions, the nurse guides the patient through the process of realistic appraisal. Giving the patient permission to discuss his or her emotions and stress may help avoid all-or-nothing thinking, overgeneralization, jumping to conclusions, mental filtering, disqualification of the positive, and magnification. The patient is allowed to talk. The patient is gently encouraged to reveal any fears. The nurse helps the patient make an association between the emotional reaction to pain and the cycle of escalating pain this can create. Drawing a picture or writing in a journal can be useful if the person is reluctant to talk. The person's ability to identify his or her emotions needs to be accepted in a nonjudgmental way. Using a real-life, real-time, stressful experience provides a rich opportunity for dialogue and for teaching concrete self-management skills.
  - Is there another way to look at the situation? Are there opportunities here? An opportunity to reconnect with what is important in life? An opportunity to learn self-management skills that can treat the underlying pathophysiology? An opportunity to break the cycle of stress–worry–chest pain–stress–worry–chest pain? This is also an opportunity for the nurse to praise the patient for doing the best that he or she could in a very stressful situation.

- **Choose:** Replace maladaptive, unrealistic, distorted thinking patterns with a more effective and realistic response. At this stage of illness, it is most helpful to focus on a plan that replaces the anxiety and tension response to chest pain with focused relaxation and affirmation. Additional coping mechanisms can be addressed later in the hospital stay or in the outpatient setting.

Evaluation

Patient outcomes that were established prior to initiating CBT and the patient's subjective experiences are used to evaluate progress toward long-term goals. To evaluate progress toward short-term goals, patient outcomes that were established prior to starting the session and the patient's subjective experiences are used. Revising and updating goals are a part of each session.

Recognizing self-defeating, automatic thoughts and silent assumptions in addition to changing longstanding health-risking behaviors is often challenging and frustrating to patients. With careful choice of interventions, honest and thoughtful feedback, and continuing support, the nurse can help patients gain significant health-affirming benefits. In turn, the nurse can realize the value of enhancing the patient's autonomy and self-confidence in healthy behavior change and self-regulation.

Conclusion

Understanding and applying the principles of CBT provides an important tool for nurses to understand and address their own reactions to stress as well as to assist patients to optimize health and/or illness across the life span. Integrating CBT into nursing practice requires an appreciation for the effect of cognition on health and illness. Simple skills such as developing an awareness of stress warning signals, automatic thoughts, and cognitive distortions, coupled with skills to choose a more effective coping strategy, can enhance the health and illness experience. Although these skills are low-tech and inexpensive, mastery of these techniques requires a skilled nurse and a committed patient. It is a subtle process. Several attempts and several different ways of looking at a situation may be required before patients can recognize the automatic thoughts and underlying beliefs involved. Once they have this insight, however, the principles can be applied broadly to the patients nurses encounter every day with powerful effect.

Directions for Future Research

1. Continue to evaluate the effectiveness of using the four-step approach of cognitive restructuring in helping patients change health-risking behaviors such as smoking, alcohol misuse, or overeating.
2. Continue to evaluate whether there are differences in the application of CBT among different genders, ages, cultural groups, or those living in underrepresented groups or developing countries.
3. Continue to investigate cognitive distortions in children. Do the distortions change or intensify as children grow? Do children with similar distortions develop similar health issues as they mature?

Nurse Healer Reflections

After reading this chapter, the nurse healer will be able to answer or to begin the process of answering the following questions:

- What are my stress warning signals?
- What are the current stressors in my life?
- Can I pinpoint my negative, automatic thoughts and silent assumptions that trigger and perpetuate my emotional upset?
- Can I use the four-step approach to help reduce my distress and effectively solve problems?
- Is there an affirmation that I can create to help me counter self-defeating, automatic thoughts and silent assumptions?

NOTES

1. G. Engel, "The Clinical Application of the Biopsychosocial Model," *American Journal of Psychiatry* 137 (1980): 535–544.

2. E. M. Stuart, J. P. Deckro, and C. L. Mandle, "Spirituality in Health and Healing: A Clinical Program," *Holistic Nursing Practice* 3, no. 3 (1989): 35–46.

3. A. T. Beck, "The Current State of Cognitive Therapy: A 40-Year Retrospective," *Archives of General Psychiatry* 62, no. 9 (2005): 953–959.

4. H. Benson and E. M. Stuart, *The Wellness Book: The Comprehensive Guide to Maintaining Health and Treating Stress-Related Illness* (New York: Fireside, 1992).

5. A. T. Beck, *Prisoners of Hate: The Cognitive Basis of Anger, Hostility, and Violence* (New York: Harper-Collins, 1999).

6. A. Ellis, *Reason and Emotion in Psychotherapy* (New York: Lyle Stuart, 1962).

7. D. D. Burns, *Feeling Good: The New Mood Therapy* (New York: William Morrow, 1999).

8. R. Manber, R. A. Bernert, S. Suh, S. Nowakowski, A. T. Siebern, and J. C. Ong, "CBT for Insomnia in Patients with High and Low Depressive Symptom Severity: Adherence and Clinical Outcomes," *Journal of Clinical Sleep Medicine* 7, no. 6 (2011): 645–652.

9. A. C. Butler, J. E. Chapman, E. M. Forman, and A. T. Beck, "The Empirical Status of Cognitive-Behavioral Therapy: A Review of Meta-Analyses," *Clinical Psychology Review* 26, no. 1 (2006): 17–31.

10. D. F. Tolin, "Is Cognitive-Behavioral Therapy More Effective Than Other Therapies? A Meta-Analytic Review," *Clinical Psychology Review* 30, no. 6 (2010): 710–720.

11. R. McKnight and J. Geddes, "Cognitive-Behavioral Therapy Improved Response and Remission at 6 and 12 Months in Treatment-Resistant Depression," *Annals of Internal Medicine* 158, no. 8 (2013): doi:10.7326/0003-4819-158-8-201304160-02007.

12. B. D. Dunn, "Helping Depressed Clients Reconnect to Positive Emotion Experience: Current Insights and Future Directions," *Clinical Psychology and Psychotherapy* 19, no. 4 (2012): 326–340.

13. H. Klumpp, D. A. Fitzgerald, and K. L. Phan, "Neural Predictors and Mechanisms of Cognitive Behavioral Therapy on Threat Processing in Social Anxiety Disorder," *Progress in Neuro-Psychopharmacology and Biology Psychiatry* 45, no. 1 (2013): 83–91.

14. H. Kornør, D. Winje, Ø. Ekeberg, L. Weisæth, I. Kirkehei, K. Johansen, and A. Steiro, "Early Trauma-Focused Cognitive-Behavioural Therapy to Prevent Chronic Post-Traumatic Stress Disorder and Related Symptoms: A Systematic Review and Meta-Analysis," *BMC Psychiatry* 8 (2008): 81.

15. E. Brunner, A. De Herdt, P. Minguet, S. S. Baldew, and M. Probst, "Can Cognitive Behavioural Therapy Based Strategies Be Integrated into Physiotherapy for the Prevention of Chronic Low Back Pain? A Systematic Review," *Disability and Rehabilitation* 35, no. 1 (2013): 1–10.

16. F. Petrak, S. Herpertz, C. Albus, N. Hermanns, C. Hiemke, W. Hiller, K. Kronfeld, et al., "Study Protocol of the Diabetes and Depression Study (DAD): A Multi-Center Randomized Controlled Trial to Compare the Efficacy of a Diabetes-Specific Cognitive Behavioral Group Therapy Versus Sertraline in Patients with Major Depression and Poorly Controlled Diabetes Mellitus," *BMC Psychiatry* 13 (2013): 206.

17. S. Zomorodi, S. Abdi, and S. K. Tabatabaee, "Comparison of Long-Term Effects of Cognitive-Behavioral Therapy Versus Mindfulness-Based Therapy on Reduction of Symptoms Among Patients Suffering from Irritable Bowel Syndrome," *Gastroenterology Hepatology from Bed to Bench* 7, no. 2 (2014): 118–124.

18. C. Wells-Federman, P. Arnstein, and M. Caudill, "Nurse-Led Pain Management Program: Effect on Self-Efficacy, Pain Intensity, Pain-Related Disability, and Depressive Symptoms in Chronic Pain Patients," *Pain Management Nursing* 3, no. 4 (2002): 131–140.

19. E. Dysvik, J. T. Kvaløy, and B. Furnes, "A Mixed-Method Study Exploring Suffering and Alleviation in Participants Attending a Chronic Pain Management Programme," *Journal of Clinical Nursing* 23, nos. 5–6 (2014): 865–876.

20. S. K. Whitten and J. Stanik-Hutt, "Group Cognitive Behavioral Therapy to Improve the Quality of Care to Opioid-Treated Patients with Chronic Noncancer Pain: A Practice Improvement Project," *Journal of the American Association of Nurse Practitioners* 25, no. 7 (2013): 368–376.

21. R. Lauche, H. Cramer, G. Dobos, J. Langhorst, and S. Schmidt, "A Systematic Review and Meta-Analysis of Mindfulness-Based Stress Reduction for the Fibromyalgia Syndrome," *Journal of Psychosomatic Research* 75, no. 6 (2013): 500–510.

22. S. Cathcart, N. Galatis, M. Immink, M. Proeve, and J. Petkov, "Brief Mindfulness-Based Therapy for Chronic Tension-Type Headache: A Randomized Controlled Pilot Study," *Behavioural and Cognitive Psychotherapy* 42, no. 1 (2014): 1–15.

23. S. Mehta, S. Orenczuk, K. T. Hansen, J. L. Aubut, S. L. Hitzig, M. Legassic, and R. W. Teasell, "An Evidence-Based Review of the Effectiveness of Cognitive Behavioral Therapy for Psychosocial Issues Post-Spinal Cord Injury," *Rehabilitation Psychology* 56, no. 1 (2011): 15–25.

24. D. Dorstyn, J. Mathias, and L. Denson, "Efficacy of Cognitive Behavior Therapy for the Management of Psychological Outcomes Following Spinal Cord Injury: A Meta-Analysis," *Journal of Health Psychology* 16, no. 2 (2011): 374–391.

25. S. Potter and R. G. Brown, "Cognitive Behavioural Therapy and Persistent Post-Concussional Symptoms: Integrating Conceptual Issues and Practical Aspects in Treatment," *Neuropsychological Rehabilitation* 22, no. 1 (2012): 1–25.

26. L. H. Goldstein, T. Chalder, C. Chigwedere, M. R. Khondoker, J. Moriarty, B. K. Toone, and J. D. Mellers, "Cognitive-Behavioral Therapy for Psychogenic Nonepileptic Seizures: A Pilot RCT," *Neurology* 74, no. 24 (2010): 1986–1994.

27. D. Stahl, K. A. Rimes, and T. Chalder, "Mechanisms of Change Underlying the Efficacy of Cognitive Behaviour Therapy for Chronic Fatigue Syndrome in a Specialist Clinic: A Mediation Analysis," *Psychological Medicine* 44, no. 6 (2014): 1331–1344.

28. A. J. Wearden, L. Riste, C. Dowrick, C. Chew-Graham, R. P. Bentall, R. K. Morriss, S. Peters, et al., "Fatigue Intervention by Nurses Evaluation—The FINE Trial. A Randomised Controlled Trial of Nurse Led Self-Help Treatment for Patients in Primary Care with Chronic Fatigue Syndrome: Study Protocol. [ISRCTN74156610]," *BMC Medicine* 4 (2006): 9–12.

29. A. Sherwood, C. M. O'Connor, F. S. Routledge, A. L. Hinderliter, L. L. Watkins, M. A. Babyak, G. G. Koch, et al., "Coping Effectively with Heart Failure (COPE-HF): Design and Rationale of a Telephone-Based Coping Skills Intervention," *Journal of Cardiac Failure* 17, no. 3 (2011): 201–207.

30. J. C. Hersey, O. Khavjou, L. B. Strange, R. L. Atkinson, S. N. Blair, S. Campbell, C. L. Hobbs, et al., "The Efficacy and Cost-Effectiveness of a Community Weight Management Intervention: A Randomized Controlled Trial of the Health Weight Management Demonstration," *Preventive Medicine* 54, no. 1 (2012): 42–49.

31. M. G. Kushner, E. W. Maurer, P. Thuras, C. Donahue, B. Frye, K. R. Menary, J. Hobbs, et al., "Hybrid Cognitive Behavioral Therapy Versus Relaxation Training for Co-Occurring Anxiety and Alcohol Disorder: A Randomized Clinical Trial," *Journal of Consulting and Clinical Psychology* 81, no. 3 (2013): 429–442.

32. C. M. Grilo, R. M. Masheb, G. T. Wilson, R. Gueorguieva, and M. A. White, "Cognitive-Behavioral Therapy, Behavioral Weight Loss, and Sequential Treatment for Obese Patients with Binge-Eating Disorder: A Randomized Controlled Trial," *Journal of Consulting and Clinical Psychology* 79, no. 5 (2011): 675–685.

33. R. F. F. Cima, G. Andersson, C. J. Schmidt, and J. A. Henry, "Cognitive-Behavioral Treatments for Tinnitus: A Review of the Literature," *Journal of the American Academy of Audiology* 25, no. 1 (2014): 29–61.

34. S. Sussman, P. Sun, and C. W. Dent, "A Meta-Analysis of Teen Cigarette Smoking Cessation," *Health Psychology* 25, no. 5 (2006): 549–557.

35. S. A. Albrecht, D. Caruthers, T. Patrick, M. Reynolds, D. Salamie, L. W. Higgins, B. Braxter, et al., "A Randomized Controlled Trial of a Smoking Cessation Intervention for Pregnant Adolescents," *Nursing Research* 55, no. 6 (2006): 402–410.

36. W. B. Cannon, "The Emergency Function of the Adrenal Medulla in Pain and the Major Emotions," *American Journal of Physiology* 33, nos. 356–372 (1914): 356–393.

37. P. Sterling, "Allostasis: A Model of Predictive Regulation," *Physiology and Behavior* 106, no. 1 (2012): 5–15.

38. J. Shelby and K. L. McCance, "Stress and Disease," in *Pathophysiology: The Biologic Basis for Disease in Adults and Children*, 3rd ed., eds. K. L. McCance and S. E. Heuther (St. Louis, MO: Mosby, 1998): 311–332.

39. G. P. Chrousos, "Stress and Disorders of the Stress System," *Nature Reviews Endocrinology* 5, no. 7 (2009): 374–381.

40. J. E. Graham, T. F. Robles, J. K. Kiecolt-Glaser, W. B. Malarkey, M. G. Bissell, and R. Glaser, "Hostility and Pain Are Related to Inflammation in Older Adults," *Brain, Behavior, and Immunity* 20, no. 4 (2006): 389–400.

41. B. S. McEwen, L. Eiland, R. G. Hunter, and M. M. Miller, "Stress and Anxiety: Structural Plasticity and Epigenetic Regulation as a Consequence of Stress," *Neuropharmacology* 62, no. 1 (2012): 3–12.

42. A. Feder, E. J. Nestler, and D. S. Charney, "Psychobiology and Molecular Genetics of Resilience," *Nature Reviews Neuroscience* 10, no. 6 (2009): 446–457.

43. N. Ranjit, A. V. Diez-Roux, S. Shea, M. Cushman, T. Seeman, S. A. Jackson, and H. Ni, "Psychosocial Factors and Inflammation in the Multi-Ethnic Study of Atherosclerosis," *Archives of Internal Medicine* 167, no. 2 (2007): 174–181.

44. T. W. McDade, L. C. Hawkley, and J. T. Cacioppo, "Psychosocial and Behavioral Predictors of Inflammation in Middle-Aged and Older Adults: The Chicago Health, Aging, and Social Relations Study," *Psychosomatic Medicine* 68, no. 3 (2006): 376–381.

45. G. M. Bartol and N. F. Courts, "The Psychophysiology of Body–Mind Healing," in *Holistic Nursing: A Handbook for Practice*, 6th ed., eds. B. M. Dossey and L. Keegan (Burlington, MA: Jones & Bartlett Learning, 2013), 705–720.

46. D. S. Krantz, M. B. Olson, J. L. Francis, C. Phankao, C. N. B. Merz, G. Sopko, D. A. Vido, et al., "Anger, Hostility, and Cardiac Symptoms in Women with Suspected Coronary Artery

Disease: The Women's Ischemia Syndrome Evaluation (WISE) Study," *Journal of Women's Health* 15, no. 10 (2006): 1214–1223.

47. L. V. Doering, D. K. Moser, W. Lemankiewicz, C. Luper, and S. Khan, "Depression, Healing, and Recovery from Coronary Artery Bypass Surgery," *American Journal of Critical Care* 14, no. 4 (2005): 316–324.

48. G. S. Alexopoulos, I. R. Katz, C. F. Reynolds, D. Carpenter, and J. P. Docherty, "The Expert Consensus Guideline Series: Pharmacotherapy of Depressive Disorders in Older Patients," *Postgraduate Medicine* Special Report (2001): 1–86.

49. S. Vocks, T. Legenbauer, A. Wächter, M. Wucherer, and J. Kosfelder, "What Happens in the Course of Body Exposure? Emotional, Cognitive, and Physiological Reactions to Mirror Confrontation in Eating Disorders," *Journal of Psychosomatic Research* 62, no. 2 (2007): 231–239.

50. C. Shennan, S. Payne, and D. Fenlon, "What Is the Evidence for the Use of Mindfulness-Based Interventions in Cancer Care? A Review," *Psycho-Oncology* 20, no. 7 (2011): 681–697.

51. P. Jones, M. Blunda, G. Biegel, L. E. Carlson, M. Biel, and L. Wiener, "Can Mindfulness-Based Interventions Help Adolescents with Cancer? *Psycho-Oncology* 22, no. 9 (2013): 2148–2151.

52. J. Piet, H. Würtzen, and R. Zachariae, "The Effect of Mindfulness-Based Therapy on Symptoms of Anxiety and Depression in Adult Cancer Patients and Survivors: A Systematic Review and Meta-Analysis," *Journal of Consulting and Clinical Psychology* 80, no. 6 (2012): 1007–1020.

53. R. K. Dissanayake and J. V. Bertouch, "Psychosocial Interventions as Adjunct Therapy for Patients with Rheumatoid Arthritis: A Systematic Review," *International Journal of Rheumatic Diseases* 13, no. 4 (2010): 324–334.

54. M. A. Caudill, *Managing Pain Before It Manages You*, 3rd ed. (New York: Guilford Press, 2009).

55. J. W. Hughes, D. M. Fresco, R. Myerscough, M. H. M. van Dulmen, L. E. Carlson, and R. Josephson, "Randomized Controlled Trial of Mindfulness-Based Stress Reduction for Prehypertension," *Psychosomatic Medicine* 75, no. 8 (2013): 721–728.

56. M. Becarevic, F. Barakovic, O. Batic-Mujanovic, and A. Beganlic, "Effect of Combination Therapy on Cardiovascular Risk in the Pit Miners with Hypertension, Metabolic Syndrome and Depression," *Materia Socio Medica* 26, no. 2 (2014): 112–115.

57. P. Palta, G. Page, R. L. Piferi, J. M. Gill, M. J. Hayat, A. B. Connolly, and S. L. Szanton, "Evaluation of a Mindfulness-Based Intervention Program to Decrease Blood Pressure in Low-Income African-American Older Adults," *Journal of Urban Health* 89, no. 2 (2012): 308–316.

58. V. M. Deshmukh, B. G. Toelle, T. Usherwood, B. O'Grady, and C. R. Jenkins, "Anxiety, Panic and Adult Asthma: A Cognitive-Behavioral Perspective," *Respiratory Medicine* 101, no. 2 (2007): 194–202.

59. A. Galhardo, M. Cunha, and J. Pinto-Gouveia, "Mindfulness-Based Program for Infertility: Efficacy Study," *Fertility and Sterility* 100, no. 4 (2013): 1059–1067.

60. K. R. Lorig, D. S. Sobel, A. L. Stewart, B. W. Brown, A. Bandura, P. Ritter, V. M. Gonzalez, et al., "Evidence Suggesting That a Chronic Disease Self-Management Program Can Improve Health Status While Reducing Hospitalization: A Randomized Trial," *Medical Care* 37, no. 1 (1999): 5–14.

61. C. L. H. Bockting, A. H. Schene, P. Spinhoven, M. W. J. Koeter, L. F. Wouters, J. Huyser, and J. H. Kamphuis, "Preventing Relapse/Recurrence in Recurrent Depression with Cognitive Therapy: A Randomized Controlled Trial," *Journal of Consulting and Clinical Psycholology* 73, no. 4 (2005): 647–657.

62. M. Tazaki and K. Landlaw, "Behavioural Mechanisms and Cognitive-Behavioural Interventions of Somatoform Disorders," *International Review of Psychiatry* 18, no. 1 (2006): 67–73.

63. T. Maruta, R. C. Colligan, M. Malinchoc, and K. P. Offord, "Optimism-Pessimism Assessed in the 1960s and Self-Reported Health Status 30 Years Later," *Mayo Clinic Proceedings* 77, no. 8 (2002): 748–753.

64. A. Steptoe, C. Wright, S. R. Kunz-Ebrecht, and S. Iliffe, "Dispositional Optimism and Health Behaviour in Community-Dwelling Older People: Associations with Healthy Ageing," *British Journal of Health Psychology* 11, no. 1 (2006): 71–84.

65. G. A. Marlatt, "Relapse Prevention: Theoretical Rationale and Overview of the Model," in *Relapse Prevention: Maintenance Strategies in the Treatment of Addictive Behaviors*, eds. G. A. Marlatt and J. R. Gordon (New York: Guilford Press, 1985): 280–350.

66. N. Frasure-Smith and F. Lespérance, "Depression and Coronary Heart Disease: Complex Synergism of Mind, Body, and Environment," *Current Directions in Psychological Science* 14, no. 1 (2005): 39–43.

67. E. D. Hodnett, S. Gates, J. Hofmeyr, and C. Sakala, "Continuous Support for Women During Childbirth," *Cochrane Database of Systematic Reviews* 7 (2013): doi:10.1002/14651858.CD003766.pub5.

68. D. A. Campbell, M. F. Lake, M. Falk, and J. R. Backstrand, "A Randomized Control Trial of Continuous Support in Labor by a Lay Doula," *Journal of Obstetric, Gynecologic, and Neonatal Nursing* 35, no. 4 (2006): 456–464.

69. D. Ornish, L. W. Scherwitz, J. H. Billings, K. L. Gould, T. A. Merritt, S. Sparler, W. T. Armstrong, et al., "Intensive Lifestyle Changes for Reversal of Coronary Heart Disease," *Journal of the American Medical Association* 280, no. 23 (1998): 2001–2007.

70. L. J. Appel, C. M. Champagne, D. W. Harsha, L. S. Cooper, E. Obarzanek, P. J. Elmer, V. J. Stevens, et al., "Effects of Comprehensive Lifestyle Modification on Blood Pressure Control: Main Results of the PREMIER Clinical Trial," *Journal of the American Medical Association* 289, no. 16 (2003): 2083–2093.

71. V. Frankl, *Man's Search for Meaning* (Boston: Beacon Press, 1963).

72. I. S. Harvey and M. Silverman, "The Role of Spirituality in the Self-Management of Chronic Illness Among Older African and Whites," *Journal of Cross-Cultural Gerontology* 22, no. 2 (2007): 205–220.

73. K. S. Masters and G. I. Spielmans, "Prayer and Health: Review, Meta-Analysis, and Research Agenda," *Journal of Behavioral Medicine* 30, no. 4 (2007): 329–338.

74. F. A. Curlin, S. A. Sellergren, J. D. Lantos, and M. H. Chin, "Physicians' Observations and Interpretations of the Influence of Religion and Spirituality on Health," *Archives of Internal Medicine* 167, no. 7 (2007): 649–654.

75. E. J. Yuen, "Spirituality, Religion, and Health," *American Journal of Medical Quality* 22, no. 2 (2007): 77–79.

76. E. L. Garland, B. Fredrickson, A. M. Kring, D. P. Johnson, P. S. Meyer, and D. L. Penn, "Upward Spirals of Positive Emotions Counter Downward Spirals of Negativity: Insights from the Broaden-and-Build Theory and Affective Neuroscience on the Treatment of Emotion Dysfunctions and Deficits in Psychopathology," *Clinical Psychology Review* 30, no. 7 (2010): 849–864.

77. J. S. Moser, R. Hartwig, T. P. Moran, A. A. Jendrusina, and E. Kross, "Neural Markers of Positive Reappraisal and Their Associations with Trait Reappraisal and Worry," *Journal of Abnormal Psychology* 123, no. 1 (2014): 91–105.

78. L. D. Butler, C. Koopman, J. Azarow, C. M. Blasey, J. C. Magdalene, S. DiMiceli, D. A. Seagraves, et al., "Psychosocial Predictors of Resilience after the September 11, 2001 Terrorist Attacks," *Journal of Nervous and Mental Disease* 197, no. 4 (2009): 266–273.

79. S. Cohen, C. M. Alper, W. J. Doyle, J. J. Treanor, and R. B. Turner, "Positive Emotional Style Predicts Resistance to Illness After Experimental Exposure to Rhinovirus or Influenza A Virus," *Psychosomatic Medicine* 68, no. 6 (2006): 809–815.

80. C. S. Carver, M. F. Scheier, and S. C. Segerstrom, "Optimism," *Clinical Psychology Review* 30, no. 7 (2010): 879–889.

81. L. I. Catalino and B. L. Fredrickson, "A Tuesday in the Life of a Flourisher: The Role of Positive Emotional Reactivity in Optimal Mental Health," *Emotion* 11, no. 4 (2011): 938–950.

82. K. J. Johnson, C. E. Waugh, and B. L. Fredrickson, "Smile to See the Forest: Facially Expressed Positive Emotions Broaden Cognition," *Cognition and Emotion* 24, no. 2 (2010): 299–321.

83. A. Webster, E. M. Stuart, and C. L. Wells-Federman, "How Thoughts Affect Health," in *The Wellness Book: The Comprehensive Guide to Maintaining Health and Treating Stress-Related Illness*, eds. H. Benson and E. M. Stuart (New York: Fireside, 1992): 189–208.

84. E. M. Stuart, A. Webster, and C. L. Wells-Federman, "Coping and Problem Solving," in *The Wellness Book: The Comprehensive Guide to Maintaining Health and Treating Stress-Related Illness*, eds. H. Benson and E. M. Stuart (New York: Fireside, 1992): 230–248.

85. Benson-Henry Institute for Mind Body Medicine, *Stress Management and Resiliency Training: Providers' Manual* (Boston: Benson-Henry Institute for Mind Body Medicine, 2014).

86. D. D. Burns, *The Feeling Good Handbook* (New York: Plume, 1999).

87. A. Ellis, *How to Make Yourself Happy and Remarkably Less Disturbable* (Lafayette, CO: Impact, 1999).

88. J. W. Pennebaker, *Opening Up: The Healing Power of Expressing Emotions* (New York: Guilford Press, 1997).

89. C. Rogers, *Client-Centered Therapy* (Boston: Houghton Mifflin, 1951).

90. J. N. Kingery, T. L. Roblek, C. Suveg, R. L. Grover, J. T. Sherrill, and R. L. Bergman, "They're Not Just "Little Adults": Developmental Considerations for Implementing Cognitive-Behavioral Therapy with Anxious Youth," *Journal of Cognitive Psychotherapy* 20, no. 3 (2006): 263–273.

91. N. J. King, D. Heyne, and T. H. Ollendick, "Cognitive-Behavioral Treatments for Anxiety and Phobic Disorders in Children and Adolescents: A Review," *Behavioral Disorders* 30, no. 3 (2005): 241–257.

92. C. A. McCarty, H. D. Violette, M. T. Duong, R. A. Cruz, and E. McCauley, "A Randomized Trial of

the Positive Thoughts and Action Program for Depression Among Early Adolescents," *Journal of Clinical Child and Adolescent Psychology* 42, no. 4 (2013): 554–563.

93. J. W. Maag, S. M. Swearer, and M. D. Toland, "Cognitive-Behavioral Interventions for Depression in Children and Adolescents: Meta-Analysis, Promising Programs, and Implications for School Personnel," in *Cognitive-Behavioral Interventions for Emotional and Behavioral Disorders: School-Based Practice*, eds. M. J. Mayer, R. Van Acker, J. E. Lochman, and F. M. Gresham (New York: Guilford Press, 2009): 235–265.

94. J. W. Maag and S. M. Swearer, "Cognitive-Behavioral Interventions for Depression: Review and Implications for School Personnel," *Behavioral Disorders* 30, no. 3 (2005): 259–276.

95. D. D. Burns, *Ten Days to Self-Esteem* (New York: William Morrow, 1993).

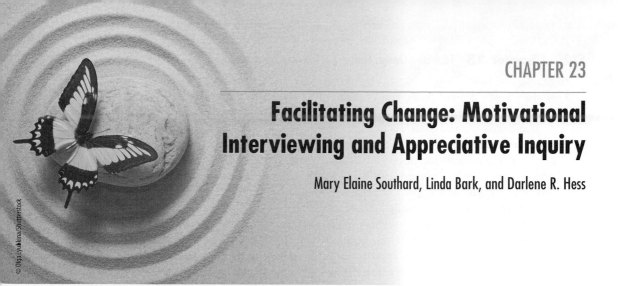

CHAPTER 23

Facilitating Change: Motivational Interviewing and Appreciative Inquiry

Mary Elaine Southard, Linda Bark, and Darlene R. Hess

Nurse Healer Objectives

Theoretical

- Describe each of the four guiding principles of motivational interviewing (MI).
- Identify eight foundational assumptions of appreciative inquiry (AI).
- Describe the 4-D cycle of AI.

Clinical

- Describe the use of AI in a patient-centered exchange.
- Describe the use of MI in a patient-centered exchange.

Personal

- Discuss how empathy is an essential component of a helping, caring relationship.
- Explore the importance of a healing presence.
- Describe how active listening enhances nurse–patient interactions.

Definitions

Appreciative inquiry (AI): Appreciative inquiry is both a philosophy and a methodology for change; the study and exploration of strengths as a way to help patients and organizations function at their best.

Instead of solving problems, AI is a process in which positive change is facilitated through identifying creative possibilities.

Empathy: An ability to "sense the patient's private world"; an essential component in understanding another person. Human sensitivity is developed by perceiving others and experiencing an awareness of the situation of the other.

Motivational interviewing (MI): Motivational interviewing is an intervention strategy for changing behavior. The central purpose of MI is to help patients explore and eventually resolve ambivalence in reference to a current health behavior; emphasizes client choice and responsibility and can be used in a variety of clinical settings.

Nurse coaching: Holistic nurse coaching is skilled, purposeful, results-oriented, and structured relationship-centered interactions with clients provided by registered nurses for the purpose of promoting the health and well-being of the whole person. Nurse coaching is grounded in the principles and core values of holistic nursing. Effective nurse coaching interactions involve the ability to create a coaching partnership, build a safe space, and be sensitive to client issues of trust and vulnerability as a basic foundation for further exploration.[1] Nurse coaches are able to structure a coaching session, explore client readiness for coaching, facilitate achievement of the client's desired goals, and co-create a means of determining and evaluating desired outcomes and goals.[2]

Therapeutic presence: Therapeutic presence is the conscious intention to be fully present for another person as a way to promote health, healing, wholeness, and well-being. *Presence* is generally defined as a multidimensional state of being available in a situation or exchange with another, acknowledging the sacred quality and interconnectedness of each person. Presence involves letting go of past or future concerns, resulting in the creation of an opening or opportunity to reveal what is needed in the moment.[3] Presence requires awareness, authenticity, and an appreciation of being in the moment.

Transtheoretical Stages of Change Model (Transtheoretical Model): The Transtheoretical Stages of Change Model is a model of behavioral change developed by Prochaska and DiClemente in 1984.[4] The five stages of the model are precontemplation, contemplation, preparation, action, and maintenance. Interventions designed to promote behavioral change are tailored to the individual's readiness for change. Relapses and recycling through the stages frequently occur. Relapse provides valuable information to assist in further change and is not viewed as a failure.

Introduction

This chapter concerns two holistic interventions that nurses can learn and use in professional nursing practice to support client behavior change to enhance client health and well-being. Nurses have always been involved in health promotion and disease prevention. As healthcare systems developed over the past 50 years, nurses have witnessed the redirection of funding from health-promotion efforts, primarily delivered through public health departments, to disease care delivered increasingly by private institutions and funded by complex payment mechanisms. Nurses have advocated for increased attention to the role that they play in assisting

clients to adopt healthier lifestyles and change unhealthy behaviors. Now policymakers, health professionals, and the general public are awakening to the fact that, unless significant changes are made, our nation will become increasingly burdened by runaway healthcare costs for treatment of conditions that could be eliminated or significantly ameliorated by behavioral changes. A report by the Kaiser Family Foundation indicates that workers are paying a notably larger share of health insurance expenses.[5] The cost of the average annual premium for a family policy increased 114% in the past decade, and worker contributions accelerated 147%. More than a quarter of insured workers—up from 10% in 2006—now have a deductible of at least $1,000 for single coverage alone. Experts forecast that out-of-pocket expenses will continue to rise.

As a result of these healthcare cost increases, employers and insurance companies are looking for ways to lessen disease progression and promote policies and create systems that lead to improved health. Health professionals are looking for effective and cost-efficient ways to help clients make health behavior changes. Hospitals are exploring and developing coordinated systems to decrease hospitalizations, reduce the use of medications and other costly treatments, and enhance the effectiveness of the care provided by health professionals. Health promotion and disease management programs now offer incentives to promote self-management. Unfortunately, many of these programs do not produce the desired results.

New approaches are needed to assist patients to achieve lasting behavior change. "Health professionals cannot assume that the only path to improving healthy lifestyles is looking for clients' problems in compliance and solving them."[6, p. S72] Ever-increasing numbers of nurses are learning evidence-based ways to assist clients to make the behavioral changes that can lead to improved health and well-being. Holistic nurse coaches are taking the lead in establishing models of coaching that are designed to engage clients in self-care and management of healthcare practices and outcomes.[2] Although there are many holistic strategies and approaches for assisting patients to reach their full potential, two accepted approaches used by many nurses are motivational interviewing and appreciative inquiry. Motivational interviewing is used when someone is ambivalent about change. Appreciative inquiry uncovers and expands what is working in a situation rather than focusing on what is not working.

Motivational Interviewing

Motivational interviewing (MI) is a well-known, research-based method of interacting with patients that was developed in the 1980s to improve outcomes associated with substance abuse.[7] Motivational interviewing is a skillful interaction for eliciting motivation for change. The fundamental premise of MI is that patients are often ambivalent to change, and ambivalence affects a patient's motivation and readiness to alter behavior.[8]

The Transtheoretical Model created by DiClemente and Prochaska guides MI.[7] DiClemente and Prochaska noticed that people frequently do not succeed in changing behavior on the first attempt and often experience numerous attempts before successfully changing. There are multiple stages, progressions, and relapses. Underlying the progressions are the patients' prior experiences with change and how they view the pros and cons of change. Patients consider whether they have the skills or resources to make a change.

Motivational interviewing is used in all aspects of behavior change, and it has been identified as an effective tool to improve medication adherence.[9] Adult patients with asthma who participated in a single session of education plus MI were more likely to show an increased level of readiness to adhere to medication regimens compared with patients receiving education alone.[10] Patients with schizophrenia who participated in eight MI sessions experienced significant improvement in overall psychotic symptoms and attitudes toward and satisfaction with medication compared with usual treatment.[11]

The application of MI in addition to a comprehensive behavioral weight loss program has been shown to aid weight loss by increasing motivation.[12] When MI was incorporated into a behavioral weight loss program, participants lost significantly more weight and engaged in significantly greater physical activity than did those in the program who did not receive MI.[13]

Numerous studies have been published indicating that the use of MI is an effective intervention to reduce smoking.[14] Motivational interviewing has been shown to be more effective with a variety of medical problems than traditional clinical advice giving, and it can help people reduce alcohol consumption, lose weight, and lower blood pressure.[15]

Guiding Principles of Motivational Interviewing

Motivational interviewing is based on four guiding principles known by the acronym RULE:[16]

- *Resist the righting reflex.* The "righting reflex" is the natural tendency of the nurse to fix a patient's problems by imposing solutions.[17] The nurse must set aside any desire to correct the course and direction of the client. If the nurse is pushing for change and the client is resisting, the nurse is in the wrong role; it is the client who should be voicing the arguments for change. The nurse must suppress what may seem like the right thing to do and instead allow the client to determine what to do.
- *Understand and explore the client's motivation.* It is the client's reasons for change, not the nurse's, that are likely to trigger change. The nurse explores the client's concerns, perceptions, and motivations. Allowing patients to tell their story and encouraging them to discuss not only their reasons for change but also how they might see themselves make those changes is the core of the partnership.
- *Listen with empathy.* Answers lie within the client, and finding them requires listening. Good listening is a complex skill; it is more than asking questions and keeping quiet long enough to hear the reply. Empathy has been defined as a complex, multidimensional phenomenon[17] but is typically understood as the ability to identify with the client's difficulties or feelings. The ability to express empathy enhances the ability

to engage patients in making necessary health changes and is a key component of MI.

- *Empower and encourage hope and optimism.* The nurse helps the client discover *how* change can happen. The nurse views the client as the expert consultant as ideas and resources for change are explored. Providing ongoing encouragement to foster the belief that the goals are achievable can help the patient carry out a plan to change behavior. Harnessing intrinsic motivation (the drive to do something because it is interesting, challenging, and absorbing) is a key component to the process and is essential for high levels of creativity.[18]

Partnering with Clients

By honoring client autonomy and effectively creating a collaborative partnership between patient and provider, nurses enable patients to become involved in identifying goals and determining how best to achieve them. Individuals are naturally motivated to improve their own well-being, and their willingness to become involved in managing their own care is closely tied to their ability to set goals and to their hopes for the future.[19] Accessing a client's hope for improved outcomes is a vital component of effective coaching for change.[20] The nurse applying an MI strategy seeks to evoke client strengths and to activate client motivation and resources for change. Helping relationships, or social support, are a vigorous predictor of behavioral success. An example of MI would be to ask the client, "Overall, how prepared or ready are you to change this behavior?" Motivational interviewing sets the stage for planning, which includes building commitment, assembling a "change team," and developing healthy alternatives to the problem.[21]

Motivational interviewing is a refined form of guiding and includes skillful informing. The process of listening to and guiding patients is a different stance from telling patients what they "should" be doing in terms of positive health-care practices. For example, telling a patient she needs to cut down on calories or providing her with a dietary referral may be a misstep or lost opportunity to engage in meaningful dialogue

that uncovers information that can enhance outcomes.

In MI, the goal of the nurse coach is not to point out discrepancies between goals and behavior but to incrementally guide the patient to self-discovery. Self-efficacy is supported when the patient realizes that behavior and goals are not congruent and makes a conscious decision to make necessary changes. Nurses who utilize MI understand that it is not the nurse's job to fix the patient or the patient's problems. To attempt to do so places responsibility on the nurse and promotes either dependency on the nurse or leads to "difficult" patients who do not listen to the information or advice provided by the nurse.[22] Nurses using MI learn to go down the patient's path rather than create the path and expect the patient to follow.

Communication Skills

To negotiate behavior change successfully, nurses must build on basic communication skills and establish a therapeutic environment. Holistic nurses understand that sacred presence is invaluable in setting the stage for exploring the change process. Coaching clients to achieve their desired goals involves developing and honing specific communication techniques such as employing reflective listening, asking open-ended questions, and using clarifying statements. Using active/reflective listening ensures that the nurse understands the patient and his or her readiness to initiate change. Open-ended questions foster dialogue and the ability to gauge deficits and strengths in relation to desired changes. Inquiring about what the patient already knows and asking if the person would like additional information show respect.

Self-awareness is a necessary component of effective partnering with clients to influence change. Communication is facilitated when the nurse is aware of his or her voice inflections, posturing, or self-talk when interacting with a patient.

Practitioner time constraints and the perception by the client of a hurried approach can be a challenge and a barrier to empathic active listening. This can lead to unintended results and patient dissatisfaction. Increased use of technology has created streamlined documentation and time-saving record keeping processes, but it also creates barriers to being fully present. However, MI can be a time saver by identifying the patient's goals, concerns, and ideas before proceeding with potentially ineffective interventions. Building MI skills takes practice and will become a cornerstone of client interactions.

Application of Motivational Interviewing in the Clinical Setting

Motivational interviewing can be used in a variety of clinical settings. The following case study illustrates how MI can be used to assist a patient to stop smoking.

Motivational Interviewing Case Study

Setting: Clinic
Patient: J. V., a 64-year-old woman with a history of severe chronic obstructive pulmonary disease (COPD)

Patterns/Challenges/Needs: Wants to stop smoking

J. V. has been diagnosed with severe COPD, has had several hospitalizations over the last 4 years, and continues to smoke heavily. Last year, she was in the precontemplation stage of smoking cessation with denial statements that ranged from "I don't have a problem" to "I don't have any willpower and I could never stop smoking." However, following her most recent hospitalization, she moved into the contemplation stage of change, realized she did have a problem and wanted to do something about it, but still she believed she could not stop smoking.

A clinic nurse decided to use MI to structure her conversation with J. V. In the left column of the following dialogue is the conversation between the patient and the nurse. In the right column are some guidelines for MI.

Patient and Nurse Conversation	Motivational Interviewing Guidelines
Nurse: Good afternoon, Mrs. V. It is good to see you again.	
J. V.: Thanks. I like seeing you, too. It's nice when I get to see the same person.	
Nurse: It's nice for me, too. It allows me to follow up with patients, and I know that last time after your hospitalization you described the pros and cons of quitting smoking.	Motivational interviewing is especially designed to deal with people who are ambivalent about making health changes.
J. V.: Oh, I hate even talking about that. I just have no idea how I would ever give up that habit. You know I have been smoking since I was 16.	
Nurse: I can understand why you feel that way, but last time you did have some interest in thinking about reducing your smoking.	Validate the patient's feelings and experiences.
J. V.: Yes, you're right. Being in the hospital was really awful, and the doctor showed me some pictures of my lungs and how my smoking makes them worse.	
Nurse: So, you actually saw with your own eyes how smoking hurts your lungs?	Reinforce reasons for change and repeat in simple, direct statements the effects of the patient's choices.
J. V.: Yes, it was quite obvious.	

(continues)

(*continued*)

Patient and Nurse Conversation	Motivational Interviewing Guidelines
Nurse: How has your decreased lung capacity affected your life?	Explore potential concerns.
J. V.: Well, it does really limit my activity. I have a grandchild who is now 2 years old and I can't keep up with him at all. I can see that my capacity to be with him is getting worse. And, of course, just shopping and other activities are limited. My family is after me all the time to quit smoking. Even my older grandchildren are starting on me.	
Nurse: It is hard to change something in your life when others are pressuring you. It's up to you to make this decision about when and if you want to make a change in this behavior. Thanks for even talking to me about this. I know it is hard for you.	Acknowledge the patient's control of the decision.
J. V.: Yes, it is, and it's nice that you know that.	
Nurse: I remember that we talked about your interest in smoking before, and using a 1 to 10 scale, you said you were at a 5. What is the number today?	Explore the patient's interest in change.
J. V.: Hum. Let me see. I guess it has moved up to a 6.	
Nurse: What does that number mean to you and how would you define it in words?	Explore meaning about change.
J. V.: Well, I guess it means that I want to stop smoking more than I don't want to. Maybe I have fallen off the fence this time, but you know I can always get back on the fence.	
Nurse: Of course, using your control to change is always your decision.	Reinforce the fact that the patient has control.
J. V.: Yes, you're right.	
Nurse: Tell me why you chose a 6 today.	Explore how things have changed.
J. V.: I just keep thinking about how my breathing limits my life and it makes me want to stop.	
Nurse: I understand how your life would be different if you changed your smoking habit.	Reinforce the concerns and the benefits of changing behaviors.
J. V.: I think about stopping, but then I get really scared and think I can't do it.	
Nurse: So, you have an interest, desire, reasons, and a need to change, but you are worried about your ability? If we were to rate your ability to change on that 1 to 10 scale, what would your number be?	Assess interest, desire, reasons, needs, ability, and commitment as appropriate.

Patient and Nurse Conversation	Motivational Interviewing Guidelines
J. V.: Now *that* is the real question. I think it is a 0. If it were higher, all those other numbers would go up too.	
Nurse: So, your belief that you can do it is really what is holding you back now. What would move you from 0 to 1?	Explore what would need to change for movement toward behavior change.
J. V.: Well, when you ask that question, it doesn't seem too hard, but I still don't know. I really don't know what would work for me to go from 0 to 1.	
Nurse: Almost every person who quits smoking starts being concerned about their ability to change their smoking habit. If it is okay, I would like to tell you some things that have helped other people.	Reframe concern about inability to change.
J. V.: Okay.	
Nurse: One of the patients who talked with me this morning began by cutting out one cigarette a day. Yesterday, a man decided not to smoke in one room of his house. Last week, a woman decided she would not smoke from 10:00 a.m. to 11:00 a.m. just to see if she could get some control of her habit.	Offer suggestions that are beginning steps for change.
J. V.: I can see how that might work for them, and something like that might work for me. Now I am almost at a 1.	
Nurse: That is great to see a change in your belief about your ability to quit smoking. I see that our time is moving to a close here. What kind of change, if any, do you want to make this next week?	Reinforce change.
J. V.: Well, I guess I could say that I won't smoke between 10:00 a.m. and 11:00 a.m. I don't think I smoke much then anyway, so I think it will be easy. I kind of feel good about some kind of beginning.	
Nurse: So, the initial goal is to limit smoking during that hour. On that old 1 to 10 scale, how committed are you to follow through on that goal?	Encourage small, initial steps. Assess commitment.
J. V.: I don't exactly know. I suppose I am pretty high . . . maybe an 8 and don't ask me how to get to a 9. I am happy with an 8.	
Nurse: An 8 is great! I am very happy for you and really look forward to talking with you about this experiment at your next appointment. Congratulations on your progress today.	Encourage small, steady steps.
J. V.: Well, to tell you the truth, it feels good to me, too. I never thought I could take this first step. And even though I asked you not to ask me about what would get me to a 9, when you called my not smoking for an hour a day an experiment, that made it sound more doable and not so scary.	

In the next session, J. V. reported that she was able to limit smoking during that hour on all the weekdays. She found the weekends harder because she had more free time. Even though she did not meet her goal of 1 hour every day, she started to feel that she had some beginning control of smoking. The nurse continued to work with her on her ability, and the patient enrolled her family for support. The patient's road to smoking cessation was long and somewhat bumpy, but after 9 months she did stop smoking and was very proud of herself. The empowerment she gained from changing that very longstanding habit allowed her to address other areas of her lifestyle with positive results.

Appreciative Inquiry

Appreciative inquiry (AI) is another increasingly popular change method that originated from organizational systems development. *To appreciate* is to see the best in a situation or another person, while *to inquire* is to explore and discover. Thus, AI is a way of asking questions that creates relationships based on the basic goodness in a person, situation, or organization. Nurses can utilize AI principles and processes to assist patients to build on their inherent strengths as a way to design and create their desired future. The main precept of AI is that individuals in relationships with one another can co-create an effective future that inspires new possibilities.[23]

Appreciative inquiry differs from other change processes by focusing on transformational change—change that transforms and energizes a person, situation, or organization. Appreciative inquiry is explicitly contrasted with problem solving, which the originators of AI describe as a deficit-based approach to change.[24] Although Cooperrider, Whitney, and Stavros describe the use of AI to effect organizational change, their discovery is that momentum for change and long-term sustainability increased the more they abandoned "delivery" ideas of action planning, monitoring progress, and building implementation strategies.[25] Such strategies are not grounded in transformational change patterns. Organizations that have utilized AI as a change strategy have achieved notable successes. Appreciative inquiry promotes a united approach to change,[26] fosters collaboration,[27, 28] and serves to build trust among workers.[29]

Rather than focusing on problems that need solving, AI focuses on imagining the best or highest outcome for the organization or client. The traditional model of disease management, for example, is in direct contrast to AI. In the disease management model, the focus is on diagnosing the problem, generating and selecting change options, and then suggesting strategies to implement the change. However, with AI, "problems" are seen as opportunities to be embraced, and the inquiry is directed toward the exploration of possibilities and the creation of a new future based on what is already working—on what is good—on what is best about the situation.

As a method of inquiry, AI has the potential to inspire patients to consider a situation previously seen as hopeless as one that can evolve to something much better. Appreciative inquiry can lead to recognition of limiting patterns of behavior so that new behaviors can be adopted. The focus is one in which the nurse holds the space for the client to see with a "new lens of perception." Appreciative inquiry provides a way to address the discouragement felt by patients when their successes and achievements are overlooked and the focus is instead on the dire consequences of their diagnosis or on things that have not gone well.

Appreciative inquiry is based on the belief that change begins the moment a question is asked. Thus, the seeds of change are implicit in the very first questions asked by the nurse. The idea is that clients will move in the direction of the questions that are asked. Holistic nurse coaches who use AI pay close attention to the exact wording and the provocative potential of the questions. They know that the words they choose have an influence far beyond the words themselves. They understand that words create worlds and that positive questions lead to positive changes. They attend carefully to the client's story, noting how language is used to convey sentiments, meanings, worldviews, and images. As they tune in to the client's reality, they ask questions that invoke new images and that serve to refashion that reality so that a new future can be brought into the present. Appreciative inquiry is based on the conviction that successful change begins with images of the future, and images of the future affect present-day performance. Hopeful and positive images lead to positive actions.

Foundational Assumptions of Appreciative Inquiry

Hammond proposes eight assumptions about AI that are useful in understanding the AI process as a vehicle for change:[30]

1. In every society, organization, or group, something works.
2. What we focus on becomes our reality.
3. Reality is created in the moment, and there are multiple realities.
4. The act of asking questions of an organization or group influences the group in some way.
5. People have more confidence and comfort to journey to the future (the unknown) when they carry forward parts of the past (the known).

6. If we carry parts of the past forward, they should be what is best about the past.
7. It is important to value differences.
8. The language we use creates our reality.

4-D Cycle of Appreciative Inquiry

The main intervention model that has come to be associated with appreciative inquiry is the 4-D cycle.[24] The model consists of four components: *Discovery* (inquiry), *Dream* (imagining what could be), *Design* (how to), and *Destiny* (what will be) (see **Figure 23-1**). The aim of the 4-D AI cycle is transformational change that originates in collaborative inquiry with participants. Use of the 4-D cycle creates a method to achieve an organic, collaborative way of working for positive and sustainable learning and change.[30]

The 4-D process enables individuals to *Discover* their foundation of strengths—their positive core. By doing this before envisioning the future (*Dream*), articulating designs for change (*Design*), and establishing a path forward (*Destiny*), they create confidence and hope for the future.[31] They experience pride and recognition

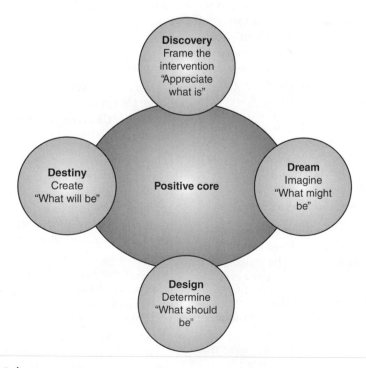

FIGURE 23-1 4-D Cycle

as they share their unique stories of success and weave them into dreams for the future. When people engage with others in conversations about what works well, they learn about capabilities and they gain confidence in their capacity for achievement. The 4-D cycle evokes and supports a life-affirming consciousness that leads to the realization of desired results. Whitney concludes that the implicit spiritual nature of AI and the 4-D cycle of inquiry has emerged as a key success factor.[32]

Discovery involves the identification of opportunities for improvement that build on previous accomplishments. The focus is on appreciating the best that the current situation has to offer. The nurse coach might ask questions such as:

- What helps you to feel happy, positive, or motivated?
- What has been most helpful to you in this situation?
- What do you do well concerning this situation?
- Based on what you already know about this condition, what else do you want to learn?

The *Dream* phase involves creatively imagining the future. In this phase, the focus is on merging the best of what is with a vision of what could be. In this phase, the client's story, insights, and viewpoint are put to constructive use to come up with a vision of how things could be better. The nurse coach might ask questions such as:

- What challenges do you anticipate and how might you meet them?
- Imagine a time when you felt healthy and energetic. What was significant to you when you felt this way?
- What possibilities do you see for yourself?

In the *Design* phase, the focus is on determining the structure for the envisioned future. Typically, choices must be made. The nurse coach might ask questions such as:

- Of all of the things you have imagined for your future, what is the one area you would like to focus on before our next visit?
- What would it take for you to make that change?

- How will you achieve that goal?
- How can you make your dream a reality for you?

The *Destiny* phase is when the nurse helps the client focus on the new future that is being created. The emphasis is on empowerment of the client and sustaining the learning that has occurred. The nurse coach might ask questions such as:

- Now that you have achieved that goal, what do you think is the most important thing you have learned?
- What will you do to celebrate now that you have accomplished your goal?
- If it is okay with you, may we talk about how you will continue to manage your diabetes?

Application of Appreciative Inquiry in the Clinical Setting

Appreciative inquiry can be applied in numerous ways, and the following case studies showcase a variety of situations. Case Study 1 illustrates the use of AI to assist unit staff to develop improved collaboration. Case Study 2 concerns the application of AI as a means to enhance self-care. Case Study 3 is about using AI to assist a patient with diabetes.

Case Study 1

Setting: Medical-surgical unit in a hospital
Client: Unit staff
Patterns/Challenges/Needs: Improved collaboration

During a staff meeting, several nurses explained that they believed that the staff did not work together well. The nurse manager decided to use appreciative inquiry as a method to address this issue. She discussed this with her supervisor, who thought it would be a good idea and was interested in how it might work in this situation. If it was successful, it could be applied to other units. She thought it could be a pilot project but said that the nurse manager would need to do this project within her regular work day. The nurse manager agreed.

First, the nurse manager initiated the *Discovery* part of appreciative inquiry, or the "appreciate the best of what is" phase, by interviewing several of the nurses who spoke in the staff meeting as well as others who did not mention the issue. The short 5- to 10-minute interviews were designed to focus on and make explicit what was working in regard to collaboration. The nurse manager explained that she was using appreciative inquiry to address the item raised by the staff and that it is based on the idea that a group grows in the direction of what it is focused on. She wanted to focus on what is going well. She further made it clear that she was not ignoring the issue: Quite the opposite, she was addressing the situation with an approach that might really benefit the staff.

The staff nurses seemed puzzled about the approach and wanted to talk about "the problem." Many said that they had never heard of looking at what was working when they were trying to solve a problem. A few thought it was an interesting idea, and most were able to mention some team situations that were effective. Several were surprised that they could come up with some positive examples and said that they had a little hope that perhaps things could change. One nurse, especially, was intrigued with this approach and came to the nurse manager several days after her interview with two more examples of things that were working. She said that she was beginning to see what the nurse manager meant about focusing on what was working because now she was more aware of positive communication and effective teamwork herself. The nurse manager was pleased with the first phase of her appreciative inquiry process because she knew this phase was more than just gathering facts: It was laying the foundation for a new way of thinking, facilitating hope about change, and building relationships and champions to maintain a positive approach.

During the next staff meeting, the nurse manager moved into the *Dreaming* phase of the appreciative inquiry process, or the "imagine what could be" part. She led 2 minutes of a relaxation meditation and then the following guided imagery:

> Imagine a time when you felt that collaboration was really working well on our unit or on some other unit where you worked in the past. Staff was supporting one another easily and things were done well—even with a sense of fun and joy. Although some things happened that could have been a problem, the team took the situations in stride and moved through them quickly, which intensified the positive spirit of the team.

She waited a couple of minutes while the staff was thinking of this image. Then, she asked each staff member to think about the following questions and write down their answers on a piece of paper: "What was significant in having this happen? How did it happen? Who was involved? What kept it going? If you could change things to your way of thinking, how would you like to see teamwork function on this unit?"

After the group had a few minutes to write down their answers, she gave them the following directions:

> Imagine it is 3 years from now, and our ability to collaborate has grown by 50 or even 100 times our current capacity. Imagine that your fondest wishes for excellent communication and teamwork have flourished. We are featured in an article in our hospital newsletter and then in a prominent nursing journal. What would the article say was happening on the unit each shift and each day? What would be described?

After this *Dreaming* period, the nurse manager asked people to share their insights and she wrote down the staff's answers on a flip chart. In this *Designing* phase, or the "determine what should be"part, the group looked for themes concerning the ways it should be. One of the topics brought up in many different ways was communication. Everyone realized that to have good teamwork, all of the team members needed the appropriate information so that they could function well as part of the team. Another issue that emerged from the discussion was the need for each team member to know exactly what was expected and when it was needed for the team to function smoothly. One of the nurses brought up the concept of unit culture. In her imagery, everyone really respected one another and she realized that was the expected group norm. The last major trend that was relayed from the exercise had to do with positive acknowledgment. Team members not only felt appreciation for one another, but they demonstrated it often during their time together.

Because it was almost time for the staff meeting to end, the nurse manager asked the staff to select one of the three major themes that had emerged (communication, role clarification, and appreciation) so that they could move into the fourth phase of appreciative inquiry, which is *Destiny*, or the "create what will be" part of the process. Then, she requested that they identify one action step. The group came up with the idea of placing sticky notes in the break room to acknowledge a team member who was working well as a good team member. A group of three staff members volunteered to create the process, manage it, and then report on the results at the next staff meeting. The nurse manager said the next staff meeting would be dedicated to planning how all insights could be turned into action steps and asked each staff member to be thinking and dreaming in the meantime for ideas. She ended the meeting by asking each member to state a "takeaway." She realized that about 90% of the comments were based on hope and promise for positive changes.

During the next staff meeting working in the *Destiny* phase of appreciative inquiry, or the "create what will be" part of the process, the Sticky Note Committee reported on the results and said that they believed that it worked some of the time but not all of the time. When it worked and staff put them up, people reported that it really felt good. Some staff reported that the more specific it was, the better it felt to them, although others said, "Great Team Member" felt good too and made their day. They thought it was a good beginning but perhaps not really manageable over time. They decided the idea could be used for short periods each month. Then, the group came up with what they called an "Appreciation Week" each month when staff would make it a priority to tell their fellow workers something they really like about them and the way they worked with the group. Even though it was only 25% of the time, they felt it would build some good habits.

Over the next year of staff meetings, three groups took over plans to design and implement the three major themes:

- *Communication*. This group developed bullet points and general scripts for shift change, handovers for break relief, and new patient admissions.
- *Role clarification*. The group that addressed this theme realized that staff already knew their clinical role. Instead, they developed a team agreement that spoke to how they treated one another. It included the following:
  - Being respectful to one another
  - Upholding identified values such as honesty, trust, and compassion
  - Agreeing to talk directly to the other person if a conflict came up between two staff members rather than involving others in the disagreement
  - Supporting direct communication for all types of communication rather than gossiping about one another
  - Having some in-service training on how to identify and express needs
  - Arriving on time
  - Helping one another complete work assignments
- *Appreciation*. This group created a variety of ways to acknowledge appreciation for one another:
  - Two-minute team huddles spontaneously during the day and at the end of shift to acknowledge one another and what worked for building team collaboration
  - Appreciation Week
  - Appreciation circles during staff meetings, where each person says something he or she appreciates about each team member
  - Appreciation log where staff and management could write down comments about good teamwork

The appreciative inquiry process was helpful in improving the unit's teamwork, and the unit's culture became more positive. Some of the dreaming is coming into fruition. The nurse manager has been asked to share her experience with other managers, and an article in the hospital newsletter is coming out soon about the results of this appreciative inquiry process.

Case Study 2

Setting: Medical-surgical unit
Client: Staff nurse
Patterns/Challenges/Needs: Self-care

C. B. is a nurse on the unit that is using appreciative inquiry to improve collaboration. She has been surprised by the improvements on the unit and enjoys the changes. She decided to use the appreciative inquiry method to look at her own self-care.

She began with the *Discovery* phase by exploring the part of her exercise program that was working, but she found it hard to come up with much. All she could see was how she was not getting exercise in her day, but then she realized that she did take the stairs instead of the elevator and that gave her a glimmer of hope and encouragement that at least she was doing something. It was a choice she made several times a day and she did feel good about herself when she was on the stairs.

Next, she took some time on her weekend off to do the *Dreaming* part of the process. She went into the "imagine what could be" phase and remembered years ago when she was trying out for a ski team and worked very hard to get in shape and build strength. She recalled how vital she felt and how people commented on her health. Even though she did not ski for very long because she ended up moving away, the way she felt was anchored in her memory. She remembered another time on a vacation when she did some hiking that involved some steep climbing. When she reached the top of the mountain, she felt very alive. She began to imagine how her life would be if she had more of those experiences. Then, she realized that she could be that healthy. She became clear about the effect that would have on both her professional and personal life. She knew she would lose some weight, which would be wonderful, and she could fit into some old clothes she saved for the time when she would be a size smaller. A shopping trip could be part of her future when she would be able to purchase some new clothes. Most of her delight in doing this imagery, though, was realizing how she would feel: alive, strong, and positive.

She began the *Design* part of the process and determined what should be in terms of her exercise program. From her past ski training phase she knew that she needed four parts to her program: cardiovascular, core building, strength, and flexibility.

Suddenly, she became excited and really felt motivated as she moved into the *Destiny* part of the appreciative inquiry process. She had received a coupon for a free week at a neighborhood gym just days before her exploration of this issue. She thought that could provide the cardiovascular training, strengthening exercises, and maybe the core building as well. A friend had been asking her to attend a yoga class and she realized that would help her with flexibility and reinforce the strengthening of her core and her muscles. She wanted to do it all but told herself to be careful and not take on more than she could complete. Her calendar was full with work and family commitments. She wanted to take slow and steady steps so that she would really make lasting changes. She put together a plan for the month that involved continuing to take the stairs and trying out the neighborhood gym. After a month, she decided that the gym really was not successful because it was not open at times that were convenient. During the times she did manage to get to the gym, she had hints of feeling alive and more vital. She knew she was on the right track.

The next month she went with her friend to the yoga studio to start a beginner's class. This did not work out well because, with her busy schedule and her friend's busy schedule, they were not able to attend the classes together. However, at the studio she found a class that had music and dancing and she loved it. She did not spend the whole time counting the minutes until the class was over. Time flew by and she felt so alive and vital. She had found something that really worked and she made a commitment to it. It was the foundation for increasing her exercise, and she realized that many errands or chores could be an excuse for another type of workout that strengthened her core, had her cardiovascular system working hard, and increased her flexibility and strength. At various times she used the four-step appreciative inquiry method to rediscover what was working, to dream of new goals, and to redesign her new destiny. She was delighted with the results.

Case Study 3

Setting: Clinic
Patient: J. W., a 56-year-old man who had recently been diagnosed with type 2 diabetes
Patterns/Challenges/Needs: Improved health and well-being

J. W. came in for his routine annual physical for work. Because of his lab results, he was diagnosed with diabetes. He attended a diabetic course that included one individual session after the second of four classes. His nurse inquired into his progress in dealing with his diabetes and learned that J. W. was feeling defeated. He felt as if he was not making any progress and he was overwhelmed with the number of changes his doctor and the nutritionists wanted him to make. His nurse believed that using the appreciative inquiry process would be helpful at this point, so she started by seeing what was working—the *Discovery* phase of appreciative inquiry. J. W. began to realize when he and the nurse reviewed the course outline that, even if he was not where he wanted to be, he had learned a great deal about his disease. He had even made some behavior changes such as eating dessert 50% less often.

Next, the nurse helped him to imagine what his goal might be. When he said he was not where he wanted to be, she asked what he meant by that. What would that look like? How would he be living his life? He described a life that had some limits in terms of what he could eat, but he began to see that not eating so much sugar would probably help him be healthier in the long run. He also began to think that he wanted to increase his exercise program because he used to be a runner when he was younger and really found that to be a great stress reliever. The *Dreaming* phase of this process continued as he wondered whether he could even return to a normal blood sugar level if he really made some significant changes.

J. W. knew that he should address his weight problem and realized that, if he was really serious about this challenge, his new diet could help him. He and the nurse explored some of the other changes that would help him move toward a healthier life in the *Design* phase of appreciative inquiry.

Then, their conversation moved to the *Destiny* stage, or the "create what will be" phase, and he put together a plan that included some simple diet changes along with a beginning walking/running program. His nurse helped him set realistic goals so that he would not become overwhelmed and feel discouraged. She set up some time in each of the remaining diabetes education classes so that he, along with other patients, could report on progress with his diet and exercise plan. By the end of his course, he was running three times a week, and although he was not feeling like his diabetes diagnosis was a positive situation in his life, he realized that he was making the best of it and making progress toward a higher level of health and well-being.

The Future

Current trends in healthcare innovations require obtaining data to support interventions that improve healthcare outcomes. Moore and Charvat pose questions regarding the use of AI with dyads, groups, or families.[6] Research studies are needed that addresses the influence of MI and AI on patients' behavior over longer lengths of time. Qualitative and quantitative studies that compare the two interventional approaches could perhaps maximize the effects of MI and AI. Studies that evaluate the long-term effectiveness of combining such interventions as MI and AI in promoting healthy behavior change would be useful.

A common concern for nurses and others is how to document and bill for nurse services. Motivational interviewing and appreciative inquiry are dynamic processes and are utilized in multiple encounters with the patient. Depending on personal style and time constraints, nurses will choose to integrate MI/AI techniques into a routine encounter or have the patient schedule specific counseling/coaching sessions. Clear documentation of length of time of visit and topics discussed will enhance future learning and reimbursement.

Because these interventions involve a philosophical approach to care that is different from customary practice in many settings, caution should be taken to adhere to the particular framework of each. Clinicians should not just insert positive questions into the traditional problem-solving mode of diagnosing and treating clients and believe that they are using these processes as they are meant to be used.[6]

The use of MI and AI to promote health and well-being for clients provides an opportunity for nurses to deliver care in a manner that is compatible with holistic nursing principles and core values.[33] By doing so, nurses may play a significant role in the transformation of healthcare delivery while simultaneously improving the effectiveness of care and reducing healthcare costs.

Conclusion

Motivational interviewing and appreciative inquiry are effective strategies for assisting clients to achieve health goals. Each is based on the ability to establish positive relationships, envision possibilities, communicate clearly, and listen attentively. The interpersonal process between each nurse and each client is a key component of MI and AI. The use of MI and AI can support a holistic model of nursing practice that incorporates creative, evidence-based approaches to facilitate change. Building MI and AI skills requires deliberate practice, critical feedback, and determined focus. Improving performance takes time and repetition, but the rewards are an exciting model of practice for the future of nursing.

Directions for Future Research

1. Determine the effectiveness of motivational interviewing (MI) and appreciative inquiry (AI) with dyads, families, and groups to sustain behavioral changes over longer periods of time.
2. Conduct qualitative and quantitative studies that compare the effects of MI and AI.
3. Evaluate the effectiveness of combining MI and AI in a coaching experience.
4. Explore the most effective ways for nurses to acquire change facilitation skills.
5. Identify ways to incorporate MI and AI into professional nursing practice.

Nurse Healer Reflections

After reading this chapter, the holistic nurse will be able to answer or to begin a process of answering the following questions:

- Am I motivated to acquire the skills necessary to become an effective practitioner of motivational interviewing (MI) or appreciative inquiry (AI)?
- How can I begin incorporating the guiding principles of MI or AI into my current nursing practice?
- Which specific communication skills can I further develop to enhance my ability to assist clients to change behavior?

NOTES

1. R. Schaub and B. G. Schaub, *The End of Fear: A Spiritual Path for Realists* (Carlsbad, CA: Hay House, 2009).
2. D. Hess, L. A. Bark, and M. E. Southard, "White Paper: Holistic Nurse Coaching" (paper presented at the National Credentialing Team for Professional Coaches in Healthcare at the Summit on Standards and Credentialing of Professional Coaches in Healthcare and Wellness, Boston, MA, September 2010).
3. M. McKivergin, "The Nurse as an Instrument of Healing," in *Holistic Nursing: A Handbook for Practice*, 5th ed., eds. B. M. Dossey and L. Keegan (Sudbury, MA: Jones and Bartlett, 2009): 721–737.
4. S. K. Leddy, *Integrative Health Promotion: Conceptual Basis for Nursing Practice*, 2nd ed. (Sudbury, MA: Jones and Bartlett, 2006).
5. G. Claxton, B. DiJulio, H. Whitmore, J. D. Pickreigh, M. McHugh, A. Osei-Anto, and B. Finder, "Health Benefits in 2010: Premiums Rise Modestly, Workers Pay More Toward Coverage," *Health Affairs* 29, no. 10 (2010): 1942–1950.
6. S. M. Moore and J. Charvat, "Promoting Health Behavior Change Using Appreciative Inquiry: Moving from Deficit Models to Affirmation Models of Care," *Family and Community Health* 30, Suppl 1 (2007): S64–S74.
7. W. R. Miller and S. Rollnick, *Motivational Interviewing: Preparing People for Change*, 2nd ed. (New York: Guilford Press, 2002).
8. B. Berger, "Motivational Interviewing Helps Patients Confront Change," *U.S. Pharmacist* 24, no. 11 (1999): 88–95.

9. H. P. McDonald, A. X. Garg, and R. B. Haynes, "Interventions to Enhance Patient Adherence to Medication Prescriptions: Scientific Review," *Journal of the American Medical Association* 288, no. 22 (2002): 2868–2879.

10. K. B. Schmaling, A. W. Blume, and N. Afari, "A Randomized Controlled Pilot Study for Motivational Interviewing to Change Attitudes About Adherence to Medications for Asthma," *Journal of Clinical Psychology Medical Settings* 8, no. 3 (2001): 167–172.

11. S. Maneesakorn, D. Robson, K. Gournay, and R. Gray, "An RCT of Adherence Therapy for People with Schizophrenia in Chiang Mai, Thailand," *Journal of Clinical Nursing* 16, no. 7 (2007): 1302–1312.

12. W. R. Miller and S. Rollnick, *Motivational Interviewing: Helping People Change*, 3rd ed. (New York: Guilford Press, 2013).

13. R. A. Carels, L. Darby, H. M. Cacciapaglia, K. Konrad, C. Coit, J. Harper, M. E. Kaplar, et al., "Using Motivational Interviewing as a Supplement to Obesity Treatment: A Stepped-Care Approach," *Health Psychology* 26, no. 3 (2007): 369–374.

14. J. E. Hettema and P. S. Hendricks, "Motivational Interviewing for Smoking Cessation: A Meta-Analytic Review," *Journal of Consulting and Clinical Psychology* 78, no. 6 (2010): 868–884.

15. Harvard Medical School, "Motivating Behavior Change," *Mental Health Letter* 27, no. 8 (2011): 1–8.

16. S. Rollnick, W. R. Miller, and C. C. Butler, *Motivational Interviewing in Health Care: Helping Patients Change Behavior* (New York: Guilford Press, 2008).

17. E. R. Levensky, A. Forcehimes, W. T. O'Donohue, and K. Beitz, "Motivational Interviewing: An Evidence-Based Approach to Counseling Helps Patients Follow Treatment Recommendations," *American Journal of Nursing* 107, no. 10 (2007): 50–58.

18. D. H. Pink, *Drive: The Surprising Truth About What Motivates Us* (New York: Riverhead Books, 2009).

19. P. McCarley, "Patient Empowerment and Motivational Interviewing: Engaging Patients to Self-Manage Their Own Care," *Nephrology Nursing Journal* 36, no. 4 (2009): 409–413.

20. K. Hammer, O. Mogensen, and E. O. Hall, "The Meaning of Hope in Nursing Research: A Meta-Synthesis," *Scandinavian Journal of Caring Sciences* 23, no. 3 (2009): 549–557.

21. J. C. Norcross, *Changeology: 5 Steps to Realizing Your Goals and Resolutions* (New York: Simon & Schuster, 2012).

22. M. A. Dart, *Motivational Interviewing in Nursing Practice* (Sudbury, MA: Jones and Bartlett, 2011).

23. M. A. Finegold, B. M. Holland, and T. Linghan, "Appreciative Inquiry and Public Dialogue: An Approach to Community Change," *Public Organization Review* 2, no. 3 (2002): 235–252.

24. D. L. Cooperrider and D. Whitney, *Appreciative Inquiry: A Positive Revolution in Change* (San Francisco: Berrett-Koehler, 2005).

25. D. L. Cooperrider, D. Whitney, and J. M. Stavros, *Appreciative Inquiry Handbook* (Brunswick, OH: Crown Custom, 2005).

26. T. Lavender and J. Chapple, "An Exploration of Midwives' Views of the Current System of Maternity Care in England," *Midwifery* 20, no. 4 (2004): 324–334.

27. A. K. Meda, "Tendercare, Inc: A Case Study Using Appreciative Inquiry," *Organizational Development Journal* 21, no. 4 (2003): 81–86.

28. J. Reed, P. Pearson, B. Douglas, S. Swinburne, and H. Wilding, "Going Home from Hospital: An Appreciative Inquiry Study," *Health and Social Care in the Community* 10, no. 1 (2002): 36–45.

29. V. George, M. Farrell, and G. Brukwitzki, "Performance Competencies of the Chief Nurse Executive in an Organized Delivery System," *Nursing Administration Quarterly* 26, no. 3 (2002): 34–43.

30. S. A. Hammond, *The Thin Book of Appreciative Inquiry*, 2nd ed. (Plano, TX: Thin Book, 1998).

31. P. Seebohm, J. Barnes, S. Yasmeen, M. Langridge, and C. Moreton-Prichard, "Using Appreciative Inquiry to Promote Choice for Older People and Their Carers," *Mental Health and Social Inclusion* 14, no. 4 (2010): 13–21.

32. D. Whitney, "Appreciative Inquiry: Creating Spiritual Resonance in the Workplace," *Journal of Management, Spirituality, and Religion* 7, no. 1 (2010): 73–88.

33. American Holistic Nurses Association and American Nurses Association, *Holistic Nursing: Scope and Standards of Practice* (Silver Spring, MD: Nursesbooks.org, 2007).

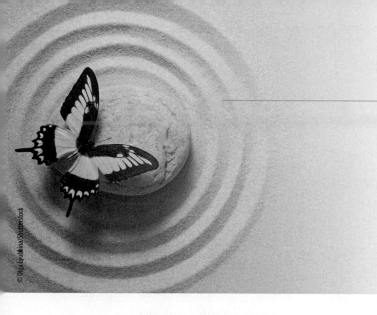

CHAPTER 24

Environmental Health

Susan Luck and Lynn Keegan

Nurse Healer Objectives

Theoretical

- Identify three principles that can direct human endeavors toward a sustainable future.
- Describe three characteristics of a sustainable community.
- Describe four ways in which substantive systems changes can diminish toxic exposures in life.

Clinical

- Examine environmental hazards and make a commitment to reducing these hazards in your home, community, and workplace.
- Examine systems changes that can reduce toxic exposures in the hospital or healthcare environment where you work.
- Subscribe or arrange to have consistent access to periodical literature specific to clinical application of environmental principles such as *Environmental Health News* (www.environmentalhealthnews.org), Health Care Without Harm (www.noharm .org), and Environmental Working Group (www.ewg.org).
- Identify and act on ways to influence environmental accountability in the workplace.
- Commit to joining an organization created to influence the direction of future sustainability in health care.

- Become sensitive to the environmental space in the institution, health agency, or clinic.
- Explore with other staff members the possibilities for creating healing environments in the workplace.

Personal

- Increase your knowledge of the relationship between health and the environment.
- Assess the health of your personal environment.
- Increase your awareness of how to reduce your environmental imprint (i.e., recycling).
- Volunteer and join local groups and organizations to support environmental efforts in your community.
- Explore what is essential about environmental relationships in your life.
- Eliminate unhealthy exposures in your personal environment (e.g., stale air, artificial lighting, subliminal noises, chemicals) whenever possible.
- Experiment with healing colors, scents, textures, sound, and lighting in your personal environment.

Definitions

Ambience: An environment or its distinct atmosphere; the totality of feeling that one experiences from a particular environment.

Anthropocentrism: The worldview that places human beings as the central fact or final aim of the universe.

Bisphenol A (BPA): An organic compound with two phenol functional groups. It is used to make polycarbonate plastic and epoxy resins, along with other applications, and since the mid-1930s is known to be estrogenic.

Chaos Theory: Sometimes called the *new science*, this theory offers a way of seeing order and patterns where formerly only the random, the erratic, and the unpredictable had been observed.

Detoxification: The metabolic process by which the toxic qualities of a poison or toxin are reduced or eliminated from the body.

Earth jurisprudence: Earth law recognizes the Earth as the primary source of law that sets human law in a context that is wider than humanity.

Ecology: The scientific study of the interrelationships between and among organisms, and among them and all aspects, living and nonliving, of their environment.

Ecominnea: The concept of an ecologically sound society.

Electromagnetic fields (EMFs): The field force in motion coupled with electric and magnetic fields that are generated by time-varying currents and accelerated charges.

Endocrine disruptors (xenoestrogens): Synthetic hormone-mimicking compounds found in many pesticides, drugs, plastics, and personal care products.

Environment: Everything that surrounds an individual or group of people: physical, social, psychological, cultural, or spiritual characteristics; external and internal features; animate and inanimate objects; climate; seen and unseen vibrations, frequencies, and energy patterns not yet understood.

Environmental ethics: A division of philosophy concerned with valuing the environment, primarily as it relates to humankind, secondarily as it relates to other creatures and to the land.

Environmental justice: A subbranch of ethics examining the innate and relational value among organisms and all aspects of their environment.

Epistemology: The branch of philosophy that addresses the origin, nature, methods, and limits of knowledge.

Ergonomics: The study and realization of the importance of human factors in engineering.

Permaculture: An approach to designing human settlements and agricultural systems that are modeled on the relationships found in natural ecologies.

Persistent organic pollutants (POPs): Chemical substances that persist in the environment, bioaccumulate through the food web, and pose a risk of causing adverse effects to human health and the environment.

Personal space: The area around an individual that should be under the control of that individual, including air, light, temperature, sound, scent, and color.

Phthalates: Classified as "plasticizers," a group of industrial chemicals used to make plastics such as polyvinyl chloride (PVC) more flexible or resilient. They are also known to be endocrine disruptors.

Precautionary principle: When an activity raises threats of harm to human health or the environment, precautionary measures shall be taken, even if some cause-and-effect relationships are not fully established scientifically.

Restorative justice: An ethical perception that directs that environmental damages not only be curtailed but also repaired and recompensed in some meaningful way.

Superfund sites: Hazardous waste landfills or abandoned manufacturing sites, names of which appear on the Environmental Protection Agency's National Priorities List.

Sustainable future: Meeting the needs of the present without compromising the needs of future generations.

Toxic substance: A substance that can cause harm to a person through either short- or long-term exposure through (1) inhalation;

(2) ingestion into the body in the form of vapors, gases, fumes, dusts, solids, liquids, or mists; or (3) skin absorption.

Xenoestrogens: Exogenous (external) substances that can interfere with the functions of the endocrine system.

Theory and Research

To engage successfully with life in modern times, we are challenged to increase awareness of how our external environment affects our health and the health of our clients/patients, families, communities, and the planet. In the spirit of Florence Nightingale, as healthcare providers and holistic nurses, how can we develop self-awareness and self-care practices that support our own internal and external healing environments? How can we integrate environmental assessment tools, education, and strategies into our professional practice and commit ourselves as Earth dwellers and Earth citizens, to the following:

- Recognize that we are the microcosm of the macrocosm—a world of vast complexity and unpredictability—and understand that our health and the health of our planet are inextricably interwoven.
- Engage in practices that create healing environments in our home, workplace, and community.
- Take the risk to challenge the existing structures and maintain values and convictions to create healthier environments.
- Reside in knowing that each individual makes a difference toward healing the global community, beginning with individual actions.
- Experience the fullness of life and the wonders of the natural world.

Environmental Leadership in Holistic Nursing

In its broadest sense, the term *environment* can mean everything, both within and external to each person. As a result, it is a challenge to determine for ourselves and others what constitutes a healing environment. In defining the constellation of environment in a grand way, five themes can be used to form a constellation—a mental map—to conceptualize the environmental world and the human place in it: (1) sharing, listening, and learning through our personal and collective life stories; (2) increasing self-awareness and self-care when living in a toxic world; (3) choosing a sustainable future; (4) building communities that support learning and positive actions for creating change: *start local, think global*; and (5) working from the inside out: healing our internal and external environments.

Telling Our Story: Local to Global

Each nurse, and each client, has a unique and personal story to tell. Everyone has an explanatory narrative that encompasses the multidimensional layers of being human. Listening to our own story and the story of others reveals the storyteller's beliefs and worldview and opens doors to exploring and expanding possibilities for growth and change in our movement toward wholeness. Within our holistic nursing worldview, we embrace the interconnectedness of body, mind, and spirit, knowing that when there is disharmony or disruption in our internal or external environment, we are out of balance. As living beings, we are a reflection of our world, and any environmental assault directly affects our energetic patterns and well-being.

When considering the environment, it is imperative to listen and respond to a larger story, not only as practitioners but also as members of humankind. This reaffirms what we deeply know through all of the senses as we ask ourselves:

- What does it mean to be human?
- What does it mean to be an Earth citizen?
- What are our beliefs about health when we tell our story?
- Do we consider all of the possible influences that affect our daily lives and those with whom we live and work?
- How can we face the great ecological crises of our time?
- How do each of our stories contribute to the larger story?
- How does changing our own story lead to planetary change?

When we embrace the matrix of our own being, we can understand, respond to, and participate in positive actions, raising the level of consciousness of our oneness with the universe.

There are two versions of the evolution of human consciousness. Both are basic truths and deep patterns in the psyche that inform an individual's day-to-day experience in various ways. One is progress and heroic advance, characterized by gradual, progressive, and familiar milestones of discovery and accomplishment: the harnessing of electricity and nuclear fission, for example. Generally, this equates with ever-increasing and refined knowledge and is thought to bring a sense of fulfillment and well-being. The scientific mind is the apex of this worldview, having its roots in ancient Greece and flourishing in the European Enlightenment of the 1700s. The modern mind is known for individualistic democracy, power, and emancipation. Inventiveness, endurance, will to succeed, and adventuresome spirit are sources of pride. The "miracles of modern medicine" are found here.

The second version of the evolution of human consciousness is the fall and tragic separation, which is a deep wounding or schism that separates humankind from nature. Manifestations of this version include exploitation of the natural environment, devastation of indigenous cultures, and an increasingly unhappy state of the human soul. Through the lens of tragic separation, humanity and nature are seen as having suffered grievously under an increasingly dualistic domination of thought and society. The worst consequences of this development are directly derived from the hegemony of modern industrial society and empowered by science and technology.

All individuals are challenged, although they may not recognize it, to reconcile these perspectives in their day-to-day lives. The two perspectives are both occurring simultaneously, although not always at the level of awareness. For example, it is possible for a family to decide to maintain heroic life support systems, beyond all parameters of the natural dignity of dying, while their deeper desire is that their loved one be at peace. Both are apprehensions of a deeper, larger, and more complex story. Gain and loss have been working together simultaneously. As nurses, we are aware of pervasive and intense suffering, not only in our own inner work but beyond, to the transpersonal and collective unconscious. Currently, the whole planet is in a transformative crisis.

Several core elements drive the multidimensional crisis. The modern mind—the mind of progress—originates in the worldview that there is a radical and irreconcilable distinction between the human self as subject and the world as object. In contrast, the primal worldview is that spirit or soul permeates the entire universe, within which the soul is embedded. The modern mind condemns this as a naïve epistemological error—childish, immature, and to be outgrown. The wisdom of the modern mind asserts that the human self is the exclusive repository of conscious intelligence; all meaning in the universe comes from the human subject. This is the classic existentialist assumption that, without humankind, the universe is meaningless.

Typically, a modern person's allegiance is to science, in the belief that science rules the cosmos and objective world, while poetry, music, and spiritual strivings inhabit the internal world. Our cherished Western autonomy, offspring of the progress perspective, has been purchased at a staggering price: gradual dilution and diminution of soul, meaning, and spirit. Thus, the purpose of the entire world is exclusive to the human self. Everything else is "out there," resulting in the demise of the metaphysical world and the disenchantment of the cosmos. Whether in conscious awareness or not, the greatest demand of modern time is to reconcile the imperatives of the two versions of what it means to be human. Modern culture itself is immersed in a rite of the most epochal and profound kind: The entire path of human civilization has placed humankind, the planet, and all of its members on a trajectory of complete alienation that is part of the mythic death and rebirth story. Something new is being formed, however, that is an innovative participative and holistic vision of the universe amply reflected by contemporary scientific and philosophic insights. In this emerging view, the human self is both highly differentiated yet reembedded in a participatory, meaning-laden universe. Throughout human history, all cultures have embedded within their collective psyche a connectedness to nature for survival not only of the human species but also for the life of planet Earth.

Holistic nursing honors human history as part of our collective story that we carry in our cellular memory, with all of its triumph and vulnerability. Holistic nurses strive for clarity of meaning, values, beliefs, and relationships. The roots and intention of nursing in caring for others is to honor the totality of the individual and support creating environments that promote healing.

Florence Nightingale as Environmentalist

Florence Nightingale, the founder of modern nursing, understood what we recognize today as ecological medicine and environmental health, involving the health not only of humans but also of all species and ecosystems with which we are connected physically, psychologically, and spiritually. Nurses have always been sensitive to environmental issues. Historically, nurses have been primarily concerned with health promotion, sanitation, and improvement in the quality of life for all people. Our modern world raises new issues and concerns for nurses, ranging from the use of increasingly toxic substances to high-technology machinery.

One of Nightingale's tenets was "the precautionary principle." It implies that when an activity raises threats of harm to human health or the environment, precautionary measures shall be taken, even if some cause-and-effect relationships are not fully established scientifically. The precautionary principle boils down to "better safe than sorry." Nightingale wrote specifically on observations of hazards in the environment and the nurse's responsibility: "If you think a patient is being poisoned by a copper kettle, cut off all possible connection to avoid further injury."[1] The essence of the precautionary principle is that if there is a suspicion about a harmful environment or exposure, even though all of the evidence is not in, remove the person from the situation or stop the use of suspected harmful exposures.

Nightingale understood that nurses have a duty as well as an ethical and moral responsibility to take anticipatory actions to prevent harm; the burden of proof for a new technology, process, activity, or chemical lies with the proponents, not with the public. The precautionary principle always inquires about alternatives. Precautionary decision making is open, informed, and democratic and must include all affected parties. The first sentence of the Preface in Nightingale's third edition of *Notes on Hospitals* (1863) reads as follows:

> It may be a strange principle to enunciate as the very first requirement in a Hospital that it should do the sick no harm. It is quite necessary, nevertheless, to lay down such a principle, because the actual mortality *in* hospitals, especially in those of large crowded cities, is very much higher than any calculation founded on the mortality of the same class of diseases among patients treated *out of* hospital would lead us to expect.[2]

Nightingale focused not only on problems, but she also sought solutions that guide us today. Nightingale engaged in what we today call risk assessment and on facts on which we base environmental decisions. Nurses are working with others to determine the degree of risk that is acceptable and asking questions such as "What is considered safe drinking water in hospitals and in homes?" "How much atmospheric pollution is safe in urban environments?"

Environmental initiatives and movements are part of a general societal intention to have a habitable planet, now and in years to come. These movements remain largely grassroots, or citizen driven, addressing their effects as they relate to humankind and Earth jurisprudence. Any benefit for the rest of the biotic community is a by-product from that frame of reference. The holistic outlook, as has been stated, recognizes all systems as interacting. If one part is affected, change of a greater or lesser magnitude occurs everywhere.

Environmental Conditions and Health

Environmental concerns range from eating contaminated poultry, hormone-fed beef, irradiated fruits and vegetables, and genetically modified foods, to living near high-voltage power lines, understanding the Antarctic atmospheric ozone hole, the threat of nuclear power plants, and coping with other new high-technology hazards that we now fully acknowledge. Noise, lighting, air quality, space allocation, and workplace toxins have all gained increasing attention as chronic stressors.

In the 1980s, the discovery of the hole in the ozone layer over Antarctica, along with escalating concern over global warming and climate change, introduced another phase of environmentalism, one that emphasized sustainability and an awareness of protecting future generations from the dangers of exceeding nature's ability to restore itself. Many people began to leave the cities, and a "back to the land" movement flourished. Other evolving perspectives addressed environmental justice and environmental ethics.

Today, a new environmental movement is rising up following 50 years of "better living through chemistry" and is gathering momentum as baby boomers, exposed to chemicals over the course of their lifetime, are exhibiting epidemic rates of cancers and Alzheimer's disease, while those just beginning life are being plagued with learning disabilities, childhood cancers, and record rates of asthma and obesity. Chemicals are the basic building blocks that make up all living and nonliving things on Earth. Many chemicals occur naturally in the environment, and many more are man-made. Chemicals can enter the air, water, and soil when they are produced, used, or discarded. Chemicals are of concern because they can work their way into the food chain and accumulate and/or persist in the environment and in our bodies for many years.

Living in a Toxic World

In June 2006, the World Health Organization (WHO) released the report *Preventing Disease Through Healthy Environments: Towards an Estimate of the Environmental Burden of Disease*, the most comprehensive and systematic study yet undertaken on how *preventable* environmental hazards contribute to a wide range of diseases and injuries.[3] By focusing on the environmental

causes of disease, and how various diseases are influenced by environmental factors, the analysis breaks new ground in understanding the interactions between environment and health. The estimate reflects how much death, illness, and disability could be realistically avoided every year as a result of better environmental management.

The report stated that nearly one-quarter of global disease is caused by environmental exposures, and "well targeted interventions can prevent much of the environmental risk," saving suffering and millions of lives every year.[4]

We can no longer deny or avoid the environmental chaos that is occurring on a planetary level in these times. We read daily about nuclear disasters, global water crises, famines from loss of land, disappearance of the Earth's rain forests, coastal devastation from toxic waste, climate change, and the long list of endangered species—that could include humans—if actions are not taken soon.

To make a list of problems or to dwell on the environmental global crises is not a solution; a more life-affirming exercise is to clarify individual and collective goals for healing our planet, beginning with our individual actions and working toward attainable goals for oneself, family, and community. Human beings are characterized by the ability to choose and change; the same minds that have created the technology and our modern world can create new solutions. Rather than continue down our current environmental path, the past need not be perpetuated. Human beings can elect and select life-affirming ways, use their inventive genius to reinvent a world that can sustain present and future generations, nurturing ourselves physically, mentally, and spiritually.

A very different world could be created by using alternative strategies and technologies that could offer the same essential services that chemicals and current energy sources provide.

Our Environmental Story

Many chemicals in use today have not yet been classified as harmful to human health, although recent reports based on current research are sounding the alarm, and many organizations are hopeful that consumer activism will gain momentum and fuel legislation for formulating a new environmental and public health policy.

To compound the problem of our toxic environment, our modern processed food supply is depleted of protective phytonutrients that can filter, neutralize, and detoxify many potentially harmful chemicals. Products too often are filled with artificial colorings, preservatives, flavorings, and many unlisted industrial ingredients. Our modern poor-quality diet, combined with agricultural pesticides and animals being raised on antibiotics, chemical feed, growth hormones, and genetically modified substances, increases our toxic body burden, stressing our immune system and our body's ability to detoxify and eliminate these harmful substances.

Children's Health

We do not inherit the Earth from our ancestors; we borrow it from our children.
—Native American Proverb

Childhood is a sequence of life stages from conception through fetal development, infancy, and adolescence, as defined by the Environmental Protection Agency (EPA). Children are the most vulnerable to environmental exposures for the following reasons:

- Their bodily systems are still developing.
- They eat more, drink more, and breathe more in proportion to their body size.
- Their behaviors can expose them more to chemicals and organisms (e.g., crawling on the ground).

Dr. Phillip Landrigan, director of the Children's Environmental Health Center, dean for Global Health, chair of Preventive Medicine, professor of Pediatrics at Mount Sinai School of Medicine, and an international leader on children's health and the environment, has written extensively and advocated for updated federal regulation of pesticides in food. He has repeatedly expressed that the public is rightly concerned about possible health effects from frequent exposures through our food supply. Industrial chemicals that injure the developing brain are sited in recent research as contributing

to the rise in prevalence of neurological problems in children. Since 2006, Landrigan and colleagues have reviewed the research on industrial chemicals as developmental neurotoxicants in children including lead, methylmercury, polychlorinated biphenyls, arsenic, and toluene. Recent epidemiological studies have documented six additional developmental neurotoxicants: manganese, fluoride, chlorpyrifos, dichlorodiphenyltrichloroethane, tetrachloroethylene, and polybrominated diphenyl ethers. To control the pandemic of developmental neurotoxicity, Landrigan and colleagues propose a global prevention strategy that advocates that untested chemicals should not be presumed to be safe to brain development, and chemicals in existing use and all new chemicals must therefore be tested for developmental neurotoxicity.[5]

Endocrine-Disrupting Compounds

A wide range of substances, both natural and man-made, is thought to cause endocrine disruption, including pharmaceuticals, polychlorinated biphenyls, DDT, dieldrin, atrazine and other pesticides and herbicides, and plasticizers such as bisphenol A (BPA) and phthalates. Endocrine disruptors are found in many everyday products, including plastic bottles, metal food cans, detergents, flame retardants, food, toys, cosmetics, pesticides, and industrial chemicals and by-products such as polychlorinated biphenyls, dioxins, and phenols. Many endocrine disruptors affect hormonal, endocrine, and reproductive function, according to findings of multigeneration animal studies. Exposure to environmental estrogens, also known as xenoestrogens, may play a causal role in the increased breast cancer incidence. Studies suggest that BPA acts through estrogen receptor pathways, directly altering gene expression and initiating a long sequence of altered morphogenetic events leading to neoplastic transformation and epigenetic changes beginning in utero with potential consequences later in life.[6]

Exposures to BPA in adulthood may also increase the growth and proliferation of existing hormone-sensitive mammary tumors, suggesting multiple mechanisms by which BPA may affect breast cancer development. This suggests that exposure to BPA in utero can be a predictor of breast cancer in adulthood in vulnerable populations.[7] BPA also has been implicated in childhood obesity and increased body mass index. The emerging literature classifies endocrine-disrupting chemicals as "obesogens" that can disrupt normal cell signaling and fat metabolism.[8]

Pesticides Permeate Our World

Early Child Development

Beginning in 2011, U.S. pediatricians called for Congress to overhaul a failed federal law that exposed millions of children, beginning in the womb, to an untold number of toxic chemicals. In its policy statement, *Chemical-Management Policy: Prioritizing Children's Health*, the American Academy of Pediatrics recommends that the 1976 Toxic Substances Control Act be substantially revised because it has "been ineffective in protecting children, pregnant women, and the general population from hazardous chemicals in the marketplace."[9, p. 983] According to the Centers for Disease Control and Prevention (CDC), approximately 13% of children have a developmental disability, ranging from language and speech impairments to serious developmental problems classified along the autism spectrum disorder.

The role of environmental factors in the development of autism is a crucial area of study. Along with genetics, the increase in autism cases has generated extreme concern over potential epigenetic changes when prenatal exposures are combined with specific genetic codes.

A study conducted by the Harvard School of Public Health linked dietary pesticide exposure to attention deficit disorders in children. The study followed more than 1,000 children and found that 94% had pesticide residues in their urine. Those with the highest levels were nearly twice as likely to have attention deficit hyperactivity disorder (ADHD).[10] The pesticide class analyzed was the common and widely used organophosphates, known to be toxic because they work by disabling a nerve chemical used to transmit signals.[11] In the study, the fruits with the highest concentration of pesticides included commercial strawberries, raspberries, and frozen blueberries. Researchers

explain that this study is important for two reasons. First, it examined children with average exposure (not those with increased exposure such as children of farm workers); second, it showed that even small and allowable amounts of pesticides can have significant effects on a developing brain. Children are at increased risk because they are exposed to higher levels of chemicals relative to their body size, and their detoxification abilities are less developed.

When it comes to pesticides, children are among the most vulnerable: Pound for pound, they drink two-and-one-half times more water, eat three to four times more food, and breathe twice as much air as adults. Exposures begin in the womb long before detoxification pathways are fully developed in a vulnerable time in growth and development.

The role of occupational exposures in both agricultural and industrial settings has been addressed in the research over many years, citing increased risk for reproductive disorders, neurological impairment, and cancers. Farm workers, who represent the backbone of our agricultural economy, are among the least protected from hazards on the job and have one of the highest rates of chemical exposures among all U.S. workers. Research on pesticide poisoning of farm workers receiving ongoing exposures has now opened a window into the lower-dose effects of pesticide exposures on the broader population. Children exposed to pesticides in utero and early childhood are at higher risk for developing not only developmental problems but also childhood cancers and leukemia.[12] Another population with high exposure to chemicals, and with little regulation, is hair and nail salon workers, who have high rates of infertility, birth defects in their offspring, and higher risks for bladder and breast cancer later in life.[13]

Nurses and other healthcare providers can play a critical role in reducing exposures to pregnant women and offspring through anticipatory, preventive guidance during preconception, prenatal, and postnatal periods.

The most challenging aspect to creating healthier environments includes discovering how to eliminate many of these compounds from the environment. The good news is that cancer and other health problems can be reduced by lifestyle interventions that can lower exposures to environmental toxicants and enhance our innate immune surveillance systems, increasing cellular energy for healthy metabolism and improving detoxification pathways through nutrition, stress reduction, and exercise.[14]

The following list shows the everyday products that contain endocrine disruptors that people can try to avoid or eliminate from their lives when possible:

- Pesticides and herbicides, including pesticide residues in soil
- Dry cleaning chemicals
- Solvents: paints, varnishes, cleaning fluids
- Spermicidal contraceptives and treated condoms
- Perfume fragrances, air fresheners, cleaning fragrances
- Car exhaust, car interiors—especially that "new car smell" (off-gassing)
- Plastics, plastic baby bottles, plastic food storage containers, Styrofoam, tin cans (BPA lining)
- PVC plumbing pipes
- Pharmaceutical runoff in the water supply
- BHA and BHT, common food preservatives
- FD&C Red No. 3, a common food dye (erythrosine)
- Personal care products that contain parabens, phthalates

Scientists and advocacy groups are informing the public and advocating for the precautionary principle while demanding health policy actions and regulation of the chemical industry.

The following is a review of the prevention strategies that we all can implement in our daily lives:

- Choose your food wisely; eat organically grown and raised foods when possible.
- Limit intake of animal fats because endocrine disruptors and heavy metals accumulate in the food chain and are stored in fat. The higher the intake of commercially raised animal products, the greater the potential for increasing toxic load.
- Choose seasonal and local foods.
- Monitor fish consumption. Large, deep-water "fatty" fish such as tuna and swordfish may contain higher levels of synthetic chemicals and heavy metals, so eat them infrequently. Better choices are wild-caught salmon, sardines, and cod.
- Avoid pesticides. If you are unable to buy all organic food, try to pick and choose. Certain crops are more heavily treated than others. The Environmental Working Group database (www.ewg.org) offers guidelines on the fruits and vegetables containing both the highest pesticide residues and the lowest. Produce containing the highest pesticide levels include peaches, apples, bell peppers, celery, nectarines, strawberries, cherries, lettuce, grapes, pears, spinach, and potatoes. Wash all fruits and vegetables thoroughly before consuming, or peel them if they are not organically grown.
- Support your body's natural ability to detoxify by exercising and sweating on a regular basis. Use a sauna or steam bath. Get regular sleep (you detoxify at night) and drink plenty of clean or filtered water.
- Consume plenty of fiber, which is found in whole grains, beans, vegetables, fruits, seeds (flax), and nuts.
- Drink beverages such as green tea that contain antioxidants and phytonutrients that can assist the body to rid itself of toxins.
- If planning a pregnancy or breastfeeding, be vigilant about chemicals and eliminate as many as possible for 1 year prior to conception. Guidelines for pregnant women on eating fish are listed at www.americanpregnancy.org/pregnancyhealth/fishmercury.htm.
- Become an environmental detective. Investigate the chemicals in your home, work, and community environments.
- Know your water supply. Determine whether your local community's water testing program checks for hormone-disrupting chemicals and heavy metals. Not all household filters work effectively on chemicals, and, unfortunately, not all bottled water is checked. Read water quality reports. If you drink purified water out of plastic bottles, do not leave the bottles in the car or the hot sun for any length of time; heat activates the molecules in the

plastic, which increases the rate at which the polycarbons leach into the water.

- Avoid using plastics. If you do use plastics, the safest plastics are marked with the recycling codes 2, 4, and 5. Never let infants chew on soft plastic toys and never microwave food in a plastic bowl or covered in plastic wrap. A good rule of thumb is that the softer the plastic, the more chemicals it contains. Buy in bulk and store foods in glass jars. Limit the use of plastic bags and cling-wrap products on your food. Assess the amount of plastic in your life and try to reduce it by five. For example, bring a reusable mug to the local coffee shop, buy a refillable glass or earthenware water jug, invest in glass food storage containers that can be washed and reused for a lifetime, and use reusable cloth totes for groceries.

- Exercise your rights as a consumer—never doubt the power of consumer demand. Ask for green products when you do not see them in your neighborhood stores. If you have a talent for organizing and recruiting people, use it to develop community groups and work with public officials to develop ordinances regarding the use of chemicals in public places. It took a while to legislate no-smoking areas; it is hoped that "chemical-free" will not be far away. Encourage youth to learn more about environmental issues and to pursue research into redesigning our future.

- Become a community advocate. Support local and federal clean air and water initiatives. Write to your local and state representatives and encourage them to vote for a healthy future. Support elected officials who make a clean environment their priority. Join national campaigns to support health policy change.

Together, we can create a healthier future for us all.

The Water We Drink

The majority of the planet is composed of water. Ninety-seven percent of this water is saltwater; the fresh water used to sustain life is only 3% of the total amount of water on Earth. The Earth has a limited supply of fresh water, stored in aquifers, surface waters, and the atmosphere. We cannot live without water. Within the next 50 years, the world population is expected to increase by another 40% to 50%. This population growth, coupled with industrialization and urbanization, will result in an increasing demand for water and will have serious consequences for human health and the environment. Currently, there is a global water shortage crisis. Here in the Western world, we face another water crisis. Chemicals leach into our urban and rural water supplies in municipalities and in wells.

A recent report by the U.S. Government Accountability Office, *Safe Drinking Water Act: Improvements in Implementation Are Needed to Better Assure the Public of Safe Drinking Water*, gave testimony to the EPA, stating that requirements for determining whether additional drinking water contaminants warrant regulation must be implemented. The number of potential drinking water contaminants is vast—tens of thousands of chemicals are used across the country, and the EPA has identified more than 6,000 chemicals that it considers to be the most likely source of human or environmental exposure. The potential health effects of exposure to most of these chemicals, and the extent of their occurrence in drinking water, are yet unknown.[15]

In early 2011, the EPA announced the agency's new Drinking Water Strategy, which aims to find ways to strengthen public health protection from contaminants in drinking water. After careful consideration, the EPA decided to address carcinogenic volatile organic compounds as a group. This new vision was intended to expand protection under existing laws and promote cost-effective new technologies to meet the needs of rural and urban communities. The EPA is investing significant resources to conduct key studies of the environmental technology available for making drinking water safer so that these processes and technologies can be developed, tested, and marketed. Effective methods must meet the following standards:

- Are sustainable and water and energy efficient
- Are cost effective for utilities and consumers

TABLE 24-1   Safe Drinking Water

Drinking Water Strategy Goal	Accomplishment(s)
Address contaminants as groups rather than one at a time so that enhancement of drinking water protection can be achieved cost effectively.	In January 2011, carcinogenic volatile organic compounds were identified as the first group that the agency plans to address.
Foster development of new drinking water technologies to address health risks posed by a broad array of contaminants.	In January 2011, the formation of a Regional Water Technology Innovation Cluster brought together public and private partners to focus on finding new ways to simultaneously treat multiple contaminants in drinking water.
Use the authority of multiple statutes to help protect drinking water.	Pesticide health benchmarks are being developed that can be used as tools in assessing the occurrence of contaminants in drinking water (when regulatory values are not available).
Partner with states to develop shared access to all public water systems monitoring data.	In 2010, a Memorandum of Understanding was developed between the EPA and state partners to facilitate sharing of drinking water monitoring data.

- Address a broad array of contaminants
- Improve public health protection

Some of the key accomplishments for each of the four goals are noted in **Table 24-1**.

New Concerns Emerge About Possible Water Contamination

At the request of Congress, the EPA is conducting a study to better understand any potential effects of hydraulic fracturing for oil and gas on drinking water resources. The scope of the "fracking" research includes the full life span of water in hydraulic fracturing, and a draft report is expected to be released for public comment and peer review in 2014.[16]

The Air We Breathe

Air pollution is a major environmental risk to health globally. According to WHO, by decreasing air pollution, countries can reduce the burden of disease, including chronic and acute respiratory disease and asthma, strokes, and cancer. The WHO estimates that some 80% of outdoor air pollution-related premature deaths are due to ischemic heart disease and strokes, while 14% of deaths are due to chronic obstructive pulmonary disease or acute lower respiratory infections, and 6% of deaths are due to lung cancer.

A 2013 assessment by WHO's International Agency for Research on Cancer concluded that outdoor air pollution is carcinogenic to humans, with the particulate matter component of air pollution most closely associated with increased cancer incidence, especially cancer of the lung. An association also has been observed between outdoor air pollution and an increase in cancer of the urinary tract/bladder.

As air pollution increases globally, studies show that nonsmoking women who live for many years in air-polluted areas have elevated risks of lung cancer. A recent study led by Harvard University researchers studied 103,650 women and examined their exposure to three airborne particulates and an increased risk of lung cancer. The study, which is the largest to date to examine the link, adds to mounting evidence that chronic exposure to soot may raise the risk of lung cancer, particularly among nonsmokers.

Since 1970, the EPA has protected public health by setting and enforcing standards to protect the quality of the air we breathe and the water we drink. Today, many older power plants and industrial facilities employ loopholes in the current regulations to allow them to pollute at much higher levels than recommended. To protect public health from these polluting plants, the EPA must require that all facilities meet the same cleaner standards. There remains resistance in government and industry to create legislation to address global warming and pollution. In 2011, diverse business organizations lobbied Congress to stop the EPA from doing its job of protecting public health by rolling back existing public health laws such as the Clean Air Act and blocking needed clean air and clean water protections. Despite the EPA's and the Clean Air Act's success, air pollution continues to be a health problem, with many types and sources of pollution left unaddressed because of loopholes or political pressure or delays. Industry and special interests must not put profits before public health, and Congress must mandate that the EPA do its job to ensure healthy air for all Americans.

World Health Organization Guidelines: March 2014

Most sources of outdoor air pollution are well beyond the control of individuals and demand action by cities, as well as national and international policymakers, in such sectors as transport, energy waste management, buildings, and agriculture. According to WHO, there are many successful policies in transport, urban planning, power generation, and industry that reduce air pollution:[17]

- *Industry:* Clean technologies that reduce industrial smokestack emissions; improved management of urban and agricultural waste, including capture of methane gas emitted from waste sites as an alternative to incineration (for use as biogas)
- *Transport:* Shifting to clean modes of power generation; prioritizing rapid urban transit, walking, and cycling networks in cities as well as rail interurban freight and passenger travel; shifting to cleaner heavy-duty diesel vehicles and low-emissions vehicles and fuels, including fuels with reduced sulfur content
- *Urban planning:* Improving the energy efficiency of buildings and making cities more compact, and thus energy efficient
- *Power generation:* Increased use of low-emissions fuels and renewable combustion-free power sources (like solar, wind,

or hydropower); co-generation of heat and power; and distributed energy generation (e.g., mini-grids and rooftop solar power generation)
- *Municipal and agricultural waste management:* Strategies for waste reduction, waste separation, recycling and reuse or waste reprocessing, as well as improved methods of biological waste management such as anaerobic waste digestion to produce biogas, are feasible, low-cost alternatives to the open incineration of solid waste; where incineration is unavoidable, then combustion technologies with strict emission controls are critical

Climate Change: Reducing Global Warming

Under the Clean Air Act, the pollution that causes global warming and climate change must be treated like any other air pollution. The Supreme Court affirmed this view in its landmark 2007 decision *Massachusetts v. EPA* and ordered the EPA to decide, based on the best available science, whether these pollutants pose a danger to public health or welfare.

Carbon dioxide and other air pollution is collecting in the atmosphere like a thickening blanket, trapping the sun's heat and causing the planet to warm up. Coal-burning power plants are the largest U.S. source of carbon dioxide pollution, producing 2.5 billion tons each year. Automobiles, the second largest source, create nearly 1.5 billion tons of carbon dioxide annually. However, technologies exist today to make cars that run cleaner and burn less gas, modernize power plants and generate electricity from nonpolluting sources, and cut our electricity use through energy efficiency. The challenge is to ensure that these solutions are implemented. A 2014 EPA report provided the following updates:[18]

- *Ocean heat.* Three separate analyses show that the amount of heat stored in the ocean has increased substantially since the 1950s. Ocean heat content not only determines sea surface temperature but also affects sea level and currents.

- *Sea surface temperature.* Ocean surface temperatures increased around the world during the 20th century. Even with some year-to-year variation, the overall increase is clear, and sea surface temperatures have been higher during the past three decades than at any other time since reliable observations began in the late 1800s.
- *Sea level.* When averaged over all of the world's oceans, sea level has increased at a rate of roughly six-tenths of an inch per decade since 1880. The rate of increase has accelerated in recent years to more than an inch per decade. Changes in sea level relative to the land vary by region. Along the U.S. coastline, sea level has risen the most along the Mid-Atlantic coast and parts of the Gulf coast, where some stations registered increases of more than 8 inches between 1960 and 2013. Sea level has decreased relative to the land in parts of Alaska and the Northwest.
- *Land loss along the Atlantic Coast.* As sea level rises, dry land and wetland can turn into open water. Along many parts of the Atlantic coast, this problem is made worse by low elevations and land that is already sinking. Between 1996 and 2011, the coastline from Florida to New York lost more land than it gained.
- *Ocean acidity.* The ocean has become more acidic over the past few centuries because of increased levels of atmospheric carbon dioxide, which dissolves in the water. Higher acidity affects the balance of minerals in the water, which can make it more difficult for certain marine animals to build their skeletons and shells.

In April 2010, the EPA took the first steps toward developing standards for vehicles, setting in motion standards for cars and light-duty trucks and separate standards for medium- and heavy-duty trucks. However, additional key public health standards must be legislated before public health safety can have the following effects:[19]

- Standards to reduce toxic pollution from the thousands of power plants nationwide could save as many as 17,000 lives each year, prevent respiratory and cardiovascular diseases, and reduce the exposure of children to mercury and lead.
- Improving emissions performance in cars and light trucks would reduce heat-trapping carbon pollution that causes global warming while saving consumers billions of dollars and cutting oil use.
- The first-ever standards to cut carbon dioxide emissions and improve fuel efficiency in medium- and heavy-duty trucks would reduce global warming pollution, save 500 million barrels of oil over the lifetimes of the trucks sold during model years 2014 to 2018, and save truck operators $49 billion over the life of the vehicles.
- Instituting standards to reduce global warming pollution from power plants would help reduce the pollution that is increasing deaths and illnesses from heat waves, air pollution, infectious diseases, and severe weather events.

Increasing Awareness for Change

Clearly, the hazards that began to be identified 50 years ago have grown exponentially. They continue to live among us despite vast concern, attempted legislation, and grassroots actions by many people and organizations. A way of life—a conscious choice—is possible only if we are willing to work, really work, to change from an industrial growth society to a life-sustaining society. It is possible to meet our needs and protect our natural resources, including the air we breathe and the water we drink, without destroying our life support system.

Lifestyle Trends

The study of chemicals in our food supply and their effects on health has fueled an informed consumer movement seeking safer food products. The U.S. Department of Agriculture issues an annual report on the amount of pesticide residue it detects in samples of fresh fruits and vegetables around the country. The EPA uses the data to monitor exposure to pesticides and enforce federal standards designed to protect infants, children, and other vulnerable people.

Sales of organic fruits and vegetables, which are grown without synthetic chemicals, are increasing exponentially. Organic produce purchases now make up an increasingly large percentage of all U.S. fruit and vegetable sales, according to the Organic Trade Association. Increasing consumer awareness has led to billions of dollars in sales annually.

As consumer awareness and knowledge expand, so does the public's influence on industry as well as retail outlets. Public awareness, especially if it is organized, can revolutionize both industry and the marketplace as demonstrated by the health food industry, which thrives in cities and small towns across the United States. Whole Foods Market, which has been outperforming competitors, plans to accelerate its growth by opening new stores in smaller markets and underserved urban locations, tripling its store count to 1,000 locations.[20] Major big-box stores, including Costco and Walmart, now carry organic food and safe cleaning products in response to consumer demand. Part of increased consumer awareness about healthy food is the movement in urban and rural areas to create local produce and community gardens and organic food cooperatives.

Community Gardens

More than 1 million acres of farmland are lost each year to urban development. The average age of the farmers in this country is older than 50 years. Over the next decade, as much as 80% of the nation's farmland will turn over, with much of it going to people who will not live on the land. At the same time, resourceful communities are creating local community gardens and farms. School-based gardens for students are a national trend that allows access to affordable organic fresh fruits and vegetables in urban communities where access has been limited, if not absent. A diverse consumer movement holds a shared philosophy that healthy soil means healthier food and healthier individuals, families, and communities. Healthy soil is free of herbicides, pesticides, and artificial fertilizers. There is a growing awareness that the Earth is a living Being and that the actions of every individual have an effect on the whole. The quality

of the soil and water are the basis of all human life, and the quality of caring for the Earth and the resulting health benefits will not only affect the people who eat the food grown sustainably today but also those who will depend on the soil in the future. A growing awareness of the proper tending of the environment is a concern and responsibility of every individual. The positive public health consequences of sustainable gardening and farming affect the long-term health of future generations.

Community workers, public health officials, and urban planners are increasingly concerned about the declining levels of physical and psychological health of city dwellers. The reasons behind this alarming trend are complex. Much of the focus is on the changing environment and factors such as car dependency, long commuter distances, and polluted and unsafe environments—all of which make it difficult for people to undertake the physical activity needed to prevent many health issues. Poor nutrition and underconsumption of clean, plant-based foods has been a significant concern in public health sectors, especially in disadvantaged communities where fresh produce is often hard to find and expensive.

Urban planners, citizens, and health professionals are working together to better understand these issues and explore solutions. As community-supported agriculture gains ground everywhere, small farmers and citizens are growing high-quality, nutritious food while preserving the health and quality of the soil. Inherent in this movement is the understanding that the Earth and its inhabitants all benefit; as the Earth heals, so do we. At the same time, the individual becomes reconnected and reintegrated into the community, healing much of the isolation and alienation experienced in modern society.

As citizens become increasingly aware of their natural environment and how it influences their health, they are making choices that will affect their future and that of future generations.

During the past 5 years there has been a significant shift toward more Americans growing their own food in home and community gardens, increasing from 36 million households in 2008 to 42 million in 2013, a 17% increase, according to a special National Gardening

Association report. In addition, young people, particularly Millennials (birth years ranging from the early 1980s to the early 2000s), are the fastest growing population segment of food gardeners. In 2008, there were 8 million Millennial food gardeners. That figure rose to 13 million in 2013, an increase of 63%.[21]

The report also found that more households with children participated in food gardening, increasing involvement during the same time period by 25%, from 12 million to 15 million.

Moreover, there was a 29% increase in food gardening by people living in urban areas, up from 7 million in 2008 to 9 million in 2013. Two million more households also reported participating in community gardening in 2013 than 2008, a 200% increase in 5 years. Additional highlights from the 5-year report include:[22]

- One in three households are now growing food—the highest overall participation and spending levels seen in a decade.
- Americans spent $3.5 billion on food gardening in 2013, up from $2.5 billion in 2008—a 40% increase in 5 years.
- Seventy-six percent of all households with a food garden grew vegetables, a 19% increase since 2008.
- From 2008 to 2013, the number of home gardens increased by 4 million to 37 million households, while community gardens tripled from 1 million to 3 million, a 200% increase.
- Households with incomes under $35,000 participating in food gardening grew to 11 million, up 38% from 2008.

Changing Public School Education

At last, environmentally conscious, scientific programs have arrived at American public and private school education. The concept called *Earth Keepers* is sweeping into curricula in the form of after-school programs, multiday weekend and summer camp opportunities, and an elective special track choice to selected students in some middle and high schools. The belief is that young people engaged daily at school with this focus will graduate with the intention to live and work to foster a cleaner, healthier world than did their parents and grandparents.

Earth Keepers offers a curriculum-based environmental science program in which students at all levels learn basic concepts such as energy flow, cycles, interrelationships, and change. Students have classroom and community experience exploring the natural world with the goal of using their knowledge and awareness to make personal commitments for environmental change. For example, the Louisiana-based program Teaching Responsible Earth Education offers a 3-day, curriculum-based, outdoor earth education program to thousands of children, parents, and teachers. Their mission is to educate children and adults about the life science processes that govern our planet, to inspire them to appreciate the natural world, and to motivate them to protect it using an innovative, instructional approach involving head, heart, and hands.[23] An Earth Keepers after-school program in Durham, North Carolina, teaches nature skills and hands-on experiential learning. Spending time outdoors in this program is linked to better performance in the classroom and a stronger lifelong connection to nature.[24]

At a middle school in Rockford, Michigan, students are tested for placement into a variety of curriculum tracks. In this school's unique Magnet Program, Earth Keepers is one of the available tracks.[25] Students in this program learn environmental science in the classroom as the topic is integrated into math, reading and writing, history, and contemporary issues. Students take field trips to community recycling centers, garbage dumps, water and waste processing centers, and other related environmental sites. It is hoped that all of these Earth Keeper students and graduates will influence their families and communities as well as help to restore our planet.

Sustainable Health Care

In the past several years in the healthcare sector, a nurse-inspired environmental health movement has emerged with outreach efforts, local to global. Health Care Without Harm (HCWH), along with its sister organizations Healthier Hospitals Initiative (http://healthier hospitals.org) and CleanMed (www.cleanmed .org), has been transforming the way hospitals are designed, built, and operated and is becoming involved with the greening of health care. According to its mission, environmentally responsible health care and its sustainable development is a concept vital to all healthcare partners: As major users of natural resources and toxic materials, hospitals make a dramatic contribution to society's ecological footprint. By using excessive amounts of energy; polluting the environment with medical supplies and materials made from plastics that include phthalates, mercury, and a multitude of other toxic chemicals; and producing waste that is burned instead of recycled, health care is ultimately compromising public health and damaging the ability of future generations to be healthy.

Hospitals all over the world are discovering that energy use can be drastically reduced, mercury can be eliminated, and better quality food for patients can be sustainably sourced. Because the purchasing power of healthcare systems is enormous, the decisions healthcare institutions make as a living cultural system can have a substantial effect on public and environmental health.

Issues to be addressed in environmentally responsible health care include waste management; elimination of toxic materials; safer cleaners, chemicals, and pesticides; healthy food systems; cleaner energy; and safe disposal of pharmaceuticals. The HCWH promotes adopting food procurement policies that are environmentally sound and socially responsible. The foods that employees and patients consume often are the very foods that the public is being warned to avoid. Adopting policies that include protecting the health of workers, patients, and communities and, by example, having a positive effect on the ecological health of the planet are moral and ethical imperatives of a healthcare model. Toward that goal, HCWH is working with hospitals to adopt food procurement policies that provide nutritionally improved food for patients, staff, visitors, and the general public and to support and create food systems that are ecologically sound, economically viable, and socially responsible.

Choosing a Sustainable Future

The fact is that growth, demographic or economic, is ultimately unsustainable; perpetual growth is mathematically impossible in a finite space such as the Earth. Sustainability demands a redefinition of consumption goals, such as use of renewable resources at a rate that does not exceed their rates of regeneration, and use of nonrenewable resources at a rate that does not exceed the rate at which sustainable, renewable substitutes are developed. The task is to confine human activity so that it can be pursued without damage to the natural systems. No goal, including sustainability, is absolute, however. For every contemplated policy or action, it is essential to consider the threat to sustainability and whether the anticipated gains are so overwhelming that they justify the action.

The Sustainable Industry Council exemplifies national industry leadership in defining the concept of high performance that focuses on the full range of sustainable/green strategies. The council is now moving to the next phase of this evolutionary process to create facilities that integrate an even more comprehensive range of design objectives into high-performing, whole system buildings. Such buildings, whether they are residential or commercial, privately or publicly owned, favor sustainability as a prominent characteristic but also are architecturally stimulating, cost effective, functional, operational, respectful of historic resources, safe, and secure.

Green Jobs Network (http://greenjobs.net) and other national organizations provide meaningful employment and training opportunities. They also connect people seeking and offering jobs that focus on environmental and social responsibility. Such organizations offer opportunities and resources and provide renewed hope for the future of the environment.

Environmental efforts are part of a general societal impetus to have a habitable planet, now and in years to come. Many of these efforts, in the aggregate, are pragmatic and based on economic interests; others are derived from a philosophic outlook such as environmental justice. Many, if not most, of the movements remain human centered, addressing their effects as they relate to humankind. Any benefit for the rest of the biotic community is a by-product from that frame of reference. The holistic outlook, as has been stated, recognizes all systems as interacting. If one part is affected, change of a greater or lesser magnitude occurs everywhere. This way of thinking is to weave the human economy back into the Earth economy.

Around the world, innovative companies and product designers are taking ecology as the basis for design, thus phasing out toxicity, cutting waste, and increasing resource efficiency. Cowan proposes strategic questions for use in evaluating which products, companies, and initiatives will lead to a less toxic world.[26] The four major categories of questions, as shown in **Exhibit 24-1**, can be asked when potential products are considered for use: substitution, stewardship, ecology, and simplicity.

For shelter, humankind originally constructed mud huts or simple structures made of found natural materials. Today, it is beyond imagination the devastation that has been inflicted on the Earth by the construction industry: Sand and water are sucked from the rivers, stones are taken from the mountains, and cement is manufactured from resources dug from the ground. In addition, carbon emission from the buildings and manufacturing of construction materials warm the air and space. To address these problems, the concept of Green Buildings has arrived. Green Buildings takes a new approach to save water, energy, and material resources in the construction and maintenance of buildings and can reduce or eliminate the adverse effects of buildings on the environment and its occupants. Green communities are planned, designed, and created to reestablish

---

EXHIBIT 24-1   Strategic Questions to Evaluate Products, Companies, and Initiatives for a Less Toxic World

Substitution of materials

- Is it synthetic? Does it biodegrade? Does it accumulate in living tissues?
- Is it a known carcinogen, mutagen, teratogen, endocrine disruptor, or acute toxin?
- When it degrades, off-gases, combusts, or reacts, does it pose any of the preceding threats?

Substitution of less toxic or nontoxic products

- How toxic is this product during its extraction, manufacturing, use, recycling, or disposal?
- Is this product durable, and is it easy to maintain, repair, reuse, remanufacture, or upgrade?
- Does it have replaceable or reusable components, parts, and materials?
- Will the manufacturer take responsibility for this product and packaging?
- Will the manufacturer completely recycle the product and packaging?
- Can the benefits of this product best be provided by turning it into a service product?

Industrial ecology

- If "waste equals food," what processes does this chemical or product feed during its entire life cycle?
- Can this entire class of chemicals or products be phased out by reconfiguring industrial ecosystems?
- At the most basic level, what services does this product provide?
- Can these services be provided by healthy ecosystems instead?

Voluntary simplicity

- Despite all efforts, does this product remain unacceptably toxic? If so, is it truly essential?
- Does the product have other purposes? Does it meet basic needs?
- What level of this product or service genuinely contributes to the quality of my life?
- Can this level of service be best supplied through my own initiative and that of my local community?

balance. Although it originally referred to restoring balance in natural ecosystems, the term *permaculture* has come to mean any system—natural, political, or cultural—that can be structured to be more self-sustaining, cooperative, and resilient. Permaculture can be applied to sustainable, human living systems.

Green Buildings Are Eco-Friendly Structures

The idea of Green Buildings evolved from an initial focus on building energy use to a broader focus on the full range of sustainable/green strategies. The Sustainable Industry Council is now moving to the next phase of this evolutionary process: going beyond green to create facilities that integrate an even more comprehensive range of design objectives into high-performing, whole buildings and providing LEED certification.[27]

Green Engineering

Green engineering advances the sustainability of manufacturing processes, construction, and infrastructure and supports research on environmentally benign manufacturing and chemical processes. Environmental sustainability encompasses consideration of more than one chemical or manufacturing process. It takes a systems or holistic approach to engineering infrastructure and buildings. Improvements in distribution and collection systems that advance smart growth strategies and ameliorate the effects of growth are research areas that are supported by environmental sustainability. Innovations include management of storm water, recycling and reuse of drinking water, and other green engineering techniques to support sustainable construction projects.

Ecological Engineering

Ecological engineering focuses on the engineering aspects of restoring ecological function to natural systems. Many communities are involved in stream restoration, revitalization of urban rivers, and rehabilitation of wetlands that require engineering input. This area addresses the fundamental engineering knowledge

necessary for ecological engineering to function sustainably.

Earth Systems Engineering

Earth systems engineering encompasses large-scale engineering projects that involve mitigation of greenhouse gas emissions, adaptation to climate change, and other global-scale concerns. Although the government provides guidelines and safeguards for the environment, these are frequently diluted or diverted by partisan or special interest groups. An environmentally responsible citizen movement in all sectors is organizing to present a clear vision with zest, care, and drive to see a more sustainable and habitable world for present and future generations.

Effective citizen involvement has the following characteristics:

- Political, corporate, and civic leadership listens to all voices in the community.
- Community activists focus on the common good.
- Media (print, television, radio, and Internet) value and commit resources to building community.
- Technology, hardware, and software are of sufficient quantity and quality to enable community and regional deliberation processes.
- Projects reflect natural ecologic and economic regions; they are not bound by traditional political jurisdictions.
- Citizen involvement in a project can continue for the long term.
- Resources are committed to enhancing community members' skills for the short and long term.
- There is an established sense of trust and mutual valuing among community members.
- Leaders recognize that needed changes are systemic, not isolated, and that both individuals and institutions are responsible for making them.

The concept of sustainability is complex and intertwined because it has to do with interrelated systems. The bottom line is wonderfully simple and straightforward, however: to live as if we belong here and are planning to stay a while.

Cultivating Healing Environments

Optimizing a healing environment in healthcare facilities has been a prevalent goal for many years. The interventions focus on environmental design and strategies, family needs interventions and presence, family visitation and partnership, family pet visiting and animal-assisted therapy, spiritual and complementary therapies, and pain management—all supported by evidence-based knowledge.

More and more hospitals are implementing "healing initiatives" that can have a transformative effect on the healthcare system. They are creating a framework of actionable practices and evaluation methods that, when implemented, lead to more cost-effective, efficient organizations in which the environment truly facilitates healing and where care providers are fully supported to reconnect to the mission at their professional roots—the mission of caring. Samueli Institute's Optimal Healing Environments (OHE) program seeks to build the knowledge base of healthcare practices that influence the healing process of recovery, repair, and return to wholeness. The OHE is unique in that it is a comprehensive approach to health care that encompasses all of the social, psychological, organizational, behavioral, and physical conditions that contribute to healing and achievement of wholeness. The OHE research is conducted in real-world settings, including hospitals, outpatient clinics, workplaces, and among specialized populations, to demonstrate how healing translates directly into current healthcare practices. In 2013, the Samueli Institute created a model for patients seeking a more healing-oriented and coordinated system of health care that focuses on the individual as a whole, where all aspects of the patient experience—physical, emotional, spiritual, behavioral, and environmental—are optimized to support and stimulate healing.[28]

With this increasing awareness of how the external environment affects the internal healing process, there is a growing movement coming from the healthcare sector and from industry to rethink how institutions that care for people can create greener sustainable buildings, including hospitals. Some of the newest technology being studied and researched to create sustainable communities includes that discussed in the following subsections.

Building Learning Communities

A learning community is a group of people who choose to enter into a discovery mode, meaning that each person is willing to teach or learn, depending on what he or she has to contribute. Characterized by safety, support, and openness, the learning community focuses on personal and societal learning. Within the context of seeking a sustainable future, the search for humankind's rightful and responsible place in the natural world fuels learning.

The community bond for many groups is the opportunity to honor deeply held values that integrate personal, social, and spiritual lives. Members enrich their inner lives while selectively engaging in some form of service work. These small grassroots efforts are conducting much of future sustainability work.

In some select instances, business communities are assuming leadership in striving toward sustainability. The trend engenders a different type of learning community, one that is integral to the preferred corporate image. Perhaps the most remarkable contemporary example is Interface (www.interface.com), a global manufacturing enterprise that produces 40% of the world's carpeting. Because of a personal, radical commitment to sustainability, its founder and chief executive officer Ray Anderson committed his company to becoming a zero-waste enterprise. It is well on its way to realizing this goal. To accomplish this immense task, involving 26 manufacturing sites delivering to 110 outlets worldwide, a very specific educational process has been initiated to engage the conscious commitment of employees at all levels over time, as well as that of stockholders. Increasingly, businesses are seeing that "green is good"—economically, socially, and sustainably.

Many facilitative and reliable resources are available to seekers and learners, from neighborhood "wise persons" to the Internet. The

Natural Resources Defense Council (www.nrdc.org), a nonpartisan international environmental advocacy group, works to protect wildlife and wild places and to ensure a healthy environment for all life on Earth. Likewise, the mission of the Environmental Working Group (www.ewg.org) is to use the power of public information to protect public health and the environment.

Sustainability includes a resolve to live in harmony with biological and physical systems and to work to create social systems that can enable us to do that. It includes a sense of connectedness and an understanding of the utter dependence of human society on the intricate web of life, a passion for environmental justice and ecological ethics, an understanding of dynamic natural balances and processes, and a recognition of the limits to growth resulting from finite resources. Our concern for sustainability recognizes our responsibility to future generations, to care for the Earth as our own home and the home of all who dwell herein. We seek a relationship between human beings and the Earth that is mutually enhancing.

Working from the Inside Out

As holistic nurses who are acutely sensitive to environmental issues, we know that the most important tool we have to offer is modeling the way we live our lives. The way we live is crafted and emerges from our day-to-day choices.

We live in a world of vast complexity and diversity. Our choice is to do whatever it takes to commit to and maintain our basic values, whatever we determine them to be. Only we can arrive at the personal meanings and understanding of relationships that provide coherence to our existence. Although we may have models, support, and assistance, each of us is called to make this determination. In our holistic practice, we assist others in examining their options and encourage them to make life-affirming choices. Our primary task is to be with our clients within their life circumstances. Often, our greatest contribution is to walk freely with our clients as they face their ordeals, joys, and transitions.

We risk everything through the clarity of our values and convictions. Being human is not for the fainthearted. Before we can take a stand or set a direction on an issue, we must reflect long and carefully about what gives meaning and brings a sense of purpose to our lives. One approach is to seek clarity within ourselves about our purpose for existence. Holistic nurses are uniquely positioned to access the fountainhead of wisdom and strength within ourselves and to assist others to reclaim their own inner strength. This work, as in all authentic endeavors, is born in silence and stillness. Striving with joy and equanimity for an environmentally conscious life means aspiring to be part of a larger whole, our inner life as a reflection of its outer manifestation.

Noise and the Stress Response

In dwelling on the importance of sound observation, it must never be lost sight of what observation is for. It is not for the sake of piling up miscellaneous information or curious facts, but for the sake of saving life and increasing health and comfort.
—Florence Nightingale

Noise pollution may be the most common modern health hazard. A growing body of data suggests a link between noise pollution and adverse mental and physical health. Elevated workplace or other noise can cause hearing impairment, hypertension, ischemic heart disease, annoyance, and sleep disturbance. Changes in the immune system and birth defects have been attributed to noise exposure, but the evidence is limited. Early studies show that noise causes changes in blood pressure, sleep patterns, and digestion, all signs of stress on the body. Studies have examined the relationship among stress and noise pollution and public health for many decades. Stress and noise pollution appear to be worse than originally thought because science now shows that noise raises stress levels to the point of causing heart and immune system problems and can alter brain chemistry in harmful ways. As part of creating healing environments, noise levels from machines to staff and their effects are being reevaluated in today's hospitals in regard to their influence on the stress levels of both patients and staff.[29]

Radiation Exposures: Living in the Modern World

We live in a radioactive world—and always have. Radiation is part of our natural environment. We are exposed to radiation from materials in the Earth itself and from the sun. With the 2011 nuclear disaster in Japan, renewed concerns over the long-term risks of radiation exposure are again on the minds of people around the world. The question becomes: How can we reduce our exposure over the course of a lifetime?

Living in today's world, we are all exposed to far more radiation than ever before, and we are only beginning to calculate the effects on our health. Estimates report that we receive up to 100,000 times more radiation than our great-grandparents did. We receive radiation exposure from routine diagnostic medical testing, including dental and chest X-rays and mammograms; from background radiation in everyday life from electromagnetic fields, microwaves, or flying in airplanes at high altitude; and from the latest technology toys. We all carry very small amounts of naturally occurring radioactive materials in our bodies.

Diagnostic Radiation

The average lifetime dose of diagnostic radiation has increased sevenfold since 1980, mostly through the use of X-rays. X-rays are energy in the form of waves, identical to visible light, the difference being that light does not have enough energy to go through the body. Some advances in equipment design reduce the radiation exposure from previous levels, such as dental X-rays. A typical dental X-ray image exposes the patient to only about 2 or 3 millirems. However, diagnostic scans are being used more routinely than ever before, especially in emergency rooms; sometimes they are ordered before the doctor has even examined the patient.

CT Scans

CT scans are an important diagnostic tool that helps physicians and healthcare providers to evaluate trauma, abdominal pain, chronic headaches, and other ailments. The fast, noninvasive CT scan offers a painless way to get three-dimensional images of the inside of the body. Since it was introduced in 1980, use of this technology has exponentially increased as a diagnostic tool. Researchers are concerned that the growing use of scanning exposes a patient to much higher doses of radiation than does a conventional X-ray. For example, one chest CT scan results in more than 100 times the radiation dose of a routine chest X-ray. CT scans provide exceptionally clear views of internal organs by combining data from multiple X-ray images. But the price for that clarity is increased exposure to X-rays.

Scanner manufacturers are designing instruments that use lower doses of radiation, but many older machines rely on higher doses. When diagnostic tests or radiation treatments are run, radiation is delivered to specific body parts and can potentially have a greater effect. Tissues that grow new cells more rapidly, such as bone marrow or the thyroid gland, are most vulnerable. The highest doses of radiation are routinely used for coronary angiography, in which cardiologists image the heart and its major blood vessels to look for blockages or other abnormalities. For women, the most frequent source of radiation exposure is the annual mammogram generally recommended for women 40 and older every one to two years based on personal history. Being an informed consumer and weighing the benefits and risks of diagnostic testing is a personal decision for women as research shows that many women are opting to receive mammograms less frequently if they are not at high risk for breast cancer based on age and family history.[30]

Airport Scanners

Recently mandated as part of the enhanced screening for travelers, body scanners are in use at many U.S. airports, and the number is expected to skyrocket over the next few years. Currently, the Transportation Security Administration (TSA) is using two types of screening machines. The millimeter wave imaging machine uses radiofrequency energy to image the body. According to TSA, these scanners deliver 10,000 times less energy than a cell phone does. The other type of machine is a backscatter X-ray, which can render a three-dimensional image of people by scanning them for as long as 8 seconds and produce a ghostly naked image. These X-rays are very low level because they bounce radiation off the skin, not penetrating organs, and back to the machine, allowing authorities to scan for dangerous items under someone's clothing. This functionality is unlike a medical X-ray, which is a higher level of radiation penetrating the skin to see bones and other tissues. Most airport scanners deliver less radiation than a passenger is likely to receive from atmospheric radiation while airborne.

The American Cancer Society recently noted that it does not anticipate airport scanners to be a serious issue for infrequent travelers. The topic remains controversial, and if made mandatory, passengers and airline crews could pass through airport screening checkpoints in the United States frequently, and some fliers could be scanned several times in one day. Frequent fliers could get hit hundreds of times each year. Pregnant women, infants, and chronically ill and immune-suppressed persons would also be exposed.

The Inter-Agency Committee on Radiation Safety recently issued a report that is restricted to the agencies concerned and not meant for public circulation. The committee, which includes the European Commission, International Atomic Energy Agency, Nuclear Energy Agency, and the World Health Organization, recommends that air passengers be made aware of the health risks of airport body screenings and that governments explain any decision to expose the public to higher levels of cancer-causing radiation. It also concludes that pregnant women and children should not be subjected to scanning, even though the radiation dose from body scanners is "extremely small." There still remain questions about health concerns and safety issues.[31]

Cell Phones

According to the communications industry, there are almost as many cell phone subscriptions (6.8 billion) as there are people on this earth (7 billion)—and it took a little more than 20 years for that to happen. In 2013, there were some 96 cell phone service subscriptions for every 100 people in the world.

Cell phones emit radiofrequency energy. Concerns have been raised that this energy from cell phones may pose a cancer risk to users. Radiofrequency energy is a form of nonionizing electromagnetic radiation; exposure depends on the technology of the phone, distance between the phone's antenna and the user, the extent and type of use, and distance of the user from base stations. Researchers are studying tumors of the brain and central nervous system and other sites of the head and neck to determine a link between cell phone use and cancer. In August 2014, the CDC issued precautionary health warnings about cell phone radiation and provided tips on how to reduce one's risk from exposure.

The CDC now asserts that "Along with many organizations worldwide, we recommend caution in cell phone use." As the lead federal health action agency, the CDC provides tips to the public on how to "reduce radio frequency radiation near your body." The CDC's latest recommendations represent a considerable improvement in the federal government's position regarding cell phone radiation health risks and the need for precaution.[32]

Researchers from the Yale School of Medicine discovered that exposing pregnant mice to radiation from a cell phone affected the behavior of their future offspring. They found that the mice exposed to radiation as fetuses were more hyperactive, had more anxiety, and had poorer memory—symptoms associated with ADHD—than mice that were not exposed to radiation. Neurological tests revealed that the radiation exposure led to abnormal development of neurons in the part of the brain linked to ADHD, leading the authors to suggest that cell phone radiation exposure may play a role in the disorder.[33] Other developing research focuses on whether radiofrequency energy can excite the brain in adults and cause acoustic neuromas.[34]

Electromagnetic Fields

Every year, more research is published about the hazards of electromagnetic pollution, more evidence is collected, and more large epidemiologic studies are conducted. The conclusion is that electromagnetic fields (EMFs) can adversely affect health, and it is important to reduce exposure to electromagnetic radiation whenever possible.

An important formula for EMF protection, and often the easiest to apply, is to know how much to increase distance from the source depending on the type of EMF hazard. For example, to halve the field intensity, a person might have to move farther away from the source of the EMF by the following distances:

- 25 meters (27 yards) for power lines and cell towers
- 30 centimeters (15 inches) for CRT computer monitors
- 5 centimeters (2 inches) for electric clocks
- 2.5 centimeters (1 inch) minimum for cell phones

To calculate exposures and risks, see www.ans .org/pi/resources/dosechart.

The following are recommendations for how people can protect themselves from radiation exposure:

- Maintain and review a personal history of diagnostic X-ray exposures to calculate risk and make informed choices moving forward.
  - Request minimal amount of X-ray during any treatment and ask for a lead shield for susceptible body parts not being scanned when possible.
  - Avoid CT scans if X-rays, magnetic resonance imaging (MRI), or other diagnostic procedures are available.
- Avoid microwaved foods (do not stand in front of the microwave while it is on; do not use plastic in the microwave).
- Keep a distance from big-screen televisions.
- Request a patdown at the airport instead of a scan if you are a frequent flyer.
- Take action and make your concerns known. The TSA consumer email address is TSA-ContactCenter@tsa.dhs.gov.
- Conduct a radiation assessment and calculate your annual dose and risk.

Detoxification

Internal biochemical processes combined with man-made chemicals can overwhelm the body's detoxification pathways and accumulate and become stored in tissues, particularly body fat. The good news is that research in the fields of human genomics, nutrition, and lifestyle choices provides new and intriguing information about how to minimize exposures and prevent toxins from wreaking havoc on immune systems and overall health.

The body has efficient mechanisms in place to detoxify harmful toxins including the lymphatic system and the most important cleansing organ, the liver. Other eliminative channels are the bowels, kidneys, skin, and lungs. When the body is doing its job and is not overburdened, the blood carries toxins to the liver, which uses enzymes, amino acids, and phytonutrients to detoxify and neutralize harmful substances, rendering them harmless by converting them into a water-soluble form to be eliminated via the urine or feces.

Carrying a large toxic body burden can stress the ability of this system, built for natural toxins and biochemical by-products, not the man-made ones people are exposed to in these modern times. If detoxification pathways in the liver are impaired, the breakdown of toxins can form intermediary metabolites that are often more toxic than the original item.

Optimizing the body's ability to detoxify, it is essential for individuals to maintain good elimination patterns, consume a whole-food diet, avoid chemicals in the food chain, and receive fresh air, natural sunlight, and exercise to support vitality and health. As a hardy and resilient species, changes we make in our lifestyles today can affect our long-term health.

Holistic Caring Process

Holistic Assessment

In preparing to exercise environmental control, the nurse assesses the following parameters as they apply to the client:

- Personal space for comfort, lighting, noise, ventilation, and privacy.
- Other people or troublesome objects that may induce anxiety.
- Awareness that environmental concerns affect individual and family coping skills.

- Awareness of objects or other environmental factors in the physical space that induce comfort or discomfort.
- Environmental concerns about the influences on health as well as the family's environmental concerns.
- Possible environmental fears (e.g., a feeling of claustrophobia from being confined to a hospital intensive care bed or intravenous lines, or a fear of death because the patient in the next bed just died).
- Grief and its relationship to environmental factors: Is the client in the same home atmosphere in which the spouse just died? Are others around the client sad and depressed? Are the colors in the environment dark and heavy?
- Personal health maintenance in relation to environmental factors: Can the client easily reach self-care hygiene items? Are throw rugs anchored? Are sunglasses worn outside to prevent glare?
- Ability to maintain and manage his or her own home.
- Risk of injury associated with factors in the environment.
- Activity deficits as a result of environmental factors.
- Home environment for its potential influence on effective parenting.
- Potential noncompliance because of environmental factors.
- Risk of impairment in physical activity because of environmental factors.
- Risk of impairment in respiratory function because of environmental factors, such as feather pillows, polluted or stale air, cigarette smoking, known or suspected allergens, or overexertion with chronic respiratory conditions.
- Possible sleep deficit because of agents in the environment, such as lighting, noise, overstimulation, overcrowding, or allergenic pillows.
- Alterations in thought processes that may be influenced by environmental factors, such as sensory bombardment with noise, lack of sleep, and transient living patterns.

Identification of Patterns/Challenges/Needs

The following patterns/challenges/needs (Chapter 8) are compatible with environmental interventions:

- Potential for ineffective choices
- Altered self-care
- Altered growth and development
- Potential for sensory perceptual alteration
- Impaired environmental interpretational syndrome
- Potential for knowledge deficit
- Altered comfort
- Altered role performance

Outcome Identification

Table 24-2 guides the nurse in client outcomes, nursing prescriptions, and evaluation for the use of the environment as a nursing intervention.

Therapeutic Care Plan and Interventions

Before the session:

- Become aware of personal thoughts, behaviors, and actions that may contribute to the coaching, teaching, counseling, or caring environment.
- Prepare the physical environment for optimal lighting, seating, air quality, and noise control.
- Consider your internal environment. Is it calm, centered, and ready to interact with others?
- Clear your mind to be fully present when meeting with the client.

At the beginning of the session:

- Take a moment to center with the client.
- Allow the client to express specific environmental concerns.
- Offer the client an environmental assessment tool (see **Table 24-2**).
- Review the assessment with the client to discover areas of concern.
- Explore how the personal environment may affect well-being (positively or negatively).

TABLE 24-2   Nursing Interventions: Environment

Client Outcomes	Nursing Prescriptions	Evaluation
The client will demonstrate awareness of environment.	Assist the client in shaping his or her own personal space environment.	The client personalized his or her own environment.
	Assist the client with choices that contribute to a positive, safe environment for those who share his or her personal and community space.	The client monitored and controlled the noise that he or she contributed to the surrounding area.
		The client respected the rights of others by not polluting air, water, and public places with wastes.
	Coach the client on creative strategies and action steps for optimizing his or her personal healing environment.	The client did not violate the personal space of others with tobacco smoke.
	Provide the client with information that helps in expanding concern for the concept of a healthy global environment.	The client participated in discussions, committees, or programs to work for a safe global environment.
The client will avoid contact and exposure to toxic substances and/or hazardous materials.	Provide the client with ideas for how to participate in safety education programs at his or her place of employment.	The client participated in his or her workplace offerings of environmental safety programs.
	Teach the client the importance of not unnecessarily handling toxic substances.	The client did not handle toxic substances unnecessarily and educated himself or herself about the dangers of hazardous materials.

- Encourage the client to write down areas of concern or areas for improvement.

During the session:

- Encourage the client to initiate specific intervention ideas in his or her personal or professional work environment.
- Explore workplace issues and possibilities for effecting change, serving on the environmental control committee, or initiating meetings with coworkers to form a committee to improve the workplace environment, including creating a healing room for staff.
- Guide the client to consider changes that would improve his or her personal and/or work environment.
- Increase awareness of sound (e.g., noise, music, machinery), air (e.g., quality, smell, circulation), and aesthetics (e.g., art, color, design, texture), as well as other areas specific to the client's overall environment.
- Educate hospitalized clients about the deleterious effects on their healing process of too much noise.

- Encourage hospitalized clients to limit the time spent watching television and instead listen to their own personal cassette players with headphones.
- Create mechanisms whereby music, imagery, relaxation, colors, aromas, and lighting can be introduced into workplace settings.

At the end of the session:

- Coach clients to learn practical ways to cope with hazards in the environment (see **Table 24-3**).
- Coach the client to write down environmental goals, action steps, and target dates.
- Provide handout materials to support established goals.
- Schedule follow-up sessions.

Specific Interventions

Personal Environment Strategies to heal the environment abound on both a personal and a professional level. Personally, we can begin to modify our own internal environment. The ability to regulate our state of consciousness,

TABLE 24-3   Coping with Environmental Hazards

Problem	Solution
Too much noise	1. Turn off radios and televisions.
	2. Lower your voice.
	3. Ask your colleagues to quiet down.
	4. Ask to serve on the agency's environmental control committee.
Inadequate lighting	1. Add more lights.
	2. Use incandescent bulbs instead of fluorescent tubes whenever possible.
	3. Open curtains and blinds whenever possible.
	4. Go outdoors for full-spectrum light breaks rather than taking cafeteria coffee breaks.
Stale air	1. Make sure agency ventilation systems work.
	2. When conducting home health visits, open the doors and windows and get fresh air and natural light into the home when appropriate.
	3. Request that broad-leaf green plants be stationed in the workplace. They are aesthetically pleasing and give off oxygen.
	4. Wear masks or protective gear if there is any risk of toxic inhalants.
Long periods at computer	1. Use a shield that cuts down glare and radiation and grounds the field of electrostatic charge.
	2. Learn some relaxation exercises to do at your desk.
	3. Ask your institution or agency to have short massage sessions available on the premises.
	4. Take frequent eye and movement breaks away from the computer screen.
	5. Use properly designed chairs.
Space allocation	1. Try to find some personal space in the workplace.
	2. Respect others' personal space. Ask before entering the client's room, closet, or dresser.
	3. Make the space you are allocated as pleasant as possible. Decorate with colorful objects, soothing scents, and aesthetic objects.

thought patterns, and reactive behaviors gives us the power to move smoothly through external crises both at work and at leisure. Approaching a hectic external environment with internal composure and tranquility makes it possible to transform crises into manageable situations. Nurturing our internal environment with food, quality sleep, supportive relationships, and joy can influence all of the external environments in which we work and live.

As we develop the optimal workplaces and living areas to foster self-actualizing conditions and maximize body–mind responses, we must continue to stay aware and informed of the effects of all aspects of the environment on human health. Many nurses find that the following exercise increases their sensitivity to the environment and its influence on their lives:

- At different times during the day, close your eyes and take a few moments to listen carefully to all of the sounds in your environment.
- Jot down the many different sounds you hear, noting which are pleasant and which are distracting or disturbing noises.
- Become aware of all of the sounds that you ordinarily hear, such as the air conditioner,

radios and televisions, the hum of fluorescent lights, the beeping and buzzing of hospital machinery, or the background music that some institutions play over the speaker system.

- Notice new smells, feelings of temperature, and so forth. There will be many sounds, smells, and sensations of which you may not previously have been aware.

Noise seems to be a major area of environmental concern that nurses can control. It is the accumulation of noises that elevates the decibels and can cause stress. By becoming increasingly sensitive to all potential environmental stressors, the nurse becomes more attuned to coaching opportunities and to offering specific interventions.

Some specific recommendations to reduce workplace noise are as follows:

- Developing staff education programs about noises, their source, and ways to quiet them
- Setting telephones and alarms to low volumes, or replacing sound devices with flashing lights
- Installing buffers in open space areas to minimize noise
- Closing the patients' doors whenever feasible
- Using bedside chairs with wheels in patient rooms with hard floors
- Choosing quieter equipment
- Placing computer printers away from patient rooms and/or installing soundproof covers
- Giving patients headphones to listen to the television or radio so that they do not disturb others
- Speaking in a softer voice

Planetary Consciousness Two points emerge as most salient within the context of nursing in general and holistic practice in particular as we consider our need to be conscious of all that we do, think, and act upon.

1. It is important to address the nature of being human and, in our Western mode, the pervasive influence of the self–other dichotomy.

2. We must be aware that we have viable choices of how we want to be and how we represent ourselves in the world.

An integration of these two points develops a personal orientation to all environmental concerns. With such an orientation, we can act from internal conviction and relatedness, rather than from institutional directives. Thus, it is up to each of us to develop an environmental sensitivity in our daily lives and become increasingly cognizant of our opportunities to institute positive change.

Case Study (Implementation)

Case Study

Setting: Outpatient clinic, or private visit
Client: A. B., a 55-year-old married man
Patterns/Challenges/Needs:

1. Altered comfort related to recurrent headaches
2. Ineffective individual coping related to environmental stress

A. B. visited the occupational health nurse because of recurrent headaches and chronic fatigue. A physical examination and laboratory tests revealed no pathology or disease, but his subjective declaration of feeling stress in the workplace warranted a closer examination of his workplace environment. A detailed history of his work hours, commuting travel, and work setting yielded evidence of environmental imbalance.

A. B. began his day with a 45-minute automobile commute through a suburban area to the inner city; he finished the day the same way. He had made this commute for years, but the traffic had lately increased and road repairs frequently slowed his pace. When he arrived at work, he went to his office, an interior room with fluorescent ceiling lights and no windows. The office walls were the standard institutional beige color; A. B. had done nothing to decorate or personalize his office. Instead of a secretary outside his office, he now had his own computer inside his office. During the company's modernization process, middle managers had been taught computer skills, and many secretarial positions had been eliminated. Each manager was now responsible for developing reports and interacting with others via personal computer terminals.

A. B.'s work routine had little variation. It consisted of meetings, telephone work, and online computer time. He kept an air freshener in his office to mask the smell of the floor cleaners that were used daily. He rarely took a lunch hour and kept a large bowl of multicolored jelly beans on his desk to fuel him throughout the day.

This information suggested that A. B. was experiencing environment-related stress, and the nurse worked with him to develop a seven-step plan of action:

1. Vary the commuting time. Begin the commute 15 minutes earlier to decrease the rushed feeling of getting to work on time. Join a health club in the city, and stay after work to exercise. The traffic would be considerably less 1 hour later, and the commute would then take only 30 minutes. Total morning and evening commute time would remain the same as before, but more would have been accomplished with less environmental stress.
2. Implement and practice computer protection skills (see **Table 24-3**).
3. Use a cordless earphone to prevent neck strain after long periods on the telephone. Use a headset on his wireless phone.
4. Personalize the office with soft, soothing colors. Add a wall picture of a mountain valley and stream that have personal significance.
5. Put an incandescent lamp on the desk, and use that rather than the overhead fluorescent lights for desk work.
6. Schedule regular lunch hour time. Replace jelly beans with healthier snacks.
7. Begin using natural aromatherapy in his office to relax him and add fragrance.

A copy of this plan was posted in a prominent place in A. B.'s home. Along with a plan for exercise and weight management (see Chapters 31 and 32) and a plan for the development of relaxation and imagery skills (see Chapters 11 and 12), this program incorporated A. B.'s need for motivation, lifestyle change, and values clarification.

When A. B. returned for his follow-up visit 2 months later, his headaches had abated, and he had made some progress toward his weight loss goals. He and his wife had redecorated his office, and on his own he had added a small cassette player to play his favorite classical music. He was bringing a healthy lunch to work and had replaced the jelly beans with a mix of nuts and dried fruit.

Six months later, A. B. was free of headaches. He asked the company director to install full-spectrum lights on all ceiling overhead panels. He also requested that unscented "natural" cleaners be brought into the unit. He felt he had regained some sense of control over his environment and was working on improvement in the other areas for which he and the nurse had developed plans.

Evaluation

How do we evaluate, for example, what may have triggered A. B.'s headaches? And what alleviated them? Could it have been a combination of factors or one specific action taken? Could his feeling empowered and supported in making changes contribute to his overall feeling of well-being and alleviation of his headache symptoms?

Trusting the client's inner wisdom, the nurse as coach can explore the chosen interventions and document changes and listen to the client's beliefs to guide future actions. For example, the nurse could ask A. B. to keep a journal to record any health changes or headache recurrences that he can relate to his environment and any alteration in the environment, including foods, stress, exercise, sleep, and any other areas that might trigger this pattern.

Each environmental intervention should be measured. The nurse can evaluate with the client the outcomes established before the implementation of any interventions (see Table 24-2). To evaluate the results further, the nurse can explore the subjective effects of the experience with the client, based on the evaluation questions in **Exhibit 24-2**. Last year's methods of handling laboratory specimens and chemotherapy preparations, for example, may be outdated next year. Nurses keep abreast of the changing

EXHIBIT 24-2   Evaluating the Client's Subjective Experience with Environmental Concerns

1. Were you aware that noise, lighting, air quality, space allocation, and workplace toxins could be chronic stressors?
2. Are any of these potential stressors in your environment? If so, can you do anything to reduce or remove them?
3. Do you realize that you can contribute to a healthier planet by virtue of changing elements in your own personal space?
4. Do you have an environmental awareness group at your workplace? If one existed, would you like to be a part of it? Would you be willing to begin one?
5. Do you feel empowered to be the person who initiates change in your work setting?
6. What are some specific things that you would like to do to create a healthier environment in your personal space or work setting?
7. What is your next step (or your plan) to integrate these changes into your life?

face of the environment to equip themselves with the newest strategies to counteract hazards. Present and future nurses would be well advised to remember and recall some of the basic nursing tenets of yesteryear that are still most relevant today. These interventions include fresh air, a comfortable climate, natural light, calming colors, and quiet (noise reduction).

Conclusion

Much of how we relate to and what we do about environmental issues is based on the development of our personal philosophy. We continue to become increasingly aware that each of the small things that we do for or against the environment has short- and long-term ramifications. Nurses want to be alert for ways to contribute to positive environmental changes for their own lives, their clients' lives, and the overall health of the planet. Environmental concerns are important to all of us, and one person's actions can have a ripple effect on many other lives. Nurses can be key agents to ensure that the environment is held sacred, supported, and tended to as it supports and gives life to all people.

Directions for Future Research

1. Evaluate the perception of quality of rest by subjects with different types of auditory stimulation.
2. Study the relationship between environmental hazards (e.g., artificial lighting,

working on video display terminals, unventilated air, shift work, high noise levels) and the rise in infertility, miscarriages, and neonate abnormalities.
3. Using an environmental assessment tool, research the health of nurses, their work environments, and health risks associated with endocrine disruptors and chemicals in the workplace and their effects on women's health.
4. Investigate the use of tactile, auditory, or olfactory stimuli on wound healing, rate of complications, length of recovery, and other health-related factors.
5. Study the effect of the environment on the reduction of stress and anxiety in ambulatory clients.
6. Become involved in local and national initiatives for creating healthier workplace environments (see https://noharm.org/).

Nurse Healer Reflections

After reading this chapter, the nurse healer will be able to answer or to begin a process of answering the following questions:

- How does the environment affect my job satisfaction?
- How does my work environment affect my health?
- What are the environmental stressors at work and at home?
- Which strategies can I incorporate into my environment to be healthier?

- Which things can I do to improve my own personal and workplace environment?
- How can I be involved with environmental issues at work and in my community?

NOTES

1. F. Nightingale, *Notes on Nursing: What It Is, and What It Is Not* (New York: Dover, 1969): 125.
2. F. Nightingale, *Notes on Hospitals*, 3rd ed. (London: Longman, Green, Longman, Roberts, and Green, 1860): iii.
3. A. Prüss-Üstün and C. Corvalán, *Preventing Disease Through Healthy Environments: Towards an Estimate of the Environmental Burden of Disease* (Geneva, Switzerland: World Health Organization, 2006).
4. World Health Organization, "Almost a Quarter of All Disease Caused by Environmental Exposure" (June 16, 2006). www.who.int /mediacentre/news/releases/2006/pr32/en/.
5. P. Grandjean and P. J. Landrigan, "Neurobehavioural Effects of Developmental Toxicity," *Lancet Neurology* 13, no. 3 (2014): 330–338.
6. M. B. Macon and S. E. Fenton, "Endocrine Disruptors and the Breast: Early Life Effects and Later Life Disease," *Journal of Mammary Gland Biology and Neoplasia* 18, no.1 (2013): 43–61.
7. E. Dhimolea, P. R. Wadia, T. J. Murray, M. L. Settles, J. D. Treitman, C. Sonnenschein, T. Shioda, et al., "Prenatal Exposure to BPA Alters the Epigenome of the Rat Mammary Gland and Increases the Propensity to Neoplastic Development," *PLoS One* 9, no. 7 (2014): 1–9.
8. K. G. Harley, R. A. Schall, R. J. Chevrier, K. Tyler, H. Aguirre, A. Bradman, N. T. Holland, et al., "Prenatal and Postnatal Bisphenol A Exposure and Body Mass Index in Childhood in the CHAMACOS Cohort," *Environmental Health Perspectives* 121, no. 4 (2013): 514–520.
9. Council on Environmental Health, "Chemical-Management Policy: Prioritizing Children's Health," *Pediatrics* 127, no. 5 (2011): 983–990.
10. B. Weiss, "Endocrine Disruptors as a Threat to Neurological Function," *Journal of Neurological Science* 305, nos. 1–2 (2011): 11–21.
11. B. M. Kuehn, "Increased Risk of ADHD Associated with Early Exposure to Pesticides, PCBs," *Journal of the American Medical Association* 304, no. 1 (2010): 27–28.
12. H. D. Bailey, L. Fritschi, C. Infante-Rivard, D. C. Glass, L. Miligi, J. D. Dockerty, T. Lightfoot, et al., "Parental Occupational Pesticide Exposure and the Risk of Childhood Leukemia in the Offspring: Findings from the Childhood Leukemia International Consortium," *International Journal of Cancer* 135, no. 9 (2014): 2157–2172.
13. V. M. Pak, M. Powers, and J. Liu, "Occupational Chemical Exposures Among Cosmetologists: Risk of Reproductive Disorders," *Workplace Health Safety* 61, no. 12 (2013): 522–552.
14. B. Sung, S. Prasad, V. R. Yadav, A. Lavasanifar, and B. B. Aggarwal, "Cancer and Diet: How Are They Related?" *Free Radical Research* 45, no. 8 (2011): 864–879.
15. U.S. Government Accountability Office, *Safe Drinking Water Act: Improvements in Implementation Are Needed to Better Assure the Public of Safe Drinking Water* (Washington, DC: U.S. Government Accountability Office, 2011).
16. B. Schumacher, J. Griggs, D. Askren, B. Litman, B. Shannon, M. Mehrhoff, A. Nelson, et al., *Development of Rapid Radiochemical Method for Gross Alpha and Gross Beta Activity Concentration in Flowback and Produced Waters from Hydraulic Fracturing Operations* (Washington, DC: U.S. Environmental Protection Agency, Office of Research and Development, 2014).
17. World Health Organization, "Ambient (Outdoor) Air Quality and Health" (March 2014). www.who.int/mediacentre/factsheets/fs313/en/.
18. U. S. Environmental Protection Agency, "Climate Change Indicators in the United States" (2014). http://epa.gov/climatechange/science/indicators/oceans/index.html.
19. H. Wilson and A. Bouchard, "Overview of the Clean Air Act and the Proposed Petroleum Refinery Sector Risk and Technology Review and New Source Performance Standards" (June 26–27, 2014). www.epa.gov/ttn/atw/petrefine/Refinery _workshop_New_Orleans_6_26-27_14.pdf.
20. L. Patton and B. Gruley, "Whole Foods Sees Stores Tripling with Embrace of Produce," *Bloomberg* (August 21, 2012). www.bloomberg .com/news/2012-08-21/whole-foods-sees-stores -tripling-with-embrace-of-produce.html.
21. National Gardening Association, *Garden to Table: A 5-Year Look at Food Gardening in America* (Williston, VT: National Gardening Association, 2014).
22. A. C. Sinnes, "Food Gardening in the U.S. at the Highest Levels in More Than a Decade According to New Report by the National Gardening Association" (April 2, 2014). www.garden.org /articles/articles.php?q=show&id=3819.
23. Teaching Responsible Earth Education, "Earthkeepers" (2011). http://treetalk.org/programs /earthkeepers.
24. Piedmont Wildlife Center, "Earth Keepers After School Program" (2014). www.piedmontwildlife center.org/earthkeepers/.

25. Rockford Public Schools, "Earth Keepers Magnet" (n.d.). https://sites.google.com/a/rockford schools.org/earth-keepers-201/home.

26. S. Cowan, "A Design Revolution," *Yes! Magazine* (June 30, 1998). www.yesmagazine.org/issues /rx-for-the-earth/829.

27. U.S. Green Building Council, "LEED Certification" (2014). www.usgbc.org/certification.

28. Samueli Institute, "Optimal Healing Environments" (2014). www.samueliinstitute.org /research-areas//optimal-healing-environments.

29. L. L. Folscher, L. N. Goldstein, M. Wells, and D. Rees, "Emergency Department Noise: Mental Activation or Mental Stress?" *Emergency Medical Journal* (2014). doi:10.1136/ emermed-2014-203735.

30. K. C. Bolton, J. L. Mace, P. M. Vacek, S. D. Herschorn, T. A. James, J. A. Tice, K. Kerlikowske, et al., "Changes in Breast Cancer Risk Distribution Among Vermont Women Using Screening Mammography," *Journal of the National Cancer Institute* 106, no. 8 (2014). doi:10.1093/jnci/dju157.

31. J. Accardo and M. A. Chaudhry. "Radiation Exposure and Privacy Concerns Surrounding Full Body Scanners in Airports," *Journal of Radiation Research and Applied Sciences* 7, no. 2 (2014): 198–200.

32. PRLog, "CDC Issues Precautionary Health Warning About Cell Phone Radiation" (August 13, 2014). www.prlog.org/12359483-cdc-issues -precautionary-health-warnings-about-cell -phone-radiation.html.

33. Environmental Health Trust, "Environmental Health Trust Experts Warn That Cell Phone Radiation Excites the Brain of Healthy Adults" (February 22, 2011). http://ehtrust .org/press-release-environmental-health-trust -experts-warn-that-cell-phone-radiation-excites -the-brain-of-healthy-adults/.

34. V. S. Benson, K. Pirie, J. Schüz, G. K. Reeves, V. Beral, and J. Green, "Mobile Phone Use and Risk of Brain Neoplasms and Other Cancers: Prospective Study," *International Journal of Epidemiology* 42, no. 3 (2013): 792–802.

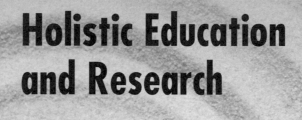

Holistic Education and Research

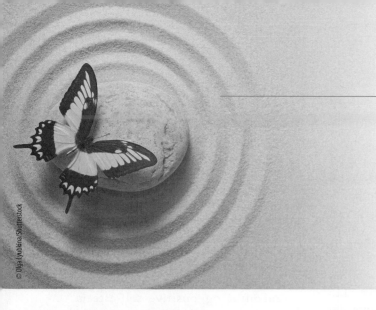

CHAPTER 25

Holistic Leadership

Veda L. Andrus and Marie M. Shanahan

Nurse Healer Objectives

Theoretical

- Identify the four characteristics of transformational leadership.
- Demonstrate integration of the three principles of influential leadership through words, actions, and leader style.
- Recognize the 10 principles of servant leadership within nursing practice.

Clinical

- Identify the seven core characteristics of a holistic leader.
- Demonstrate holistic philosophy, knowledge, and skill when mentoring colleagues.
- Develop strategies to link the caring case and business case of healthcare transformation.

Personal

- Identify gaps in holistic leadership competencies.
- Develop strategies to incorporate the principles of holistic leadership into practice.

Definitions

Appreciative inquiry: An asset-based approach built on the assumption that every organization has positive elements and processes and that these strengths can be the starting point for positive change.

Cultural transformational agent: An individual who holds the vision for and works to actualize a plan to transform the culture of an organization to become a caring, healing environment.

Holistic leadership: A participative leadership model in which people, regardless of formal titles, engage in a constructive process as equal partners to influence an affirming, sustainable, and humanistic outcome.

Influential leadership: A leadership style that seeks to understand human behavior and employ that understanding to drive effective performance. Three principles of influential leadership are self-awareness, collaboration, connectivity.

Intention: Focused, thoughtful attention directed toward a desired object, idea, or action. Used by holistic leaders to "engage the field" prior to designing and implementing an action plan.

Narrative research inquiry: A research method that includes the written and/or spoken word or visual (art, photography) representation of an individual's story.

Nurse empowerment: A state in which nurses assume control over their practice, enabling successful fulfillment of professional nursing responsibilities.[1]

Nurse engagement: A positive state of fulfillment and satisfaction experienced by nurses at work. When nurses are engaged they feel energetic and dedicated to their work and become immersed in work activities.

Servant leadership: A servant leader focuses primarily on the growth and well-being of people and the communities to which they belong. The servant leader shares power, puts the needs of others first, and helps people develop and perform as effectively as possible.

Structural empowerment: Work environment structures and processes designed to promote innovative high performance and professional practice.

Therapeutic healing environment: A milieu consciously created by a holistic healthcare professional(s) to promote the outcomes of health, healing, and well-being.

Transformational leadership: A style of leadership in which the individual identifies the needed change and (co)creates a clearly articulated vision to guide the change through inspiration, integrity, and mutual respect. The change is accomplished with the commitment of the group members and by maximizing human potential and mentorship.

Transparency: An intentional, ethical choice to be clear, plain, forthright, and above board.

Vision statement: An inspiring, compelling, clear, and direct statement of intention that guides the fulfillment of the purpose of an individual or organization.

Visionary: Having or marked by foresight and imagination.[2]

General Leadership Frameworks

The holistic leadership model draws its inspiration from three general progressive leadership frameworks that have informed its development. These frameworks have, at their roots, common conceptual perspectives that focus on principles that serve as the container and guiding light for leader actions. The principles become the foundation and springboard for the leader's relationship with self, others, and the organization, and then, by extension, become the keys to influence and manifest change.

Transformational Leadership

The concept of transformational leadership was introduced by Robert MacGregor Burns in 1978 as a leadership style in which the formal leader influences high performance by developing and articulating a compelling vision that inspires, motivates, and empowers followers to work toward fulfillment of a common goal.

> The roles of the transformational leader in the healthcare setting include promoting teamwork among staff, encouraging positive self-esteem, motivating staff to function at a high level of performance, and empowering staff to become more involved in the development and implementation of policies and procedures. The transformational leader portrays trustworthiness and serves as an inspiration to others, possessing an optimistic, positive, and encouraging outlook.[3]

The following are the core characteristics of transformational leadership:[4]

- *Idealized influence.* The leader possesses and models self-confidence, inspires trust and encouragement for followers to bring forth their best selves, and provides mentorship that enhances nurse engagement.
- *Inspiration and vision.* The leader develops, articulates, and models a compelling vision that inspires followers to passionately execute the vision.
- *Intellectual stimulation.* The leader respects the follower's creativity through identification of co-created goals, encourages identification and actualization of innovative solutions, and guides followers to find meaning and purpose in their work.
- *Individual consideration.* The leader maintains open, clear, and effective communication; fosters quality relationships with followers; and offers support, encouragement, and recognition.

Transformational leadership is one of the five components of the American Nurses Credentialing Center's Magnet Recognition Program® Model. This component was selected with the understanding that nurse leaders today must provide the necessary leadership to prepare organizations to meet the current and future demands of healthcare reform. "Unlike yesterday's leadership requirement for stabilization and growth, today's leaders must transform their organization's values, beliefs, and behaviors."[5]

Influential Leadership

The influential leadership framework, introduced by Michael Frisina in 2011, identifies three fundamental principles that facilitate effective performance for making a sustainable difference within organizations. The first principle, *self-awareness*, is viewed as the *basic competency* for influential leaders, recognizing that when learning about themselves, leaders are then able to serve as inspiring role models and supportive mentors for others.

> By learning about the self, leaders become comfortable with their internal thought processes, values, beliefs, preferences, and emotions. They become self-managers, careful about how they present themselves and respond to the outside world. A self-aware leader, then, is in a better position to collaborate and connect with others.[6, p. 4]

The second principle, *collaboration*, is viewed as the *duty* and a performance improvement strategy for influential leaders, with the understanding that creating a common goal through partnering with others allows for greater trust, accountability, and harmony. Collaborative action provides a climate for dynamic transformation from a competitive, power-over environment to a cooperative, power-with organizational culture. Sustainable collaboration draws on the expertise, knowledge, and strengths of each team member, allowing for collective decision making, cultivation of strong relationships, and acknowledgment that every person provides a unique talent and contribution to the creation of a high-performing organization.

Connection is the third principle of influential leadership and is regarded as a core *strategy* to build and strengthen a compassionate culture that promotes effective relationships and "raises everyone's level of energy, engagement, motivation, and performance."[6, p. 160] Sharing meaningful experiences through authentic connection fosters organizational commitment and drives performance excellence.

Servant Leadership

Servant leadership, introduced by Robert Greenleaf in 1970, is a values-based style of leadership in which leaders place the needs of others ahead of their own interests in order to share power and be effective.

> The servant-leader is *servant* first.... It begins with the natural feeling that one wants to serve, to serve *first*. Then conscious choice brings one to aspire to lead. That person is sharply different from one who is *leader* first.[7]

The primary focus is on the growth, well-being, and autonomy of others, which, in nursing, holds the promise of leading to enhanced quality of care, improved nursing satisfaction, and assisting nurses in finding meaning in their work.

Neill and Saunders applied the Ten Principles of Servant Leadership to the practice of nursing to enhance both patient and nurse satisfaction and nurse–person engagement.[8]

1. *Listening.* Commitment to reflection and receptive listening with the recognition that everyone has a contribution.
2. *Empathy.* Understands the circumstances of others. Recognizes and accepts others for their unique contributions.
3. *Healing.* Healing relationships become a transformative process within an organization.
4. *Awareness.* Has a strong sense of the healthcare setting and looks for input to develop meaningful solutions to challenges.
5. *Persuasion.* Engages in shared decision making and is effective at building consensus within groups.
6. *Conceptualization.* Sees the big picture while seeking a delicate balance between conceptualization and a day-to-day focus.

7. *Foresight.* Anticipates outcomes yet remains open to how decisions made in the present may influence the future.
8. *Stewardship.* Responsibility for preparing an organization to fulfill its mission and contribute to the betterment of society.
9. *Growth.* Has a strong commitment to the growth of people and works to help them reach their true potential, personally and professionally.
10. *Building community.* Is inclusive rather than competitive by identifying shared values and a common sense of purpose.

Greenleaf recognized that *organizations* could also be viewed as servant leaders by developing a mission that encompasses creating a healing environment for patients and care providers, along with contributing to the growth and transformation of the community and society at large.

Professional Practice Models

Professional practice models provide a container to operationalize theoretical frameworks within a course of action. Most practice models encompass an amalgam of theories that serve as an anchor to support nursing practice. Three professional practice models have been selected to support holistic leadership as a leadership model: the BirchTree Center Model™, the Quality-Caring Model©, and the Caring in Nursing Administration Model.

BirchTree Center Model™

The BirchTree Center Model™ (or Renaissance Caring Model) was developed by Marie Shanahan and Veda Andrus in 2005. It is an integrative, interdisciplinary, progressive practice model of personal and professional transformation that promotes consistent and sustainable holistic practice in nursing and health care (see **Figure 25-1**). In this model, as individuals build the capacity for developing a caring, healing ethic to transform their practice, organizations build the capacity for developing a caring, healing work environment to transform the organizational culture.[9]

Engagement with the BirchTree Center Model™ begins with the relationship one has with self. Through self-reflection, individuals come to realize that self-care and renewal are essential to their effectiveness in therapeutic relationships. Engagement in self-renewal practices expands and enhances their ability to be a healing presence with others, and caring for oneself is thus properly reframed as integral with compassionate, professional care for others. Holistic leaders model self-awareness and renewal in professional settings and identify them as an essential leadership competency, indicating the importance of these behaviors in contributing to a therapeutic healing environment.

The model is used within healthcare settings to reorient the values, behaviors, actions, and practice ethic toward healing and caring through greater awareness of a shared humanity. When compassion is appropriately linked with organizational excellence, the intrinsic motivation to be/provide caring creates deeper engagement with the mission of the organization. As the field of compassion expands, the shift in organizational identity begins. The identification of compassion as a cultural anchor linked to performance fosters a sustainable transformation.

The model is represented in the image of an open basket. The open basket imagery "holds space" for the practitioner and the organization to recognize, develop, and allow an ever-increasing capacity to heal and be healed; to receive new gifts, knowledge, and understanding; to let go of that which no longer is needed; and to transform and lead transformation with others. The concept of an open basket is intended to challenge the long-held image of a practitioner's "toolkit." The open basket of the BirchTree Center Model™ invites the concept of holding all possibilities for a healing process, going well beyond a practitioner tending to the person to encompass such notions as the practitioner's own well-being and potential for influencing organizational and community health. By shifting to the image of an open basket, the potential to hold healing energy for ourselves, our patients, our fellow coworkers, and the healthcare system is engaged.[10]

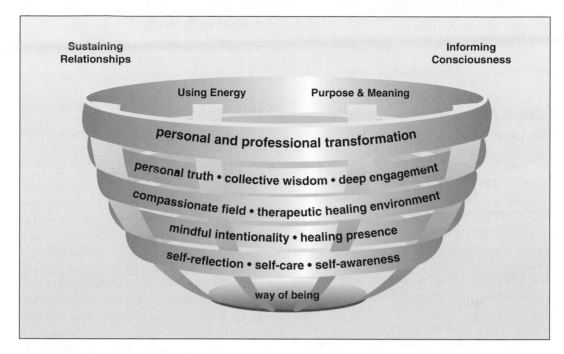

FIGURE 25-1 The BirchTree Center Model™

Source: BirchTree Center Press

Quality-Caring Model©

The Quality-Caring Model© was developed by Joanne Duffy in 2003 with the intention of integrating caring processes with quality concepts to promote excellence in nursing practice. "The major proposition of the model is that caring relationships influence attainment of positive health outcomes for patients/families, health care providers, and health care systems."[11, p. 35] The model is based on the three primary components of Donabedian's classic healthcare quality framework: structure, process, and outcomes.[12]

The *structure* component of Duffy's model includes all of the elements that are involved in delivering health care: the care provider (life experiences, skills, attitudes), patients/family (life stories, current illnesses, relationships), and the healthcare organization/system (organizational culture, available resources, community reputation). Each structure contributes to a unique configuration that defines the healthcare experience.

The *process* component of the model is relationship centered and encompasses the relationship the care provider has with the patient/family as well as the relationships between care providers. Caring values, attitudes, and behaviors inform all professional encounters with the intention that all interactions are grounded in caring actions. Nurses form caring relationships with patients/families and collaborative relationships with other care team members while upholding the mission/vision of the healthcare organization.

The *outcomes* component of the model has an affirming effect on all three components of the framework. The care provider experiences increased satisfaction, professional growth, and improved clinical and service outcomes; the patient/family experiences increased satisfaction with their care, a safe healing environment, and enhanced knowledge and understanding of their health concerns; and, the organization/system experiences cost containment, better utilization of resources, and enhanced quality and safety.

"Nursing leaders must own and genuinely connect to the practice of nursing using caring relationships as the underlying foundation."[11, p. 115] It is essential that leaders value all relationships by building a caring professional practice environment and culture through maximizing time spent in relationships. "Using a caring ethic as a basis for decision making and recognizing caring as having economic value, nurse leaders can positively enhance quality care."[11, p. 115]

Caring in Nursing Administration Model

The Caring in Nursing Administration professional practice model was introduced by Jan Nyberg in 1998 and presents a model for identifying the practices, effects, domains, and outcomes of caring in nursing administration, demonstrated through leadership actions.[13]

To truly execute this model, all leadership actions are rooted in a foundation of caring *philosophy* and caring *theory*, modeled and articulated through caring *ethics*, and substantiated within a framework of evidence-informed caring *research*. The nurse leader promotes and supports research that showcases caring and healing with an emphasis on unit-based, nurse-led quality improvement demonstration projects.

Nursing administrators engage in and model self-care practices, developing skills of caring presence and caring relationships to create a healing work environment. They evaluate and document the relationship between and among caring practices and nurse retention, patient–nurse satisfaction, healing outcomes, and cost.

With "incongruities between the staff nurses' caring ethic and the health care industry's focus on competition, profit, and productivity,"[14, p. 7] nursing administrators become stewards of life-sustaining caring economics by incorporating caring as a valuable economic resource to change the conversation of transformation within nursing practice.

Research

The concept and language of holistic leadership is on the cutting edge of a new paradigm of leadership. There is ample research available in the literature that substantiates the implementation of transformational leadership; however, holistic leadership, as presented in this chapter, currently does not have a research base that substantiates outcomes. An inclusion of various research methodological models that reflect the principles of holistic leadership must be considered.

Quantitative Research

Quantitative research is an objective, systematic form of research that is a reductionist approach used to measure nursing *science*.

Qualitative Research

Qualitative research is a subjective form of research that describes life experiences and provides meaning. This research methodology measures both the *art* and the *science* of holistic inquiry.

Narrative Research Inquiry

Narrative research inquiry is a collection of approaches that includes the written and/or spoken word or visual (art, photography) representation of an individual's story. Through sharing a lived/living story, there is an opportunity for self-reflection, allowing the individual to understand and bring personal meaning to his or her experience in a relational manner and for the narrative inquirer to gain insight into the individual's life journey. Within the process of giving voice to the story, the individual may experience an epiphany, a moment of insight, significance, and personal revelation.[15]

A key component of narrative inquiry is the role of the narrative inquirer who, through posing reflective questions and engaging in deep listening and full presence, provides an occasion where the individual can be truly listened to and heard. Through co-creating the opportunity of listening/receiving the individual's story, the narrative inquirer may also have the opportunity to engage in his or her own self-reflection.

Appreciative Inquiry

Appreciative inquiry is an asset-based approach built on the assumption that every organization has things that work well and that these strengths can be the starting point for positive change.

> Every human system has something that works right—things that give it life when it is vital, effective, and successful. Appreciative inquiry begins by identifying this positive core and connecting to it in ways that heighten energy, sharpen vision, and inspire action for change.[16]

This is a shift from the traditional deficit-based problem-solving approach to change and group engagement by studying what *does* work, building solutions from this knowledge base, unlocking innovation, and yielding greater creativity.

The 5-D model of appreciative inquiry includes the following cycle processes:[17]

1. *Definition*. Reframe focus of the inquiry in the affirmative and on topics valuable to the people involved.
2. *Discovery*. A collaborative search for "the best of what is" that already provides optimal performance. Discovery involves meaningful conversations.
3. *Dream*. Dialogue, reflection, envisioning. An exploration of "what might be," where people collectively explore their hopes and dreams.
4. *Design*. Co-constructing the vision created in the *Dream* phase into specific changes to create a preferred future.
5. *Destiny*. Focuses on personal commitments and implementation of innovation.

Appreciative inquiry is a cycle: When *Destiny* is implemented, the cycle starts again with *Definition*.

The process of appreciative inquiry fosters excitement, enthusiasm, and commitment among nursing personnel through inclusivity of those who may have the best insights into solutions. This enhances nurse engagement, encourages identification of strengths and resources, stimulates optimal performance, and assists in recognizing what the organization does best.

Characteristics of a Holistic Leader

To manage is to control; to lead is to liberate.[18]*

Holistic leadership is a synthesis of participative leadership models with the recognition that it is imperative to redefine and expand the concept of leadership to meet the future directions within nursing and health care. With the introduction in 2010 of the Patient Protection and Affordable Care Act (commonly known as the Affordable Care Act), nurses hold the potential to play key roles in the rollout of healthcare reform and must assume leadership roles that align with a new model of holistic leadership. When approaching leadership roles from a holistic–integrative perspective, nurses, as holistic leaders, will position themselves to assume innovative roles as the edge runners of healthcare change.

There is one assumption to embrace: Everyone is a leader. This means that every nurse, whether holding a formal leadership title or not, has a responsibility to influence the advancement of the nursing profession. A shift in language from *follower*, as noted in the transformational leadership model, to *partner*, as presented in the holistic leadership model, is essential to authentically demonstrate that everyone is, indeed, a leader. It is critical not to underestimate the compelling value proposition of nursing as being a prime contributor of healthcare transformation.

There are seven core characteristics of a holistic leader:[10]

1. Visionary
2. Inspirational presence
3. Role model
4. Mentor
5. Champion for clinical excellence
6. Courageous advocate
7. Cultural transformational agent

Although these seven characteristics will be presented individually, it is important to recognize that they are interrelated and integral to one another. The thread that weaves them together radiates from a foundation of competence, heart-centered collaboration, and self-awareness as the essence of a leader's way of being, personally and professionally.

Holistic Leader as Visionary

There are two ways of spreading light—to be the candle or the mirror that reflects it."
—Edith Wharton[19]

---

*Above quote reprinted with permission of the publisher. From The Spirit of Leadership: Liberating the Leader in Each of Us, copyright © 1999 by H. Owen, Berrett-Koehler Publishers, Inc., San Francisco, CA. All rights reserved. www.bkconnection.com.

A visionary is conventionally defined as "a person with original ideas about what the future will or could be like."[20] When defined in concert with the concept of holistic leadership, the future is co-created in a collaborative manner through the recognition that everyone is a leader and that drawing out each person's creative potential calls forth the best in people, bringing them together around a shared sense of purpose. The holistic visionary leader is open to learning from other points of view through evolving the art of full presence, deep listening, and a nonjudgmental attitude.

There is an inherent need on the part of human beings for their work to serve as an avenue for the fulfillment of purpose and meaning. A visionary leader understands the deeper spiritual needs of people by caring for the souls of individuals as well as the soul of the organization. It is through this awareness that leaders align with a higher purpose for themselves, their coworkers, the organization, and the greater community.

As architects of change (change agents), seeing the big picture and utilizing out-of-the-box thinking allows for innovative co-participative strategic actions. This is not done in isolation. The visionary leader is often a catalyst for innovation, working with imagination, insight, and boldness through a partnership approach with other nurse colleagues and in concert with the multidisciplinary team.

Vision Statement Development

The co-creation of a nursing vision statement serves as both a solid foundation and a guiding compass for nursing practice. The key word is *co-creation*. A vision statement is developed as a collaborative and inclusive process that serves as an energetic directive of shared purpose and direction. In a conventional mode, it is often the nursing executive team that develops the vision and sets standards for nursing practice. Within a holistic paradigmatic mode, the holistic leader identifies and utilizes a creative approach to include all nurses to have an active voice in the development process.

The vision statement must be inspiring, compelling, clear, direct, and communicated in a manner that brings the vision into reality as a guide for professional practice. Revisiting the vision statement annually is imperative to

assure it continues to align with purpose, meaning, and the current trajectory of nursing practice for the organization.

It is also important to create an avenue by which all nurses have an understanding of and relationship with the vision statement as the foundation for their nursing practice. Presenting the nursing vision statement and what it means to the organization is essential to incorporate into all new nurse orientation sessions. Posting the vision statement on each hospital unit will remind nurses of the purpose and meaning of their practice. Creating opportunities for nurses to dialogue about how they are clinically operationalizing the nursing vision serves to keep the vision alive and aligns all nurses with a common foundation and direction for their practice.

Holistic Leader as Inspirational Presence

Leaders cannot demand inspiration from others; they must create the environment *that encourages such inspiration.*[21, p. 152]

The holistic leader has a role in creating a vibrant environment that *inspires* people to be their best selves through inclusion, respect, caring, and acknowledgement. The physical environment in which many nurses work may not be particularly inspiring in design and function; however, the culture of the work environment can always foster creativity, insight, and engagement. The holistic leader, through his or her very presence, can cultivate commitment and passion in the workplace where nurses and members of the multidisciplinary team are encouraged to grow, learn, and develop as care providers and as human beings.

As an inspirational presence, the holistic leader performs an important role in creating a positive and engaging environment. *Inspiration* is described as "emotions and behaviors determined by powers from within. Inspired people arouse the hearts of others."[21, p. 51] When the heart is aroused, people become enthusiastic, knowing their participation is invited as a contribution to the developing landscape of their work environment.

The holistic leader understands that an expression of positive energy and vitality has an affirming correlation with indicators such as productivity and job performance. Although the primary focus may not be on these specific indicators, through an inspiring environment that fosters collaboration, teamwork, and shared information, the holistic leader conveys an air of confidence that the right energetic environment will support greater productivity and improved job performance.

An inspirational leader embodies a sense of personal integrity that radiates to others as respect, kindness, and genuine, authentic caring. The words *genuine* and *authentic* are essential because words and actions, including genuine celebration of accomplishments and successes, that come from this place of true caring are acknowledged and appreciated by others.

Holistic Leader as Role Model

The responsibility of a role model is to set standards of excellence in clinical nursing in concert with exemplifying both the vision and values that are fundamental within the organization. The central intention of being a role model is to serve as a positive example for other nurses to follow and emulate.

Core Principles

There are four core principles that serve as pillars for role modeling holistic leadership: maintaining integrity, upholding ethical standards, demonstrating bold and courageous actions, and being visible-approachable-accessible.

1. *Integrity.* Adheres to superior moral principles and professional standards; not willing to trade integrity for personal advancement. Holistic leaders choose not to compromise their integrity with behaviors that do not align with their sense of right action.
2. *Ethical.* Models a professional code of holistic nursing ethics that includes being a therapeutic, caring presence; facilitating healing and wholeness; practicing loving kindness; and sustaining honesty. "Holistic nurses [may] assume a leadership position to guide the profession towards holism"[22] through integration of Holistic Nursing Core Value 1: *Holistic Philosophy, Theories, and Ethics.*[23, p. 9]

3. *Bold and courageous.* Stands firmly in own truth and knowing; is confident and bold in speaking out in support of holistic nursing practice. Holistic leaders access their courage and assume the responsibility to take risks to advance nursing excellence.
4. *Visible-approachable-accessible.* Values meaningful connection with nurse colleagues and other care providers; intentionally maintains an open heart and mind, without judgment, to enhance engagement, communication, and exploration. Holistic leaders demonstrate a passion for nursing and a love of the profession, igniting the soul of nursing and exhibiting excitement for what the future will bring for the profession.

Artistry of Authentic Communication

Holistic leaders must be aware of and sensitive to the diversity of communication styles and present information in a manner that is clear, direct, and genuine. Presenting information in a way that others can best receive it is an art that takes practice and reflection. The practice of taking a breath as a momentary pause prior to presenting information can demonstrate role modeling an authentic communication style.

Holistic leaders model respectful holistic communication by:

- Making no assumptions: creating a culture where asking questions is an acceptable practice
- Fostering nonjudgmental behavior and actions
- Choosing to be compassionate and sincere
- Drawing information from a broad range of sources
- Engaging in deep listening (heart/mind) through full presence
- Acting in a manner that is reflective and responsive, rather than reactive
- Modeling transparency through open and honest dialogue

Self-Reflection and Self-Care

One of the core values that is foundational to holistic nursing practice is "*Holistic Nurse Self-Reflection and Self-Care.*"[23, pp. 20–21] Engaging in self-care practices, both personally and professionally, can be a challenge for many nurses because affirming models for self-care in their families and within the practice environment are frequently absent.

It is the responsibility of holistic leaders to model self-reflection and self-care on a regular and consistent basis with the intention of building their own resiliency and demonstrating support and encouragement for others to care well for themselves.

In a professional work environment, self-reflective and self-care practices may include taking lunch breaks, utilizing reflective time for decision making, and departing the workplace in a timely manner at the end of the day. Participating in these and other self-care activities demonstrates that the holistic leader values these practices, and, through role modeling, provides permission for others to do the same.

The use of grounding and centering techniques, such as taking a few deeps breaths prior to attending meetings, during all interactions, and in transitions from one activity to the next, models a process to help others cope with workplace stressors.

Holistic Leader as Mentor

Individualized, tailor-made, one-on-one environments for giving and receiving the gift of wisdom.[24]*

This description provides a unique perspective for mentorship, one that may stretch the common image that a mentor is the person replete with skills, information, and knowledge, negating the recognition that mentorship can be an exchange of ideas and experience. Holistic leaders view mentorship as a mutually beneficial shared, rather than hierarchical, process where both people, as partners, learn and grow from one another's insights and wisdom.

Through cultivation of a mentorship culture, holistic leaders guide/facilitate projects for skill development that demonstrate a commitment to

*Brief quote from p. xi from MENTORING: THE TAO OF GIVING AND RECEIVING WISDOM by CHUNGLIANG AL HUANG and JERRY LYNCH. Copyright © 1995 by Chungliang Al Huang and Jerry Lynch. Reprinted by permission of HarperCollins Publishers.

lifelong learning. This environment fosters ongoing professional growth and continued career advancement in nursing leadership, strengthens confidence and competence, and enhances nurse engagement through a co-participative model.

Giving and receiving, working together as partners, becomes the acceptable norm, allowing for acceptance, cooperation, appreciation, and inclusivity—a circle of influence.

Holistic Leader as Champion for Clinical Excellence

A number of barriers prevent nurses from being able to respond effectively to rapidly changing health care settings and an evolving health care system. These barriers need to be overcome to ensure that nurses are well-positioned to lead change and advance health.[25]

Serving as a champion for clinical excellence is a critical role for holistic nursing leaders in today's healthcare climate. This has always been an important role for nurse leaders; however, with the introduction of the Medicare Hospital Value-Based Purchasing Program[26] and the HCAHPS (Hospital Consumer Assessment of Healthcare Providers and Systems) survey,[27] it has become even more critical for holistic leaders to concentrate on clinical excellence and view this as a central construct for a new value proposition for nursing.

To begin, holistic leaders must become articulate in linking the *caring case* of bedside care with the *business case* of healthcare transformation—and require clinical nurses to do the same. This can be accomplished by promoting education and learning at every level, where nurses understand how their role as care providers has a direct relationship with the business case. The next step is to hold nurses accountable for clinical excellence as demonstrated by exceptional quality patient care, purposeful nurse–patient engagement, genuine peer-to-peer caring, personal self-care practices to enhance resiliency, and appreciation for the larger role their organization plays as an instrument of change within the community and the broader healthcare environment.

Innovative Strategies for Clinical Excellence

Holistic leaders are intentional about selecting and implementing progressive, innovative strategies that will achieve clinical excellence within a healthy, supportive work environment. The American Association of Critical-Care Nurses' Synergy Model for Patient Care states that "when nurse competencies stem from patient needs and the characteristics of the nurse and patient synergize, optimal patient outcomes can result."[28, p. 1] Accessible provision of relevant professional development education to improve competency levels in knowledge development, clinical skills expertise, and critical thinking is an avenue that supports and fosters optimal clinical outcomes.

Cultivation of true collaboration among clinical nurses, across the multidisciplinary team, with inclusion of patients and their families, promotes clinical excellence when creative opportunities for communication and learning are employed. In this integrative approach, the knowledge and abilities of each professional and patient are respected to achieve safe, quality care. Implementation of bedside shift report, shared decision making, and interprofessional rounds are examples of true collaboration that can enhance the quality of the patient experience and outcomes.

"Bedside shift report has been shown to empower staff, improve patient involvement, and allow for a safe transition of care between providers."[29, p. 16] This effective communication mode for transferring information creates a strong interprofessional team approach and includes the patients as active participants in contributing to and knowing their plan of care.

Shared decision making, a quality measure for accountable care organizations, is a "collaborative process in which patients and providers make health care decisions together, weighing the medical evidence of various options, and considering the patient's values and preferences."[30, p. 28] Three key questions to consider with shared decision making are: Is the patient informed? Did the patient get the treatment that best matched his or her goals? Was the patient meaningfully involved in the decision? Shared decision-making survey tools are being integrated into care pathways with the intention of enhancing patient engagement.

Interprofessional rounds provide a venue for collaboration where interdisciplinary healthcare professionals (conventional medical and complementary care providers) dialogue together, share their knowledge and skills, and co-participate in decision making, all with the objective of providing excellent patient care. Although quality patient care is the primary consideration of interprofessional rounds, additional outcomes include development of cooperation, mutual respect, and a deeper understanding of how each discipline contributes to the delivery of holistic and integrative care.

The Broader Context of Professionalism

Holistic leaders elevate the professionalism of nurses by encouraging and supporting ongoing professional development and clinical competence through advanced degrees and certifications. As a result of advancing their education and career, nurses are recognized and rewarded in a manner that demonstrates how this personal accomplishment also advances nursing within the specific healthcare organization and, by extension, within the overall profession.

Membership in professional organizations is promoted, viewing this as essential to support professional growth and serving as an avenue to effect change through a reshaping of the broader healthcare environment. This involvement empowers clinical nurses to "find their voice" and discover what they can do to further the profession.

Holistic leaders, with an eye on accessing national comparative data with other hospitals, participate in the National Database of Nursing Quality Indicators (NDNQI®) Program, which provides unit-level performance data for quality improvement and data measurement of nursing-sensitive indicators to improve patient care and outcomes.[31]

Holistic Leader as Courageous Advocate

Courage: Mental or moral strength to venture, persevere, and withstand danger, fear, or difficulty.[32]

Advocate: A person who pleads on someone else's behalf.[33]

As courageous advocates, holistic leaders exhibit an unwavering commitment to support and enrich all dimensions of holistic nursing practice, from bedside to boardroom, for nurses and for the planet. This is a tall order. However, the realm of advocacy must be inclusive of all areas in which nurses are influential, and it takes courage to be a progressive thinker and an innovative change agent to facilitate nursing in achieving its full potential.

For the Advancement of Holistic Nursing and the Nursing Profession

Holistic leaders are visible and vocal advocates for holistic nursing. They are active (visible) in professional organizations (e.g., American Holistic Nurses Association, American Organization of Nurse Executives, Sigma Theta Tau International), not only as members but also as spokespersons (vocal) for framing nursing practice in holistic nursing principles, philosophy, and theory. They choose to be informed on healthcare policy and financing with an intention of aligning current models to a holistic paradigm—building a business *and* a caring case for nursing and health care.

For Nurses

Creating a work environment and culture that fosters caring for nurses is foundational to holistic leaders who regard nurse self-care as a clinical competency. Inclusion of a self-care reflection on the annual performance review demonstrates that self-care within the work environment is valued and viewed as a benchmark of clinical excellence.

Holistic leaders endorse nurses taking their breaks and choose to fund the creation of workplace renewal spaces for rest, rejuvenation, and reflection. There is a reinforcement of unit-based, self-care activities (e.g., afternoon tea time, hand/foot massage) along with the development of nurse-initiated wellness-related activities (e.g., stair-climbing for aerobic exercise, aromatherapy for stress reduction).

Upholding *The Future of Nursing* report recommendations from the Institute of Medicine is considered foundational when advocating for nursing excellence. The key messages from the report are:[34]

- Nurses should practice to the full extent of their education and training.

- Nurses should achieve higher levels of education and training through an improved education system that promotes seamless academic progression.
- Nurses should be full partners, with physicians and other health care professionals, in redesigning health care in the United States.
- Effective workforce planning and policymaking require better data collection and an improved information infrastructure.

These key messages are promoted by holistic leaders through ongoing organizational support for clinical nurses and creative, cutting-edge implementation to advance nursing practice.

For Patients

First and foremost, holistic leaders uphold a culture of quality and safety through reduction of interruptions and noisy, distracting work environments. Quiet time, when lights are lowered and a peaceful environment is employed, creates a healing healthcare environment that benefits both patients and nurses.[35] It serves as an opportunity for patients to rest and for nurses to have a respite from continuous activity.

An innovative culture and workplace environment that enhances the patient experience and patient satisfaction is developed that embraces enrichment of the nurse–patient engagement. One way in which this can be demonstrated is through the delivery of integrative therapies at the bedside. Also, a subtle shift in language from *patient-centered care* to *person-centered care* assists in viewing patients (persons) as whole human beings with rich life stories and serves to include them as partners in their plan of care.

For the Community

Holistic leaders see beyond the borders of their healthcare organization by building collaborative relationships and partnerships with community organizations. This is done by recognizing the importance of forming networks with other organizational leaders to promote community-based health and wellness educational programs and services. With the aging population and increase in chronic care needs, there must be reengineered pathways to fill this current "chasm of care."[36]

For the Earth

The American Nurses Association, with a focus on population health, added an environmental standard to the *Scope and Standards of Practice*, stating that "the registered nurse integrates the principles of environmental health for nursing in all areas of practice."[23, p. 57] Holistic leaders demonstrate awareness of the influence their organization has on the health of the community and planet Earth by taking the bold, progressive stance of including environmental health as a nurse competency. For example, clinical nurses are expected to promote "a practice environment that reduces environmental health risks of workers and healthcare consumers" and participate "in strategies to promote healthy communities."[37]

Actions in support of a healthful environment include (1) fostering environmental education and resources for nurses, (2) encouraging awareness regarding environmental factors (e.g., noise, lights, use of toxic cleaning materials), and (3) implementing organizational programs for the care of the Earth (e.g., unit-based and whole organization recycling programs).[38]

Holistic Leader as Cultural Transformational Agent

Moving from a "chain of command" to a "web of influence."[39]

A cultural transformational agent, as defined at the start of this chapter, is an individual who holds the vision for and works to actualize a plan to transform the culture of an organization to become a caring, healing environment. An embodiment and actualization of all of the identified core characteristics of a holistic leader are critical to effect organizational culture change: visionary, inspirational presence, role model, mentor, champion for clinical excellence, and courageous advocate—all with the intention of co-creating an inspiring and engaging work environment that supports nurse well-being, nurse–patient engagement, and a collaborative partnership among healthcare providers.

The overarching key to cultural transformation is the cultivation of a therapeutic healing environment for nurses and patients in which fostering quality relationships becomes the primary focus: the relationship nurses have with themselves, their colleagues, their patients, and with the profession of nursing.

Holistic leaders create avenues and opportunities for *nurse empowerment* by encouraging autonomy through shifting the outmoded language of viewing nurses as *followers* to relating to them as *partners* who are vibrant contributors to evolving the culture of the organization. Participatory management through active involvement in a shared governance professional practice model is promoted to empower nurses and to enhance nurse satisfaction.

Holistic leaders develop an infrastructure for an innovative, collaborative practice environment by providing *structural empowerment*.[5] When nurses have a positive perception of organizational support and the work environment inspires caring and healing, they are able to place their attention on intentional engagement with their patients and colleagues. When highly engaged, nurses become partners in workforce transformation, which reignites their passion for nursing.

Holistic Caring Process

Case Study (Overview)

Dana has been a nurse manager on a busy medical-surgical unit in a 450-bed inner-city hospital for the past 2 years. She has been slowly, and intentionally, building team cohesiveness since her arrival and introducing holistic leadership as the leadership style for the unit.

An innovative hospital-wide initiative has been introduced to improve HCAHPS scores with a rollout time of 3 months. The unit nurses are feeling stressed about implementing the new initiative and are complaining about having something else to add to their already busy work assignments.

Dana views the new initiative as an avenue to continue to strengthen her team and to practice the key principles of holistic leadership. Prior to introducing it to her staff, she prepared herself by taking quiet time to reflect on how best to present the initiative, understanding that how it is presented will make all the difference in receptivity. She chose to introduce the initiative in an affirming manner, inspiring everyone to approach it as an opportunity to enhance engagement and improve the quality of patient care.

This case study will be viewed through the lens of the holistic caring process.

Holistic Assessment

- Engage in an inclusive, collaborative reflection and assessment:
  - Include full-time, part-time, day/night shift clinical nurses and nursing assistants as colleagues-partners-community in the process
  - Yield a shared sense of purpose
- Facilitate a time-regulated opportunity for colleagues to express concerns about the initiative and rollout time frame (reacting) and redirect to a proactive approach to identify a creative process for the rollout (responding).
- Empower the community to infuse the initiative with loving kindness, viewing it in a positive light and as an opportunity for professional growth and development
- Set a team-inspired intention for the project:
  - Experience as an opportunity for grounding and centering, rather than approaching the initiative only as a task to be completed
    - Envision successful process/outcome
    - Complete rollout plan on time
    - Work collaboratively together with ease, support, and joy
- Review/assess past and current unit HCAHPS scores, without judgment, with rekindled interest in identifying new strategies to enhance engagement and improve quality of patient care
- Inspire colleagues to view the initiative as an opportunity for change, not as a criticism of their practice
- Collaboratively apply the *Definition* step of the 5-D model of appreciative inquiry:

- Define/describe the purpose and content of the initiative in commonly understood language
- Frame the initiative in an affirming light
- Assess elements of structural empowerment:
  - Review policies, programs, and organizational structure that will support fulfillment of the initiative
- Align with the care model and theory to provide a framework for assessing the initiative

Identification of Patterns/ Challenges/Needs

- Collaboratively apply the *Discovery* step of the 5-D model of appreciative inquiry:
  - (Re)discover what already provides optimal performance
  - Acknowledge strengths and challenges as growing edges
- Foster inspired engagement through inclusivity of reflections and insights:
  - Creatively include all colleagues
- Co-create questions that inspire courageous conversations
- Listen to experience, contribution, and insight from each person
- Identify resources/infrastructure (people, services, technology) that will support the initiative:
  - Required attendance at the Professional Holistic Nurse Practice Council meeting to network with other clinical nurses
    - Select/mentor unit representatives: one registered nurse day shift, registered nurse night shift, nursing assistant
  - Select/mentor a three-person team to review National Database of Nursing Quality Indicators data for quality improvement nurse-sensitive indicator information to inform the rollout plan

Outcome Identification

- Collaboratively apply the *Dream* step of the 5-D model of appreciative inquiry:
  - Reflection, dialogue, envisioning

- Invite storytelling to inspire new creativity
- Explore evidence-based and evidence-informed best practices:
  - Select/mentor a four-person team for research (webinars, hospital library)
    - Provide unit coverage to support research process
- Utilize out-of-the-box creative and critical thinking:
  - Record ideas and insights: story boards, vision boards

Therapeutic Care Plan and Interventions

- Collaboratively apply the *Design* step of the 5-D model of appreciative inquiry:
  - Co-participation in shared decision making of unit-based rollout plan
- Unit representatives present to Professional Holistic Nurse Practice Council for feedback
- Caring and business cases are identified and both considered integral within rollout plan
- Co-creation of a project-based vision statement:
  - Vision statement posted in strategic locations on the unit

Case Study (Implementation)

- Collaboratively apply the *Destiny* step of the 5-D model of appreciative inquiry:
  - Implementation of rollout plan
- Implement with enthusiasm, confidence, and commitment
- Model and uphold self-care practices for resiliency:
  - Breaks, hand massages, tea time, aromatherapy
  - Grounding and centering practices
- Foster engagement, partnership, personal/professional empowerment

Evaluation

- Collaboratively reflect on the process, remaining open to revision as needed

- Acknowledge and celebrate the process and outcome
- Recognize each person for his or her valuable contribution
- Include as an exemplar in the mentorship program
- Consider the possibility for unit-based research, poster presentation, and publication
- Apply the *Definition* step of the 5-D model of appreciative inquiry:
  - Begin cycle again with intention of refining the process and preparing for future initiatives

Next Steps

Becoming a holistic leader is a *process* that takes *practice, patience*, and *reflection*. Although the core characteristics of holistic leadership, as identified in this chapter, are fundamentally interrelated and integral with one another, consider selecting one of these characteristics each week and focus on strategic integration of that characteristic within nursing practice. At the end of the week, create the opportunity for reflection, considering what went well, what needs change, and how to best enrich the practice environment with creative approaches. Then, the next week, select another characteristic and continue through all the core characteristics, repeating the cycle with the intention to develop a "felt experience" of holistic leadership as a progressive leadership model and framework.

The development of an innovative and compelling value proposition for nursing requires nurses to play key roles in healthcare transformation. Nurses, as holistic leaders, are catalysts and architects-of-change, who, through the cultivation of true collaboration, contribute to the creation of an enlightened therapeutic healing environment.

Directions for Future Research

1. Explore the relationship between integration of the characteristics of holistic leadership and nurse satisfaction, nurse retention, and nurse-partner-colleague communication and engagement.

2. Utilize the principles of holistic leadership to increase nursing structural empowerment.

3. Implement various unit-based research models (narrative research inquiry, appreciative inquiry) to measure the effects and outcomes of holistic leadership integration.

4. Evaluate how holistic leadership creates opportunities for nurse empowerment, autonomy, and collegiality.

Nurse Healer Reflections

After reading this chapter, the nurse healer will be able to answer or begin a process of answering the following questions:

- How am I integrating the seven core characteristics of holistic leadership within my nursing practice?
- Am I practicing and role modeling the AHNA Core Value 5: *Holistic Nurse Self-Reflection and Self-Care* as a holistic leader? How have my self-care practices influenced and supported me personally and professionally?
- What gaps do I see in my holistic leadership competencies?
- How do I inspire and collaborate with my partners and colleagues to "bring their best selves" to the workplace?
- What professional practice model am I utilizing as a container for my practice as a holistic leader? What is my theoretical framework?
- In what ways has my role as a holistic leader impacted the elevation and advancement of the nursing profession? Of healthcare reform? Of global health?

NOTES

1. A. Rao, "The Contemporary Construction of Nurse Empowerment," *Journal of Nursing Scholarship* 44, no. 4 (2012): 396–402.
2. Merriam-Webster, "Visionary" (2014). www.merriam-webster.com/dictionary/visionary.
3. M. Atkinson, "Magnet Hospital: Are You a Transformational Leader?" *Nursing Management* 42, no. 9 (2011): 44–50.
4. E. S. Marshall, *Transformational Leadership in Nursing: From Expert Clinician to Influential Leader* (New York: Springer, 2011): 4–6.
5. American Nurses Credentialing Center, "Magnet Recognition Program® Model" (2014). www.nursecredentialing.org/magnet/programoverview/new-magnet-model.
6. M. Frisina, *Influential Leadership: Change Your Behavior, Change Your Organization, Change Health Care* (Chicago: American Hospital Association, 2011).
7. Greenleaf Center for Servant Leadership, "What Is Servant Leadership?" (n.d.). https://greenleaf.org/what-is-servant-leadership/.
8. M. Neill and N. Saunders, "Servant Leadership: Enhancing Quality Care and Staff Satisfaction," *Journal of Nursing Administration* 28, no. 9 (2008): 395–400.
9. V. Andrus and M. Shanahan, "Holistic Leadership," in *Core Curriculum for Holistic Nursing*, 2nd ed., eds. M. Helming, C. Barrere, K. Avino, and D. Shields (Burlington, MA: Jones & Bartlett Learning, 2014): 61–72.
10. M. Shanahan, "The BirchTree Center Model: Transforming the Healthcare System with Heart!" *Beginnings* 34, no. 3 (2014): 6–9, 30.
11. J. Duffy, *Quality Caring in Nursing: Applying Theory to Clinical Practice, Education, and Leadership* (New York: Springer, 2009).
12. A. Donabedian, "Methods for Deriving Criteria for Assessing the Quality of Medical Care," *Medical Care Review* 37, no. 7 (1980): 653–698.
13. J. Nyberg, *A Caring Approach in Nursing Administration* (Boulder, CO: University Press of Colorado, 1998).
14. C. Chantal, J. Nyberg, and S. Brousseau, "Fostering the Coexistence of Caring Philosophy and Economics in Today's Health Care System," *Nursing Administration Quarterly* 35, no. 1 (2011): 6–14.
15. D. J. Clandinin and J. Huber, "Narrative Inquiry," in *International Encyclopedia of Education*, 3rd ed., eds. B. McGaw, E. Baker, and P. P. Peterson (New York: Elsevier, in press).
16. Center for Appreciative Inquiry, "What Is Appreciative Inquiry (AI)?" (2014). www.centerforappreciativeinquiry.net/more-on-ai/what-is-appreciative-inquiry-ai/.
17. Center for Appreciative Inquiry, "Generic Processes of Appreciative Inquiry" (2014). www.centerforappreciativeinquiry.net/more-on-ai/the-generic-processes-of-appreciative-inquiry/.

18. H. Owen, *The Spirit of Leadership: Liberating the Leader in Each of Us* (San Francisco: Berrett-Koehler, 1999): 53.

19. E. Wharton. "Vesalius in Zante (1564)" in *North American Review* (November, 1902, p. 631.).

20. Oxford Dictionaries, "Visionary" (2014). www.oxforddictionaries.com/definition/american_english/visionary.

21. L. Secretan, *Inspirational Leadership: Destiny, Calling and Cause* (Toronto, Ontario: MacMillan Canada, 1999).

22. American Holistic Nurses Association, *Position Statement on Holistic Nursing Ethics* (Flagstaff, AZ: American Holistic Nurses Association, revised and approved 2012).

23. American Holistic Nurses Association and American Nurses Association, *Holistic Nursing: Scope and Standards of Practice*, 2nd ed. (Silver Spring, MD: Nursesbooks.org, 2013).

24. C. A. Huang and J. Lynch, *Tao Mentoring* (New York: Marlowe, 1999): xi.

25. Institute of Medicine, *The Future of Nursing: Leading Change, Advancing Health*, Report Brief (Washington, DC: National Academies Press, 2010): 1.

26. Centers for Medicare and Medicaid Services, "Hospital Value-Based Purchasing" (2014). www.cms.gov/Medicare/Quality-Initiatives-Patient-Assessment-Instruments/hospital-value-based-purchasing/index.html?redirect=/hospital-value-based-purchasing.

27. Centers for Medicare and Medicaid Services, "Hospital Consumer Assessment of Healthcare Providers and Systems" (2014). www.hcahpsonline.org/home.aspx.

28. American Association of Critical-Care Nurses, "The AACN Synergy Model for Patient Care" (2014). www.aacn.org/wd/certifications/docs/synergymodelforpatientcare.pdf.

29. D. Reinbeck and V. Fitzsimons, "Improving the Patient Experience Through Bedside Shift Report," *Nursing Management* 44, no. 2 (2013): 16–17.

30. L. Butcher, "Shared Decision-Making: Giving the Patient a Say. No, Really," *Hospitals and Health Networks* 87, no. 5 (2013): 26–31.

31. Press Ganey Associates, "Press Ganey Acquired National Database of Nursing Quality Indicators (NDNQI®)" (June 10, 2014). www.pressganey.com/newsLanding/2014/06/10/press-ganey-acquires-national-database-of-nursing-quality-indicators-(ndnqi-).

32. Merriam-Webster, "Courage" (2014). www.merriam-webster.com/dictionary/courage.

33. Merriam-Webster, "Advocate" (2014). www.merriam-webster.com/dictionary/advocate.

34. Institute of Medicine, *The Future of Nursing: Leading Change, Advancing Health* (Washington, DC: National Academies Press, 2010): S3.

35. H. Boehm and S. Morast, "Quiet Time: A Daily Period Without Distractions Benefits Both Patients and Nurses," *American Journal of Nursing* 109, Suppl 11 (2009): 29–32.

36. S. Nahm and G. Mack, "Goodbye, Post-Acute Care," *Modern Healthcare* 43, no. 3 (2013): 26.

37. R. Gilden, "Desired Environmental Health Competencies for Registered Nurses" (2010). http://envirn.org/pg/groups/3755/environmental-health-scope-and-standards-of-practice/.

38. C. M. Smith, "Why Nurses Are Involved with Environmental Health" (June 1, 2010). http://envirn.org/pg/pages/view/1781/why-nurses-are-involved-with-environmental-health.

39. V. L. Andrus, "Transformational Leadership for Organizational Change," in *The Integrative Healing Arts Program Training Manual: Session One* (Florence, MA: BirchTree Center Press, 2011): p. 55.

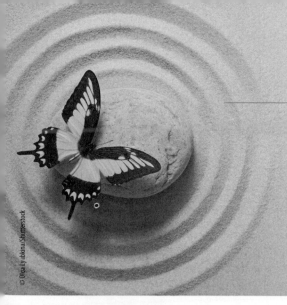

CHAPTER 26

Holistic Nursing Education

Karen M. Avino, Mary A. Helming, Deborah A. Shields, and Mary Ann Cordeau

Nurse Healer Objectives

Theoretical

- Compare and contrast various methods of curriculum integration.
- Name the theoretical basis for clinical simulation in nursing.

Clinical

- Discuss a variety of means to integrate holistic content into clinical and experiential learning experiences.
- Create opportunities to integrate holistic concepts into patient care.

Personal

- Reflect on methods of learning for self-growth in holism.
- Describe how to apply for holistic endorsement of a nursing education program.

Definitions

Clinical scenario: The plan of an expected and potential course of events for a simulated clinical experience. The clinical scenario provides the context for the simulation and can vary in length and complexity, depending on the objectives. The clinical scenario design includes participant preparation; prebriefing (review of objectives, instructions prior to implementation of scenario, questions, or other resources used in the scenario): patient information describing the situation to be managed; participant objectives; environmental conditions, including mannequin, setting, or standardized patient preparation; related equipment, props, and tools or resources for assessing and managing the simulated experience to increase the realism; roles, expectations, or limitations of each role to be played by participants; a progression outline including a beginning and an ending; debriefing; and evaluation criteria.[1, pp. S4–S5]

Curriculum: A formal set of content and outcomes to be mastered with identification of the learning activities designed to reach specific educational goals.

Fidelity: Believability, or the degree to which a simulated experience approaches reality; as fidelity increases, realism increases. The level of fidelity is determined by the environment, the tools and resources used, and the many factors associated with the participants. Fidelity can involve a variety of dimensions, including physical factors such as environment, equipment, and related tools; psychological factors such as emotions, beliefs, and self-awareness of participants; social factors such as participant and instructor motivation and goals; culture of the group; and degree of openness and trust, as well as participants' modes of thinking.[1, p. S6]

Levels of fidelity: Low-fidelity simulation involves task trainers or static mannequins used for teaching specific skills. Moderate-fidelity simulation involves more realistic mannequins with breath and heart sounds used for problem solving or teaching assessment skills. High-fidelity simulation involves the use of computerized mannequins or standardized patients in realistic environments and can be used in teaching the cognitive, affective, and psychomotor skills needed for professional practice.

Simulated-based learning experiences: An array of structured activities that represent actual or potential situations in education and practice and allow participants to develop or enhance knowledge, skills, and attitudes or analyze and respond to realistic situations in a simulated environment or through an unfolding case study.[1, p. S9]

Skill acquisition (skill attainment): After instruction, the ability to integrate the knowledge, skills (technical and nontechnical), and attitudes necessary to provide safe patient care. The individual progresses through five stages of proficiency: novice, advanced beginner, competent, proficient, and expert.[1, p. S9]

Standardized patient: A person trained to consistently portray a patient or other individual in a scripted scenario for the purposes of instruction, practice, or evaluation.[1, p. S9]

Introduction

Once upon a time, holism was a core component of nursing practice. An emphasis on technology tipped the scale to a focus on the science of nursing and the tasks of "doing." Acknowledging this imbalance, an interest in bringing the art back into nursing spurred the development of the American Holistic Nurses Association (AHNA) in 1981. A review of the 1980s literature confirmed that there were many articles written about the need for change.[2-8]

From 1990 to 2000, schools of nursing began to discuss and publish how to integrate holistic nursing into a concept-packed curriculum.[9-18]

More recent articles discuss specific competencies of holistic nursing and how to transfer this knowledge into actual nursing practice using simulation and experiential learning.[19-22] Articles that now address curriculum integration originate from outside the United States in such countries as Scotland, West Africa, China, and others.[23-25] This chapter will provide the details of curriculum integration and the transfer of holistic nursing knowledge into practice. Program exemplars will be given to help guide others on this journey.

The Need

Professional nursing practice uses standards to guide its practice and curricula. The Commission on Collegiate Nursing Education provides standards for professional nursing practice and also recommends that nursing programs adopt the American Association of Colleges of Nursing's *Essentials of Baccalaureate Education* to guide nursing curriculum development.[26] Concepts of holistic nursing are woven as recommendations throughout the *Essentials* document, such as caring, healing techniques, compassionate care, complementary and alternative therapies, health promotion, culturally diverse care, and spiritual care.

Presently, nursing specialty organizations develop additional standards to emphasize practice in a particular area. *Holistic Nursing: Scope and Standards of Practice, Second Edition*, serves as a foundation for holistic nursing practice.[27] The five AHNA Core Values from the Scope and Standards of Practice guided the development of this textbook to provide a comprehensive foundation for practice knowledge content that includes knowledge competencies, holistic theories, and supportive research.

Undergraduate Curriculum: University of Delaware, Newark, DE

Curriculum is commonly known as a formal set of goals, content, and outcomes to be mastered. Curriculum identifies the learning activities designed to reach specific educational goals.

Nelms said it best when stating that curriculum is to be viewed holistically as

> the educational journey, in an educational environment in which the biography of the person interacts with the history of the culture of nursing through the biography of another person to create meaning and release potential in the lives of all participants.[28, p. 6]

It is important to educate students as well as all faculty on the holistic concepts and complementary and integrative therapies to ensure that values and beliefs are conveyed to students not only through formal teaching but in hidden curriculum methods such as verbal and nonverbal communication. There have been curricular concerns about the need to include education in the concepts of holistic nursing rather than just providing content on specific complementary therapies, which are often associated with holistic nursing practice. Developing a holistic perspective of patient care is the core of nursing practice that can be expressed through complementary therapies. Using the five AHNA Core Values of holistic nursing ensures this.

Concept Map

Nurses can become confident in holistic nursing practice and providing appropriate complementary and integrative therapies when it is put into the context of the professional nursing practice qualities of assessment, reflection, and holism. The first step is to identify the AHNA Core Values and their placement and progression in the curriculum. As the AHNA Core Values become an integral part of the curriculum, knowledge development in complementary therapies will naturally follow. As an example, a concept map is proposed for use by the University of Delaware School of Nursing. Undergraduate course numbers can be placed in **Table 26-1** to correspond to placement of the five AHNA Core Value concepts in the curriculum.

Complementary Therapies and Scope of Practice

There is a wide range of complementary therapies available to consumers. It is within nursing's scope of practice as stated in the Board of Registered Nursing's Nurse Practice Act to provide care and comfort to patients through a variety of nursing interventions. It is commonly known that many nurses are unsure of which complementary therapies are permitted within their scope of practice. An accepted approach to integration of complementary therapies in curriculum is to review each individual state's Nurse Practice Act to identify accepted holistic nursing practice (see the AHNA website www.ahna.org/Resources/Publications/State-Practice-Acts for more information).

Most states have no mention of the words *holism/holistic* or recognition of holistic nursing as a specialty. However, 17 states have separate documents or statements regarding complementary therapies including Arkansas, California, Colorado, Florida, Kentucky, Louisiana, Maine, Massachusetts, Minnesota, New Hampshire, New York, North Carolina, North Dakota, Oregon, Pennsylvania, Texas, and Vermont. Education regarding scope of practice should include information to review the Board of Registered Nursing's Practice Act, recognition of basic care and comfort as a nursing intervention, and use of quality resources, critical thinking ability, and decision-making skills for determining appropriate care for clients. It should be emphasized to students that proper credentialing and patient consent are important. Nurses use complementary therapies to meet their clients' needs to promote healing, wellness, relaxation, and balance. As long as the evidence supports safe practice, and no additional licensure, credentials, or training is required to provide a complementary therapy, care is provided as a basic care and comfort nursing intervention.

In 2001, Frisch first clarified how holistic nursing interventions can be integrated into care and identified as professional nursing practice.[13] Developing nursing diagnosis provides a framework for naming and documenting a patient's lived experience. Nursing diagnoses are statements of problems or risks for and/or identification of openness and opportunities to enhance an individual's health status. **Table 26-2** provides possible NANDA and holistic practice pairings. This could be a useful and accepted way for

TABLE 26-1   Concepts of the American Holistic Nurses Association Core Values Across Three Levels of Baccalaureate Nursing Courses

Core Value 1	Sophomore Level	Junior Level	Senior Level
Holistic Philosophy	Writes personal philosophy based on knowledge of holistic practice.	Applies philosophy.	Reflects and revises personal philosophy for practice.
University of Delaware undergraduate courses	2XX	3XX	4XX
Theory	Remembers theoretical perspectives.	Applies theory to practice; compares/contrasts theories.	Synthesizes theory in practice settings.
University of Delaware undergraduate courses	2XX	3XX	4XX
Ethics	Remembers ethical theory.	Applies ethical principles in practice.	Internalizes ethical principles for beginning professional practice.
University of Delaware undergraduate courses	2XX	3XX	4XX
Core Value 2	**Sophomore Level**	**Junior Level**	**Senior Level**
Holistic Caring Process	Initiates nursing practice based on the process.	Moves practice to increasing levels of complexity and diversity in keeping with standards of holistic practice.	Moves practice to increasing levels of complexity and diversity in keeping with standards of holistic practice.
University of Delaware undergraduate courses	2XX	3XX	4XX
Core Value 3	**Sophomore Level**	**Junior Level**	**Senior Level**
Holistic Communication	Demonstrates professional and cultural competence in communication.	Demonstrates therapeutic communication.	Extends communication skills to community/group settings.
University of Delaware undergraduate courses	2XX	3XX	4XX
Therapeutic Environment	Maintains an environment conducive to healing in structural settings.	Maintains an environment conducive to healing in increasingly unpredictable and unstructured settings.	Maintains an environment conducive to healing in increasingly unpredictable and unstructured settings.
University of Delaware undergraduate courses	2XX	3XX	4XX
Cultural Diversity	Describes similarities and differences among people.	Uses knowledge in practice decisions of increasing complexity.	Uses knowledge in practice decisions of increasing complexity.
University of Delaware undergraduate courses	2XX	3XX	4XX
Core Value 4	**Sophomore Level**	**Junior Level**	**Senior Level**
Holistic Education	Values ways of knowing and learning.	Applies a wide range of norms and practices to a variety of backgrounds.	Collaborates to guide individuals/ families in healthcare decisions and options.

TABLE 26-1   Concepts of the American Holistic Nurses Association Core Values Across Three Levels of Baccalaureate Nursing Courses (*continued*)

Core Value 4 (*continued*)	Sophomore Level	Junior Level	Senior Level
University of Delaware undergraduate courses	2XX	3XX	4XX
Research	Acknowledges the need for evidence in practice decisions.	Reads and critiques research articles.	Uses published research findings as evidence for practice decisions.
University of Delaware undergraduate courses	2XX	3XX	4XX

Core Value 5	Sophomore Level	Junior Level	Senior Level
Holistic Nurse Self-Care	Creates self-care techniques and practice plans and applies techniques throughout the education program.	Maintains self-care techniques and practice plans.	Maintains self-care techniques and practice plans.
University of Delaware undergraduate courses	2XX	3XX	4XX

Source: Modified from AHNA.

TABLE 26-2   Nursing Diagnosis and Holistic Nursing Interventions

Nursing Diagnosis/ Concern	Nursing Intervention(s)	Rationale
Impaired comfort	Acupressure, Therapeutic Touch	To decrease perceived pain
Disturbed sleep pattern	Massage	To promote relaxation, rest
Social isolation	Animal-assisted therapy	To provide affection
Impaired coping	Humor	To facilitate appreciation of that which is funny, to relieve tension
Hopelessness	Hope instillation	To promote a positive sense of the future
Spiritual distress	Spiritual support	To facilitate a sense of inner peace
Spiritual well-being	Spiritual growth facilitation	To support growth/reflection and reexamination of values
Anxiety or fear	Guided imagery, relaxation therapy, biofeedback, calming techniques	To reduce sense of anxiety
Impaired communication	Art therapy	To facilitate expression
Disturbed energy field	Therapeutic Touch	To facilitate self-healing
Stress overload	Stress management, breathing techniques	To promote self-care
Self-health management	Nurse coaching	To facilitate self-discovery

faculty to easily integrate holistic nursing practices into their courses.

Curriculum Development

Ideally, opportunities for complementary therapy experiences should be integrated throughout the curriculum. In order for students to develop a holistic vision for their nursing practice, self-development is necessary and requires time for reflection and experiential opportunities for self-discovery. By first incorporating the body-mind-spirit aspects of care for self, this then transfers to understanding holistic care of individuals, families, and communities. Undergraduate students should become familiar with a broad range of complementary therapies to become a health-promotion resource. Students learn the concepts that underlie complementary therapies practices, develop awareness of specific therapies, and develop skill in holistically assessing, evaluating, and referring patients to the interprofessional team members. This also broadens the student's cultural practices awareness and acceptance of individuals' belief systems.

Some curriculum topics include the following:

- The role of nurses in the Affordable Care Act related to health promotion
- The holistic concepts that guide Eastern medicine and cultures
- Psychoneuroimmunology: the stress response and immune function
- Holistic nursing theorists and systems theory
- Evaluation of safety and efficacy and referral of complementary therapies as nursing interventions
- Self-care plan and vision development for holistic nursing practice

Experiential learning, discussion groups, and skill development can be used to facilitate this process. Experiential learning involves exposure to educational experiences that include hands-on training, observation, and personal participation. Effective time-saving faculty utilization measures could include the use of videotaped demonstrations of therapies and didactic lectures to be viewed before discussion in class. The University of Minnesota's Center for Spirituality and Healing offers a free online Healthcare Professional Series on complementary therapies that can be used to provide students with background information (see www.csh.umn.edu/modules/index.html). In addition, videotaping guest lecturers on various specialized topics to be used in future semesters is one way to avoid duplication of effort and burnout of volunteer speakers.

Providing holistic care includes critical thinking and taking into account the patient's beliefs, values, and cultural environment. It is not obvious to students with little life experience to recognize and make meaning out of the various factors that can affect healing in clients. To create practice experiences for students with little clinical experience, the Healthcare Theater at the University of Delaware provides an experiential learning opportunity. The course NURS 235, Health: Promotion and Vulnerability, includes four scenarios related to the topics of culture, folk medicine, homelessness, and physical disability.

Chlan and colleagues developed undergraduate competencies in complementary therapies.[20] The intention of competencies is to offer direction to faculty in providing content. Students should achieve these competencies after progressing through the entire curriculum (see **Table 26-3**). Competencies are integrated into identified courses as individual course outcomes and noted in the course syllabi. Table 26-3 has been updated to fit the needs of the School of Nursing at the University of Delaware and proposed for use.

Undergraduate Curriculum: Quinnipiac, Hamden, CT

At Quinnipiac University (QU) in Hamden, Connecticut, the Bachelor of Science in Nursing (BSN)—basic, generic, and accelerated—and Master of Science in Nursing (MSN) programs are currently endorsed by the American Holistic Nurses Certification Corporation (AHNCC). Additional new programs at QU include the Doctor of Nursing Practice (DNP) graduate programs, post-BSN and post-MSN, the Certified Nurse Anesthesia DNP program, and the online RN to BSN program. Initial holistic endorsement was applied for following the AHNCC

TABLE 26-3   University of Delaware School of Nursing Undergraduate Complementary and Integrative Therapy Competencies

Complementary Therapy Competency	Nursing-Specific Competency	Course #
1. Create an environment where patients openly discuss their use of complementary therapies	1A. Obtain information from all patients/clients on the use of any integrative modalities.	2XX
	1B. Recognize how your own cultural and spiritual beliefs may affect one's interaction with patients/clients/families.	2XX
	1C. Practice deep listening/presence when interacting with patients/clients/families.	3XX
	1D. Interact with all patients/clients/families in a nonjudgmental manner if different healthcare practices or non-Western healthcare/healing systems are practiced by clients.	3XX
2. Evaluate the safety and efficiency of selected complementary therapies for patient/client use.	2A. Demonstrate knowledge of the range of therapies included in the five complementary therapy domains including the historical and cultural context, scientific rationale for use, and supporting evidence: ■ Alternative healing systems ■ Mind–body interventions ■ Energy therapies ■ Manipulative/body-based therapies ■ Biologically based therapies	3XX
	2B. Conduct research-based integrative literature reviews on representative complementary therapies for symptoms and patient problems amenable to nursing intervention.	4XX
3. Advise patients regarding their use of complementary therapies from an evidence-based perspective.	3A. Have knowledge of appropriate Web-based and print sources for reliable and scientific information on complementary therapies.	4XX
	3B. Demonstrate knowledge and understanding of the evidence base on those complementary therapy interventions integral to bachelor of science nursing practice (see competency 5).	4XX
4. Work within an interdisciplinary team that includes complementary therapy practitioners.	4A. Demonstrate the ability and skill to be a contributing member of an interdisciplinary care team that includes complementary therapy practitioners in all leadership-focused courses.	4XX
	4B. Integrate provision of complementary therapies by appropriate practitioners into a patient/client care plan as desired or indicated.	4XX

(continues)

TABLE 26-3   University of Delaware School of Nursing Undergraduate Complementary and Integrative Therapy Competencies (*continued*)

Complementary Therapy Competency	Nursing-Specific Competency	Course #
5. Incorporate appropriate complementary therapies into practice or provide appropriate referrals.	5A. Demonstrate knowledge and beginning skills in the following complementary interventions: ▪ Acupressure (i.e., P6 for nausea) ▪ Music ▪ Nutrition counseling ▪ Aromatherapy ▪ Guided imagery ▪ Meditation ▪ Simple muscle relaxation ▪ Healing/touch therapies ▪ Presence/deep listening	4XX
	5B. Provide referral to licensed complementary therapy practitioners as indicated.	4XX
6. Integrate self-reflection and self-care into personal health and wellness.	6A. Learn and practice one self-care technique while a student, which will form the basis for lifelong self-care practices.	2XX
	6B. Participate in School of Nursing self-care activities scheduled throughout the curriculum.	All levels
	6C. Include self-care practices and reflections on self-care in all clinical log assignments.	4XX

Source: Reproduced from University of Delaware, School of Nursing, Undergraduate CAM Competencies.

guidelines, which can be found at http://ahncc .org/. The undergraduate and MSN program applications for holistic endorsement were prepared and submitted simultaneously in 2010. A holistic endorsement subcommittee with four faculty members planned and prepared this major application. A thorough review of all BSN and MSN course content was made, and holistic content was identified. A series of student and faculty exemplars that demonstrated holistic nursing practices were collected and some were submitted to AHNCC as evidence. Two faculty members were certified as advanced holistic nurses, thus meeting the requirements for at least one AHNCC-certified faculty member per program. The following discussion of

the coursework in the generic and accelerated BSN programs exemplifies a variety of courses, objectives, projects, and assigned readings that are holistic in nature. This discussion is not all inclusive; however, the aim is to give the reader a sense of how holistic nursing content can be incorporated into undergraduate curricula.

Quinnipiac University BSN students are accepted into the nursing program in the freshman year, or they transfer internally or externally into nursing in their junior year. The freshman and sophomore years at QU are dedicated to learning the basic fundamental core curriculum designated by both the university and the School of Nursing (SON). The junior and senior undergraduate years are almost entirely composed of nursing courses that are considered the professional component. Clinical practica are included beginning in the fall semester of the junior year, and the clinical, laboratory, and didactic coursework is carefully integrated so that students essentially have the opportunity to practice what they have just learned. An integrated simulation curriculum is included, and more information on holistic practice in simulation is described elsewhere in this chapter.

The SON mission "is to provide leadership in nursing and healthcare through innovative undergraduate and graduate education that embraces holism, interprofessionalism and inclusivity." The vision statement is "to prepare transformational leaders in healthcare." The SON website (www.quinnipiac.edu/academics /colleges-schools-and-departments/school-of -nursing/) highlights the following motto and explanations:

> Caring To Make a Difference: Nursing is a profession based on science, a culture of compassion, commitment to best practices, and connection to individuals. The practice of nursing is research-based, goal-directed, creative and concerned with the health and dignity of the whole person. The art of delivering quality nursing care depends upon the successful mastery and application of intellectually rigorous nursing knowledge.

The BSN program website (www.quinnipiac .edu/academics/colleges-schools-departments /school-of-nursing/programs-of-study/programs -of-study/bs-in-nursing/) includes the following emphasis on holistic nursing:

> The School of Nursing prepares nursing students for entry-level professional nursing practice as skilled providers of holistic care for families and individuals of all ages and diverse cultural backgrounds. Since nursing involves a wide range of responsibilities caring for patients across their life spans, the program utilizes a holistic framework throughout the curriculum.

The undergraduate nursing program at QU "prepares students with the knowledge, skills, and attitudes to provide holistic care for diverse individuals, families, and populations across the lifespan." Prospective students also learn about the SON's holistic endorsement, and an explanation of holistic nursing is provided at open houses.

A primary textbook that is fundamental to and required in many of the undergraduate courses is the sixth edition of Dossey and Keegan's *Holistic Nursing: A Handbook for Practice*,[29] hereafter referred to as the *Handbook*. The BSN students understand that QU features holistic nursing as essential to its objectives and that this textbook is fundamental for much of their holistic coursework. The following discussion provides examples of selected junior- and senior-year nursing courses and the ways holistic content is included in them.

NUR 300, Core Concepts in Nursing, notes in its description that "The delivery of safe, evidence-based, holistic, patient-centered care is emphasized." Overall content includes defining nursing roles, the Nurse Practice Act, the Institute of Medicine reports, the interprofessional team, and holistic nursing inclusive of its evolution and scope. Holistic content includes holistic communication, the CLEAR technique ("**C**enter Yourself, **L**isten Wholeheartedly, **E**mpathize, **A**ttention, Being Fully Present, and **R**espect"), and both therapeutic and nontherapeutic relationships and communication. Students are assigned to read "Evolving from Therapeutic to Holistic Communication" in the *Handbook*, and an in-class therapeutic communication assignment is completed. Another unit comprehensively covers holistic nursing, with assigned readings in guided imagery for pain management, as well as the AHNA Core Values and Standards of Practice. Concepts of the nurse as an instrument of healing, centering, therapeutic presence, sacred space, acceptance, transpersonal human caring, and self-reflection are included, with readings from the *Handbook*. Complementary and alternative modalities are also described, including music therapy, humor, meditation, imagery, and a variety of interventions, such as massage, Reiki, Therapeutic Touch, acupressure, and reflexology. Approximately 12 chapters from the *Handbook* are assigned. Occasionally, chapters in other course textbooks that are holistic in nature or that describe complementary and integrative therapies are also assigned readings. For example, the Assessment Technologies Institute coursework to prepare for the National Council Licensure Examination, which is threaded throughout the undergraduate BSN curricula, also has chapters with holistic content, and these are assigned as well.

In the prior year, another NUR 300 professor included two holistic student projects. For end-of-life care, a reading of the "Dying in Peace" chapter in the *Handbook* accompanied an end-of-life group assignment. The groups watched videos about a young woman dying and then an old man dying, and students discussed the differences between the two cases and how these might influence nursing care, comfort, and compassion. Another creative assignment for this course included having students write letters to themselves regarding their past selves, present selves, and future selves as they looked at life goals from a holistic standpoint. Music therapy was included, with the professor playing different genres of music to demonstrate how each brought on different emotions. Finally, students observed a photo of a piece of art representing the Irish famine and had a group discussion about its meaning, helping them to understand how art can be healing.

The junior-level BSN course NUR 302, Nursing Science and Information Literacy, "examines historical and contemporary nursing science [and] students are introduced to patterns of knowing, clinical reasoning, and select disciplinary and interdisciplinary concepts and theories useful in nursing practice." Included in the course content are concepts from the *Handbook*, including the holistic model, healing, the nurse as an instrument of healing, centering, intentionality, unconditional acceptance, and caring. The AHNA's Scope and Standards of Practice guidelines are discussed; students read the chapter on this topic and also read the "Transpersonal Human Caring and Healing" chapter. Additional holistic concepts covered include the AHNA Core Values, Kolcaba's Theory of Comfort, suffering, Watson's Philosophy

and Theory of Transpersonal Caring, sacred space, and delivering culturally relevant care. Holistically applied ethical principles are also addressed. Students complete an assignment to research and present a complementary therapy practice in the classroom. Students also are asked to identify how a nurse in a movie applies holistic concepts to patient care.

A first-semester junior-level course is NUR 304, Health Promotion and Wellness. The course description includes a focus "on health promotion, wellness, and disease and injury prevention across the lifespan." Content includes a variety of holistic topics, and numerous chapters in the *Handbook* are assigned. Healthy nutrition is discussed, and students conduct a problem-based learning project on rapid eating. Another unit covers both stress management and substance abuse. Considerable emphasis on self-care and stress management for nurses is included. Other units cover exercise, movement, and weight management. Holistically focused problem-based learning assignments, mostly done in class, include body image assessment and self-care assessment. Loss and grief are included, with a focus on the "good death" and appropriate communication skills to help care for the dying patient and deal with family members. Spirituality and prayer are discussed, especially as they relate to care of the dying patient. Therapeutic, holistic communication and developing cultural competence are also addressed. Finally, an entire class is devoted to complementary therapies in health promotion and disease prevention. Covered concepts include a variety of complementary therapies as well as herbal medications and over-the-counter supplements; students create an herb information card for problem-based learning. Guided imagery, breathing and relaxation techniques, aromatherapy, and touch and energetic therapies are covered.

NUR 307, Core Nursing Practicum, is taken concurrently with junior-level didactic classes. As part of the clinical practice, students work on therapeutic communication skills and do an oral presentation on complementary therapies with older adults, focusing especially on pet, art, music, and dance therapies. Quality and safety in nursing, covered in the *Handbook*, is also a related topic. NUR 330L, Holistic Nursing Integration Lab I, is a clinical laboratory class that includes physical assessment practice. Holistic content includes practice with therapeutic communication and evaluation of alternative and homeopathic healthcare practices (e.g., massage therapy, acupuncture, herbal medicine, and mineral supplements).

The senior-year course NUR 400, Psychiatric-Mental Health Nursing, "examines concepts of nursing management for individuals with psychiatric-mental health needs across the lifespan. The delivery of safe, evidence-based, holistic, patient-centered care is emphasized." Cultural implications of nursing care, communication skills, therapeutic relationships, therapeutic environment, and stress management are among the topics with holistic influence. Cognitive behavioral therapy and behavior modification techniques, covered in the *Handbook*, are included. This course describes spiritual distress, substance abuse and recovery, and incorporating cultural practices and beliefs, all topics included in the *Handbook*.

NUR 424, Care of Adults with Complex Health Needs II, a senior-level course, includes the following description of its content: "This course examines concepts of nursing management for adults with complex, high acuity healthcare needs requiring sophisticated patient care technologies. The delivery of safe, evidence-based, holistic, patient-centered care is emphasized." A significant component of this course involves nursing end-of-life care, including care of the caregivers. Concepts from the End-of-Life Nursing Education Consortium guide are included to augment the basic holistic principles of care of the dying and hospice care. Nonpharmacological, holistic palliative care measures are described.

Another example of a final-year nursing clinical laboratory course is NUR 430L, Holistic Nursing Integration Lab III. An important topic that is covered holistically is care of the depressed patient, including one with suicidal ideation. Therapeutic communication and a clinical scenario, using simulated, high-fidelity mannequins, are included to teach senior students how to manage the depressed patient from a holistic viewpoint.

NUR 426, Pathophysiology and Pharmacology II, a combined course, includes faculty reading of topically relevant poetry written by another faculty member who is a nurse–poet. For example, a poem describing a nurse's reaction to her blood exposure with HIV-positive (human immunodeficiency virus) blood is included. Holistic nursing integrates with the humanities as well; for example, in past courses, nursing students have practiced creating mandalas and writing holistically focused poetry.

Quinnipiac University also has a new RN–BSN program. An example of one of its online courses, NUR 382, which includes holistic content, will be discussed. It has similar content to the NUR 302 on-ground course described previously, but one assignment for these students is to describe how they use or could use the holistic model in their practices. It was discovered that many nurses in practice do not truly understand the holistic model, so the students were excited to have this new knowledge.

Finally, to segue into the following section describing how numerous high-fidelity simulation scenarios that include providing holistic care to "patients" have been created, a complex, interprofessional simulation scenario on end-of-life care was created by nursing faculty and other healthcare professionals from the Interprofessional Simulation Learning and Assessment Committee. Quinnipiac University is committed to interprofessional education and practice and has established the Center for Interprofessional Healthcare Education. This 4-week interprofessional scenario utilized students from nursing, DNP, physician assistant, athletic training, occupational therapy, physical therapy, and Master of Social Work programs. The scenario is described in the following manner:

Week 1:

- Part 1: Held outside on the front green of the school. Josh (played by a student) is a 16-year-old soccer player injured on the soccer field. Emergency Medical Services (played by an athletic training [AT] student) and a physician's assistant ([PA] played by a PA student) assess him, splint his leg for possible femur fracture, put him on a backboard and stretcher, and transfer him to the simulation suite (4th floor, nursing). Scene ends.

- Part 2: Josh (portrayed by a mannequin) is in the emergency room. The PA and nursing student assess him. Josh's mother (played by a faculty member) comes into the room distraught. A social work (SW) student is there to help her. Josh needs surgery. Scene ends.
- Part 3: In the postanesthesia care unit. Josh (as a mannequin) just came out of surgery. His parents (played by faculty) are at his bedside. Occupational therapy (OT), physical therapy (PT), SW, PA, nursing, and perfusion (cardio perfusion) students are also at his bedside. Josh is on a ventilator and extracorporeal membrane oxygenation machine. The surgeon found something suspicious during surgery and biopsied it. The team needs to tell the family.

Week 2:

- In the simulation lab, orthopedic unit. Josh (as a mannequin) has his parents at his bedside (played by a faculty member and a student). The healthcare team (NP, nursing, OT, PT, and SW) needs to tell them that the biopsy came back positive for osteosarcoma.

Week 3:

- Hospice homecare. Josh is home (mannequin in simulation lab). His mother (played by a faculty member) is in the room distraught and anxious because she is unable to handle Josh's increasing pain. The healthcare team of OT, PT, SW, nursing, and NP are in the room offering support and assistance.

Week 4:

- Part 1: Hospice. Josh is actively dying (mannequin in simulation lab). His parents are at his bedside. Nursing and NP are there as well. Josh dies. Pronounced by NP. Care is given. Parents view body. Parents meet with SW about arrangements.
- Part 2: Classroom setting. The OT, PT, NP, and AT need to tell their teammates that

Josh has died. The teammates (played by faculty) are sitting around the table. They each have a different reaction to the news, and members of the team must address their needs.

Using Simulated-Based Learning Experiences for Teaching Holistic Nursing Principles and Core Values: Quinnipiac University

Twenty-first century nurses are expected to provide holistic patient-centered care.[29] Students must be provided learning experiences that foster the development of the knowledge, skills, and attitudes needed for holistic nursing care. Students gain the knowledge needed in the classroom and the psychomotor skills in the laboratory. However, students need the opportunity to incorporate and practice what was learned in the classroom and skills laboratory while developing the affective domain. Clinical scenarios provide the opportunity for students to develop knowledge in all three domains in a safe, realistic, learning environment. The National League for Nursing[30] and the American Association of Colleges of Nursing[26] support the use of clinical simulation as a teaching/learning strategy for nursing education. This section discusses how clinical scenarios can be used to teach holistic nursing principles and core values.

Theory Related to Simulation-Based Learning

Educators use various theories to guide simulation-based learning. Jeffries and Rogers developed the Nursing Education Simulation Framework as a model for clinical simulation.[31] This comprehensive framework takes into account the student, teacher, and educational practices, along with outcomes and simulation design characteristics.[32] Noting that the literature did not fully examine the qualitative aspect of clinical simulation, Cordeau conducted research related to the learner experience of clinical simulation and developed a substantive theory, "Linking the Transition," that describes how "Clinical simulation fosters the situational transition from student to professional nurse by providing students with the opportunity to care for simulated patients."[32, p. E90] This theory can be used to develop clinical scenarios that foster the transition from student to professional nurse. According to Cordeau, linking is a four-stage process of managing sim-hype, encountering barriers, integrating the self, and interconnecting.[33] Cordeau discussed how nurse educators can foster student success during each stage.[33] In Stage 1, managing sim-hype, facilitators must engage in prebriefing, which includes orientation to the mannequin, environment, and scenario.[33] During this stage, it is very important to assist the student in assigning significance to the experience, which promotes optimum engagement and learning.[34] Viewing the simulation experience as having value for learning or viewing the mannequin as an actual patient requiring nursing care are two ways of assigning significance. The barriers encountered during Stage 2 can be minimized through integrating the self by focusing or zoning in. It is through interconnection or integration of the cognitive, affective, and psychomotor domains that the student learns to provide holistic nursing care.

Quinnipiac University Clinical Simulation Laboratory

Quinnipiac University has several low- and moderate-fidelity laboratories as well as a high-fidelity simulation suite. Low and moderate laboratories have multiple beds with equipment such as suction machines and simulated oxygen for each bed. The simulation suite has five patient rooms connected by a hallway. Each room is divided into two sections, a patient section and a control room. From the control room, facilitators run the clinical scenarios and observe learners through a one-way mirror. The university has three adult high-fidelity mannequins, one high-fidelity birthing mannequin, one high-fidelity newborn mannequin, and one high-fidelity pediatric mannequin. Cognitive, psychomotor, and affective skills are learned and practiced in each of the laboratory settings. With appropriate props, acute, long-term, or community setting

environments can be created in each laboratory. Streaming from the high-fidelity laboratory to the classroom is possible. Streaming allows students sitting in a classroom to observe a clinical scenario in the simulation laboratory. Faculty can also bring standardized patients and moderate- or high-fidelity mannequins into the classroom. Both of these multimodality strategies are used to teach a particular concept or multiple concepts, such as a client newly diagnosed with cancer who is demonstrating spiritual distress, thus enhancing student learning.

Clinical Simulation Process

The majority of simulation-based learning at Quinnipiac University follows the standard practice of running a clinical scenario. Prior to participating in clinical simulation experiences, students are given an orientation to the simulation suite, process, and ground rules. Common ground rules include respect for the mannequin as a patient needing holistic care, viewing the self as a student learning to practice holistic nursing, respect for classmates' learning, and adherence to Quinnipiac University's academic integrity policy. Fidelity is very important when using clinical simulation as a teaching–learning strategy. An unrealistic learning environment interferes with learning because students focus more on trying to figure out what is part of the scenario and what is not rather than on the clinical scenario experience.

Currently, simulated-learning experiences are developed to meet individual course and integrated laboratory outcomes and are conducted during the junior and senior years; however, consideration is being given to offering a course during the sophomore year. A clinical simulation experience offered during the sophomore year is an excellent teaching–learning strategy for introducing students to holistic nursing. The integrated laboratory covers content from all courses taught during the semester and provides students with the opportunity to see the connection between the didactic, laboratory, and clinical aspects of their education. Depending on the outcomes, low-, moderate-, and high-fidelity scenarios are used as well as standardized patients. One-on-one, small-group (four to five learners), and large-group streaming from the simulation laboratory to the classroom can be employed.

Holistic Nursing Core Values Scenario Development

When developing scenarios for teaching holistic nursing core values, it is important that the learner is able to experience the interconnectedness of the body-mind-emotion-spirit-environmental principles while providing care within the framework of the core values. Although holistic nursing focuses on caring for the whole person, this can be very difficult for the beginning learner. For the beginner, it is better to introduce one or two holistic principles in a single clinical simulation experience. The ability to integrate more than two holistic principles into the same scenario should be an expectation of the more experienced student. This section provides examples of which kind(s) of scenarios are most appropriate for teaching specific holistic nursing principles and provides outcomes for teaching the core values. Scenarios can take place in acute care, long-term care, home, or community settings. Although this discussion focuses on individual principles for clarity, Cordeau has discussed how more than one principle can be taught during a single clinical simulation experience.[33]

Simple or complex scenarios should be used for knowledge and skill acquisition related to physiology. Scenario outcome(s) determine the level of fidelity needed for the scenario. Bed bath, medication administration, urinary catheterization, and wound care are skills that can be taught using task trainers or low-fidelity scenarios. Assessing breath sounds or vital signs is best accomplished using a moderate-fidelity scenario. Managing the patient during a cardiac arrest or code requires the use of high-fidelity scenarios. Patient education related to a specific task such as insulin administration is best accomplished using standardized patients. The mannequins do not have electronic ability to perform the skill and, because of this, the scenario is very unrealistic and frustrating for the learner.

Promoting the knowledge and skill acquisition related to the mind, spirit, culture, and environment is best accomplished using high-fidelity mannequins, with the facilitator speaking as the patient or using a standardized patient. When using high-fidelity mannequins to teach emotion, it is important that the facilitator expresses emotion through tone of voice because there are no other cues for the student to observe. Students often state that they connect to the patient through the voice and that is what helps them imagine the mannequin as an actual patient needing care. Props such as prayer beads, a patient journal, coffee cups, food, empty alcoholic beverage containers, and books on complementary modalities or spirituality are useful for fidelity and engaging the student. When simulating a community setting, appropriate props are needed to simulate the home, community center, or other environment. Patient statements such as "I'm feeling very anxious today" or "I feel like no one understands me" or "Why is God punishing me this way?" or "Can you tell me about energy healing?" or "I don't feel safe returning to my home" interjected at appropriate times help direct the scenario.

Developed scenarios such as those found on the National League for Nursing's Advancing Care Excellence for Seniors website (www .nln.org/facultyprograms/facultyresources /aces/index.htm) can be used as presented or be adapted to meet core values. Other developed scenarios can be found in published textbooks.[35] There are several ways to employ clinical simulation to meet holistic nursing core values. Students can participate in several different individual and group scenarios to meet specific outcomes, or students can meet outcomes through caring for one or two "patients" during their nursing program. However, students could also be assigned to care for two to three patients as unfolding cases during the program. Students could "meet" their first simulated patient early in their educational experience. This can happen during a course offered to sophomore students or during a class meeting. A photo of the mannequin dressed as the patient (wig, glasses, makeup, etc.) and a voice recording of the patient narrative help connect students to the patient. The photo and voice recording can be posted on a website for future reference. A graded or nongraded assignment based on cultural diversity and care (Core Value 5) could be given to the students. This provides an introduction to holistic nursing. Throughout the student's educational experience, individual or group clinical simulations using the same patient(s) should be assigned to promote the incorporation of holistic nursing content with practice. A list of possible outcomes for the beginner (level 1) and more experienced (level 2) students are provided in **Table 26-4**.

TABLE 26-4   Outcomes to Foster the Knowledge, Skills, and Attitudes for Core Values

Possible Outcomes for AHNA Core Value 1

Level 1 Student	Level 2 Student
Describes the role of the nurse as a member of the interprofessional healthcare team.	Contacts the primary care provider to describe a changing patient condition needing attention.
Demonstrates awareness of the client's narrative.	Incorporates client's narrative when providing care.
Identifies and meets client needs in two holistic principles when providing client care.	Identifies and meets client needs related to all holistic principles when providing care.
Applies a holistic-focused midrange theory when providing care.	Applies a holistic-focused grand theory when providing care.
Identifies a moral or ethical dilemma when providing care.	Applies the Holistic Nursing Code of Ethics to a moral or ethical dilemma.

Possible Outcomes for Core Value 2

Level 1 Student	Level 2 Student
Applies the holistic nursing process to meet patient needs related to one or two holistic nursing principles.	Engages in structured reflection during debriefing.
Identifies patient patterns/challenges/needs related to motivational interviewing.	Demonstrates motivational interviewing when caring for a patient.
Demonstrates the use of one complementary therapy when providing patient care.	Provides patient education related to the use of complementary therapies.
Identifies needs and appropriate resources when caring for a patient receiving hospice care.	Provides holistic care for a dying patient and family/significant others.

Possible Outcomes for Core Value 3

Level 1 Student	Level 2 Student
Demonstrates therapeutic communication when caring for a patient.	Demonstrates holistic communication when caring for a patient.
Incorporates patient's beliefs and values when providing care in an acute/long-term care setting.	Incorporates patient's beliefs and values when providing care in the community.

Possible Outcomes for Core Value 4

Level 1 Student	Level 2 Student
Identifies patient's spiritual preferences and needs.	Demonstrates understanding of the relationship between spirituality and health.
Demonstrates listening and intentional presence when caring for a patient.	Discusses energy healing with a patient.
Meets patient's spiritual needs.	

Source: Data from Mary Ann Cordeau.

At Quinnipiac University, students are introduced to clinical simulation during the fall semester of the junior year when they participate in small-group simulations. During the fall semester of the senior year, students participate in mock codes. During the spring semester of the senior year, students take Holistic Nursing Integration Lab IV. The outcomes for this lab are student proficiency in their role as care provider, manager and coordinator of care, and member of a profession. Graded clinical simulation using low- and high-fidelity mannequins as well as standardized patients (faculty, students, and staff serve as standardized patients) is used to meet course outcomes. Scenarios include holistic care of a diabetic patient in the community, a patient with congestive heart failure in the acute care and community settings, a patient with a threatened abortion in an acute care setting, a veteran with posttraumatic stress disorder in the community, an infant with abusive head trauma in an emergency room, and caring for an adolescent in a home and inpatient hospice setting.

The scenario and assigned preparation for each week are listed in the syllabus; students do not know who will be assigned to care for the patient until the day of the clinical simulation. All students participate as nurses and observers at least once during the semester. During the first 15 minutes of class, all students are given reports and must formulate a care plan. Each week, three students are assigned to the simulated patient and three students are assigned to lead, with facilitator assistance, the debriefing session for the entire class. Once care plans have been formulated and the three nurses are prebriefed, the scenario begins with the nurses providing care while the three observers and the entire class watch the scenario as it is streamed from the simulation laboratory or acted out in the classroom live. The observers use the observation guidelines (see **Table 26-5**) to critique the nurses' performance. The scenario is designed to last approximately 20 minutes. Once the scenario is over, the observers are given time to address each question from the observation guidelines and plan for the debriefing.

TABLE 26-5   Observer Debriefing Guide
Was care patient centered?   Give evidence for answering why or why not.   Which improvements, if needed, should be implemented?
Was care delivered using holistic concepts?   Give evidence for answering why or why not.   Which improvements, if necessary, should be implemented?
Were there any safety issues?   Give evidence for answering why or why not.   Which improvements, if needed, should be implemented?
Was the nursing diagnosis appropriate?   Give evidence for answering why or why not.   Which improvements, if needed, should be implemented?   Which other nursing diagnoses would be appropriate?
Were outcomes appropriate for the patient situation?   Give evidence for answering why or why not.   Which improvements, if needed, should be implemented?   Which other outcomes would be appropriate?
Did interventions meet patient needs?   Give evidence for answering why or why not.   Which improvements, if needed, should be implemented?   Which other interventions would be appropriate?
How well did the group work as a team?   Give examples of good teamwork and teamwork that needs improvement.

Source: Data from Mary Ann Cordeau.

The instructors/facilitators use the assessment rubric (see **Table 26-6**) to grade the nurses and the debriefing rubric (see **Table 26-7**) to grade the observers.[36] Student evaluation of this course has been positive: 99% of the students who completed evaluations agreed or strongly agreed that simulated clinical experiences enhanced learning and helped prepare them for clinical practice.

TABLE 26-6   Clinical Simulation Assessment Rubric

	Very Good 4	Good 3	Needs Much Improvement 2	N/A
Patient-Centered Care				
Provided care using holistic concepts.				
Used the clinical reasoning process to develop a patient-centered care plan for assigned patient.				
Used appropriate nursing diagnosis/diagnoses.				
Determined appropriate outcomes.				
Applied appropriate interventions.				
Modified care based on patient situation.				
Elicited patient values, preferences, and expressed needs as part of the interview, implementation of care, and evaluation of care.				
Provided patient-centered care with sensitivity and respect for the diversity of human experience.				
Communicated patient values, preferences, and expressed needs to other members of the healthcare team.				
Assessed presence and extent of pain and suffering.				
Assessed levels of physical and emotional comfort.				
Elicited expectations of patient and family for relief of pain, discomfort, or suffering.				
Initiated effective treatments to relieve pain and suffering in light of patient values, preferences, and expressed needs.				
Removed barriers to presence of families and other designated surrogates based on patient preferences.				
Assessed level of patient's decisional conflict and provided access to resources.				
Engaged patients or designated surrogates in active partnerships that promote health, safety, well-being, and self-care management.				
Facilitated informed patient consent for care.				
Teamwork and Collaboration				
Demonstrated awareness of own strengths and limitations as a team member.				
Acted with integrity, consistency, and respect for differing views.				
Initiated request for help when appropriate to the situation.				
Clarified roles and accountabilities under conditions of potential overlap in team-member functioning.				

(continues)

	Very Good 4	Good 3	Needs Much Improvement 2	N/A
Teamwork and Collaboration (*continued*)				
Solicited input from other team members to improve individual and team performance				
Safety				
Demonstrated effective use of technology and standardized practices that support safety and quality.				
Demonstrated effective use of strategies to reduce risk of harm to self or others.				
Used appropriate strategies to reduce reliance on memory (checklists).				
Communicated observations or concerns related to hazards and errors to families and the healthcare team.				
Informatics				
Navigated the electronic health record.				
Documented and planned patient care in an electronic health record.				
Employed communication technologies to coordinate care for patients.				

TABLE 26-6   Clinical Simulation Assessment Rubric (*continued*)

Source: Modified from QSEN.

The Journey of Holistic Education: Entering and Beyond: Capital University, Columbus, OH

Capital University was founded in 1860 as a Lutheran School of Theology in a suburb of Columbus, Ohio. Over the years, it has transitioned to a liberal arts university while keeping the theological program intact. The baccalaureate nursing program was founded in 1950; an early revision of the curriculum incorporated holistic health concepts into all courses. The philosophy of holism, which continues today, is a valued part of the curriculum.

Capital University's Department of Nursing has four distinct programs: a traditional undergraduate program; an accelerated program for students who hold a BS in another area; a BSN completion and MSN program with concentrated areas of study that include nursing education, administration, an Adult-Gerontology Clinical Nurse Specialist program and dual degrees in nursing and business and nursing. All of the nursing programs were originally endorsed by the AHNCC in 2009 and reaccredited in 2014. The entire Capital University community is deeply honored and proud of this continuing recognition and remains committed to co-creating caring, healing learning communities.

The faculty of the Department of Nursing embraces the core values of holistic nursing as the fundamental tenets within the discipline of nursing. The AHNA Core Values and *Holistic Nursing: Scope and Standards of Practice, Second Edition*, are introduced in the entry courses in each program. Integral self-development, self-reflection, holistic communication, and therapeutic presence are foundational concepts that

TABLE 26-7 Debriefing Rubric	Very Good	Good	Needs Much Improvement
Patient-Centered Care: Aesthetic Knowing			
Used clinical reasoning process to develop care plan.	14	12	10
Peer Critique: Aesthetic Knowing			
Quality critique of patient-centered care.	12	10	9
Provided evidence for critique.			
Quality of suggested improvements.			
Quality of critique of use of holistic nursing.	14	12	10
Provided evidence for critique.			
Quality of suggested improvements.			
Quality of safety critique.	12	10	9
Provided evidence for critique.			
Quality of suggested improvements.			
Quality of critique of nursing diagnosis.	12	10	9
Provided evidence for critique.			
Appropriateness of suggested nursing diagnosis.			
Quality of critique of outcomes.	12	10	9
Provided evidence for critique.			
Appropriateness of suggested outcomes.			
Quality of critique of interventions.	12	10	9
Provided evidence for critique.			
Appropriateness of suggested outcomes.			
Quality of critique of teamwork.	12	10	9
Provided examples of good teamwork and teamwork that needs improvement.			

Source: Data from Mary Ann Cordeau.

are cultivated and nurtured throughout the students' time at Capital and beyond. Within nursing coursework, students become competent with a variety of skills and learn to make clinical judgments based on a holistic analysis of evidence and the individual context for each patient. Reflective practice underlies all didactic and clinical experiences; students engage in a variety of activities and truly experience nursing as an art and a science. The faculty believe in the importance of service and provide many opportunities for students to discover the joy of giving and receiving. Interdisciplinary engagement is seminal in creating a broadened lens through which to view the world. The goal in nursing is to support students who will graduate with a solid foundation in holism, able to articulate the importance of this philosophy, bring their caring presence into the diverse world of health care, and, ultimately, contribute to healthcare transformation.

Education at Capital University is approached from a holistic paradigm that integrates unitary and biomedical science (see Chapter 29 for specific details). This model represents a whole worldview of nursing that does not elevate one aspect to a position of dominance but rather creates an understanding and appreciation of the importance of both. In this way, the faculty believe that students will develop their abilities as nursing scientists and artists. Two textbooks that are required and used in both the pre- and postlicensure programs are *Holistic Nursing: A Handbook for Practice*[29] and *Holistic Nursing: Scope and Standards of Practice, Second Edition.*[27]

Within this broad philosophical perspective, the reader may wonder how these ideas are actualized: How do the students at Capital experience holism? What do courses and assignments look like? Are the graduates prepared for the required licensing and credentialing examinations? These are excellent questions, and what follows exemplifies some of the ways in which holism is manifest at Capital. While this discussion is not all inclusive, it is hoped that through the exploration of five curricular threads the reader can more deeply envision how holistic content can be woven into nursing curricula in both pre- and postlicensure programs.

Integral Self-Development

Integral self-development (holistic self-care) is a lifelong commitment to and process of actualizing one's potential for well-being. The core of self-development is developing the Beingness of the nurse through the intentional development of self-awareness, self-reflection, and commitment to a higher purpose.[37] Self-care activities, then, are activities that individuals initiate and perform on their own behalf to maintain their own health and well-being.[37] This commitment to self-development is taken very seriously and is, perhaps, the solid foundation on which all other components of the curricula develop. This process begins on day one and continues until graduation—and after, the faculty hope,

as graduates take their place in the nursing community.

In introducing the concept of self-development, students are initially taught about the gift of stillness—of quieting the mind and beginning to listen deeply. This is laying the groundwork for the cultivation of a discipline of contemplative practice. While many believe that this practice refers to prayer or meditation, the faculty believe that it is the engagement of reflective activities that help a person be quiet—still. For many, this at first seems like an unknown idea but, often, students discover that they have been engaged in some form of quieting through such activities as faith traditions, sports, or dance.

It is in this early time that students are also introduced to the practice of mindfulness—living in the moment, aware and present. The attitudes of mindfulness by Kabat-Zinn are explored,[38] and students consider these in their own lives. Discussions and sharing are powerful ways in which to co-create communities of discovery; they are also strategies that require patience and commitment as members find their way.

Quieting and mindfulness, then, are practiced. All classes begin with an activity such as breath awareness, which is often combined with a movement—students are encouraged to be gentle with themselves as they "learn" about stillness and to deeply sense in their bodies what they are feeling. Practice outside of class is essential, beginning with 3 to 5 minutes daily, increasing the time of their practice. Students adopt an attitude of mindfulness—to pay attention to without judging. All of this is designed to both increase students' self-awareness and ability to be still and to cultivate the discipline essential for holistic self-care. It is, in essence, the cultivation of a lifeway.

As students are more able to find their stillness, they are invited to take some time (usually 1 to 2 weeks) and complete a holistic self-assessment using the Integrative Health and Wellness Assessment located in Chapter 30. They complete the entire assessment, identify goals, and then decide which one goal is speaking the most loudly to them; for this goal, the student develops a plan with outcomes in order to achieve it. Over the years, the faculty have revised their expectations; at first, the students were asked to develop a whole plan, but that was found to be overwhelming and ineffective. Because this assessment and plan follows the students throughout their entire educational program, there is adequate time to revise and reshape, and thus it has been transformed into a lived experience. Faculty in all courses check on the progress and support students as indicated.

Integral self-development is a part of every course; over time, students are introduced to a variety of quieting activities. For example, in one course students create a mandala; in another, they color one that they locate; in more than one course, students take mindfulness walks and also walk in the neighborhood labyrinth. In another course, students read a book and facilitate a "book club," a moving and reflective experience. Most important, the reader can see that self-development, grounded in contemplative practice, is initiated at the outset, continued in each course, reflected in the personality of that particular learning community, and deepened over time. The process is supported by faculty and, as students become increasingly engaged, they support one another as partners/coaches—it always *is*. To share the words from one student:

> My practice of deep breathing, which I thought in the beginning to be such a cliché, has led to so many insights for me. . . . Practice has given me the gift of healing.

Integral self-development—a beautiful process of self-awareness, quiet, and gentleness to self—is discussed in depth in Chapter 29. It is a discipline and, the faculty believe, foundational in the development of a healing consciousness.

Reflective Practice

Nursing is a discipline of knowledge grounded in holistic values, principles, and caring, which incorporates an area of scholarly study and an expert, complex field of professional practice.[39] The focus of nursing as a discipline and a profession is, according to Boykin and Schoenhofer, to promote the processes of being and becoming through caring.[40]

Reflective practice is part of classroom and clinical experiences. In the classroom, students participate in a variety of activities and reflect

on them. For example, in one assessment course, the students do a group project related to men's and women's health; they decide how the project will unfold, all of the nuances, and, upon completion, share their reflections about the experience. In clinical experiences, students are introduced to ways of becoming present and focused on the moment. Hand washing is suggested by many faculty as a ritual of being in the moment. The important point is that students are being taught to be attentive and focused; it is such a critically important part of practice.

The faculty believe that reflective practice is an expression of the holistic nurse that the student is. It is a weaving together of reflection on and within experience—an exploration of self as the student deepens his or her holistic nursing practice. It might be thought of as a lifeway grounded in compassionate self-inquiry, self-awareness, and mindfulness, and, as such, a part of our continuous becoming.

> Reflection is living through our everyday experiences towards realizing one's vision of desirable practice as a lived reality. . . . It is a critical and reflective process of self-inquiry and transformation of being and becoming the practitioner you desire to be.[41]

> Reproduced from C. Johns Reflection as a way of being in practice. In H. L. Erickson (Ed.), Modeling and role-modeling at work, (2010). (pp. 311–328). Cedar Park, Texas: Unicorns Unlimited.

Reflective practice invites us to be open to all viewpoints, nonjudging and willing to change. From this place we can, as caring nurses, bear witness and interweave into our practice all ways of knowing, clear on the value of each. According to Johns, "Being mindful is the quintessential nature of reflective practice."[42, p. 313] Toward that end, students are asked to journal and share their practice through narrative, art, poetry, or whichever way is the best for them to do this.

Guidelines for journaling vary; the following are a few examples of ways reflective practice is incorporated into courses:

- *BSNC course.* A mindfulness meditation journal is due biweekly in class. This assignment is designed to increase your ability to be mindful for self-care, improved communication, and safe nursing practice. We will examine the seven attitudinal foundations of mindfulness practice. In 2-week increments you will be introduced to one or two foundations. In your journal you will reflect on those attitudes and your 5-minute meditation; two reflections per week are required.

- *Accelerated class.* To develop the ability to be mindful in self-care and nursing practices. This assignment is worth 20% of the course grade. The journal is due weekly throughout the semester. This assignment is designed to increase your ability to be mindful for self-care, improved communication, and safe nursing practice. Each week you will reflect on mindfulness practices in your daily rounds related to self-care, communication, and nursing practice. You may also journal on observations of others' use of mindfulness practices.

- *Graduate CNS: first clinical course.* Your reflective journal is divided into two sections: One section focuses specifically on your continuing self-care and mindfulness practice, while the second section focuses on your clinical experiences. Although at first glance this may seem like two independent activities, you will likely discover the integrating thread that immersion in reflective practice offers to help you connect what you are learning in the classroom with your experience. As you track your personal and professional growth over the semester you might ask: (1) What insights am I discovering? (2) Where are my strengths? (3) Where might I grow? and (4) How am I living in this transformation?

There is a cadre of rich resources available to readers who are interested in integrating reflective practice into nursing curricula—or, perhaps, even into your own practice. You are encouraged to find ones that resonate with where you are. Most models are uniquely developed from the expert resources combined with the context of the experience. The model for the brand-new student will look different than that of one ready to graduate; remember that one key reason for reflective practice is to create the space and the discipline for holistic nurses to reflect

both in and on practice—in a way, to reflect on the holistic paradigm of care—without harsh judgment but rather with an attitude of exploration that helps us grow as nurses and deepen our practice.

Holistic Communication

While all students learn about therapeutic communication, they also spend time exploring the ideas presented in Chapter 19 on holistic communication. Course faculty develop activities based on the students' experience and the overall focus of the course. For example, the scenarios in the course related to mental health are different than those in pediatrics. However, what is not different are the principles underlying holistic communication, including the recognition that we are always communicating, being authentic, centering, setting intention, being present, and meeting people where they are—respectfully, heeding your intuition, and listening as well as hearing.

One example of supporting the student's ability to listen is the listening exercises that are conducted in several courses. These have been very powerful and revealing. In a senior prelicensure course there is a module on death and dying. At the end of the discussion, students pair up and, for 5 minutes, tell the other about a loss they have experienced; there is no writing, no questioning—only listening. Then, to the extent that they are comfortable, the pairs share with the group what it has been like to listen so deeply. A similar activity is done in a graduate course, but this time pairs are asked to share a poignant moment from their clinical practice.

Student feedback from the exercises on communication have been affirming; students are developing an awareness of their skills and areas ripe for growth. This is important in practice and in life; the adage "Say what you mean and mean what you say" can mean the difference between a healing or a less-than-healing encounter with another.

Evidence

The healthcare world is abuzz with evidence, and it is essential that nurses make decisions based on the best evidence. How does this happen? What is the difference between quality research and evidence-based practice? Chapters 27 and 28 present a comprehensive discussion about each of these, and the reader will find much information that will be helpful in developing both. As faculty, how do we support students in better understanding the world of evidence? At Capital, faculty members are committed to supporting students as they look at evidence for practice holistically.

Students are introduced to ideas about evidence in their first course, which is integrated into each and every experience thereafter. It might remind us of the questions when we were in school: What is your rationale? Why are you doing it? As they become more immersed in clinical, students always have questions; these, then, are developed more fully in that particular course and also in the research course, which is taken by every student.

The process of evidence appraisal is introduced, and students engage in this activity over a full term. They learn that the best evidence is that which supports their question; while the value of large trials are honored, so, too, are well-done qualitative studies as evidence in meaningful queries. In many courses—from the first skills lab course before beginning clinical and extending all the way to graduation with a MSN—students develop a poster or presentation related to a beginning search of evidence that supports a question they have. Examples of these include:

- *Senior prelicensure.* Gastric tube verification; exercise as part of care for people living with cancer, especially related to depression and anxiety reduction; kangaroo care for premature babies related to physiological stability; turning intervals, and skin preservation; evidence-based strategies for creating a culture of evidence-based practice; and exercise for children with type 2 diabetes.
- *BSNC.* The meaning of family presence during resuscitation for the family; the effect of no time to debrief after a traumatic event on the self-care of nurses and safety of patients; early referral to palliative care and quality of life; and biofield therapies

in healing in people who have joint replacements.
- *Graduate.* Music therapy for postoperative pain relief; suicide prevention in the homeless; medication compliance in the homeless; music therapy for laboring mothers; medication interventions for postoperative pain (intravenous acetaminophen); strategies for hand-hygiene compliance; nurse–family partnerships for teen mothers; play therapy for preoperative children; and touch therapies for people living with cancer.

Evidence is so important, and we have a responsibility to patients and students to ensure that it is used and understood. This is an example of evaluating the evidence holistically, as explained by a faculty member:

> As I mature as a teacher and become increasingly comfortable with the content, it is my goal that Capital nursing students would have exceptional EBP [evidence-based practice] skills and could generate intervention EBP projects using our rich base of Qualitative Research to inform the practice change and to impact affective learning. Lincoln and Guba have taught that Qualitative research can and should be used to affect decision-making and policy. It is my goal that our students learn how to do this—to provide momentum for EBP by effectively appealing to the heart of both nurses and policy-makers.[43]

Interdisciplinary Education

One of the exciting ways that holism is lived is the opportunity for nursing students from any program to be part of the interdisciplinary community in the course Interdisciplinary Explorations of Human Experience. This course was developed by a group of faculty in 2012 who believe that the opportunity to see through another lens is a powerful experience and, as such, supports the deepening of us all. It is guided by two lead faculty with assistance from other faculty members in such disciplines as art therapy, business, music, nursing, religion and philosophy, psychology, and social work. The current exploration is of hope.

Endemic to human experience, the topic chosen for exploration engages students in various learning modalities. Class discussions, scholarly readings, and research assignments are designed to deepen self-reflection and awareness. Music playlists, artistic expressions, empirical research projects, critical reading and writing, and a required abstract for submission to the Undergraduate Scholarship Symposium are hallmarks of this course. See **Table 26-8** for an overview of the specific course activities.

TABLE 26-8 Learning Objectives, Course Activities, and Assessment

Knowledge	Learning Objectives	Course Activities	Assessment
Foundational	Describe definitions of hope; Create a personal definition of hope; Appreciate the complexity of hope	Read professional literature; Discuss professional literature; Written assignments	Contribution to discussion; Journal submissions; Significant project
Application	Apply "hope" to personal development; Apply "hope" to discipline; Apply "hope" to potential career	Discussion; Written assignments; Artistic works	Contribution to discussion; Journal submissions
Integration	Examine cross-disciplinary connections of hope; Explore hope in relation to other classes	Read professional literature; Interview professionals	Contribution to discussion; Significant project
Human dimension	Inspire hope in oneself and/or in others	Create a playlist of hopeful music; Develop and implement an action plan for inspiring hope	Journal submissions; Action plan and outcome of implementing action plan
Caring	Recognize and appreciate your own gifts, contributions; Recognize and appreciate others' gifts, contributions	Discussion; Written assignments; Artistic works	Contribution to discussion; Journal submissions
Lifelong learning	Conduct interdisciplinary research on an abstract concept	Interview professionals; Analyze, synthesize, and interpret interview data in the context of the literature; Integrate the interpretation into a significant project	Significant project

Source: Reproduced from L. D. Fink (2003). *Creating Significant Learning Experiences: An Integrated Approach to Designing College Courses.* San Francisco, CA: John Wiley & Sons.

The feedback from those who have taken this interdisciplinary course has been wonderful. Capstone projects are amazing and, in many ways, life transforming. We all come to understand more about the idea we are exploring and, importantly, more about one another.

There are many exciting ways in which holism lives at Capital University. There is a bulletin board that is filled with news from AHNA and the *Beginnings* journal, as well as photographs, reflections, affirmations, and pieces of art. The walls are alive with posters, artwork, healing flags, and photos of colleagues and friends. Students and faculty alike have great opportunities for service both nationally and internationally. Faculty research is ongoing and currently examining (1) a survey of graduates and their ability to live holism in practice, (2) the lived experience of being a faculty member in an endorsed program, (3) the experiences of reflective practice as shared in narrative, and (4) the experience of being a student in a holistic nursing program. We want to keep on growing! This brief introduction illuminates a few ways in which holism is lived and nurtured.

Conclusion

This chapter demonstrates the variety of ways that holistic nursing is integrated into nursing education. Each school has developed unique methods of confirming that holistic nursing content is delivered in a consistent approach to all students rather than based on individual faculty interests. The recommendations and requirements from licensure, professional organizations, and accrediting bodies are that holistic nursing core values are an essential component to nursing education.

Directions for Future Research

1. Compare and contrast the various methods of integrating holistic nursing core values in the curriculum.
2. Measure the effect of holistic nursing education on daily nursing practice.
3. Examine the effect of pedagogical methods on student and faculty satisfaction.

4. Explore the impact of teaching in a holistically grounded program on faculty "burnout."

Nurse Healer Reflections

After reading this chapter, the holistic nurse will be able to answer or to begin a process of answering the following questions:

- How can I model holistic nursing core values to nursing students and colleagues?
- What are the next steps to ensure holistic nursing is integrated in the curriculum?
- How do I ensure that faculty beliefs are aligned?

NOTES

1. C. Meakim, T. Boese, S. Decker, A. E. Franklin, D. Gloe, L. Lioce, C. R. Sando, et al., "Standards of Best Practice: Simulation Standard I: Terminology," *Clinical Simulation in Nursing* 9, no. 6S (2013): S3–S11.
2. B. Dossey, "Holistic Nursing: How to Make It Work for You," *NursingLife* 1 (1981): 40–45.
3. B. Dossey, "Holistic Nursing: How to Make It Work for You," *Journal of Holistic Nursing* 1, no. 1 (1983): 32–36.
4. L. Keegan, "Holistic Nursing: An Approach to Patient and Self-Care," *AORN Journal* 46, no. 3 (1987): 499–506.
5. B. Dossey, "Holistic Nursing: What Is It?" *Journal of Holistic Nursing* 1, no. 1 (1983): 37–38.
6. M. G. Nagai-Jacobson and M. A. Burkhardt, "Spirituality: Cornerstone of Holistic Nursing Practice," *Holistic Nursing Practice* 3, no. 3 (1989): 18–26.
7. C. Sims, "Spiritual Care as a Part of Holistic Nursing," *Imprint* 34, no. 4 (1987): 63–67.
8. H. Yura, "Human Needs and Holistic Nursing Practice," *Journal of Holistic Nursing* 4, no. 1 (1986): 14–15.
9. B. Berman, "Complementary Medicine and Medical Education: Teaching Complementary Medicine Offers a Way of Making Teaching More Holistic," *British Medical Journal* 322, no. 7279 (2001): 121–122.
10. E. O. Bevis, "Nursing Curriculum as Professional Education," in *Toward a Caring Curriculum: A New Pedagogy for Nursing*, E. O. Bevis and J. Watson (Washington, DC: National League for Nursing, 2000): 74–77.

11. B. M. Dossey, *Core Curriculum for Holistic Nursing* (Sudbury, MA: Jones & Bartlett, 1997).

12. M. V. Fenton and D. L. Morris, "The Integration of Holistic Nursing Practices and Complementary and Alternative Modalities into Curricula of Schools of Nursing," *Alternative Therapies in Health and Medicine* 9, no. 4 (2003): 62–67.

13. N. C. Frisch, "Nursing as Context for Alternative/Complementary Modalities," *Online Journal of Issues in Nursing* 6, no. 2 (2001): 2.

14. N. C. Frisch, "Standards of Holistic Nursing Practice as Guidelines for Quality Undergraduate Nursing Curricula," *Journal of Professional Nursing* 19, no. 6 (2003): 382–386.

15. H. L. Barbato Gaydos, "Complementary and Alternative Therapies in Nursing Education: Trends and Issues," *Online Journal of Issues in Nursing* 6, no. 2 (2001): 5.

16. L. L. Halcon, B. Leonard, M. Snyder, A. Garwick, and M. J. Kreitzer, "Incorporating Alternative and Complementary Health Practices Within University-Based Nursing Education," *Journal of Evidence-Based Complementary and Alternative Medicine* 6, no. 2 (2001): 127–135.

17. S. F. Richardson, "Complementary Health and Healing in Nursing Education," *Journal of Holistic Nursing* 21, no. 1 (2003): 20–35.

18. S. R. Sok, J. A. Erlen, and K. B. Kim, "Complementary and Alternative Therapies in Nursing Curricula: A New Direction for Nurse Educators," *Journal of Nursing Education* 43, no. 9 (2004): 401–405.

19. K. Avino, "Knowledge, Attitudes, and Practices of Nursing Faculty and Students Related to Complementary and Alternative Medicine: A Statewide Look," *Holistic Nursing Practice* 25 no. 6 (2011): 280–288.

20. L. Chlan, L. Halcon, M. J. Kreitzer, and B. Leonard, "Influence of an Experiential Education Session on Nursing Students' Confidence Levels in Performing Selected Complementary Therapy Skills," *Journal of Evidence-Based Complementary and Alternative Medicine* 10, no. 3 (2005): 189–201.

21. M. Wallace, S. Campbell, S. C. Grossman, J. M. Shea, J. W. Lange, and T. T. Quell, "Integrating Spirituality into Undergraduate Nursing Curricula," *International Journal of Nursing Education Scholarship* 5, no. 1 (2008): 1–13.

22. N. Johnson, J. List-Ivankovic, W. O. Eboh, J. Ireland, D. Adams, E. Mowatt, and S. Martindale, "Research and Evidence Based Practice: Using a Blended Approach to Teaching and Learning in Undergraduate Nurse Education," *Nurse Education in Practice* 10, no. 1 (2010): 43–47.

23. S. Buchan, M. Shakeel, A. Trinidade, D. Buchan, and K. Ah-See. "The Use of Complementary and Alternative Medicine by Nurses," *British Journal of Nursing* 21, no. 11 (2012): 672–674.

24. M. Popoola, "Popoola Holistic Practice Model—A Framework for Curriculum Development," *West African Journal of Nursing* 23, no. 2 (2012): 43–56.

25. H. L. Wung, H. L. Chen, and Y. J. Hwu, "Teaching Patient-Centered Holistic Care," *Journal of Nursing* 54, no. 3 (2007): 27–32.

26. American Association of Colleges of Nursing, *The Essentials of Baccalaureate Education for Professional Nursing Practice* (Washington, DC: American Association of Colleges of Nursing, 2008).

27. American Holistic Nurses Association and American Nurses Association, *Holistic Nursing: Scope and Standards of Practice*, 2nd ed. (Silver Spring, MD: Nursesbooks.org, 2013).

28. T. P. Nelms, "Has the Curriculum Revolution Revolutionized the Definition of Curriculum?" *Journal of Nursing Education* 30, no. 1 (1991): 5–8.

29. B. M. Dossey and L. Keegan, eds., *Holistic Nursing: A Handbook for Practice*, 6th ed. (Burlington, MA: Jones & Bartlett Learning, 2013).

30. National League for Nursing, "Simulation and Technology" (2013). www.nln.org/faculty programs/simulation_tech.htm.

31. P. Jeffries, *Simulation in Nursing Education* (Washington, DC: National League for Nursing, 2007).

32. M. A. Cordeau, "Linking the Transition: A Substantive Theory of High-Stakes Clinical Simulation," *Advances in Nursing Science* 35, no. 3 (2012): E90–E102.

33. M. A. Cordeau, "Teaching Holistic Nursing Using Clinical Simulation: A Pedagogical Essay," *Journal of Nursing Education and Practice* 3, no. 4 (2013): 40–50.

34. National League for Nursing, "Unfolding Cases" (2010). www.nln.org/facultyprograms/faculty resources/aces/unfolding_cases.htm.

35. S. H. Campbell and K. M. Daley, *Simulation Scenarios for Nursing Educators: Making It Real*, 2nd ed. (New York: Springer, 2013).

36. L. Cronenwett, G. Sherwood, J. Barnsteiner, J. Disch, J. Johnson, P. Mitchell, D. T. Sullivan, et al., "Quality and Safety Education for Nurses," *Nursing Outlook* 55, no. 3 (2007): 122–131.

37. D. Shields and S. Stout-Shaffer, "Self-Development: The Foundation of Holistic Self-Care," in *Holistic Nursing: A Handbook for Practice*, 7th ed., eds. B. M. Dossey and L. Keegan (Burlington, MA: Jones & Bartlett Learning, 2015).

38. J. Kabat-Zinn, *Coming to Our Senses: Healing Ourselves and the World Through Mindfulness* (New York: Hyperion, 2005).

39. T. Touhy and A. Boykin, "Caring as the Central Domain in Nursing Education," *International Journal for Human Caring* 12, no. 2 (2008): 8–15.

40. A. Boykin and S. O. Schoenhofer, *Nursing as Caring: A Model for Transforming Practice* (Washington, DC: National League for Nursing, 2001).

41. C. Johns, *Becoming a Reflective Practitioner*, 3rd ed. (West Sussex, UK: Wiley-Blackwell, 2009): 3.

42. C. Johns, "Reflection as a Way of Being in Practice," in *Modeling and Role-Modeling at Work*, ed. H. L. Erickson (Cedar Park, TX: Unicorns Unlimited, 2010): 311–328.

43. Personal communication.

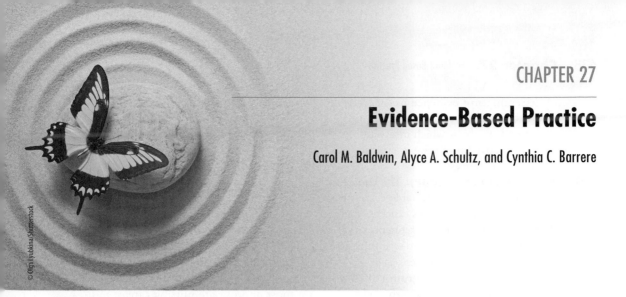

Evidence-Based Practice

Carol M. Baldwin, Alyce A. Schultz, and Cynthia C. Barrere

Nurse Healer Objectives

Theoretical

- Explore the concept of evidence-based practice (EBP).
- Review the historical underpinnings of EBP.
- Compare and discriminate between individual and system-wide models of EBP.
- Discuss ways in which EBP has redirected priorities for evaluating best practices in nursing research.
- Compare and contrast the barriers to and strengths of evidence-based care.
- Examine international approaches to EBP in holistic nursing practice.
- Define and describe evidence-based practice programs (EBPP).
- Examine ways in which EBPPs can be utilized within the holistic caring process.

Clinical

- Describe the EBP process for translating best evidence into practice.
- Apply the EBP process to a peer-reviewed journal article and assess the evidence for making a decision or practice change.
- Identify resources that can be used to incorporate EBP into clinical settings.
- Define and describe ways in which EBP informs comparative effectiveness research.

- Describe the concept of protocol-driven EBPPs and their application to clinical practice.

Personal

- Set aside time to learn more about how EBP can enhance the holistic caring process.
- Attend an EBP conference or workshop.
- Develop expertise in EBP through an online course or program of study.
- Search online resources to appreciate the application of EBP and EBPPs in clinical practice nationally and internationally.
- Discuss ways in which EBP can be adapted at your clinical setting to enhance best practices in the holistic caring process.
- Practice framing a clinical issue of interest into a standardized clinical question, such as the PICOT format in your clinical setting.

Definitions

Comparative effectiveness research (CER): The conduct and synthesis of research that compares the benefits and harms of various interventions and strategies for preventing, diagnosing, treating, and monitoring health conditions in real-world settings. The purpose of this research is to improve health outcomes by developing and disseminating evidence-based information to patients, clinicians, and other decision makers about which interventions are most effective for which patients under specific circumstances.

Evidence-based practice (EBP): The conscientious use of the best available evidence combined with the clinician's expertise and judgment and the patient's preferences and values to arrive at the best decision that leads to high-quality outcomes.

Evidence-based practice program (EBPP): A protocol-driven "packaged" program targeting outcomes specific to persons, families, schools, and communities that have been found to be effective based on the results of rigorous evaluations.

Patient-Centered Outcomes Research Institute (PCORI): Created as part of the Patient Protection and Affordable Care Act of 2010 by the U.S. Congress, it is a private, independent, nonprofit institute to fund innovative, comparative, clinical effectiveness research to assist patients, caregivers, clinicians, and others in making evidence-based health decisions.

PICOT: A standardized format for asking the searchable, answerable question: the population of interest (P); the intervention or issue of interest (I); the comparison intervention (C), if relevant; the outcome (O); and the time frame (T), if relevant.

Holistic Nursing and Evidence-Based Practice

The science and art of holistic nursing honor an individual's subjective experience about health, health beliefs, and values and develop therapeutic partnerships with individuals, families, and communities that are grounded in nursing knowledge, theories, research expertise, intuition, and creativity.[1] Sigma Theta Tau International (STTI), the only nursing honor society, defines evidence-based nursing practice as

> an integration of the best evidence available, nursing expertise, and the values and preferences of the individuals,

families and communities who are served. This assumes that optimal nursing care is provided when nurses and health care decision makers have access to a synthesis of the latest research, a consensus of expert opinion, and are thus able to exercise their judgment as they plan and provide care that takes into account cultural and personal values and preferences. This approach to nursing care bridges the gap between the best evidence available and the most appropriate nursing care of individuals, groups and populations with varied needs.[2]

Schultz provides an alternative yet complementary definition that encompasses nursing and other care disciplines to promote change within organizations defined as

> an interdisciplinary approach to healthcare practice that bases decisions and practice strategies on the best available evidence including: research findings, quality improvement data, clinical expertise, and patient/family (recipient) values; considering feasibility, risk or harm, and costs, for the purpose of improving patient, administrative, and environmental outcomes. It requires creative, critical thinkers and the support and flexibility of management to implement and evaluate change and innovation in clinical practice.[3,4]

Historical Underpinnings of Current Evidence-Based Practice

Knowledge translation or the use of research evidence to improve clinical outcomes is not a 21st-century phenomenon; neither is the difficulty with or resistance to the application of new scientific knowledge to practice. For example, the usefulness of citrus juice for the treatment of scurvy was noted in the 16th century, although it would be another 100 years for these findings to be put into practice by the British Admiralty.[5] Another example is that of the work of Ignatz Semmelweis, who recognized that obstetricians were carrying the contagion for puerperal fever from the morgue to the delivery room.[5] His recommendation to reduce maternal mortality by hand washing was rejected by the Viennese medical society in the mid-18th century with a mantra used today that contradicts evidence to practice: "Because we've always done it that way."

As the disease transmission theory was being rejected by practicing physicians, Florence Nightingale, as a nurse in the Crimean War (1853–1856), found that washing hands between patients, along with other public health measures, reduced morbidity and mortality among the soldiers.[6] Recognized as the first nurse to conduct and use research, Nightingale showed that the quality of care can be improved through sanitary conditions, careful data collection, and critical thinking.[7] More than 150 years later, Nightingale's insight into the need for research laid the groundwork for EBP in holistic nursing when she wrote:

> In dwelling upon the vital importance of *sound* observation, it must never be lost sight of what observation is for. It is not for the sake of piling up miscellaneous information or curious facts, but for the sake of saving life and increasing health and comfort.[8]

Nursing Research into Evidence-Based Practice

For 75 years, research has been recognized as important for improving nursing education and practice. The STTI offered the first nursing research grant in 1936. Thirty-five years later, research became a required course in baccalaureate nursing programs. As research skills and knowledge became a requirement for the professional nurse, concern for use of research findings in practice and strategies to increase research utilization became a top priority. In the mid-1970s, federal grants supported the Western Interstate Commission on Higher Education's Regional Program for Nursing Research Development, the Conduct and Utilization of Research in Nursing (CURN), and Nursing

Child Assessment Satellite Training (NCAST).[9] The Regional Program for Nursing Research Development was conducted in the 13 western states to teach practicing nurses how to identify researchable practice issues, critique the current research literature, initiate and lead practice changes, and evaluate their outcomes.[10] The CURN project was designed to develop practice protocols based on the synthesis of the best available science. Ten research-based protocols were completed and evaluated for their applicability.[11] The NCAST, based on the early findings of Dr. Kathryn Barnard, focused on teaching cues to maternal–child interaction to nurses in Washington state using the new satellite system. Stetler and Marram, as young doctoral students, published the original version of their research utilization model for use by advanced practice nurses as leaders and mentors for changing clinical nursing practice.[12] An early meta-analysis showed that patients who received research-based interventions experienced outcomes that were 28% better than patients receiving routine care.[13] These findings strongly supported the efforts to increase the use of research by direct care providers.

Despite this foundation of nursing knowledge built on practice based on evidence, Ketefian concluded that nurses who conducted research and nurses who practiced at the bedside lived in separate "subcultures" and that, to narrow this gap, researchers must publish research findings in a format that practicing nurses could read and use.[14] It was apparent that even though individual nurses learned and supported the concepts of research utilization, there were many barriers to actually implementing and maintaining research-based practice changes.[15-17]

Further studies exploring barriers to and facilitators of research use were conducted in the 1980s and 1990s, and studies continue today.[9, 18] Funk and colleagues, using the concepts within Rogers's Diffusion of Innovation Theory, explored the individual and organizational challenges to the use of research in the early 1990s. They reported barriers associated with the characteristics of the adopter, the organization, the innovation itself, and the communication and dissemination of the findings.

These findings encouraged the development of models and programs addressing organizational and dissemination barriers. Using the Dissemination Model, the authors held a series of national conferences on the use of research in practice.[19] Cronenwett implemented research utilization conferences at Dartmouth-Hitchcock Medical Center that focused on integrative reviews for promoting research use by direct care nurses.[20] An early model for addressing organizational challenges was implemented in a rural Iowa hospital that was later adapted at the University of Iowa Hospitals and Clinics.[21] Four educational videos on research utilization for direct care nurses were developed to support the Organizational Process Research Utilization Model.[22-25] Titler and colleagues expanded on this organizational model in their development of the Iowa Model for Research in Practice.[26] Rutledge and Donaldson received federal funding to develop and implement the Orange County Research Utilization in Nursing project, focusing on building organizational capacity as a tool for increasing research utilization.[27]

As it became evident that much of nursing care was based on best practice and the methodology for and emphasis on quality improvement was increasing, more forms of evidence began to be used as the basis for practice. In the early 1990s, Sackett and colleagues coined the term *evidence-based medicine* to add credibility to internal quality improvement data and common practices that were providing good patient outcomes.[28] *Evidence-based practice* soon became the term used to describe practices by all healthcare professionals. One of the early interdisciplinary models for EBP was developed at the University of Colorado to provide the framework for quality improvement activities.[29] From the mid-1990s to the present, several new quality improvement and EBP models and frameworks have been developed.

Conceptual Models for Evidence-Based Practice

From these early underpinnings, a variety of conceptual models have emerged for EBP, including models that focus on the EBP process for individuals and teams of clinicians, such as the model of DiCenso and colleagues,[30] the Stetler Model,[31] the Clinical Scholar Model,[32] the Iowa Model,[33] the Promoting Action on Research Implementation in Health Services (PARIHS) Model,[34] and the Johns Hopkins Nursing Evidence-Based Practice (JHNEBP) Model,[35] which, like all the models, is intended to change a system-wide culture. Although these models are useful in conceptually guiding the implementation of EBP for individuals and within systems, there is a pressing need for further testing to support them empirically. Exemplars for these models are described in this chapter.

Exemplar: The DiCenso Model

The DiCenso Model of EBP,[30] adapted from Haynes and colleagues,[36] promotes the use of research findings within the context of an evidence-based decision-making framework.[3, 4] The individual clinician integrates the best research evidence with the patient's clinical status, preferences, actions, circumstances, available healthcare resources, and clinical expertise to decide on the interventions or the type of care to be delivered.

Exemplar: The Clinical Scholar Model and Program

Clinical scholars are agents of change whether through promoting the spirit of inquiry in the areas in which they work, translating new knowledge into practice using internal and external evidence, or generating new knowledge through the conduct of research. The Clinical Scholar Model and Program provides a framework and process for these agents of change. Aspects of this approach are described using a clinical scenario and an exemplar analysis when the principles of the EBP process are used to critically appraise an article from the *Research in Gerontological Nursing* journal later in this chapter.

Seeds for the Clinical Scholar Model were sown in 1980 when Dr. Janelle Krueger, in her keynote address at one of the first national nursing research conferences, Promoting

Nursing Research as a Staff Nursing Function, emphasized that staff nurses could "use" and "do" research.[10] She argued that research utilization and conduct should be an expectation of bedside nurses because they are the link between research and practice and can identify problems that need to be researched. During the 1990s, teams of staff nurses at Maine Medical Center in Portland, with the mentorship of a doctorally prepared nurse researcher, learned how to apply research findings to practice and answer their own clinical questions by conducting studies and subsequently disseminating their results nationally and internationally.

The Clinical Scholar Model is inductive, decentralized, and predicated on "building a community" of clinical scholars to serve as mentors anywhere patient care is provided.[32] The clinical scholar is always questioning whether a procedure needs to be performed at all and, if so, whether there is a more efficient and effective way of providing the same care. Clinical scholarship, as described in an STTI position paper,[37] is an intellectual process, steeped in curiosity that challenges traditional nursing practice through Observation, Analysis, Synthesis, Application and Evaluation, and Dissemination, concepts that were adapted to form the structure of the Clinical Scholar Model.[32, 38] Reflective thinking and clinical judgment are required within each concept as the evidence-based process unfolds. Qualitative and quantitative studies and internal evidence are reviewed for applicability to practice, and knowledge generation research designs are based on the clinical inquiry. Clinical scholars recognize that the most efficient approach to care requires that the delivery of care is based on sound scientific evidence and the continuous implementation and evaluation of effective practices. The Clinical Scholar Program was developed to facilitate larger cohorts of professional nurses who were interested in improving quality of care through the use of internal and external evidence. The program, based on the Clinical Scholar Model, is a series of six interdisciplinary all-day workshops, generally presented one month apart. The goals of the program are to (1) promote a culture of EBP and clinical scholarship through a program of interdisciplinary clinical research and EBP at the

bedside, extending work that has already been initiated in a clinical setting; and (2) to prepare a cadre of direct care providers as clinical scholars to implement change and evaluate practice based on evidence. The clinical scholars serve as mentors/champions to other staff.

The Clinical Scholar Model serves as the framework for several academic and community healthcare facilities across the country including Scottsdale Healthcare System; John C. Lincoln North Mountain Hospital; Ministry St. Joseph's Hospital in Marshfield, Wisconsin; Maine Medical Center; St. Joseph Medical Center in Kansas City, Missouri; the James Comprehensive Cancer Center at The Ohio State University; and Phoenix Children's Hospital.[39-41] Concepts of the Clinical Scholar Model have been adapted into models within nursing departments at Baylor Health Care System and Mayo Clinic and also serve as the underlying framework for the Maine Nursing Practice Consortium in northern Maine and the Texas Christian University Evidence-Based Practice and Research Collaborative among urban hospitals in the Dallas-Fort Worth area.[42, 43]

Exemplar: Promoting Action on Research Implementation in Health Services Model

If implementation were straightforward, the production and dissemination of evidence in the form of guidelines, followed by an education or teaching package, would lead to an expectation that practitioners would automatically integrate them into their everyday practice. Politically and educationally, there has been a focus on developing the skills and knowledge of individual practitioners to appraise research and make rational decisions. As such, the emphasis has been placed on developing the skills of individual nurses to be able to find and critically appraise research evidence in the hope that this will influence its use in practice.

Despite these efforts and considerable investment, for the most part research evidence is still not used routinely in practice. Over recent years, it has been recognized that the process of implementing evidence into practice is more complex than some rational or linear models and approaches to implementation imply. The individual nurse cannot be isolated from all of the bureaucratic, political, organizational, and social factors that affect change.[44-48] The implementation of research-based practice depends on an ability to achieve significant and planned behavior change involving individuals, teams, and organizations.[49]

Stetler and colleagues conducted a study in which the importance of organizational context in the routine use of EBP was highlighted.[48, 50] Their research shows that some key contextual features enable the institutionalization of EBP. These features include leadership in EBP at all levels of the organization from chief nursing officer to staff nurse, a supportive organizational culture, effective multidisciplinary teamwork, and coherent policies and procedures. This research supports the idea that although it is critical to have reflective and inquiring nurses, their ability to practice in an evidence-based way may be more or less facilitated by the context in which they work.

The PARIHS framework was developed to represent the complexities involved in implementing evidence into practice.[19, 34] The successful implementation (SI) of evidence into practice is a function (f) of the nature and type of evidence (E), the qualities of the context (C) in which the evidence is to be implemented, and the way the process is facilitated (F); therefore, SI = f (E,C,F). It provides a practical and conceptual heuristic to guide implementation and practice improvement activity, which takes multiple factors into account and acknowledges the dynamism in implementation processes. This conceptual and theoretical framework has been used for research and evaluation, as the basis for tool development, for modeling research utilization, and for evaluating the facilitation of interventions.[34]

Exemplar: The Iowa Model of Evidence-Based Practice to Promote Quality Care

One of the earliest models for addressing the utilization of research in practice was initiated in rural hospitals in Iowa in the late 1980s as the Organizational Process Research Utilization Model.[21] As a doctoral student, Marita Titler[26] developed the first Iowa Model for Research

in Practice, which was later revised as the Iowa Model of Evidence-Based Practice to Promote Quality Care.[33] The Iowa Model is a multiphase decision-making model with feedback loops for making informed recommendations for practice and administrative changes. It has been widely used nationally and internationally by nursing and interdisciplinary healthcare teams.

Using the Iowa Model, the process begins with knowledge-focused or problem-focused "triggers." If the change suggested by the "trigger" is an organizational priority, a team is formed followed by a search for the applicable research and a subsequent critique and synthesis of the findings. Based on the research synthesis, a recommendation is made to continue with a pilot change project or the conduct of a research study. Conduct and evaluation of the pilot project may result in modifications of the practice change and/or adoption on a wider scale. Results are disseminated, and outcomes of the practice change are continuously monitored until sustainability is achieved.[33]

With the successful longevity of the Iowa Model, multiple practice changes have been recommended and implemented. For more than 20 years, a national conference on EBP has been held in Iowa. Multiple EBP resources are available on the University of Iowa's website (www.uihealthcare.org/nursing-research-and-evidence-based-practice).

Exemplar: The Johns Hopkins Nursing Evidence-Based Practice Model

The JHNEBP model is based on the foundation for professional nursing and is represented by a triad of important concepts: practice, education, and research.[35] The purpose of the model is to facilitate the translation of research and nonresearch evidence into nursing practice. Implementation of the model is influenced by internal factors, such as organizational culture, leadership support, supportive resources, and organizational policies, procedures, and protocols, and external factors including accreditation bodies, state and national legislation, quality standards, and state practice acts.

The JHNEBP implementation process is described by practice, evidence, and translation.

Within this process are 18 prescriptive steps. The process begins with identification and delineation of the practice question, issue, or concern. Once the question is clear, a team is formed and a search for the evidence is conducted. Evidence includes the appraisal and evaluation of internal (e.g., quality improvement data) and external (e.g., research) evidence. Appraisal tools have been developed to assist the team with this step in the process.[35] Recommendations for change are based on the overall strength and quality of the evidence. Translation, the third step in the process, is when the team determines if the changes are feasible in the target setting. If so, the translation plan is incorporated into the quality improvement framework, followed by implementation, evaluation, and dissemination.

Challenges to and Strengths of Evidence-Based Care

There are several barriers to providing care based on the latest evidence, including lack of searching skills, inability to critically appraise studies, insufficient institutional support, and negative attitudes toward research. Based on a nationwide sample of 1,097 randomly selected registered nurses in the United States, the Nursing Informatics Expert Panel of the American Academy of Nursing found that almost half of the respondents were not familiar with the terms *evidence-based practice* and *EBP*, more than half of the respondents reported that they did not believe their colleagues used research findings in practice, only 27% of the respondents had been taught how to use electronic databases, most of the respondents did not search information databases (e.g., MEDLINE and CINAHL) to gather practice information, and respondents who did search these resources did not believe they had adequate searching skills.[51]

Similar survey data have been collected at several Pan American Health Organization (PAHO)-sponsored conferences in Argentina, Ecuador, Panama, and Spain.[51] The leading individual barriers reported by U.S. nurses include lack of value for research in practice, lack of knowledge of electronic database organization and structure, and difficulty accessing research materials. Pan American nurses rated lack of research knowledge, synthesis skills, and library access as their leading individual barriers. Both U.S. and Pan American nurses rated presence of goals with higher priority and organization budget for acquisition of information resources as their first and third leading institutional barriers, whereas U.S. nurses rated difficulty in recruiting and retaining nursing staff as second compared to Pan American nurses rating the organization's perception of lack of nurse preparation for EBP as second among institutional barriers.[52]

For several years, however, empirical evidence has shown that patient outcomes are at least 28% better when clinical care is based on rigorously designed research studies rather than care that is steeped in tradition.[13] Studies also suggest that clinicians who use research evidence in their practice are more satisfied with their roles.[53-54] Anecdotal reports indicate that evidence-based care renews the professional spirit of the nurse, a key variable in professional satisfaction. Nurses who incorporate EBP into their care report that it gives them a voice, allows them to reclaim their authentic selves as real nurses, and supports them in becoming patient advocates to improve the quality of care given to patients and families.[55] As holistic nurses embrace EBP, it will be important for them to have a sound understanding of strategies to reduce barriers when implementing EBP to nurture the holistic caring process based on evidence that can empirically support the science and art of holistic nursing.[56]

Magnet Recognition and Evidence-Based Practice

The Magnet Recognition Program®, developed in the early 1990s by the American Nurses Credentialing Center (ANCC), added impetus to the EBP movement, particularly in nursing.[57] Originally, the Magnet Recognition Program® was based on 14 "Forces of Magnetism" derived from research findings characterizing hospital nursing departments that were able to attract and retain excellent nurses during a time of nursing shortage.[58] From its beginning, the

Magnet Recognition Program® expectations were based on the American Nurses Association's (ANA) *Nursing Administration: Scope and Standards of Practice*.[58] These standards of practice have always expected that nurses will be involved in the conduct and utilization of research. The expectation for nurses in ANCC Magnet-recognized facilities to be actively generating new knowledge through the conduct of research has increased in the past decade.[57] Likewise, there is the expectation that nurses at all levels of practice will apply research-based evidence (the science) and utilize practice-based evidence as appropriate. Practice-based evidence is defined in the Magnet Recognition Program® as interventions that have been shown effective in improving outcomes but have not been scientifically validated.[59] The emphasis on the improvement of dynamic and measurable outcomes has markedly increased with the 2014 Magnet application manual. The number of Magnet-recognized facilities around the globe is just over 400, including designated facilities in Lebanon, Singapore, Saudi Arabia, New Zealand, and Australia.[60] Magnet designation requires that organizations develop, disseminate, and enculturate evidence-based criteria and continuously promote patient care, safety, and satisfaction, resulting in a positive work environment for nurses and all employees.[60]

Applying Evidence-Based Practice to the Holistic Caring Process with the Clinical Scholar Model

Holistic nurses may believe that barriers, such as time, search skills, knowledge of research, or minimal support in their working environment, may preclude them from incorporating EBP into their professional practice. The Clinical Scholar EBP process (see **Exhibit 27-1**), however, can become as natural a part of holistic nursing care as it is to utilize a 5-minute relaxation technique. The EBP process requires that

---

EXHIBIT 27-1   The Clinical Scholar Evidence-Based Practice Process

1. **OBSERVE Curiosity and Reflective Thinking**
   - Observe a family/patient, knowledge-driven, staff/practice, or data-driven issue.
   - Determine its significance to practitioners and/or the organization, independent or interdependent nursing action, key stakeholders, outcome of interest, feasibility, cost benefit, and risk benefit.
   - Develop a clinically relevant, researchable question for the issue.

2. **ANALYZE Evidence**
   - Search for the best external (science) and internal evidence to answer the question.
   - Critically appraise the evidence.

3. **SYNTHESIZE Evidence for Completeness, Quality, and Strength**
   - If synthesis results in incomplete or weakly supported evidence, prepare a research proposal.
   - If synthesis results in well-supported evidence, prepare an evidence-based pilot project.

4. **APPLY and EVALUATE the Practice Change**
   - Conduct a pilot project; monitor and evaluate the outcomes.
   - Based on results, adapt and adopt on a wider scale or discard.

5. **DISSEMINATE Broadly**
   - Present findings (internally/externally, nationally/internationally).
   - Publish an article on results as related to practice, education, administration, or policy.

the holistic nurse (1) *observes* with an inquiring mind using reflective thinking to identify a patient/family or community issue and formulate a researchable, relevant clinical question; (2) *analyzes* and searches for the best internal and external evidence that answers the question; (3) *synthesizes* the evidence for completeness, quality, and strength; (4) *implements* and *evaluates* the practice change if the evidence supports a change or conducts a research study; and (5) *disseminates* the findings, positive or negative, to a wide audience and publishes results that influence practice, education, administration, and/or policy.[38, 61] This is not unlike the holistic caring process.[62] To help you understand the EBP process, this chapter includes a peer-reviewed publication drawn from the *Research in Gerontological Nursing* journal to provide a scenario[63] and an exemplar journal article appraisal[64] for applying the five phases according to the Clinical Scholar Model.[39-41]

Clinical Scenario: Chair Yoga for Older Adults with Moderate and Severe Alzheimer's Disease[63]

1. OBSERVE Curiosity and Reflective Thinking

Observe a family/patient, knowledge-driven, staff/practice, or data-driven issue. Imagine a clinical scenario in which the holistic nurse, caring for patients in the home setting, is assessing a new patient diagnosed with Alzheimer's disease (AD). The patient is an 87-year-old man who uses the support of a walker to ambulate. A month ago, the patient had fallen and sustained bruises; however, he did not need hospitalization. The patient's wife is present during the assessment and verbalizes concern that her husband might fall again. She is very supportive and wants to keep her husband safe.

The holistic nurse is aware of the many challenges the couple will face as this patient's dementia progresses. She reflects on this situation and wonders if there is any additional supportive measure that might help decrease this patient's fall risk potential. The nurse knows that AD affects an estimated 5 million Americans.[65] To maintain quality of life for AD patients, symptom management is the focus of

care because there are few effective treatment options for this patient population. The holistic nurse believes that it is important for this patient to remain at home with his wife as long as possible. The nurse is also aware that there is considerable evidence to indicate that physical activity enhances balance and strength for all age groups, including individuals with cognitive impairments.[66, 67]

The nurse recently attended a holistic conference in which she learned about chair yoga. She remembered the yoga instructor mentioning the possible benefits of chair yoga for individuals who were unable to practice standing yoga positions. Clinical judgment leads the holistic nurse to believe that there may be a positive connection between chair yoga and the physical functioning of patients with AD. Chair yoga is easy to learn, has minimal associated costs, and has low potential risk benefits.[68] The home-care agency in which the nurse works supports inquiry. She understands that the EBP process can assist in finding answers for best practices in providing holistic care.

The holistic nurse also recognizes that to implement a new program into the clinical setting, the nurse first must identify if the outcome to be achieved is significant not only to nurses, patients, and families but also to members of other healthcare disciplines. This decision will help determine who will be needed as stakeholders on the team and for support. The holistic nurse will consider the costs, benefits, and potential risks of the practice change very early in the planning. Early consideration of these issues can help prepare the nurse for challenges that will need to be addressed during implementation.

The final step in the observation phase of the EBP process—developing the clinically relevant, researchable question—is the step in which the holistic nurse is encouraged to use a standardized format when clarifying the clinical issue of interest.[69] The PICOT is one such recommended format that consists of the population of interest (P); the intervention or issue of interest (I); the comparison intervention or current practice (C); the outcome (O); and the time frame (T), if relevant (see **Table 27-1**). For this clinical scenario, time frame is not relevant; thus,

TABLE 27-1 Applying the Standardized Format (PICOT) for Formulating a Searchable, Answerable Question

PICO Format	Clinical Scenario
Population of interest	Patients with Alzheimer's disease
Intervention of interest	Chair yoga
Comparison of interest	Current standard of practice
Outcome of interest	Improved balance, strength, ambulation (walking and speed)
Time frame	N/A

the clinical question using the PICO format is: "For patients with AD (P), does chair yoga (I) as compared to the current standard of practice (C) improve physical functioning (O) as measured by improved balance, strength, and ambulation?"

2. ANALYZE Evidence

To find the best external (science) and internal evidence to answer the sample question, the nurse implements a thorough, efficient search.[61] Holistic nurses would also explore whether any internal data had been gathered on other strategies to address AD patients' physical functioning needs. In this clinical scenario, chair yoga was used by community-dwelling patients who were cared for in an adult day care center. When examining whether chair yoga techniques may lead to the most desired outcome in addressing AD patients' physical functioning, a systematic review or meta-analysis of all relevant randomized controlled trials (RCTs) or practice guidelines based on RCTs of Level 1 evidence would provide the strongest evidence to guide practice. Levels of evidence are ranked by the type of design or methodology that answers the question with the least amount of error and provides the most reliable findings.[61, 69] Level 2 evidence derives from at least one well-designed

RCT; Level 3 from controlled trials without randomization; Level 4 from case-control or cohort studies; Level 5 from descriptive and qualitative systematic reviews; Level 6 from a single descriptive or qualitative study; and Level 7 from expert opinion or committee reports.[61, 69] For example, epidemiological studies are best suited to questions about disease risk (Level 4 or 5), while qualitative or descriptive studies might best answer questions of personal meaning or experience (Level 5, 6, or 7).

Frequently, RCTs are not available to answer intervention questions in holistic nursing literature; however, other evidence may be helpful in guiding holistic practice. The initial search begins with the keywords from the PICOT question. For this scenario, the keywords are *AD*, *chair yoga*, *physical functioning*, *balance and strength*, and *ambulation*. It is important for the holistic nurse to choose databases carefully to gather all relevant evidence such as found in the Cochrane Database of Systematic Reviews, MEDLINE, CINAHL, PsycINFO, and other search engines using keywords and controlled vocabulary headings that provide mechanisms to gather more relevant evidence.[3, 4, 61, 64] In the search, the nurse begins with single keywords, such as *AD*, *chair yoga*, or *physical functioning*, and then combines the search results of keywords to specifically answer the PICOT question and reduce the number of studies gathered to answer the question.[69]

The purpose of evaluating single primary studies is to establish if there is enough scientific evidence (also known as empirical or external evidence) to change practice without increasing the potential for risk or harm to the recipient, whether the recipient is a patient, nurse, or community group. Critiquing primary studies can be time consuming, but it is necessary to assess the soundness of the outcomes, determine their importance to EBP, and synthesize the findings of multiple studies. In time, the holistic nurse will likely be able to complete a synthesis without doing individual evaluations on each primary study.

The overall purpose of the individual evaluations is to identify the clinically relevant and statistically significant findings for each study. The holistic nurse should also look for elements of the study that may apply in work; for example, a clear definition of an outcome variable is important for further research and EBP. The holistic nurse begins the critique by reading the abstract to determine if the article is worthy of further examination. Does the purpose of the study, the setting, the sample, and the major variables answer the PICOT question? If so, continue with the evaluation. If not, the nurse should not spend any additional time on the research article. While reviewing the results of the search, the holistic nurse identifies a study that examined the use of chair yoga to improve physical functioning in nine older adults with moderate to severe AD who are cared for in an adult day care center.[63]

The most effective way to critically analyze research studies is to use a standardized and consistent process and format. **Exhibit 27-2** asks specific questions to help guide the nurse's critique. The first question that the holistic nurse considers when reading the study is whether the study answers an important variable in the PICOT question. If the study does not, time should not be spent on its critique. The nurse then focuses on only the major variables of interest that answer the PICOT question instead of all of the variables described, such as intervening or demographic variables. This is particularly important when scrutinizing and documenting the statistical results. When documenting important statistical results, the nurse includes only the outcomes that answer the PICOT question. The documentation must include the actual numbers as in this study: the numerical results at each point in time for the Six-Minute Walk Test and their statistical significance. Recording the actual findings allows for comparison of results across studies. The final consideration in evaluation of this study by the holistic nurse is to contemplate the feasibility of implementing the Sit 'N' Fit Chair Yoga Program into clinical practice and its value to patients and families.

The research study is a quasi-experimental, single-group design that could provide an answer to the clinical question.[63] It is important for the nurse to determine the best available evidence and related implications for holistic practice; therefore, the nurse carefully reviews all of the evidence collected for consideration.

The holistic nurse finds that this Level-3, quasi-experimental, single-group study examined the feasibility of older adults with AD to complete the Sit 'N' Fit Chair Yoga Program. The research question was: "What is the effect of the 8-week Sit 'N' Fit Chair Yoga Program on the gait and balance in older adults with moderate to severe AD?" Nine older adults with AD participated in this 8-week program at an adult day care center. Physical outcomes were measured at pre-intervention, 4 weeks, 8 weeks, and 1 month after program completion and included the Six-Minute Walk Test (6MWT), the Gait Speed Test (GST), and the Berg Balance Scale (BBS).

The quality of evidence in the study is also evaluated by using **Table 27-2**. An introduction described the significance and prevalence of AD in the United States, the difficulty of symptom management as AD progresses, and the substantial evidence indicating how physical activity can enhance balance and strength, among other positive effects. Yoga was noted as one such form of physical activity that may be beneficial. A thorough literature review gave a current synopsis of the physical and cognitive benefits of yoga as well as the recent studies conducted to examine chair yoga.

The quality of evidence in this study is further reflected in the reported information on the sample and the rationale for its small size for this feasibility study, the sample selection, the psychometric testing for the three outcome measures, the clearly described intervention, the researcher's observation of each session to determine instructor fidelity (assuring consistency of the instruction), the appropriateness of the repeated measures, analysis of variance performed on the data collected in relation to the small sample size, the easy to understand tables that highlighted important comparative content, and the follow-up measures at all time points as planned.

The study findings were presented clearly, and the conclusions were based on the study results. Findings revealed that older adults with moderate to severe AD could complete a twice weekly chair yoga program (see Table 27-2). Positive changes were found in all three physical measures; however, only the change in balance attained statistical significance ($p = .034$) with

EXHIBIT 27-2   Quantitative Study Evaluation Checklist

	Yes	No	N/A	Unknown
1. Are the study findings valid?				
▪ Does the study answer your PICOT question?	☐	☐	☐	☐
▪ Were the subjects randomly assigned to the experimental and control groups?	☐	☐	☐	☐
▪ Were the researchers, subjects, and providers kept blind to the study group(s)?	☐	☐	☐	☐
▪ Did at least 80% of the subjects complete the study? (Attrition)	☐	☐	☐	☐
▪ Were the subjects analyzed in the group to which they were randomly assigned? (Statistical assumptions)	☐	☐	☐	☐
▪ Was the sample size large enough to detect statistical significance if present? (Power analysis)	☐	☐	☐	☐
▪ Were the subjects in each of the groups similar on demographic and baseline clinical variables?	☐	☐	☐	☐
▪ Were the instruments used to measure the outcomes valid and reliable? (Psychometric evaluation)	☐	☐	☐	☐
▪ Was the study protocol carefully followed for the intervention/program? (Fidelity)	☐	☐	☐	☐
▪ Were the follow-up assessments conducted long enough to fully study the effects of the intervention?	☐	☐	☐	☐
▪ Was the data collection protocol followed? (Fidelity)	☐	☐	☐	☐
2. Are the results of the study important?				
▪ Does the study design provide evidence to change practice?	☐	☐	☐	☐
▪ Are the actual numerical results reported?	☐	☐	☐	☐
▪ Is there a medium to large treatment effect? (Effect size)	☐	☐	☐	☐
▪ Were the results statistically significant?	☐	☐	☐	☐
▪ Are there other possible explanations for the findings?	☐	☐	☐	☐
3. Will the findings apply in caring for patients?				
▪ Are the results applicable to your clients?	☐	☐	☐	☐
▪ Were all clinically important outcomes measured?	☐	☐	☐	☐
▪ Were the results clinically significant?	☐	☐	☐	☐
▪ Are there potential risks if the treatment or program is implemented?	☐	☐	☐	☐
▪ Are there potential benefits if the treatment or program is implemented?	☐	☐	☐	☐
▪ Is implementation of the treatment or program feasible in your clinical setting?	☐	☐	☐	☐
▪ Are the results of the study valuable to your client/family/community?	☐	☐	☐	☐

Source: Clinical Scholar Toolkit©, Alyce A. Schultz & Associates, EBP Concepts, LLC. Adapted from the Centre for Evidence-Based Medicine, Toronto.

TABLE 27-2 Important Outcome Results for the Sit 'N' Fit Chair Yoga Program Measure of Physical Function at Baseline, 4 Weeks, 8 Weeks, and 1-Month Follow Up				
	Six-Minute Walk Test[a]	Gait Speed Test[b]	Berg Balance Scale[c]	
Collection Point	Mean (SD)	Mean (SD)	Mean (SD)	p value
Baseline	492.40 (237.10)	10.76 (7.86)	40.46 (13.34)	
4 weeks	516.30 (330.00)	8.90 (6.21)	42.00 (14.83)	.937
8 weeks	482.00 (308.30)	7.86 (3.50)	43.00 (13.59)	.696
1-month follow up	500.00 (359.00)	8.50 (4.36)	45.13 (14.34)	.034

[a]Measured in feet

[b]Measured in seconds

[c]14-item, 5-point Likert scale

a pretest BBS mean score of 40.46, increasing to 45.13 at the 1-month follow up. The GST improvement was clinically significant, thus demonstrating positive changes, but it was not statistically significant. At pretest, GST showed a mean of 10.76 seconds to walk 20 feet, decreasing to a mean of 4.36 seconds at the end of the program but increasing to a mean of 8.5 seconds at the 1-month follow up. This was a moderate effect size of 0.495. At pretest, the average distance walked in 6 minutes was 492.40 feet. After participation in the chair yoga intervention program, the average distance increased to 516.30 feet in 6 minutes, at 8 weeks the distance decreased to 482 feet, and at the 1-month follow up, the distance improved to 500 feet in 6 minutes. Limitations such as the small sample size and single, nonrandom, noncontrol design were noted, and recommendations were made for future studies.

It is important to note that the researchers incorporated measures to create a comfortable environment for participants (assistance to the bathroom was provided prior to the session; sessions took place after breakfast, in a well-lit, warm room with soft, calming music; pillows were placed under the feet of those whose feet did not touch the floor; and time was allowed to warm up in an unhurried manner). Findings were reported as supporting the implementation of the Sit 'N' Fit Chair Yoga Program; however, larger RCTs are needed to substantiate this recommendation. After reading the study and appraising the evidence, the holistic nurse determines that this study may apply to holistic practice, but additional evidence is needed.

Holistic nurses also use qualitative studies to enhance the implementation and feasibility of any practice change. Qualitative studies are analyzed similar to quantitative studies, but different evaluation questions are used (see **Exhibit 27-3**). Qualitative studies can also be synthesized by examining the similarities among the identified themes across studies asking similar research questions.

3. SYNTHESIZE Evidence for Completeness, Quality, and Strength

The essential step after the appraisal phase is synthesis. Synthesis in the EBP process highlights the integration of evidence obtained from the critical appraisal of more than one study and any internal evidence combined with the holistic nurse's clinical expertise and patient preferences and values to make a practice decision or change. The holistic nurse knows that

EXHIBIT 27-3   Qualitative Evaluation Checklist

	Yes	No	N/A	Unknown
1. Are the study findings valid?				
■ Does the study answer your PICOT question?	☐	☐	☐	☐
■ Does the study question match the study design?	☐	☐	☐	☐
■ Does the study design fit the purpose?	☐	☐	☐	☐
■ Was the sample size appropriate for the study design?	☐	☐	☐	☐
■ Were additional subjects added to saturate data?	☐	☐	☐	☐
■ Was the data collection method appropriate?	☐	☐	☐	☐
■ Were there an adequate number of observations or interviews?	☐	☐	☐	☐
■ Was the duration of study adequate?	☐	☐	☐	☐
■ Were multiple observers or interviewers used?	☐	☐	☐	☐
■ Was the data analysis method appropriate?	☐	☐	☐	☐
2. Are the results of the study "trustworthy"?				
a. Are the themes in the study credible?				
■ Was there prolonged engagement?	☐	☐	☐	☐
■ Was there persistent observation?	☐	☐	☐	☐
■ Was there triangulation of investigators, settings, and/or data examination?	☐	☐	☐	☐
■ Were there external checks?	☐	☐	☐	☐
■ Was there a search for disconfirming evidence?	☐	☐	☐	☐
■ Were the researchers credible?	☐	☐	☐	☐
b. Are the results dependable?				
■ Were there independent inquiries of data by different researchers?	☐	☐	☐	☐
■ Was there an inquiry audit by an outside reviewer?	☐	☐	☐	☐
c. Was there confirmability?				
■ Was there an audit trail of a systematic collection of materials and documentation?	☐	☐	☐	☐
d. Are the findings transferable?				
■ Do the quotes fit the findings?	☐	☐	☐	☐
■ Are the results plausible and believable?	☐	☐	☐	☐
■ Can the themes be used across the healthcare spectrum?	☐	☐	☐	☐
3. Will the findings apply in caring for patients?				
■ Do the findings apply to your patients?	☐	☐	☐	☐
■ Are there potential risks if the treatment or program is implemented?	☐	☐	☐	☐
■ Are there potential benefits if the treatment or program is implemented?	☐	☐	☐	☐
■ Is implementation of the treatment or program feasible in your clinical setting?	☐	☐	☐	☐
■ Are the results of the study valuable to your client/family/community?	☐	☐	☐	☐

Source: Clinical Scholar Toolkit©, Alyce A. Schultz & Associates, EBP Concepts, LLC. Trustworthiness of results adapted from Y. S. Lincoln and E. G. Guba, *Naturalistic Inquiry* (Beverly Hills, CA: Sage, 1985).

AD is progressive and that physical functioning slowly declines, which negatively affects quality of life; thus, improvement in movement and activity is desirable. The holistic nurse recognizes that there are numerous approaches to increasing activity, such as physical therapy, occupational therapy, walking with assistance/assistive devices, water therapy, tai chi, energy healing, and qi gong. Regardless of the modality, each approach would require empirical support to determine its effectiveness in improving physical functioning in patients with AD, as well as the patient's and caregiver's perception of the intervention. The holistic nurse is aware that several of these holistic interventions require advanced education and/or certification, and the holistic nurse may or may not have the required training. However, the chair yoga program used in the study was acceptable to the patients because all of them attended and participated in all of the sessions. Chair yoga is also safe and easy to implement.

For the holistic nurse to be able to synthesize the evidence, results of two or more studies that provide outcomes on the same data measures and over the same time period must be appraised and reported. In this example, changes in scores following physical functioning in other studies can then be compared. Studies that report only the statistical results and not the actual numerical findings do not provide the evidence needed for synthesis. Qualitative studies also provide information that lends insight into the lived experiences of AD patients and can enhance the understanding of quantitative findings. The quantitative findings in this small pilot study were in part both statistically and clinically significant over a 3-month period, which was somewhat encouraging; however, the outcomes did not result in strong enough evidence for the nurse to make an informed decision regarding the use of chair yoga in patients with AD from this single study. Because the results were clinically significant, the holistic nurse can weigh the results in terms of Sit 'N' Fit Chair Yoga Program costs and feasibility because there is little to no risk to the patients with its implementation, and the early results were promising. The holistic nurse also appreciates the importance of patient values as used in this study where participants willingly attended all of the chair yoga sessions.

4. APPLY and EVALUATE the Practice Change

The holistic nurse is cognizant of the fact that incorporating interventions, such as the Sit 'N' Fit Chair Yoga Program, into clinical practice requires additional well-supported evidence.[61] The nurse, or team of nurses, should return to Phase 2 and continue to search for additional scientific evidence or design their own study (Phase 3). The outcome indicators will assist in evaluating the success of or need for changes in the patient-preferred chair yoga therapy program. The holistic nurse also recognizes that chair yoga may have actions other than providing nurses with an intervention to addressing patients' balance and strengthening needs. Perhaps nurses will find that patients' quality of life and cognitive skills will be enhanced as well. Using clinical expertise, the holistic nurse searches for empirical evidence to further establish the relationships among chair yoga as an intervention for patients diagnosed with AD, such as a decrease in patient falls, an increase in patients remaining safely at home with a primary caregiver, and other clinical outcome indicators. The nurse may also add these indicators to a new study.

When the holistic nurse has synthesized enough empirical and practice-based evidence to safely implement a change in practice, a team of nurses and other healthcare providers should be convened to pilot the change in a single facility or on a single AD unit. As part of the pilot project, the nurse will carefully monitor the fidelity of the change through observation and documentation of the program, the Sit 'N' Fit Chair Yoga Program, for example. Fidelity must be monitored to determine whether the success of the change is due to the new program; if it is not successful, verify whether the program was implemented correctly. The program outcomes should use the same outcome measures as in the clinical trials.

5. DISSEMINATE Broadly

The holistic nurse knows that implementing a practice change or decision is not the sum total of the EBP process. A critical component of the EBP process for the nurse, both professionally and personally, is that of disseminating the change to colleagues, the organization, and peers nationally and, if culturally relevant, internationally.[61] Venues that the holistic nurse can utilize for disseminating the outcomes of the practice change include conducting organizational in-services, giving paper and poster presentations at the American Holistic Nurses Association annual conference, publishing an article on the change in the *Journal of Holistic Nursing*, and presenting the practice change at the annual STTI Nursing Research Conference. It is important for holistic nurses to disseminate their results, positive or negative, to a broad audience, and to consider whether their findings will influence not only practice but also education, administration, or policy.

Evidence-Based Practice and Holistic Nursing Practice, Education, and Scholarship

On average, it takes 17 years to translate research findings into clinical practice.[70] Based on this report, leading professional and healthcare organizations and policymakers have placed a major emphasis on accelerating EBP in the educational, practice, and research settings. In the landmark document *Crossing the Quality Chasm*, the Institute of Medicine (IOM) emphasized that one of the 10 "rules for health care" is evidence-based decision making.[71] In addition, the five core competencies for educational programs for healthcare professionals deemed essential by the IOM's Health Professions Educational Summit include employing EBP.[72] The EBP must be the foundation of practice, education, and research. Holistic nursing requires valid EBP that is conducted to assist clinicians at the point of care to have the latest and best information on which to base their care.[10]

Global Health, Holistic Culture Care, and Evidence-Based Practice

The teaching, implementation, and application of EBP are shared concerns globally, according

to the STTI *Resource Paper on Global Health and Nursing Research Priorities*.[73] In addition to EBP, the global development initiative outlines common priorities among regions, such as health promotion, health policy, advocacy, patient-centered care, palliative care, genetic testing, and professional issues, that are relevant to transcultural and international care from a holistic nursing perspective. Each of these priorities would benefit from an understanding and application of EBP principles and practices. To guide all nurses toward understanding the implications and applications of EBP internationally, the peer-reviewed journal *Worldviews on Evidence-Based Nursing* is an informational resource for nurses worldwide that is published on a quarterly basis under the auspices of STTI. The Joanna Briggs Institute is an international nonprofit research and development organization based within the Faculty of Health Sciences at the University of Adelaide, South Australia.[74] The institute collaborates internationally with more than 60 entities around the world, including centers in Singapore, Canada, China, and the United States. The institute and its collaborating entities promote and support the synthesis, transfer, and utilization of evidence through identifying feasible, appropriate, meaningful, and effective healthcare practices to assist in the improvement of healthcare outcomes globally. The EBP process has been disseminated throughout the Americas via a technical agreement between the PAHO and the Arizona State University College of Nursing and Health Innovation. Pre-colloquiums and paper and poster presentations held in such PAHO-determined venues as Mexico, Central and South America, and Spain highlight the emphasis placed on the role of EBP in the global arena and support best practices for holistically based culture care.[52] The Clinical Scholar Program conducted through Boromarajonani College of Nursing, Nakhon Lampang, Thailand, under the auspices of a Fulbright program, resulted in 40 ongoing evidence-based clinical practice projects in hospitals in northern Thailand.[75] In 2013, the Clinical Scholar Program, again supported by the Fulbright program, was delivered at St. Louis University in Bagio, Philippines, resulting in 17 collaborative academic-practice team EBP projects.[76] Components of the model formed the basis for evidence-based applications in Bogota, Colombia, and Santiago, Chile. As the Iowa Model, Clinical Scholar Model, PARIHS, and other models are adapted as frameworks for EBP and clinical research around the globe, more empirical research regarding clinician and patient outcomes as well as organizational changes are needed.

The PAHO Evidence Informed Policy Network (EVIPNet) is also involved in facilitating knowledge transfer or translation, researcher and decision-maker interaction, and translation of research into policies, programs, and law.[77] The key elements of developing these policies, programs, and laws are grounded in the EBP synthesis and analysis process. By 2010, the EVIPNet Americas included the development of national multidisciplinary teams in Brazil, Paraguay, Mexico, the United States, and Tobago and Trinidad; by 2012, eight EVIPNet workshops were held that included 16 countries and 277 subjects with outcomes that resulted in 8 evidence-based policy briefs and another 16 under development.[77]

Evidence-Based Practice and Comparative Effectiveness Research

It is important for holistic nurses to know the advances in moving evidence forward to inform national and global health policy and to support informed consumer choices.[78, 79] In these matters, EBP and comparative effectiveness research (CER) are not mutually exclusive. Initiated as a focal activity by the National Institutes of Health and the IOM in 2009,[80, 81] the purpose of CER is to improve health outcomes by developing and disseminating evidence-based information to patients, clinicians, and other decision makers about which interventions are most effective for which patients under specific circumstances at individual and population levels.[79]

Characteristics of CER studies include but are not limited to (1) directly informing clinical or health policy decisions; (2) comparing at least two alternatives, each with the potential to be best practices; (3) generating results at population and subgroup levels; (4) outcome measures that are important to patients; (5) methods and data sources (qualitative and/or quantitative) that are appropriate for the decision of interest; and (6) employing real-world settings.[82] Interventions may include medications, procedures, medical and assistive devices and technologies, diagnostic testing, holistic practices, behavioral change, and delivery system strategies. The implementation of CER necessitates the development, expansion, and use of a variety of data sources and methods to assess comparative effectiveness and disseminate the results. The Society for Prevention Research has published criteria for determining effective prevention programs that may be efficacious, effective, or ready for dissemination.[83]

With the advent of the Patient Protection and Affordable Care Act of 2010, the Patient-Centered Outcomes Research Institute (PCORI), authorized by the U.S. Congress, was established as a nonpartisan, private, independent, nonprofit institute to represent the needs and perspectives of the healthcare community and as a trusted source of information.[84] The focus of PCORI is to fund comparative clinical effectiveness research to evaluate the risks and benefits of interventions, procedures, medical devices, and diagnostic tools; healthcare promotion; management and delivery programs; complementary, alternative, and integrative practices; and other evidence-based strategies used in the prevention, treatment, and management of disease and health promotion.[84, 85] Sample topics relevant to holistic nursing might include a comparison of the clinical effectiveness of primary prevention methods, such as tai chi exercise and balance training versus clinical treatments in preventing falls in older adults with varying degrees of risk. At the organizational level, a sample topic might compare the clinical effectiveness of comprehensive care coordination programs, such as the medical home, and usual care in managing children and adults with severe chronic disease, especially in populations with known health disparities. A focus of CER is to implement practice- and cost-effective interventions to improve health outcomes in large patient populations.

Evidence-Based Programs

Evidence-based practice programs (EBPP) target outcomes specific to persons, families, schools, and communities that have been found to be effective based on the results of rigorous evaluations. Criteria that must be met for a program to be considered evidence-based include evaluation research (e.g., clinical trials, CER) indicating that the programs produced predictable positive results, the outcomes/results are attributed to the programs rather than other factors, the programs are peer reviewed by experts in the field, and the programs are endorsed by a federal agency (e.g., Centers for Disease Control and Prevention, Department of Health and Human Services) or a highly regarded research organization (e.g., National Council on Aging, Substance Abuse and Mental Health Services Administration).[86] In addition to the criteria to adjudge whether a program is evidence based, Cooney and colleagues provide a comprehensive overview to include program advantages and disadvantages, "evidence" versus "research" based programs, and searching for and implementing an EBPP. To be designated as an EBPP, the program must demonstrate through rigorous methodology that it provides effective results in addition to research-based content.[86] A primary objective of an EBPP is to support the three aims of (1) improving health care, (2) improving health, and (3) improving the values that undergird the Affordable Care Act.[87] These aims are in concert with holistic nursing and the holistic nursing process.

Several programs have recently emerged that meet the criteria of an EBPP. For example, CarePRO: Care Partners Reaching Out is an evidence-based treatment program that supports caregivers of persons with AD through a partnership among the local Alzheimer's Association chapters, local area agencies on aging, and state units on aging in Arizona and Nevada to train and supervise agency staff to deliver psychoeducational skill training to more than 600 family caregivers in a 3-year project.[88] The CarePRO EBPP was awarded the 2013 Rosalynn Carter National Leadership in Caregiving Award given its positive effect on a variety of outcomes (e.g., depression, coping, burden, behavior problems) and its group-based delivery designed to reduce agency costs and enhance sustainability. Coon and colleagues provide a cogent and extended overview of the development of empirically based family caregiver programs like CarePRO and all that it entails to become an EBPP.[88] Holistic nurses can use this material as a template in the development of holistic nursing-based EBPPs.

Lorig and her team have also addressed health equity in their Chronic Disease Self-Management Program with translation of their programs into Spanish.[89] An emerging program grounded in holistic nursing principles and practices is that of a sleep training module for Spanish-speaking lay health workers (promotores) and a separate manual for health providers. The sleep component for promotores has been incorporated into a manual, *Camino a la Salud* (Road to Health), published in 2014, that provides health promotion information and guidelines on diet, physical activity, mental health, relaxation techniques, diabetes, heart disease, and sleep to enhance health equity among underserved Spanish-speaking populations along the U.S.–Mexico border.[90]

Baldwin and colleagues have validated the sleep component and have pre- and posttested the training with promotores working along the border.[91] Next steps are to further test for outcomes relevant to patient populations and cost savings with the lay health manual, as well as to test the training manual for health providers and outcomes on patient populations following training. The sleep training for health providers will be translated into and validated in several languages, including Portuguese and Korean in addition to the existing Spanish and English, in order for this "train the trainer" program to remain consistent across populations while addressing culture care within specific populations. There are several resources listed at the end of this chapter for holistic nurses to pursue if they wish to become trained and skilled in a particular program.

Conclusion

Holistic nursing scholarship grounded in empiricism is necessary to determine "(1) basic mechanisms of nursing actions and integrative therapies; (2) clinical safety, efficacy, and treatment outcomes of holistic modalities; and (3) the interactive nature of body-mind-spirit."[1] The EBP supports a culture of best practices across multiple settings within a holistic nursing framework to improve health care, client outcomes, and systems. It is essential for holistic nursing to adopt EBP as a culture in education, practice, and research for the ultimate purposes of improving the quality of health care and patient outcomes, as well as empowering holistic nurses to implement best practices, which result in a higher level of professional care and personal satisfaction. Future directions for EBP in holistic nursing practice include the understanding and application of EBP into CER for health policy changes at the national and global levels.

Directions for Future Research

1. Using the evidence-based practice (EBP) process, evaluate holistic, complementary, alternative, integrative, and folk therapies that may promote healthy lifestyles based on client preferences in specific client populations.
2. Using the EBP process, synthesize evidence from literature searches on such topics as body-mind-spirit healing modalities to determine statistically significant and clinically meaningful best practices.
3. Implement quantitative and/or qualitative studies of nurse retention, satisfaction, creativity, and well-being in clinical settings that have and have not implemented system-wide EBP.
4. Implement quantitative and/or qualitative studies of patient and family satisfaction, well-being, and outcomes in clinical settings that have and have not implemented system-wide EBP.
5. Examine the quality of health care, healthcare delivery, and health outcomes from a global perspective as EBP becomes utilized by nurses around the globe as the gold standard for best practices.
6. Develop a working knowledge of ways in which EBP and comparative effectiveness research (CER) work in concert to make policy changes at the national and global levels, taking into consideration the needs and preferences of diverse populations.
7. Determine ways in which complementary, alternative, and integrative approaches to holistic care may be implemented as culturally responsive evidence-based practice programs for individuals, families, communities, and organizations to promote health and reduce healthcare costs.

Nurse Healer Reflections

After reading this chapter, the nurse healer will be able to answer or to begin a process of answering the following questions:

- What is my role in establishing an evidence-based holistic nursing practice?
- How do I feel about the importance of EBP in advancing holistic nursing practice?
- What are my personal and clinical barriers to adopting EBP, and what can I do to reduce these barriers?
- What are my personal and clinical strengths that would support EBP, and what can I do to enhance these strengths?
- Which models are suited to my private or clinical practice, and how can I facilitate the interweaving of a model to improve holistic clinical care?
- How can I become more involved in EBP?
- How can I become more involved in CER to effect policy change?

NOTES

1. American Holistic Nurses Association, "What Is Holistic Nursing?" (2014). www.ahna.org /AboutUs/WhatisHolisticNursing/tabid/1165 /Default.aspx.
2. Sigma Theta Tau International, "Evidence-Based Nursing Position Statement" (2014). www .nursingsociety.org/aboutus/PositionPapers /Pages/EBN_positionpaper.aspx.
3. A. A. Schultz, "Evidence Based Practice: Listening with an Inquiring Mind" (presentation at the Maine Medical Center Outreach Program, Portland, May 25, 2003).

4. A. A. Schultz, "Innovations for Evidence-Based Practice: A Blueprint for the Future" (keynote address at the 19th National Evidence-Based Practice Conference: Remaking Health Care, University of Iowa, Ames, May 4, 2012).

5. S. Doherty, "History of Evidence-Based Medicine. Oranges, Chloride of Lime and Leeches: Barriers to Teaching Old Dogs New Tricks," *Emergency Medicine Australasia* 17, no. 4 (2005): 314–321.

6. B. M. Dossey, *Florence Nightingale: Mystic, Visionary, Healer,* Commemorative ed. (Philadelphia: F. A. Davis, 2010).

7. H. Stringer, "The Evolution of Evidence-Based Practice," *Nursing Spectrum/NurseWeek: Commemorating Nightingale's Legacy* (2010): 70–72.

8. F. Nightingale, *Notes on Nursing: What It Is, and What It Is Not* (New York: Dover, 1969): 125.

9. S. G. Funk, E. M. Tornquist, and M. T. Champagne, "Barriers and Facilitators of Research Utilization: An Integrative Review," *Nursing Clinics of North America* 30, no. 3 (1995): 395–407.

10. J. C. Krueger, "Utilization of Nursing Research: The Planning Process," *Journal of Nursing Administration* 8, no. 1 (1978): 6–9.

11. J. A. Horsley, *Using Research to Improve Nursing Practice: A Guide* (Orlando, FL: Green & Stratton, 1983).

12. C. B. Stetler and G. Marram, "Evaluating Research Findings for Applicability to Practice," *Nursing Outlook* 24, no. 9 (1976): 559–563.

13. B. S. Heater, A. M. Becker, and R. K. Olsen, "Nursing Intervention and Patient Outcomes: A Meta-Analysis of Studies," *Nursing Research* 37, no. 5 (1988): 303–307.

14. S. Ketefian, "Application of Selected Nursing Research Findings into Nursing Practice: A Pilot Study," *Nursing Research* 24 (1975): 89–92.

15. K. T. Kirchhoff, "Using Research in Clinical Practice: Should Staff Nurses Be Expected to Use Research?" *Western Journal of Nursing Research* 5 (1983): 245–247.

16. C. A. Lindeman, "Priorities in Clinical Nursing Research," *Nursing Outlook* 23 (1975): 693–698.

17. J. R. Miller and S. R. Messenger, "Obstacles to Applying Nursing Research Findings," *American Journal of Nursing* 78, no. 4 (1978): 632–634.

18. S. G. Funk, E. M. Tornquist, and M. T. Champagne, "Application and Evaluation of the Dissemination Model," *Western Journal of Nursing Research* 11, no. 4 (1989): 486–491.

19. J. Rycroft-Malone, G. Harvey, K. Seers, A. Kitson, B. McCormack, and A. Titchen, "An Exploration of the Factors That Influence the Implementation of Evidence into Practice," *Journal of Clinical Nursing* 13, no. 8 (2004): 913–924.

20. L. R. Cronenwett, "Research Utilization in a Practice Setting," *Journal of Nursing Administration* 17, nos. 7–8 (1987): 9–10.

21. C. J. Goode and G. M. Bulechek, "Research Utilization: An Organizational Process That Enhances Quality of Care," *Journal of Nursing Care Quality* (1992): 27–35.

22. C. J. Goode, *Using Research in Clinical Nursing Practice* [Videotape] (Ida Grove, IA: Horn Video Productions, 1987).

23. C. J. Goode and J. Cipperley, *Research Utilization: A Process of Organizational Change* [Videotape] (Ida Grove, IA: Horn Video Productions, 1989).

24. C. J. Goode, *Research Utilization: A Study Guide* [Videotape] (Ida Grove, IA: Horn Video Productions, 1991).

25. C. J. Goode and J. Cipperley, *Reading and Critiquing a Research Report* [Videotape] (Ida Grove, IA: Horn Video Productions, 1991).

26. M. G. Titler, C. Kleiber, V. Steelman, C. Goode, B. Rakel, J. Barry-Walker, S. Small, et al., "Infusing Research into Practice to Promote Quality Care," *Nursing Research* 43, no. 5 (1994): 307–313.

27. D. N. Rutledge and N. E. Donaldson, "Building Organizational Capacity to Engage in Research Utilization," *Journal of Nursing Administration* 25, no. 10 (1995): 12–16.

28. D. L. Sackett, S. E. Straus, W. S. Richardson, W. Rosenberg, and R. B. Haynes, *Evidence-Based Medicine: How to Practice and Teach EBM,* 2nd ed. (New York: Churchill Livingstone, 2000).

29. C. J. Goode and F. Piedalue, "Evidence-Based Clinical Practice," *Journal of Nursing Administration* 29, no. 6 (1999): 15–21.

30. A. DiCenso, G. Guyatt, and D. Ciliska, *Evidence-Based Nursing: A Guide to Clinical Practice* (St. Louis, MO: Mosby, 2005).

31. C. B. Stetler, "Updating the Stetler Model of Research Utilization to Facilitate Evidence-Based Practice," *Nursing Outlook* 49, no. 6 (2001): 272–278.

32. A. A. Schultz, "Clinical Scholars at the Bedside: An EBP Mentorship Model for Today," *Online Journal of Excellence in Nursing Knowledge* (2005): 8 pp.

33. M. G. Titler, "Use of Research in Practice," in *Nursing Research: Methods, Critical Appraisal, and Utilization,* 5th ed., eds. G. LoBiondo-Wood and J. Haber (St. Louis, MO: Mosby, 2002):385–403.

34. J. Rycroft-Malone, "Promoting Action on Research Implementation in Health Services (PARIHS)," in *Models and Frameworks for Implementing Evidence-Based Practice: Linking Evidence to Action,* eds. J. Rycroft-Malone and T. Bucknall (Oxford, UK: Wiley Blackwell, 2010): 109–136.

35. R. P. Newhouse, S. Dearholt, S. Poe, L. C. Pugh, and K. M. White, "Organizational Change

Strategies for Evidence-Based Practice," *Journal of Nursing Administration* 37, no. 12 (2007): 552–557.

36. R. B. Haynes, P. J. Devereaux, and G. H. Guyatt, "Clinical Expertise in the Era of Evidence-Based Medicine and Patient Choice," *ACP Journal Club* 136, no. 2 (2002): A11–A14.

37. Clinical Scholarship Task Force, "Clinical Scholarship Research Paper" (1999). www.nursing society.org/aboutus/PositionPapers/Documents /clinical_scholarship_paper.pdf.

38. T. D. Strout, K. Lancaster, and A. A. Schultz, "Development and Implementation of an Inductive Model for Evidence-Based Practice: A Grassroots Approach for Building Evidence-Based Practice Capacity in Staff Nurses," *Nursing Clinics of North America* 44, no. 1 (2009): 93–102.

39. B. B. Brewer, M. A. Brewer, and A. A. Schultz, "A Collaborative Approach to Building the Capacity for Research and Evidence-Based Practice in Community Hospitals," *Nursing Clinics of North America* 44, no. 1 (2009): 11–25.

40. C. Honess, P. Gallant, and K. Keane, "The Clinical Scholar Model: Evidence Based Practice at the Bedside," *Nursing Clinics of North America* 44, no. 1 (2009): 117–130.

41. C. Mulvenon and M. K. Brewer, "From the Bedside to the Boardroom: Resuscitating Nursing Research," *Nursing Clinics of North America* 44, no. 1 (2009): 145–152.

42. A. E. Sossong, S. Cullen, P. Theriault, A. Stetson, B. Higgins, S. Roche, S. Ellis-Hermansen, et al., "Renewing the Spirit of Nursing by Embracing Evidence-Based Practice," *Nursing Clinics of North America* 44, no. 1 (2009): 33–42.

43. S. M. Weeks, J. Marshall, and P. Burns, "Development of an Evidence-Based Practice and Research Collaborative Among Urban Hospitals," *Nursing Clinics of North America* 44, no. 1 (2009): 27–31.

44. S. Dopson and L. Fitzgerald, eds., *Knowledge into Action: Evidence-Based Health Care in Context* (Oxford, UK: Oxford University Press, 2005).

45. J. Gabbay, A. le May, H. Jefferson, D. Webb, R. Lovelock, J. Powell, and J. Lathlean, "A Case Study of Knowledge Management in Multiagency Consumer-Informed 'Communities of Practice': Implications for Evidence-Based Policy Development in Health and Social Services," *Health* 7, no. 3 (2003): 283–310.

46. T. Greenhalgh, G. Robert, F. Macfarlane, P. Bate, and O. Kyriakidou, "Diffusion of Innovations in Service Organizations: Systematic Review and Recommendations," *Milbank Quarterly* 82, no. 4 (2004): 584–629.

47. J. Rycroft-Malone, "Evidence-Informed Practice: From Individual to Context," *Journal of Nursing Management* 16, no. 4 (2008): 404–408.

48. C. B. Stetler, J. A. Ritchie, J. Rycroft-Malone, A. A. Schultz, and M. P. Charns, "Institutionalizing Evidence-Based Practice: An Organizational Case Study Using a Model of Strategic Change," *Implementation Science* 4 (2009): 78.

49. J. Rycroft-Malone, "The Politics of Evidence-Based Practice: Legacies and Current Challenges," *Journal of Research in Nursing* 11, no. 2 (2006): 95–108.

50. C. B. Stetler, J. A. Ritchie, J. Rycroft-Malone, A. A. Schultz, and M. P. Charns, "Improving Quality of Care Through Routine, Successful Implementation of Evidence-Based Practice at the Bedside: An Organizational Case Study Protocol Using the Pettigrew and Whipp Model of Strategic Change," *Implementation Science* 2 (2007): 3.

51. D. S. Pravikoff, S. T. Pierce, and A. Tanner, "Evidence-Based Practice Readiness Study Supported by Academy Nursing Informatics Expert Panel," *Nursing Outlook* 53, no. 1 (2005): 49–50.

52. C. M. Baldwin, B. M. Melnyk, E. Fineout-Overholt, M. C. Cometto, and G. Avila, "Individual and Institutional Barriers to Implementing EBP in Clinical Practice: A Comparison of Pan American and U.S. Nurses" (paper presented at the 10th Annual National/International Evidence-Based Practice Conference, Phoenix, AZ, February 20, 2009).

53. R. Maljanian, L. Caramanica, S. K. Taylor, J. B. MacRea, and D. K. Beland, "Evidence-Based Nursing Practice, Part 2: Building Skills Through Research Roundtables," *Journal of Nursing Administration* 32, no. 2 (2002): 85–90.

54. A. Retsas, "Barriers to Using Research Evidence in Nursing Practice," *Journal of Advanced Nursing* 31, no. 3 (2000): 599–606.

55. T. Strout, "Curiosity and Reflective Thinking: Renewal of the Spirit," *Online Journal of Excellence in Nursing Knowledge* 2 (2005): 39.

56. B. Melnyk, "Calling All Educators to Teach and Model Evidence-Based Practice in Academic Settings," *Worldviews on Evidence-Based Nursing* 3, no. 3 (2006): 93–94.

57. B. S. Reigle, K. R. Stevens, J. V. Belcher, M. M. Huth, E. McGuire, D. Mais, and T. Volz, "Evidence-Based Practice and the Road to Magnet Status," *Journal of Nursing Administration* 38, no. 2 (2008): 97–102.

58. M. L. McClure, M. Poulin, M. D. Sovie, and M. A. Wandelt, *Magnet Hospitals: Attraction and Retention of Professional Nurses* (Washington, DC: American Nurses Association, 1983).

59. American Nurses Credentialing Center, *2014 Magnet Application Manual* (Silver Spring, MD: American Nurses Credentialing Center, 2014).

60. American Nurses Credentialing Center, "ANCC Magnet Recognition Program®" (2014). www .nursecredentialing.org/Magnet.aspx.

61. R. W. Puddy and N. Wilkins, *Understanding Evidence Part 1: Best Available Research Evidence. A Guide to the Continuum of Evidence of Effectiveness* (Atlanta, GA: Centers for Disease Control and Prevention, 2011).

62. C. M. Baldwin and E. Fineout-Overholt, "Evidence-Based Practice as Holistic Nursing Research," *Beginnings* 25, no. 3 (2005): 16.

63. R. McCaffrey, J. Park, D. Newman, and D. Hagen, "The Effect of Chair Yoga in Older Adults with Moderate and Severe Alzheimer's Disease," *Research in Gerontological Nursing* 7, no. 4 (2014): 171–177.

64. C. M. Baldwin, "Práctica Basada en la Evidencia (PBE): Una Introducción a la Revisión de la Evidencia para Mejorar el Resultado en los Pacientes (Evidence-Based Practice (EBP): An Introduction to Reviewing the Evidence to Improve Patient Outcomes) [Abstract]," in *Proceedings of the 10th Coloquio Panamericano de Investigacion en Enfermeria* (Buenos Aires, Argentina: Office of Pan American Health Organization, 2006): 41.

65. Alzheimer's Association Report, "2013 Alzheimer's Disease Facts and Figures," *Alzheimer's and Dementia* 9, no. 2 (2013): 208–245.

66. K. Y. Liang, M. A. Mintun, A. M. Fagan, A. M. Goate, J. M. Bugg, D. M. Holtzman, J. C. Morris, et al., "Exercise and Alzheimer's Disease Biomarkers in Cognitively Normal Older Adults," *Annals of Neurology* 63, no. 3 (2010): 311–318.

67. M. C. McCall, "How Might Yoga Work? An Overview of Potential Underlying Mechanisms," *Journal of Yoga and Physical Therapy* 3, no. 1 (2013): 1–6.

68. L. G. Litchke, J. S. Hodges, and R. F. Reardon, "Benefits of Chair Yoga for Persons with Mild to Severe Alzheimer's Disease," *Activities, Adaptation, and Aging* 36, no. 4 (2012): 317–328.

69. B. M. Melnyk and E. Fineout-Overholt, "Key Steps in Implementing Evidence-Based Practice: Asking Compelling, Searchable Questions and Searching for the Best Evidence," *Pediatric Nursing* 28, no. 3 (2002): 262–263, 266.

70. E. A. Balas and S. A. Boren, "Managing Clinical Knowledge for Health Care Improvement," in *Yearbook of Medical Informatics 2000: Patient-Centered Systems*, eds. J. Bemmel and A. T. McCray (Stuttgart, Germany: Schattauer Verlagsgesellschaft, 2000): 65–70.

71. Committee on Quality of Health Care in America, Institute of Medicine, *Crossing the Quality Chasm: A New Health System for the 21st Century* (Washington, DC: National Academies Press, 2001).

72. A. Greiner and E. Knebel, eds., *Health Professions Education: A Bridge to Quality* (Washington, DC: National Academies Press, 2003).

73. Sigma Theta Tau International, "Global Development Position Statement" (2005). www.nursingsociety.org/aboutus/PositionPapers/Documents/policy_development.pdf.

74. Joanna Briggs Institute, "About JBI" (2014). http://joannabriggs.org/about.html.

75. A. A. Schultz, "The Clinical Scholar Program: A Fulbright Collaboration in Northern Thailand" (paper presented at the 41st Biennial Convention, Sigma Theta Tau International, Grapevine, TX, November 2, 2011).

76. A. A. Schultz, "The Clinical Scholar Program: A Fulbright Collaboration in Northern Philippines" (paper presented at the Western Institute of Nursing 47th Annual Communicating Nursing Research Conference, Seattle, WA, April 10, 2014).

77. E. Chapman, "Evaluation of the Evidence Informed Policy Networks (EVIPNet)" (August 2010–July 2012). www.who.int/evidence/EvaluationEVIPNetAmericas.pdf.

78. J. G. Bauer and F. Chiappelli, "Transforming Scientific Evidence into Better Consumer Choices," *Bioinformation* 5, no. 7 (2011): 297–299.

79. K. Chalkidou, S. Tunis, R. Lopert, P. T. Sawicki, M. Nasser, and B. Xerri, "Comparative Effectiveness Research and Evidence-Based Health Policy: Experience from Four Countries," *Milbank Quarterly* 87, no. 2 (2009): 339–367.

80. J. K. Iglehart, "Prioritizing Comparative Effectiveness Research: IOM Recommendations," *New England Journal of Medicine* 361, no. 4 (2009): 325–328.

81. E. Nabel, "Role of the NIH in Comparative Effectiveness Research" (presentation at the National Comparative Effectiveness Research Summit, Washington, DC, September 16, 2009).

82. S. L. West, G. Gartlehner, A. J. Mansfield, C. Poole, E. Tant, N. Lenfestey, L. J. Lux, et al., *Comparative Effectiveness Review Methods: Clinical Heterogeneity*, AHRQ Publication No. 10-EHC070-EF (Research Triangle Park: TRI International, University of North Carolina Evidence-Based Practice Center, 2010).

83. Society for Prevention Research, "Standards of Evidence: Criteria for Efficacy, Effectiveness and Dissemination" (2005). www.preventionresearch.org/StandardsofEvidencebook.pdf.

84. D. J. Barksdale, R. Newhouse, and J. A. Miller, "The Patient-Centered Outcomes Research Institute (PCORI): Information for Academic Nursing," *Nursing Outlook* 62, no. 3 (2014): 192–200.

85. K. Stevens, "The Impact of Evidence-Based Practice in Nursing and the Next Big Ideas," *OJIN: The Online Journal of Issues in Nursing* 18, no. 2 (May 31, 2013): Manuscript 4.

86. S. M. Cooney, M. Huser, S. Small, and C. O'Connor, "Evidence-Based Programs: An Overview," *What Works, Wisconsin–Research to Practice Series* 6 (2007): 1–8.

87. D. M. Berwick, T. W. Nolan, and J. Whittington, "The Triple Aim: Care, Health, and Cost," *Health Affairs* 27, no. 3 (2008): 759–769.

88. D. W. Coon, M. Keaveny, I. R. Valverde, S. Dadvar, and D. Gallagher-Thompson, "Evidence-Based Psychological Treatments for Distress in Family Caregivers of Older Adults," in *Making Evidence-Based Psychological Treatments Work with Older Adults*, eds. F. Scogin and A. Shah (Washington, DC: American Psychological Association, 2012): 225–284.

89. K. R. Lorig, P. L. Ritter, and V. M. González, "Hispanic Chronic Disease Self-Management: A Randomized Community-Based Outcome Trial," *Nursing Research* 52, no. 6 (2003): 361–369.

90. Pan American Health Organization, *Camino a la Salud (Su corazón, su vida) Manual para Promotoras y Promotores* (Washington, DC: Pan American Health Organization, 2014).

91. C. M. Baldwin, M. Choi, M. T. Cerqueira, C. Urista-Solomon, L. Reynaga-Ornelas, S. F. Quan. "Linking Research with Practice and Health Equity: Implementation and Evaluation of a Spanish-Language Sleep Promotion Manual for Lay Health Workers" (paper presented at the IV Congress of Research in Nursing of Ibero-American and Portuguese Speaking Countries and X Conference of the Global Network of World Health Organization Collaborating Centers in Nursing and Midwifery, Coimbra, Portugal, July 21–25, 2014).

EVIDENCE-BASED PRACTICE RESOURCES

Annual national and international EBP conferences and workshops offer intensive sessions on EBP. Some of these venues include STTI's yearly international EBP/research congress, annual EBP conferences held by the Academic Center for Evidence-Based Practice at the University of Texas Health Science Center's San Antonio School of Nursing, and the University of Iowa Hospitals and Clinics. The following is a selection of national and international EBP, EBPP, and Magnet online resources:

- Academic Center for Evidence-Based Practice, University of Texas www.acestar.uthscsa.edu/
- Active for Life www.activeforlife.info
- Agency for Healthcare Research and Quality Evidence-Based Practice Centers www.ahrq.gov/clinic/epc/
- Chronic Disease Self-Management Program http://patienteducation.stanford.edu/programs/cdsmp.html
- The Cochrane Collaboration www.cochrane.org/
- Joanna Briggs Institute http://joannabriggs.org
- Magnet Recognition Program® www.nursecredentialing.org/Magnet.aspx
- Medications Management Improvement System www.homemeds.org
- National Institutes of Health Library, Evidence Based Practice Resources http://nihlibrary.ors.nih.gov/jw/ebp.html
- Evidence-Informed Policy Network (EVIPNet) http://global.evipnet.org
- EPIS Center, Evidence-Based Programs www.episcenter.psu.edu/ebp
- Sigma Theta Tau International, Evidence-Based Nursing Position Statement www.nursingsociety.org/aboutus/Position Papers/Pages/EBN_positionpaper.aspx
- Tai Chi: Moving for Better Balance www.taichimovingforbetterbalance.org
- University of Iowa Hospitals and Clinics, Nursing Research and Evidence-Based Practice www.uihealthcare.org/nursing-research-and-evidence-based-practice

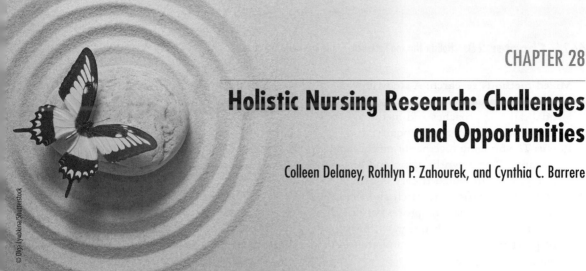

CHAPTER 28

Holistic Nursing Research: Challenges and Opportunities

Colleen Delaney, Rothlyn P. Zahourek, and Cynthia C. Barrere

Nurse Healer Objectives

Theoretical

- Discuss ways holistic philosophy and theoretical frameworks are reflected in holistic nursing research.
- Define holistic nursing research.
- Compare and contrast a variety of research methods used to examine different aspects of holistic nursing practice.
- Explore the challenges and future trends affecting holistic nursing research.

Clinical

- Explore how holistic nursing research questions can be developed in your clinical setting.
- Read a research article related to a core concept/modality you use in your holistic nursing practice.
- Discuss ways to enhance practice through holistic research with colleagues and nurse researchers.
- Devise a holistic nursing research question and propose a method of research that would best explore that question.

Personal

- Contemplate how a conceptual framework of holism is the foundation for holistic nursing research and practice.

- Consider that you do research every day in clinical practice as you assess patients and their situations, make diagnoses, plan and follow through on actions, and evaluate those actions.
- Plan time to learn how to form a research question.
- Attend a research conference or a section on research at the American Holistic Nurses Association annual conference or at a local networking meeting or other research conference and reflect on how the content relates to you and to your practice.

Definitions

Bracketing: A characteristic of qualitative research. The researcher outlines in writing his or her philosophies, biases, or concerns and expectations about the research project process and/or outcome.

Credibility: A term used in qualitative research that accounts for the researcher's trustworthiness in demonstrating the process of data collection and interpretation of results.

Empirical: A means of gaining knowledge based on experience or observation.

Meta-analysis: A statistical technique that combines the results of many studies related to one topic to establish an overall estimate of the therapeutic effectiveness of an intervention.

Mixed methods research: A study in which the investigator uses both quantitative and qualitative approaches and methods in a single study or program of inquiry.

Praxis: The bringing together of practice and research. It is a synthesizing and reflective process in which theory is dynamic and practice reflects research and theory in a unified whole. The process of reflection in action that fully integrates the roles of practitioner, researcher, and educator within a single nurse.

Qualitative research: A systematic, subjective research approach that describes life experiences and searches for how participants find meaning in their experiences; based on philosophical, psychological, and sociological theory; focuses on understanding the whole, which is consistent with the philosophy of holistic nursing.

Quantitative research: A systematic, formal objective approach in which numerical data are used to obtain and interpret information about the world. It embodies the principles of the scientific method, which describes variables, examines relationships among variables, determines cause-and-effect interactions between variables, and predicts future responses.

Reliability: Generally associated with quantitative research and the ability of a scale or a tool to consistently measure a phenomenon when used repeatedly.

Research: A diligent, systematic inquiry or investigation that uses disciplined methods to answer questions or solve problems.

Saturation: Relates to the data collection process of a qualitative study in which the researcher determines that responses are repetitive and no new information is being generated.

Systematic review: A specific form of review of research studies that yields more convincing evidence. Several methods exist; these are invaluable in determining what has already been discovered about a particular phenomenon.

Translational research: Taking basic bench, highly reductionist (molecular or cellular) research and translating that into clinical application. It generates new research questions that are fed back to the bench. More broadly, translating any research into practice.

Trustworthiness: A term used in qualitative research similar to credibility, dependability, and transferability. Ensures that the researcher has fully explained the sample and circumstances of the research and has bracketed prior preconceived notions and expectations.

Validity: Generally associated with quantitative research; internal and external; relates to the interpretation of data; meaningful, appropriate, and useful results are required for validity. Internal validity is related to the controls placed on the research design and process and ensures that the effects of the independent variable are causing the results in the dependent variable. External validity ensures that the results are generalizable to other populations, settings, and times and depends on internal validity.

What Is Holistic Nursing Research?

The field of holistic nursing is growing rapidly due to the changing healthcare climate and a recognition of the benefits of integrating conventional traditional health care, as well as complementary and alternative modalities, with patient-centered approaches that are focused on health and healing. With the increased interest in integrative care, holistic nursing has risen in visibility and importance to both patients and practitioners alike. Consequently, there is a growing need for research studies that provide evidence of the positive health-related outcomes associated with holistic nursing care. The need for research is imperative for holistic care to thrive and fully develop in healthcare delivery systems.

How do holistic nurses understand and connect science and spirit? How do they explore the healing relationship and healing itself? What is holistic nursing research? The American Holistic Nurses Association (AHNA) embraces and supports all research that has holism as a foundation.[1] Holistic nursing research (HNR) is grounded in the belief that humans are whole and complete and must be studied as such. Holistic research focuses on creating evidence of the mind-body-spirit connection and unity in health and the ability of humans to intentionally practice self-healing as well as participate in healing others and society. To create a strong body of evidence for holistic nursing, research in this area encompasses all modes of inquiry, including quantitative, qualitative, and mixed methods, as well as such unique approaches as aesthetic inquiry and interpretations and transpersonal approaches to posing research questions and data analysis.[2] Zahourek emphasized that for nursing research to be considered "holistic nursing research" it must occur within a framework that acknowledges, utilizes, and/or integrates a concept of holism and/or has holistic nursing implications.[3]

This chapter provides a context for understanding the multiplicity of research methods used to describe and explore relevant concepts and modalities specific to holistic nursing practice. The various philosophical and theoretical frameworks that provide a foundation for HNR are discussed, along with the current status of this evolving area of research. Exemplars, challenges, implications, and future directions for HNR are presented.

Setting the Foundation for Holistic Nursing Research: Philosophical and Theoretical Underpinnings

Philosophy

The philosophical legacy for HNR spans centuries of thought ranging from 17th-century Cartesian logic and the scientific method, which historically separates parts from the whole and "soul from body," to 20th-century complex quantum physics and 21st-century complexity theory, both of which view a unified universe in which parts cannot be separated. The logic of the scientific method requires that A plus B has to equal C; these logical relationships must behave predictably to be considered credible and valid. This philosophy is the basis of quantitative research and the prevailing gold standard of research—the randomized controlled trial. The more subtle concepts held particularly dear in holistic nursing, such as spirituality, caring, presence, intention and intentionality, and "subtle energies," create research challenges because of the difficulty in both definition and measurement. (Previous chapters in this text present these concepts, including research and research implications.) While those concepts can be, and are, researched successfully through quantitative research, qualitative research methods have found a home in describing and creating theory about such phenomena. Although holistic nurses believe in the power of spirit, energies, and unexplained forces, such as presence and intentionality, holistic nurses have a duty to understand the nature of such phenomena and to ethically demonstrate their safety, efficacy, and effectiveness. A scholarly body of credible, reliable, and valid research that has implications for practice, education, and continued scholarship must be developed.

Specific Frameworks of Holistic Nursing Research

All research is based on a philosophy or worldview. Relevant nursing theories and a philosophy of holism form the foundation of HNR. Holistic worldviews range from a holographic perspective (neuroscientist Karl Pribram)[4] to the postmodern view of the quantum nature of holism (David Bohm)[5] to complexity science and chaos theory.[6] According to the Bristol Center for Complexity Science, some view complexity as each scientific branch having its own complex investigative system and that complexity science itself "refutes the approach of traditional science according to which a system's behaviour can be understood by studying the system's parts independently."[7] These highly abstract and theoretical perspectives propose an unbroken, entangled wholeness of the universe. These theories help explain approaches that are grounded in the appreciation of the body-mind-spirit-environment-energy union.

Theoretical frameworks provide a structure for research approaches. Hagedorn and Zahourek developed an integrated model for understanding both quantitative and qualitative designs.[2] They emphasize that although holistic nurses use a variety of integrative and complementary modalities, HNR must occur within a framework of theory and practice that considers holism. The research question, method, analysis, and interpretation of findings depend on a worldview and/or paradigmatic framework.

The following frameworks are related in their model:

- The AHNA's definitions of holism (*integral* and *unitary*)[8]
- Carper's classic ways of knowing (*subjective* and *objective*, *individual* and *intrapersonal*, *interpersonal* and *cultural*, *aesthetic* and *ethical*)[9]
- Classic paradigms developed by Newman and enlarged by Fawcett (*particulate–deterministic*, *interactive–integrative*, *unitary–transformative*)[10, 11]
- Mariano's five attributes of holistic scholarship[12]

Figure 28-1 presents the framework for HNR.

AHNA Definition of Holism

- *Integral.* The interrelationships of the bio-psycho-social-spiritual dimensions of the person make up the whole, which is viewed as greater than a relational integration of parts.
- *Unitary.* The individual is a whole in mutual process with the environment and not separate from but greater than the parts.

Carper's Ways of Knowing

- *Empirical.* Objective, logical, and positivistic science.
- *Ethical.* Obligations, what should be done in a given situation; what is acceptable practice; requires openness to differences in philosophical positions.
- *Personal.* Self-knowledge; determined by the ability to self-actualize; comfort with ambiguity; commitment to patience and self-care.
- *Aesthetic.* Artful knowledge; abstract; defies formal description and measurement; understanding of subjective experiences; creative pattern.

Three Competing Paradigms (Newman and Fawcett)

- *Particulate–deterministic.* Reductionist view of parts as isolatable and reducible and separate as related to the whole; change is predictable and may be controlled; concrete.
- *Interactive–integrative.* Reality is experiential, multidimensional, and contextual; reciprocal relationships comprise the whole; more abstract.
- *Unitary–transformative.* Human beings are unitary, evolving, self-organizing fields, the whole is defined by pattern; change is increasingly complex and unpredictable; highly abstract.

Mariano: Attributes of Holistic Scholarship

- *Openness.* Thoughtful about all possibilities.
- *Keeping wide awake.* Attending to others and conscious of one's experiences.
- *Reflectivity.* Critical ethical thinking; displaying to self and others one's thought process.
- *Caring.* Knowledge related to caring, passion, humility, courage, empathy, and fair-mindedness.
- *Humor.* Embracing the unexpected as opportunity; seeing oneself and one's work in perspective.

Theory

Several nursing theories relevant to holistic nursing practice incorporate abstract concepts drawn from theoretical frameworks such as quantum physics, systems theory, and post modernism. (See Chapter 5 for a full discussion of nurse theorists.) Theories associated with holism continue to develop, such as Dossey's Theory of Integrative Nursing[13] (see Chapter 1), Pamela Reed's Self Transcendence,[14] and Zahourek's Intentionality: The Matrix of Healing.[15] However, the major theorists usually associated with holistic nursing include but are not limited to Martha Rogers,[16] Margaret Newman,[10] Rosemarie Parse,[17] Jean Watson,[18] Helen Erickson,[19] and Madeleine Leininger.[20] These nurses have developed a wealth of both *integral* and *unitary* theories related to caring, healing, culture, and the nature of the whole in the human–person

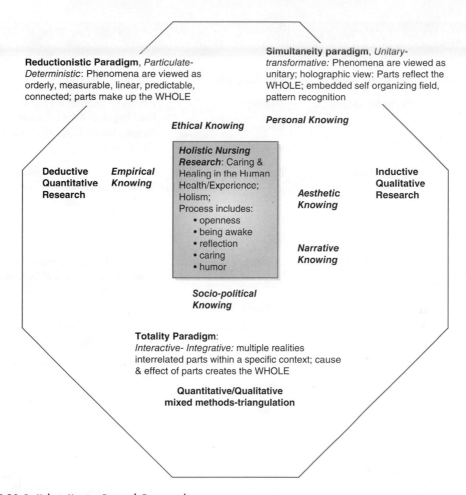

FIGURE 28-1 Holistic Nursing Research Framework

Source: Reproduced from M. Enzman-Hagedorn and R. P. Zahourek, Research Paradigms and Methods for Investigating Holistic Nursing Concerns, Nursing Clinics of North America 42, no. 2 (2007): 335–353.

environment. In addition, they and other scholars have created methodologies and tools to conduct research. For example, Margaret Newman (unitary theory: Health as Expanding Consciousness) proposes a qualitative "hermeneutic, dialectic method" that allows "the pattern of the person and environment to reveal itself without disrupting the unity of the pattern. The process culminates in intuitive apprehension and expression."[10] For Newman, research is *praxis* and based in practice. Research emanates from the nurse's engagement with participants during important events and within significant relationships; pattern recognition acknowledges the whole.[21] **Table 28-1** displays recent studies based on holistic nursing theories.

As evidence of the evolution of holistic nursing, nurse scholars have developed research instruments to document holistic nursing phenomena. Examples of such instruments include:

- Jean Watson, Theory of Transpersonal Caring: The Caring Factor Survey.[18, 28]
- Elizabeth Barrett, Rogerian Power Theory: A quantitative measurement tool for power as knowing participation in change.[29]
- Rosemarie Parse, Theory of Human Becoming: A specific phenomenological method to explore the universal lived experiences of health through the process of dialogical engagement, extraction-synthesis, and heuristic interpretation.[17, p 62]

TABLE 28-1	Examples of Theory-Based Research Relevant to Holistic Nursing		
Theorist	**Model or Theory**	**Key Concepts**	**Research Example**
Rogers	Unitary Human Beings	Resonancy	J. Hubbard, "Evaluation of a Brief Mindfulness-Based Program on Recall and Sense of Well-Being in a Sample of Older African Americans"[22]
		Helicy	
		Integrality	
Newman	Health as Expanding Consciousness	Health	M. Smith, "Integrative Review of Research Related to Margaret Newman's Theory of Health as Expanding Consciousness"[23]
		Consciousness	
		Patterns of movement	
		Space–time	
Parse	Theory of Human Becoming	Meaning	H. Y. Chen, "The Lived Experience of Moving Forward for Clients with Spinal Cord Injury: A Parse Research Method Study"[24]
		Rhythmicity	
		Transcendence	
Watson	Theory of Human Caring	10 caritas factors	J. Nelson and J. Watson, *Measuring Caring: International Research on Caritas as Healing*[25]
Erickson	Modeling and Role-Modeling Theory	Modeling	M. E. Koren and C. Papadimitiou, "Spirituality of Staff Nurses: Application of Modeling and Role Modeling Theory"[26]
		Role modeling	
		Arousal	
		Equilibrium	
		Impoverishment	
Leininger	Transcultural Nursing	Cultural preservation or maintenance	M. Bengtsson, K. Ulander, E. Börgdal, and B. Ohlsson, "A Holistic Approach for Planning Care of Patients with Irritable Bowel Syndrome"[27]
		Cultural care accommodation or negotiation	
		Cultural care repatterning or restructuring	

Holistic Research Methods and Designs

Research is diligent, systematic inquiry to validate and refine existing knowledge and to generate new knowledge.[30] No longer limited to qualitative and quantitative approaches, methods now include triangulation and mixed methods, aesthetic, postmodern, feminist, reflective, narrative, participatory action, transpersonal, systemic reviews, meta-analyses, and methods based on specific nurse theorists such as Parse, Watson, and Newman (see Chapter 5) as well as others. This section provides (1) a brief review

of the two most conventional research methods (quantitative and qualitative), (2) the key steps of quantitative and qualitative methods, and (3) additional approaches relevant to HNR. Readers are encouraged to explore various methods and philosophical bases with experienced nurse researchers and social scientists, keeping in mind the need for a unitary or integral perspective. An important point to remember is that the research question determines the method.

Quantitative Research Designs

Quantitative research is a systematic, formal, objective process based on the scientific method in which numerical data are used to obtain information about the world. Quantitative research involves the following designs.

Experimental Designs

1. *Experimental.* Also referred to as randomized controlled trial. A true experiment has three properties: (1) manipulation—researchers introduce an intervention, (2) control—researchers use a control group and other controls over variables in the study, and (3) randomization—researchers randomly assign participants to a control or intervention group.
2. *Quasi-experimental.* Lacks randomization but involves manipulation in which researchers introduce an intervention. Quasi-experimental studies may also include a control group, but the distinguishing characteristic is lack of randomization.
3. *Pre-experimental.* Introduces an intervention without a control group or randomization.

Non-experimental Designs

1. *Correlational.* Studies that examine relationships among variables.
2. *Descriptive.* Studies that attempt to observe, describe, and document phenomena or experiences. Often used as a starting point for future research and generation of hypotheses.

Applying the Five Phases of the Quantitative Research Process in Holistic Nursing Practice

Quantitative research studies typically follow a five-phase process.[30] These activities usually occur in a linear fashion, and in some studies, these steps overlap. This section illustrates the application of these steps and describes the timeline of a quantitative study conducted by the first author of this chapter.[31]

Phase I: The Conceptual Phase

In Phase I of the research process, the holistic nurse ponders a research question based on a foundation of holism. During this thinking phase, questions are reflected on such as: Why am I drawn to study? How will this work contribute to the advancement of holistic nursing and/or improved patient outcomes? Holistic nurses are encouraged to review the related literature on their selected topic to understand the current state of the science. It is often helpful to create a table with all related studies to compare designs and methods. This phase concludes with development of the research question.

Example This first phase spanned about 6 months. During this time, the researcher reviewed interdisciplinary research in spirituality, developed conceptual definitions, and drafted the items on the Spirituality Scale (SS). Spirituality was conceptualized as having three dimensions: personal, interpersonal, and transpersonal. The instrument was reviewed by a group of content experts and revisions were made based on their suggestions. The research questions guiding the study were: What is the content validity of the SS? What is the factorial structure of the SS? What is the alpha internal consistency of the SS? What is the 2-week test–retest reliability of the SS?

Phase II: Design and Planning

Once a research question is determined, the holistic nurse selects a research design to best answer the question. Activities in this stage include selecting a research design, developing study protocols, selecting the population and sampling plan, identifying measurement instruments, and human subject considerations.

Example This phase was completed in 2 months. A methodological research design was used in this study. During this phase, the researcher finalized the SS; gained access to inpatient, outpatient, and community settings in two hospitals, one assisted living facility, and two home care agencies; and obtained human subjects protection through Institutional Review Board (IRB) approval from the university and permission letters from the research committees at the participating data collection sites. The researcher met with a statistical consultant several times. The target population selected for this study was adults with chronic illness.

Phase III: Empirical

In this phase, the holistic nurse collects data and prepares the data for analysis. This phase typically takes the most time in studies.

Example   Data collection took about 8 months to complete. The research design required a minimum sample size of 190, as there should be at least five times as many participants as items, or at least 200 respondents.

Phase IV: Analytic

During this phase, the holistic nurse analyzes and interprets the data. A statistician should be used to assist with analysis.

Example   This phase occurred over 2 months. Two hundred twenty-six participants completed the study. Statistical tests were performed to evaluate the psychometric properties of the SS. Validity was examined with exploratory factor analysis and content validity. Factor analysis revealed three factors consistent with the theoretical framework. Content validity of the SS was .94, or 94% agreement among the content experts. These tests supported the validity of the SS. Internal reliability and test–retest reliability findings also supported the reliability of the SS.

Phase V: Dissemination

In this phase, the holistic nurse communicates the research findings through publications and professional presentations. Consideration for utilizing findings in practice also occurs at this time.

Example   This phase was the longest. The study manuscript was prepared and accepted for publication by the *Journal of Holistic Nursing*. During this time, the study was presented at regional and national conferences. Since its publication in 2005, the SS has been requested by researchers in 12 countries and translated into 6 languages.

Qualitative Research

Holistic nurses embrace several philosophies of science and research methods that are compatible with investigating humanistic, unitary, and integral phenomena. Qualitative methods are appropriate when little information is known about a phenomenon or when phenomena are difficult to measure.[32] Qualitative research systematically describes and promotes understanding of human experiences such as health, healing, energy, intention, caring, comfort, and

meaning. The context of this approach is meaning of observed patterns. The goal is to discover and communicate rich, articulate, in-depth, and coherent understanding of phenomena.

The following are considered to be the five basic traditions in qualitative research.[32] There are many others that utilize various approaches as well as methods of analysis including transpersonal, feminist, descriptive, narrative, content analysis, participatory inquiry, and aesthetic forms of inquiry. Each of the five traditions is grounded in a specific philosophical framework and includes guidelines for data analysis.[32, p. 37]

1. *Phenomenology*. Strongly based in philosophy and focuses on experience as the whole person lives it.
2. *Ethnography*. A highly detailed description of a culture and roles of the people and their culture.
3. *Grounded theory*. A systematic investigation in which constructs and theories related to psychosocial problems and how people manage are developed.
4. *Historical research*. Focuses on a biography of an individual and/or describes or analyzes past events to better understand the present.
5. *Case study*. Focuses on an in-depth study of the context and time of a single "case," which may be an individual or group in a "bounded system" (limited in time and place).

Applying the Four Phases of the Qualitative Research Process in Holistic Nursing Practice

Qualitative studies typically follow a four-phase process.[30] In contrast to quantitative studies, qualitative studies are best described as a circular process as there is a continual exchange between analyzing and interpreting data and deciding on how to proceed based on current findings. This section illustrates the steps and timeline by using a qualitative study conducted by the second author of this chapter.[15]

Phase I: Planning the Study

Phase I of the qualitative process is both similar to and different from the quantitative process.

Both processes begin with reflection, identification of the research problem, and deciding on an overall approach. In addition, ethical considerations for the protection of human subjects is an essential aspect of all research studies. In qualitative studies, reflection is a key component of the initial phase of the study and continues throughout the four phases. Important activities are journaling and memoing. The researcher outlines in writing his or her philosophies, biases, or concerns and expectations about the research project process and/or outcome (a process called *bracketing*). Further differences are found in performing literature reviews and developing research questions. In some qualitative studies a literature review may be delayed until after data collection to avoid influencing the researcher's conceptualization of the phenomenon of interest. Qualitative studies may or may not develop refined research questions at this stage; instead, a broad topic area is developed that is later narrowed down once the study is in progress.

Example The grounded theory study of Healing Through the Lens of Intentionality is a secondary analysis of an original study that focused on the concept of intentionality in healing. During this phase the researcher reviewed her passion for understanding the process of healing and the role of intention and intentionality. In the first study she had developed a theory about the role of intentionality in the context of healing.[15] But the question remained: How did her participants view and experience healing? The researcher believed that an increased understanding of healing was central to holistic nursing theory and practice as well as for all of nursing. The IRB had been obtained for the original study but, because this was a reanalysis of previous data with no participant contact, no new IRB was sought.

Phase II: Design and Planning

The researcher chooses the most appropriate approach to qualitative research based on the research question and desired end result.

Example In this example, grounded theory (the design of the original study) and a secondary analysis of the original data were chosen. As in quantitative research, developing data collection strategies is the next phase in which the qualitative researcher determines the type of data to be collected, how the data will be collected, and from whom the data will be collected and develops protocols to enhance the trustworthiness and credibility of the data.

Example For the original study, literature was reviewed from various fields, including complementary alternative therapies, philosophy, psychology, and nursing, to determine the need for and potential value of the study. The results of the original study were reviewed in addition to the literature on healing. Theoretical sampling was used in which the researcher may return to the literature or other sources of data for comparisons with the identified categories and themes. The convenience sample included six expert female nurses and six female patients. The participants were interviewed as individuals and, when possible, as a dyad (patient and nurse) prior to the treatment and after. The treatment was observed and videotaped. Material was transcribed.

Phase III: Empirical: Gathering and Analyzing Data

Activities in this phase include collecting and organizing data, evaluating data and making modifications to data collection strategies when indicated, and determining if data saturation has been achieved (themes and categories are repeated). Inherent in qualitative studies is flexibility in approach in direct contrast to the strict adherence to predefined protocols characteristic of quantitative studies.

Example For this secondary analysis, the transcribed interview data from the original study was analyzed by rereading transcripts and conducting computer searches for specific words in the documents, again looking for references to healing and any concepts that participants connected to healing. The constant comparison method was used for back-and-forth coding among all transcripts. Data analysis also included writing personal reactions, process observations, theory hunches, and methodological issues as memos. Gradually, themes, core concepts, and definitions of healing began to emerge. As the analysis progressed, a process of how healing happens was identified that included mediating factors. Because participants had previously reacted to the summaries of their interviews, and those summaries included definitions of healing, it was accepted that member checks for credibility and trustworthiness done in the first study applied to this current study.

Phase IV: Disseminating Findings

Analogous to Phase V of the quantitative process, the holistic nurse communicates research findings through publications and presentations. Study findings are used to make recommendations for practice changes and future research.

Example   The study was written for publication and accepted in two journals, presented at national and international conferences, and incorporated into literature reviews in additional studies related to both intentionality and healing. See **Table 28-2** for HNR examples.

TABLE 28-2	Examples of Holistic Nursing Research

Study Design	Research Example	Summary
Quantitative Designs		
Randomized controlled trial	J. E. Bormann, S. R. Thorp, J. L. Wetherell, S. L. Golshan, and J. Ariel, "Meditation-Based Mantram Intervention for Veterans with Posttraumatic Stress Disorder: A Randomized Trial"[33]	**Purpose:** To establish the efficacy of the Mantram Repetition Program (MRP), a portable practice of repeating a mantram or sacred word or phrase, slowing down, and practicing one-pointed attention as an evidence-based intervention for veterans with posttraumatic stress disorder (PTSD). **Method:** Veteran participants diagnosed with PTSD were randomly assigned to MRP (n = 25) or present-centered therapy (PCT) (n = 20), both delivered in an individual treatment format according to standard protocols in 8 weekly, 60-minute sessions. **Results:** Veterans randomized to MRP experienced a significantly greater reduction of PTSD symptoms relative to veterans who received PCT (p = .003).
Quasi-experimental	J. Park, R. McCaffrey, D. Newman, C. Cheung, and D. Hagen, "The Effect of Sit 'n' Fit Chair Yoga Among Community-Dwelling Older Adults with Osteoarthritis"[34]	**Purpose:** To examine the effects of Sit 'n' Fit chair yoga in decreasing pain and improving physical function and psychosocial well-being in older adults with osteoarthritis. **Method:** Thirty-nine participants were randomly assigned to the intervention or attention control groups. A randomized controlled trial could not be used; participants in the Alzheimer's disease unit were excluded from randomization. **Results:** Participants in the yoga group experienced a greater improvement in depression (p = .263) and life satisfaction (p = .012) compared to control group participants.
Pre-experimental	L. Kluepfel, T. Ward, R. Yehuda, E. Dimoulas, A. Smith, and K. Daly, "The Evaluation of Mindfulness-Based Stress Reduction for Veterans with Mental Health Conditions"[35]	**Purpose:** To assess the feasibility of mindfulness-based stress reduction (MBSR) for veterans with mental health conditions and evaluate its efficacy on psychological well-being and stress reduction. **Method:** Thirty veterans in a mental health clinic of a Veterans Administration medical center were enrolled in an 8-week standard MBSR program. Perceived stress, sleep, mindfulness, and depression were measured via self-reports at baseline and study end. **Results:** Scores on the Perceived Stress Scale (p =.002) and Beck Depression Inventory-II (p = .005) were significantly reduced (p = .002). The global measure for sleep from the Pittsburgh Sleep Quality Index improved significantly (p = .035).

TABLE 28-2   Examples of Holistic Nursing Research (*continued*)

Study Design	Research Example	Summary
Quantitative Designs		
Correlational	S. Cutshall, D. Dercheid, A. G. Miers, S. Ruegg, B. J. Schroeder, S. Tucker, and L. Wentworth, "Knowledge, Attitudes, and Use of Complementary and Alternative Therapies Among Clinical Nurse Specialists in an Academic Medical Center"[36]	***Purpose:*** To describe the knowledge, attitudes, and use of complementary and alternative medicine (CAM) by clinical nurse specialists (CNSs) in a large Midwestern medical center. ***Method:*** Seventy-six CNSs who work in various inpatient and outpatient units within this medical facility were surveyed using a 26-item questionnaire developed by the research team. ***Results:*** The CNSs at this academic medical center use several CAM therapies for their personal use and for professional practice with patients. The top therapies that CNSs personally used were humor, massage, spirituality/prayer, music therapy, and relaxed breathing. The top therapies requested most by patients were massage, spirituality/prayer, Healing Touch, acupuncture, and music therapy.
Descriptive	B. S. Gallison, Y. Xu, C. Y. Jurgens, and S. M. Boyle, "Acute Care Nurses' Spiritual Care Practices"[37]	***Purpose:*** To identify barriers in providing spiritual care to hospitalized patients. A convenience sample (N = 271) was recruited at an academic medical center in New York City. ***Method:*** The Spiritual Care Practice (SCP) questionnaire assesses spiritual care practices and perceived barriers to spiritual care. ***Results:*** Sixty-one percent scored less than the ideal mean on the SCP. Although 96% (N = 114) believe that addressing patients' spiritual needs are within their role, nearly half (48%) report rarely participating in spiritual practices. The greatest perceived barriers were beliefs that patients' spirituality is private, insufficient time, difficulty distinguishing proselytizing from spiritual care, and difficulty meeting patient needs when spiritual beliefs were different from their own.
Qualitative Designs		
Phenomenology	D. Leone, S. Ray, and M. Evans, "The Lived Experience of Anxiety Among Late Adolescents During High School: An Interpretive Phenomenological Inquiry"[38]	***Purpose:*** To understand everyday anxiety among late adolescents during high school. ***Method:*** A purposive sample of eight males and females in late adolescence with everyday anxiety were interviewed. ***Results:*** Themes reflective of the lived body in time and space and in relation with others. The three themes were the embodied experience of anxiety; feeling uncomfortable in the lived space of school; and life at home.
Qualitative descriptive	A. Liptak, J. Tate, J. Flatt, M. Oakley, and J. Lingler, "Humor and Laughter in Persons with Cognitive Impairment and Their Caregivers"[39]	***Purpose:*** To describe humor and laughter in persons with cognitive impairment and caregivers who were recalling a shared experience in a focus group. ***Method:*** Twenty participants attended an Art Engagement Activity, which included a guided tour and an art project. Four focus groups were conducted, and transcripts of audio-recorded sessions were transferred to a qualitative software program. ***Results:*** Humor and laughter were present in all four focus groups. Emerging themes of humor included silliness, sarcasm, and commenting about the hardships of dementia. Laughter was identified in segments with and without humor.

(*continues*)

	TABLE 28-2 Examples of Holistic Nursing Research (*continued*)

Study Design	Research Example	Summary
		Qualitative Designs
Ethnography	M. Poole, J. Bond, C. Emmett, H. Greener, S. Louw, L. Robinson, and J. Hughes, "Going Home? An Ethnographic Study of Assessment of Capacity and Best Interests in People with Dementia Being Discharged from Hospital"[40]	**Purpose:** To understand how medical wards make judgments about capacity and how best interests are determined for people with dementia and their families. **Method:** Award-based ethnography. Observational data were captured through detailed field notes, in-depth interviews, medical record review, and focus groups. **Results:** Five key themes emerged from the data: the complexity of borderline decisions, the requirement for better understanding of assessment approaches regarding residence capacity, the need for better documentation, the importance of narrative, and the crucial relevance of time and timing in making these decisions.
Grounded theory	P. Cone and T. Giske, "Teaching Spiritual Care—A Grounded Theory Study Among Undergraduate Nursing Educators"[41]	**Purpose:** To explore teachers' understanding of spirituality and how they prepare undergraduate nursing students to recognize spiritual cues and learn to assess and provide spiritual care. **Method:** Data collected during semi-structured interviews at three Norwegian university colleges in five focus groups with 19 undergraduate nursing teachers. **Results:** The participants' main concern was how to help students recognize cues and ways of providing spiritual care. This basic social process has three iterative phases that develop throughout the nursing program: raising student awareness to recognize the essence of spirituality, assisting students to overcome personal barriers, and mentoring students' competency in spiritual care.
Historical	D. Wagner and B. Whaite, "An Exploration of the Nature of Caring Relationships in the Writings of Florence Nightingale"[42]	**Purpose:** To identify the nature and attributes of caring relationships in Florence Nightingale's writings. **Method:** Historical field study, content analysis, and Watson's carative factors used as cross-validation. **Results:** Five themes representing caring congruent with Nightingale's threefold concept of nursing: attend to, attention to, nurture, competent, and genuine. Caring relationships are part of nursing history.
Case study	J. C. Gershon, "Healing the Healer: One Step at a Time"[43]	Provides an in-depth presentation and analysis of a 6-week program to help health caregivers manage stress. It describes and examines the structure, purpose, and design of the course. Results are theory based and supported by the case presentation.

Broadening the Scope of Holistic Research

Mixed Methods

Mixed methods research is research in which the investigator collects and analyzes data, integrates the findings, and draws inferences using both quantitative and qualitative approaches and methods in a single study or program of inquiry.[44] Mixed methods research is gaining popularity as the value of both quantitative and qualitative methods are recognized and as HNR continues to develop. A mixed methods study might use a quantifiable survey instrument on which participants indicate their answers on a Likert scale (1 equals "strongly disagree";

4 equals "strongly agree"). The qualitative component of this same study might ask participants to write their thoughts to an open-ended question. The narrative responses can be analyzed using a qualitative research data analysis method such as content analysis.

Mixed methods inquiry provides objective data as well as clinically relevant subjective data that the nurse may consider when evaluating the evidence for practice. For example, pain management is an elusive and challenging phenomenon to study, as demonstrated by Coleman.[45] She was interested in the routine use of Spring Forest Qigong (SFQ) and if it might alleviate perceived emotional and/or physical discomfort for persons with chronic pain She designed a mixed methods pilot study to investigate the effects of routine, independent SFQ practice on chronic pain reduction in 86 participants. Pre- and posttest quantitative measures included the standardized, self-rated Visual Analog Scale to measure intensity of perceived pain and emotional distress. Coleman also developed a symptom survey tool to evaluate changes in pain and distress-related symptoms. In addition to these outcomes measures, anecdotal narratives were captured through participants' comments on their experiences using SFQ. Even though the objective analyses revealed a significant decrease in the perception of physical pain and emotional distress as well as improvement in selected related symptoms in the majority of participants, the anecdotal narratives provided description and richness to the objective analysis. There are several study limitations for consideration when designing future mixed methods studies; however, the combination of methodologies used presents a clearer clinical picture of results and understanding of the potential for use of SFQ in practice.

Additional Methods: Aesthetic, Transpersonal

Numerous approaches to research exist and should be considered by holistic nurse researchers. The caveat remains: The method evolves from the question being asked and what the researcher hopes to find as an outcome. Holistic nurses have been embracing several versions of qualitative research in addition to mixed methods that include quantitative approaches. For example, narrative inquiries describe nurses' stories of healing,[46, 47] through participatory inquiry women describe their experiences with despair,[48] and other descriptive approaches frequently use qualitative methods. On occasion, the specific qualitative tradition is not identified, but the question is formed descriptively and data are analyzed using text or observations that are coded, categorized, and then thematized into a whole.

Aesthetic methods are methodologies that value the researcher's reactions as well as interpretation of data. Margo Ely and colleagues[49] and Lee Gaydos[50] developed classic aesthetic methods that are incorporated into data collection and interpretation. Butcher developed the "field pattern portrait" as an aesthetic way of knowing.[51] Aesthetic expressions (poetry, painting, music) can be used to explain ineffable phenomena such as healing and caring. Purnell and Locsin developed the *Journal of Art and Aesthetics in Nursing and Health Sciences* (http://nursing.fau.edu/JAANHS), a free-access, online journal in which creative expressions of nursing experiences are presented. Lange, Zahourek, and Mariano used the aesthetic approach to present the results of their historical narrative study with elders from AHNA.[52] The aesthetic approach included presenting a "snapshot" of each participant, a pastiche poem that summarized participants' experiences, and a collage that described the meanings and implications gleaned from each researchers' reflections.

The *transpersonal* approach championed by Braud and Anderson is a worldview that recognizes, values, and seeks to understand individuals' fundamental oneness with one another and with all of life.[53, 54] Implicit in this approach is a sense of "wonderment about the commonplace, an acceptance of life as precious, and recognition of the miraculous strata of all experiences."[53, p. xxii] The authors describe a research process that

> can be accompanied by increased self-awareness, enhanced psycho-spiritual growth and development, and other personal changes of great consequence to the individuals involved . . .

a qualitative shift in one's lifeview and/or worldview . . . one's perspective, understandings, attitudes, ways of knowing and doing, and way of being in the world. It may be recognized by changes in one's body, feelings and emotions, ways of thinking, forms of expression, and relationships with others and with the world. This approach includes intuition, storytelling, imagery, meditation, direct knowing, dreams, trance states, and describing uncommon experiences that are used as possible strategies and procedures at all phases of the research inquiry.[54, p. xxx]

An example of this method can be found in a poem Zahourek wrote following a dream, which illuminates concepts from the data that later became part of her Theory of Intentionality in Healing.[55] Because these approaches are currently out of the norm for research methodology, it is less likely that traditional funding agencies would consider such methodology valid.

Methods: Synthesis, Systematic Reviews, and Meta-analysis

Increasingly, meta-analyses, systematic reviews, and syntheses of research studies are published. At the top of the hierarchy of evidence are the systematic reviews and meta-analyses. According to Rew:

> A systematic review of literature is done not only to provide the evidence to guide current practice, but it is also an essential step in conducting research on new and innovative ideas for practice. In particular, conducting a systematic review of literature can be helpful in identifying tools to measure specific constructs in a planned study.[56, p. 3]

Anderson and Taylor conducted a systematic review of Healing Touch.[57] They noted that Healing Touch was practiced in a variety of settings and led to reports of improved outcomes such as reduced anxiety, increased relaxation, decreased pain, diminished depression, and an enhanced sense of well-being. Their systematic review critically evaluated data from randomized clinical trials examining the clinical effectiveness of Healing Touch. They began with an electronic database search of MEDLINE, CINAHL, and ClinicalTrials.gov, along with a supplemental manual database search using the search term *healing touch* to locate potentially relevant articles. Two reviewers independently validated, extracted, and recorded data using predetermined criteria. The methodological quality was then scored by the reviewers—again independently. A total of 322 articles were identified, of which 5 were randomized controlled trials. The studies support potential clinical effectiveness of Healing Touch in improving healthcare quality of life in chronic disease management; however, there were limitations in the research design methodologies used in each study. Examples of limitations found were the examination of Healing Touch but without the inclusion of a comparison group receiving the usual standard of care or of another alternative therapy that may evoke relaxation such as music during a Healing Touch intervention. In addition, there were general problematic issues found with the studies, such as minimal study descriptions, which prevent replication studies to confirm clinical results. Examples of descriptions that were lacking were treatment duration and number of treatments, along with a clear rationale for each. Also important to include in future studies is the level of experience of the Healing Touch practitioner. The investigators highlight the need for sound, scientific research that will demonstrate the effectiveness and potential therapeutic use of Healing Touch. Holistic nurses are challenged to design clinical trials that will address these methodological issues.

Holistic Nursing Research: Exemplars and Challenges

It is imperative that holistic nursing continue to advance the scientific knowledge base of evidence for holistic practice. Embracing the application of evidence-based nursing research to practice was one of the important responses by nursing and healthcare organizations to the Institute of Medicine report *The Future of Nursing: Leading Change, Advancing Health*.[58] Healthcare professionals need such quality information to provide evidence-based, comprehensive care that encourages a focus on healing and recognizes the importance of compassion and caring. The varied settings in which holistic nurses practice offer many opportunities to conduct meaningful research to address clinically relevant issues for holistic patient-centered care and improving patient outcomes.

Many strides have been made in selected areas of holistic practice that provide exemplars of research efforts and evidence for the effectiveness of holistic interventions. Recent examples of such exemplars include mindfulness meditation to relieve stress in patients diagnosed with diabetes or coronary heart disease,[59] loving kindness meditation to immediately reduce migraine headaches and alleviate emotional tension,[60] music to promote relaxation and alleviate pain in a variety of individuals,[61] and imagery as a simple, economical intervention to treat fatigue.[62] Studies have also been conducted to examine the effects of holistic interventions such as art therapy to aid in the healing process, increase relaxation, and decrease pain;[63] qi gong and tai chi have demonstrated positive effects on cancer-related quality of life, fatigue, immune function, and cortisol levels of cancer patients;[64] and tai chi has also been shown to improve balance, glucose control, neuropathy scores, and quality of life in diabetic patients.[65] Spirituality, once vague and difficult to define, now has a significant body of literature examining this essential holistic aspect of care.[66] The growing acceptance of integrative care has led nurses to design protocols and examine the effect of spiritual care interventions.[67] Self-care research has also come to the forefront by showcasing positive outcomes for patients with heart failure[68] as well as self-care strategies for use by nurses.[69]

Research challenges present themselves in selected areas of holistic care; these remain abstract and difficult to define and measure.

Authentic presence is central to holistic nursing and pertinent to all care, yet little research has been conducted to demonstrate evidence of its effectiveness or to more fully describe "consciously staying in the present moment."[70] Also core to holistic nursing practice is the expectation of nurses to transform healthcare settings into healing environments to provide quality patient care and realize positive outcomes for patients.[71] Holistic nurse researchers are challenged to examine what constitutes a healing environment, determine how faculty teach nursing students to create healing environments, and evaluate the effectiveness of a healing environment.

More recent research challenges have arisen as holistic nursing expands. Nurse coaches work with individuals and groups in all practice areas to create coaching partnerships.[72] Nurse coaching shows promise in improving overall health, life balance, and well-being in persons with chronic conditions.[73] Additional research on the effectiveness of nurse coaching will better support the success of best practice coaching interventions. Much of healthcare uses a team approach to care; research efforts need to evaluate patient outcomes of the team approach such as collaborating in providing end-of-life care[74] and persistence in overcoming issues encountered working with vulnerable palliative care populations coupled with conducting studies in research-naïve clinical settings.[75]

Another research gap identified in the literature is evidence supporting effective pedagogies for teaching holistic care. Research is needed that examines optimal ways to teach various aspects of holistic nursing.[76-79] Research examining the outcomes of teaching approaches used will assist faculty when planning curricula and nurse educators when developing programs. As an example, the End-of-Life Nursing Education Consortium (ELNEC) developed a comprehensive education program to teach nurses and nursing students about care of the dying.[80] A phenomenological study, conducted by the third author of this chapter and a colleague, examined the lived experiences of 12 recent graduates from a baccalaureate nursing school in which the ELNEC program was integrated throughout the curriculum.[81] These new nurses shared their experiences about caring for patients at the end of life during their first year in clinical practice. Four themes emerged.

1. *Facilitating a good death*. Nurses felt their holistic presence was key to truly "being present" with patients in a genuine and caring way.
2. *Experiencing intrinsic rewards*. Caring for patients at end of life often involved opportunities for new nurses to develop close relationships with patients and families.
3. *Learning through impressionable experiences*. The most memorable learning experience was their first experience providing care for a terminal patient, at which point they felt unprepared.
4. *Maintaining a balance*. The nurses learned to set individual emotional boundaries to cope with the sadness.

A pervading sentiment among the new nurses was not knowing what to say to offer comfort. The detailed accounts of opportunities for caring and healing provided from this research have implications for faculty designing end-of-life curricula and for nurse educators designing new nurse orientation programs.

Holistic nurse researchers must persist in efforts to find innovative ways to study health and healing aimed at building the base of evidence to convince third-party payers about the cost effectiveness of holistic care, how holistic practice enhances quality patient outcomes, and how authentic caring increases patient satisfaction scores. Creatively designed and rigorous quantitative and qualitative research, including larger, multisite studies, to examine holistic caring interventions and the effects these interventions have will highlight the essential role of holistic nursing.

Implications for Holistic Nursing

Every holistic nurse has a responsibility to engage in what has been described as the consumer–producer continuum in nursing research.[8] At one end of the continuum are nurse consumers of nursing research who review and critique research for evidence-based practice. At the other end are producers of nursing research who actively engage in generating evidence. Along this continuum lies a rich variety of activities in which holistic nurses may engage. A few examples include the following:

- Forming or participating in a journal club to review holistic-based research.
- Using holistic research findings to make clinical decisions.
- Collaborating on ideas for developing a holistic nursing research study.
- Becoming a member of a multidisciplinary team.
- Discussing the implications and relevance of HNR and CAM findings with patients.

Conclusion

What will the future bring? More research in multidisciplinary teams? Investigators working on a similar problem or concept at multiple sites? It will bring a marriage between highly technical and skilled research that maps our molecular–chemical selves and our energetic makeup with a more profound appreciation for and understanding of the range of human experience in which we participate and hope to enhance and repair to promote growth and healing. The challenges continue to be great, and the opportunities to explore new frontiers of investigation and understanding of HNR are enlivening.

Directions for Future Research

1. Evaluate a holistic nursing therapy that may promote wellness and healing in a specific client population.
2. Ask both healers and the ones being healed how they experience and understand healing and the healing relationship.
3. Determine whether holistic therapies can be combined to augment their effectiveness in achieving desired client outcomes (e.g., combine Reiki with imagery or music therapy with therapeutic touch).

4. Determine the most effective ways to integrate holistic therapies with traditional modes of therapy to achieve optimal outcomes.

5. Identify which standard health-related outcomes (e.g., in cardiology, rehabilitation, or during pregnancy) are most influenced by a healing relationship.

Nurse Healer Reflections

After reading this chapter, the nurse healer will be able to answer or to begin a process of answering the following questions:

- How do I view healing and holism?
- How do I feel about the importance of research in advancing holistic nursing practice?
- What is my role in nursing research?
- How can I become more involved in holistic clinical research?

NOTES

1. American Holistic Nurses Association, *Position Statement on Holistic Nursing Research and Scholarship* (Flagstaff, AZ: American Holistic Nurses Association, revised and approved 2006).
2. M. Enzman-Hagedorn and R. P. Zahourek, "Research Paradigms and Methods for Investigating Holistic Nursing Concerns," *Nursing Clinics of North America* 42, no. 2 (2007): 335–353.
3. R. P. Zahourek, "What Is Holistic Nursing Research? Is It Different?" *Beginnings* 26, no. 5 (2006): 4–6.
4. K. Pribram, "What the Fuss Is All About," in *The Holographic Paradigm and Other Paradoxes*, ed. K. Wilder (Boston: Shambhala, 1982): 29–34.
5. D. Bohm, *Wholeness and the Implicate Order* (New York: Rutledge & Kegan Paul, 1980).
6. J. Briggs and F. D. Peat, *The Turbulent Mirror: An Illustrated Guide to Chaos Theory and the Science of Wholeness* (New York: Harper & Row, 1989).
7. University of Bristol, "What Is Complexity Sciences?" (2014). www.bristol.ac.uk/bccs/whatis/.
8. American Holistic Nurses Association, "What Is Holistic Nursing," in *AHNA Leadership Council Handbook* (Flagstaff, AZ: American Holistic Nurses Association: 2006).
9. B. Carper, "Fundamental Patterns of Knowing in Nursing," *Advances in Nursing Science* 1, no. 1 (1978): 13–24.
10. M. A. Newman, "Health as Expanding Consciousness" (2014). www.healthasexpandingconsciousness.org.
11. J. Fawcett, *Analysis and Evaluation of Nursing Theories* (Philadelphia: F. A. Davis, 1993).
12. C. Mariano, "The Many Faces of Scholarship," *Beginnings* 26, no. 5 (2009): 3–18.
13. B. M. Dossey, "Nursing: Integral, Integrative, and Holistic—Local to Global," in *Holistic Nursing: A Handbook for Practice*, 6th ed., eds. B. M. Dossey and L. Keegan (Burlington, MA: Jones & Bartlett Learning, 2013): 3–58.
14. P. G. Reed, "Toward a Nursing Theory of Self-Transcendence: Deductive Reformulation Using Developmental Theories," *Advances in Nursing Science* 13, no. 4 (1991): 64–77.
15. R. P. Zahourek, "Healing: Through the Lens of Intentionality," *Holistic Nursing Practice* 21, no. 1 (2012): 6–21.
16. M. E. Rogers, "Nursing: A Science of Unitary Man," in *Conceptual Models for Nursing Practice*, 2nd ed., eds. J. P. Reihl and C. Roy (New York: Appleton-Century-Crofts, 1980): 329–337.
17. R. R. Parse, *Human Becoming School of Thought: A Perspective for Nurses and Other Health Professionals* (Thousand Oaks, CA: Sage., 1998).
18. J. Watson, *Nursing: Human Science and Human Care: A Theory of Nursing* (Sudbury, MA: Jones and Bartlett, 2007).
19. H. C. Erickson, E. M. Tomlin, and M. A. Swain, *Modeling and Role Modeling: A Theory and Paradigm for Nursing* (Englewood Cliffs, NJ: Prentice Hall, 1983).
20. M. Leininger and M. McFarland, *Transcultural Nursing: Concepts, Theory, Research, and Practice* (New York: McGraw-Hill Professional, 2002).
21. D. A. Jones, "The Impact of HEC: Concluding Thoughts and Future Directions," in *Giving Voice to What We Know: Margaret Newman's Theory of Health as Expanding Consciousness in Nursing Practice, Research, and Education*, eds. C. Picard and D. Jones (Sudbury, MA: Jones and Bartlett, 2005): 219–228.
22. J. Hubbard, "Evaluation of a Brief Mindfulness-Based Program on Recall and Sense of Well-Being in a Sample of Older African Americans," *Visions: The Journal of Rogerian Nursing Science* 18, no. 1 (2011): 22–41.
23. M. Smith, "Integrative Review of Research Related to Margaret Newman's Theory of Health as Expanding Consciousness," *Nursing Science Quarterly* 24, no. 3 (2011): 256–272.

24. H. Y. Chen, "The Lived Experience of Moving Forward for Clients with Spinal Cord Injury: A Parse Research Method Study," *Journal of Advanced Nursing* 66, no. 5 (2010): 1132–1141.

25. J. Nelson and J. Watson, *Measuring Caring: International Research on Caritas as Healing* (New York: Springer, 2012).

26. M. E. Koren and C. Papadimitiou, "Spirituality of Staff Nurses: Application of Modeling and Role Modeling Theory," *Holistic Nursing Practice* 27, no. 1 (2013): 37–44.

27. M. Bengtsson, K. Ulander, E. Börgdal, and B. Ohlsson, "A Holistic Approach for Planning Care of Patients with Irritable Bowel Syndrome," *Gastroenterology Nursing* 33, no. 2 (2010): 98–108.

28. P. P. DiNapoli, J. Nelson, M. Turkel, and J. Watson, "Measuring the Caritas Process: Caring Factor Survey," *International Journal of Human Caring* 14, no. 3 (2010): 16–21.

29. E. A. M. Barrett, "A Measure of Power as Knowing Participation in Change," *Measurement of Nursing Outcomes*, 2nd ed., Vol. 3, eds. O. Strickland and C. Dilorio (New York: Springer, 2003): 21–39.

30. D. F. Polit and C. T. Beck, *Nursing Research: Generating and Assessing Evidence for Nursing Practice* (Philadelphia: Lippincott Williams & Wilkins, 2012).

31. C. Delaney, "The Spirituality Scale: Development and Psychometric Testing of a Holistic Instrument to Assess the Human Spiritual Dimension," *Journal of Holistic Nursing* 23, no. 2 (2005): 145–167.

32. J. W. Creswell, *Qualitative Inquiry and Research Design: Choosing Among the Five Traditions* (Thousand Oaks, CA: Sage, 1998).

33. J. E. Bormann, S. R. Thorp, J. L. Wetherell, S. L. Golshan, and J. Ariel, "Meditation-Based Mantram Intervention for Veterans with Posttraumatic Stress Disorder: A Randomized Trial," *Psychological Trauma: Theory, Research, Practice, and Policy* 5, no. 3 (2013): 259–267.

34. J. Park, R. McCaffrey, D. Newman, C. Cheung, and D. Hagen, "The Effect of Sit 'n' Fit Chair Yoga Among Community-Dwelling Older Adults with Osteoarthritis," *Holistic Nursing Practice* 28, no. 4 (2014): 247–257.

35. L. Kluepfel, T. Ward, R. Yehuda, E. Dimoulas, A. Smith, and K. Daly, "The Evaluation of Mindfulness-Based Stress Reduction for Veterans with Mental Health Conditions," *Journal of Holistic Nursing* 31, no. 4 (2013): 248–255.

36. S. Cutshall, D. Dercheid, A. G. Miers, S. Ruegg, B. J. Schroeder, S. Tucker, and L. Wentworth, "Knowledge, Attitudes, and Use of Complementary and Alternative Therapies Among Clinical Nurse Specialists in an Academic Medical Center," *Clinical Nurse Specialist* 24, no. 3 (2010): 125–131.

37. B. S. Gallison, Y. Xu, C. Y. Jurgens, and S. M. Boyle, "Acute Care Nurses' Spiritual Care Practices," *Journal of Holistic Nursing* 31, no. 2 (2013): 95–103.

38. D. Leone, S. Ray, and M. Evans, "The Lived Experience of Anxiety Among Late Adolescents During High School: An Interpretive Phenomenological Inquiry," *Journal of Holistic Nursing* 31, no. 3 (2013): 188–197.

39. A. Liptak, J. Tate, J. Flatt, M. Oakley, and J. Lingler, "Humor and Laughter in Persons with Cognitive Impairment and Their Caregivers," *Journal of Holistic Nursing* 31, no. 1 (2014): 25–34.

40. M. Poole, J. Bond, C. Emmett, H. Greener, S. Louw, L. Robinson, and J. Hughes, "Going Home? An Ethnographic Study of Assessment of Capacity and Best Interests in People with Dementia Being Discharged from Hospital," *BMC Geriatrics* 14 (2014): 56.

41. P. Cone and T. Giske, "Teaching Spiritual Care—A Grounded Theory Study Among Undergraduate Nursing Educators," *Journal of Clinical Nursing* 22, nos. 13–14 (2013): 1951–1960.

42. D. Wagner and B. Whaite, "An Exploration of the Nature of Caring Relationships in the Writings of Florence Nightingale," *Journal of Holistic Nursing* 28, no. 4 (2010): 225–234.

43. J. C. Gershon, "Healing the Healer: One Step at a Time," *Journal of Holistic Nursing* 32, no. 1 (2014): 6–15.

44. C. Boswell and S. Cannon, *Introduction to Nursing Research: Incorporating Evidence-Based Practice* (Burlington, MA: Jones & Bartlett Learning, 2014).

45. J. F. Coleman, "Spring Forest Qigong and Chronic Pain: Making a Difference," *Journal of Holistic Nursing* 29, no. 2 (2011): 118–128.

46. M. C. Smith, R. Zahourek, M. E. Hines, J. Engebretson, and D. D Wardell, "Holistic Nurses' Stories of Personal Healing," *Journal of Holistic Nursing* 31, no. 3 (2013): 173–187.

47. M. E. Hines, D. W. Wardell, J. Engebretson, R. Zahourek, and M. C. Smith, "Holistic Nurses' Stories of Healing of Another," *Journal of Holistic Nursing* (May 30, 2014). doi:10.1177/0898010114536925.

48. W. R. Cowling, "Despairing Women and Healing Outcomes: A Unitary Appreciative Nursing Perspective," *Advances in Nursing Science* 28, no. 2 (2005): 94–106.

49. M. Ely, *On Writing Qualitative Research: Living by Words* (New York: Psychology Press, 1997).

50. H. L. Gaydos, "Making Special: A Framework for Understanding the Art of Holistic Nursing," *Journal of Holistic Nursing* 22, no. 2 (2004): 152–163.

51. H. K. Butcher, "The Unitary Field Pattern Portrait Research Method: Facets, Processes, and Findings," *Nursing Science Quarterly* 1, no. 4 (2005): 293–297.

52. B. Lange, R. Zahourek, and C. Mariano, "Legacy Building Model for Holistic Nursing," *Journal of Holistic Nursing* 32, no. 2 (2014): 116–125.

53. W. Braud and R. Andersen, *Transpersonal Research Methods for the Social Sciences: Honoring Human Experience* (Thousand Oaks, CA: Sage, 1998).

54. R. Anderson and W. Braud, *Transforming Self and Others Through Research: Transpersonal Research Methods and Skills for the Human Sciences and Humanities* (Albany: State University of New York Press, 2011).

55. R. Zahourek, *Intentionality: The Matrix of Healing: A Qualitative Theory for Research, Education and Practice* (Saarbrucken, Germany: VDM Verlag, 2009).

56. L. Rew, "How to Conduct a Systematic Review of Literature," *American Holistic Nurses Association Research eNews* (April 2010). www.ahna.org /Portals/4/docs/Research/Library/Conduct -systematic-review.pdf.

57. J. G. Anderson and A. G. Taylor, "Effects of Healing Touch in Clinical Practice: A Systematic Review of Randomized Clinical Trials," *Journal of Holistic Nursing* 29, no. 3 (2011): 221–228.

58. S. Ellerbe and D. Regen, "Responding to Health Care Reform by Addressing the Institute of Medicine Report on the Future of Nursing," *Nursing Administration Quarterly* 36, no. 3 (2012): 210–216.

59. C. Keyworth, J. Knopp, K. Roughley, C. Dickens, S. Bold, and P. Coventry, "A Mixed-Methods Pilot Study of the Acceptability and Effectiveness of a Brief Meditation and Mindfulness Intervention for People with Diabetes and Coronary Heart Disease," *Behavioral Medicine* 40, no. 2 (2014): 53–64.

60. M. E. Tonelli and A. B. Wachholtz, "Meditation-Based Treatment Yielding Immediate Relief for Meditation-Naïve Migraineurs," *Pain Management Nursing* 15, no. 1 (2014): 36–40.

61. G. C. Chi and A. Young, "Selection of Music for Inducing Relaxation and Alleviating Pain: Literature Review," *Holistic Nursing Practice* 25, no. 3 (2011): 127–135.

62. V. Menzies and N. Jallo, "Guided Imagery as a Treatment Option for Fatigue: A Literature Review," *Journal of Holistic Nursing* 29, no. 4 (2011): 279–286.

63. C. E. Hurdle and M. M. Quinlan, "A Transpersonal Approach to Care: A Qualitative Study of Performers' Experiences with Door to Door, a Hospital-Based Arts Program," *Journal of Holistic Nursing* 32, no. 2 (2014): 78–88.

64. Y. Zeng, T. Luo, H. Xie, M. Huang, and A. S. K. Cheng, "Health Benefits of Qigong or Tai Chi for Cancer Patients: A Systematic Review and Meta-Analysis," *Complementary Therapies in Medicine* 22, no. 1 (2014): 173–186.

65. S. Ahn and R. Song, "Effects of Tai Chi Exercise on Glucose Control, Neuropathy Scores, Balance, and Quality of Life in Patients with Type 2 Diabetes and Neuropathy," *Journal of Complementary and Alternative Medicine* 18, no. 12 (2012): 1172–1178.

66. N. Cockell and W. Mcsherry, "Spiritual Care in Nursing: An Overview of Published International Research," *Journal of Nursing Management* 20, no. 8 (2012): 958–969.

67. R. R. Chan, "Mantra Meditation as a Bedside Spiritual Intervention," *MEDSURG Nursing* 23, no. 2 (2014): 84–100.

68. S. Barnason, L. Zimmerman, and L. Young, "An Integrative Review of Interventions Promoting Self-Care of Patients with Heart Failure," *Journal of Clinical Nursing* 21, nos. 3–4 (2012): 448–475.

69. D. McElligott, K. Capitulo, D. L. Morris, and E. R. Click, "The Effect of a Holistic Program on Health Promoting Behaviors in Hospital Registered Nurses," *Journal of Holistic Nursing* 28, no. 3 (2010): 175–183.

70. D. R. Hess and N. A. Klebanoff, "Holistic Perioperative Nursing: Part 1—Presence," *OR Nurse* 18, no. 1 (2014): 48.

71. N. E. M. France, D. Byers, B. Kearney, and S. U. Myatt, "Creating a Healing Environment: Nurse-to-Nurse Caring in the Critical Care Unit," *International Journal of Human Caring* 15, no. 1 (2011): 44–48.

72. D. Hess and B. M. Dossey, "The Emerging Role of the Nurse Coach," *New Mexico Nurse* 2 (2013): 8.

73. A. E. Vincent and A. C. Birkhead, "Evaluation of the Effectiveness of Nurse Coaching in Improving Health Outcomes in Chronic Conditions," *Holistic Nursing Practice* 27, no. 3 (2013): 148–161.

74. M. A. Halm, R. Evans, A. Wittenberg, and E. Wilgus, "Broadening Cultural Sensitivity at the End of Life," *Holistic Nursing Practice* 26, no. 6 (2012): 335–349.

75. T. Bullen, K. Maher, J. P. Rosenberg, and B. Smith, "Establishing Research in a Palliative Care Clinical Setting: Perceived Barriers and Implemented Strategies," *Applied Nursing Research* 27, no. 1 (2014): 78–83.

76. K. Brykczynski, "Clarifying, Affirming, and Preserving the Nurse in Nurse Practitioner Education and Practice," *Journal of the American Academy of Nurse Practitioners* 24, no. 9 (2012): 554–564.

77. M. A. Cordeau, "Teaching Holistic Nursing Using Simulation: A Pedagogical Essay," *Journal of Nursing Education and Practice* 3, no. 4 (2013): 40–50.

78. T. Giske and P. H. Cone, "Opening Up to Learning Spiritual Care of Patients: A Grounded Theory Study of Nursing Students," *Journal of Clinical Nursing* 21, nos. 13–14 (2012): 2006–2015.

79. F. Timmins and F. Neill, "Teaching Nursing Students About Spiritual Care—A Review of the Literature," *Nurse Education in Practice* 13, no. 6 (2013): 499–505.

80. American Association of Colleges of Nursing, "Peaceful Death: Recommended Competencies and Curricular Guidelines for End-of-Life Nursing Care" (2014). www.aacn.nche.edu/elnec/publications/peaceful-death.

81. C. Barrere and A. Durkin, "Finding the Right Words: The Experience of New Nurses After ELNEC Education Integration into a BSN Curriculum," *MEDSURG Nursing* 23, no. 1 (2014): 35–43, 53.

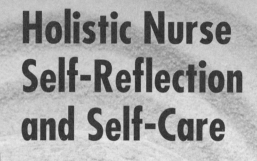

Holistic Nurse Self-Reflection and Self-Care

CHAPTER 29

Self-Development: The Foundation of Holistic Self-Care

Deborah A. Shields and Sharon Stout-Shaffer

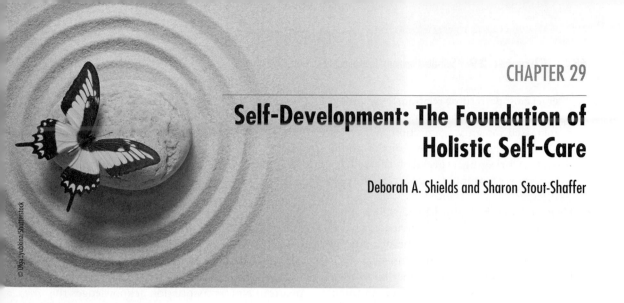

Morning mists enveloping earth
veil indigo skies of dawn
Bali
easing slowly upward
sprinkles light beams into the fog
revealing glimpses
the unfolding of new adventures . . .

Nurse Healer Objectives

Theoretical

- Review key theories that support nurse self-development as foundational to healing relationships, use of self as an instrument of healing, and implementation of integrative interventions.
- Relate essential self-development practices to their theoretical foundations.
- Understand current evidence that supports self-development of the nurse as important to maintaining holistic practice and healing environments.

Clinical

- Value self-development as foundational to holistic nursing practice.
- Identify components of holistic self-assessment and the care plan.
- Apply what is learned from your own self-development to clinical scenarios and your own clinical practice.

Personal

- Explore contemplative practices as a path to your personal stillpoint.
- Choose one or two contemplative practices to integrate into your own self-development plan.
- Use the holistic self-assessment tool to identify your own patterns and develop a realistic self-development plan.
- Reflect on the process of self-development, including self-awareness, patterns, presence, intuition, and healing attitudes.
- Identify and mobilize self-care resources and rituals.
- Commit to behavior patterns consistent with self-development as a holistic nurse.

Definitions

Caring (healing) consciousness: A "deeper" level where the nurse is mindful, intentional, and present and chooses how he or she portrays "being" in the interaction (achieved through centering).[1]

Centering: The process of being present to oneself;[2] a mind-body-spirit activity (breathing, exercise, meditation) to prepare the body to enter into, prepare for, and begin caring consciousness in relationships.[1]

Healing: A process of bringing aspects of oneself into harmony and inner knowing that leads to integration;[3] involves an emerging pattern of relationships among elements of the whole person, leading to increased integrity, connection, and cohesion;[4] an emergent process of the whole system bringing aspects of the self to deeper levels of inner knowing, leading to integration and balance.[5]

Health: An individually defined state or process in which the person experiences a sense of well-being, harmony, and unity; a process of becoming an expanding consciousness.[5]

Inner wisdom: The innate inner knowledge or knowing that one can access through meditation, mindfulness, and other methods that expand conscious awareness.

Intention: Every action starts from an intention in the implicate order; behavior that can move one into conscious relationships; the active part of "attention."[2]

Self: An individual expression or hologram of the whole; a Universal Being that serves as an interface between part (individual being) and whole (universal being), between personal consciousness and universal consciousness.[6,7]

Self-care: Activities that individuals initiate and perform on their own behalf to maintain their own health and well-being.[8]

Self-development (holistic self-care): The lifelong commitment to and process of actualizing one's potential for well-being. The core of self-development is developing the Beingness of the nurse through the intentional development of self-awareness, self-reflection, and commitment to higher purpose.

self or "I": The *self* is a personal center of pure conscious awareness and *will* that acts as a unifying center to integrate parts of the self to develop more wholeness; serves to connect personal consciousness and universal consciousness.[6,9]

Transpersonal: A personal experience that transcends the boundaries of an individual ego identity to acknowledge and appreciate something greater than the personal self.[5]

Well-being: An inner attitude of acceptance of the wholeness of one's Being. Integrated, congruent functioning to achieve one's highest potential.[10]

Introduction

This chapter integrates material from other sections of this text so that readers can apply the content and strategies to develop the lifestyle practices required of holistic practitioners. Holistic nursing requires developing consciousness of one's inner being, the capacity for supporting well-being of oneself and commitment to personal self-healing as an ethic of care. The *Scope and Standards of Practice, Second Edition*, of the American Holistic Nurses Association and American Nurses Association acknowledges the primacy of self-care if nurses are to fully connect with and support the healing of others. Attending to one's personal self-development as a lifestyle pattern is foundational to fully practice from a caring science/unitary philosophy; to act with compassion; to serve as an instrument of healing; to develop therapeutic listening, communication, and coaching skills; to implement evidence-based pharmacologic and nonpharmacologic integrative interventions; and to create healing environments.

Core Value 5: Holistic Nurse Self-Reflection and Self-Care requires self-assessment, self-reflection, and self-responsibility to adopt a lifestyle that supports all dimensions of well-being, including the physical, emotional, mental, and spiritual aspects of oneself as well as relationships with others and with the environment, to create life balance and satisfaction. While the concept of self-care is defined as holistic in the core value, many of us approach self-care as something we do or do not do to support our physical, mental–emotional, and spiritual health for the purpose of personal wellness. This dimension of self-care is critically important to our overall being; however, it is not sufficient from a holistic standpoint. The term *self-development* as defined in this chapter suggests a more holistic understanding of self-care that involves the process of developing self-awareness, self-reflection, self-responsibility, and the healing consciousness required to care for others. It expands the traditional view of self-care to include development of the healing consciousness inherent to our inner being and connection to a source of wisdom greater than our personal self. Self-development, then, is synonymous with holistic self-care. The purpose of self-development is not only to adopt personal health promotion behaviors and manage stress but also to connect us with the larger purpose of our lives as healers. It is a lifelong process of developing one's being. Self-development requires an integration of rational and paradoxical consciousness, or the "doing" and "being" dimensions of healing. **Reflective Exercise 29-1** will help you to review and integrate these concepts into your conscious awareness.

Reflective Exercise 29-1

Review the discussion of Rational Versus Paradoxical Healing in Chapter 1 and then complete this exercise.

1. Center your attention and take a deep centering breath.
2. Imagine yourself involved in (doing) self-care for the purpose of personal health, and make some notes on what you noticed.
3. Imagine being involved in self-development to develop your being/well-being for the purpose of caring for others, and make some notes on what you noticed.
4. How were your images of self-care and self-development similar? How were they different?
5. How important to you is self-development to your practice?

Development of a healing consciousness requires a lifelong commitment to contemplative practice and personal integration that enables intentional action or doing from an inner healing consciousness, our being. It requires capacity for self-awareness, intentionality, connection to unitive consciousness, and the ability to repattern and identify with our wholeness.[2] Thus, self-development requires an understanding of unitary science and is based on the following theoretical assumptions:

Assumption 1. There is a core essence to our being experienced as a point of stillness (stillpoint) that connects us directly to expanded levels of consciousness.

Assumption 2. Connecting with this core essence allows us to connect with and actualize the authentic purpose of our lives.

Assumption 3. A discipline of contemplative practice is required for self-development.

The theoretical roots of these assumptions will be explored more fully through the exercises in this chapter. The intent of these exercises is to assist readers to apply what has been presented about holistic nursing in other chapters of this text to develop their own personal well-being and healing consciousness. These exercises invite you to enter into a new, lifelong process to uncover those energetic patterns of thought, attitude, emotion, and behavior that are no longer useful and to intentionally develop new patterns that support holistic practice. Enjoy your journey and be well.

International and National Trends

A thorough discussion of the national and international issues and trends related to health care is provided in Chapters 1 and 3. The following review of four distinct trends summarizes some of the main points that relate directly to the importance of holistic nurses assuming responsibility for their own self-development as defined in this chapter.

1. Health promotion, self-care of individuals and communities, and health coaching are key nursing roles. Numerous national goals and initiatives support the movement toward health promotion/self-responsibility for health in the United States, including *Healthy People 2020*, the Institute of Medicine, the *National Prevention Strategy* created by the Surgeon General's National Prevention and Health Promotion Council, the more recent Wellness Initiative for the Nation, and the Patient Protection and Affordable Care Act. As suggested in Chapter 3, these initiatives clearly indicate the need to shift our nation from a focus on sickness and disease care to one based on wellness and prevention. Nursing has espoused "caring of the whole being"; however, it is difficult for nurses to relate to patients as whole while practicing in a paradigm that views health as the absence of disease. The gradual shift from

an illness-based system to a system focused on newer definitions of health is encouraging to the long-term development of truly holistic practice. Thus, this trend is clearly significant.

2. At an international level, health is also increasingly emphasized. The United Nations Millennium Declaration of 2000 is directed toward global health problems and aims to improve well-being by 2015 in eight different areas: poverty and hunger, gender equality and empowerment of women, child mortality, maternal health, HIV/AIDS, environmental sustainability, and development of global partnerships.[11-14]

3. Stress is a significant health issue for clients and family caregivers.[5, 15] The psychophysiological effects of chronic stress are now known to contribute to at least 80% of the chronic healthcare issues in the United States. In addition, stress associated with caregiving for family members who experience long-term chronic disease is increasingly recognized to affect both short- and long-term caregiver health. Thus, developing a lifestyle that downregulates the effects of stress is recognized as an important aspect of self-responsibility for patients and their caregivers.[16] What is less visible is the underlying need to maintain the health of nurses as caregivers. To teach self-care to patients and family caregivers, nurses must own responsibility for their own self-care and model behaviors/lifestyle practices to others. Ask yourself the following question: How effective can you really be in helping others take responsibility for their self-care if you are not able to set your own health and care of your well-being as a priority and model this for others?

Nursing is a highly stressful profession. McElligott has written extensively about the crucial requirement of nurses to develop resilience to stress through meditation and other self-care practices in order to develop themselves as instruments of healing.[17] Symptoms resulting from the stressors involved in caregiving include caregiver burnout (cumulative work demands and stress); moral distress (perceived inability

to act from caring values and patient needs); horizontal hostility (behavioral control, devaluating or diminishing a peer or group); secondary trauma/compassion fatigue (dysfunction from exposure to pain and suffering of others); and structural violence (systematic group or individual discrimination).[18,19] In this context, hospitals, particularly those achieving magnet status, expect nurses to implement caring, healing practices required of relationship-based care, improve patient outcomes and satisfaction, and strengthen team communication required for quality and safety. Thus, attention to the health and well-being of the nurse is increasingly recognized as a critical variance for safe, relationship-based care,[20] and self-development as outlined in this chapter is considered to be an ethic of holistic practice. Please take some time now to complete **Reflective Exercise 29-2**.

Reflective Exercise 29-2

Review Table 1-4, Optimal Healing Environments, from Chapter 1 and reflect on the following questions. Note that the "Core Internal Healing Environment" required for a healer includes healing intention and personal wellness.

1. How do these qualities relate to your images of self-development in the previous exercise?
2. What does developing a core inner environment mean for your practice? For your self-development?
3. Ask if you care for yourself as much as you do your patients.

---

4. Integrative therapies are rapidly increasing as research evidence documents the effectiveness of many of these lifestyle patterns on well-being. Review Exhibit 3-1, The White House Commission on Complementary Alternative Medicine Policy Guiding Principles, and Exhibit 3-2, Themes of the Summit on Integrative Medicine and the Health of the Public, in Chapter 3 and reflect on what these mean to your practice of holistic nursing. As the public use of complementary and integrative therapies expands into areas of health promotion

and management of chronic illness, it is critical for nurses to develop the personal knowledge underlying these practices; to practice integrative therapies correctly requires the development of the healing consciousness of the practitioner. Thus, self-development is critical for nurses as they learn to teach and practice evidence-based interventions such as yoga, relaxation, meditation, imagery, and coaching.

Theoretical Foundations of Self-Development

The eras of medicine currently operational in Western biomedicine are described in Chapter 1. As the biomedical paradigm has shifted from Era I to Era II and Era III paradigms, the role of consciousness in healing has become increasingly defined. This shift has allowed for alignment of biomedical science and unitary science, which is largely reflected in nursing theory. With the movement into the Era III paradigm, many of nursing's most significant theoretical underpinnings are recognized as important to the healing practice of nurses, as well as to physicians and other health providers.

Take a moment to review the discussion of eras of medicine in Chapter 1. Next, review the key ideas of unitary science described in Chapter 4 and in Exhibit 4-1: Ways of Being with People Seeking Help. As you review, notice the shift in our understanding from a purely biomedical view, Era I, "getting the job done," to the expanded worldview of the universe that assumes a nonlocal nature of consciousness and posits a human energy field that connects with the environment, "holding sacred space." Key concepts differentiating biomedical and unitary worldviews are summarized in **Table 29-1**. Understanding these basic concepts is crucial to interpret the nursing theories that underpin

---

TABLE 29-1   Self-Care, Self-Development, and Scientific Worldviews

Key Concepts	Biomedical Science: Eras I and II	Unitary Science: Era III
Nature of self	Physical body	Energy field
	Body–mind	
Nature of consciousness	Local consciousness: personal	Nonlocal consciousness: transpersonal
Methods of science	Empiric observation and measurement	Intuitive pattern recognition
	Evidence based	Unfolding process
	Rational	Paradoxical
Outcome	Curing, fixing parts	Experience/process of healing
	May be recognition or role of mind in healing but not primary	Wholeness
Caring	Leading: power over	Guiding, coaching, allowing
	Doing to or for the person	Being with
Responsibility of caregiver	Outcome	Competent practice
Focus of self-care	Personal	Holistic process: self-development, mindful awareness, attention, intention, self-reflection
	Doing for body–mind: nutrition, exercise, work–life balance, sleep	

Source: © Shields & Stout-Shaffer, 2013

self-development and the relationship between self-development and one's ability to fully engage in healing.

The critical nature of self-development to nursing practice is grounded in all traditional nursing theory. Florence Nightingale emphasized the creation of an environment so that natural healing could take place; she also defined the need for nurses to develop a sacred space through reflection to gain support from a Being greater than themselves.[21] Based on Nightingale's ideas, one can logically assume that her theory suggests that development of

nurses' internal environment and identification with their inner essence was an important component of creating an external healing environment and ability to see or connect with the being in each person.

Numerous other nursing theorists, individually and collectively, imply the primacy of healing consciousness and attention to self as a foundation of practice. Several of these important theories and their potential influence on nursing practice are reviewed in Chapter 5. **Table 29-2** offers a brief summary of these theoretical assumptions from key theories as they

---

TABLE 29-2　Theoretical Foundations of Self-Development

Theorist/Theory	Key Points
Dossey: Theory of Integral Nursing	▪ Healing is the central core concept and includes knowing, doing, and being; we are born with healing capacity.
	▪ Requires development of different patterns of knowing.
	▪ The process requires development of the "I," is built on "we," and requires behavior and skill development and the ability to deal with systems and structures.
Erickson, Tomlin, and Swain: Modeling and Role-Modeling	▪ Client self-knowledge should be the nurse's primary source of information.
	▪ Holistic nurses must discover their gift to their clients—the gift of themselves.
	▪ Self-nurturance, self-discovery, and self-growth are conditions of holistic nursing that become a way of living.
Newman: Health as Expanding Consciousness	▪ Consciousness is the information capacity of the system.
	▪ Health and illness are a unitary process of order and disorder; health (observable) is a manifestation of the underlying energetic pattern.
	▪ The focus of nursing is to recognize life patterns and how they manifest.
	▪ A sense of disorder (choice point) precedes a transformation to higher consciousness.
Parse: Theory of Human Becoming	▪ Nursing is guiding individuals to choose possibilities in changing the health process.
	▪ Health as a synthesis of values, a way of living; hopes, meaning, dreams.
	▪ True presence, a way of "being with" another, requires preparation and focused attention.

TABLE 29-2 Theoretical Foundations of Self-Development (*Continued*)	
Theorist/Theory	**Key Points**
Quinn: Transpersonal Human Caring and Healing	▪ Caring is the context and healing is the goal of nursing; the direction of healing is always toward self-transcendence.
	▪ Learning to shift consciousness into a healing state is basic to healing; nurses are integral to the patient's environment.
Rogers: Science of Unitary Human Beings	▪ Identifies the person as an energy field; a unified whole.
	▪ Nursing is the scientific study of human and environmental energy fields.
	▪ Our thoughts and feelings affect ourselves and others simultaneously; thoughts are action.
Waters and Daubenmire: Therapeutic Capacity: The Critical Variance in Nursing Practice	▪ The essence of nursing is to create a healing environment and engage the patient's consciousness in the healing process.
	▪ Centering, the process of being present to oneself, intentionality, connecting, and repatterning is essential to one's therapeutic capacity; these skills are required to evoke the endogenous healing process of the client.
Watson: Theory of Transpersonal Caring and Caring Science	▪ Emphasizes the relational aspects of nursing combined with scientific knowledge.
	▪ Expanding unitary energetic worldview with a relational caring ethic; caring presence where the nurse acknowledges and appreciates the total body, mind, and spirit connection between each interaction with self and others.

Source: © Shields & Stout-Shaffer, 2014

relate to self-development of the nurse. True understanding of nursing theories that underpin self-development requires careful examination of your perspective of wholeness. Notice the similarities in the theories as they relate to development of a healing consciousness.

In summary, from a unitary worldview there is no separation between internal and external consciousness; from an energetic/consciousness perspective, boundaries are false. We are not physical beings who have consciousness; instead, we are conscious beings who are embodied. Caregiving is considered a dynamic, reciprocal process rooted in compassion and responsiveness to the suffering of others and requires the ability to intentionally act from a healing consciousness.

Healing is considered a repatterning of consciousness, an allowing for new patterns to emerge in the moment and the ability to be with or guide another to deeper levels of inner knowing to create a greater wholeness. Relational connection and compassionate presence or "use of self" is a nursing intervention that supports repatterning the physiological challenges, emotional fear, and suffering and social disruption that come with any threat to well-being.[2, 4] From this unitary worldview, developing the personal knowledge and intuition to "hold sacred space" is no less important than scientific, measurable empiric knowledge for professional nursing practice.[22] Please take some time now to complete **Reflective Exercise 29-3**.

Reflective Exercise 29-3

Path to Center

Before reading further, you are invited to review the relaxation exercises outlined in Chapter 11. Select one of the breathing exercises and focus on awareness of the breath for several minutes. As your body—mind begins to relax, review the following script in your imagination. When you are finished, make some notes on your experience of this centered state of awareness.

Get in a comfortable position and take a moment to just look around the room. Really see the light . . . the colors . . . the people. Now, take a deep breath, close your eyes, and let all of the visual awareness go . . .

As your visual awareness fades, be aware of the sounds in the room. . . . Attend only to the sounds that surround you . . . noticing what you hear. Now, take a deep breath and let go of all sounds as you move your awareness more deeply into center . . .

Lightly scan your body from head to toe . . . very gently . . . and if you need to move to be more comfortable, do that now. With the next breath, let go of your body awareness and pay attention only to the breath. . . . Just be aware of your breathing without trying to change it . . .

As you focus on the breath, notice any thoughts or feelings that arise and let them go. . . . Do not hold onto them. . . . Just let them pass through . . . and with each breath breathe yourself more deeply into your center of silence. . . . Breathe into your stillpoint. . . . Breathe in the peace and silence of this center . . . still . . . calm . . . deepening. . . .

And now notice how it feels to be you in this moment.

The Concept of Self: Who Am I and Why Am I Here?

Assumption 1. There is a core essence to our being experienced as a point of stillness (stillpoint) that connects us directly to expanded levels of consciousness.

Assumption 2. Connecting with this core essence allows us to connect with and actualize the authentic purpose of our lives.

Assumptions 1 and 2 require an understanding of one's self in relation to others and the environment and a worldview of self based on consciousness. For many of us, self or "I" is associated with the physical body and mental-emotional-spiritual personality rather than with a deeper state of conscious being. The work of Roberto Assagioli, the founder of psychosynthesis, offers another view. Assagioli's work relates to using the mind through imagery and intention to positively affect psychospiritual growth. The use of imagery to affect integration toward wholeness is one major contribution of his work.

Assagioli noticed a recurring theme in Eastern and Western philosophy regarding the essence of a *self* as an integrating center that *is* the essential individual. As a synonym for human growth, psychosynthesis views the self as the most elementary and distinctive part of our being—in other words, its core. This core is entirely different in nature from all elements (physical sensations, feelings, thoughts, desires, intuition, and so on) that make up our personality. Therefore, it acts as a unifying center, directing those elements and bringing them into unity and wholeness.[9]

The *self* or "I" is a personal center (conscious space) of pure awareness and *will*. Will is a fundamental inner power with tremendous unrealized potency, and it is considered the most direct expression of self. One can consciously experience the self as a center of pure awareness, and from this center we make the intentional choices that determine our life direction. With experience and practice people are able to develop their awareness and remain "centered" in the face of extreme hardship. This experience is of being—unshaken by changes in the body, feelings, mind, or environment and always self-aware and capable of choice. The self, then, represents our inner being and is experienced as we make choices from the point of inner stillness.

The *self,* lowercase, is understood to be a manifestation of a Higher Self, or *Self,* uppercase, described as an energetic source that is rarely experienced directly, is unaffected by the flow of the mind-stream or by daily conditions, and can only be reflected or expressed in the personal self, which is accessible to direct experience.[7] In other words, the Self is transpersonal and yet can become embodied through the personal choices an individual makes through activation of personal will. Just as there is a personal *will*, there is a Transpersonal Will, the *Will* to transcend the limitations of our personal self and unite with higher levels of consciousness to express Self more fully in the world; this can be equated with Maslow's self-actualization.

Assagioli suggests that the purpose of life is basically to find forms for expressing the qualities emanating from the Self; this is achieved as we align our personal and Transpersonal Will to express our higher potentials. Awareness, acceptance, and integration of material from the higher levels of consciousness is as vital to our self-development as is processing material from the lower unconsciousness. This process may be experienced as a "Calling" or vocation.

Finally, the *Self* is thought to be an individual expression of the whole, a Universal Being. *Self* is a hologram of the Universal Being and serves as in interface between part (individual being) and whole (universal being). Higher unconscious energies store tremendous potential for love, compassion, forgiveness, and other expressions of Self. The goal of psychosynthesis could be described as bridging spirit and matter, as creating a world at the personality level that is fully expressive of the person's spiritual being.[23, 24] Self-development, then, from the psychosynthesis view, requires training of our awareness and will to bring our personality functions into right relationship with Self and with one another. As we integrate and express Self through our personal self, we discover our basic interdependency, our essential unity with one another, and we expand our healing consciousness.

Figure 29-1 provides an image of the major concepts in Assagioli's system of thought.[6]

Assumption 3. A discipline of contemplative practice is required for holistic self-development.

From a psychosynthesis perspective, self-development requires practice of key skills because knowledge and control of our inner being remains very limited.[7] Human beings have a limited field of conscious awareness; feelings, patterns, relationships, attitudes, and memories are largely not part of our direct awareness, yet they control a large part of our behavior and choice in daily living. We react based on long-established patterns of thought and feeling that may not be applicable to our current situation. Learning to live with less reactivity, from our center of conscious awareness and choice, requires practice in paying attention to the self, the choices we make, and self-reflection. Awareness can take the form of intellectual insight or experiential awareness; however, there is a major difference between intellectual insight and the direct conscious experience of a state of being. Direct conscious experience requires a discipline of contemplative practice.

The process of identification is at the heart of all self-development. Who or what aspect of our personality we identify with either limits or challenges us to expand our capacities. Growth occurs as we disidentify from past limited perceptions of ourselves and our world and identify with new, more integrating ones. When we are identified with our mind, our emotions, or

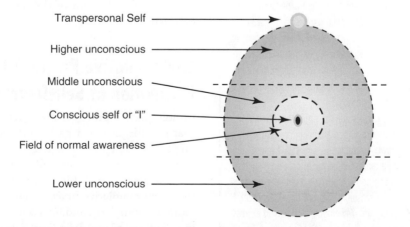

FIGURE 29-1 Oval Diagram: Relationship between personal self and Higher Self

Source: Data from Assagioli, R. (1981). *Psychosynthesis: A manual of principles and techniques.* Middlesex, England; New York: Penguin Books.

our body, these thoughts, feelings, attitudes, physical sensations, and desires define who we think we are. Self-development, learning to act from a centered state of awareness, requires that we disidentify with these limiting parts of ourselves and integrate these parts (thought patterns, images, etc.) into a larger consciousness of self. This process of consistent identification with our center allows for development of connection among or between parts of the whole. We develop right relationship with self, and, as Quinn suggests, right relationship to self leads to increased energy, coherence, and creativity in the body–mind system.[4]

Reflective Exercise 29-4 is a method of letting go of limiting ideas of oneself and finding a deep sense of who one really is; through this process, we develop the freedom of choice to be who we really are; we can more fully appreciate and use the power of our mind, body, and feelings rather than being controlled by the ever-changing nature of our thoughts and sensations.[24] Please take some time now to complete Reflective Exercise 29-4.

Reflective Exercise 29-4

Identification

Sit comfortably, relax your body, and allow your breathing to become slow and deep as you move into center. Read each paragraph slowly and then close your eyes and pay attention to your inner responses.

I have a body and I value my body. I experience sensations of my body through different experiences of sickness and health, activity and rest, vigor and tiredness. My body is my precious instrument of experience and of action and so I treat it well and seek to keep it in good health. My body affects and expresses who I am, but it is not my self. I have a body, but I am not only a body.

I have emotions and I value my emotions. My feelings are countless, contradictory, and changing, yet while they change I know I always remain "I," my self. I remain my self in times of hope or despair, in joy or pain, in a state of irritation or calm. Because I can observe and understand my emotions, and then increasingly embrace and direct them, I know they are not my self. My emotions affect and express who I am, but I am not only my emotions.

I have a thinking mind and I value my thinking mind. It is a primary tool of discovery and expression, constantly changing with new ideas, beliefs, knowledge, and experience. My mind is not the essence of my being, however, because I remain essentially my self through all of my mind's changes. My mind affects and expresses who I am, but it does not determine who I am. I have a thinking mind, but I am not only my thinking mind.

I have a body, emotions, and a thinking mind, and yet I am not only these. Who am I? I am a center of consciousness and will, distinct but not separate from my body, feelings, and mind. I am "I," capable of observing, harmonizing, and making choices about my life, my attitudes, and my actions. I am the one who is aware, the one who chooses.

Take time to honor all of your experiences in this exercise. Make some notes about your experience.

Source: Based on Brown, M. (1983). *The unfolding self: Psychosynthesis and counseling.* Los Angeles: Psychosynthesis Press.

Self-development, then, begins with an ever-expansive awareness of and a deepening relationship with self. Reflective dialogue invites us to explore the potential meaning of the truths we discover on this lifelong journey and to consider patterns that support as well as hinder our growth as individuals and as holistic nurses. It might be thought of as a space like no other, a sacred space of unity and stillness— our stillpoint. How might we reach that space? We suggest that the cultivation of contemplative practice is foundational in this quest and forms the root system of the self-development experience.

Contemplative Practice: The Foundation of Self-Development

Contemplative practices are quieting practices that can illuminate a path to the stillpoint of our being. They are practices that are intentional, requiring choice and will; as we cultivate the discipline within ourselves to engage in them, contemplative practices allow us to relax more into ourselves and, in a sense, become still in the storm of our daily lives. Through regular practice we develop a relationship between our ego and our higher self and a unity of self–Self. Our awareness of our being—our inner I AM—becomes more expansive and open, and we are reminded of what is meaningful to us in our lives. What is our purpose? What do we value most?

Contemplative practice is not easy. It is a journey of uncovering, much like lifting off the stones on the cairns of our lives. Within the cairns we find joy, discomfort, *aha* moments, challenges, and so much more. We remember, though, that the practice is enfolded in equanimity and compassion, and we trust. The practice can be transformative. With deepening reflection we are able to meet ourselves where we are and listen, without judging and harshness; within the stillpoint we are open to sense unitary connections that support healing and our wholeness.

When we hear the word *contemplative*, we often think of meditation and prayer as the practice. We believe that contemplative practices are whatever you choose that creates the space for quiet within you. There is no right or wrong practice; each is as unique as each of you. The power of the practice is your intention and your willingness to stay the course. In our busy world it is easy to become distracted and guilty—and even to give up. Remember, contemplative practice is a gentle discipline; notice that when you stray a bit you return with love, not self-criticism. **Reflective Exercise 29-5** is designed to help you get started.

Reflective Exercise 29-5

Planting

Find a space that is comfortable and nourishing to you. Settle in and be for a few moments. Look around and notice what you see; listen to the space. What do you hear? Are there any aromas? Be sure to adjust yourself so that you are deeply comfortable and feel grounded. When you are ready, we invite you to:

1. Center your attention and take a deep centering breath.
2. Imagine yourself holding a seed; take a moment to gaze upon it. Notice how it looks and feels, what color

it is. What senses do you experience as you explore the seed?
3. As your eyes move upward, you notice a beautiful field of soil—verdant, rich, fertile. You are drawn to the earth; smell the richness of the dirt.
4. Walk to the field; in a gentle, comfortable way, lean over and scoop up a handful of soil. Let it crumble through your fingers—notice the texture, the temperature, the moisture.
5. Envision the soil as receptive—a vessel of equanimity and compassion. Sense how that knowing feels deep within you.
6. Take your seed now and nestle it into the awaiting earthen bed. Choose the depth, the position, the space of your seed.
7. Take a moment to offer nourishment to your seed: water, love, intention to grow.
8. Stay in the field as long as you should. You will know what is right for you.
9. Take a deep breath.
10. Imagine that the seed you have planted is your being, nestled in your stillpoint—safe and open—surrounded by compassion and equanimity.
11. How does this feel? Can you envision weaving a contemplative practice into your life?

Table 29-3 offers some examples of contemplative practices that you might consider; this is not an exhaustive list, and we encourage you to find what works for you. You might also discover ideas in other chapters of this text (e.g., Chapters 11 and 14) or by visiting the Center for Contemplative Mind in Society at www.contemplativemind.org/.

Research: What Do We Know About Contemplative Practices?

The body of evidence related to the positive outcomes of contemplative practices is increasing, nudging us from considering only the negative effects of stress (which are plentiful) to proactive explorations of strategies to modulate it. The more evidence we generate, the more likely it is that self-development will become a priority both individually and organizationally.

TABLE 29-3 Types of Contemplative Practices	
Contemplative Practice Category (examples)	**Practices (examples)**
Quieting practices	Silence and breath awareness
	Centering
	Meditation (all types)
	Prayer
	Imagery and relaxation exercises (all forms)
	Ritual
Creative expression	Art
	Writing: narrative, story, poetry, journaling
	Mandala
	Music
	Improvisation
Movement	Walking
	Running
	Yoga, tai chi, qi gong, Aikido
	Dance
Nourishment	Mindful eating
	Mindful drinking
Nature	Walking the labyrinth
	Medicine walk

Source: © Shields & Stout-Shaffer, 2014

Mindfulness meditation has been widely studied, and the results overwhelmingly support the positive effects of this contemplative practice in a variety of situations. Developed by Jon Kabat-Zinn in 1979, mindfulness-based stress-reduction programs are integrated into the personal and professional lives of individuals and organizations all over the world. According to the Foundation for a Mindfulness Society at the University of Massachusetts, mindfulness is "the intention to pay attention to each and every moment of our life, non-judgmentally."[25] Mindfulness practices are introduced in Chapter 11.

In the health policy paper "The Role of Mindfulness in Healthcare Reform," Ruff and Mackenzie present compelling evidence that mindfulness improves health and quality of life and is cost effective.[26] In the studies cited, participants reported decreased pain perception, stress, anxiety, depression, and use of medication; increased pain tolerance, decision making, social and interpersonal connection, and ability to adhere to lifestyle changes; and enhanced neuroendocrine and immune system function. The authors posit strategies that could be used in researching and implementing mindfulness training programs in different settings. These specific areas are not reviewed here but could be useful for anyone interested in further investigation.

The Contemplative Sciences Center at the University of Virginia is engaged in numerous initiatives exploring contemplative practice. Interdisciplinary and interprofessional research teams are examining, for example:[27]

- *Landscapes of longevity.* An exploration of the role that cultural landscapes and public space play in fostering healthy aging.
- *Post-television executive function depletion in young children.* An examination of whether contemplative practices can help to repair and restore the cognitive activity associated with Executive Function (EF) in young children. Executive Function describes the higher cognitive processes that enable goal-directed behaviors—processes that enable us to inhibit automatic responses, to follow rules, and to hold and manipulate information in the conscious mind (working memory). Because such processes allow us to follow directions, plan, and regulate our behavior, EF is considered to be crucial for healthy cognitive and social functioning and is strongly associated with children's success in school, itself a basic predictor of overall health and well-being into adulthood. Children today frequently engage with media that depletes their EF.

- *Mindfulness-based relapse prevention.* A study of the benefits of mindfulness-based stress reduction techniques in assisting people recovering from alcohol use disorders.
- *Contemplation and contexts.* An observation of how philosophical, social, aesthetic, environmental, and other contexts are centrally constitutive of the nature, dynamics, and influence of any given contemplative practice, rather than being incidental.

These highlights are offered to the reader as a sampling of the work being done in contemplative practice in the hope that you will visit the websites located in the Notes section and discover much more. Importantly, it is hoped that exploring the evidence will excite and encourage you to begin, return to, or continue contemplative practice as a foundation for your self-development. Indeed, the root system is deeply anchoring the seed of you—you, who through the journey, transform into a beautiful flower. Please take some time now to complete **Reflective Exercise 29-6**.

Reflective Exercise 29-6

Choosing

Find a space that is comfortable and nourishing to you. Settle in and be for a few moments. Look around and notice what you see; listen to the space. What do you hear? Are there any aromas? Be sure to adjust yourself so that you are deeply comfortable and feel grounded. When you are ready, we invite you to:

1. Center your attention and take a deep centering breath.
2. Imagine the seed you have planted earlier, your being, nestled in your stillpoint—safe and open—surrounded by compassion and equanimity.
3. Choose a contemplative practice that resonates with you.
4. See yourself engaged in that practice every day.

Notice that, every day, there are more and more roots emanating from your seed—from you. They are spreading and rooting deeply into the soil of equanimity and compassion. How does that feel?

Holistic Caring Process: Continuing the Path of Self-Development

When self-care is viewed from the perspective of holism, the practice is an integration of being and doing for the purpose of nurturing the well-being of the whole. Without this perspective, the behaviors might be good for us in some ways (e.g., daily running, weight management) but there is a risk that they become a habit pattern that provides only a superficial nurturing. Self-development means that we are choosing what we do from our stillpoint, where we are aware of our felt senses and possibilities and connected to higher consciousness. This journey is continuous throughout our life.

Few of us are taught to recognize and understand our own experience of being aware.[28] Learning to self-regulate our attention and intention is a fundamental self-development skill. In addition, listening, knowingly choosing, reflection, and presence are seminal in your unfolding. Continuing now to cultivate self-development practices built on the foundation of contemplative practice is your opportunity to transform your discoveries into actions that promote your well-being.

As with any trip you take, you need to prepare. You must be clear on your purpose, your reason for taking the trip. This will influence your planning—what you need, what you must take with you, how to prepare. Next, you assess where you are and select what you need to focus on: what you need to pack, how long you anticipate being gone. You are then able to be intentional as you plan the trip and travel with confidence. Of course, you evaluate the experience and note what worked well and how you might need to modify your planning in the future as you enjoy the travel.

The holistic caring process requires the same attention to detail and intentional action. It involves being present to yourself, clarifying your *purpose*, *assessing* where you are and setting an *intention* and *plan* for the journey, and *evaluating* or monitoring outcomes for ongoing revisions. As you begin your process, ensure that you are comfortable and safe, that you are not time-rushed, and that you are ready. Take a few breaths to become present and focused . . . and begin.

Assessment

There are numerous tools available for your use in self-assessment; we suggest that you use the Integrative Health and Wellness Assessment located in Chapter 30. This tool invites you to reflect on eight dimensions of health and wellness, consider where you are in your life, and, from there, determine where you would like to be. In essence, you are able to gently and non-judgmentally meet yourself where you are in this moment. Take your time and thoughtfully complete your self-assessment; try to not leave any area blank. If you feel it best, put it down and return to it, but please do return. This is your dialogue with yourself and it offers you a place to begin.

As you review your self-assessment, you will likely notice your individual patterns. Reflect on any sensations you experience as you bring to your awareness a pattern—you might feel, for example, vibrant, energized, uncomfortable, guilty, tired, steady, or anxious. Your awareness is so important. Experiencing an embodied sense or felt sense of how these patterns affect your consciousness and behavior helps you to better understand how your patterns are energetically affecting you. Remember that self-development invites you to accept yourself and to learn to embrace your patterns and choose actions to modify or strengthen them.

Throughout your self-assessment, we invite you to pause for a moment and notice. You might benefit from making notes about your experience that you can refer to later. Importantly, follow your inner knowing about what is best for you.

Purpose, Intention, Plan, Evaluation

Identification of your patterns leads to defining the intention and actions you want to take for self-development; this is a dynamic process and we are unfolding it all of the time. Depending on your patterns, you may choose actions to modulate (tone down) them so that they do not have power over the choices your make and/or choose actions to strengthen patterns that help you to behave from more holistic/prosocial levels of awareness. You will also become more aware of these patterns that truly serve you well—embrace these!

In developing your unique self-development plan, you may choose to work in one health and wellness dimension to begin. Your goals should be realistic in how much you can achieve; set yourself up for success! Clear, specific goals with actions and mental desire and commitment enables action (intention); it activates our will so that we choose to follow our plan.

Intervention (action) should be chosen mindfully and connected to our purpose. Self-care behaviors can become patterned responses that may or may not serve our development over time—the key is attending mindfully to what occurs in your being. Give the plan a chance to work; you are not likely to lose 30 pounds in 2 or 3 weeks or run a marathon without training if you have not ever run a block. If, however, you find that an action is not working, revise it. Always strive to notice the felt sense—the energetic response—that you are experiencing with your self-development actions.

The evaluation of your self-development plan can include both short-term (immediate feelings that reinforce your specific behavior—the bubble bath was relaxing in the moment) and longer-term (recognizing that my goal of deep relaxation and sleep is occurring as I take bubble baths every night) results. Mindful observation and reflection on your progress enhance your self-awareness; subsequently, you are more able to self-correct and discern how your development is progressing. As you stay the course, you become more and more observant and responsive to patterns; your embodied sense—felt sense—is shifting within you.

Approach your self-development with an attitude of gentle discipline; if you stray from your desired plan, appreciate what that might mean and return to your path. Remember that contemplative practice is the foundation for self-development. We recommend that you have a coach to support you; importantly, recognize whether you may want to seek professional help if your patterns are particularly hard to break or difficult for you to see how to approach them. You must accept who you are, where you are.

Holistic self-development activities are plentiful and it is important to choose those that resonate with you. There are numerous chapters in this text that can offer you solid ideas as you develop your plan, and we encourage you to use them. Today is your day!

Staying the Course: Thoughts to Sustain YOU on Your Self-Development Journey

A garden of possibilities awaiting discovery
panoramic beauty
so many paths to choose from
which one?
Trusting . . . stepping in . . . trusting . . .
Beingcare

Self-development is a complex, exciting, and challenging undertaking. It involves a myriad of activities, woven into a plan that is right for you. While there are moments of pure joy and celebration, there can be bumps and detours along the way. We offer the following thoughts that you may find helpful as you stay the course, never giving up on YOU!

1. Recognize that contemplative practice is foundational to self-development; it is the path to your stillpoint. Explore quieting activities, and select one or two that speak to you; choose activities that are spiritually comfortable and interesting to you.

2. Begin a daily practice. It is helpful to carve out a bit of time on a fairly regular schedule to practice; initially, that may be for just a few minutes daily. Try not to get caught in the linear time roadblock, but rather immerse yourself in the experience. Be aware of what you are noticing: What is your felt sense? What does stillness feel like for you?

3. Consider where you practice. What is comfortable for you? Can you name a designated space that would support you on your path to stillness? The environment is important, but, again, try to avoid those roadblocks of "needing" certain props; you know where you feel best. This is the perfect place to begin your practice.

4. Notice when thoughts of guilt (for taking this time when "there is so much to do"), need (more time, equipment, space), and even frustration ("I cannot quiet my mind," "I am never going to get this," "I am not an artist," "I cannot even draw a straight line") appear. Bear witness to your discomfort: What are you discovering about you?

5. When you are ready, begin your self-assessment and create your plan for self-development. Remember that, whichever action(s) you undertake, your contemplative practice is the foundation. If, for example, you determine that you are going to work in one dimension, that of movement and exercise, you choose a goal to walk for 30 minutes daily 5 days per week; currently, you do not walk at all. You develop a plan that integrates a walking practice into your life, beginning with 10 minutes and gradually increasing to your goal of 30 minutes. You are ready, and, as you begin, begin from your stillpoint. Weave your contemplative practice into the fabric of your chosen activity (walking) and notice your felt sense of the experience from a gentle, nonjudging place.

6. Take the time to see how your plan is working (evaluate it); revise it as you deem important.

There are a few other tips that may be helpful to you to stay the course of your self-development. Again, this is not an exhaustive list but rather some ideas.

1. *Breath breaks.* When it is difficult to carve out time—or even as you move through your day—begin to appreciate the stillness and immediate connection to your being that is offered with a few deep breaths. The beauty of this is that we must breathe, so this is a matter of momentarily shifting

our attention to stillness in order to reap the benefits of the breath break.

2. *Journal.* There is much power in writing and/or drawing your practice experience. This might take the form of narrative, poetry, or some other creative expression. It is a record of *your* journey—for you. Often, rereading our journals illuminates deeper understanding and insights.

3. *Your setting.* A designated practice space is helpful; it is also true that you may benefit from trying other spaces—for example, stepping out into nature. As with all parts of your self-development, you are aware of and sense how this affects you.

4. *Community.* Although self-development is a personal journey, your ability to stay the course may be strengthened by joining with others who share the same goal. The walker mentioned earlier may benefit from having a walking partner or from becoming part of a group activity (e.g., triweekly walks along the local bike path or at the local gym).

5. *Retreats.* These getaways are valuable if they are within your desire and ability to participate in them. There are numerous retreat venues; some are for quiet practice, others are with activities in mind, and many integrate both.

6. *Coach, guide, friend.* It is, for many, wonderful to have the support of another as you live your self-development experience. It is also important to seek professional counseling when you need this; sometimes our coaches and friends realize this is needed and guide us toward appropriate resources.

Just as the journey begins with one step, the commitment of individuals to self-development will create pathways to support change in our practice and the healthcare environment. Holistic nurses understand the importance of supporting others in their self-development journey. With increasing self-awareness and commitment to the discipline of self-development, we begin to consider the ways in which we might integrate knowledge and skills into our holistic nursing practice. Clearly, being present to colleagues, those we serve in our practice and our Earth, is essential in health promotion and well-being.

The Importance of Self-Development on Nursing Practice and the Environment

There is a growing body of research on the effects of contemplative practice and other self-development activities in general; however, much less has been studied to determine how these practices may affect the well-being of caregivers working in challenging environments. The demands of caregiving are stressful; we must acknowledge that fact and begin to view self-development as critical to practice, teach self-development strategies to students and practitioners, and evaluate the outcomes.

Reports of the potential benefits of teaching self-care for physicians, nurses, and consumers at major university medical centers began to appear several years ago.[29-31] However, little has been done to support educators to integrate self-development into curricula on a widespread scale. There is, however, a developing body of research that suggests an important contribution of contemplative practice for caregivers and students. **Table 29-4** summarizes the psychological, physiological, and organizational outcomes of nine recently published studies that deal specifically with self-care and contemplative practices for nurses and nursing students.

As shown in Table 29-4, perceived stress and burnout were reduced and perceived resilience was increased in all of the studies that measured these variables. Other outcomes, including anxiety, compassion, and sense of well-being, were also documented. Taken together, these studies begin to demonstrate the potential influence of contemplative practices on the well-being of nurses as caregivers. It is an exciting beginning.

Continuing the journey of self-development, holistic nurses are ever aware of the effects of the environment on health and well-being as well as the influence of behaviors on the Earth. In the quest to create caring, healing spaces, the importance of mindful living is appreciated. We know that resources are limited and respect what we are offered. Holistic nurses actively advocate for the health of the environment and participate in initiatives designed to nurture the Earth. We are reminded of the words of Joanna

TABLE 29-4   Synthesis Table of Self-Care Research for Nurses and Nursing Students, 2011–2014

Outcomes		1	2	3	4	5	6	7	8	9
				Research Studies						
Psychological	Stress/burnout	↓			↓	↓	↓		↓	↓*
	Attention/awareness				↑*	↑	↑	↑	↑	↑*
	Resilience							↑		
	Anxiety/depression			↓* 1					↓	
	Self-compassion/connect				↑	↑				↑*
	Well-being		↑*							
Physiological	Systolic blood pressure/ diastolic blood pressure			↓* 2						
	Heart rate			↔						
	Cortisol/telomerase									
	Patient safety events				↓					
	Sleep								↑	
Organizational	Unplanned/illness	↓								
	Turnover/absenteeism	↔								
	Workplace relationships							↑		

* *p* = .05; 1 = anxiety only; 2 = systolic blood pressure only
Source: Data from 1. Hoolahan, Greenhouse, Hoffmann, and Lehman, 2012;[32] 2. Pal, 2011;[33] 3. Chen, Yang, Wang, and Zhang, 2013;[34] 4. Brady, O'Connor, Burgermeister, and Hanson, 2011;[35] 5. Horner, Piercy, Eure, and Woodard, 2014;[36] 6. Foureur, Besley, Burton, Yu, and Crisp, 2013;[37] 7. McDonald, Jackson, Wilkes, and Vickers, 2013;[38] 8. Alexander, 2013;[39] 9. Newsome, Waldo, and Gruszka, 2012.[40]

Macy: "When we open our eyes to what is happening, even when it breaks our hearts, we discover our true size; for our heart, when it breaks open, can hold the whole universe."[41]

Conclusion

Self-development is a rhythm, and you are invited to find yours. There are ups and downs and that is okay. Practices are challenging, and we learn from these experiences. As we move to that place of being able to "let go"—to not be attached to the outcomes—we live the experience.

As Dr. Emoto shares:[42]

If you feel lost, disappointed, hesitant, or weak, return to yourself,
to who you are, here and now. And when you get there, you will discover yourself,
like a lotus flower in full bloom,
even in a muddy pond, beautiful and strong.

Credit: M. Emoto, Office Masaru Emoto, LLC. Used with permission.

Please take some time to complete **Reflective Exercise 29-7**. You are, now, the blossoming flower grown from the seed that you planted earlier in the rich soil of equanimity and compassion. Celebrate that! Congratulations on choosing YOU!

Reflective Exercise 29-7

Developing

Find a space that is comfortable and nourishing to you. Settle in and be for a few moments. Look around and notice

---

Reflective Exercise 29-7 (*continued*)

what you see; listen to the space. What do you hear? Are there any aromas? Be sure to adjust yourself so that you are deeply comfortable and feel grounded. When you are ready, we invite you to:

1. Center your attention and take a deep centering breath.
2. Imagine the seed you have planted with all of its roots, your being, nestled in your stillpoint—safe and open—surrounded by compassion and equanimity.
3. Imagine completing a holistic self-assessment—notice what speaks to you. Are there any patterns being revealed?
4. Choose a holistic self-care action that resonates with you.
5. See yourself engaged in that action every day.
6. Notice that, every day, you are emerging higher and higher from the soil; see yourself as a flower bud, beginning to open, ever expansive.
7. See the beautiful flower that you are.

How does that feel?

Directions for Future Research

1. Create qualitative design studies that document the experience of nurse caregivers and nursing students as they commit to self-development.
2. Develop qualitative research that captures the experience of caregiver–patient dyads.
3. Document the need for more consistency in programmatic methods and outcome measures, as well as instrumentation for nursing education.
4. Expand outcome measures to include more physiological data and environmental measures including safety, communication with peers, and teamwork.
5. Determine ways in which mindfulness and other self-development practices can be supported over time and measure long-term outcomes.
6. Identify the types of contemplative practices most used in the acute care setting and most foundational to self-development

Nurse Healer Reflections

After reading this chapter, the nurse healer will be able to answer or to begin a process of answering the following questions:

- What are the four most important messages I have received from completing the exercises in this chapter?
- What intention will I set for my self-development over the next month?
- Do I believe that developing a contemplative practice is an ethic of care?
- How might I use the skills of centering and intention when I am coaching patients and others on their self-care needs?
- How might I use the skills of centering and intention in interactions with coworkers?
- Are there advanced practice nurses or nurse researchers in my organization who would help me to design and evaluate a self-development program for nurses on my unit?
- How can I capture and analyze data about changes in myself, my practice, and my relationships with coworkers as I continue my self-development?
- Are there coworkers who may be interested in helping me to gather ongoing current evidence about the effect of self-development on nursing care? Could this become an evidence-based practice project?

Flocks of geese soar
into rosygolden horizons
of the setting sun
they dance in the brilliance
unique . . . unified
reminding us . . .
the adventure is life-long
All is . . .

NOTES

1. S. S. S. Ingersoll and A. Schaper, "Music: A Caring, Healing Modality," in *Holistic Nursing: A Handbook for Practice*, 6th ed., eds. B. M. Dossey and L. Keegan (Burlington, MA: Jones & Bartlett Learning, 2013): 397–415.
2. P. Waters and M. J. Daubenmire, "Therapeutic Capacity: The Critical Variance in Nursing Practice," in *Reflections on Healing: A Central Nursing*

Construct, ed. P. Kritek (New York: National League for Nursing, 1997): 55–67.

3. B. M. Dossey, "Nursing: Integral, Integrative, and Holistic—Local to Global," in *Holistic Nursing: A Handbook for Practice*, 6th ed., eds. B. M. Dossey and L. Keegan (Burlington, MA: Jones & Bartlett Learning, 2013): 3–58.

4. J. F. Quinn, "Transpersonal Human Caring and Healing," in *Holistic Nursing: A Handbook for Practice*, 6th ed., eds. B. M. Dossey and L. Keegan (Burlington, MA: Jones & Bartlett Learning, 2013): 107–116.

5. C. Mariano, "Holistic Nursing: Scope and Standards of Practice," in *Holistic Nursing: A Handbook for Practice*, 6th ed., eds. B. M. Dossey and L. Keegan (Burlington, MA: Jones & Bartlett Learning, 2013): 59–84.

6. R. Assagioli, *Psychosynthesis: A Manual of Principles and Techniques* (New York: Hobbs, Dorman, 1965).

7. R. Assagioli, *The Act of Will* (New York: Viking Press, 1973).

8. D. Orem, *Nursing: Concepts of Practice*, 6th ed. (St. Louis, MO: Mosby, 2011).

9. P. Ferrucci, *What We May Be: Techniques for Psychological and Spiritual Growth* (Los Angeles: J. P. Tarcher, 1982).

10. American Holistic Nurses Association and American Nurses Association, *Holistic Nursing: Scope and Standards of Practice* (Silver Spring, MD: Nursesbooks.org, 2007).

11. Centers for Disease Control and Prevention, "Chronic Disease Prevention and Health Promotion" (2014). www.cdc.gov/chronicdisease/index.htm.

12. Institute of Medicine, *Summit on Integrative Medicine and the Health of the Public* (Washington, DC: National Academies Press, 2009): 1–2.

13. U.S. Department of Health and Human Services, *Healthy People 2020* (Washington, DC: U.S. Department of Health and Human Services, 2010).

14. World Health Organization, "Millennium Developmental Goals (MDGs)" (2014). www.who.int/topics/millennium_development_goals/en/.

15. G. Bartol, "The Psychophysiology of Body–Mind Healing," in *Holistic Nursing: A Handbook for Practice*, 7th ed., eds. B. M. Dossey and L. Keegan (Burlington, MA: Jones & Bartlett Learning, 2015).

16. R. R. Whitebird, M. Kreitzer, and A. L. Crain, "Mindfulness-Based Stress Reduction for Family Caregivers: A Randomized Controlled Trial," *Gerontologist* 53, no. 4 (2013): 676–686.

17. D. McElligott, "The Nurse as an Instrument of Healing," in *Holistic Nursing: A Handbook for Practice*, 6th ed., eds. B. M. Dossey and L. Keegan (Burlington, MA: Jones & Bartlett Learning, 2013): 327–342.

18. J. Borysenko, *Fried: Why You Burn Out and How to Revive* (New York: Hay House, 2011).

19. J. Halifax, "The Precious Necessity of Compassion," *Journal of Pain and Symptom Management* 41, no. 1 (2011): 146–153.

20. The Joint Commission, "National Patient Safety Goals" (2015). http://www.jointcommission.org/standards_information/npsgs.aspx.

21. B. M. Dossey, L. C. Selanders, D. M. Beck, and A. Attewell, *Florence Nightingale Today: Healing, Leadership, Global Action* (Silver Spring, MD: American Nurses Association, 2005).

22. P. Chinn and M. K. Kramer, *Integrated Knowledge Development in Nursing* (St. Louis, MO: Mosby, 2004).

23. M. Crampton, *Psychosynthesis: Some Key Aspects of Theory and Practice* (Montreal: Canadian Institute of Psychosynthesis, 1977).

24. M. Brown, *The Unfolding Self: Psychosynthesis and Counseling* (Los Angeles: Psychosynthesis Press, 1983).

25. Foundation for a Mindful Society, "Center for Mindfulness in Medicine, Health Care and Society" (2012). www.mindful.org/our-partners/the-center-for-mindfulness-in-medicine-health-care-and-society.

26. K. M. Ruff and E. R. MacKenzie, "The Role of Mindfulness in Healthcare Reform," *EXPLORE: The Journal of Science and Healing* 5, no. 6 (2009): 313–317.

27. Contemplative Sciences Center, University of Virginia, "School of Nursing" (n.d.). www.uvacontemplation.org/content/school-nursing.

28. R. Moss, *The Mandala of Being: Discovering the Power of Awareness* (Novato, CA: New World Library, 2007).

29. M. Brodsky, C. Fung, V. Dirtpins, and M. J. Kreitzer, "Teaching Self-Care at UCLA Medical School," *EXPLORE: The Journal of Science and Healing* 5, no. 1 (2009): 61–62.

30. M. J. Kreitzer, V. S. Sierpina, M. Traub, and K. Riff, "Transformational Learning: An Immersion Course on the Big Island of Hawaii," *EXPLORE: The Journal of Science and Healing* 4, no. 5 (2008): 335–337.

31. D. McElligott, "An Intervention to Increase Health Promotion in Hospital Nurses," (unpublished doctoral dissertation, Frances Payne Bolton School of Nursing, Case Western Reserve University, Cleveland, OH, 2009).

32. S. E. Hoolahan, P. K. Greenhouse, R. L. Hoffmann, and L. A. Lehman, "Energy Capacity Model for Nurses: The Impact of Relaxation and Restoration," *Journal of Nursing Administration* 42, no. 2 (2012): 103–109.

33. A. Pal, "Effect of Meditation on Wellbeing of Nursing Students," *Nursing Journal of India* 102, no. 10 (2011): 1–3.

34. Y. Chen, X. Yang, L. Wang, and X. Zhang, "A Randomized Controlled Trial of the Effects of Brief Mindfulness Meditation on Anxiety Symptoms and Systolic Blood Pressure in Chinese Nursing Students," *Nurse Education Today* 33, no. 10 (2013): 1166–1172.

35. S. Brady, N. O'Connor, D. Burgermeister, and P. Hanson, "The Impact of Mindfulness Meditation in Promoting a Culture of Safety on an Acute Psychiatric Unit," *Perspectives in Psychiatric Care* 48, no. 3 (2011): 129–137.

36. J. K. Horner, B. S. Piercy, L. Eure, and E. K. Woodard, "A Pilot Study to Evaluate Mindfulness as a Strategy to Improve Inpatient Nurse and Patient Experiences," *Applied Nursing Research* 27, no. 3 (2014): 198–201.

37. M. Foureur, K. Besley, G. Burton, N. Yu, and J. Crisp, "Enhancing the Resilience of Nurses and Midwives: Pilot of a Mindfulness-Based Program for Increased Health, Sense of Coherence and Decreased Depression, Anxiety and Stress," *Contemporary Nurse: A Journal for the Australian Nursing Profession* 45, no. 1 (2013): 114–125.

38. G. McDonald, D. Jackson, L. Wilkes, and M. Vickers, "Personal Resilience in Nurses and Midwives: Effects of a Work-Based Educational Intervention," *Contemporary Nurse: A Journal for the Australian Nursing Profession* 44, no. 1 (2013): 134–143.

39. G. Alexander, "Self-Care and Yoga–Academic-Practice Collaboration for Occupational Health," *Workplace Health and Safety* 61, no. 12 (2013): 510–513.

40. S. Newsome, M. Waldo, and C. Gruszka, "Mindfulness Group Work: Preventing Stress and Increasing Self-Compassion Among Helping Professionals in Training," *Journal for Specialists in Group Work* 37, no. 4 (2012): 297–311.

41. J. Macy, "The Greatest Danger," *Yes! Magazine* (February 1, 2008). www.yesmagazine.org /issues/climate-solutions/the-greatest-danger.

42. M. Emoto, *Secret Life of Water* (London: Simon & Schuster, 2006): 172.

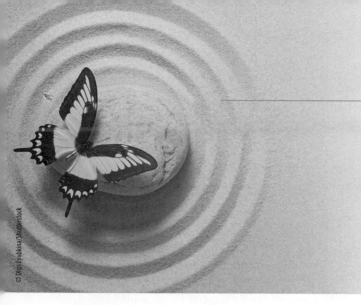

CHAPTER 30

Self-Assessments

Barbara Montgomery Dossey and Susan Luck

Nurse Healer Objectives

Theoretical

- Explore the *Healthy People 2020* initiative and its application for holistic nurses.
- Examine the Integrative Health and Wellness Assessment (IHWA) and its eight categories.

Clinical

- Use the IHWA with clients who wish to learn new healthcare behaviors.
- Incorporate the IHWA into clinical practice.

Personal

- Complete the IHWA.
- Identify your readiness to change related to your desired health goals.

---

*Contact the International Nurse Coach Association at http://inursecoach.com/contact/contact-us/ for use of the Integrative Health and Wellness Assessment (short form and long form) and for the survey software.

**This chapter is adapted from B. M. Dossey, "Integrative Health and Wellness Assessment," in *Nurse Coaching: Integrative Approaches for Health and Wellbeing*, B. M. Dossey, S. Luck, and B. G. Schaub (North Miami, FL: International Nurse Coach Association, 2015): 109–122.

***www. [CA2]See online Integrative Health and Wellness Assessment (long form).

- Create personal action plan goals that lead to new health behaviors.
- Increase your awareness of ways to gain access to your inner healing process.

Definitions

Healing: A process of understanding and integrating the many aspects of self, leading to a deep connection with inner wisdom and an experience of balance and wholeness.

Healing awareness: A person's conscious recognition of and focused attention on intuitions, subtle feelings, conditions, and circumstances relating to the needs of self or clients.

Health: An individual's (nurse, client, family, group, or community) subjective sense of well-being, harmony, and unity that is supported by the experience of health beliefs and values being honored; a process of opening and widening of awareness and consciousness.

Nurse healer: A professional nurse who supports and facilitates a person's process of growth and experience of wholeness through an integration of body, mind, and spirit and/or who assists in the recovery from illness or in the transition to peaceful death.

Process: The continual changing and evolution of one's self through life that includes reflecting on meaning and purpose in living.

Self-efficacy: The belief that one has the capability of initiating and sustaining desired behaviors with a sense of empowerment and ability to make healthful choices that lead to enduring change.

Transpersonal self: The self that transcends personal, individual identity and meaning and opens to connecting with purpose, meaning, values, unitive experiences, and universal principles.

Transpersonal view: The state that occurs during a person's life maturity, whereby a sense of self expands.

Wellness: An integrated, congruent functioning toward reaching one's highest potential.

Holistic Nurses, Healthy People, and a Healthy World

Many 21st-century conversations and initiatives focus on health promotion, health maintenance, disease prevention, and prevention of the catastrophic effect of diseases. Holistic nurses are leaders practicing at the forefront of this initiative. As change agents, their objective is to increase the health of the nation, focusing on addressing the wellness and "health span" of people. They are sharing this information with other nurses and healthcare colleagues around the world. Their endeavors include using health and wellness assessments, assessing readiness to change, and implementing action plans for healthy lifestyle behaviors and approaches that will lead to healthy people living in a healthy nation and on a healthy planet by 2020.

In the United States, actual solutions to health problems guide holistic nurses and healthcare professionals. The *Healthy People 2020* initiative continues the work started in 2000 with the *Healthy People 2010* initiative for improving the nation's health. *Healthy People 2020* is the result of a multiyear process that reflects input from a diverse group of individuals and organizations.[1] The leading health indicators are increased physical activity; reduced obesity, tobacco use, substance abuse, injury, and violence; increased

responsibility in sexual behavior; and improved mental health, environmental quality, immunizations, and access to health care. These health indicators were selected on the basis of their ability to motivate action, the availability of data to measure progress, and their importance as public health issues.

The *Healthy People 2010* vision, mission, and overarching goals provide structure and guidance for achieving the *Healthy People 2020* objectives.[2] Although general in nature, they offer specific, important areas of emphasis where action must be taken if the United States is to achieve better health by the year 2020. Developed under the leadership of the Federal Interagency Workgroup, the *Healthy People 2020* framework is the product of an exhaustive collaborative process among the U.S. Department of Health and Human Services and other federal agencies, public stakeholders, and the advisory committee. The *Healthy People 2020* mission strives to accomplish the following:[1]

- Identify nationwide health improvement priorities.
- Increase public awareness and understanding of the determinants of health, disease, and disability and the opportunities for progress.
- Provide measurable objectives and goals that are applicable at the national, state, and local levels.
- Engage multiple sectors to take actions to strengthen policies and improve practices that are driven by the best available evidence and knowledge.
- Identify critical research, evaluation, and data collection needs.

Overall goals of the *Healthy People 2020* mission include the following:[1]

- Attain high-quality, longer lives free of preventable disease, disability, injury, and premature death.
- Achieve health equity, eliminate disparities, and improve the health of all groups.
- Create social and physical environments that promote good health for all.
- Promote quality of life, healthy development, and healthy behaviors across all life stages.

Other important endeavors in national health are the Patient Protection and Affordable Care Act[2] and the *National Prevention Strategy*.[3] The following section addresses the use of the Integrative Health and Wellness Assessment in coaching clients to be active participants in increasing health-promoting behaviors, assessing readiness to change, and establishing action plans and goals.

Integrative Health and Wellness Assessment

Holistic nurses use self-assessments and other strategies to assist individuals to learn how to prefer wellness to unhealthy habits. They are assuming a leadership role in the health and wellness coaching movement as "pioneers on the vast frontier of our nation's health care reform."[4, p. 78] The Integrative Health and Wellness Assessment (IHWA) was developed and is based on 35 years of the authors' holistic nursing clinical practices, education, and research with clients and patients in changing lifestyle behaviors, health promotion, health maintenance, and disease prevention.[5]* This includes coaching and supporting clients who are learning new self-management skills in living with an acute or chronic illness and/or symptoms. It is expanded from Self-Care Assessments.[6]

The circle is an ancient symbol of wholeness. As shown in **Figure 30-1**, the IHWA wheel has eight components: (1) life balance and satisfaction, (2) relationships, (3) spirituality, (4) mental, (5) emotional, (6) physical (nutrition, exercise, weight management), (7) environmental, and (8) health responsibility. All are important components of the self that are interwoven and constantly interacting.

The IHWA (see **Figure 30-2**) assists people in becoming aware of their human potentials in each of these categories, identifying strengths

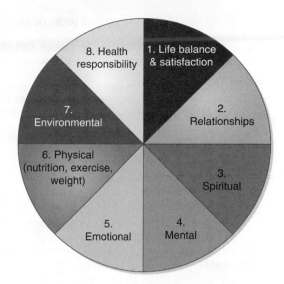

FIGURE 30-1 Integrative Health and Wellness Assessment Wheel

Source: Used with permission. B. M. Dossey, S. Luck, and B. G. Schaub, *Nurse Coaching: Integrative Approaches for Health and Wellbeing* (North Miami, FL: International Nurse Coach Association, 2015): 434–437. www.iNurseCoach .com.

and weaknesses and considering and creating new health goals.

The IHWA is an effective coaching tool for holistic nurses and is designed to increase both nurse self-development (self-reflection, self-assessment, self-evaluation, self-care) and client self-development. It is essential that holistic nurses deepen their personal exploration of self (see Chapters 1, 4, 7, 9, 21, and 29), examine their vulnerabilities (see Chapter 33), and explore their wellness from an integrative lifestyle health perspective (see Chapters 24 and 31). This also includes looking at their life balance and satisfaction, as well as recognizing which factors are contributing to imbalance(s) and how they affect well-being. Creating the time for nurse self-development through integrating body, mind, spirit skills, integrative health knowledge, and nutritional, psychological, and other integrative resources is essential for becoming an effective nurse coach.[7, 8]

In using the IHWA, the holistic nurse skillfully creates and holds sacred space in which the client feels trust, respect, listened to, and not judged. Depending on the clinical situation, the

---

Disclaimer: The Integrative Health and Wellness Assessment (IHWA) is intended for informational purposes only. It is not a substitute for professional medical advice, diagnosis, or treatment.

INTEGRATIVE HEALTH AND WELLNESS ASSESSMENT™

This **INTEGRATIVE HEALTH** and **WELLNESS ASSESSMENT** (short form) is intended for informational purposes only. It is not a substitute for professional medical advice, diagnosis or treatment.

DIRECTIONS: This questionnaire contains statements about your present way of life, feelings, and personal habits. Please respond to each item as accurately as possible, and try not to skip any item. Indicate the frequency with which you engage in each item by shading (●) one of the following:

1 = Never   2 = Rarely   3 = Occasionally   4 = Frequently   5 = Always

	/ 20	①	②	③	④	⑤
Life Balance/Statisfaction						
1. I have balance between my work, family, friends, and self.		○	○	○	○	○
2. I can release anxiety, worry, and fear in a healthy way.		○	○	○	○	○
3. I use strategies (breathing, stretching, relaxation, mediation and imagery) to manage stress daily.		○	○	○	○	○
4. I recognize negative thoughts and reframe them.		○	○	○	○	○
Relationships	/ 15					
5. I create and participate in satisfying relationships.		○	○	○	○	○
6. I feel comfortable sharing my feelings/opinion without feeling guilty.		○	○	○	○	○
7. I easily express love and concern to those I care about.		○	○	○	○	○
Spiritual	/ 15					
8. I feel that my life has meaning, value, and purpose.		○	○	○	○	○
9. I feel connected to a force greater than myself.		○	○	○	○	○
10. I make time for reflective practice (affirmation, prayer, meditation).		○	○	○	○	○
Mental	/ 15					
11. I prioritize my work and set realistic goals.		○	○	○	○	○
12. I ask for help/assistance when needed.		○	○	○	○	○
13. I can accept circumstances and events that are beyond my control.		○	○	○	○	○

FIGURE 30-2 Integrative Health and Wellness Assessment: Short Form

Emotional	/ 20	①	②	③	④	⑤
14. I recognize my own feelings and emotions.		○	○	○	○	○
15. I express my feelings in appropriate ways.		○	○	○	○	○
16. I practice forgiveness.		○	○	○	○	○
17. I listen to and respect the feelings of others.		○	○	○	○	○

Physical/Nutrition	/ 20					
18. I eat at least 5 servings of fruits and vegetables, and recommended whole foods (beans, nuts, etc.) daily.		○	○	○	○	○
19. I drink 6-8 glasses of water daily.		○	○	○	○	○
20. I eat real food.		○	○	○	○	○
21. I eat mindfully (concentrate on eating and not multi-tasking or eating in front of the TV).		○	○	○	○	○

Physical/Exercise	/ 15					
22. I do stretching or flexibility activities 2 or more days a week.		○	○	○	○	○
23. I do muscle-strengthening activities (i.e., free-weights, machines, resistance bands, body weight exercises, or carrying heavy loads) for all major muscle groups (legs, back, core, chest, arms) 2 or more days a week.		○	○	○	○	○
24. I do moderate-intensity aerobic activity (i.e., brisk walking, or any activity that makes you breathe harder with an increased heart rate) for at least 150 minutes (2 hours and 30 minutes) a week.		○	○	○	○	○

Physical/Weight	/ 10					
25. I maintain an ideal weight.		○	○	○	○	○
26. I have gained no more than 11 pounds in adulthood.		○	○	○	○	○

Environmental	/ 15					
27. I have a healthy non-toxic home environment.		○	○	○	○	○
28. I have a healthy non-toxic work environment.		○	○	○	○	○
29. I am aware of how my external environment affects my health and wellbeing.		○	○	○	○	○

②

FIGURE 30-2 Integrative Health and Wellness Assessment: Short Form (*continued*)

Health Responsibility	/ 35	1	2	3	4	5
30. I believe I am key to my wellbeing and overall health, and address symptoms as they arise.		○	○	○	○	○
31. I know my blood pressure, triglycerides, cholesterol and glucose levels.		○	○	○	○	○
32. I am aware of my risk factors for disease.		○	○	○	○	○
33. I am not addicted to a substance or behavior (alcohol, drugs, sex, food, gambling, shopping, exercise, internet).		○	○	○	○	○
34. I can work and do regular activities of daily life.		○	○	○	○	○
35. I avoid smoking or using smokeless tobacco.		○	○	○	○	○
36. I discuss/formulate a wellness plan with my primary healthcare provider, and if needed, take and know prescribed medications and possible side effects.		○	○	○	○	○

Total Score	/ 180

3

FIGURE 30-2 Integrative Health and Wellness Assessment: Short Form (*continued*)

AREAS TO ADDRESS	SCORE	MY READINESS TO CHANGE 1 = In one year 2 = Within 6 months 3 = Next month 4 = In two weeks 5 = Now	PRIORITY FOR MAKING CHANGE (1–5) 1 = Never a priority 2 = Very low priority 3 = Medium priority 4 = Priority 5 = Highest priority	CONFIDENCE IN MY ABILITY TO DO IT (1–5) 1 = Not at all confident 2 = Not very confident 3 = Somewhat confident 4 = Confident 5 = Very confident
Life Balance/Satisfaction	/ 20			
Relationship	/ 15			
Spiritual	/ 15			
Mental	/ 15			
Emotional	/ 20			
Physical/Nutrition	/ 20			
Physical/Exercise	/ 15			
Physical/Weight	/ 10			
Environment	/ 15			
Health Responsibility	/ 35			

④

FIGURE 30-2 Integrative Health and Wellness Assessment: Short Form (*continued*)

ACTION PLAN

Please list 3 changes that you can implement into your current lifestyle over the next 3 months:

1. _____
_____
_____
_____
_____
_____
_____

2. _____
_____
_____
_____
_____
_____
_____

3. _____
_____
_____
_____
_____
_____

Additional changes, comments, thoughts:
_____
_____
_____
_____
_____
_____
_____
_____
_____

⑤

FIGURE 30-2 Integrative Health and Wellness Assessment: Short Form (*continued*)

tool can be provided at one time for the client to complete in advance of a session or it can be used one section at a time. It is a useful guide in assisting individuals to change health behaviors. In the following sections, each of the eight IHWA components is explored.

Life Balance and Satisfaction

Assessing our life balance and satisfaction (see the Life Balance and Satisfaction section in Figure 30-2) strengthens our capacities and human potentials. It attunes us to our healing awareness that is the innate quality with which all people are born. Healing is recognizing our feelings, attitudes, and emotions, which are not isolated but that are literally translated into body changes. Images cause internal events through mind modulation that simultaneously affect the autonomic, endocrine, immune, and neuropeptide systems (see Chapter 12). Everyone has the capacity to, and can choose to, tap into this innate healing potential. Healing is more likely to occur on many levels when we attend to our life balance and satisfaction. During times of stress and crisis, focusing only on all of the things that are wrong each day can block self-healing. Therefore, it is necessary to continually assess and reassess our wholeness, which includes attention to stress management, time management, and adequate sleep. Recognizing and celebrating the joys and good things in life add to experiencing life balance and satisfaction. Life is a journey. Willingness to be present for all that this life journey brings, cultivating the ability to be fully in the moment with "what is," is a component of a transformative healing process.

Assessing our life balance and satisfaction acknowledges our capacity for both conscious and unconscious choices in our lives. Conscious choices involve awareness and skills such as self-reflection, self-care, discipline, persistence, goal setting, priority setting, action steps, discerning best options, and acknowledging and trusting perceptions. We can be active participants in daily living, not passive observers who hope that life will be good to us.

The unconscious also plays a major role in our choices. Jung conceived of the unconscious as a series of layers.[9] The layers closest to our awareness may become known; those farthest away are, in principle, inaccessible to our awareness and operate autonomously. Jung saw the unconscious as the home of timeless psychic forces that he called *archetypes*, which generally are invariant throughout all cultures and eras. He felt that every psychic force has its opposite in the unconsciousness—the force of light is always counterposed with that of darkness, good with evil, love with hate, and so on. Jung believed that any psychic energy can become unbalanced. Therefore, one of life's greatest challenges is to achieve a dynamic balance of the innate opposites and make this balancing process as conscious as possible.

Relationships

Healthy people live in intricate networks of relationships (see the Relationships section in Figure 30-2) and are always in search of new, unifying concepts of the universe and social order (see Chapter 20). Learning how to understand and nurture our relationships assists us in creating and sustaining meaningful relationships. A healthy person cannot live in isolation. In a given day, we interact with many people: immediate family, extended family, colleagues at work, neighbors in the community, numerous people in organizations, and now, through the ever-expanding web of electronic connection, friends, colleagues, and others around the world.

Relationships have different levels of meaning, from the superficial to the deeply connected. The challenges in relationships are multifaceted. First, we must recognize what we personally are hoping for and what we are bringing to the variety of relationships in which we engage. How do we discern and decide when we feel willing to exchange feelings of honesty, trust, intimacy, compassion, openness, and harmony? Many, if not most, people spend at least half of their waking hours at work with colleagues. Within the context of a work environment, we must support and nourish these relationships as well.

Sharing life processes requires truthful and caring self-reflection and communication with others. This includes meaningful dialogues around end-of-life care. These conversations require deep, personal contemplation about what is desired and hoped for. The dialogue may begin with the family and/or friends most intimately involved and may need to extend beyond to colleagues, clients, and the community at large.

It is essential that we identify both the cohesiveness and the disharmony in our relationships. We must be aware of the effect that we have on clients, family, and friends. Something always happens when people meet and spend time together, for life is never a neutral event. Our attitudes, healing awareness, and concern for self and others have a direct effect on the outcome of all of our encounters. We also must extend our networks to include our immediate environment and consider that what we do locally has an influence on our larger community—the nation and planet Earth (see Chapter 24). Each of us can take an active role in developing local networks of relationships that can have a ripple effect on local to global health concerns.

Spirituality

Throughout history, there has been a quest to understand the purpose of the human life experience. Assessing aspects of our spiritual nature (see the Spirituality section in Figure 30-2) can be a profound learning opportunity (see Chapters 4 and 7). Spirit comes from our roots— it is a universal need to understand the human experience. It is a vital element and driving force in how we live our lives. It affects every aspect of our life balance and satisfaction, as well as the degree to which we develop our human potentials. Usually, though not universally, spirituality is considered to involve a sense of connection with an absolute, imminent, or transcendent spiritual force, however named. It includes the conviction that ethical values, direction, meaning, and purpose are valid aspects of the individual and universe. It is the essence of being and relatedness that permeates all of life and is manifested in one's knowing, doing, and being. This interconnectedness with self, others, Nature, and God/Life Force/Absolute/Transcendent is not necessarily synonymous with religion. Religion is the codified and ritualized beliefs and behaviors of those involved in spirituality,

usually taking place within a community of like-minded individuals.

Spirit involves the development of our higher self, also referred to as the transpersonal self. A transpersonal experience (i.e., transcendence) is described as a feeling of oneness, inner peace, harmony, wholeness, and connection with the universe. The meaning and joy that flow from developing this aspect of our human potential allow us to have a transpersonal view. Some of the ways we may come to know this transcendence are through prayer, meditation, organized religion, philosophy, science, poetry, music, inspired friends, and group work.

Our spiritual potential does not develop without some attention. Every day, with each of our experiences, we must acknowledge that our spirit potential is essential to the development of a healthy value system. We shape our perception of the world through our value system, and our perceptions influence whether we have positive or negative experiences. Even through the pain of a negative experience (which may be physical, mental, emotional, relational, or spiritual), we have the ability to learn. Pain can be a great teacher. On the other side of the experience we may find new wisdom, self-discovery, and the opportunity to make new choices based on freshly acquired knowledge.

Mental

Assessing our mental capacity (see the Mental section in Figure 30-2) helps us to examine our belief systems. In our early life, we had role models who influenced our beliefs, thoughts, behaviors, and values. With maturity and as a result of life experiences, we begin to recognize shifts that occur in regard to these same beliefs, thoughts, behaviors, and values. We may experience conflicts when we do not take the time to examine our changing perspectives, beliefs, and values.

Our challenge is to use our cognitive capacities to perceive the world with greater clarity. This includes recognizing, to the best of our ability, the variety of perspectives that we are presented with both personally and in the world in general (see Chapter 1 and the description of the Theory of Integral Nursing). Through both logical and nonlogical mental processes, we become aware of a broad range of subjects that have the potential to enhance our full appreciation of the many great pleasures in life. We can also build our capacity to notice, process, and integrate both logical thought and intuitive awareness.

With interventions such as relaxation and imagery, we learn to be present in the moment. It is during these moments that we can notice and release the incessant, self-judging, critical inner voice that is constantly engaging in self-dialogue. These are the moments when we expand our mental knowing. We become more capable of focusing our attention away from fear-based, negative thought patterns and become more open and receptive to life-affirming information and patterns of thought. In this way, mental growth can occur. Every aspect of our life is a learning experience and becomes part of a lesson in change.

Emotional

Assessing our emotional potential (see the Emotional section in Figure 30-2) assists us in our willingness to acknowledge the presence of feelings, value them as important information to notice, and express them (see Chapters 7, 22, and 29). Emotional health implies that we have the choice and freedom to process and/or express the full spectrum of emotions, including love, joy, guilt, forgiveness, fear, and anger. The expression of these emotions can give us immediate feedback about our inner state, which may be crying out for a new way of being.

Emotions are responses to the events in our lives. We are living systems that are constantly exchanging with our environment. All life events affect our emotions and general well-being. We have the potential to lessen varying degrees of chronic anxiety, depression, worry, fear, guilt, anger, denial, failure, or repression and to experience true healing when we are willing to confront our emotions.

As we start to live in a more balanced way, we allow our humanness to develop. We reach out and ask for human dialogue that is meaningful. Increasing emotional potential allows openness, creativity, and spontaneity to be experienced. This contributes to the emergence of a positive, healthy zest for living. We can learn to take responsibility for allowing this part of us, our spirit and intuition, to blossom and fully bloom.

Emotions are gifts. Frequently, a first step toward releasing a burden in a relationship is to share deep feelings with another. There is no such thing as a good or bad emotion; each is part of the human condition. Emotions exist as the light and shadow of the self; thus, we must acknowledge all of them. The only reason that we can identify the light is that we know its opposite, the shadow. When we recognize the value in both types of emotions, we are in a position of new insight and understanding, and we can make more effective choices. As we increase our attention to body-mind-spirit interrelationships, we can focus on the emotions that move us toward wholeness and inner understanding.

Physical

All humans share the common biological experiences of birth, gender, growth, aging, and death. When a person's basic biological needs for food, shelter, and clothing have been met, there are many ways to seek wholeness of physical potential. Assessing our physical potential (see the Physical section in Figure 30-2) includes many elements, with three major areas being nutrition (see Chapter 31), exercise (see Chapter 32), and weight management (see Chapter 34). Many people have become obsessed with these elements of the physical potential but have failed to recognize that they are not separate from—or more important than—the other potentials. Health is more than just physical and the absence of pain and symptoms, and it is present when there is balance. As we assess biological needs, we also must take into consideration our perceptions of these areas. Many illnesses have been documented as stress related because our consciousness plays a major role in health and physical potential.[10]

Our body is a gift to nurture and respect. As we nurture ourselves, we increase our uniqueness in energy, sexuality, vitality, capacity for language, and connection with our other potentials. This nurturance strengthens our self-image, which, in turn, causes several things to happen. First, our bodymindspirit responds in a positive and integrated fashion. Second, we become a role model with a positive influence on others. Finally, we enhance our general feeling of well-being, gaining strengths and becoming empowered. The resulting effect is a greater sense of balance and an openness to more fully realized potentials.

Environmental

Assessing our environment (see the Environmental section in Figure 30-2) increases our awareness of its effect on our health and well-being (see Chapter 24). The environment is the context or habitat within which all living systems participate and interact. This includes the physical body and its physical habitat; cultural, psychological, social, and historical influences; and both the external physical space and a person's internal space (physical, mental, emotional, social, and spiritual experiences). A healing environment includes everything that surrounds the nurse, healthcare practitioner, and student, and the patient/client, family, community, and significant others, as well as patterns not yet understood.

Florence Nightingale was an environmentalist who wrote about the effects of polluted homes and environments and the importance of avoiding anything that makes one ill or may be considered toxic. Today, this is recognized as the "precautionary principle," which states that when an activity raises threats of harm to human health or the environment, precautionary measures shall be taken, even if some cause-and-effect relationships are not fully established scientifically—or "better safe than sorry."[11] If there is a suspicion about a harmful environment or substance, even though all of the evidence is not in, remove the person from the situation or stop the use of suspected harmful substances. The emphasis is on *zero* contamination and pollution of our environments as acceptable, not minimal/moderate.

Health Responsibility

Health responsibility (see the Health Responsibility section in Figure 30-2) occurs when an individual takes an active role in making lifestyle choices to protect and improve his or her health. These actions and behaviors that enhance health and well-being are explored in the IHWA.

Health responsibility includes having physical examinations and eye examinations as recommended for one's age and health status by qualified healthcare practitioners. A personal health record includes all baseline personal physiologic parameters, personal history, family history, and any current symptoms. In addition, all medications and supplements that are being taken should be noted and evaluated in terms of any potential interactions of the pharmaceuticals with the supplements. Allergies, hospitalizations, surgeries, and other specific medical factors are also important to note.

In health care, we may hear that a client/patient is noncompliant with medical orders. This is often a misnomer because there are many reasons why an individual may not follow medical recommendations. Some common reasons for this "noncompliance" include too much information given at one time; lack of fully understanding the recommendations and having unanswered questions; language barriers or cognitive limitations; fear(s); denial; previous lack of commitment or lack of success (e.g., weight management, smoking cessation); side effects of medications; financial constraints; religious beliefs; disabilities; and lack of support from significant others. In addition, there is usually an inadequate amount of time for effective patient education in clinics, doctors' offices, hospitals when providing discharge information, and other healthcare settings.

Conclusion

Use of the IHWA can engage both clients and nurses in self-development. Holistic nurses are challenged to learn new nurse coaching knowledge and skills to assist clients and self in new health behaviors and how to sustain them. If one IHWA category is not assessed or is left undeveloped, things will not seem to be as good as they could be. When one strives to develop in one or several areas, a sense of wholeness emerges, one's self-worth increases, and action plans for healthier lifestyle behaviors and goals are actualized. Being alive becomes more exciting, rewarding, and fulfilling. By taking an active role in health promotion, health maintenance, and disease management, clients can integrate strengths, action plans, and affirmations and can continue on a creative journey of healing. By changing our perceptions and beliefs and empowering ourselves for effective change, we become healthier.

Directions for Future Research

1. Determine whether the percentage of desired client outcomes increases when the nurse uses the Integrative Health and Wellness Assessment (IHWA) as a coaching tool.
2. Determine whether the client's self-efficacy and self-esteem increase with use of the IHWA.
3. Evaluate changes in health behavior and perceived quality of life when assessing the IHWA's eight categories.

Nurse Healer Reflections

After reading this chapter, the nurse healer will be able to answer or to begin a process of answering the following questions:

- What is my process when I complete the Integrative Health and Wellness Assessment?
- Am I consciously aware of the daily opportunity to increase my health and well-being?
- What can I do to increase my conscious awareness of fully participating in my life?
- What do I experience when I acknowledge my healing potential?

NOTES

1. U.S. Department of Health and Human Services, *Healthy People 2020* (Washington, DC: U.S. Department of Health and Human Services, 2010).
2. Office of the Legislative Council, "Compilation of Patient Protection and Affordable Care Act" (May 1, 2010). http://docs.house.gov/energycommerce/ppacacon.pdf.
3. U.S. Department of Health and Human Services, "Obama Administration Releases National Prevention Strategy" (June 16, 2011). www.businesswire.com/news/home/20110616005341/en/Obama-Administration-Releases-National-Prevention-Strategy#.VHUQrIuKxtd.
4. S. Luck, "Changing the Health of Our Nation: The Role of Nurse Coaches," *Alternative Therapies in Health and Medicine* 16, no. 5 (2010): 78–80.
5. B. M. Dossey, S. Luck, and B. G. Schaub, *Nurse Coaching: Integrative Approaches for Health and Well-being* (North Miami, FL: International Nurse Coach Association, 2015).
6. L. Keegan and B. Dossey, *Self Care: A Program to Improve Your Life* (Port Angeles, WA: Holistic Nursing Consultants, 2007).
7. R. DiClemente, L. Salazar, and R. Crosby, *Health Behavior Theory for Public Health: Principles, Foundations, and Applications* (Burlington, MA: Jones & Bartlett Learning, 2013).
8. S. Weinstein, *B Is for Balance: A Nurse's Guide for Enjoying Life at Work and at Home*, 2nd ed. (Indianapolis, IN: Sigma Theta Tau International, 2014).
9. C. Jung, "Archetypes of the Collective Unconscious," in *Collected Works of C. G. Jung*, Vol. 9, Part 1, trans. R. F. C. Hull (Princeton, NJ: Princeton University Press, 1980): 3–41.
10. C. C. Clark and K. K. Paraska, *Health Promotion for Nurses: A Practical Guide* (Burlington, MA: Jones & Bartlett Learning, 2014).
11. C. Raffensperger and J. Tickner, *Protecting Public Health and the Environment: Implementing the Precautionary Principle* (Washington, DC: Island Press, 1999).

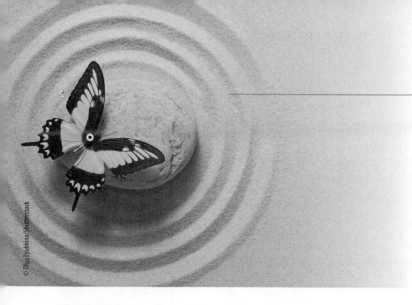

© Olga Lyubkina/Shutterstock

CHAPTER 31

Nutrition

Susan Luck and Karen M. Avino

Nurse Healer Objectives

Theoretical

- Learn the definitions of terms in this chapter.
- Differentiate between the Recommended Dietary Allowance and the optimal daily allowance.
- Develop a plan that combines good nutrition with a healthy lifestyle.
- Learn the benefits of healthy eating for wellness promotion and disease prevention.
- Explore the nurse's role as coach in behavioral and dietary change.

Clinical

- Explore the meaning of foods in different cultural traditions.
- Listen to the client/patient story around health and nutrition.
- Identify nutritional foods that support the client/patient healing process.
- Use open-ended questions to learn more from clients about eating habits and health behaviors.
- Increase your knowledge of current nutrition research.

Personal

- Assess the quality of your food intake and note how it increases or decreases your energy level at work.

- Heighten your awareness of the way in which what you eat affects how you feel.
- Examine your eating patterns and the meaning of food in your life.
- Explore new foods and food preparation to support your health and well-being.
- Plan a day's menu, asking yourself, "What does my body need to enhance my wellness?"
- Explore mindful eating practices.
- Prepare foods to bring to your workplace to support your health goals.
- Find a nurse coach and enter into a coaching agreement to reach desired nutrition goals.
- Employ strategies to improve nutrition in your workplace.

Definitions

Antioxidants: Substances that limit free radical formation and damage by stabilizing or deactivating free radicals before they attack cells.

Diabesity: A popular term for the common clinical association of type 2 diabetes mellitus and obesity.

Epigenetics: The study of changes produced in gene expression caused by mechanisms other than changes in the underlying DNA sequence.

Free radicals: Electrically charged molecules with an unpaired electron capable of attacking healthy cells in the body, causing them to lose their structure and function.

Glycemic index: An index that classifies carbohydrate foods according to their glycemic response (effect on blood glucose levels), which varies with fiber content, starch structure, food processing, and presence of proteins and fats.

High-density lipoprotein (HDL): A form of cholesterol associated with reduced risk of atherosclerosis.

Homocysteine: An amino acid found in the blood and an intermediate product of methionine metabolism.

Leptin: A peptide hormone neurotransmitter produced by fat cells and involved in the regulation of appetite.

Low-density lipoprotein (LDL): A form of cholesterol strongly associated with increased risk of atherosclerosis.

Metabolic syndrome: A collection of heart disease risk factors that increase the chance of developing heart disease, stroke, and diabetes. The condition is also known by other names including Syndrome X and cardiometabolic and insulin resistance syndrome.

Mineral: An inorganic trace element or compound that works in synergy with other compounds and is essential for human life.

Nutraceuticals: Food, or parts of food, that provide medical or health benefits, including the prevention and treatment of disease.

Nutrigenomics: The study of the effects of foods and food constituents on gene expression; how our DNA is transcribed into mRNA and then to proteins to provide a basis for understanding the biological activity of food components.

Obesogens: Identifiable industrial pollutants contributing to the obesity epidemic by increasing fat cells in the body and altering metabolism and feelings of hunger and fullness.

Optimal nutrition: The adequate intake of nutrients for health promotion and disease prevention.

Organic food: Food from plants and animals that has been grown without the use of synthetic fertilizers or pesticides and without antibiotics, growth hormones, and feed additives.

Phytochemicals: Biologically active compounds found in foods and plants.

Phytoestrogens: A family of compounds found in plants that have some estrogenic or antiestrogenic activity.

Probiotic: A formulation containing beneficial living microorganisms that maintain health as part of the internal ecology of the digestive tract.

Vitamin: An organic substance necessary for normal growth, metabolism, and development of the body; acts as a catalyst and coenzyme, assisting in many chemical reactions while nourishing the body.

Xenoestrogens: Synthetic, environmental, hormone-mimicking compounds found in many pesticides, drugs, plastics, and personal care products.

Current Nutrition Theory and Research

Nutrition is integral to maintaining health throughout the life cycle and has a profound influence on disease prevention, health maintenance, and the aging process. By including nutrition into a holistic approach we acknowledge the individual's physiologic, psychological, social, genetic, cultural, religious, economic, and environmental needs. The individual's eating patterns, food preferences, motivation, attitudes, and beliefs are all part of nutrition coaching, counseling, and education.

Dietary habits play a central role in almost all health conditions seen today, including inflammation and pain, digestive and gastrointestinal disturbances, allergies and food sensitivities, fatigue, mood disorders, and immune dysfunction. Food and nutrients are no longer viewed merely as providing substances whose absence would produce disease but as having a positive effect on an individual's overall health, including physical performance, aging process, cognitive function, energy levels, and daily quality of life.

It is common knowledge that foods produced today are processed and denatured, depleted of nutrients, and often contain toxic chemicals including additives, preservatives, pesticides, hormones, antibiotics, and many other residues. The changes to our food supply contribute to a rising number of chronic health issues including learning disabilities, obesity, diabetes, atherosclerosis, heart disease, hypertension, immune and autoimmune diseases, and various cancers.[1] Examining the methods used to produce crops is important for health. A meta-analysis found the nutritional and food safety benefits of organic farming to provide a rich source of antioxidants with few pesticides.[2]

According to several recently published studies, evidence-based guidelines regarding recommendations on lifestyle and healthy nutrition as a primary preventive intervention demonstrate consistent results. Furthermore, the cost effectiveness of primary prevention services is proven. Health promotion and disease prevention are emerging as a national strategy, and nurses in all healthcare settings are in a key position to use their professional skills to coach and educate individuals and communities in nutrition and lifestyle changes that affect long-term health goals and health policy. Integrating nurse coaching into clinical practice is a new direction for nurses in a patient-centered care model.

A personalized comprehensive approach that examines the complex interactions among a combination of factors, including the individual's genetics and diet, appears to have more influence on life span and is more effective than looking at single factors.[3] For example, researchers found that a new gene variant increases the risk of colorectal cancer if eating processed meat.[4] Understanding the effect of interactions of our individual biology can lead to future targeted prevention strategies. The evidence-based science of nutrition and lifestyle interventions for preventing or treating chronic disease demonstrates the powerful, cost-effective, and critical role that nutrition plays in the promotion and restoration of health. Current research supports healthful dietary patterns, such as the Mediterranean diet, which includes whole grains, legumes, nuts, vegetables, fruits, olive oil, and fish and is associated with a decrease in chronic disease and death from all causes. The harmful effects of trans and certain saturated fats, refined carbohydrates, high fructose corn syrup, and many food additives are well documented in the medical literature.[5]

Current Global Health Crisis

In 2013, an American Heart Association report stated that the economic costs of cardiovascular disease and stroke in the United States was estimated to be $656 billion in the year 2015 and expected to grow to $1208 billion by 2030. In this report, cardiovascular disease was highlighted as complex, with genetic, environmental, and epigenetic factors influencing disease progression.[6]

In a comprehensive global study of more than 188 countries, researchers found that over the past 3 decades there has been a startling increase of greater than 27.5% in overweight and obese people. More than half of these people live in 10 countries, including the United States, China, Russia, Brazil, Mexico, Egypt, Germany, Pakistan, and Indonesia.[7] In the United States, more than one-third (34.9%) of adults were obese in 2011–2012.[8]

Obesity and metabolic syndrome have the potential to affect the incidence and severity of cardiovascular pathologies and to increase diabetes and present implications for worldwide healthcare systems. The metabolic syndrome is characterized by visceral obesity, insulin resistance, hypertension, chronic inflammation, and thrombotic disorders contributing to endothelial dysfunction and, subsequently, to accelerated atherosclerosis. Obesity is a key component in the development of the metabolic syndrome, and it is becoming increasingly clear that a central factor in this is the production by adipose cells of bioactive substances that directly influence insulin sensitivity and vascular injury.

According to the Centers for Disease Control and Prevention (CDC), *overweight* and *obese* are labels for ranges of weight that are greater than what is generally considered healthy for a given height. It can also be defined as weighing in excess of 40 pounds more than ideal body weight. The national prevalence of overweight and obesity is monitored using data from the National Health and Nutrition Examination Survey. *Healthy People 2020* identified obesity as a problem throughout the entire population. However, among adults, the prevalence is highest for middle-aged people and for non-Hispanic black and Mexican American women. Among children and adolescents, the prevalence of obesity is highest among older and Mexican American children and non-Hispanic black girls.[9] The association of income with obesity varies by age, gender, and race/ethnicity.[10] Obesity reduces life expectancy while increasing the risk of illness and death from a range of other diseases. It is now so common in adults and children that the World Health Organization characterizes this condition as a global epidemic.

Type 2 diabetes mellitus is a preventable disease and a growing public health problem. Epidemiologic and interventional studies suggest that weight loss is the main driving force to reduce diabetes risk. Landmark clinical trials of lifestyle changes in subjects with prediabetes have shown that combining changes in eating patterns and behaviors with exercise promotes weight loss and consistently reduces the incidence of diabetes.[11]

Energy imbalance is an immediate trigger of obesity: a combination of excess calories and a lack of physical activity. Sugar intake significantly contributes to compromised health and raises triglycerides and cholesterol levels. Hypertriglyceridemia is a common lipid abnormality in persons with visceral obesity, metabolic syndrome, and type 2 diabetes.[12] In pregnant women whose dietary pattern mainly consisted of discretionary foods including sugar, a correlation was found between preterm delivery and shorter birth length.[13]

Researchers at Emory University and the CDC examined the added sugar intake and blood fat levels in more than 6,100 adults. Participants consumed an average of 21.4 teaspoons of added sugars a day, or more than 320 calories a day from these sources.[11] According to the report, type 2 diabetes and obesity hold long-term health implications for the U.S. population: Obesity is a contributing cause of many health problems, including heart disease, stroke, diabetes, and some types of cancer. Researchers in Germany at the University Children's Hospital in Leipzig compared fat cell composition and biology in lean and obese children and adolescents. They found that when children become obese, beginning as early as age 6, there was an increase in the number of adipose cells, which were larger in size than the cells found in the bodies of lean children. The researchers also found evidence of dysfunction in the fat cells of obese children, including signs of inflammation, which can lead to insulin resistance, diabetes, and other problems, such as high blood pressure. Statistically, these are some of the leading causes of death in the United States.[14]

Other symptoms and health risks attributed to obesity include sleep apnea, asthma and breathing problems, limited mobility, inflammation, early deterioration of joints leading to arthritis, and osteoporosis and hip fractures. Obesity can cause problems during pregnancy and indicates a higher risk for obesity in children of obese parents.[15]

Emerging Research in the Study of Obesity and the Environment

Current research focuses on how environmental toxins, described as obesogens, are stored in fat tissue and can influence and interfere with healthy fat cell signaling and fat metabolism and with cell signaling messengers that control feelings of satiety after eating. For healthy fat metabolism, leptin, an adipocyte-derived hormone, plays an essential role in the maintenance of normal body weight and energy expenditure, as well as glucose homeostasis. Leptin resistance occurs in those who are chronically overweight. The role of leptin in fat cells is to reduce appetite and stimulate fat burning. The relationship between leptin and perceived hunger, and on the eating behavior of leptin-deficient individuals, appears to be blocked in chronically overweight individuals as they develop leptin resistance, making losing weight increasingly difficult, if not impossible.[16]

Fat also regulates the processes by which the body burns fuel for energy, especially in muscle. Adiponectin, another hormone-like chemical, plays a central role in the biology of fat and is normally produced to curb appetite and spark the burning of fat. But unlike leptin, which remains present but stops functioning, chronically overweight individuals have an adiponectin deficiency. Many adipokines are also mediators of inflammation and promote and encourage the inflammatory response, which further affects fat metabolism and homeostasis.[17] Weight loss is associated with reduced inflammation systemically.[18]

Routine exposures to human-made chemicals may also increase an individual's risk of obesity. The obesogen hypothesis proposes that perturbations in metabolic signaling that result from exposure to environmental chemicals known as endocrine disrupting chemicals are stored in the body's adipose tissue and may further exacerbate the effects of imbalances, resulting in an increased susceptibility to obesity and obesity-related disorders.[19] These markers indicate the potential for nutritional coaching for behavioral change to improve metabolism and cellular communication and to promote healthier choices for long-term health.

Obesity is on the minds of health policy analysts and healthcare providers both nationally and globally. According to a CDC report, obesity is a complex problem that requires both personal and community action.[20] The report goes on to mandate that people in all communities should be able to make healthy choices.

As part of a health strategy and health care policy to promote lifestyle behavioral change, nurses as coaches are in a prime position to guide and motivate individuals toward healthy behaviors. Effective health promotion programs include awareness practices, exercise, behavioral motivation for change, nutrition and environmental health education. . . . Comprehensive effective nutrition programs integrate coaching skills for the patient/client to set attainable goals. This process is a gradual and highly individualized process for reversing patterns that can lead to chronic disease.

Effective therapeutic nutritional guidelines honor the totality of the individual. An individual's metabolism, environment, genetics, emotional health, social networks, and life stressors must be considered in evaluating nutritional needs and nutritional goals. Beliefs, attitudes, eating patterns, food choices and culinary styles are deeply embedded in one's cultural, physiological, psychological, emotional, spiritual, and socioeconomic needs and must be considered for whole person healing. Listening to an individual's story is central to guiding behavioral change around food.[20]

From an evolutionary and cultural perspective, our modern-day food supply has been dramatically altered, although our biological nutrient needs have not. The human diet remained constant for thousands of years but has radically changed in the past few decades. It is now painfully clear that our modern dietary habits influence our health and well-being. For example, we know that food composition and macronutrient content are essential for biochemical processes, working synergistically to produce energy on a cellular level. Without proper nutrient synergy and healthy cellular communication, the end result is diminished function that often causes decreased energy output, inflammation, and lowered immune response. Essential macronutrients and micronutrients include carbohydrates, proteins, fats, vitamins and minerals, and essential fatty acids.[20]

Food as Energy

The body is an energy flow system, and cells must live in harmony in the extracellular matrix. Over time, nutritional deficiencies create disharmony within the cellular structure and diminish energy exchange within cells, essential for healthy cell signaling and function. Overt symptoms of nutrient deficiency are the result of a long chain of reactions in the body. When an individual consumes a nutrient-deficient diet, the initial reactions occur on a molecular level. First, enzymes that are dependent on the deficient nutrients become depleted. This depletion brings about changes within cells. The deficiencies may continue for many years until the body can no longer carry out its normal functions. Eventually, overt signs and symptoms appear, even though the deficiency may still be considered subclinical because routine laboratory tests do not necessarily uncover nutritional deficiencies. Nevertheless, these unseen deficiencies can lead to a broad range of nonspecific conditions that can diminish an individual's overall quality of life. Undiagnosed, nutrient deficiencies over many years leave the body more vulnerable to illnesses to which the individual may be genetically predisposed and to immune system compromise. Yet, as resilient beings, even when health is compromised, we can reprogram our cells and create an internal and external healing environment to restore health and balance.[21]

Debate continues over the most efficient "diet" for weight loss and overall health. Advocates of diverse approaches include the high-fat, low-carbohydrate Atkins diet and the high-protein, low-carbohydrate Paleo Diet, which are challenged by vegan-type diets consisting of high amounts of complex carbohydrates and high intake of fruits and vegetables. A study of more than 100,000 people over more than 20 years—the Nurses' Health Study—concludes that a low-carbohydrate diet high in vegetables and with a larger proportion of proteins and fats coming mostly from plant sources decreases mortality. In contrast, a low-carbohydrate diet with largely animal sources of protein and fat increases mortality.[22]

An Integrative Health and Well-Being Model

In a nutritional coaching model, the client moves beyond the concept of a "diet" to set attainable goals leading to a healthier lifestyle, new behaviors, and improved health outcomes. As nutrition research and information reach the public and the existing healthcare model, there is a hunger for a new paradigm that explores and examines the underlying causes of disease. Functional medicine is an emerging field with an emphasis on personalized nutrition and lifestyle interventions. For holistic nurses, in a patient-centered care model, health is viewed as a positive vitality, representing more than the absence of disease. By maintaining balance of a complex web of physiologic, cognitive/emotional, and physical processes, health and well-being can be achieved.

Adapted from functional medicine, an Integrative Lifestyle Health and Well-Being Model (ILHWB) is congruent and compatible with holistic nursing philosophy and practice. The ILHWB is a unique nursing model that expands on functional medicine, integrating the art and science of nursing and nursing theories, and builds on the holistic nursing process. The ILHWB model views health and balance as a dynamic interaction and an interconnectedness within an individual's internal and external environment. Coaching strategies for a healthy lifestyle integrate nutritional knowledge and nutritional coaching; they are opportunities for nurses to bring new skills and tools to the art and science of nursing. This model moves nurses beyond understanding a client's chemistry, diagnosis, and ailments from a medical construct and views health, energy, and balance through an expanded, holistic, integral, and integrative perspective. The physical and social environment in which symptoms occur; the dietary habits of the person (present and past); the environment in which the person lives; his or her beliefs about health, illness, and diagnosis; and the combined effect of these factors on social, physical, and psychological function are all interconnected to one's lifestyle choices and influence health outcomes. Discovery of the factors that aggravate or ameliorate symptoms and that predispose the client to illness or facilitate recovery provides for the possibilities of co-creating lifestyle and behavioral changes and establishing an integrative care plan. The nurse coach's collaborative relationship recognizes and acknowledges the individual's experience of health or illness and explores the totality of the individual by deeply listening to the client's story.

Within this larger context of the whole person, nurses as educators increase their knowledge, understand the current nutrition science and research, and stay informed. Increasing awareness, assessing the client's relationship to nutrition and food, evaluating the client's eating patterns and nutritional needs, assisting in developing a personalized nutrition plan and goals, and implementing effective nutritional guidelines and strategies for enhancing wellness are all part of the role of the nurse as coach.

Foundations of a Nurse-Based Integrative Lifestyle Health and Well-Being Model

- *Interconnectedness.* This includes the mind, body, and spiritual dimensions of physiologic factors. An abundance of research now supports the view that the human body functions as an orchestrated network of interconnected systems rather than as individual systems that function autonomously and without effect on one another.

- *Energy field principles and dynamics.* An understanding of how thoughts, stress, toxic environments, and a nutrient-deficient diet can disrupt human energy fields, impair optimal functioning, and contribute to disease.
- *Patient centeredness.* Honors and emphasizes the individual's unique history, beliefs, and story rather than a medical diagnosis and disease orientation.
- *Biochemical individuality.* Recognizes the importance of variations in metabolic function that derive from unique genetic and environmental vulnerabilities and strengths among individuals.
- *Health on a wellness continuum.* Views health as a dynamic balance on multiple levels and seeks to identify, restore, and support our innate reserve as the means to enhance well-being and healing throughout the life cycle.
- *Optimization of our internal and external healing environments.* Holds the worldview that human health is the microcosm of the macrocosm in the web of life.

Source: Copyright © 2015. Adapted by S. Luck. Nutritional Health (pp. 147–183). In Dossey, B. M., Luck, S. and Schaub, B. G., *Nurse Coaching: Integrative Approaches for Health and Wellbeing.* North Miami, FL: International Nurse Coach Association. www.iNurseCoach .com

Overview of Clinical Nutrition

The Standard American Diet

Nutrient deficiencies most often result from a high intake of processed and refined foods. According to a report from the 2005–2010 National Health and Nutrition Examination Survey, Americans eat about 20 teaspoons of sugar a day. Most of the sugar is from foods (not beverages) that contain sugar and high fructose corn syrup, hidden in packaged products and consumed at home.[23] High fructose corn syrup is produced by chemically converting the starch in corn to a substance that is about 90% fructose, a sugar that is sweeter than the glucose that fuels body cells and that is processed differently by the body. Fructose is metabolized primarily in the liver, which favors the formation of fats and results in elevated triglycerides, one of the markers for increased risk of metabolic syndrome. It is estimated that more than 28% of calories in the standard American diet consist of refined products such as white bread and white rice, which are deficient in 28 essential nutrients including essential vitamins (in particular the B vitamins), minerals, protein, and fiber, all contained in the whole grain prior to processing.

With more than one-third of children and more than two-thirds of adults in the United States overweight or obese, the seventh edition of the U.S. Department of Agriculture's *Dietary Guidelines for Americans* places stronger emphasis on reducing calorie consumption and increasing physical activity.

For the first time in more than 40 years, the U.S. Department of Agriculture has reissued its guidelines for nutrient needs, originally defined as the Recommended Daily Allowances (RDAs) by the U.S. Food and Nutrition Board. The RDA guidelines specified the levels of nutrients required to prevent overt symptoms of deficiency. In 2010, to meet the growing healthcare crisis, the new guidelines known as Dietary Reference Intakes, or DRIs, address the questions that have been asked by experts in the field.[24]

Clinical Nutrition Research

As nurses expand their knowledge of nutrition, they can assist clients in their decision-making processes, including lifestyle and nutritional choices. Americans spend an estimated $22 billion a year out of pocket on nutrition-related products, according to a 2009 National Health Statistics report. The introduction of pharmaceutical-grade omega-3 essential fatty acids is an example of a nutraceutical recently recommended by the American Heart Association. Omega-3 essential fatty acids, deficient in our modern food supply, play an important role in immune function, brain health, prevention of cardiovascular disease and stroke, and in inhibiting the development of macular degeneration given the growing epidemic predicted to increase to 50% in the elderly by the year 2020.[25] Omega-3 essential fatty acids have been well researched in the treatment of arthritis, diabetes, obesity, cancer, immune and autoimmune disorders, cognitive function, and a variety of women's health problems.[26]

Many epidemiologic studies report strong correlations between Western diseases and dietary habits (see **Exhibit 31-1** for guidelines to assist in weight loss, blood glucose regulation, energy maintenance, nutrient needs, and satiety.). Mortality rates for certain cancers, as well as the incidence of cardiovascular disease, are higher among those who consume the standard American diet than among those who consume Asian, Scandinavian, or Mediterranean diets.[27] A meta-analysis reported that nut intake can actually prevent cardiovascular diseases and improve mortality rates.[28] (See the Mediterranean food pyramid in **Figure 31-1**.)

A growing body of research indicates that elevated homocysteine levels result from subclinical deficiencies of the B vitamins, including folic acid, vitamin B_6, and vitamin B_{12}. Knowledge about nutrient deficiencies and their potentially life-threatening consequences is slowly being integrated into routine physical examinations and health assessments. Two articles in the *New England Journal of Medicine* report that high plasma homocysteine concentrations and low concentrations of folate and vitamin B_6 play roles in homocysteine metabolism, inflammation, and cardiovascular health. Deficiencies in many of these nutrients are also associated with diabetes, heart disease, depression, anxiety, and premenstrual syndrome.[29]

Heart disease is responsible for 45% of all deaths among women, and nearly 40% of all females are expected to develop cancer at some point in their lifetime. Coaching women to make healthy dietary and lifestyle choices can have a significant, positive effect on their health. Recent research demonstrates the cardioprotective effects of several dietary nutrients, including fiber (both soluble and insoluble), antioxidants (vitamins C and E, beta-carotene, selenium, coenzyme Q10), folic acid, and omega-3 essential fatty acids. According to several recent studies, women can lower their risk of heart disease and heart attacks by improving their blood lipid and fatty acid profiles by consuming a combination of essential fatty acids derived primarily

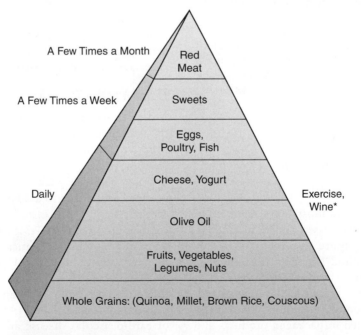

*Daily, wine in moderation

FIGURE 31-1 Mediterranean Food Pyramid

EXHIBIT 31-1   Hypoglycemic Food Plan

These guidelines can assist in weight loss, blood glucose regulation, energy maintenance, nutrient needs, and satiety.

- Eliminate caffeine, soda, fruit juice, white sugar, white flour, white rice, artificial sweeteners, and white bread.
- Limit fruits—two per day and divide into four portions. Avoid grapes and bananas (high in sugar).
- Throughout the day, consume several small meals consisting of protein with vegetables and complex carbohydrates if needed.
- Vegetables—unlimited—raw or cooked depending on your preference (and digestion); limit beets, peas, and carrots.

SAMPLE FOODS TO INCLUDE

Protein

Fish	Wild Alaskan salmon (or canned); sardines; broiled, baked, steamed fish
Chicken	Baked, broiled; remove skin; white meat (free range if available)
Turkey	Fresh turkey, white meat
Beans*	Lentils (best for improving blood sugar regulation), soy (tofu), black beans, red beans, garbanzo beans, hummus, tempeh
Whole grains*	Quinoa, millet, buckwheat (kasha), brown rice, oatmeal (if not gluten intolerant), barley, whole wheat, spelt, amaranth

Whole Grains + Beans = Complete Protein

Seeds and nuts* (2-tablespoon servings)	Almonds, sunflower seeds, walnuts, pumpkin seeds, nut butters (almond, sesame; raw, unsalted)
Eggs	Boiled, poached (free range or organic if available)
Dairy	Low-fat plain yogurt, skim-milk ricotta or mozzarella cheese, goat feta, yogurt (plain and if not lactose intolerant)

Vegetables 5–7 servings daily

Salads

Steamed vegetables; fresh or frozen; avoid canned

Sample Menu

- Salad with grilled chicken or fish
- Hummus and vegetables in whole-wheat pita
- Lentil soup with gluten-free rice crackers or whole grains (millet, brown rice, quinoa, whole wheat pita)
- Grilled skinless chicken breast with 0.5 cup brown rice or quinoa and steamed vegetables
- Tofu or black beans with brown rice and steamed vegetables
- Grilled fish with half baked sweet potato and salad

Snacks: *Small meals to have between meals, midmorning and midafternoon*

- Low-fat plain yogurt with 0.5 cup fresh fruit, whole-wheat or gluten-free rice crackers with tuna salad, hummus with whole-wheat pita or vegetables
- 1 to 2 tablespoons almonds or sunflower seeds, or nut butter (almond or sesame tahini) on whole-wheat or rice crackers, leftover lunch portion
- Protein shake (whey, rice, hemp, pea, or soy protein)

Source: Copyright © 2015. Adapted by S. Luck. Hypoglycemic Food Plan (p. 477). In Dossey, B. M., Luck, S. and Schaub, B. G. *Nurse Coaching: Integrative Approaches for Health and Wellbeing.* North Miami, FL: International Nurse Coach Association. www.iNurseCoach.com

from fish oils and seed-based oils. Researchers estimate that this combination produces a 43% risk reduction over a 10-year period.[30]

Review of Nutrient Sources

Carbohydrates

Carbohydrates provide a main source of energy for all body functions, aiding in digestion, assimilation, and metabolism of proteins and fats. Carbohydrates are classified as simple and complex. Simple carbohydrates include refined white flour products, white rice, white table sugar (dextrose), honey, fruit sugars (fructose), and milk sugars (lactose). Complex carbohydrates are found in whole grains, legumes, seeds, nuts, and vegetables and contain protein, vitamins, minerals, and fiber. Throughout human history, foods that contain complex carbohydrates have been important staples in diverse cultures. Complex carbohydrates supply the body with essential nutrients and protein amino acids and provide longer-lasting energy than do simple carbohydrates.[31] All animal proteins are complete, including red meat, poultry, seafood, eggs, and dairy. Complete proteins can also be obtained through plant foods as when combining lentils, quinoa, or black beans with brown rice.

Fiber

Dietary fiber is plant material that is left undigested after passing through the body's digestive system. Fiber contains polysaccharides and can be subdivided into insoluble fiber and soluble fiber, each with a different mixture of compounds. Food sources of dietary fiber are often classified according to whether they contain predominantly soluble or insoluble fiber. Plant foods usually contain a combination of both types of fiber in varying degrees, according to the plant's characteristics. Insoluble fiber includes pectin and cellulose, hemicellulose, and lignins.[32] Insoluble fiber is present in fruits, leafy vegetables, whole grains, and beans. Soluble fiber is a gelatin-like substance, such as the mucilage found in oatmeal and legumes.

Research clearly documents that the modern Western diet with its low-fiber content has led to an increase in digestive problems, including diverticulitis, constipation, colon cancer, gallstone formation, and other gastrointestinal disturbances. Although dietary fiber is not digested, it increases fecal bulk and weight, making the passage of waste products more efficient and assists in carrying toxins and metabolic by-products through the intestines to be eliminated quickly from the system. Fiber also is important in modulating insulin response and stabilizing blood glucose levels and as a fuel for healthy intestinal flora. In recent years, research into the benefits of dietary fiber has led many practitioners to recommend a low-fat, high-fiber diet for prevention of heart disease, diabetes, obesity, digestive disorders, and cancer.

A diet high in saturated animal fat and low in fiber has been shown to increase the risk of colon cancer. Complex-carbohydrate foods offer fiber and are also good sources of protein, vitamins, and minerals.[33] Fiber-rich diets help lower blood cholesterol levels and stabilize blood glucose levels and are considered heart healthy by multiple research studies. According to the *Dietary Guidelines for Americans 2015*, at least half of all grains consumed daily should be whole and unrefined. The goal for fiber is 25 grams per day for women and 28 grams per day for men. Achieving these goals may reduce a person's risk of dying from heart disease, infections, and respiratory diseases.[34]

Protein

Protein is the second most plentiful substance in the body (after water) and constitutes approximately one-fifth of the body's weight. Protein is the basic building block of the body and makes up the rigid structures such as bone, solid organs, and blood vessels. It is essential for the growth and maintenance of all body tissues, including muscle, skin, hair, nails, and eyes. Hormones, chemicals such as antibodies, and enzymes are composed of protein. Protein molecules, essentially composed of amino acids, form long chains and branched structures. Amino acids contain nitrogen, carbon, hydrogen, and sometimes sulfur. Twenty-two amino acids are required to build protein; half of these are produced in the body when adequate nutrients are available, and eight are considered essential.

Excessive protein consumption can stress the kidneys and digestive system. Protein requirements depend on an individual's activity level, energy requirements, age, and digestive health. The recommended protein allowance for health maintenance in the United States is 0.8 grams per kilogram of body weight per day. Men and women who body build require up to 1.2 grams per kilogram of body weight per day.[35]

Lipids

Lipids are a group of fats and fatlike substances, including essential fatty acids, that account for more than 10% of body weight in most adults. The principal function of fats is to serve as a source of energy. Stored fats also act as a thermal blanket, insulating the body and providing a protective cushion for many tissues and organs. According to the third National Health and Nutrition Examination Survey, Americans are eating less fat than they were 10 years ago. Americans now average 34% of their total daily calories (82 grams) from fat, with approximately 12% (29 grams) from saturated fats. Current dietary recommendations call for 20% of total calories from fat and less than 10% from saturated fats. The RDA for dietary fat is suggested to be 25 grams to ensure the intake of essential fatty acids. Unsaturated fats are usually liquid at room temperature and are derived from vegetables, nuts, seeds, and olives. Saturated fats— found in animal products, including meat and dairy products—are generally associated with an increased risk of cancer and cardiovascular disease. Foods often contain a mixture of saturated and unsaturated fatty acids. Fats are calorie rich and contain approximately 9 calories per gram, almost twice the calories of carbohydrates and proteins.

Essential fatty acids are found in both monosaturated and polyunsaturated fats. Monosaturated fats include olive, peanut, avocado, and canola oils. Polyunsaturated fats are found in safflower, sunflower, corn, sesame, and soy oils. Fats can be further divided into two main classes: omega-3 fatty acids and omega-6 fatty acids. Essential fatty acids form a structural part of all cell membranes and create electrical potentials across the membrane, facilitating the generation of bioelectrical currents that transmit messages. Certain essential fatty acids substantially shorten the time required for the recovery of fatigued muscles after exercise by facilitating the conversion of lactic acid to water and carbon dioxide.[36] Essential fatty acids act as precursors for a family of hormone-like substances called *prostaglandins*, which regulate many functions in the body, including inflammatory processes and immune responses. Omega-3 essential fatty acids are immune enhancing and are often deficient in the modern diet. They contain high concentrations of linoleic acid and are necessary for normal growth and development throughout the life cycle. Omega-3 essential fatty acids are found in high concentrations in fish, fish oils, flaxseeds, and walnuts. High concentrations of docosahexaenoic acid are found in the brain, and a deficiency of this omega-3 essential fatty acid component can lead to impaired learning and decreased cognitive function beginning in utero and is needed in large amounts during development. Other essential fatty acid deficiency symptoms include poor immune response, dry skin and hair, behavioral changes, menstrual irregularities, and arthritic and inflammatory conditions. **Exhibit 31-2** serves as a guide for general dietary goals and recommendations.[37]

Vitamins

Vitamins are nutrients essential to life. They contribute to good health by regulating the metabolism and assisting in biochemical processes that release energy from digested food. Vitamins function mostly as coenzymes that activate the chemical reactions continually occurring in the body. Vitamins are the foundation for all aspects of body function, from nervous system transmission to proper composition of bodily fluids. Vitamins are divided into two major groups: water soluble and fat soluble. Water-soluble vitamins must be taken into the body daily and are excreted within 1 to 4 days. They include vitamin C and the B-complex vitamins. Because excessive quantities are excreted rather than stored, water-soluble vitamins are seldom associated with toxicity problems. Fat-soluble vitamins are absorbed into the blood along with dietary fats. Because they are insoluble in water, they are transported via the lymphatic vessels and are stored in the body's adipose tissue and in the liver. Fat-soluble

---

EXHIBIT 31-2   Healthy Lifestyle Nutrition Guidelines

- Choose a predominantly plant-based diet rich in a variety of vegetables and fruits (organic or local and seasonal).
- Avoid being underweight or overweight, and limit weight gain in adulthood to less than 11 pounds.
  - Limit meats, especially sandwich meats (ham, salami, bacon, sausage).
  - Increase fish, chicken, turkey (white meat) — free range or organic when possible.
  - Use cold-pressed, unprocessed oils — olive, coconut, canola, sesame.
  - Avoid fried and greasy foods.
  - Use low-fat dairy products (organic when available).
  - Bake, broil, steam, or poach food.
  - Avoid refined sugars — soft drinks, pastries, white sugar, corn syrup solids.
  - Eliminate refined carbohydrates and processed foods — white rice, white bread, pasta.
- Remember to read ingredients on labels.

Source: Copyright © 2015. Adapted by S. Luck. Nutritional Health, (pp. 147–183). In Dossey, B. M., Luck, S. and Schaub, B. G. *Nurse Coaching: Integrative Approaches for Health and Wellbeing.* North Miami, FL: International Nurse Coach Association. www.iNurseCoach.com

---

vitamins include vitamins A, D, E, and K.[38] **Table 31-1** provides more information about vitamins and their food sources.

Minerals

Minerals are naturally occurring elements or compounds found in the Earth. Minerals are essential components of all cells and function as coenzymes. They are necessary for proper composition of body fluids, formation of blood and bone, and maintenance of healthy nerve function. Once a mineral is absorbed, it must be carried from the blood to the cells and then transported across the cell membrane in a form that can be utilized by the cell. Minerals, like vitamins, work in combination with other nutrients and have both synergistic and antagonistic effects. Some minerals compete with one another for absorption, while others enhance the absorption of other minerals. For example, too much calcium can decrease the absorption of magnesium; therefore, these minerals should be consumed in the proper ratio to maintain balance.

Minerals are classified as either major minerals or trace minerals; however, this classification does not reflect their importance. A deficiency of either type of mineral can have a deleterious effect on health. To be classified as a major mineral, the mineral must make up no less than 0.01% of body weight. Major minerals include calcium, magnesium, phosphorus, potassium, sodium, and chloride. Trace minerals include arsenic, boron, chromium, cobalt, copper, fluoride, iodine, iron, manganese, molybdenum, nickel, selenium, silicon, tin, vanadium, and zinc.[39]

Although normal dietary intake of trace nutrients poses no threat to human health, long-term therapeutic doses of one or more minerals at the expense of other minerals may result in secondary deficiencies that could impair immunological or antioxidant processes. Even borderline levels of certain minerals can suppress a variety of immune responses. Cell-mediated immunity, antibody response, and other immune responses may be impaired by marginal deficiencies in trace minerals. For example, borderline zinc deficiency is associated with depletion of lymphocytes and lymphoid tissue atrophy. Excessive long-term consumption of competing minerals, such as iron, may suppress immune response by producing a secondary deficiency of zinc.

Bioavailability and supplementation are some of the most controversial areas in nutrition

TABLE 31-1   Fat-Soluble and Water-Soluble Vitamins

Vitamin	Function	Food Source
Fat-Soluble Vitamins		
Vitamin A (retinol)	Antioxidant. Aids in maintenance and repair of mucous membranes and epithelial tissue. Assists in growth and development of bones.	All orange and yellow fruits and vegetables (sweet potatoes, squash, yams, carrots, pumpkin, parsley, mango, apricots), dark leafy greens (kale, spinach, broccoli), salmon, fish oils.
Carotenoids (carotenes, lycopenes)	Antioxidant. Enhances cell communication and immune competence.	Orange, yellow, and dark green fruits and vegetables.
Vitamin D	Aids in transport of calcium. Promotes intestinal and renal absorption of phosphorus. Aids in growth of bones and teeth and neuromuscular function. Immunoprotective.	Egg yolks, alfalfa, dairy products, fish, especially fatty fish such as halibut, salmon, and sardines.
Vitamin E	Antioxidant. Promotes wound healing. Protects cell membranes against lipid perioxidation and destruction. Improves circulation.	Cold-pressed vegetable oils, whole grains, dark leafy green vegetables, nuts and seeds, legumes, wheat germ, oatmeal.
Vitamin K	Aids in blood clotting. Promotes formation and maintenance of healthy bone.	Green leafy vegetables, egg yolks.
Water-Soluble Vitamins		
Vitamin B_1 (thiamine)	Coenzyme in oxidation of glucose. Assists in production of hydrochloric acid.	Dried beans, brown rice, egg yolks, fish, chicken, peanuts.
Vitamin B_2 (riboflavin)	Assists in red blood cell formation. Aids in metabolism of carbohydrates, fats, and proteins.	Beans, eggs, fish, poultry, meat, spinach, yogurt, asparagus, avocado.
Vitamin B_3 (niacin)	Promotes healthy skin and nervous system. Lowers cholesterol, improves circulation.	Fish, eggs, beef, cheese, potatoes, whole wheat.
Vitamin B_5 (pantothenic acid)	"Antistress" vitamin. Aids in production of adrenal hormones. Assists in formation of antibodies and protein metabolism.	Beans, beef, eggs, mother's milk, fresh vegetables, whole wheat, pork, saltwater fish.
Vitamin B_6 (pyridoxine)	Acts as a coenzyme in the metabolism of amino acids and essential fatty acids necessary for production of serotonin and other neurotransmitters. Essential for healthy nervous system. Assists in converting iron to hemoglobin.	Eggs, fish, spinach, peas, meat, nuts, carrots, poultry, soybeans, bananas, avocados, whole-grain cereals, prunes.
Vitamin B_{12} (cobalamin)	Aids in synthesis of red blood cells. Required for proper digestion and absorption of foods. Prevents nerve damage.	Beef, herring, cheese, sardines, salmon, tempeh, miso, tofu, eggs, dairy products.
Folic acid	Participates in amino acid conversion, manufacture of neurotransmitters. Cardioprotective.	Dark green vegetables, kidney beans, asparagus, broccoli, whole grains, cereals.
Vitamin C (ascorbic acid)	Antioxidant. Aids in collagen formation, absorption of iron, interferon production. Promotes capillary integrity. Aids in release of stress hormones.	Citrus fruits, papaya, parsley, watercress, berries, tomatoes, broccoli, Brussels sprouts.

Source: Copyright © 2015. Adapted by S. Luck, Nutritional Health, (pp. 147–183). In Dossey, B. M., Luck, S. and Schaub, B. G. *Nurse Coaching: Integrative Approaches for Health and Wellbeing.* North Miami, FL: International Nurse Coach Association. www.iNurseCoach.com

research and practice. Nutrient intake through food consumption depends on many factors, including the quality of the soil in which the foods were grown, use of fertilizers, and genetic engineering of foods, to name a few. Other considerations include digestive function, medications (e.g., proton-pump inhibitors), and the gut microbiome. Consumption of a wide variety of fresh fruits and vegetables and unprocessed whole foods, locally grown and organic whenever possible, is recommended. **Table 31-2** provides further information on minerals and their food sources.

Antioxidants

Some vitamins and minerals function as antioxidants. These include vitamins C and E, beta-carotene (a precursor of vitamin A), coenzyme Q10, alpha lipoic acid, vitamin D, and the trace mineral selenium. Antioxidants protect the body from the formation of free radicals. Free radicals are electrically charged molecules that have

---

TABLE 31-2   Major Minerals and Trace Elements

Mineral	Function	Food Source
Calcium	Formation of strong bones, transmission of nerve impulses, muscle growth, and movement. Blood clotting. Prevention of hypertension.	Dairy products, salmon, sardines, green leafy vegetables, seeds and nuts, tofu, blackstrap molasses, seaweed.
Chromium	Metabolism of glucose. Stabilization of blood sugar levels. Synthesis of cholesterol, fats, and proteins.	Brewer's yeast, brown rice, cheese, whole grains, beans, mushrooms, potatoes.
Copper	Formation of bone, hemoglobin, red blood cells. Healing process.	Whole grains, avocados, oyster, lobster, dandelion greens, mushrooms, blackstrap molasses, seeds and nuts, soybeans.
Iodine	Energy production. Body temperature regulation, thyroid gland health.	Seaweed, iodized salt, dairy products, seafood, saltwater fish, garlic, Swiss chard, summer squash.
Iron	Hemoglobin production. Stress and disease resistance. Energy production. Immune system health.	Eggs, fish, poultry, dark leafy greens, blackstrap molasses, almonds, seaweed.
Magnesium	Formation of bone. Carbohydrate and mineral metabolism. Maintenance of proper pH balance. Immune function.	Dairy products, fish, seafood, blackstrap molasses, garlic, whole grains, seeds, tofu, green leafy vegetables, nuts.
Manganese	Enzyme activation. Sex hormone production. Nerve health. Energy production.	Avocados, nuts, seeds, seaweed, whole grains.
Phosphorus	Bone and teeth formation. Cell growth. Contraction of heart muscle. Kidney function.	Asparagus, brewer's yeast, fish, dried fruits, garlic, legumes, seeds and nuts.
Potassium	Healthy nervous system. Regulation of body fluids with sodium, pH balance.	Apricots, bananas, potatoes, sunflower seeds, blackstrap molasses, sprouts, broccoli.
Selenium	Antioxidant function. Immune system protection, cancer prevention.	Brazil nuts, brewer's yeast, brown rice, dairy products, garlic, onions, whole grains.
Sodium	With potassium, regulation of body fluids necessary for nerve and muscle function.	Table salt, seaweed.
Zinc	Burn and wound healing. Carbohydrate digestion. Prostate function, reproductive organ growth and development. Immune system health, production of antibodies.	Sardines and other fish, legumes, gland poultry, meat, egg yolks, beans, pumpkin and sunflower seeds.

an unpaired electron. Free radicals can damage healthy cells. They can also stress the immune system and suppress its ability to defend the host adequately against organisms, toxins, and metabolic by-products, all of which can lead to degenerative or infectious disease states. Antioxidants can stabilize or deactivate free radicals before the latter attack cells. Antioxidants are critical for maintaining optimal cellular and systemic health and well-being.[40] In a meta-analysis of more than 17,000 cancer patients, researchers found that high levels of vitamin D in conjunction with a cancer diagnosis are associated with improved remission and survival rates.[41] In adults, lower levels of vitamin D were linked to a higher premature death rate.[41, 42]

Vitamin D is especially critical during pregnancy and the first year of life. Researchers found that most U.S. infants are not consuming adequate amounts of vitamin D, according to the 2008 American Academy of Pediatrics recommendation of 400 IU/day. Breastfeeding infants get their vitamin D from their mother's reserves. However, researchers found that there are suboptimal levels of vitamin D in most pregnant women. Pediatricians and healthcare providers should encourage parents of infants who are either breastfed or consuming <1 L/day of infant formula to give their infants an oral vitamin D_3 supplement.[43]

The body can manufacture its own antioxidant, glutathione. Glutathione is a powerful antioxidant composed of the amino acids cysteine, glycine, and glutamic acid. It is activated and recycled by other antioxidants, including vitamin C, selenium, alpha lipoic acid, and coenzyme Q10. It is synthesized and most concentrated in the liver, where it is involved in detoxification pathways and protects against free radical damage. Glutathione helps to recycle other antioxidants,[44] and it is involved in the synthesis and repair of DNA. Decline in glutathione concentrations in intracellular fluids correlates directly with indicators of immunological function and longevity. Liver stores of glutathione can be depleted by disease processes, malnutrition, and poor-quality nutrient intake. Dietary amino acids are essential to glutathione synthesis. Lifestyle factors that affect efficient utilization of glutathione include stress, alcohol, cigarette smoking, excessive pharmaceutical use, drug abuse, and aging.[45]

Phytonutrients

Plant-based chemicals and nutrients have been used throughout human evolution to benefit health. Many phytochemicals contain protective, disease-preventing compounds, and their discovery has been the basis for many pharmaceuticals in use today. Although phytochemicals are not yet classified as nutrients—"substances necessary for sustaining life"—they have been identified as having properties that support health. Plant nutrients and their bioactive components have been studied for the treatment of cancer, diabetes, cardiovascular disease, and hypertension. They have been shown to exhibit potent antioxidant properties and modulate many processes including cellular protection, healthy cell signaling, cancer cell replication, and apoptosis (cancer cell death), and they can decrease cholesterol levels.[46]

One of the interesting observations in nature has been the role that these chemical components play in providing built-in protection from disease, injuries, insects, drought, excessive heat, ultraviolet rays, and poisons or pollutants in the air or soil. They appear to form part of plants' immune system. Current research is exploring the mechanisms of these compounds to affect immunological and epigenetic changes in humans, an emerging field in cancer research and in the application of novel chemotherapeutic interventions,[47] as well as the potential synergistic effects of phytochemicals used in combination with current chemotherapy.[48]

To ensure that adequate amounts of nutrients and phytochemicals are obtained from fruits and vegetables, it is recommended that people eat a minimum of five to seven portions daily of a variety of foods from the following color groups:

Red: Beets, red cabbage, cherries, cranberries, pink grapefruit, red grapes, red peppers, pomegranates, red potatoes, radishes, raspberries, rhubarb, strawberries, tomatoes, watermelon
Orange: Apricots, butternut squash, cantaloupe, carrots, mangoes, nectarines, oranges, papayas, peaches, persimmons, pumpkin, tangerines

Yellow-green: Green apples, artichokes, asparagus, avocados, green beans, broccoli, Brussels sprouts, green cabbage, cucumbers, green grapes, honeydew melon, kiwi, lettuce, lemons, limes, green onions, peas, green pepper, spinach, zucchini

Blue-purple: Purple kale, purple cabbage, purple potatoes, eggplant, purple grapes, blueberries, blackberries, boysenberries, raspberries, raisins, figs, plums

Sample a variety of flavors. By consuming small amounts of nature's diverse foods and flavors, you can enhance taste and pleasure while benefiting from phytochemicals that support your health.

Digestion, Absorption, and Assimilation

Assessing nutrition includes not only examining what people eat but how they digest, absorb, assimilate, and eliminate foods—all essential for good health. Diet is the food we eat. Nutrition is the study of what happens after we eat it.

Optimal absorption of nutrients depends on the integrity of the digestive system. Good health requires proper digestion and absorption. Digestion is the mechanical and chemical breakdown of the food we eat. Digestion is initiated when we chew food and begin to break it down with digestive enzymes. As food is digested, it must be absorbed. Absorption is the process of bringing the nutrients from the gastrointestinal tract to the rest of the body's tissues. The entire gastrointestinal tract is lined with mucosal tissue that secretes enzymes and multiple protective antibodies, an essential part of our immune defense. The gastrointestinal tract also contains trillions of friendly microflora known as the microbiome and begins during the birth process. These microorganisms assist in metabolic processes while maintaining the integrity of the mucosal lining and overall health.[49]

Digestion in the stomach occurs as food is churned and mixed with hydrochloric acid and various enzymes, which prepares it for entry into the small intestine via the duodenum. In the small intestine, digestive enzymes from the liver, gallbladder, and pancreas are added to the partially digested food. The pancreas secretes amylase, lipase, protease, and chymotrypsin, while the liver and gallbladder secrete bile to aid in the digestion of fats and the absorption of essential fatty acids and fat-soluble vitamins. Food spends 1 to 4 hours in the small intestine, which is approximately 25 feet long. As food is digested, it is absorbed into small blood vessels in the lining of the intestine. Toxins and waste products enter the large intestine to be excreted as fecal matter. The large intestine processes primarily fiber and water. The proper absorption and utilization of nutrients depends on a complex orchestration of processes in the digestive tract, and therefore it is essential to maintain the health and balance of this system.[50]

The friendly bacteria that live in the gastrointestinal tract, including strains of *Lactobacillus* and *acidophilus*, have many beneficial effects on health. They assist in synthesizing B vitamins, digesting proteins, balancing intestinal pH, reducing serum cholesterol, strengthening the immune system in the gut, preventing parasites and overgrowth of yeast, and maintaining bowel regularity. The most common reason for the destruction of friendly bacteria in the gastrointestinal tract is from the use of antibiotics and from ingestion through consumption of antibiotic-treated animal products. Leaky gut syndrome or gut permeability can occur with the loss of integrity of the mucosal lining. Studies indicate that beneficial bacteria must be replaced by probiotic supplementation following antibiotic therapy to prevent symptoms of dysbiosis and leaky gut syndrome that manifest as fatigue, bloating, gas, diarrhea, constipation, food allergies, inflammatory disorders, migraine headache, yeast overgrowth, and weight gain.[51] Mycrobial dysbiosis of the human body has recently been associated with obesity, diabetes, and colon and breast cancers. Dysbiosis is associated with a decreased survival rate in women with breast cancer.[52]

The use of probiotics in infants (1 to 3 months old) was found effective in preventing gastrointestinal disorders such as infantile colic, gastroesophageal reflux, and constipation. As a result, the infants had 44% fewer medical visits, 82% fewer lost parental work days, less use of prescribed or over-the-counter medications, and 71% fewer emergency room visits.[53]

An awareness of food sensitivity has grown. The United Kingdom has seen a fourfold increase in the diagnosis rate of celiac disease.[9] Improving digestion includes dietary modification, such as the elimination of fried foods, sugars, and any foods that stress an individual's digestive system. Keeping a food journal and then following an elimination diet is helpful in identifying foods that may trigger digestive disorders, food allergies, and autoimmune responses. Removing "triggers" from the diet for a minimum of 21 days can be an important dietary intervention for those with food sensitivities and can assist with weight loss. Wheat, gluten, lactose, and casein products are the most common foods to eliminate and often can relieve many common gastrointestinal problems including constipation, bloating after consuming, and irritable bowel syndrome.[54] The individual can slowly reintroduce the food item and observe whether symptoms return. Each person has a unique relationship with food and its chemical properties, and therefore nutritional assessment and dietary recommendations are based on biochemical individuality. Assessing the unique needs of each individual and offering health education, coaching, and self-care tools can affect the health and well-being of the individual over time.

Eating to Promote Health

Increasing awareness of how food can affect health and well-being is an essential component in nutrition coaching and education. Nurses can use the following questions as a guideline.

Sit down in a quiet place and plan a day's menu by asking yourself these questions:

- What does my body need to enhance wellness?
- What are my past eating patterns? Which do I want to keep? Which do I want to change?
- What are my activity levels, and how should I include foods that meet my needs?
- How do I need to plan for psychological factors?
- Which factors, unique to me, influence my food planning and food choices?

Stress and Nutrient Needs

The consequences of stress in our lives and its effect on our health can be mediated through increasing nutrient intake to support normalization of stress-induced biochemical changes, increased nutrient needs, and natural resistance to stress responses. Research increasingly supports the critical role in disease played by stress-induced hormones, including elevated cortisol levels, which induces inflammation, sleep disturbances, and obesity. Inflammation is part of the body's natural response to infection, injury, allergens, and other foreign substances in the body, including chemicals in the environment. Removing inflammatory triggers is an important intervention to calm the inflammatory chemicals and cytokines produced. Chronic inflammation plays a role in diabetes, osteoporosis, hypertension, cardiovascular disease, infectious disease, gastric ulcer, cancer, immune system disturbances, and gastrointestinal, skin, endocrine, and neurologic disorders. Researchers found that a low-carbohydrate diet reduced inflammation in type 2 diabetes more than a low-fat diet.[10] The vulnerability of a particular bodily system to stress varies from one individual to another, is determined by genetic makeup and constitution, and may be influenced by nutritional and environmental factors. A healthy diet rich in whole foods that contain antioxidants, B vitamins, essential fatty acids, and trace minerals can mediate the stress response and support overall health and well-being throughout life.

Eco Nutrition

Breast cancer is the second most common cause of cancer-related deaths in women in the United States. Research indicates that low nutrient intake, chronic stress, inflammatory processes, and obesity are all risk factors. Mounting evidence shows that chemical exposure to xenotoxins is another risk factor for breast cancer.[55] Environmental xenoestrogens—synthetic hormone-mimicking compounds found in many food products including pesticides, colorings and preservatives, drugs, and plastics—may play a role in the etiology of breast cancer.[56]

Xenoestrogens accumulate in the fatty tissues of the body and may interact at estrogen receptor sites in the breast, trigging breast cell changes. Also, women with breast cancer often have higher concentrations of pesticides in their blood and fatty tissues than do healthy women.[57]

Many epidemiologic studies associate a high-fat, low-fiber diet with an increased risk of developing cancer of the colon, prostate, and breast. A review of the literature also suggests an inverse relationship between the quantity of fresh fruits and vegetables consumed and the incidence of cancer. Weight loss plans that support a low-fat, high-fiber, whole foods diet, stress reduction, and exercise are part of a comprehensive health approach for the prevention of cardiovascular disease and breast cancer in women.

Fruits and vegetables are rich in fiber, antioxidants, and other plant-derived substances, or phytonutrients, believed to protect against disease and contain cancer-protective properties. The risk of developing type 2 diabetes can be reduced by eating more fruits and vegetables.[58]

Fiber is thought to influence hormone levels by facilitating the fecal excretion of estrogen metabolites, which at high levels can pose a risk for many women.[59] Other ingredients that contain potential anticancer compounds include cruciferous vegetables (watercress, broccoli, cauliflower, Brussels sprouts), which contain isothiocynates, such as sulforophane. These substances assist in liver detoxification, aid in the removal of environmental toxins, and play a role in cancer prevention.[60, 61] Soy products that contain natural plant phytoestrogens (genistein and daidzen) called *isoflavones* may play a significant role in the prevention, and possibly the treatment, of some hormone-related diseases, although this remains controversial in the literature.[62] Curcumin and resveratrol are phytonutrients that demonstrate both antioxidant and anti-inflammatory properties, and they appear to be immunoprotective and chemopreventive. These phytonutrients also appear to be protective against both breast cancer and prostate cancer.[63]

The following guidelines ensure optimal digestion, absorption, and elimination and promote optimal health and well-being. This approach offers a hypoallergenic and anti-inflammatory response to optimize cellular energy.

Whole Food Nutrition Plan

- *Plant-based diet:* Whole, unprocessed, predominately plant-based diet
- *Low glycemic load:* Foods that slow the speed at which the blood glucose level is raised
- *Proper fatty acid composition:* High levels of healthy omega-3 essential fatty acids including walnuts, flaxseeds, avocados, and fish oils
- *High phytonutrient density:* High levels of phytonutrients and antioxidants
- *Healthy protein:* Lean, healthy, predominately plant-based proteins or pasture-raised, chemical-free animal products
- *High micronutrient density:* High amounts of vitamins and minerals
- *Low allergenic burden:* Low in foods that are highly allergenic (based on individual)
- *Elimination plan:* Gluten- and casein-free diet for a minimum of 3 weeks
- *Low toxic burden:* Minimizes toxic burden of food: no added hormones, pesticides, antibiotics, or any other artificial additives or preservatives
- *Organic fruits, vegetables, and animal products:* Whenever possible, high in organic products; local produce is the next best choice
- *Healthy pH balance:* Provides proper balance between acidity and alkalinity
- *High fiber content:* High in fiber to help slow the insulin response and optimize digestive health, detoxification
- *Optimized elimination pathways*

Source: Copyright © 2015. Adapted by S. Luck. Nutritional Health (pp. 147–183). In Dossey, B. M., Luck, S. and Schaub, B. G., *Nurse Coaching: Integrative Approaches for Health and Wellbeing.* North Miami, FL: International Nurse Coach Association. www.iNurseCoach .com

Osteoporosis

The best treatment for osteoporosis is prevention. Along with lack of exercise, osteoporosis often is the result of deficiencies of several key nutrients, of which calcium is but one. Research indicates that other essential nutrients, including vitamin D_3, vitamin K, magnesium, boron, and other trace minerals must be available in the proper balance to facilitate calcium resorption and uptake into the bone. In multiple studies, supplementation has been shown to be effective in preventing fractures in both men and women.[64]

Beyond maintaining healthy bones (and preventing rickets), research on the role of vitamin D in maintaining health has exploded in recent years. Vitamin D is not only a vitamin but a prohormone that has hundreds of receptor sites on every cell. Emerging nutritional science is rethinking the need for vitamin D_3 and reexamining the optimal levels needed for supporting immune health, cognitive function, and cancer prevention.[65] Vitamin D deficiency in adults is reported to exacerbate osteopenia, osteoporosis, muscle weakness, fractures, common cancers including prostate and breast,[66] autoimmune diseases, infectious diseases, cognitive impairment and Alzheimer's disease,[67] and cardiovascular disease. The vitamin may reduce the incidence of several types of cancer and type 1 diabetes.[68] Recent research has explored vitamin D_3 deficiency and the increased risk of multiple sclerosis.[69]

Common Dietary Risk Factors for Osteoporosis

- Low intake of vitamin D, calcium, magnesium, and trace minerals (note that vitamin D is now first in this list)
- High intake of animal protein
- High intake of caffeine
- Excessive intake of carbonated beverages
- High intake of sodium
- High intake of refined sugar
- Lack of exercise
- Lack of sunlight exposure
- Excessive intake of alcohol
- Hypochlorhydria (low hydrochloric stomach acid), which can occur with aging and intake of antacids

Guidelines for Healthy Bones

- Increase consumption of calcium-rich foods, including green leafy vegetables, whole grains, beans, tofu, dairy products, nuts, and seeds.
- Increase weight-bearing exercise, such as walking.
- Decrease consumption of soda, caffeine, and alcohol.
- Check vitamin D levels (25-hydroxyvitamin D).
- Spend at least 15 minutes a day exposed to direct sunlight.

Supplement Recommendations for Healthy Bones

The current RDA for calcium is 800 to 1200 milligrams per day of elemental calcium. Magnesium and calcium function in balance. The recommended ratio of calcium to magnesium is usually 2:1; thus, the recommended dosage of magnesium is 400 to 600 milligrams per day. According to new research, the daily amount of vitamin D, taken in as vitamin D_3, depends on exposure to sunlight, genetics, skin pigmentation, geographical location, and individual physiologic requirements. Testing 25-hydroxyvitamin D levels is recommended prior to and during supplementation. Compelling research suggests that vitamin D levels be maintained above 40, and supplementation is recommended to achieve this level. Other nutrients that help maintain bone mass include vitamin K, boron, vitamin B_6, manganese, folic acid, vitamin C, and zinc.[70]

Nutrition and Healthy Aging

According to the U.S. Census Bureau, by the year 2025, with the aging of the baby boomers, there will be more people older than 60 than younger than 25 for the first time in this nation's history.

Nutrition practices play a fundamental role in and greatly influence the aging process. Research reveals the health benefits of improving nutrition anywhere in the life cycle, including in the older years, which can affect and prevent much of the decline associated with aging. Older adults are vulnerable to the cumulative health effects of inadequate nutrition. The National Health and Nutrition Examination Surveys, conducted by the Department of Health and Human Services, reveal that the nation's older citizens remain at high risk of macronutrient and micronutrient deficiencies.

Inadequate nutrition and protein deficiencies, for example, can lead to increased muscle loss, cognitive decline, fatigue, and immune system impairment. Medical foods such as whey protein powder, high in glutamine and other amino acids, have been shown to improve protein stores and rebuild muscle mass.[71] Untreated and often undiagnosed deficiencies take a heavy toll on older people, resulting in accelerated aging. Research over the past decade clearly shows that many of the ailments previously thought to be an inevitable result of old age can be prevented by aggressive detection and treatment of subclinical nutrient deficits.[72]

Oxidative stress without adequate repair mechanisms may contribute to the onset of Alzheimer's disease, and the risk of Alzheimer's disease may be reduced by intake of antioxidants that counteract the detrimental effects of oxidative stress.[73] Regardless of a person's age, calcium, vitamin D_3, and trace nutrients are essential for maintaining bone mass and overall good health. Recent research indicates that vitamin D may be involved in neuroprotection, control of pro-inflammatory, cytokine-induced cognitive dysfunction, and synthesis of calcium-binding proteins.[74] The role of vitamin D receptors in the pathophysiology of cognitive decline, incidence of Alzheimer's disease, and vascular dementia and/or cognitive decline with respect to previous plasma 25-hydroxyvitamin D concentration has been observed in several studies.[75]

Although elderly individuals must be evaluated individually, many psychosocial factors need to be considered when addressing nutrition needs and goals, including economics, ability to shop for and prepare meals, and social support networks. Many older adults suffer from vitamin B_{12} deficiency as a result of impaired absorption of micronutrients. Other issues that interfere with nutrient intake include chewing difficulties, impaired cognitive function and forgetting to eat, social isolation and apathy in food preparation, and inability to shop or carry packages. Impaired memory in elderly people often is related to the effect of B vitamins, vitamin D, antioxidants, and essential fatty acid deficiencies.

Undetected hypochlorhydria, a deficiency of hydrochloric acid in the stomach, leads to bacterial overgrowth in the small bowel and results in impaired digestion and absorption of essential nutrients, including vitamins B_6 and B_{12}.[76] Americans older than age 65 consume 30% of the over-the-counter drugs sold in the United States. Many of these medications are known to impair absorption and metabolism of nutrients and act as nutrient antagonists. The most commonly used over-the-counter drugs among older adults are laxatives, which can impair the status of the fat-soluble vitamins A, E, D, and K. Vitamin deficiencies remain subclinical in older adults and are the result of inadequate nutrient stores over many years. One of the hallmarks of biologic aging is altered glucose metabolism, which affects many age-related diseases, including heart disease, inflammatory disorders, dementia, and diabetes. Those who ate a healthy diet in midlife, including vegetables, fruits and berries, fish and unsaturated fats, had a 90% lower risk for dementia.[77] Establishing a reservoir of nutrients and eating a healthy diet throughout the life cycle is key for healthy aging.

Successful weight loss and improvements in health are achieved and maintained with a regular exercise program, psychological support, and a personal commitment to wellness. Working with a coach supports goals and plans to achieve desired results. Healthy food choices along with caloric restriction promote healthy aging and longevity.[45, 78, 79]

Weight Management Guidelines

- Recognize management of obesity as a lifelong commitment that requires lifestyle changes.
- Set realistic goals for weight loss.
- Implement meal planning with daily menus.
- Serve smaller portions (use smaller plates).
- Avoid keeping ready-to-eat snack food around the house.
- Prepare grocery shopping from a list and not on an empty stomach.
- Do all eating in one room and focus on eating without distractions.
- Increase intake of vegetables ("free" foods).
- Leave a small amount of food on the plate.
- Increase activity level.
- Avoid skipping meals.

- Avoid late-night eating.
- Drink at least six glasses of water daily.
- Try a food allergy elimination diet.
- Eliminate all junk foods (processed, refined foods) from the diet.

Eating with Awareness

Taking time for the eating experience can help to reduce cravings, control portion sizes, enhance the eating experience, improve digestion and overall health, and engender a sense of well-being. Nurse coaches can recommend the following guidelines to their clients:

1. *Eat in a setting where you feel relaxed.* This practice helps with the digestive process, including absorption to assimilation of nutrients. Create healing environments at home and in the workplace.
2. *Chew thoroughly.* The process of digestion begins in the mouth where enzymes are secreted in saliva to break down food. Explore the texture in your mouth. If we do not properly chew and make our food morsels smaller, indigestion and other digestive problems can occur. The act of eating allows us to be mindful, and in the moment, of the exchange of energy in the food.
3. *Eat mindfully.* Become increasingly aware of how what you eat nurtures your body–mind. At the end of each meal, leave a small amount of food on your plate. Take the time to feel your satiety. Step away from the table. Observe your physical sensations. With gratitude and a sense of abundance, know you have nurtured and cared for yourself.
4. *Choose foods to support your health and well-being.* Avoid processed, packaged, fast, and prepared foods. Broil, steam, and bake to avoid fried foods. Fresh is always best. Choose organic or local produce whenever possible.

Source: Copyright © 2015. Adapted by S. Luck. Nutritional Health (pp. 147–183). In Dossey, B. M., Luck, S. and Schaub, B. G., *Nurse Coaching: Integrative Approaches for Health and Wellbeing.* North Miami, FL: International Nurse Coach Association. www.iNurseCoach .com

Foods to Avoid

- *Sugars:* Cookies, soda, candy, jelly, syrup, corn syrup
- *Processed foods:* Additives, preservatives, artificial colorings, flavorings, artificial sugars including aspartame (Equal, diet sodas)
- *Canned foods:* Fresh is best, frozen is next best
- *Refined hydrogenated oils:* Crisco, palm oil, cottonseed oil
- *Fast foods and junk foods*

Nutrition Guidelines for Maintaining Healthy Cholesterol Levels

1. *Oatmeal, oat bran, and high-fiber foods.* Oatmeal contains soluble fiber, which reduces low-density lipoprotein (LDL). Soluble fiber is also found in such foods as kidney beans, apples, pears, barley, and prunes. Five to 10 grams or more of soluble fiber a day decreases LDL cholesterol. Eating 1.5 cups of cooked oatmeal provides 6 grams of fiber.
2. *Fish and omega-3 fatty acids.* Eating fatty fish can be heart healthy with its high levels of omega-3 fatty acids. In people with a history of heart attacks, fish oil or omega-3 fatty acids reduce the risk of sudden death. The highest levels of omega-3 fatty acids are in the following types of fish:
   - Mackerel
   - Lake trout
   - Herring
   - Sardines
   - Wild salmon
   - Halibut

   Bake or grill to avoid adding unhealthy fats or heated oils. Most farm-raised fish are high in chemicals, including hormones and antibiotics. Other plant sources of omega-3 essential fatty acids are walnuts and ground flaxseeds.
3. *Walnuts, almonds, and other nuts.* Walnuts, almonds, and other nuts can reduce blood cholesterol. Rich in polyunsaturated fatty acids, walnuts also help keep blood vessels healthy. According to the Food and Drug Administration, eating about a handful (1.5 ounces, or 42.5 grams) a day of most

nuts, such as almonds, hazelnuts, peanuts, pecans, some pine nuts, pistachio nuts, and walnuts, may reduce the risk of heart disease. Nuts should be raw if possible and without additional oils added. All nuts are high in calories, so a handful will do. Replace foods high in saturated fat with nuts.

4. *Olive oil.* Olive oil contains a potent mix of antioxidants that can lower "bad" (LDL) cholesterol but leave "good" (HDL) cholesterol untouched. Evidence from epidemiologic studies also suggests that a higher proportion of monounsaturated fats in the diet is linked to a reduction in the risk of coronary heart disease. This is significant because olive oil is considerably rich in monounsaturated fats, most notably oleic acid.

Olive oil contains a wide variety of valuable antioxidants that are not found in other oils. Hydroxytyrosol is thought to be the main antioxidant compound in olives and is believed to play a significant role in the many health benefits attributed to olive oil. The Food and Drug Administration recommends using about 2 tablespoons (23 grams) of olive oil a day in place of other fats to receive heart-healthy benefits. To add olive oil to your diet, you can sauté vegetables in it, add it to a marinade, or mix it with vinegar as a salad dressing. The cholesterol-lowering effects of olive oil are even greater in cold-pressed extra-virgin olive oil, meaning the oil is less processed and contains more heart-healthy antioxidants, than in other types of olive oils that are processed differently.[80] For example, "light" olive oils are usually more processed than are extra-virgin or virgin olive oils and are lighter in color but not in fat or calories.

Other Important Health-Promoting Tips

- Drink four to six glasses of liquid daily—spring or filtered water or herbal teas.
- Cook and prepare food in cast-iron or stainless steel cookware (avoid aluminum).
- Chew foods slowly and thoroughly.
- Eat smaller, simpler meals.
- Include fiber with each meal.
- Exercise daily—walk, bicycle, jog, dance, swim, stretch.

- Reduce stress through yoga, meditation, deep breathing, relaxation practice, and visualization.
- Avoid alcohol, caffeine, smoking, recreational drugs, and over-the-counter drugs.
- Get sufficient rest and sleep.

Holistic Caring Process

The nurse as coach restores balance and improves overall health and well-being by managing complex, chronic illnesses and facilitating and deepening awareness of the relationship between nutrition and well-being. The nurse as coach:

- Explores the totality of the individual
- Explores the beliefs and meaning, relationship, and behaviors around food
- Assesses the client's nutritional patterns, including food choices, food preparation, meal planning, food budget, and accessibility
- Evaluates the client's nutritional needs
- Guides the client in developing a personalized nutrition food plan
- Increases understanding of effective nutritional guidelines for enhancing wellness
- Increases awareness of environmental factors that influence health
- Offers information, handouts, and guidelines in the role of the nurse coach/expert

Source: Adapted from S. Luck, "Nutritional Health," in *Nurse Coaching: Integrative Approaches for Health and Well-being,* B. M. Dossey, S. Luck, and B. G. Schaub (North Miami, FL: International Nurse Coach Association, 2015): 147–183. www.iNurseCoach.com. Used with permission.

Holistic Assessment

Nurse Coaching in Behavioral and Lifestyle Change

In preparing to use nutrition interventions, the nurse assesses the following parameters:

- The client's relationship to nutrition and diet: biochemical, genetic, cultural, social, emotional, religious/spiritual, economic, environmental, and physiologic components

- The client's eating habits, food preferences, and nutritional needs
- The client's motivation and ability to make the necessary dietary and lifestyle changes
- The client's understanding that changing food and eating patterns is part of a wellness process

Identification of Patterns/ Challenges/Needs

The patterns/challenges/needs (see Chapter 8) compatible with nutrition interventions are as follows:

- Altered nutrition
- Altered circulation
- Altered oxygenation
- Altered energy
- Altered coping
- Altered physical mobility
- Sleep pattern disturbances
- Altered patterns of daily living
- Disturbance in body image
- Disturbance in self-esteem
- Potential hopelessness
- Potential powerlessness
- Knowledge deficit
- Pain
- Anxiety

- Grieving
- Depression
- Fear

Outcome Identification

Table 31-3 guides the nurse in client outcomes, nurse coaching, and evaluation of changes in awareness, eating patterns, relationship to food, healthier food choices, and overall health using standard evaluations including weight, body mass index, bioelectrical impedance analysis, and laboratory testing. Integrating nurse coaching with nutrition education is an effective nursing intervention.

Therapeutic Care Plan and Interventions

The nurse coach can implement the following activities over one session or several sessions.

Before the session:

- Prepare yourself to be fully present with the client.
- Create an environment in which the client feels comfortable discussing beliefs about health and exploring his or her relationship to food.
- Listen deeply to the client's story.
- Prepare assessment tools.

TABLE 31-3 Nursing Interventions: Nutrition		
Client Outcomes	**Nursing Prescriptions**	**Evaluation**
The client will be motivated to improve nutrition.	Assist the client in a personal self-assessment.	The client completed a self-assessment form.
	Encourage the client to participate with the nurse to develop goals and action plans. Prepare the client to follow through with the nurse on evaluation and formulation of new goals.	The client participated with the nurse to develop a personalized program. The client met with the nurse for program evaluation.
The client will demonstrate knowledge of healthful nutrition.	Motivate the client to contribute to discussions about his or her program.	The client participated in the session discussion.
	Encourage the client to learn more about healthful behaviors as he or she works with the nurse.	The client demonstrated new knowledge.

Source: Copyright © 2015. Adapted by S. Luck. Nutritional Health (pp. 147–183). In Dossey, B. M., Luck, S. and Schaub, B. G., *Nurse Coaching: Integrative Approaches for Health and Wellbeing.* North Miami, FL: International Nurse Coach Association. www.iNurseCoach.com

- Focus on the client's nutritional and physical needs.
- Prepare educational materials.

At the beginning of the session:

- Introduce relaxation and centering techniques.
- Take and record the necessary physical assessment data (e.g., weight, bioelectrical impedance analysis, body mass index, skinfold thickness measurements).
- Guide the client to disclose past habits and patterns that affect eating behaviors.
- Engage the client in sharing his or her association between food and feelings of well-being or distress.
- Ask the client to describe food intake in a typical day.
- Assist the client in creating a sample menu or food plan.
- Encourage the client to participate in setting nutritional goals and action plans.
- Present specific nutritional guidelines for the client to follow.
- Direct the client to keep a food journal to present at a follow-up session.

During the session:

- Serve as a coach, guiding the process.
- Emphasize the connection between nutrition and whole-person health.
- Guide the client to develop strategies for changing nutrition habits, nutrient intake, and eating patterns and behaviors.

- Assist the client in optimizing nutrition choices by doing the following:
  - Creating an image of food as a healing energy
  - Reframing the nutrition process into a positive action
  - Reframing nutrition and food as an empowerment tool
  - Illustrating how external nutrition changes promote internal healing responses
  - Reinforcing the client's positive changes in nutrition as part of the healing process
  - Ending sessions with images of the desired state of well-being.

At the end of the session:

- The client identifies the options presented that best fit with his or her lifestyle.
- Invite the client to create an action plan with an attainable goal.
- Work with the client to write down goals and target dates.
- Encourage the client to create specific affirmations to support these goals.
- Give the client handout materials to reinforce the teaching.
- Reinforce the client's plan and positive outcomes that were established before each session (see Exhibit 13-2) and listen to the client's subjective experiences (see **Exhibit 31-3**) to evaluate the session and deepen the process.
- Schedule a follow-up session.

EXHIBIT 31-3   Evaluation of the Client's Subjective Experience with Nutrition

1. Is this the first time you have considered the effects of healing nutrition from a holistic perspective?
2. Have you discovered ways you can eat for increased vitality and vibrant living?
3. Do you believe there are any links between your food choices and development of health-related concerns or current symptoms?
4. Is your life filled with healing foods? Do you want it to be?
5. What support systems would help you develop and adhere to a lifestyle that includes healing foods?
6. Can you think of anything else that would help you to maintain a routine that includes healing nutrition?
7. What is your next step (or your plan) to integrate these experiences on a daily basis?

Possible Supportive Interventions for Optimal Nutrition

To optimize nutrient intake, the nurse as coach supports the client in the following interventions for optimal nutrition:

- Offers guidelines for a mindfulness eating practice
- Encourages keeping a food journal for 1 week to increase awareness of food choices, patterns, and behaviors and observe emotional and stress triggers
- Reinforces the benefits of adhering to the recommended healthy food plan and of observing changes, challenges, and benefits
- Offers relaxation techniques to integrate into daily practice
- Includes an exercise plan following evaluation by a trained professional

As health educators, nurses can share information and research data on the health benefits of phytonutrients, antioxidants, and food components known to assist balancing the body in supporting the healing process.

When developing a new menu plan to fit the client's particular needs, the following is part of a whole-person assessment:

- Daily activity status
- Current health status
- Physical limitations
- Economic considerations
- Social and cultural influences
- Emotional state of being
- Individual differences, including food preferences and religious dietary customs

To motivate and assist the client, the nurse coach can do the following:

- Encourage the client to keep a daily food journal.
- Encourage the client to develop mindful eating practices.
- Demonstrate the daily practice of asking the body what it needs to be healthy.
- Create daily menus using healthy choices that are mutually agreed upon.
- Explore health goals
- Establish attainable goals

- Guide the client to self-assess health changes that occur with dietary interventions.
- Encourage the client who is currently using nutritional supplementation to organize a routine to optimize compliance and benefits.

The nurse coach can use open-ended questions, images, journal writing, drawing, and other creative strategies to integrate nutrition into the client's daily life to close the session.

Case Study (Implementation)

Case Study

Setting: An integrative medicine/wellness center
Client: B. V., a 40-year-old married woman seeking counseling for weight loss
Patterns/Challenges/Needs:

1. Altered nutrition (more than body requirements) related to improper eating and lack of exercise
2. Altered self-esteem related to obesity
3. Ineffective reversal/prevention of coronary artery disease risk factors (hypertension, hypercholesterolemia, obesity) related to stress and low self-esteem

B. V. came to the wellness center after having a physical examination by her primary care physician and being told for the sixth straight year that she needs to lose weight. Her total cholesterol is 340 milligrams per deciliter, blood pressure is 180/100 mm Hg, height is 5'7", and weight is 220 pounds. She is a nurse and seeks help from a nurse colleague at the wellness center because her elevated cholesterol level has finally motivated her to lose weight. Her husband has been encouraging this for years, but she just cannot seem to make it happen.

During the initial session, the nurse takes a food intake history and does a nutrition assessment (see **Figure 31-2**). Like most self-referrals for weight loss, B. V. is knowledgeable about various diet programs and has tried different plans for several years. She has a pattern of losing and then regaining up to 50 pounds on each attempt. At this point, she is willing to try anything. The nurse discovers during the interview

—— **INTEGRATIVE HEALTH and WELLNESS ASSESSMENT**™ ——

This **INTEGRATIVE HEALTH and WELLNESS ASSESSMENT** is intended for informational purposes only. It is not a substitute for professional medical advice, diagnosis, or treatment.

DIRECTIONS: This questionnaire contains statements about your present way of life, feelings, and personal habits. Please respond to each item as accurately as possible, and try not to skip any item. Indicate the frequency with which you engage in each item by checking (✓) one of the following:

PHYSICAL	Never	Almost Never	Once in a While	Almost Always	Always
1. I eat a nutritious breakfast daily.	❏	❏	❏	❏	❏
NUTRITION					
2. I eat at least five servings of vegetables and fruits daily.	❏	❏	❏	❏	❏
3. I eat whole foods (grains, beans, seeds, and nuts).	❏	❏	❏	❏	❏
4. I eat low-fat foods (fish, low-fat dairy, beans, skinless chicken).	❏	❏	❏	❏	❏
5. I avoid red meat or eat it only a few times a week.	❏	❏	❏	❏	❏
6. I decrease high-fat foods (hot dogs, steaks, cheese, ice cream, whole milk, cakes, sweets, fried foods, butter).	❏	❏	❏	❏	❏
7. I avoid sugar.	❏	❏	❏	❏	❏
8. I avoid junk food.	❏	❏	❏	❏	❏
9. I avoid regular soda drinks with sugar or diet drinks with artificial sweeteners.	❏	❏	❏	❏	❏
10. I drink six to eight glasses of water daily.	❏	❏	❏	❏	❏
11. I read labels for ingredients.	❏	❏	❏	❏	❏
12. I avoid food colorings, flavoring, and additives in my foods.	❏	❏	❏	❏	❏
13. I avoid canned and processed foods.	❏	❏	❏	❏	❏
14. I eat organic and/or local produce.	❏	❏	❏	❏	❏
15. I eat my meals at home.	❏	❏	❏	❏	❏
16. I prepare my meals in an oven or on stove top burners.	❏	❏	❏	❏	❏
17. I have access to healthy food choices.	❏	❏	❏	❏	❏
18. I purchase healthy foods.	❏	❏	❏	❏	❏
19. I experience pain or inflammation in my body.	❏	❏	❏	❏	❏

FIGURE 31-2 Nutrition Assessment

NUTRITION *(continued)*	Never	Almost Never	Once in a While	Almost Always	Always
20. I experience digestive discomfort.	❏	❏	❏	❏	❏
21. I am aware of foods that affect my digestion.	❏	❏	❏	❏	❏
22. I feel bloated after eating.	❏	❏	❏	❏	❏
23. I take medication for digestive reasons.	❏	❏	❏	❏	❏
24. I am aware of any food sensitivities or food allergies.	❏	❏	❏	❏	❏
25. I have a bowel movement daily.	❏	❏	❏	❏	❏
26. I chew my food thoroughly.	❏	❏	❏	❏	❏
27. I eat mindfully (concentrate on my eating, not multitasking or eating in front of the television).	❏	❏	❏	❏	❏
28. I eat late at night.	❏	❏	❏	❏	❏
29. I crave sweets.	❏	❏	❏	❏	❏
30. I eat larger portions than I need.	❏	❏	❏	❏	❏
31. I feel energy after eating.	❏	❏	❏	❏	❏
32. I feel tired after eating.	❏	❏	❏	❏	❏

For items 33–35, check (✓) the response that most closely resembles how you feel about making changes or improvements to your NUTRITION.

33. My readiness for change is

❏ Now   ❏ Within 2 weeks   ❏ Next month   ❏ In 6 months
❏ In a year or more

34. My priority for making change is

❏ Highest priority   ❏ Priority   ❏ Medium priority
❏ Very low priority   ❏ Never a priority

35. My confidence in my ability to make a positive change is

❏ Very confident   ❏ Confident   ❏ Somewhat confident
❏ Not very confident   ❏ Not at all confident

NUTRITION ACTION PLAN. Please list three changes that you can implement into your current lifestyle over the next 3 months:

1. _____

2. _____

3. _____

Additional changes, comments, thoughts:

_____

FIGURE 31-2 Nutrition Assessment *(continued)*

	Never	Almost Never	Once in a While	Almost Always	Always
EXERCISE (Know your limitations)					
1. I do **aerobic exercise** (jogging, swimming, fitness walking using arms, aerobic dance, active sports) regularly. (*Vigorous intensity*—at least 20 minutes 3 or more days a week; *Moderate intensity*—at least 30 minutes per week)	❏	❏	❏	❏	❏
2. I do **strength exercises** (use strength-training equipment, sit-ups, push-ups) regularly.	❏	❏	❏	❏	❏
3. I do **stretching or flexibility exercises** (head, neck, shoulders, back, legs) for at least 5 minutes 3 days a week.	❏	❏	❏	❏	❏

For items 4–6, check (✓) the response that most closely resembles how you feel about making changes or improvements to your EXERCISE.

4. My readiness for change is
   ❏ Now   ❏ Within 2 weeks   ❏ Next month   ❏ In 6 months
   ❏ In a year or more

5. My priority for making change is
   ❏ Highest priority   ❏ Priority   ❏ Medium priority
   ❏ Very low priority   ❏ Never a priority

6. My confidence in my ability to make a positive change is
   ❏ Very confident   ❏ Confident   ❏ Somewhat confident
   ❏ Not very confident   ❏ Not at all confident

EXERCISE ACTION PLAN. Please list 3 changes that you can implement into your current lifestyle over the next 3 months:

1. _____

2. _____

3. _____

Additional changes, comments, thoughts:

_____

	Never	Almost Never	Once in a While	Almost Always	Always
WEIGHT					
1. I maintain my ideal weight.	❏	❏	❏	❏	❏
2. I have gained no more than 11 pounds in adulthood.	❏	❏	❏	❏	❏

For item 3–5, check (✓) the response that most closely resembles how you feel about making changes or improvements to your WEIGHT.

3. My readiness for change is
   ❏ Now   ❏ Within 2 weeks   ❏ Next month   ❏ In 6 months   ❏ In a year

FIGURE 31-2 Nutrition Assessment (*continued*)

4. My priority for making change is
   ❏ Highest priority   ❏ Priority   ❏ Medium priority
   ❏ Very low priority   ❏ Never a priority

5. My confidence in my ability to make a positive change is
   ❏ Very confident   ❏ Confident   ❏ Somewhat confident
   ❏ Not very confident ❏ Not at all confident

WEIGHT MANAGEMENT ACTION PLAN. Please list 3 changes that you can implement into your current lifestyle over the next 3 months:

1. _____

2. _____

3. _____

Additional changes, comments, thoughts:

_____

Source: "Integrative Health and Wellness Assessment," in *Nurse Coaching: Integrative Approaches for Health and Wellbeing*, B. M. Dossey, S. Luck, and B. G. Schaub (North Miami, FL: International Nurse Coach Association, 2015): 442–443. www.iNurseCoach.com. Used with permission.

FIGURE 31-2 Nutrition Assessment (*continued*)

that B. V. has been on numerous antihypertensive drugs for 10 years without attaining consistent control. The assessment shows that, in general, B. V. is physically out of shape and emotionally depressed and discouraged.

After establishing 6-week and 6-month goals, B. V. and the nurse schedule weekly sessions. At the next session, B. V. reviews what she has discovered about her eating patterns and food choices and reflects on changes as compared to the initial nutrition assessment. Rather than be given a standard weekly diet, the nurse as coach encourages B. V. to explore the steps to reach her desired outcome and her challenges to reaching her goals. B. V. discusses her desire to begin to exercise and how her emotions affect her activities and her food choices. The nurse asks her to write down everything she eats, as well as the feeling that she has before, during, and after eating, for the week leading up to her follow-up visit.

In the second session, B. V. and the nurse review her eating/feeling diary and discuss what she has observed and where significant relationships between feelings and eating are observed. During this and subsequent sessions, it is important to explore and acknowledge B. V.'s feelings that are closely tied to her eating behaviors. In addition, the nurse records the physical parameters of weight and body fat calibration measurements for B. V.

Goals that are too difficult to achieve can discourage the client. Therefore, during each session, B. V. sets several small, attainable goals for the following week. Exercise is one of her goals, and she chooses to begin with taking the stairs in her apartment building. At the next session, she reports feeling more energy and that she is using the stairs daily. She also reports that she is controlling her portion size, and she notes that her eating patterns are shifting for the first time in years. She states that she is feeling more in control.

B. V. meets with the nurse coach on a regular basis for 6 months. During that time, she joins a gym and works out in a regular aerobic exercise program three to four times a week. She reports an interest in nutrition and has begun reading nutrition books, increasing her knowledge and interest in healthful food consumption. At the end of this period, she has reduced her weight to 160 pounds (approximately 10 pounds monthly). B. V. shares that with a new self-image she has begun to look for a new job that will allow her time to care for herself. At her 6-month medical checkup, her labs are normal and she is taken off of her blood pressure and cholesterol-lowering medications. B. V. and her nurse coach agree to move to monthly visits for the next three sessions and plan for termination of the appointments at that time, with the knowledge that B. V. can return for a "check in" as needed.

Evaluation

In a patient-centered model, the client and the nurse as coach and educator develop a nutrition program based on the client establishing goals and action steps. This process in the nurse coach model establishes SMART goals—integrative goals that are *s*pecific, *m*easurable, *a*ction based, *r*ealistic, have a *t*imeline, and are attainable and sustainable.

A client decides on the next step in moving closer to the desired health goals that he or she has established through using a series of tools, practices, and processes for increasing awareness, implementing change (Exhibit 31-2), and achieving goals. To evaluate the session further, the nurse may again explore with the client the subjective effects of the experience using the evaluation questions in Exhibit 31-3.

Conclusion

Nurses always chart all information they share with the client, as well as an evaluation of the session. When the nurse works in an inpatient facility, other staff must be informed of the program and its progress. Nurses who work in wellness centers, in centers using integrative models, and in private practice also keep records for each client and need to include nursing diagnoses, coaching tools employed, educational and counseling interventions, and the effectiveness of each session, along with the overall plan, goals, and next steps. Embedded within the holistic nursing and integrative nurse coach process is the implementation of self-care practices including developing nutrition goals and plans for health and wellness.

Directions for Future Research

1. Investigate the hypothesis that those who eat a nutritionally balanced diet live longer.
2. Continue the investigation on how a healthy diet and lifestyle affect a person's sense of well-being and quality of life.
3. Study the role of the nurse coach in guiding nutritional changes and eating behaviors and the effect on health outcomes.
4. Investigate the role of vitamin and mineral supplementation in disease prevention and health promotion.
5. Analyze the qualities of effective nutrition programs in diverse cultural and ethnic groups in a community setting.
6. Study and analyze health outcomes and cost savings for patients receiving integrative nurse coaching sessions.

Nurse Healer Reflections

After reading this chapter, the nurse healer will be able to answer or to begin the process of answering the following questions:

- Which sensations accompany physical well-being because of my improved nutrition?
- What composes healthy eating for me and my clients?
- How can I model healthy nutrition practices?
- What are my next steps in coaching myself to create nutritional goals and an action plan?

NOTES

1. M. Miller, N. J. Stone, C. Ballantyne, V. Bittner, M. H. Criqui, H. N. Ginsberg, A. C. Goldberg, et al., "Triglycerides and Cardiovascular Disease: A Scientific Statement from the American Heart Association," *Circulation* 123, no. 20 (2011): 2292–2333.
2. C. Smith-Spangler, M. L. Brandeau, G. E. Hunter, C. Bavinger, M. Pearson, P. J. Eschbach, V. Sundaram, et al., "Are Organic Foods Safer or Healthier Than Conventional Alternatives? A Systematic Review," *Annals of Internal Medicine* 157, no. 5 (2012): 1–24.

3. C. T. Zhu, P. Ingelmo, and D. M. Rand, "G×G×E for Lifespan in *Drosophila*: Mitochondrial, Nuclear, and Dietary Interactions That Modify Longevity," *PLoS Genetics* 10, no. 5 (2014): e1004354. doi:10.1371/journal.pgen.1004354.

4. J. C. Figueiredo, L. Hsu, C. M. Hutter, Y. Lin, P. T. Campbell, J. A. Baron, S. I. Berndt, et al., "Genome-Wide Diet-Gene Interaction Analyses for Risk of Colorectal Cancer," *PLoS Genetics* 10, no. 4 (2014): e1004228. doi:10.1371/journal.pgen.1004228.

5. R. Solá, M. Fitó, R. Estruch, J. Salas-Salvadó, D. Corella, R. de La Torre, M. A. Muñoz, et al., "Effect of a Traditional Mediterranean Diet on Apolipoproteins B. A-I, and Their Ratio: A Randomized, Controlled Trial," *Atherosclerosis* 218, no. 1 (2011): 174–180.

6. A. S. Go, D. Mozaffarian, V. L. Roger, E. J. Benjamin, J. D. Berry, M. J. Blaha, S. Dai, et al., "Heart Disease and Stroke Statistics—2014 Update: A Report from the American Heart Association," *Circulation* (2014): doi:10.1161/01.cir.0000441139.02102.80.

7. M. Ng, T. Fleming, M. Robinson, B. Thomson, N. Graetz, C. Margono, E. C. Mullany, et al., "Global, Regional, and National Prevalence of Overweight and Obesity in Children and Adults During 1980–2013: A Systematic Analysis for the Global Burden of Disease Study 2013," *The Lancet* 384, no. 9945 (2014): 766–781.

8. C. L. Ogden, M. D. Carroll, B. K. Kit, and K. M. Flegal, "Prevalence of Obesity Among Adults: United States, 2011–2012," *NCHS Data Brief No. 131* (October 2013). www.cdc.gov/nchs/data/databriefs/db131.htm.

9. J. West, K. M. Fleming, L. J. Tata, T. R. Card, and C. J. Crooks, "Incidence and Prevalence of Celiac Disease and Dermatitis Herpetiformis in the UK Over Two Decades: Population-Based Study," *American Journal of Gastroenterology* 109, no. 5 (2014): 757–768.

10. L. Jonasson, H. Gullbrand, A. K. Lundberg, and F. H. Nyström, "Advice to Follow a Low-Carbohydrate Diet Has a Favourable Impact on Low-Grade Inflammation in Type 2 Diabetes Compared with Advice to Follow a Low-Fat Diet," *Annals of Medicine* 46, no. 3 (2014): 182–187.

11. D. Lloyd-Jones, R. Adams, M. Carnethon, G. De Simone, B. Ferguson, K. Flegal, E. Ford, et al., "Heart Disease and Stroke Statistics—2009 Update: A Report from the American Heart Association Statistics Committee and Stroke Statistics Subcommittee," *Circulation* 119 (2009): e21–e181.

12. L. E. Cahill, A. Pan, S. E. Chiuve, Q. Sun, W. C. Willett, F. B. Hu, and E. B. Rimm, "Fried-Food Consumption and Risk of Type 2 Diabetes and Coronary Artery Disease: A Prospective Study in 2 Cohorts of US Women and Men," *American Journal of Clinical Nutrition* 100 (2014): 667–675.

13. J. A. Grieger, L. E. Grzeskowiak, and V. L. Clifton, "Preconception Dietary Patterns in Human Pregnancies Are Associated with Preterm Delivery," *Journal of Nutrition* (April 30, 2014): doi:10.3945/jn.114.190686.

14. A. Körner, "Obesity in Children Is Associated with Early Alterations in Adipose Tissue Biology" (paper presented at the American Diabetes Association 2014 Scientific Sessions, San Francisco, CA, June 15, 2014).

15. C. G. Perrine, A. J. Sharma, M. E. Jefferds, M. K. Serdula, and K. S. Scanlon, "Adherence to Vitamin D Recommendations Among U.S. Infants," *Pediatrics* 125, no. 4 (2010): 627–632.

16. T. T. Fung, R. M. van Dam, S. E. Hankinson, M. Stampfer, W. C. Willett, and F. B. Hu, "Low-Carbohydrate Diets and All-Cause and Cause-Specific Mortality: Two Cohort Studies," *Annals of Internal Medicine* 153, no. 5 (2010): 289–298.

17. J. Levi, S. L. Gray, M. Speck, F. K. Huynh, S. L. Babich, W. T. Gibson, and T. J. Kieffer, "Acute Disruption of Leptin Signaling In Vivo Leads to Increased Insulin Levels and Insulin Resistance," *Endocrinology* 152, no. 9 (2011): 3385–3395.

18. O. K. Basoglu, F. Sarac, S. Sarac, H. Uluer, and C. Yilmaz, "Metabolic Syndrome, Insulin Resistance, Fibrinogen, Homocysteine, Leptin, and C-Reactive Protein in Obese Patients with Obstructive Sleep Apnea Syndrome," *Annals of Thoracic Medicine* 6, no. 3 (2011): 120–125.

19. F. Grün and B. Blumberg, "Minireview: The Case for Obesogens," *Molecular Endocrinology* 23, no. 8 (2009): 1127–1134.

20. B. M. Dossey, S. Luck, and B. G. Schaub, "Nutritional Health," in *Nurse Coaching: Integrative Approaches for Health and Wellbeing* (North Miami, FL: International Nurse Coach Association, 2015): 148.

21. M. C. de Oliveira Otto, A. Alonso, D. H. Lee, G. L. Delclos, N. S. Jenny, R. Jiang, J. A. Lima, et al., "Dietary Micronutrient Intakes Are Associated with Markers of Inflammation but Not with Markers of Subclinical Atherosclerosis," *Journal of Nutrition* 141, no. 8 (2011): 1508–1515.

22. J. L. Jones, M. Comperatore, J. Barona, M. C. Calle, C. Andersen, M. McIntosh, W. Najm, et al., "A Mediterranean-Style, Low-Glycemic-Load Diet Decreases Atherogenic Lipoproteins and Reduces Lipoprotein (a) and Oxidized Low-Density Lipoprotein in Women with Metabolic Syndrome," *Metabolism* 61, no. 3 (2012): 366–372.

23. R. B. Ervin and C. L. Ogden, "Consumption of Added Sugars Among U.S. Adults, 2005–2010,"

NCHS Data Brief No. 122 (May 2013). www.cdc.gov/nchs/data/databriefs/db122.pdf.

24. National Research Council, *Recommended Daily Allowance*, 10th ed. (Washington, DC: National Academies Press, 1989).

25. R. Yanai, L. Mulki, E. Hasegawa, K. Takeuchi, H. Sweigard, J. Suzuki, P. Gaissert, et al., "Cytochrome P450-Generated Metabolites Derived from ω-3 Fatty Acids Attenuate Neovascularization," *Proceedings of the National Academy of Sciences* 111, no. 26 (2014): 9603–9608.

26. J. Salas-Salvadó, M. Bulló, N. Babio, M. A. Martínez-González, N. Ibarrola-Jurado J. Basora, R. Estruch, et al., "Reduction in the Incidence of Type 2 Diabetes with the Mediterranean Diet," *Diabetes Care* 34, no. 1 (2011): 14–19.

27. J. L. Jones, M. L. Fernandez, M. S. McIntosh, W. Najm, M. C. Calle, C. Kalynych, C. Vukich, et al., "Mediterranean-Style Low-Glycemic-Load Diet Improves Variables of Metabolic Syndrome in Women, and Addition of a Phytochemical-Rich Medical Food Enhances Benefits on Lipoprotein Metabolism," *Journal of Clinical Lipidology* 5, no. 3 (2011): 188–196.

28. C. Luo, Y. Zhang, Y. Ding, Z. Shan, S. Chen, M. Yu, F. B. Hu, et al., "Nut Consumption and Risk of Type 2 Diabetes, Cardiovascular Disease, and All-Cause Mortality: A Systematic Review and Meta-Analysis," *American Journal of Clinical Nutrition* 100, no. 1 (2014): 256–269.

29. R. Clarke, "Homocysteine, B Vitamins, and the Risk of Cardiovascular Disease," *Clinical Chemistry* 57, no. 8 (2011): 1201–1202.

30. C. Galli and P. Risé, "Fish Consumption, Omega 3 Fatty Acids and Cardiovascular Disease: The Science and the Clinical Trials," *Nutrition and Health* 20, no. 1 (2009): 11–20.

31. P. J. Boyle and J. Zrebiec, "Management of Diabetes-Related Hypoglycemia," *Southern Medical Journal* 100, no. 2 (2007): 183–194.

32. A. Mente, L. de Koning, H. S. Shannon, and S. S. Anand, "A Systematic Review of the Evidence Supporting a Causal Link Between Dietary Factors and Coronary Heart Disease," *Archives of Internal Medicine* 169, no. 7 (2009): 659–669.

33. M. S. Touillaud, A. C. Thiébaut, A. Fournier, M. Niravong, M. C. Boutron-Ruault, and F. Clavel-Chapelon, "Dietary Lignan Intake and Postmenopausal Breast Cancer Risk by Estrogen and Progesterone Receptor Status," *Journal of the National Cancer Institute* 99, no. 6 (2007): 475–486.

34. Y. Park, A. F. Subar, A. Hollenbeck, and A. Schatzkin, "Dietary Fiber Intake and Mortality in the NIH-AARP Diet and Health Study," *Archives of Internal Medicine* 171, no. 12 (2011): 1061–1068.

35. R. Deminice, G. V. Portari, J. S. Marchini, H. Vannucchi, and A. A. Jordao, "Effects of a Low-Protein Diet on Plasma Amino Acid and Homocysteine Levels and Oxidative Status in Rats," *Annals of Nutrition and Metabolism* 54, no. 3 (2009): 202–207.

36. M. Fotuhi, P. Mohassel, and K. Yaffe, "Fish Consumption, Long-Chain Omega-3 Fatty Acids and Risk of Cognitive Decline or Alzheimer Disease: A Complex Association," *Nature Clinical Practice Neurology* 5, no. 3 (2009): 140–152.

37. P. Barberger-Gateau, C. Samieri, C. Féart, and M. Plourde, "Dietary Omega 3 Polyunsaturated Fatty Acids and Alzheimer's Disease: Interaction with Apolipoprotein E Genotype," *Current Alzheimer Research* 8, no. 5 (2011): 479–491.

38. B. N. Ames, "Optimal Micronutrients Delay Mitochondrial Decay and Age-Associated Diseases," *Mechanisms of Ageing and Development* 131, nos. 7–8 (2010): 473–479.

39. J. Thompson, "Vitamins, Minerals and Supplements: Overview of Vitamin C (5)," *Community Practice* 80, no. 1 (2007): 35–36.

40. G. J. Dusting and C. Triggle, "Are We Over Oxidized? Oxidative Stress, Cardiovascular Disease, and the Future of Intervention Studies with Antioxidants," *Vascular Health Risk Management* 1, no. 2 (2005): 93–97.

41. M. Li, P. Chen, J. Li, R. Chu, D. Xie, and H. Wang, "Review: The Impacts of Circulating 25-Hydroxyvitamin D Levels on Cancer Patient Outcomes: A Systematic Review and Meta-Analysis," *Journal of Clinical Endocrinology and Metabolism* 99, no. 7 (2014): 2327–2336.

42. C. F. Garland, J. J. Kim, S. B. Mohr, E. D. Gorham, W. B. Grant, E. L. Giovannucci, L. Baggerly, et al., "Meta-Analysis of All-Cause Mortality According to Serum 25-Hydroxyvitamin D," *American Journal of Public Health* 104, no. 8 (2014): e43–e50.

43. W. Li, T. J. Green, S. M. Innis, S. I. Barr, S. J. Whiting, A. Shand, and P. von Dadelszen, "Suboptimal Vitamin D Levels in Pregnant Women Despite Supplement Use," *Canada Journal of Public Health* 102, no. 4 (2011): 308–312.

44. P. Chen, J. Stone, G. Sullivan, J. A. Drisko, and Q. Chen, "Anti-Cancer Effect of Pharmacologic Ascorbate and Its Interaction with Supplementary Parenteral Glutathione in Preclinical Cancer Models," *Free Radical Biology and Medicine* 51, no. 3 (2011): 681–687.

45. M. Meydani, S. Das, M. Band, S. Epstein, and S. Roberts, "The Effect of Caloric Restriction and Glycemic Load on Measures of Oxidative Stress and Antioxidants in Humans: Results from the CALERIE Trial of Human Caloric Restriction,"

Journal of Nutrition and Healthy Aging 15, no. 6 (2011): 456–460.

46. C. Martin, E. Butelli, K. Petroni, and C. Toneli, "How Can Research on Plants Contribute to Promoting Human Health?" *Plant Cell* 23, no. 5 (2011): 1685–1699.

47. S. Reuter, S. C. Gupta, B. Park, A. Goel, and B. B. Aggarwal, "Epigenetic Changes Induced by Curcumin and Other Natural Compounds," *Genes and Nutrition* 6, no. 2 (2011): 93–108.

48. A. Malhotra, P. Nair, and D. K. Dhawan, "Curcumin and Resveratrol Synergistically Stimulate p21 and Regulate Cox-2 by Maintaining Adequate Zinc Levels During Lung Carcinogenesis," *European Journal of Cancer Prevention* 20, no. 5 (2011): 411–416.

49. A. Di Mauro, J. Neu, G. Riezzo, F. Raimondi, D. Martinelli, R. Francavilla, and F. Indrio, "Gastrointestinal Function Development and Microbiota," *Italian Journal of Pediatrics* 39 (2013): 15.

50. W. Deechakawan, K. C. Cain, M. E. Jarrett, R. L. Burr, and M. M. Heitkemper, "Effect of Self-Management Intervention on Cortisol and Daily Stress Levels in Irritable Bowel Syndrome," *Biological Research for Nursing* 15, no. 1 (2013): 26–36.

51. R. A. Rudel, S. E. Fenton, J. M. Ackerman, S. Y. Euling, and S. L. Makris, "Environmental Exposures and Mammary Gland Development: State of the Science, Public Health Implications, and Research Recommendations," *Environmental Health Perspectives* 119, no. 8 (2011): 1053–1061.

52. C. Xuan, J. M. Shamonki, A. Chung, M. L. DiNome, M. Chung, P. A. Sieling, and D. J. Lee, "Microbial Dysbiosis Is Associated with Human Breast Cancer," *PLoS One* 9, no. 1 (2014): e83744. doi:10.1371/journal.pone.0083744.

53. B. P. Chumpitazi and R. J. Shulman, "Five Probiotic Drops a Day to Keep Infantile Colic Away?" *Pediatrics* 168, no. 3 (2014): 204–205.

54. S. Guandalini and C. Newland, "Differentiating Food Allergies from Food Intolerances," *Current Gastroenterology Reports* 13, no. 5 (2011): 426–434.

55. Z. Nahleh, "Breast Cancer, Obesity and Hormonal Imbalance: A Worrisome Trend," *Expert Review of Anticancer Therapy* 11, no. 6 (2011): 817–819.

56. F. Labrèche, M. S. Goldberg, M. F. Valois, and L. Nadon, "Postmenopausal Breast Cancer and Occupational Exposures," *Occupational and Environmental Medicine* 67, no. 4 (2010): 263–269.

57. S. L. Teitelbaum, M. D. Gammon, J. A. Britton, A. I. Neugut, B. Levin, and S. D. Stellman, "Reported Residential Pesticide Use and Breast Cancer Risk on Long Island, New York," *American Journal of Epidemiology* 165, no. 6 (2007): 643–651.

58. C. R. Hofe, L. Feng, D. Zephyr, A. J. Stromberg, B. Hennig, and L. M. Gaetke, "Fruit and Vegetable Intake, as Reflected by Serum Carotenoid Concentrations, Predicts Reduced Probability of Polychlorinated Biphenyl-Associated Risk for Type 2 Diabetes: National Health and Nutrition Examination Survey 2003–2004," *Nutrition Research* 34, no. 4 (2014): 285–293.

59. E. Sonestedt, B. Gullberg, and E. Wirfält, "Both Food Habit Change in the Past and Obesity Status May Influence the Association Between Dietary Factors and Postmenopausal Breast Cancer," *Public Health Nutrition* 10, no. 8 (2007): 769–779.

60. V. Hanf and U. Gonder, "Nutrition and Primary Prevention of Breast Cancer: Foods, Nutrients and Breast Cancer Risk," *European Journal of Obstetrics and Gynecology and Reproductive Biology* 123, no. 2 (2005): 139–149.

61. American Institute for Cancer Research, "AICR's Foods That Fight Cancer" (2014). www.aicr.org /foods-that-fight-cancer/.

62. H. B. Patisaul and W. Jefferson, "The Pros and Cons of Phytoestrogens," *Frontiers in Neuroendocrinology* 31, no. 4 (2010): 400–419.

63. L. Nonn, D. Duong, and D. M. Peehl, "Chemopreventive Anti-Inflammatory Activities of Curcumin and Other Phytochemicals Mediated by MAP Kinase Phosphatase-5 in Prostate Cells," *Carcinogenesis* 28, no. 6 (2007): 1188–1196.

64. E. Warensjö, L. Byberg, H. Melhus, R. Gedeborg, H. Mallmin, A. Wolk, and K. Michaëlsson, "Dietary Calcium Intake and Risk of Fracture and Osteoporosis: Prospective Longitudinal Cohort Study," *British Medical Journal* 342 (2011): d1473. doi:10.1136/bmj.d1473.

65. R. Scragg, "Vitamin D and Public Health: An Overview of Recent Research on Common Diseases and Mortality in Adulthood," *Public Health Nutrition* 14, no. 9 (2011): 1515–1532.

66. J. Welsh, "Vitamin D Metabolism in Mammary Gland and Breast Cancer," *Molecular and Cellular Endocrinology* 347, nos. 1–2 (2011): 55–60.

67. T. Constans, K. Mondon, C. Annweiler, and C. Hommet, "Vitamin D and Cognition in the Elderly," *Gériatrie et Psychologie Neuropsychiatrie du Vieillissement* 8, no. 4 (2010): 255–262.

68. N. Binkley, R. Novotny, D. Krueger, T. Kawahara, Y. G. Daida, G. Lensmeyer, B. W. Hollis, et al., "Low Vitamin D Status Despite Abundant Sun Exposure," *Journal of Clinical Endocrinology and Metabolism* 92, no. 6 (2007): 2130–2135.

69. A. Ascherio, K. L. Munger, and K. C. Simon, "Vitamin D and Multiple Sclerosis," *Lancet Neurology* 9, no. 6 (2010): 599–612.

70. K. Barnard and C. Colón-Emeric, "Extraskeletal Effects of Vitamin D in Older Adults:

Cardiovascular Disease, Mortality, Mood, and Cognition," *American Journal of Geriatric Pharmacotherapy* 8, no. 1 (2010): 4–33.

71. C. S. Katsanos, D. L. Chinkes, D. Paddon-Jones, X. J. Zhang, A. Aarsland, and R. R. Wolfe, "Whey Protein Ingestion in Elderly Persons Results in Greater Muscle Protein Accrual Than Ingestion of Its Constituent Essential Amino Acid Content," *Nutrition Research* 28, no. 10 (2008): 651–658.

72. G. Buhr and C. W. Bales, "Nutritional Supplements for Older Adults: Review and Recommendations—Part I," *Journal of Nutrition for the Elderly* 28, no. 1 (2009): 5–29.

73. M. S. Wellan, "Prevention, Prevention, Prevention: Nutrition for Successful Aging," *Journal of the American Dietetic Association* 107, no. 5 (2007): 741–743.

74. Q. Liu, F. Xie, R. Rolston, P. I. Moreira, A. Nunomura, X. Zhu, M. A. Smith, et al., "Prevention and Treatment of Alzheimer Disease and Aging: Antioxidants," *Mini Reviews in Medicinal Chemistry* 7, no. 2 (2007): 171–180.

75. L. M. Donini, M. R. De Felice, and C. Cannella, "Nutritional Status Determinants and Cognition in the Elderly," *Archives of Gerontology and Geriatrics* 44, suppl 1 (2007): 143–153.

76. M. S. Morris, P. F. Jacques, I. H. Rosenberg, and J. Selhub, "Folate and Vitamin B-12 Status in Relation to Anemia, Macrocytosis, and Cognitive Impairment in Older Americans in the Age of Folic Acid Fortification," *American Journal of Clinical Nutrition* 85, no. 1 (2007): 193–200.

77. M. Eskelinen, "The Effects of Midlife Diet on Late-Life Cognition: An Epidemiological Approach," *Dissertations in Health Sciences No. 220* (May 2014). http://epublications.uef.fi/pub/urn_isbn_978-952-61-1394-4/urn_isbn_978-952-61-1394-4.pdf.

78. C. Mason, L. Xiao, I. Imayama, C. R. Duggan, C. Bain, K. E. Foster-Schubert, A. Kong, et al., "Effects of Weight Loss on Serum Vitamin D in Postmenopausal Women," *American Journal of Clinical Nutrition* 94, no. 1 (2011): 95–103.

79. L. Fontana and S. Klein, "Aging, Adiposity, and Calorie Restriction," *Journal of the American Medical Association* 297, no. 9 (2007): 986–994.

80. M. I. Covas, V. Konstantinidou, and M. Fitó, "Olive Oil and Cardiovascular Health," *Journal of Cardiovascular Pharmacology* 54, no. 6 (2009): 477–482.

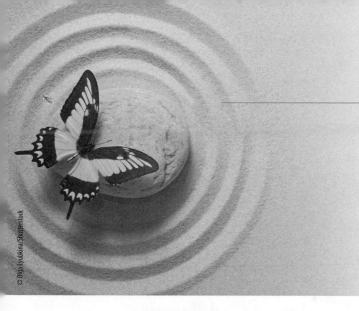

CHAPTER 32

Exercise and Movement

Francie Halderman and Christina Jackson

Nurse Healer Objectives

Theoretical

- Describe how exercise and movement support the innate healing mechanisms of the whole person.
- Identify how holistic nursing supports salutogenesis across the lifespan.
- Comprehend the benefits of mindful movement practices.
- Identify recommended amounts of exercise for various age groups.
- Discuss the benefits of exercise and movement both in illness and in health.
- Understand psychological, environmental, and other types of barriers to starting a personal fitness program.
- Discern between a compliance/achievement model of fitness and a model of engagement and adherence based on holistic nursing competencies.

Clinical

- Assess exercise and movement when working with individuals across the life span.
- Involve clients in self-assessment of their movement and exercise patterns as a routine part of health promotion and as a strategy for management and recovery from illness.

- Seek current clinical research regarding special health concerns and the recommendations for therapeutic exercise and movement, and make the information available to clients.
- Learn about a wide variety of exercise and movement modalities and their efficacies and provide education to clients that will expand their options for activity.
- Collaborate with clients to develop an individualized fitness plan that combines mindful movement and exercise.
- Become aware of community-based health programs that support exercise and movement for various populations and age groups and disseminate this information as appropriate.
- Act as a role model for daily movement and exercise.

Personal

- Assess your activities and patterns related to both exercise and movement.
- Experiment with new modalities of exercise and movement.
- Practice mindful exercise and movement to increase self-awareness.
- Practice centering techniques to become fully present when working with clients.
- Cultivate equanimity and respect for every individual's innate wisdom and timing of their unique process related to physical activity.

Definitions

Aerobic exercise: Sustained muscle activity within the target heart rate range that challenges the cardiovascular system to meet the muscles' needs for oxygen.

Co-vitalities: Various practices and conditions that, in combination, produce health; the opposite of comorbidities.

Endurance: The period of time the body can sustain exercise or movement.

Fitness: The ability to carry out daily tasks with vigor and alertness, without undue fatigue, and with ample reserve to enjoy leisure pursuits. It is the ability to respond to physical and emotional stress without an excessive increase in heart rate and blood pressure. Fitness comprises flexibility, endurance, strength, and balance.

Flexibility: The ability to use a joint throughout its full range of motion and to maintain some degree of elasticity of major muscle groups.

Innate healing mechanisms: Inherent processes that have the potential to promote health and healing that are already within, but may need to be evoked or supported.

Kinesthetic: The felt sense that detects bodily position, weight, or movement of the body.

Maximal heart rate: The rate of the heart when the body is engaged in intense physical activity.

Mindful movement: Movement with intention to notice present moment sensations, thoughts, feelings, and emotions with a nonjudgmental and compassionate attitude. A focus on full, rhythmic breathing is incorporated to enhance mindful awareness.

Moderate-intensity activity: That which induces an intermediate change in breathing and heart rate.

Posture: Pose or placement of parts of the body in spatial relationships.

Resistance training: The use of weights or opposing forces to strengthen muscle groups.

Resting heart rate: The heart's rate when the body is at rest.

Strength: The power of muscle groups.

Salutogenesis: The origin of health; the opposite of pathogenesis.

Target heart rate: The safe rate for the heart during exercise that produces health benefits.

Training: Repetitive bouts of exercise over a period of time with the intention of developing fitness.

Vigorous-intensity activity: That which induces large changes in breathing and heart rate.

Exercise and Movement

Few lifestyle practices have such large-scale effects on health and well-being as exercise and movement. Physical activity is more effective at preventively reducing morbidity and premature mortality than medications or procedures. Exercise and movement can positively influence physical, mental, and behavioral health, emotional well-being, and cognitive function.[1] Furthermore, they can produce positive effects in populations with and without existing disease.[2] In combination with nutrition and other lifestyle practices, exercise and movement comprise highly effective ways to maintain or regain optimal health and functioning where possible.

Exercise and Innate Healing Mechanisms

Exercise and movement are integral to the holistic paradigm that supports the *innate* healing mechanisms of the client.[3] Research shows that even discussing innate healing mechanisms with clients can begin to engage them in a new way.[4] A client's consciousness is expanded when he or she learns about the inherent healing capacities already within. This has the potential to change self-perception and ultimately one's subjective meaning of and relationship to health and illness.

There are multiple healing mechanisms by which exercise influences positive change. Endorphins are released creating positive neurohormonal cascades that decrease anxiety and depression and improve mental outlook.[2] It is well established that exercise can decrease risk and/or severity of cardiovascular disease, cancer, type 2 diabetes, and other chronic and degenerative diseases.[1] Inflammation has been identified as playing a component in these and many other physical and cognitive problems. The anti-inflammatory effects of exercise explain possible benefits of its use for these conditions.[5] In addition, exercise affects substance P, a neurotransmitter and neuromodulator involved with inflammation and pain perception. This may explain why longitudinal research concludes that exercise is associated with lower levels of pain.[6] Recent findings from the field of epigenetics describe how exercise can positively alter gene expression and cellular metabolism, helping people genetically predisposed to certain diseases avoid their actual development.[7] Moreover, exercise improves immune function, helping to prevent infectious disease.[8] Mindful breathing with movement directly mediates the nervous system and can stimulate positive parasympathetic responses that reduce stress.[9] Mindful movement and exercise can generate a sense of flow and interconnectedness with implications for spirituality and psychosocial health.

Despite the well-established benefits of exercise, fewer than 20% of American meet the U.S. Physical Activity Guidelines for exercise (see Table 32-2 later in the chapter). Research shows that patients are more likely to engage in exercise and movement when prescribers provide an exercise plan to them.[10] However, most primary health providers practicing from the predominant biomedical model of care do not routinely review exercise with their patients. Although 80% of U.S. adults are seen by a care provider at least once a year, fewer than 1 in 3 have been given exercise advice on physical activity.[11] There are many missed opportunities to discuss this lifestyle intervention with patients.

The failure of care providers to routinely prescribe exercise is part of a systemic problem that must be addressed. Research on establishing exercise as a vital sign concluded that programs that elevate exercise as an essential metric to be evaluated during outpatient visits is a valuable next step.[12] However, these programs must also begin to embrace holistic communication skills in order to truly engage patients. A population study found that healthcare provider biases around weight and lack of exercise contribute to unskillful interactions with overweight patients. This can inadvertently contribute to the "fat-shaming" phenomenon, which is not only ineffective for motivating patients but actually linked to additional weight gain from attempts to self-soothe the shameful feelings by eating more.[13]

Clearly, a healthcare system is needed that not only routinely addresses exercise and movement with patients but also equips healthcare providers with the knowledge and communication tools to engage and motivate them. The holistic nursing model provides a comprehensive approach to engage patients using advanced communication skills for behavior change, such as appreciative inquiry and motivational interviewing, and is rooted in a foundation of respect and caring for the patient. In addition, holistic nurses identify personal biases and address them through self-reflection, leading to greater self-awareness and maintenance of respect for the patient. The knowledge, skills, and attitudes of the holistic nurse are based on the Holistic Nursing Scope and Standards and serve as an exemplar that all healthcare providers can strive to model when engaging patients in positive behavior change.[3]

Advancing a Paradigm Shift

The biomedical model of *reactively* treating disease with medications, procedures, surgeries, and hospitalizations is costly and fraught with untoward reactions and complications. In addition, this model is ill-equipped to manage the rapid rise in obesity, chronic illness, and age-related conditions that are increasing due to the aging of the American population. Annual medical costs related to obesity alone recently exceeded $147 billion.[14] The current biomedical model does not, in practice, routinely address exercise for most adults. In contrast, the integral nursing model embraces appropriate use of biomedical treatment options while partnering with patients to promote exercise and movement along with other healing and health-sustaining practices. Holistic and integrative nurse coaches have additional expertise in these areas.

The biomedical model of care focuses on comorbidities and examines simultaneously occurring illnesses and their interactions with one another and how their combination affects the prognosis or course of disease. Conversely, a holistic approach brings a systemic focus on covitalities to ask: Which combination of lifestyle practices and environmental, relational, or other factors synergistically promotes vitality, health, and well-being in people? Salutogenesis is the study of the origin of health and the covitalities that contribute to it.[15] It is a prospective approach that studies how to create health and well-being for the whole person. As the study of salutogenesis matures, important gains will be made that inform how to keep people healthy, support populations with illness to heal and regain their highest level of possible health, and help all people maintain well-being throughout the health–illness continuum across the life span.

In a holistic nursing model, exercise is not a singular approach but ideally is combined with nutrition, healthy relationships, community connectedness, and other lifestyle practices that constitute covitalities. **Table 32-1** contrasts the old and new paradigms related to fitness.

The primary purpose of exercise is to produce health and fitness in the whole person. The following are the four basic components of fitness:

1. Flexibility is the ability to use a joint throughout its full range of motion and to maintain some degree of elasticity of major muscle groups. It is important for the following reasons:
   - It provides increased resistance to muscle and joint injury.
   - It helps prevent mild muscle soreness if flexibility exercises are done before and after vigorous activity.
2. Muscle strength is the contracting power of a muscle. It is important for the following reasons:
   - Daily activities become less strenuous as muscles become stronger.

TABLE 32-1   Fitness Paradigms for Exercise and Movement

Old Fitness Paradigm	New Fitness Paradigm
Compliance Model	Engagement and Adherence Model
Sense of obligation or dread	Enjoyable and fun
Rigorous and punitive	Mindful and reflective
Competitive with comparison to others	Self-aware with goal for personal best
Body focused and achievement oriented	Integration of bodymindspirit
Uses breathing to control the body and mind	Mindful breathing is cultivated to energize, calm, and bring greater awareness of the whole person
Regimented routines with little variety	Encompassing many types of activities, including interactive video games, aerobic and nonaerobic, group and individual practices
Compartmentalized time of the day or week dedicated to fitness: "all or nothing" view	Awareness of cumulative effects of activities throughout the week: "some better than none"
Providers view clients as resistant	Holistic practitioners understand that ambivalence is the core issue, not resistance, and use motivational interviewing to support clients
Providers identify weaknesses and barriers	Holistic practitioners use appreciative inquiry to identify strengths and build on past successes
Exercise viewed as a singular intervention	Exercise viewed as one aspect of a comprehensive lifestyle plan for health and well-being

- Strong abdominal and lower back muscles help prevent lower back problems.
- Appearance improves as muscles become firmer.

3. Cardiorespiratory endurance is the ability of the circulatory and respiratory systems to maintain blood and oxygen delivery to the exercising muscles. It is important for the following reasons:
   - It increases resistance to cardiovascular diseases.
   - It improves the ability to maintain activity levels (endurance).
   - It allows for a high-energy return from daily activities.

4. Postural stability is the body's ability to balance and stay balanced during dynamic action. This ability declines naturally with age. Exercise and movement practices such as yoga, standing Pilates, and tai chi assist with fall prevention through integration of neuromuscular and sensory responses.

Flexibility, strength, endurance, and balance refer not only to the physical body but also to the whole person and bodymindspirit. Movement practices from Eastern traditions have embraced this understanding for several thousand years and, in this sense, the paradigm is not new. However, adaptations of these traditions have developed as the practices came to the West. There are many styles of yoga that range from meditative and restorative to athletic and achievement-oriented practice. Research is currently under way to evaluate the particular benefits of various types of yoga. In general, styles with pacing of movements and postures that are slow, flowing, meditative, and mindful may be more conducive to relaxation and positive parasympathetic response while promoting endurance, balance, strength, and flexibility.[2]

Movement Modalities

Movement practices promote health, wellness, and disease prevention. Modalities from Eastern traditions such as yoga, tai chi, and qi gong have become increasingly available and help cultivate mindfulness in movement. These practices employ rhythmic patterns and sequences of movement and/or holding postures or poses along with mindful breathing. They help enhance present moment awareness of what is happening in one's interior environment of sensations, thoughts, emotions, feelings, and energy flow, as well as awareness in the exterior environment. A greater sense of connection with oneself can be cultivated as well as a sense of being part of a greater unity and flow of life.

A comparison review of 81 scientific and nursing journal articles found that yoga was as effective or better than other forms of exercise in improving various health metrics such as glucose regulation, reduction of depression, pain and fatigue, improved balance and flexibility, and stress reduction. Movement that involves slow, rhythmic patterns, breath work, and holding postures may regulate the body's hormonal response to stress and improve health outcomes in ways equal to or better than exercise in populations with and without disease.[2] However, aerobic exercise and movement that is more physically active, such as dancing, is more effective in improving cardiorespiratory fitness. A routine that integrates aerobic exercise, strength training, and mindful movement practices can provide variety and enjoyment that leads to sustained behavior change over time.

Recommendations for Physical Activity

In 2008, the U.S. Department of Health and Human Services released the Physical Activity Guidelines for Americans that serve as the first-ever national guidelines for exercise and movement. **Table 32-2** illustrates weekly recommendations of aerobic activity and muscle strengthening activity according to age group.

In addition to these guidelines, research supports a new trend in cardiovascular fitness called *high-intensity interval training*, which has been shown to be an effective and efficient means to achieve aerobic fitness. By intermittently taking the body up to peak heart rate and respiratory rate for short bursts of 1 to 3 minutes, and then allowing an interval of reduced effort, the muscle cells develop more mitochondria, which allow the muscles to use energy more efficiently.

TABLE 32-2	National Physical Activity Guidelines for Americans		

Age	Weekly Aerobic Exercise Recommendations	Weekly Muscle Strengthening Recommendations
Children (aged 6–17 years)	Moderate intensity: 60 minutes 4 days per week AND Vigorous activity: 60 minutes 3 days per week or more	3 days per week of muscle and bone strengthening activity (biking, running, jumping rope)
Adults (aged 18–64 years)	Moderate intensity: 2 hours and 30 minutes a week OR Vigorous intensity: 1 hour and 15 minutes a week	2 or more days per week Include all major muscle groups: legs, hips, back, chest, stomach, shoulders, arms Repeat 8 to 12 times per session
Older Adults (65 years and older)	Follow adult guidelines: adjust as appropriate to abilities	Choose activities that maintain or improve balance if there is a risk of falling

Source: Modified from U.S. Department of Health and Human Services, Office of Disease Prevention and Health Promotion, "2008 Physical Activity Guidelines for Americans," *ODPHP Publication No. U0036* (October 2008). www.health.gov/paguidelines/pdf/paguide.pdf.

The body achieves aerobic metabolism with less time expenditure and increases endurance in the process. Typically, one will go through several cycles of brief peak effort followed by several minutes of reduced effort. In this way, one can experience a complete and productive aerobic workout in 20 minutes. In the absence of contraindications, high-intensity interval training is a recommended method for all populations to achieve maximum health benefits in a minimal amount of time.[16]

Exercise has a point of diminishing returns, whereby its benefits decrease with too much intensity and amount. It is well established that immune function is negatively affected by exercise that is too rigorous and long.[5] In addition, pre-aging and oxidative stress result from extreme overexertion.[17] Overexercise syndrome and exercise dependence are issues that can be related to eating disorders and psychological issues that may require intervention and the support of a mental health professional.[18]

Adherence

Fewer than 20% of adult Americans meet the U.S. Physical Activity Guidelines for both aerobic and muscle-strengthening activities.[1] Individual barriers to physical activity may vary but often include "lack of time." The benefits of exercise are cumulative, and just 10 minutes of sustained vigorous activity can be beneficial and count cumulatively toward the weekly guideline totals.

The nurse can use motivational interviewing techniques to assess the person's phase of readiness and level of intrinsic motivation. It is important to understand the common factors that enhance adherence for many people as well as to learn the unique motivations of each individual. Multiple studies show that exercise adherence in adults is greatly enhanced by the following: the enjoyment derived from using a variety of activities; the ability to self-select the level, intensity, and type of exercise; and the establishment of a regular routine.[10] The holistic nurse can empower the person to explore types and levels of activity that are uniquely appealing to him or her and find creative ways to implement them. This individualized approach will increase the likelihood of engagement and adherence over time.

The Interconnectedness of Interventions

Exercise and movement are the physical expressions of the whole person. A major tenet of holistic nursing is that *making changes in one part changes the whole*.[3] Body-mind-emotion-spirit-environment comprise some of the interwoven aspects of being human. A change in any one of these areas can affect the rest in seen and/or unseen ways. Holistic nurses understand that any aspect can be an entry point for helping a client move toward healing and positive growth. Every client is unique and there is no *universal* hierarchy of entry point in working with a client (i.e., using a mind approach over a body approach) because they are interconnected. The old maxim of "mind over matter" is best understood when remembering that, conversely, making changes in the body can also dramatically affect the mind. Exercise and movement may be initially thought of as a "body approach" but they inextricably affect mind, spirit, and emotion as well, and change can be omnidirectional in all of these domains.

Small changes in body habitus (how one is embodied and positioned) can lead to powerful changes in a very short time. Research shows that holding a "power pose" for as little as 1 minute reduced cortisol and increased healthy levels of testosterone. This resulted in improved feeling and thinking states that, in turn, promoted adaptive and positive behavior changes.[19] The power pose is described as confidently holding the arms over the head in a "V" or a solid stance with legs slightly spread and the hands firmly on the hips in a Wonder Woman–type pose for 1 to 3 minutes. Practitioners of yoga and other movement therapies may recognize striking similarities that power poses share with various poses or asanas within their practice.

Like the power pose research, yoga postures are also held for maximum benefit. Teaching a client about the practice of power posing at strategic times (before a significant event or interpersonal interaction) gives him or her a self-empowering tool that can be used to maximize performance and reduce stress.

When working collectively, a nurse and client *partner together* to address where to start. Exercise and movement may be part of a comprehensive health evaluation and lifestyle plan that a client is seeking, or they may be an entry point for initial healing in a specific area. For example, a client who wants to address stress and anxiety but is reluctant to talk about significant family issues may be receptive to discussing exercise and movement. Both are evidence-based approaches that can be highly effective for stress, anxiety, and depression.[2] In this scenario, a change in the body through mild aerobics and yoga may create a positive cascade of neurohormonal changes that improve mood, positive outlook, mental clarity, and sense of well-being. Change may go far beyond these metrics because the whole is greater than the sum of the parts of body-mind-spirit. Helping a client with even one behavior change may result in unseen effects down the road, with benefits that unfold over time. The nurse recognizes the holistic nursing principle that interventions may not be immediately visible, yet could have meaningful and systemic repercussions over time, and brings this awareness to clients as well.[3]

Exercise Across the Life Span

Maternal–Infant Benefits

Exercise provides significant health benefits across the life span, beginning in the womb (see Table 32-2). Research studies examining exercise in pregnancy demonstrate important physical and emotional benefits to the mother and the newborn after delivery. Healthy pregnant women who engaged in moderate intensity exercise throughout pregnancy are less likely to have Cesarean and instrumental deliveries.[20] The risk for preterm delivery is also reduced by prenatal exercise and a lower body mass index.[21] Women with gestational diabetes who exercise during pregnancy decrease the risk of having babies with macrosomia and have reduced rates of Cesarean deliveries.[22] Significant maternal weight gain during pregnancy (>40 pounds), in and of itself, has been associated with increased risk of childhood obesity. Children born to women who had significant weight gain during pregnancy had an 8% greater risk of obesity.[23]

Pregnant women feel healthier when they exercise regularly. A study revealed significant decreases in depression, anger, tension, fatigue, and anxiety and increased energy in those who exercised moderately to vigorously for 30 minutes on a regular basis.[24] In addition, pregnant women who exercised regularly using resistance (strength) training reported less nausea, back pain, and fatigue. Sleep patterns and general well-being also improved with prenatal exercise.[25]

Benefits for Children

The prevalence of obesity in children is estimated at 23.6% and is linked to the development of diabetes and metabolic syndrome. Children with developmental disabilities can be at higher risk for low levels of fitness.[26] Consumption of processed, calorie-dense foods along with increased time spent in sedentary activities fuel this disturbing trend among youth. Social determinants of health such as poverty, education, food deserts, and lack of green spaces and playgrounds underlie this trend of childhood obesity.[10]

There is increasing evidence that yoga for children and adolescents is an effective method to calm the mind and increase health and well-being. A feasibility study of yoga for urban youth with emotional and behavioral issues found that the children had improved attention in class and adaptive skills, reduced depressive symptoms, and fewer negative behavioral occurrences.[27] Recommendations to increase school-based programs to raise awareness of physical activity and improve nutrition abound, and robust data from many studies demonstrate significant improvements to health (including musculoskeletal strength, cardiorespiratory function, body mass index, and adiposity) as a result of these targeted programs in both typical and developmentally disabled cohorts.[26]

Benefits for the Elderly

The benefits of exercise in the elderly population (healthy as well as those with chronic illness) are well documented, and data show significant improvements in lean body mass, skeletal muscle mass, exercise capacity, cardiorespiratory function, chronic knee pain, balance, mood, self-confidence, and cognitive function in those who exercise regularly.[28-33] Many of these studies measure outcomes after 8 to 12 weeks of exercise, though participants perceive benefits sooner. Research showed that a regular walking program for elderly people with diabetes significantly improved daily physical activity levels, physical strength, energy consumption, fasting blood glucose, glycated hemoglobin, total cholesterol, and triglyceride levels.[34] Another study found that walking combined with meditative activities resulted in improved mood and immune function.[35] Much of the research demonstrates that elderly do well with gentle approaches to exercise that involve social engagement.

Cultural and Socioeconomic Considerations

A person's cultural background includes his or her beliefs, practices, values, and preferences. The meaning and purpose of exercise may be culturally and economically influenced. The preference to play a team sport, for example, may come from the desire for community and connection with others and/or may be a result of limited access to health facilities.[36] Conversely, an individual working out in a health club may be purposefully working toward health maintenance and has the financial means to do so. When working with clients, the holistic nurse discusses relevant cultural and economic factors that may affect choice of activities. Where economic disparities exist, the nurse finds creative ways to meet clients' needs. Community centers and churches may offer free programs for those who are motivated to exercise in groups. Public television and basic cable channels frequently offer yoga and cardiovascular workout programs for those who are motivated to exercise individually or who may otherwise need to work out at home. Libraries frequently offer free DVD rentals including those for health and fitness. High-quality exercise and movement classes can be easily found online as well as support groups and blogs that foster community and virtual connections with others. As with any exercise class, online classes (such as YouTube videos) should be evaluated for quality of instruction and safety of movements.

Healthy People 2020 identifies the most common factors that positively and negatively affect adult exercise adherence (see **Table 32-3**) and offers several new objectives that reflect a multidisciplinary approach to promote exercise for all. It also addresses the underlying disparities regarding access to environments that support physical activity including the availability of parks, sidewalks, and the presence of policies in the worksite, schools, and communities that promote fitness.[1]

Nurses can advocate for justice to reduce disparities in access to healthy environments and resources for exercise and movement.

Employers and Exercise

Employers benefit from creating environments that support fitness among their employees. Workplace programs can decrease direct and indirect healthcare costs, reduce absenteeism, prevent illness and injury, and increase morale and quality of work.[37] Workplace exercise programs have been shown to reduce total cholesterol, body fat, and diastolic blood pressure, thereby reducing the cardiovascular risk factors of employees.[38] As part of an integrated health strategy, exercise has helped some cancer survivors return to work faster, improve cognitive functioning and productivity, and engage in long-term adherence to exercise that may influence quality of life for survivors.[39]

One study of an incentive-based employer exercise program found that participation was affected by employee attitudes around the beliefs about the benefits of exercise as well as perceived barriers. In addition, proximity and access to facilities, preference for exercising at a fitness center, and prior experiences with exercising were related to adoption and maintenance of an employer-sponsored program.[40] A randomized controlled pilot showed that a worksite yoga and mindfulness program resulted in employee improvements in perceived stress, sleep quality, and autonomic balance as measured by heart rate variability.[41]

TABLE 32-3 Adherence Factors	
Factors That Positively Affect Exercise Adherence in Adults	**Factors That Negatively Affect Exercise Adherence in Adults**
Education beyond high school	Advancing age
Higher income	Low income
Enjoyment of exercise	Lack of time
Expectation of benefits	Low motivation
Belief in ability to exercise	Rural residency
History of activity in adulthood	Belief that great effort is needed to exercise
Social support from peers, family, or spouse	Overweight or obese
Access to acceptable facilities	Perception of poor health
Pleasant scenery in environment	Disability
Safe neighborhood	

Source: Modfied from U.S. Department of Health and Human Services, Office of Disease Prevention and Health Promotion, "2008 Physical Activity Guidelines for Americans," *ODPHP Publication No. U0036* (October 2008). www.health.gov/paguidelines/pdf/paguide.pdf.

Holistic Caring Process

When discussing exercise and movement with clients, the holistic nurse employs holistic nursing competencies and relational communication skills to create an environment that fosters trust and positive behavior change. The nurse who regards the client as already whole is contributing to an environment conducive to healing, which is another holistic nursing competency. By regarding clients as already whole, holistic nurses communicate unconditional acceptance and meet the clients where they are while simultaneously partnering with them to support change.

Holistic Assessment

The holistic caring process is an all-at-once process, whereby the nurse simultaneously assesses, accesses the client's patterns/challenges/needs, diagnoses as appropriate, co-plans, and assists clients with implementing plans for exercise and movement. With this nonlinear, iterative approach, the nurse is fully present and open to all ways of knowing that may inform interaction with the client. In preparing to use exercise and movement interventions, the nurse assesses the following parameters:

- The client's motivation, phase of readiness, and ability to make the necessary lifestyle changes in the areas of exercise and movement
- The client's history of exercise and movement, any positive associations and past enjoyment of activities, and any modalities about which the client might be curious
- Perception of barriers to perform exercise and movement
- Cultural, socioeconomic, and environmental factors
- Support systems that may enhance adherence

Identification of Patterns/ Challenges/Needs

The following are patterns/challenges/ needs affected by exercise and movement interventions:

- Altered nutrition
- Altered circulation
- Altered oxygenation
- Altered coping
- Altered physical mobility
- Sleep pattern disturbance
- Altered activities of daily living
- Disturbance in body image
- Disturbance in self-esteem
- Potential hopelessness
- Potential powerlessness
- Pain
- Anxiety

Outcome Identification

Table 32-4 guides the nurse in client outcomes, nursing prescriptions, and evaluation for the use of exercise and movement as nursing interventions.

Therapeutic Care Plan and Interventions

Before the session:

- Create a safe environment in which the client feels comfortable discussing the needs of his or her physical body from a physical movement perspective.
- Clear your mind of other client or personal encounters to be fully present when meeting with the client.
- Bring intention for wholeness and highest good of the person to the session and respect for his or her healing process and choice.

At the beginning of the session:

- Take and record any necessary physical assessment data (e.g., height, weight, skinfold thickness measurements, hip–waist ratio, blood pressure, and data on range of motion and mobility limitations, postural assessment).
- Guide the client as he or she discloses past habit patterns that affect exercise behavior.
- Assess the client's phase of readiness and level of motivation.

During the session:

- Ascertain the client's current weekly exercise pattern and practice.
- Be alert to psychological clues that may relate to exercise behavior or extremes (i.e., completely sedentary or excessive exercise dependence).
- Help the client identify any barriers that prevent starting or maintaining a program.

TABLE 32-4   Nursing Interventions: Exercise and Movement

Client Outcomes	Nursing Prescriptions	Evaluation
The client will demonstrate knowledge of healthful exercise and movement programs and resources.	Engage the client to discuss his or her program.	The client participated in the session discussions.
The client will develop a personal fitness plan.	Assist the client in identifying resources for healthful exercise and movement.	The client demonstrated content knowledge and resource acquisition for using new behaviors in exercise.
The client will engage in exercise and movement practice and meet with the nurse for evaluation of goals.	Assist the client in a personal self-assessment. Encourage the client to participate with the nurse to develop goals and action plans. Prepare the client to start his or her personal fitness plan and establish follow-up meetings.	The client completed a self-assessment. The client participated with the nurse to develop a personalized program of exercise and movement. The client started his or her fitness plan and met with the nurse to discuss outcomes and follow up.
The client will be aware of the potential benefits of exercise and movement practice.	Encourage the client to journal or reflect on his or her experience with exercise and movement in a direction of healing.	The client links exercise and movement with changes in patterns/challenges/needs such as mood, sleep, energy level, and body image.

Guide his or her exploration of creative solutions and available resources.

- Assist the client to explore multiple types of activities that are enjoyable and cumulative throughout the week.
- Discuss rhythmic breathing and awareness of full breathing during movement to increase attention to mindful movement practice.
- Support the client to develop an individualized exercise and movement program.
- Ensure that the teaching is at the client's cognitive and emotional levels.

At the end of the session:

- Have the client identify the options presented that best fit his or her lifestyle.
- Work with the client to establish written attainable goals and target dates.
- Give the client specific affirmations to use to support these goals.
- Give the client handout materials or refer to pertinent resources to reinforce the teaching.

- Use the client outcomes that were established before the session and the client's subjective experiences to evaluate the session (see **Exhibit 32-1**).
- Schedule a follow-up session.

Getting Started

Beginning the fitness regimen in a disciplined manner increases the chances of maintaining the program. Thus, before beginning an exercise program, an individual should be encouraged to follow these basic guidelines:

- Learn about the different types of exercise and movement programs available in the area.
- Consult a physician or exercise authority. If you are older than 35 years, have never seriously exercised, have a disability or chronic illness, or are pregnant, obtain guidance to avoid injuries or complications.
- Warm up and cool down. Stretching exercises are essential before and after each activity or period of exercise.

EXHIBIT 32-1   Evaluation of the Client's Subjective Experience with Exercise and Movement Interventions

1. How has your fitness program been going in general?
2. Do you have any concerns or questions about the program or your response to it?
3. Has your vitality increased since beginning regular exercise?
4. Does exercise give you a sense of reduced stress in your life?
5. Do you find time during your normal day to integrate mindful movement and breathing techniques?
6. Would you like to learn more ways to incorporate movement into your work environment?
7. What support systems have you discovered that assist you with maintaining and developing your exercise regimen?
8. Is there some other support that you need to assist you in adhering to your new exercise regimen?
9. What is your next step for integrating exercise and therapeutic movement into your daily life?
10. Do you need help in obtaining more resources for this final step?

- Wear shoes with proper support for the activity and choose proper ground surfaces for activities.
- Establish an exercise routine.
- Evaluate your program periodically. Determine if you are making progress. If you want to go further, set new goals.
- Create competition for yourself only if it benefits you. If you have allowed too much competition, exercise may become more of a burden than a joy.

Many rewards of exercise and physical activity do begin immediately. Mental and spiritual improvements include beneficial changes in the following areas:

- Mental attitude and outlook on life
- Ability to cope with stress
- Ability to avoid or control mild depression
- Sleep patterns
- Strength and endurance
- Eating habits
- Appearance and vitality
- Posture
- Physical stamina as you age

To reduce the risks associated with exercise, clients must know not only how often and how long to exercise but also how vigorously to exercise. Although the target pulse range allows for a heart rate within 60% to 80% of maximal capacity, the American Heart Association guidelines state that regular exercise of a moderate level, or from 50% to 75% of maximal capacity, appears to be sufficient. Maintaining the target pulse rate during physical exercise for 15 to 30 minutes three to five times per week reduces the risk of overexertion, enhances enjoyment, and results in cardiovascular fitness. Each person can discern whether activity is vigorous or moderate based on his or her body's response. If one can talk but not sing while exercising, that person has reached moderate intensity. If one can say only a few words and then needs to catch his or her breath while exercising, that person has reached vigorous intensity.

Because uncontrolled exercising may result in injury, it is wise to follow these guidelines:

- Always warm up for at least 5 to 10 minutes.
- If you are tired, stop.
- If something hurts, stop.
- If you feel dizzy or nauseated, stop.
- Take your pulse at regular intervals.
- Cool down after exercising.

To ease your heart rate into the training range, clients should begin with 10 minutes of low-intensity, warm-up exercise. To cool down, they should do 10 minutes of the same slow activity.

Case Study (Implementation)

The nurse determines with the client whether the client goals for exercise and movement were successfully achieved. To evaluate the session further, the nurse may again explore the subjective effects of the experience with the client. Whenever possible, every healthcare encounter with all populations should include discussions and documentation about exercise and movement for health promotion and disease prevention.

Case Study

Setting: School of nursing
Client: J. C., a 32–year-old nursing student who is a single mother of an active toddler
Patterns/Challenges/Needs:

1. Altered physical mobility (less than body requirements) related to lifestyle changes
2. Altered nutrition (more than body requirements) related to excessive intake and improper eating patterns
3. Sleep pattern disturbance related to self-care deficit

J. C. is a 32-year-old nursing student who is a single mother of an active toddler. Her general health is sound, but recently she is experiencing high levels of stress related to the demands of nursing school and single parenting. With little time, her nutritional and exercise behaviors have become a lower priority. Her food consumption is mostly of packaged, processed food for convenience. She has become sedentary from studying and gained 15 pounds over the past 6 months. After growing concerned about her weight gain, she began to run for several weeks but failed to do proper warm-up stretching or use proper shoe support and developed extremely sore feet and then stopped. Concerned about her health and fitness, she met with the university health services nurse for guidance, relating, "I'm pulled in so many different directions and don't feel like I'm doing anything well." She is interested in becoming more physically active but does not believe she can adjust her diet right now. Recently, she began to have trouble falling asleep and she feels that it is related to not having any time to herself. The nurse listened

with open presence and then helped her explore a self-assessment and self-care plan. It was identified that her physical and social aspects are most in need of attention.

The interview revealed that J. C. loved to dance but has not been able to since her daughter was born. Since starting nursing school a year ago, she has lost contact with other friends who are mothers of young children like herself. J. C. states she feels guilty about relying on the television to entertain her daughter and wished she felt more present with her. She describes a decreased ability to focus while studying and a general sense of feeling overwhelmed. At night when trying to sleep she feels a sense of loneliness and disconnection.

The nurse helped J. C. begin to explore ways of adding movement and exercise that would support her bodymindspirit by incorporating activities she loves to meet her unique needs. Together they found a 20-minute mother–child dance cardio DVD that she could play three times per week that would utilize her exercise time as a means to also connect with her daughter. She has been wanting to try yoga and a biweekly class was discovered at a nearby YMCA that also offers affordable child care. They reviewed how to stretch before exercising and how to incorporate warm-up and cool-down periods. The nurse identified the free resource of the university gym at J. C.'s school of nursing, and a plan was made for her to attend twice a week (right before her nursing classes) and work out with weights for strength training, as well as park in the farthest parking lot to promote walking and take stairs at all times. She believed other nursing students in her cohort might want to join her for both the yoga class and the weight training and a plan was made to invite them. The nurse suggested that J. C. create a written self-care contract that includes the steps discussed and share it with another person to enhance accountability. J. C. wanted to lose eight pounds in the next 4 weeks, and a follow-up visit was planned for 1 month to review the status of the exercise and movement plan.

J. C. returned to the health services department for her follow-up visit and had a five-pound weight loss over the past month. She reported that she is feeling "so much more upbeat and clear" since starting a yoga class and playing with her daughter while exercising together with the cardio DVD. She found two nursing cohort friends who have joined her for a community yoga class and strength training at the university gym before classes, and she exchanged a self-care contract with one of them. She is feeling motivated to eat differently and desires to improve her nutritional intake as well as her daughter's. She describes being better able to concentrate on her studies as well as being more present for her daughter. Her sleep has improved and she reports that the feelings of loneliness and being overwhelmed have significantly decreased. The stretching has eased the soreness in her feet and she feels motivated to step up her fitness program.

Together they discussed strategies to obtain additional videos for her and her daughter to avoid boredom and ways to include outdoor activity such as bicycling instead of just going for walks to maximize aerobic conditioning. J. C. established a new goal to lose the remaining 10 pounds, and the nurse provided J. C. with a link to a free Internet video that reviews peak interval training. The nurse will also begin focused nutritional counseling with J. C.

Evaluation

The nurse determines with the client whether the client outcomes for exercise and movement were successfully achieved. To evaluate the session further, the nurse may again explore the subjective effects of the experience with the client.

Conclusion

Nurses should chart the information they impart to the client as well as the evaluation of the session. When the nurse works in an inpatient facility, other staff must be apprised of the program and the client's progress. Nurses who work in wellness centers, independent practices, or other areas in which counseling sessions are the primary care modality should keep records for each client that state the nursing diagnosis, type of counseling employed, and effectiveness of each session. Whenever possible, every healthcare encounter with all populations should

include discussions and documentation about exercise and movement for health promotion and disease prevention.

Directions for Future Research

1. Further investigate the benefit of various types of movement modalities for specific disease states.
2. Continue investigating ways in which the lifestyle behaviors of exercise and movement affect a person's well-being and optimal health as well as act as an intervention for disease.
3. Study the specific factors that are important in tailoring exercise programs to ethnic and cultural groups as well as aging populations.
4. Identify the most effective means to shift nursing practice so that all populations receive teaching on exercise and movement at every possible healthcare encounter.
5. Determine how to close the research–practice gap regarding lack of exercise prescriptions by health providers.
6. Translate evidence into practice so that exercise is prescribed and assessed routinely across the life span as part of a comprehensive lifestyle overview.

Nurse Healer Reflections

After reading this chapter, the nurse healer will be able to answer or to begin the process of answering the following questions:

- Do I strive to identify personal biases regarding the weight of patients, and do I practice self-reflection and holistic strategies to address them?
- How would I describe the meaning and practice of exercise and movement in my life today?
- Do I meet or exceed the recommended weekly Physical Activity Guidelines?
- Are there any barriers that interfere with my own practice of exercise and movement?
- What exercise and movement changes can I incorporate that will improve my fitness

and bring pleasure and enjoyment into my life?

- How does fitness affect my experience of bodymindspirit, sense of self, and others?
- Do I view myself and others as already whole, with an innate ability to heal, throughout all of the stages of readiness regarding exercise?
- How can I best learn, practice, and model healthy exercise and movement?

NOTES

1. U.S. Department of Health and Human Services, *Healthy People 2020* (Washington, DC: U.S. Department of Health and Human Services, 2010).

2. A. Ross and S. Thomas, "The Health Benefits of Yoga and Exercise: A Review of Comparison Studies," *Journal of Alternative and Complementary Medicine* 16, no. 1 (2010): 3–12.

3. American Holistic Nurses Association and American Nurses Association, *Holistic Nursing: Scope and Standards of Practice*, 2nd ed. (Silver Spring, MD: Nursesbooks.org, 2013).

4. J. S. Prager and J. Acosta, *Verbal First Aid: Help Your Kids Heal from Fear and Pain—and Come Out Strong* (New York: Berkley, 2010).

5. M. Gleeson, N. Bishop, D. Stensel, M. Lindley, S. Mastana, and M. Nimmo, "The Anti-Inflammatory Effects of Exercise: Mechanisms and Implications for the Prevention and Treatment of Disease," *Nature Review Immunology* 11 (2011): 607–615.

6. T. Landmark, P. Romundstat, P. Borchgrevink, S. Kaasa, and O. Dale, "Longitudinal Associations Between Exercise and Pain in the General Population—The HUNT Pain Study," *Public Library of Science* 8, no. 6 (2013): 1–6.

7. C. Ling and T. Rönn, "Epigenetic Adaptation to Regular Exercise in Humans," *Drug Discovery Today* 19, no. 7 (2014): 1015–1018.

8. D. C. Nieman, D. A. Henson, M. D. Austin, and W. Sha, "Upper Respiratory Tract Infection Is Reduced in Physically Fit and Active Adults," *British Journal of Sports Medicine* 45, no. 12 (2010): 987–992.

9. T. Field, "Yoga Clinical Research Review," *Complementary Therapies in Clinical Practice* 17, no. 1 (2011): 1–8.

10. J. S. Larson and M. Winn, "Health Policy and Exercise: A Brief BRFSS Study and Recommendations," *Health Promotion Practice* 11, no. 2 (2010): 268–274.

11. P. M. Barnes and C. A. Schoenborn, "Trends in Adults Receiving a Recommendation for Exercise or Other Physical Activity from a Physician or Other Health Professional," *NCHS Statistics Data Brief No. 86* (February 2012). www.cdc.gov /nchs/data/databriefs/db86.htm.

12. R. Grant, J. Schmittdiel, R. Neugebauer, C. Uratsu, and B. Sternfeld, "Exercise as a Vital Sign: A Quasi-Experimental Analysis of a Health System Intervention to Collect Patient-Reported Exercise Levels," *Journal of General Internal Medicine* 29, no. 2 (2013): 341–348.

13. S. Jackson, R. Beeken, and J. Wardle, "Perceived Weight Discrimination and Changes in Weight, Waist Circumference, and Weight Status," *Obesity* 22, no. 12 (2014): 2485–2488.

14. Centers for Disease Control and Prevention, "Adult Obesity Facts" (2012). www.cdc.gov /obesity/data/adult.html.

15. C. M. Becker, M. A. Glascoff, and W. M. Felts, "Salutogenesis 30 Years Later: Where Do We Go from Here?" *International Electronic Journal of Health Education* 13 (2010): 25–32.

16. G. Reynolds, *The First 20 Minutes: Surprising Science Reveals How We Can Exercise Better, Train Smarter, Live Longer* (New York: Hudson Street Press, 2012).

17. K. A. Brooks and J. G. Carter, "Overtraining, Exercise, and Adrenal Insufficiency," *Journal of Novel Physiotherapies* 16, no. 3 (2012): 1–8.

18. E. Landolfi, "Exercise Addictions," *Sports Medicine* 43, no. 2 (2013): 111–119.

19. D. Carney, A. Cuddy, and A. Yap, "Power Posing: Brief Nonverbal Displays Affect Neuroendocrine Levels and Risk Tolerance," *Psychological Science* 21, no. 10 (2010): 1363–1368.

20. R. Barakat, C. Pelaez, R. Montjo, and J. Coteron, "Exercise During Pregnancy Reduces the Rate of Cesarean and Instrumental Deliveries: Results of a Randomized Controlled Trial," *Journal of Maternal-Fetal and Neonatal Medicine* 25, no. 11 (2012): 2372–2376.

21. S. Guendelman, M. Pearl, J. Kosa, S. Graham, B. Abrams, and M. Kharrazi, "Association Between Preterm Delivery and Pre-Pregnancy Body Mass (BMI), Exercise and Sleep During Pregnancy Among Working Women in Southern California," *Maternal Child Health Journal* 17, no. 4 (2013): 723–731.

22. R. Barakat, M. Pelaez, C. Lopez, A. Lucia, and J. Ruiz, "Exercise During Pregnancy and Gestational Diabetes-Related Adverse Effects: A Randomized, Controlled Trial," *British Journal of Sports Medicine* 47, no. 10 (2013): 630–636.

23. J. Bainbridge, "Weight Gain During Pregnancy Linked to Childhood Obesity," *British Journal of Midwifery* 22, no. 1 (2014): 66–67.

24. A. Gaston and H. Prapavessis, "Tired, Moody and Pregnant? Exercise May Be the Answer," *Psychology and Health* 28, no. 12 (2013): 1353–1369.

25. K. Fieril, M. Olsen, A. Glantz, and M. Larsson, "Experiences of Exercise During Pregnancy Among Women Who Perform Regular Resistance Training: A Qualitative Study," *Physical Therapy* 94, no. 8 (2014): 1135–1143.

26. S. Srinivasan, L. Pescatello, and A. Bhat, "Current Perspectives on Physical Activity and Exercise Recommendations for Children and Adolescents with Autism Spectrum Disorders," *Physical Therapy* 94, no. 6 (2014): 875–889.

27. N. Steiner, T. Sidhu, P. Pop, E. Frenette, and E. Perrin, "Yoga in an Urban School for Children with Emotional and Behavioral Disorders: A Feasibility Study," *Journal of Child and Family Studies* 22, no. 6 (2013): 815–826.

28. W. Kemmler and S. von Stengel, "Exercise Frequency, Health Risk Factors, and Diseases of the Elderly," *Archives of Physical Medicine and Rehabilitation* 94, no. 11 (2013): 2046–2053.

29. M. Mador, M. Krauza, and M. Shaffer, "Effect of Exercise Training in Patients with Chronic Obstructive Pulmonary Disease Compared with Healthy Subjects," *Journal of Cardiopulmonary Rehabilitation and Prevention* 32, no. 3 (2012): 155–162.

30. H. Ikeda, F. Ishizaki, M. Shiokawa, S. Aoi, T. Iida, C. Chiho, N. Tamura, et al., "Correlations Between Walking Exercise and Each of Bone Density, Muscle Volume, Fluctuation of the Center of Gravity, and Dementia in Middle-Aged and Elderly Women," *International Medical Journal* 19, no. 2 (2012): 154–157.

31. J. Kloubec, M. Rozga, and M. Block, "Balance Improvement in Independent-Living Elderly Adults Following a 12-Week Structured Exercise Program," *Activities, Adaptation and Aging* 36, no. 2 (2012): 167–178.

32. M. Hasegawa, S. Yamazaki, M. Kimura, K. Nakano, and S. Yasumura, "Community-Based Exercise Program Reduces Chronic Knee Pain in Elderly Japanese Women at High Risk of Requiring Long-Term Care: A Non-Randomized Controlled Trial," *Geriatrics and Gerontology International* 13, no. 1 (2013): 167–174.

33. T. Kamegaya, Y. Maki, T. Yamagami, T. Yamaguchi, T. Murai, and H. Yamaguchi, "Pleasant Physical Exercise Program for Prevention of Cognitive Decline in Community-Dwelling Elderly with Subjective Memory Complaints," *Geriatrics and Gerontology International* 12, no. 4 (2012): 673–679.

34. K. Sung and S. Bae, "Effects of a Regular Walking Exercise Program on Behavioral and Biochemical Aspects in Elderly People with Type II Diabetes," *Nursing and Health Sciences* 14, no. 4 (2012): 438–445.

35. S. Prakhinkit, S. Suppapitiporn, H. Tanaka, and D. Suksom, "Effects of Buddhism Walking Meditation on Depression, Functional Fitness, and Endothelium-Dependent Vasodilation in Depressed Elderly," *Journal of Alternative and Complementary Medicine* 20, no. 5 (2014): 411–416.

36. J. M. Saint Onge and P. M. Krueger, "Education and Racial-Ethnic Differences in Types of Exercise in the United States," *Journal of Health and Social Behavior* 52, no. 2 (2011): 197–211.

37. C. Michaels and A. Greene, "Worksite Wellness: Increasing Adoption of Workplace Health Promotion Programs," *Health Promotion Practice* 14, no. 4 (2013): 473–479.

38. A. Osiecki, R. Osiecki, L. Timossi, L. Rossetin, T. Machado, S. Góes, and N. Leite, "Effects of Workplace Based Exercises on the Lipid Profile, Systemic Blood Pressure, and Body Fat of Female Workers," *Journal of Exercise Physiology* 16, no. 3 (2013): 69–75.

39. I. Groeneveld, A. de Boer, and M. Frings-Dresen, "Physical Exercise and Return to Work: Cancer Survivors' Experiences," *Journal of Cancer Survivorship* 7, no. 2 (2013): 237–246.

40. L. Andersen, "Influence of Psychosocial Work Environment on Adherence to Workplace Exercise," *Journal of Occupational and Environmental Medicine* 53, no. 2 (2011): 182–184.

41. R. Wolever, K. Bobinet, K. McCabe, L. MacKenzie, E. Fekete, C. Kusnick, and M. Baime, "Effective and Viable Mind-Body Stress Reduction in the Workplace: Two RCTs," *BMC Complementary and Alternative Medicine* 12, Suppl 1 (2012): 87.

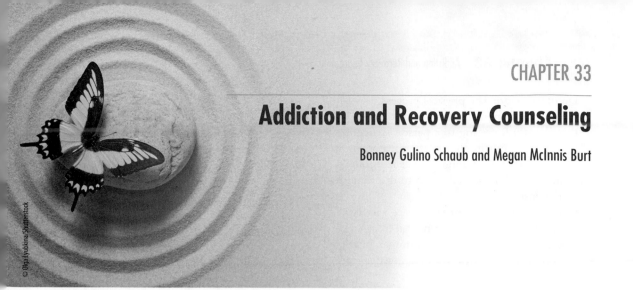

CHAPTER 33

Addiction and Recovery Counseling

Bonney Gulino Schaub and Megan McInnis Burt

Nurse Healer Objectives

Theoretical

- Discuss the factors leading to addiction.
- Identify patterns of thinking and behavior associated with addictions.
- Identify the reasons that spiritual development is important in long-term recovery.

Clinical

- Develop skills in assessing clients' relationships to drugs, alcohol, and addictive patterns of behavior.
- Learn to recognize the patterns of denial that perpetuate and protect addictive behaviors.
- Become knowledgeable about the long-term issues in recovery and relapse prevention.
- Identify support systems within the community for the person in recovery, such as support groups, psychotherapists knowledgeable about issues in recovery, meditation or prayer groups, and other resources for spiritual development.

Personal

- Take the self-assessment about problem drinking (Exhibit 33-4) and determine if drinking is a problem in your life.
- Assess your responses to stress from the perspective of addictive patterns of behavior (e.g., alcohol or drug use, smoking, excessive sugar consumption), and learn more effective stress management strategies.
- Recognize your own feelings of vulnerability and your characteristic responses to these feelings.
- Assess your environment, and determine whether there are any people with addictions in your personal or work life; notice whether you have any patterns of denial and enabling in relating to them.

Definitions

Addiction: A physiologic or psychological dependence on a substance (e.g., alcohol, cocaine) or behavior (e.g., gambling, sex, eating).

Alcohol use disorder (AUD): A wide spectrum of negative patterns of alcohol use that includes emotional and psychological dependence, binge drinking, excessive consumption, and physical addiction. Men consuming on average more than 15 drinks a week and women more than 8 are considered at risk for negative effects from alcohol.

Denial: A major dynamic in the process of addiction in which the person willfully refuses to accept the reality of his or her behavior and its effect on self and others.

Detoxification: The physical process of withdrawing from using drugs or alcohol.

Dry drunk: Referring to a person struggling with alcoholism, *dry* means the person is not currently drinking but has maintained all of the attitudes that led to drinking in the past.

Entheogenic substances: A wide variety of substances that have been used in ceremonies and rituals throughout human history and many cultures to evoke mystical and spiritual experiences.

New consciousness: A concept used in Alcoholics Anonymous that refers to a movement away from addictive thinking and toward an understanding of one's life purpose or spiritual purpose.

Psychosynthesis: The developmental and transpersonal psychology of Roberto Assagioli.[1,2]

Recovery: The mental, emotional, physical, and spiritual actions that support conscious living and freedom from addictive behaviors.

Relapse: A return to addictive behavior.

Smart drugs: Stimulant drugs such as Ritalin, Dexedrine, and Adderal that are used because they are believed to improve mental function by increasing working memory, motivation, and attention; referred to as nootropic drugs.

Spiritual awakening: An expansion of awareness that results in a realization that the isolated individual is, in fact, participating in a universe of divine intention and order.

Substance use disorder (SUD): The continued use of one or more substances such as alcohol, cigarettes, or other nonmedically indicated drugs. This term is currently used as an alternative to substance abuse.

Transpersonal development: The words *transpersonal* and *spiritual* are used interchangeably in this chapter. Transpersonal development involves cultivation of the human resources of peace, wisdom, purpose, and oneness.

Transpersonal experiences: Direct personal experiences of inner peace and wisdom and connecting with a deeper sense of purpose and oneness.

Theory and Research

Drug misuse and addiction have negative consequences for individuals and for society. Estimates of the total overall costs of substance misuse in the United States, including health, productivity, and crime-related costs, exceed $600 billion annually. This includes approximately $181 billion for illicit drugs, $193 billion for tobacco, and $235 billion for alcohol. Almost 60% of this cost is borne by the government and other members of society, with almost 70% of it attributable to loss of productivity. As staggering as these numbers are, they do not fully describe the breadth of destructive public health and safety implications of drug misuse and addiction. Excessive drinking can lead to a broad range of health problems including heart disease; sexually transmitted diseases; fetal alcohol spectrum disorder; sudden infant death syndrome; cancers such as breast, head and neck, and liver; and unintended pregnancy. In addition, it contributes to family disintegration, loss of employment, failure in school, domestic violence, and child abuse. It is generally accepted that chemical dependency, along with associated mental health disorders, has become one of the most severe health and social problems facing the United States.[3,4]

It is estimated that 38 million adults in the United States drink excessively, resulting in about 88,000 deaths a year. It is significant to note that research shows that only 1 in 6 patients are asked about their alcohol use by their primary healthcare provider. Alcohol screening and brief counseling have been proven to be effective, reducing the amount that a person consumes by 25%. It is recommended that it be a part of routine screening as is blood pressure, cholesterol, and breast cancer. The Affordable Care Act requires that new health insurance plans cover this service without a copayment.[5]

There are three simple screening tools that are recognized by the National Institute on Alcohol Abuse and Alcoholism (NIAAA) that are readily available online. The first is referred to as AUDIT (Alcohol Use Disorder Identification Test). The others are known by their acronyms, CAGE and T-ACE. These screening tools can be obtained at the NIAAA website.[6]

It is important to note that these screening tools look at a spectrum of substance use/misuse behaviors, not just addiction. For instance, binge drinking may be overlooked if the screening is only evaluating the daily use of a substance that is considered an aspect of addiction. The National Institutes of Health developed a helpful, free booklet, *Rethinking Drinking: Alcohol and Your Health*, that is available electronically.[7] These tools and guidelines are also relevant to other kinds of substance use/misuse.

It is estimated that more than 28 million children are living in homes with adults who have alcohol use disorders.[8,9] Children raised in homes with substance-abusing parents are at increased risk for chronic anxiety disorders and social phobias as well as increased risk for their own substance misuse.[10] In the United States in 2008, almost one-third of adolescents aged 12 to 17 drank alcohol in the past year, around one-fifth used an illicit drug, and almost one-sixth smoked cigarettes. Caffeine is a widely used psychoactive substance that is legal, easy to obtain, and socially acceptable to consume. Although once relatively restricted to use among adults, caffeine-containing drinks are now consumed regularly by children. Children and adolescents are the fastest growing population of caffeine users, with an increase of 70% in the past 30 years. Energy drinks sales have grown by more than 50% since 2005 and represent the fastest growing segment of the beverage industry.[11]

Because of the prevalence of alcoholism and other addictions, nurses in every practice setting inevitably will work with individuals who are addicted, who are in recovery, or whose lives are affected by the addiction of a friend or family member.

Addiction Defined

Alcoholics Anonymous (AA), in its basic book (referred to by people in AA as the "Big Book"), describes alcoholism as a "mental obsession and a physical compulsion."[12] This description of a pattern of thinking and behaving applies to many things besides alcohol, most obviously the use of other substances such as cocaine, heroin, methamphetamine, and marijuana. The elements of obsession and compulsion are evident in the actions of people with unhealthy relationships to food, exercise, work, gambling, Internet and smartphone use, television viewing, shopping, sexual behaviors (including compulsive use of pornography), and other activities. Recent studies show that the use of tanning beds can be addictive. Researchers proposed that tanning beds that emit ultraviolet rays caused a release of cutaneous endorphins that created a sense of well-being in the tanner. When opioid antagonists were administered this feeling was blocked.[13] Indoor tanning is seen as a common adolescent risk behavior, and the mood-altering effect of the ultraviolet rays is a factor that motivates maintenance of the behavior.[14]

Certain elements distinguish the process of addiction from the healthy or recreational use of any of these substances or behaviors. The key difference is in the individual's relationship to the substance or behavior. In the addictive process, the element of choice is absent. A woman no longer chooses to relax with a glass of wine at a dinner party—she goes to the party because it is an opportunity to drink a great deal. A man no longer enjoys watching a sporting event—he watches it only because he has a bet on it. A young college student takes up running to lose weight and feels compelled to go for a run despite her knee injury because she will be depressed and obsessing about her weight without a run of at least 5 miles a day. In other words, the mental obsession has overruled the ability to reflect on behavior and has bypassed any self-awareness that could lead to alternative behaviors. These addictive behaviors often coexist with various forms of substance misuse. The addictive use of any of these activities serves the same purpose as alcohol or drugs: The person is seeking relief and distraction from painful, unsafe, and vulnerable feelings.

The Cycle of Addiction

All addictions have a basic cycle. Understanding this cycle makes it possible to understand the specific kinds of help that a person with an addiction needs to facilitate the healing process. In the early stage of addiction, people use a substance or substances or activity as a means of changing unsafe or vulnerable feelings. Some commonly heard descriptions of these vulnerable feelings include, "I feel like I don't have any skin," "Everything gets to me," and "Everything is just too much." Typically, there are physical signs of anxiety such as lightheadedness, palpitations, painful levels of self-consciousness and social discomfort, and generally heightened degrees of agitation or irritability.

Vulnerability is a normal human emotion that everyone has experienced, but the person vulnerable to addictive behaviors feels it more intensely and more frequently. Characteristics such as low frustration tolerance, low pain threshold, and a need for instant gratification go along with this vulnerability. These characteristics present challenges for nurses when caring for addicted clients.

Most people who have become addicted to a substance have a vivid memory of their first experience of relief from the feelings of discomfort as a result of using the substance. This first encounter typically occurs in early adolescence, a time of normal emotional turmoil and struggle for social identity and acceptance. Use of the substance may have alleviated social anxiety or the pain of family conflicts. The incidence of substance misuse is high among young people in conflict about their sexual identity because they often lack support and positive role models in their life. For some young people, sharing drugs or alcohol becomes a way of being accepted into a peer group and it changes the feeling that they do not feel that they "fit in." Thus, the stage is set for dependence and progression to addiction. The process of building emotional and social skills, which is a major developmental task of adolescence, stops because an instant solution has been found. Picking up where they have left off in this process of emotional and social skill building is one of the major challenges for people in recovery.

The Early Stage of the Addictive Cycle

In the early stage of addiction, a person has some awareness of seeking relief from discomfort. It may simply be an awareness of feeling stressed, anxious, or self-conscious. The following is a typical progression of feelings and responses in the early stage of addiction:[15, p. 5]

1. Unsafe feelings
2. Mental focus on the feelings
3. A desire to get rid of the feelings
4. The use of chemicals to get rid of the feelings
5. Nervous system disturbance caused by the chemicals
6. The return of unsafe feelings

The Middle Stage of the Addictive Cycle

In the middle stage of addiction, the unsafe feeling is not experienced as a thought. It is experienced only as danger or discomfort. The person knows that immediate relief comes with use of the substance. The following is the typical progression and recurring pattern in the middle stage of addiction:[15, p. 8]

1. Unsafe feelings
2. The use of chemicals to get rid of the feelings
3. Nervous system disturbance caused by the chemicals
4. Unsafe feelings

The Late Stage of the Addictive Cycle

People in the depths of addiction rarely talk about feeling high. The need is more frequently described as a desire to feel "normal." The impulse is to escape a feeling that is intolerable. At the late stage of addiction, physical instability replaces the emotional vulnerability. The addiction has come full circle. What was initially used as an answer to unsafe feelings has become the source of unsafe feelings. Mental instability and confusion, mental terrors and paranoia, and hallucinations or feelings of unreality are all possible results of the neurological damage from the substances. The following is the recurring pattern of the late stage of addiction:[15, p. 11]

1. Nervous system disturbance
2. The use of chemicals
3. The return of nervous system disturbance

Models of Addiction

Many models have been put forth to explain why a person develops an addiction. Any nurse who has worked with addicted patients can recognize recurring themes such as familial and environmental patterns of addiction or early childhood trauma and loss. Clearly, addiction defies simple explanation. Each of these models offers a piece of a complex puzzle.

Medical Model

In the medical model, the emphasis is on the physiologic effect of the substance itself. The body's tolerance for the drug leads to the need for greater and greater amounts to achieve the desired effect, which results in addiction. The absence of the drug leads to cravings, and then to a withdrawal or abstinence syndrome characterized by symptoms such as fever, nausea, seizures, chills, hallucinations, and delirium tremens. In this model, the progression toward addiction is a property of the drug's effect. Those in the media often demonstrate this attitude toward addiction when they describe a celebrity who has attended a 30-day alcohol or drug rehabilitation program as "free" of drugs. In fact, 30 days is just the beginning of treatment. Most drugs of misuse directly or indirectly target the brain's reward system by flooding the circuit with dopamine. Dopamine is a neurotransmitter present in regions of the brain that regulate movement, emotion, cognition, motivation, and feelings of pleasure. The overstimulation of this system, which rewards our natural behaviors, produces the euphoric effects sought by people who misuse drugs and teaches them to repeat the behavior.

Genetic Disease Model

In this model, addiction is a chronic, often relapsing brain disease that causes compulsive drug seeking and use, despite harmful consequences to the addicted individual and to those around him or her. Although the initial decision to take drugs is voluntary for most people, the brain changes that occur over time challenge a person's self-control and ability to resist intense impulses, urging him or her to take drugs.

It can be wrongfully assumed that drug misusers lack moral principles or willpower and that they could stop using drugs simply by choosing to change their behavior. In reality, drug addiction is a complex disease, and quitting takes more than good intentions. In fact, because drugs change the brain in ways that foster compulsive drug misuse, quitting is difficult, even for those who are ready to do so.

Much research points to strong patterns of alcoholism within biologically linked families. For example, adoption studies show a three times greater incidence of alcoholism in children of alcoholics, even if they have been raised in a nonalcoholic family.[16] The possibility that genetics plays a role in a greater vulnerability to addiction in some individuals aligns with the idea that differences in brain biochemistry are a factor in being susceptible to addiction.

The emerging field of epigenetics is further advancing our understanding of the role of genetics in addictions. Epigenetics is the study of changes in the regulation of gene expression and gene activity. The field of epigenetics studies how the development, functioning, and evolution of biological systems are influenced by forces operating outside the DNA sequence, such as environmental and energetic influences. Studies indicate that there is an alteration in gene expression by repeated substance misuse that can produce lasting changes in gene expression within the reward pathways of the brain. Drugs of misuse such as cocaine trigger epigenetic changes in certain brain regions, affecting hundreds of genes at a time. Some of these changes remain long after the drug has been cleared from the system. Research in this area suggests that some of the long-term effects of drug misuse and addiction (including high rates of relapse) may be written in epigenetic code. Insights into the long-lasting gene adaptations that underlie the chronic relapsing nature of addiction are on the cutting edge of research and have implications for new treatments.[17-19]

Dysfunctional Family System Model

The frequent appearance of addictions within the families of addicts may indicate that substance misuse can be a learned behavior. In effect, children learn by daily close observation of the adults in their environment that conflicts and stressors are to be dealt with by using drugs and alcohol. Children usually do not have a conscious awareness of this message. They may not have a full understanding of the role that addiction played in their home life until they reach adulthood and begin their own recovery. It is important to acknowledge that many other people who have grown up in such an environment are aware of the damage done and make a conscious choice to abstain from alcohol or other substances.

Self-Medication Model

According to the self-medication model, the addict has an underlying psychiatric disorder and is, in effect, self-prescribing to alleviate symptoms. For example, in a Canadian survey of more than 14,000 residents aged 18 to 76, there was a significantly greater use of alcohol among those who were suffering from depression.[20] Addicts characteristically have tried a variety of substances and have found that they have a strong preference for a particular category of drug and drug effect. It is not unusual for addicts to say that their preferred substance makes them feel "normal."

Significant vulnerability to substance use disorders is present in those suffering from posttraumatic stress disorder (PTSD). Returning veterans who have been receiving pain medication for physical injuries are particularly vulnerable. Other vulnerable PTSD survivors are those suffering the depression, anxiety, and emotional devastation of childhood violence and sexual abuse as well as other experiences of violence.[9,21-23]

Psychosexual, Psychoanalytic Model

Emerging from Freud's conceptualization of psychosexual stages of development, addiction appears to be a fixation at the oral stage of development. In the psychosexual, psychoanalytic model, an infant or child whose basic needs are unmet becomes focused on seeking gratification of those unmet needs. Emotional development becomes fixated at the age of this early trauma.[15, p. 23]

Oral gratification is the most basic need of the infant, as seen in the way an infant receives nourishment and pleasure through sucking. In adulthood, people continue to seek comfort and pleasure from gratification of oral needs through behaviors such as eating, smoking, talking, touching their mouth, and various chewing behaviors. Whereas healthy human activity includes some limited seeking of oral gratification, the addict is fixated at this developmental phase. The compelling need for comfort derived

from oral gratification then becomes focused on the consumption of substances.

Ego Psychology Model

Also emerging from Freudian theory, ego psychology suggests that when an infant's or child's environment does not provide an adequate degree of nurturance and acknowledgment, the child grows into adulthood with an impaired sense of self. This results in feelings of emptiness and hypersensitivity that lead to a self-absorbed and narcissistic relationship with the world. The addict's behaviors are then seen as self-soothing attempts to relieve the basic feelings of emptiness.[15, p. 24]

Cultural Model

Our culture may be a contributing factor in addiction because it teaches us to seek materialistic answers outside ourselves to experience well-being. People in the United States are confronted with a relentless message of consumerism and quick fixes. This then leads to a society of consumers with impulse disorders who seek instant gratification and believe that there is a pill for every ill.

In recent years, media advertising has bombarded people with messages about both over-the-counter and prescription medications. In light of this, it is interesting to note the following information. The total number of drug-related emergency department (ED) visits increased 81% from 2004 (2.5 million) to 2009 (4.6 million). The ED visits involving nonmedical use of pharmaceuticals increased 98.4% over the same period, from 627,291 visits to 1,244,679. The largest pharmaceutical increases were observed for oxycodone products (242.2% increase), alprazolam (148.3% increase), and hydrocodone products (124.5% increase). Among ED visits involving illicit drugs, only those involving Ecstasy increased more than 100% from 2004 to 2009 (123.2% increase). For patients aged 20 or younger, ED visits resulting from nonmedical use of pharmaceuticals increased 45.4% between 2004 and 2009 (116,644 and 169,589 visits, respectively). Among patients aged 21 or older, there was an increase of 111.0%.[24,25] In the United States in 2012, healthcare providers prescribed

259 million prescriptions for painkillers, enough for every adult to have a bottle of pills. This is more than twice as many pills per person as is prescribed in Canada.[5]

Another area of increasing substance misuse is seen in the use of stimulants by students. Approximately 30% of middle school and high school students have stimulants prescribed to them. There is a selective use of stimulants only during the school year with a significant decrease during the summer. Socioeconomically advantaged children are more likely to be receiving these prescriptions. This difference along socioeconomic status persists when studying children seeing the same healthcare provider. This practice is most evident in states with the highest level of academic accountability.[26]

The use of these drugs for neuroenhancement (NE) extends beyond compliance with prescriptions, resulting in the availability of "smart drugs" to share with or sell to fellow students. Nonmedical prescription stimulants are widely used in the United States, but usage is higher at colleges in the northeastern United States and at schools with higher admissions standards. In a study in Germany where more than 1,300 college students were screened, the primary motive for use was for improving concentration (55%) and increasing vigilance (49%). The primary motivation given for NE use was high levels of stress and large academic workload. In both the United States and Germany, students using substances for NE were more likely to use marijuana, Ecstasy, cocaine, and cigarettes and to indulge in other risky behaviors.[27]

In considering this profile of student substance misusers, we can identify strong cultural elements: (1) the tremendous pressure on students within some communities to excel in school and to succeed academically and professionally, and (2) the peer pressure in schools to fit in and be accepted. These elements contribute to the substance misuse behaviors regardless of their dangers.[28]

Group support is an important element in the recovery process, whether it is through involvement in AA, other 12-step programs, or group support through a treatment program. It is particularly challenging for young students who

are in recovery when they go to college and live on campus. This is a vulnerable time for most young people because it is a time of questioning identity and learning how to fit in to a new peer group and community. Some schools have established "chemical free" dorms to provide a healthy, supportive environment, one that is open not only to students in recovery but also to those wanting to be in a healthier environment.[29]

There is also an increased awareness of substance misuse among athletes. Their primary misuse is of "recreational" drugs such as cocaine and alcohol. There is a significant increase in the use of performance-enhancing (i.e., ergogenic) drugs such as amphetamines, as well as "designer" stimulants such as Ecstasy (i.e., methylenedioxymethamphetamine, or MDMA). Two readily available drugs that mimic amphetamine when taken in high doses are pseudoephedrine, available in cold medications, and ephedrine marketed as a dietary supplement. Anabolic steroids and other drugs are taken in an attempt to enhance performance and build muscle mass. In addition, human growth hormone precursors are marketed in various forms, promising increased muscle mass, heightened energy, and performance enhancement.[30] This is another situation in which to consider the role of the media and other cultural influences in the patterns of misuse and choice of substances.

Character Defect Model of AA

Alcoholics and other addicts are seen as having different characters and morals from nonaddicts in the character defect model of AA. Although the idea of a "moral" defect is not used extensively in addiction treatment settings, it is a concept that pervades the AA literature. Those in recovery may explain their "character defect" as the reason for their difficulty in making behavioral and attitudinal changes.

Trance Model

Derived from learning theory and the principles of hypnosis, the trance model proposes that the memory of the intense pleasure experienced in response to a substance is never forgotten. The experience is recorded by the pleasure-seeking, pain-avoiding part of the brain and remains, in effect, a deeply planted, posthypnotic suggestion that repeatedly seeks expression. The addict essentially falls in love with the feelings that the addictive behaviors produced. The AA literature speaks to this idea in stating,

> The urge to repeat the experience of becoming "high" is so strong that we will forsake . . . our responsibilities and values, . . . our families, our jobs, our personal welfare, our respect, and our integrity . . . to satisfy the urge.[31]

Transpersonal Intoxication Model

According to the transpersonal intoxication model, the desire to break free of a limited, time-bound, socially defined sense of self as well as the desire to expand consciousness are the driving forces in addiction. Many people have experimented with lysergic acid diethylamide (LSD), marijuana, psilocybin mushrooms, peyote cactus, and other psychedelic substances and have experienced expanded states of awareness that have resulted in spiritual and creative breakthroughs. The challenge, then, is to integrate these insights into daily life.

Throughout human history people have used hallucinogenic and consciousness altering substances to produce mystical and visionary experiences. They have been used as sacraments in the context of spiritual and religious rituals and ceremonies. These substances are called *entheogens*, meaning bringing forth the god within. In the 1960s, there was a counterculture that promoted substances such as psilocybin and other mushrooms, peyote, and LSD.

Currently, there is a resurgence of interest in psychoactive drugs. The desire for a "spiritual awakening of self-awareness and liberation" was identified as a motivator in a study of the users of two drugs popularly made available at dance parties, ketamine and Ecstasy.[32]

There is a significant degree of substance misuse and addiction among artists, writers, performers, and musicians. This model suggests that their desire to break free of mental and emotional limitations is at the heart of their substance use. One part of the artistic process is about finding a way to express the most intimate, subtle, personal, and spiritual aspects of human experience. Artists often mention a fear of losing this creative capacity—of becoming "ordinary"—as they enter recovery. They have given the creative power to the substance rather than trusting that it resides within themselves. The ability to practice their creative endeavor while sober then becomes a major milestone in the recovery process.

Transpersonal–Existential Model

In the transpersonal–existential model, the human condition is such that humans are inherently anxious because they have knowledge of their mortality. Psychiatrist Aaron Beck, the renowned innovator in the development of cognitive therapy, views fear of death as the cause of all anxiety disorders, including generalized anxiety disorder, panic disorder, obsessive-compulsive disorder, and phobias.[33] However, during intense vulnerability, even death itself (the imagined end of all feeling) can be desired over the continuation of the vulnerability. This perspective helps us understand the extreme self-destructive behaviors that can be observed in many individuals lost in their addictions.

Everyone finds ways to bypass or deny this awareness of reality. Ernest Becker, in a book authored when he was dying of cancer, wrote that a person

> has to protect himself against the world, and he can do this only as any other animal would—by . . . shutting off experience and developing an obliviousness both to the terrors of the world and to his own anxieties. Otherwise he would be crippled for action . . . some people have more trouble with their lies than others. The world is too much with them.[34]

This heightened awareness and sensitivity to the human condition can lead to addiction as a solution to the existential pain.

Vulnerability Model of Recovery from Addiction

A model of the recovery process that resonates with a holistic nursing perspective is the Vulnerability Model of Recovery. This model honors the biological, emotional, social, familial, neurochemical, and spiritual aspects of addiction. It focuses on the lived experience of the addict, which is that of essential vulnerability. The model points to specific ways that the holistic nurse can facilitate the healing journey of full bio-psycho-social-spiritual recovery. The basic points are presented in **Exhibit 33-1**.

Recognition of Addiction

Given the prevalence of alcoholism and other addictions, it can be assumed that nurses in every clinical area are working with people whose lives are affected by this problem—even when the issue is never directly addressed. Therefore, it is essential that all nurses become skilled in assessing

the possibility of addiction, as well as recognizing the risk factors and behaviors suggestive of substance misuse. Nurses must first examine any preconceived notions that they may have about what an addict or alcoholic looks like. Addiction is a problem that occurs in every profession, in every educational and socioeconomic group, in every ethnic group, and in every age group from early adolescence through senescence.

Fifty percent of patients admitted to trauma centers are intoxicated with alcohol. Studies have shown that alcohol interventions initiated in these settings result in a 50% reduction in reinjury rates and a 66% reduction of drunk driving arrests. In addition, introducing alcohol intervention is extremely cost effective, saving $4 for every dollar spent.[35]

EXHIBIT 33-1   The Vulnerability Model of Recovery

- Addiction is a repetitive, maladaptive, avoidant, substitutive process of getting rid of vulnerability.

- This addictive process is triggered by an experience of vulnerability that is believed to be intolerable.

- Vulnerability is anxiety ultimately rooted in the human condition of being conscious, separate, and mortal. As such, this vulnerability is a normal emotion and an elemental aspect of our actual human situation.

- People who have a greater degree of vulnerability (explanations for which include genetic, biochemical, characterological, familial, cultural, and spiritual) have a greater degree of need to get rid of it.

- Getting rid of vulnerability is accomplished by trying to feel powerful or by trying to feel numb. Trying to feel powerful is an act of willfulness. Trying to feel numb is an act of will-lessness. Drugs are selected to help produce these results. Trying to feel powerful and trying to feel numb are both choices. Made repeatedly, they become addictive, producing predictable but brief episodes of relief from vulnerability.

- People in recovery from addiction begin to heal their feelings by recognizing and respecting their vulnerability.

- Continued recovery is based on developing new, nonavoidant responses to vulnerability.

- However, this vulnerability cannot be effectively addressed on a long-term basis by the separate, ego-level, temporary sense of self because it is that sense of self that is at the very root of the vulnerability.

- Advanced recovery therefore requires the development of an expanded sense of self that is communal and spiritual in awareness. Such spiritual development is a normal aspect of adult development, despite the fact that it is ignored by most Western psychology.

- Communal awareness is provided by Alcoholics Anonymous and other 12-step programs through fellowship and service to others in recovery. Spiritual awareness requires development, which has been studied by the world's wisdom traditions and, more recently, by transpersonal psychology.

- Many people in recovery do not experience spiritual awareness because this aspect of human nature has been neglected and poorly understood in modern culture. Pioneering transpersonal psychiatrist Roberto Assagioli referred to this issue as "repression of the sublime."

- Transpersonal approaches offer insights and practices that can lift repression of the sublime, energize spiritual awareness and increase inner peace, and work at the deepest root of the addictive process.

Source: Reproduced by permission. Healing Addictions by Schaub and Schaub. Delmar Publishers, Albany, NY. 1997.

The most challenging, and potentially frustrating, aspect of working with people at the stage of active addiction is their pervasive denial of the problem, even when confronted with blatant evidence of their addiction. Alcoholics Anonymous uses the phrase "self-will run riot" in describing this behavior. It is the key obstacle to entering into the healing process of recovery. See **Exhibit 33-2** for definitions of denial.

The addict's loyalty to the substance is profound. It surpasses loyalty to family and friends and is the cause of the addict's manipulations. The nurse should not personalize these manipulations. Attempts to be of help often meet outright rejection or failure. The root of the addict's behaviors is an intense fear of living without the mood-altering effects of the alcohol or drugs. The behaviors are attempts to control the world and avoid painful feelings. The first step of recovery is relinquishing this control effort and admitting to oneself and others that the addictive process is not working, that it is actually making everything worse, that he or she does not know what to do, and that he or she must learn a new way to be in the world. This new way means a change in attitude to recognize that people who want to help stop the addictive behaviors are acting from a place of caring.

Detoxification

The simplest, most straightforward aspect of the recovery process is detoxification. When medical management of detoxification is necessary, brief inpatient or outpatient treatment is available in many hospitals and addiction treatment centers. Auricular acupuncture has been successfully used in detoxifying people from alcohol, heroin, nicotine, and other drugs. Its use was pioneered in New York City in the 1970s by Dr. Michael O. Smith. In recent years, it has gained wider acceptance and has been found to be an effective, natural treatment that is simple, safe, and inexpensive by improving patient outcomes in terms of program retention and reductions in cravings, anxiety, sleep disturbance, and need for pharmaceuticals.[36,37]

Alcoholics Anonymous

With its 12-step, self-help treatment approach, AA offers one of the most important, effective, and widely accepted interventions in addiction treatment. The 12 steps of Alcoholics Anonymous put forth a systematic progression of actions to take that, when followed, will assist the person in recovery to find a new way to be

---

EXHIBIT 33-2   Definitions of Denial

- Continuous negative behavior in the face of obvious negative physical, emotional, and social consequences, as in "My girlfriend is constantly bugging me and threatening to break up with me because of my drinking. She's really got hang-ups about drinking because her father is an alcoholic."

- Prideful insistence that he or she has control of behaviors that are out of control, as in "I didn't get into that car accident because of the coke. I actually am a better driver when I've done a few lines. It keeps me alert and my reflexes are better."

- A maladaptive strategy for achieving security, as in "I don't really have a problem with alcohol. I just need a few drinks when I get home from work because I work the evening shift. My job is very stressful and it's hard to relax enough to fall asleep."

- The energy used to maintain a destructive lie, as in "I only use drugs because my girlfriend does. I can stop whenever I want."

- A narrowing of awareness to shut out anything that makes the person vulnerable, as in "When I get high I just don't give a damn. All this crap just fades away."

- An unwillingness to experience the feelings the truth provokes, as in "My boss was a total hypocrite. He was always on my case. All the guys have a few beers at lunch time. He fired me because he never liked me."

Source: Reproduced by permission. Healing Addictions by Schaub and Schaub. Delmar Publishers, Albany, NY. 1997.

EXHIBIT 33-3   The 12 Steps of Alcoholics Anonymous

1. We admitted we were powerless over alcohol — that our lives had become unmanageable.
2. Came to believe that a power greater than ourselves could restore us to sanity.
3. Made a decision to turn our will and our lives over to the care of God as we understood Him.
4. Made a searching and fearless moral inventory of ourselves.
5. Admitted to God, to ourselves, and to another human being the exact nature of our wrongs.
6. Were entirely ready to have God remove all these defects of character.
7. Humbly asked Him to remove our shortcomings.
8. Made a list of all persons we had harmed, and became willing to make amends to them all.
9. Made direct amends to such people whenever possible, except when to do so would injure them or others.
10. Continued to take personal inventory, and when we were wrong promptly admitted it.
11. Sought through prayer and meditation to improve our conscious contact with God as we understood Him, praying only for knowledge of His will for us and the power to carry that out.
12. Having had a spiritual awakening as the result of these steps, we tried to carry this message to others, and to practice these principles in all our affairs.

Source: The Twelve Steps are reprinted with permission of Alcoholics Anonymous World Services, Inc. ("AAWS"). Permission to reprint the Twelve Steps does not mean that AAWS has reviewed or approved the contents of this publication, or that AAWS necessarily agrees with the views expressed herein. AA is a program of recovery from alcoholism only - use of the Twelve Steps in connection with programs and activities which are patterned after AA, but which address other problems, or in any other non-AA context, does not imply otherwise.

---

in the world (see **Exhibit 33-3**). Ongoing peer support as well as support for spiritual development were cited as significant factors in the effectiveness of this program.[38–40]

An important element in AA is the practice of providing service to other members of the program by becoming a sponsor. Members who have achieved a strong recovery are encouraged to be available to newer participants to help them in their sobriety. They may attend meetings with the new participant, be available by phone on a regular basis, and generally serve as a role model and guide toward effective use of the program.

Family Awareness

A person in the addictive process has fears about change, and the people closest to him or her usually have fears as well. It is in the nature of the addictive process that the people living and working closest to the person with the addiction have made accommodations to compensate for and cover up the addicted person's behaviors. The nurse who takes on the role of working with a person in recovery will find it necessary to help the people closest to the person change their behavior as well. The individuals in this close circle need to look at their own patterns of enabling the addicted person's behavior and be willing to keep the focus on their own process of growth and change.

Al-Anon is a self-help program for the friends and family members of alcoholics and other substance misusers. Family members, particularly spouses and partners, who have undoubtedly expended much energy in trying to help the addicted person, learn in Al-Anon how to accept their powerlessness to control others. The emphasis of Al-Anon is on reorienting priorities and supporting the group members to focus energy on making positive life changes for themselves.

Early Recovery

Detoxification is the initial step in early recovery, and it is just the beginning of the addicted person's process of making new choices, moment by moment, hour by hour, and day by day. The nurse can help the person in recovery to make healthy choices through intensive questioning of old patterns of substance misuse and other behaviors. This information can then be used to develop new ways of responding. Because behaviors associated with addiction are totally integrated into the person's life, he or she needs help in recognizing them and accepting the fact that they are no longer possible. The following are some important questions for the nurse to ask:

- Where did the addictive behavior take place? Some people stay isolated in their home or car when using drugs, while others prefer social settings such as bars, clubs, or the work environment.
- What special rituals were a part of the addictive behavior? People typically have a routine associated with their substance use. For example, a marijuana misuser may purchase her favorite foods in anticipation of using the substance.
- What locations served as cues for the addictive behavior? For the alcoholic, particular liquor stores or bars may have strong memories and pulls. A particular street sign or exit on the expressway may trigger the desire to go to the neighborhood where drugs were bought and shared.
- What people in the environment were associated with the addictive behavior? The person in recovery may come to realize that everyone he or she knows is associated with the drug use. People in recovery often cannot name a single person they can count on to be drug free. The feeling of loss of family and friends associated with this realization can be profound.

Nutritional Factors

Alcohol has high caloric content, but it is useless as a source of nutrients. Malnutrition is common in alcoholics because they often fail to consume adequate amounts of food. In addition, alcohol interferes with the absorption of vitamins and minerals. Alcoholics typically are deficient in B vitamins, especially thiamine, pyridoxine, and vitamins B_{12} and folate. There is also some evidence that the B vitamin deficiency itself may increase alcohol cravings. There is

an increased risk of developing alcohol-related complications, such as osteopenia/osteoporosis and weakened muscle strength, when malnutrition is present. For this reason, specific screening and a targeted plan of treatment of nutritional deficits is an important component of care in the recovery process.[41] Avoiding caffeine, drinking plenty of water and soothing herbal teas, exercising, and taking warm baths or showers are all helpful during this period when the body is literally releasing and cleansing itself of a build-up of toxins.

Some studies indicate that alcoholics who followed healthy dietary plans that included both nutritional and vitamin supplementation, along with nutrition education, were more successful at maintaining sobriety.[42] The effectiveness of this approach may be attributed not only to the actual physiologic effect of improved nutrition but also to the individual's commitment to making significant lifestyle changes. As stated earlier, recovery is a process of repeatedly choosing healthy, life-affirming actions.

For the recovering alcoholic or other addict, working with a holistic nurse to develop a nutritious eating plan may be an important first step on the path to restoring health. As with any treatment plan, the key to its success depends on compliance. Having a variety of approaches helps to develop personalized care and increases the likelihood of acceptance.

Bodywork and Energy Work

In the early phase of recovery, shortly after cessation of use and resolution of any primary withdrawal symptoms, the person in recovery may experience difficulty sleeping, general agitation, and irritability. Acupuncture has been found to be helpful in the reduction of withdrawal symptoms and in the overall rebalancing of the physical system. Other types of bodywork, such as Reiki, therapeutic touch, massage, and reflexology, can be of help in calming the body. Modalities offering direct physical touch or energy work are of value in the very early stages of recovery.

The energy-based approach of Healing Touch has been effectively used with patients in recovery from alcoholism.[43] The person in recovery from an addiction typically experiences irritability, anxiety, tremors, and weakness, among other symptoms. In addition, there is the stigma associated with addiction that is usually internalized by the person in recovery. Healing Touch is seen as promoting self-healing and integration of mind, body, and spirit. Another innovative practitioner has introduced the use of drumming circles into recovery work. One aspect of this treatment's effectiveness is in creating a sense of connectedness with self and others.[44]

Relapse

A person can achieve abstinence and still not make life changes at the level of emotions and spirit. A person can, in fact, stop drinking and continue to be hostile, rageful, blameful, and irresponsible. These people are controlling their behavior through force of will. Alcoholics Anonymous refers to these individuals as "dry drunks." The person functioning in recovery in this way is at greater risk for relapse.

Relapse is an ongoing issue in every stage of recovery. Many people stop completely without treatment, or with very brief intervention, but others relapse repeatedly. In AA, there is a saying, "The further you are from your last drink, the closer you are to your next." It is helpful to differentiate between someone who very briefly returns to drinking and then returns to abstinence versus someone who resumes heavy drinking. The brief episode is referred to as a lapse rather than a full relapse. This distinction is important to avoid the all-or-nothing, black-and-white thinking that can sabotage the process of recovery.

It is estimated that up to 75% of people in recovery relapse within the first year. It is significant to note that this figure is estimated to be even higher, up to 90%, for women with a history of sexual abuse and trauma. This information points back to the Vulnerability Model. If sexual abuse and trauma caused the unbearable feelings of vulnerability that led to the person's addiction, then abstaining from the substances that served as the emotional anesthesia results in a return of these feelings. It becomes important to connect the painful feelings to the trauma rather than to attribute them all to the absence of the substance. This opens the door to the need for a second recovery process—the treatment and recovery from trauma.[15, p. 75]

Alcoholics Anonymous has a helpful acronym that identifies the times that a person in recovery may be most vulnerable to drinking: HALT. This is shorthand for hungry, angry, lonely, tired. If the person in recovery notices the impulse to drink, it is advised that he or she stop and take the time to determine whether any of these factors are creating this feeling. It is also advised to avoid, whenever possible, letting these situations develop. This simple advice is a very helpful tool for a person in recovery.

Gorski and Miller outline the signs that lead back toward addiction.[45] Nurses can use this list to evaluate a relapse trend in the person's recovery process. Paraphrased from Gorski and Miller, the signs leading to relapse include the following:

- Active denial in many areas of life
- Efforts to convince others of their need for sobriety, referred to in AA as taking someone else's inventory
- Compulsive behaviors
- Impulsive behaviors
- Tendencies toward isolation and bitterness
- Failure to see the big picture
- Idle daydreaming with wishful and magical answers to complex problems
- Helplessness and hopelessness
- An immature wish to be happy always
- Frequent episodes of confusion
- Tendency to judge other people
- Quick anger
- Irregular eating habits
- Listlessness
- Irregular sleeping habits
- Progressive loss of daily structure
- Irregular attendance at treatment meetings
- Development of an "I don't care" attitude
- Open rejection of help
- Self-pity
- Opinion that social drinking is manageable
- Conscious lying
- Complete loss of self-confidence

These are simply warning signs, not inevitable signs of relapse, and constructive responses are possible. The person in recovery will have these thoughts and feelings, to one degree or another, on a recurring basis throughout his or her life. Each time the person lives through the experience and finds that it passes, and each time the person tolerates the feeling effectively and responds to it in a healthy manner, recovery and satisfaction in living deepen.

Deepening of the Recovery Process

Choosing to take new actions in response to vulnerability is the key to recovery. If the element of choice is absent in the obsession and compulsion of addiction, then reclaiming the ability to make life-affirming choices—reclaiming free will—is the essence of recovery. The use of will can be considered the use of one's life energy. If someone is "willing" to do something, he or she is choosing to give energy to the task at hand. If he or she is "unwilling" to do something, he or she is withholding life energy. There are three different ways to use energy: willfully, will-lessly, and willingly. "Willingness and willfulness become possibilities every time we truly engage life. There is only one other option—to avoid engagement entirely [will-lessness]."[46]

The energy of willfulness is reflected in behaviors of force, exertion, strain, contraction, constriction, violence, manipulation, controlling actions, and drive. It is the fight aspect of the fight-or-flight response to perceived danger. Will-lessness—the withdrawal of energy—is seen in behaviors reflecting withdrawal, escape, giving up, immobilization, collapse, and numbness. Will-lessness is the flight response to fear and vulnerability.

Every person tends to favor one of these patterns of behavior. Typically, a person who is predominantly willful eventually becomes exhausted and collapses into will-less behaviors. A person following a very restrictive and rigid weight loss diet, for example, ultimately binges. In contrast, a person who has fallen into a pattern of total will-lessness (e.g., has gone on an extended alcohol binge) suddenly becomes scared, vows to stop drinking, and goes on a "health kick." This grasp of control cannot be sustained because it is not grounded in any deeper changes. Consequently, the person swings back to the will-less behavior.

The array of behaviors that can be identified as willful and will-less is shown in **Figures 33-1** and **33-2**. These models are useful in teaching a person in recovery about patterns of behavior. People readily recognize and identify with these descriptions, and they generally appreciate the nonjudgmental presentation. As can be seen in these images, these behaviors can be observed in every aspect of a person's life—in the physical, mental, emotional, and spiritual realms.

Willfulness and will-lessness are extreme uses of energy. They each represent an energetic state of imbalance. The goal in recovery from addictions is to lead a life of balance, harmony, and increasing serenity. Willingness is the active state of living life from the place of dynamic balance, as opposed to the extremes. It can be likened to the ideal of many of the world's wisdom traditions. It is spoken of in the Buddhist path of the middle way, in the Taoist concept of the balance of yin and yang energies, in the Greek ideal of the golden mean, and in the common sense of moderation in all things. The qualities of life lived from this ideal are depicted in **Figure 33-3**.

Transpersonal/Spiritual Development and Transformation

Transpersonal/spiritual development is an innate evolutionary capacity within all people.[47] It is not a concept but is instead a process of learning about love, caring, empathy, and meaning in life (see Chapter 7). This process leads a person to join with his or her psyche, soul, or spirit and to have a lived experience of inner peace and connection with inner wisdom or guidance that evokes a correlation to a deeper purpose and feelings of oneness.

Participants in AA and other 12-step programs are encouraged to seek spiritual growth and connection with their own higher power. Studies have shown that people in recovery who score higher in standardized spirituality measures are more successful in maintaining abstinence than those with lower scores. Spirituality in these studies was not equated with participation in religion. Rather, individuals in treatment spoke of experiencing a turning point in their life, feeling "protection and support from a higher power, guidance of an inner

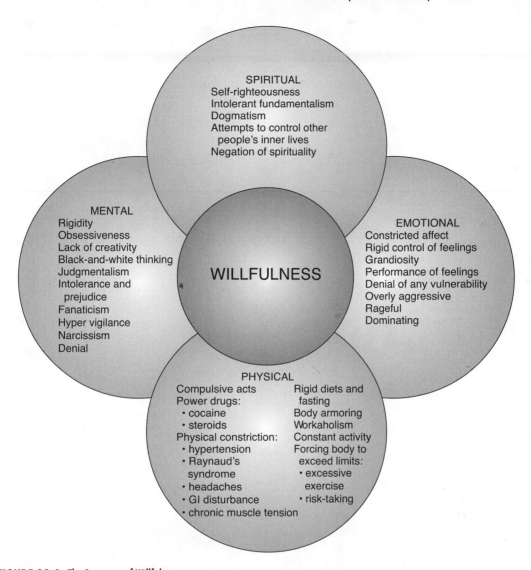

FIGURE 33-1 The Spectrum of Willfulness

Source: Reproduced by permission. Healing Addictions by Schaub and Schaub. Delmar Publishers, Albany, NY. Copyright 1997.

voice, life meaning, gratitude, and an appreciation of service work."[48, p. 58] These experiences reflect the fact that long-term recovery is a process that goes beyond abstinence and can lead to deep healing and an enriched sense of meaning and purpose.[49,50] In a study that examined a deeper understanding of the process of recovery, 9,341 people (54% female) who self-identified as being in recovery responded to an Internet-based survey. The findings showed that there are important elements in recovery that must be addressed and supported beyond the basic issue

of abstinence. Some of the most important elements were identified as self-care, compassion and concern for others, personal growth, and developing ways of being that sustain the process of recovery.[51]

In a qualitative phenomenological study conducted by Bowden, eight recovering alcoholics described the importance of integrating spiritual practices into their daily lives.[52] In addition to developing self-acceptance, those who were doing well in recovery were also participating in an ongoing search for connections with the

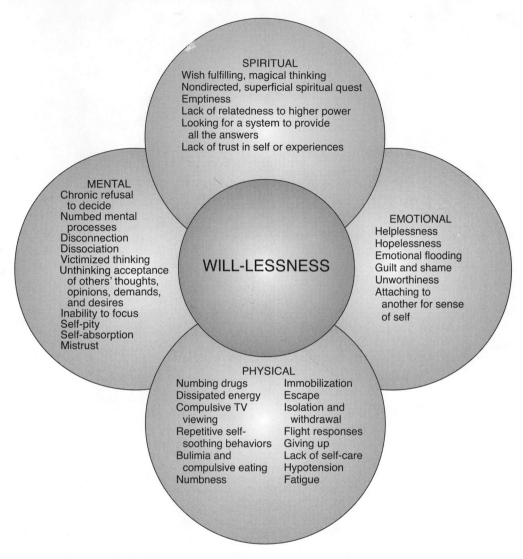

FIGURE 33-2 The Spectrum of Will-lessness

Source: Reproduced by permission. Healing Addictions by Schaub and Schaub. Delmar Publishers, Albany, NY. Copyright 1997.

transpersonal realm. This information confirms that it is important to encourage the person in recovery to explore his or her transpersonal/spiritual nature (see Exhibit 33-1).

There is much cynicism and discouragement in addiction treatment because professionals in rehabilitation and treatment centers often witness the "revolving door syndrome." Yet, unlike so many other conditions with which nurses work, addiction is completely reversible. There is a real possibility for a person to transform his or her life dramatically and to begin living a healthy and sane life.

Because of their compatibility with 12-step programs and the AA philosophy, psychological models such as psychosynthesis—that recognize and understand the individual's transpersonal nature—are important components of care. Central concepts of psychosynthesis include self-knowledge, awareness and choice, and spiritual development. These all contribute to the effectiveness of a person's recovery from addiction.[53,54] Addiction treatment is one of the few areas in health care where spiritual development and exploration are not only openly addressed but are recognized as an integral aspect of care.

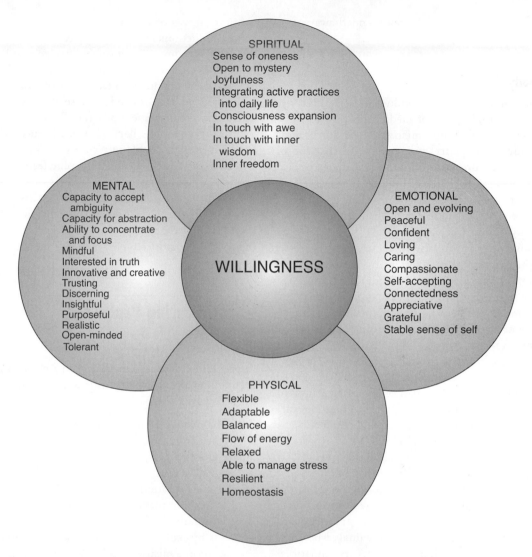

FIGURE 33-3 The Spectrum of Willingness

Source: Reproduced by permission. Healing Addictions by Schaub and Schaub. Delmar Publishers, Albany, NY. Copyright 1997.

As nurses and other healthcare professionals interested in addictions counseling explore their own attitudes, experiences, and beliefs, they can serve as role models for grounding spirituality in real, human terms.

No single nurse or therapist can provide enough support and reinforcement for the recovery process. Thus, the nurse must be aware of a client's degree of participation in AA and any resistance to the transpersonal/spiritual aspect of the AA meetings. A person who feels alienated by this component of AA is unlikely to participate in meetings. Some individuals hear the words *God* or *Higher Power* in meetings and begin to reject AA's "God talk." If this is the case, the nurse can determine if there is a way that the person can translate these concepts into personally acceptable ideas to facilitate a broader approach to spirituality. For some people, the idea of a higher power can be translated into Mother Nature, or the healing energy and intention of the people in their AA group. Clients may benefit from developing a more open view of spirituality by seeking out books on different philosophies or exploring spiritual practices such as yoga, tai chi, or meditation that offer people ways to experience expanded awareness (see Chapter 11).

Body–Mind Responses

Benson and Wallace conducted a classic study on the application of meditation to the treatment of substance misuse. Their study had 1,862 participants, and they found that those who used prescription and illicit drugs began reducing their intake of drugs as they learned to enter a deep state of relaxation. After 21 months of regular meditation, most had stopped using drugs completely. The investigators looked closely at alcohol use in these same subjects. They classified drinkers as light users (three times a month or less), medium users (once to six times a week), and heavy users (once a day or more). After 21 months of meditation, heavy use of alcohol had dropped from 2.7% to 0.6%, medium use dropped from 15.8% to 3.7%, and light use dropped from 41.4% to 25.8%. The percentage of nonusers of alcohol rose from 40.1% to 69.9%. More than half of the participants in this study, 61.1%, reported that meditation was "extremely important" in helping to reduce their alcohol consumption. The more the participants meditated, the less they drank.[55]

A study at the Addictive Behaviors Research Center at the University of Washington in Seattle explored whether Vipassana meditation (VM), a Buddhist mindfulness-based practice, can provide an alternative for individuals who find traditional addiction treatments incompatible or unattractive. The investigators evaluated the effectiveness of a VM course on substance use and psychosocial outcomes in an incarcerated population. Results indicated that after release from jail, participants in the VM course, as compared with those in a treatment-as-usual control condition, showed significant reductions in alcohol, marijuana, and crack cocaine use.[56]

Researchers at the University of Maryland School of Medicine in Baltimore investigated the efficacy of adding Qi Gong to a residential treatment program for substance misuse. Qi Gong, which blends relaxation, breathing, guided imagery, inward attention, and mindfulness to elicit a tranquil, healing state, was introduced into a short-term residential treatment program. Participants whose Qi Gong meditation was of acceptable quality reported greater reductions in craving, anxiety, and withdrawal symptoms. The investigators conclude that Qi Gong meditation appears to contribute positively to addiction treatment outcomes, with results at least as good as those of an established stress management program.[57]

Brain-wave biofeedback also has been used successfully with people in recovery. It is a process in which electroencephalographic feedback helps participants go into deep states of relaxation. This heightened awareness also assists clients in recognizing their feelings of tension and then learning that deep relaxation can replace the chemically induced relief gained from addictive substances.[58]

Holistic Caring Process

Holistic Assessment

In preparing to use strategies to assist clients in overcoming alcoholism, the nurse should assess the following:

- The client's characteristics that may suggest alcoholism:
  - Restlessness, impulsiveness, anxiety
  - Selfishness, self-centeredness, lack of consideration
  - Stubbornness, irritability, anger, rage, ill humor
  - Physical cruelty, brawling, child and spouse misuse
  - Depression, isolation, self-destructiveness
  - Aggressive sexuality, often accompanied by infidelity, which may give way to sexual disinterest or impotence
  - Arrogance that may lead to aggression, coldness, or withdrawal
  - Low self-esteem, shame, guilt, remorse, loneliness
  - Reduced mental and physical function leading to eventual blackouts
  - Susceptibility to other disease
  - Lying, deceit, broken promises
  - Denial that there is a drinking problem
  - Projection of blame onto people, places, and things
- The client's current drinking patterns (**Exhibit 33-4** provides a self-scoring test that

can be taken by a client or a family member or friend concerned about the client's drinking.)

- The client's attitudes, beliefs, and motivation to learn interventions to become nonaddicted
- The client's available family and friends
- The client's eating and exercise patterns
- The client's existing stress management strategies
- The client's willingness to join a support group

Identification of Patterns/ Challenges/Needs

The patterns/challenges/needs (see Chapter 8) compatible with addiction interventions are as follows:

- Altered nutrition (more or less than body requirements)
- High risk for trauma
- Impaired verbal communication
- Altered social interaction
- Altered family processes
- Altered sexuality patterns
- Spiritual distress
- Ineffective individual and family coping

- Noncompliance
- Health-seeking behaviors
- Decreased physical mobility
- Sleep pattern disturbance
- Disturbance in self-esteem
- Disturbance in personal identity
- Hopelessness
- Powerlessness
- Knowledge deficit
- Altered thought processes
- Anxiety
- Potential for violence
- Fear

Outcome Identification

Table 33-1 guides the nurse in client outcomes, nursing prescriptions, and evaluation for overcoming addictions.

Therapeutic Care Plan and Interventions

Before the session:

- Spend a few moments centering yourself, connecting with your inner wisdom and intention to facilitate healing.
- Create a quiet place to begin guiding the client in strategies to overcome addiction(s).

EXHIBIT 33-4   Are You a Problem Drinker?

1. Have you ever tried to stop drinking for a week (or longer), only to fall short of your goal?
2. Do you resent the advice of others who try to get you to stop drinking?
3. Have you ever tried to control your drinking by switching from one alcoholic beverage to another?
4. Have you taken a morning drink during the past year?
5. Do you envy people who can drink without getting into trouble?
6. Has your drinking problem become progressively more serious during the past year?
7. Has your drinking created problems at home?
8. At social affairs where drinking is limited, do you try to obtain "extra" drinks?
9. Despite evidence to the contrary, have you continued to assert that you can stop drinking "on your own" whenever you wish?
10. During the past year, have you missed time from work as a result of your drinking?
11. Have you ever "blacked out" (had a loss of memory) during your drinking?
12. Have you ever felt you could do more with your life if you did not drink?

Did you answer YES four or more times? If so, chances are you have a serious drinking problem or may have one in the future.

Source: The preceding twelve questions have been excerpted from material appearing in the pamphlet, "*Is A.A. For You?*" and has been reprinted with permission of Alcoholics Anonymous World Services, Inc. ("AAWS"). Permission to reprint this material does not mean that AAWS has reviewed and/or endorses this publication. AA is a program of recovery from alcoholism only — use of AA material in any non-AA context does not imply otherwise.

TABLE 33-1 Nursing Interventions: Overcoming Addictions

Client Outcomes	Nursing Prescriptions	Evaluation
The client demonstrated attitudes, beliefs, and actions that reflect an intention to overcome addiction.	The client set realistic plans for overcoming addiction as evidenced by the following actions:	The client will demonstrate attitudes, beliefs, and behaviors that result in overcoming addictions.
	■ Accepted support of healthy family or friends	Determine the client's intention to overcome addiction by assessing completion of the following actions:
	■ Attended AA daily	■ Seeking support from healthy family and friends
	■ Contacted an AA sponsor regularly	■ Attending AA meetings
	■ Detoxified self and environment of drugs and alcohol	■ Seeking support of a sponsor
	■ Practiced relaxation and imagery daily	■ Detoxifying self and environment of alcohol and drugs
	■ Integrated behavioral changes on a daily basis	■ Practicing relaxation and imagery
	■ Rewarded self for attaining set goals	■ Integrating behavioral changes
		■ Selecting ways to reward self for attaining goals

At the beginning of the session:

- Review the results of the self-assessment.
- Reinforce the concept that overcoming addictions is a process requiring commitment, new behavioral skills, and support from peers, friends, and/or family.
- Ask the client to tell his or her personal story.
- Assist the client in identifying the steps necessary for overcoming addictions. If necessary, assist the client in going through detoxification.

During the session:

- Teach the client general relaxation and imagery exercises that focus on awareness of body sensations and their connection to feelings.
- Help the client to identify specific imagery practices that enhance healing (see Chapter 12). These could include the following:
  1. *Active images.* Images such as cleansing the body of impurities, possibly by a gentle waterfall; creating a safe place where the client can feel secure and comfortable; and using a protective shield to let the client receive what is needed from others and to block out negative images, such as alcohol or drug signals, places, or events.
  2. *End-state images.* Images of feeling healthy, of living with a sense of accomplishment and satisfaction, and of having healthy, supportive relationships.
  3. *Healing images.* Images such as connecting the inner healer, inner wisdom, and spiritual resources.
  4. *Process images.* Imagining successfully overcoming drink or drug signals and making healthy, alternative choices.
- Teach the client to reframe current situations and problems. For example, instead of the client saying, "I can't admit publicly that I'm an alcoholic," help the client rehearse being at a 12-step meeting and saying, "Thank you for letting me share my story with you. I have been an alcoholic for 10 years, and I am ready to quit."
- Teach the client to use HALT, checking to notice if being hungry, angry, lonely, or tired is a contributing factor when experiencing alcohol or drug signals. Encourage the client to avoid these conditions whenever possible.

- Encourage the development of creative skills as a means of working with strong emotions and experiences. This may include actively working with dreams; journal keeping; letter writing (see Chapter 14); using artistic expressions by drawing, painting, or sculpting with clay; and playing evocative music to enhance images or dance with the emotions (see Chapter 32).
- Have the client identify his or her habit breakers (see Chapter 35).
- Help the client to learn forgiveness (see Chapter 7).

At the end of the session:

- Encourage the client to explore the value of a 12-step program as an adjunct to treatment.
- Emphasize the value of selecting someone in the program as a sponsor so that a support person is available to be contacted on a daily basis.
- Reinforce the idea that the client can learn to recognize high-risk situations and make healthy choices.
- Reinforce the value of using HALT when experiencing signals for substance use. Is hunger, anger, loneliness, or tiredness contributing to these feelings? Encourage the client to make a list of particular high-risk situations and decide in advance quick action steps to prevent relapse.
- Reinforce the importance of integrating healthful habits into daily life. Encourage the client to select one or two practices to which he or she is willing to make a commitment to include in daily life. Imagery, breathing exercises, meditation, yoga, jogging or other physical activities, and dietary changes are all of value.
- Use the client outcomes (see Exhibit 33-5) that were established before the session to evaluate the session.
- Schedule a follow-up session.

Holistic Interventions

Imagery and Creative Imagination Processes As previously noted, substance misusing individuals are not in touch with their bodies or feelings. Basic relaxation and imagery training can help them to experience themselves with new awareness. The daily practice of relaxation and imagery exercises not only reverses stress and depression but also increases clients' recognition of inner knowledge. People who have been addicted have lost trust in themselves because of all the poor choices they have made while in their addiction. In addition, they experience a deep shame when thinking of all the people they have hurt or disappointed. There is a harsh, condemning, inner voice with which these clients must contend.

Clients must become aware of their physical responses to stress (e.g., heart palpitations, muscle tightness, headaches, stomachaches). The misuse of alcohol, drugs, food, or other substances or behaviors numbs awareness of body responses, short-circuiting mind–body communication. Clients must learn to practice stress management skills daily rather than waiting until a vulnerable moment occurs. For example, the nurse can teach diaphragmatic breathing as a very basic skill. Shallow chest and shoulder breathing is a common stress response, one that often becomes chronic. Simply breathing diaphragmatically can bring about significant physiologic and psychological responses. Changing to this breath pattern efficiently slows the heart rate, increases oxygenation of the blood, strengthens weak intestinal and abdominal muscles, and can bring about a sense of well-being and inner calm.

Teaching a client the concept of "constant instant practice" is a way of linking a new behavior to an activity that is done repeatedly during the course of the day. For example, if the person spends a great deal of time on the telephone, he or she can let the telephone be the reminder to take a few deep, cleansing breaths. If the telephone is ringing, the person can let it ring a few extra times and take a deep breath before answering. This practice can be linked with any activity that occurs frequently during the client's day.

The mind responds best when it is given positive images about new ideas and new behavior patterns. A nurse may start by guiding clients in rhythmic breathing exercises. When the clients are in a quieted state, they can be guided to imagine being clean and sober and walking down a street where they went to use drugs or alcohol with friends, now experiencing this place from a sober perspective. The image of experiencing their world from a new perspective can then be practiced and reinforced, resulting in the breakdown of addictive responses and the strengthening of positive coping strategies.

Imagery Practices To assist in the client's recovery process, the nurse can take time to create special relaxation and imagery tapes that the client can listen to several times a day. The following three imagery practices focus on substance misuse, but they can be modified for other addictions. A relaxation exercise from Chapter 11 may be recorded for 5 to 10 minutes, followed by one or several of the scripts for overcoming addictions for 15 minutes or longer.

Consider these imagery processes as suggestions. The most effective imagery tapes take advantage of the nurse's creativity, intuition, and clinical insights—in combination with words and images the client has used—to create an imagery script that is designed for a particular person (see Chapter 12). It is best to start with the simplest suggestions. Just beginning to be able to notice distraction is progress. This is challenging for all of us and someone who has put so much effort in to not being aware of difficult thoughts and feelings needs to feel encouraged by small successes.

link them at all. Do what feels best to you.

7. Slowly repeat this phrase over and over in your mind. Whenever you find a thought entering your awareness, just return to your "let go" practice.

8. Continue this practice for a few minutes and then let go of the words and notice how you are.

Adapted with permission from R. Schaub and B. G. Schaub, *Transpersonal Development: Cultivating the Human Resources of Peace, Wisdom, Purpose and Oneness* (Huntington, NY: Florence Press, 2013).

This "let go" practice, because of its simplicity, often surprises clients with its effect. Often, the person will be surprised at how quickly he or she was able to experience a shift to a feeling of deep calm. This state of inner quiet, for some, is what they seek in getting "stoned." This then becomes a teachable moment when people learn that they have skills and inner resources that can connect them with inner calm. This feeling most likely will be transient, but it will be able to reoccur with further practice.

Practice: "Let Go"

1. Close your eyes, or lower your eyes and find a place on the ground to focus on.
2. Now give way to the chair you are in. Let it hold you.
3. Now let your shoulders drop . . .
4. Now I am going to ask you to repeat a three-word phrase over and over again in your mind.
5. The first word is your first name, and the next two words are "let go." Your first name followed by "let go" . . .
6. You can link these three words to your in breath or your out breath, or not

Practice: Centering and Naming

1. Gently shake your hands for a while.
2. Now place one hand just under your navel and place your other hand on top of the first hand.
3. Slowly let your awareness go down to your hands and notice the sensations of one hand touching the other.
4. Now begin to notice the rising and falling of your belly underneath your hands.
5. Let yourself become interested in the sensations of the rising and falling. . . . Nothing else to do. . . . Nothing special has to happen . . . just notice the rising and falling.

6. If a thought or sensation or other distraction pulls you away from focusing on your belly, name the thought or sensation and then return to noticing the rising and falling.

In this "centering and naming" practice, the focus is on the rising and falling of the belly with each breath rather than on breath passing through the nostrils. This brings attention away from the head, making it easier for the person to not focus on thoughts when his or her concentration is on the tactile sensation of hands and away from the head.

Adapted with permission from R. Schaub and B. G. Schaub, *Transpersonal Development: Cultivating the Human Resources of Peace, Wisdom, Purpose and Oneness* (Huntington, NY: Florence Press, 2013).

Practice: Evocative Words

The first step in using evocative words is to choose the word or words that best express the specific new quality you want to energize in your mind. You are using the transformational principle that you solve problems by energizing the answers.

Alcoholics Anonymous uses short slogans such as "Easy does it" or "Let go and let God" for this purpose. You can apply evocative words practice to any pattern of addiction or compulsion, with the goal of replacing needy addictive thinking. With healthy, peaceful thinking, old habits remain in the mind, especially when we are under stress, long after the actual behavior has stopped. Evocative words help to create a new mental climate.

Once you have chosen your evocative word or words, write each word or phrase on a blank filing card. Place these cards throughout your environment—on your desk, your mirror, the refrigerator door—so that you see them frequently throughout your day as reminders. These words will serve as an antidote to the destructive mental obsession of the addictive process.

When you have decided on the evocative word or words you want to energize, try this practice:

1. Sit on a comfortable chair and let your muscles relax. Let the chair hold you.
2. Place the evocative word in your mind and focus on it as best you can. Do not be discouraged if other thoughts distract you—that is normal; just return to your word.
3. If ideas and images connected to the word come to you, watch them for a while and then return to the evocative word.

These evocative word cards provide people with a tangible reminder of what they want to reinforce in their thinking. They can become subtle cue cards that can be carried with the person or placed on noticeable surfaces such as on a mirror at home, on the refrigerator, by the home telephone or computer, on a desk at work, and at other suitable places.

Adapted with permission from B. G. Schaub and R. Schaub, *Dante's Path: Vulnerability and the Spiritual Journey* (Huntington, NY: Florence Press, 2014).

Case Study (Implementation)

Case Study

Setting: AA meeting

Client: S. W., a 45-year-old successful, married professional with two children. At the time he told us his story, he had been free of alcohol and amphetamines for 3 months and had begun his path toward recovery.

Patterns/Challenges/Needs: Health maintenance related to engaging in actions supportive of remaining free of addiction

"My healing began when I finally admitted to myself, my family, and my friends that I was addicted to alcohol and drugs. I began to explore and own my dark side. I've created some wonderful healing rituals, which include getting the nerve up to attend my first AA meeting—which gave me the opportunity to hear other people tell their stories. I've been regularly attending AA meetings and have a sponsor who I've called several times when I felt myself slipping. I realized I didn't know how to do anything to relax except drink. If I needed energy, I didn't know any way to get it but to take speed. So, I've learned relaxation and imagery skills, started an exercise program, and am taking time for myself.

"Here I was at 45 feeling lost and wondering if this was all life had to offer. How could I feel lost? I had so much. My career was going well. I had good kids, a loving and supportive wife, good looks, and I was involved in several civic projects. Everyone was always telling me how wonderful I was and stressing my contributions to the community. But I was searching for more to fulfill my life. I had been a secret drinker and had taken speed off and on since college in order to do all that I needed to accomplish. Everybody saw me as perfect, but I could feel my world falling apart. I got scared.

"For the past 5 years or so my wife had said that she thought I was drinking too much, which had recently become a source of tension between us. I told my wife to take the kids and go on a holiday while I worked at home alone. As soon as they left, I got drunk. When I fractured my ankle from a fall in my own house the

first day they were gone, I really began to look at my life. I suffered a month of deep depression. During that time, my inner voice was screaming at me about all the misuse I was into. It was as if I was having a conversation with a part of myself that I had never heard. The message was so clear I could not turn it off.

"I'm not like many addicts who lose family, money, jobs, and friends. During a month of struggling to perform and continuing to hear my inner dialogue, one day my depression lifted enough for me to find a local AA meeting and hear myself say, 'I've had it; I need help.' I finally admitted in public that I was addicted to alcohol and drugs and used them to be successful. I began educating myself about addictions. I asked for help. What I recognized was that previously I sought ways to connect with sources outside of myself to make me feel good. The real healing came when I learned to connect with the core of my spirit, which awakened my inner resources for feelings of wholeness."

Evaluation

With the client, the nurse determines whether the client outcomes for overcoming addictions were achieved. To evaluate the session further, the nurse may explore the subjective effects of the experience with the client (see **Exhibit 33-5**).

EXHIBIT 33-5   Evaluating the Client's Subjective Experience with Overcoming Addictions

1. What new awarenesses have you had today?
2. Do you understand how to keep a journal of your habits?
3. Can you identify two habit-breaker strategies that you are planning to utilize?
4. Are you aware of your body–mind's signals of wanting a drink?
5. Which relaxation exercises are you finding most beneficial?
6. Do you have any questions on how best to practice your imagery and meditation?
7. Which physical activities are you including in your daily routine?
8. Have you been monitoring the pattern of your craving by using HALT?
9. Which words of affirmation are you working with to reinforce your intentions to be conscious and sober?
10. What have you observed about your patterns of response to vulnerability? Do you tend toward willfulness or will-lessness?
11. What have you discovered is your preferred way of connecting with your spiritual nature?
12. What is your next step?

Conclusion

The evaluation and treatment of addictions have progressed rapidly over the past few years. The science of addictive behaviors is growing. This is a very important area of science and practice that is relevant to holistic nurses.

Directions for Future Research

1. Determine the effectiveness of imagery and breathing techniques in assisting clients to manage cravings.
2. Determine the effectiveness of cognitive strategies (e.g., teaching about willfulness and will-lessness, using HALT) in helping clients to manage feelings of vulnerability.
3. Study the role of spiritual perspective and practice in long-term recovery.

Nurse Healer Reflections

After reading this chapter, the nurse healer will be able to answer or to begin a process of answering the following questions:

- Which addictive patterns do I recognize in my own life?
- Which patterns of response to vulnerability do I observe in myself?
- Which practices and changes am I willing to bring into my life to encourage my own healing?
- Who are the people in my life who would support me in making healthy changes?
- Can I allow an image to emerge that represents my inner wisdom?
- Can I identify what interferes with my connection to my inner wisdom?
- How do I connect with my spiritual nature and how do I support this in my daily life?

NOTES

1. R. Assagioli, *Psychosynthesis: A Manual of Principles and Techniques* (New York: Hobbs, Dorman, 1965).

2. R. Assagioli, *The Act of Will* (New York: Viking Press, 1973).

3. J. Rehm, C. Mathers, S. Popova, M. Thavorncharoensap, Y. Teerawattananon, and J. Patra, "Global Burden of Disease and Injury and Economic Cost Attributable to Alcohol Use and Alcohol-Use Disorders," *The Lancet* 373, no. 9682 (2009): 2223–2233.

4. J. J. Sacks, J. Roeber, E. E. Boucherev, K. Gonzales, F. J. Chaloupka, and R. D. Brewer, "State Costs of Excessive Alcohol Consumption, 2006," *American Journal of Preventive Medicine* 45, no. 4 (2013): 474–485.

5. Centers for Disease Control and Prevention, "Alcohol Screening and Counseling," *Vital Signs* (January 2014). www.cdc.gov/vitalsigns /alcohol-screening-counseling/.

6. National Institute on Alcohol Abuse and Alcoholism, "Screening Tests" (n.d.). http://pubs .niaaa.nih.gov/publications/arh28-2/78-79.htm.

7. National Institutes of Health, "Rethinking Drinking: Alcohol and Your Health," *NIH Publication No. 13-3770* (2010). http://pubs.niaaa.nih .gov/publications/RethinkingDrinking /Rethinking_Drinking.pdf.

8. C. E. Rice, D. Dandreaux, E. D. Handley, and L. Chassin, "Children of Alcoholics: Risk and Resilience," *Prevention Researcher* 13, no. 4 (2006): 3–6.

9. L. Keyser-Marcus, A. Alvanzo, T. Rieckmann, L. Thacker, A. Sepulveda, A. Forcehimes, L. Z. Islam, et al., "Trauma, Gender, and Mental Health Symptoms in Individuals with Substance Use Disorders," *Journal of Interpersonal Violence* 30, no. 1 (2015): 3–24.

10. M. E. Pagano, R. Rende, B. F. Rodriguez, E. L. Hargraves, A. T. Moskowitz, and M. B. Keller, "Impact of Parental History of Substance Use Disorders on the Clinical Course of Anxiety Disorders," *Substance Abuse Treatment, Prevention, and Policy* 2 (2007): 13.

11. Substance Abuse and Mental Health Services Administration, *Results from the 2008 National Survey on Drug Use and Health: National Findings*, HHS Publication No. SMA 09-4434 (Rockville, MD: Substance Abuse and Mental Health Services Administration, 2009).

12. Alcoholics Anonymous, *Alcoholics Anonymous* (New York: Alcoholics Anonymous World Services, 1976).

13. M. Kaur, A. Liguori, W. Lang, S. R. Rapp, A. B. Fleischer, Jr., and S. R. Feldman, "Induction of Withdrawal-Like Symptoms in a Small Randomized, Controlled Trial of Opioid Blockade in Frequent Tanners," *Journal of the American Academy of Dermatology* 54, no. 4 (2006): 709–711.

14. C. R. Harrington, T. C. Beswick, J. Leitenberger, A. Minhajuddin, H. T. Jacobe, and B. Adinoff, "Addictive-Like Behaviours to Ultraviolet Light Among Frequent Indoor Tanners," *Clinical and Experimental Dermatology* 36, no. 1 (2011): 33–38.

15. B. Schaub and R. Schaub, *Healing Addictions: The Vulnerability Model of Recovery* (Albany, NY: Delmar, 1997).

16. American Psychiatric Association, *Diagnostic and Statistical Manual of Mental Disorders-TR* (Washington, DC: American Psychiatric Association, 2000).

17. A. Kumar, K. H. Choi, W. Renthal, N. M. Tsankova, D. E. Theobald, H. T. Truong, S. J. Russo, et al., "Chromatin Remodeling Is a Key Mechanism Underlying Cocaine-Induced Plasticity in Striatum," *Neuron* 48, no. 2 (2005): 303–314.

18. I. Maze and E. J. Nestler, "The Epigenetic Landscape of Addiction," *Annals of the New York Academy of Sciences* 1216 (2011): 99–113.

19. S. C. McQuown and M. A. Wood, "Epigenetic Regulation in Substance Use Disorders," *Current Psychiatry Report* 12, no. 2 (2010): 145–153.

20. K. Graham and A. Massak, "Alcohol Consumption and the Use of Antidepressants," *Canadian Medical Association Journal* 176, no. 5 (2007): 633–637.

21. M. Leeies, J. Pagura, J. Sareen, and J. M. Bolton, "The Use of Alcohol and Drugs to Self-Medicate Symptoms of Posttraumatic Stress Disorder," *Depression and Anxiety* 27, no. 8 (2010): 731–736.

22. L. Khoury, Y. L. Tang, B. Bradley, J. F. Cubells, and K. J. Ressler, "Substance Use, Childhood Traumatic Experience, and Posttraumatic Stress Disorder in an Urban Civilian Population," *Depression and Anxiety* 27, no. 12 (2010): 1077–1086.

23. H. Vest, C. Kane, J. DeMarce, E. Barbero, R. Harmon, J. Hawley, and L. Lehman, "Outcomes Following Treatment of Veterans for Substance and Tobacco Addiction," *Archives of Psychiatric Nursing* 28, no. 5 (2014): 333–338.

24. Center for Behavioral Health Statistics and Quality, *The DAWN Report: Highlights of the 2009 Drug Abuse Warning Network (DAWN) Findings on Drug-Related Emergency Department Visits* (Rockville, MD: Substance Abuse and Mental Health Services Administration, 2010).

25. Substance Abuse and Mental Health Services Administration, "Emergency Department Data/DAWN" (2014). www.samhsa.gov/data/emergency-department-data-dawn.

26. S. E. McCabe, J. R. Knight, C. J. Teter, and H. Wechser, "Non-Medical Use of Prescription Stimulants Among US College Students: Prevalence and Correlates from a National Survey," *Addiction* 100, no. 1 (2005): 96–106.

27. P. Eickenhorst, K. Vitzhum, B. F. Klapp, D. Groneberg, and S. Mache, "Neuroenhancement Among German University Students: Motives, Expectations, and Relationship with Psychoactive Lifestyle Drugs," *Journal of Psychoactive Drugs* 44, no. 5 (2012): 418–427.

28. M. D. King, J. Jennings, and J. M. Fletcher, "Medical Adaptation to Academic Pressure: Schooling, Stimulant Use, and Socioeconomic Status," *American Sociological Review* (October 13, 2014): doi:10:1177/0003122414553657.

29. H. H. Cleveland, K. S. Harris, A. K. Baker, R. Herbert, and L. R. Dean, "Characteristics of a Collegiate Recovery Community: Maintaining Recovery in an Abstinence-Hostile Environment," *Journal of Substance Abuse Treatment* 33, no. 1 (2007): 13–23.

30. P. Agostino, "Unsportsmanlike Conduct," *NurseWeek* (April 25, 2005): 5–7.

31. Hazelden Foundation, *The Twelve Steps of Alcoholics Anonymous* (New York: Harper/Hazelden, 1987): 2.

32. K. Joe-Laidler and G. Hunt, "Unlocking the Spiritual with Club Drugs: A Case Study of Two Youth Cultures," *Substance Use and Misuse* 48, no. 12 (2013): 1099–1108.

33. A. Beck and G. Emery, *Anxiety Disorders and Phobias: A Cognitive Perspective* (New York: Basic Books, 1985).

34. E. Becker, *The Denial of Death* (New York: The Free Press, 1973): 178.

35. L. M. Gentilello, "Let's Diagnose Alcohol Problems in the ER and Successfully Intervene," *Medscape General Medicine* 8, no. 1 (2006): 1.

36. T. T. Liu, J. Shi, D. H. Epstein, Y. P. Bao, and L. Lu, "A Meta-Analysis of Acupuncture Combined with Opioid Receptor Agonists for Treatment of Opiate-Withdrawal Symptoms," *Cellular Molecular Neurobiology* 29, no. 4 (2009): 449–454.

37. B. Chang and E. Sommers, "Acupuncture and Relaxation Response for Craving and Anxiety Reduction Among Military Veterans in Recovery from Substance Use Disorder," *American Journal on Addictions* 23, no. 2 (2014): 129–136.

38. E. A. Robinson, A. R. Krentzman, J. R. Webb, and K. J. Brower, "Six-Month Changes in Spirituality and Religiousness in Alcoholics Predict Drinking Outcomes at Nine Months," *Journal of Studies on Alcohol and Drugs* 72, no. 4 (2011): 660–668.

39. C. A. Bradley, "Women in AA: 'Sharing Experience, Strength and Hope': The Relational Nature of Spirituality," *Journal of Religion and Spirituality in Social Work* 30, no. 2 (2011): 89–112.

40. S. A. Straussner and H. Byrne, "Alcoholics Anonymous: Key Research Findings from 2002–2007," *Alcoholism Treatment Quarterly* 27, no. 4 (2009): 349–367.

41. W. Knudsen, J. E. Jensen, I. Nordgaard-Lassen, T. Almdal, J. Kondrup, and U. Becker, "Nutritional Intake and Status in Persons with Alcohol Dependency: Data from an Outpatient Treatment Programme," *European Journal of Nutrition* 53, no. 7 (2014): 1483–1492.

42. M. R. Werbach, *Nutritional Influences on Mental Illness* (Tarzana, CA: Third Line Press, 1991): 15.

43. R. J. DuBrey, "The Role of Healing Touch in the Treatment of Persons in Recovery from Alcoholism," *Counselor: The Magazine for Addiction Professionals* 7, no. 6 (2006): 58–64.

44. M. Winkelman, "Complementary Therapy for Addiction: 'Drumming Out Drugs,'" *American Journal of Public Health* 93, no. 4 (2003): 647–651.

45. T. T. Gorski and M. Miller, *Counseling for Relapse Prevention* (Independence, MO: Independence Press, 1982).

46. G. G. May, *Addiction and Grace* (New York: HarperCollins, 1991): 104.

47. R. Schaub and B. G. Schaub, *Transpersonal Development: Cultivating the Human Resources of Peace, Wisdom, Purpose and Oneness* (Huntington, NY: Florence Press, 2013).

48. W. White and A. Laudet, "Spirituality, Science and Addiction," *Counselor: The Magazine for Addiction Professionals* 7, no. 1 (2006): 56–59.

49. A. B. Laudet, K. Morgen, and W. L. White, "The Role of Social Supports, Spirituality, Religiousness, Life Meaning and Affiliation with 12-Step Fellowships in Quality of Life Satisfaction Among Individuals in Recovery from Alcohol and Drug Problems," *Alcohol Treatment Quarterly* 24, nos. 1–2 (2006): 33–73.

50. E. A. R. Robinson, J. A. Cranford, J. R. Webb, and K. J. Brower, "Six-Month Changes in Spirituality, Religiousness, and Heavy Drinking in a Treatment-Seeking Sample," *Journal of Studies on Alcohol and Drugs* 68, no. 2 (2007): 282–290.

51. L. A. Kaskutas, T. J. Borkman, A. Laudet, L. A. Ritter, J. Witbrodt, M. S. Subbaraman, A. Stunz, et al., "Elements That Define Recovery: The Experiential Perspective," *Journal of Studies on Alcohol and Drugs* 75, no. 6 (2014): 999–1010.

52. J. W. Bowden, "Recovery from Alcoholism: A Spiritual Journey," *Issues in Mental Health Nursing* 19, no. 4 (1998): 337–352.

53. R. Schaub, "Spirituality and the Health Professional," *Substance Use and Misuse* 48, no. 12 (2013): 1174–1179.

54. R. Schaub and B. G. Schaub, "Psychosynthesis and the Addictions Recovery Process," in *Essays on the Theory and Practice of a Psychospiritual Psychology*, Vol. 2, eds. S. Simpson, J. Evans, and R. Evans (London: Institute of Psychosynthesis, 2014): 79–91.

55. H. Benson and R. K. Wallace, "Decreased Drug Abuse with Transcendental Meditation: A Study of 1,862 Subjects," *Drug Abuse: Proceedings of the International Conference*, ed. C. J. D. Zarafonetis (Philadelphia: Lea & Febiger, 1972): 369–376.

56. S. Bowen, K. Witkiewitz, T. M. Dillworth, N. Chawla, T. L. Simpson, B. D. Ostafin, M. E. Larimer, et al., "Mindfulness Meditation and Substance Use in an Incarcerated Population," *Psychology of Addictive Behaviors* 20, no. 3 (2006): 343–347.

57. K. W. Chen, A. Comerford, P. Shinnick, and D. M. Ziedonis, "Introducing Qigong Meditation into Residential Addiction Treatment: A Pilot Study Where Gender Makes a Difference," *Journal of Alternative and Complementary Medicine* 16, no. 8 (2010): 875–882.

58. T. M. Sokhadze, R. L. Cannon, and D. L. Trudeau, "EEG Biofeedback as a Treatment for Substance Use Disorders: Review, Rating of Efficacy, and Recommendations for Further Research," *Applied Psychophysiology and Biofeedback* 33, no. 1 (2008): 1–28.

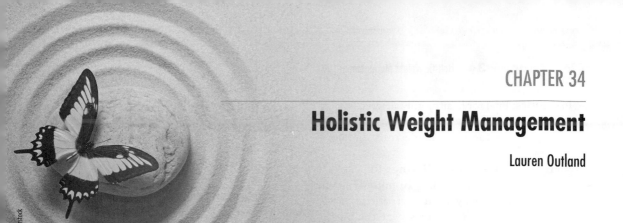

CHAPTER 34

Holistic Weight Management

Lauren Outland

© Olga Lyubkina/Shutterstock

Nurse Healer Objectives

Theoretical

- List two contributing factors to the obesity epidemic in addition to sedentary lifestyle and fast food.
- Identify a negative health consequence of weight cycling.
- Explain how hunger triggered by dieting disrupts homeostasis.
- Describe the pathogenesis behind a lowered metabolism.
- List two ways to improve gut microbiota.

Clinical

- Discuss the benefits of eating only and always when hungry.
- List the four ways in which hunger and fullness can be overridden (e.g., delaying meals).
- Explain why overeating is not always caused by lack of willpower.
- Explain the role of adequate sleep and a healthy gut in weight management.

Personal

- Discuss the benefits of intuitive eating.
- Describe how eating in response to hunger and fullness is perceived by the psyche.

Definitions

Anorexigenic: Appetite depressing.

Bingeing: Eating a large number of calories at one time in response to emotional needs.

Calorie: As opposed to calorie, a Calorie is a unit of consumable energy equal to a kilocalorie (kcal).

Ghrelin: An orexigenic hormone produced by gut mucosa.

Gut microbiome: The community of bacteria residing in the intestinal tract.

Holism: A perspective that views the human organism as a physical, emotional, and spiritual being.

Intuitive eating: Tuning into internal cues of hunger and fullness to guide when and how much to eat.

Leptin: An anorexigenic hormone produced by adipocytes; communicates status of fat stores to the hypothalamus.

Neuropeptide Y: A central nervous system hunger hormone.

Nutrition transition: The transition from food scarcity and traditional diets high in cereal and fiber to relative food and calorie abundance, especially foods high in fat, sugar, and animal protein.

Orexigenic: Appetite stimulating.

Overeating: Eating when not hungry or eating more than is required to satisfy hunger.

Peptide YY (3–36): An anorexigenic hormone.

Prebiotics: Fuel for healthy gut bacteria.

Probiotics: Healthy gut bacteria that are present in foods or made into dietary supplements.

Weight cycling/yo-yo dieting: Repeated weight loss greater than 10 pounds followed by weight gain, in a repetitive pattern, three or more times over the past 2 years.

Weight homeostasis: The vast biochemical and hormonal responses involved in maintaining a healthy weight and/or to prevent starvation.

Theory and Research

The Obesity Epidemic

More people are overweight in the United States and many parts of the developed and developing world than ever before. This climb began in the middle of the 20th century, after the industrialized world's move through the nutrition transition. In the 1950s, fewer than 10% of people in the United States were obese. This number has grown sharply so that by 2010 more than one-third of Americans were obese.[1, 2] Many developing countries began going through the nutrition transition decades later. Transitioning from food scarcity to excess is so challenging to the maintenance of a healthy weight that it is predicted that, by 2030, 1.12 billion people worldwide will be obese.[3] Mexico in particular has experienced one of the largest increases in obesity in the world from 1990 to 2010.[4]

One interesting point about the rapid increase in obesity is that the growth in dieting has been as equally rapid. Although it may be presumed that dieting is in response to an expanding waistline, new evidence is showing that dieting may in part be causing some of the epidemic.[5-7] Perhaps part if this apparent paradox can be explained by the harsh effects of dieting, which disrupt homeostasis. As this chapter explains, going hungry as a solution for excess weight disturbs the body, mind, and spirit. It is antithetical to a holistic approach to weight control.

Toward Holistic, Homeostasis-Based Eating and Moving

Perhaps in no other realm of health have we in nursing neglected as many components of holism as in weight management. In all other areas of health, recommendations and actions have worked to restore homeostasis and reassure patients at the physical, emotional, and spiritual realms. For example, the postoperative patient who is shivering with cold gets warm blankets. This action physically restores heat homeostasis, emotionally makes the patient feel cared for, and spiritually supports a sense of a gentle and caring universe.

More often than not, the overweight patient presenting for her yearly physical is reminded that she should "lose weight." This is often done before checking for physical impediments to a healthy weight, exploring her eating and moving habits, and learning her beliefs about herself and her desired weight. The overwhelming majority of overweight patients believe that they "should lose weight" and exercise more. Most of these patients dread the shame they feel when stepping on the scale and the discussion that will follow.

Unfortunately, while reducing caloric consumption by 20% to 50% will result in short-term weight loss, this very same weight loss may be setting the stage for future weight cycling and metabolic irregularities. Far from being a purely caloric receptacle, adding and subtracting calories to achieve a particular weight, there are homeostatic mechanisms that will work invisibly to add calories and prevent their loss.[8]

Homeostasis and Weight

Although the possible physiologic mechanisms for weight control were speculated about in scientific journals written as early as 1969, ironically, it was not until the rise in obesity and the search for medical solutions that what is known about weight homeostasis exploded.[9] Early on, Hervey proposed that somehow the central nervous system must have an idea about how much stored energy is available. However, it was not until 1998 before the exact hormone that did this was discovered.[10] Leptin, a hormone produced by the fat cells themselves, proved to be the messenger relaying stored energy information to the hypothalamus. Initially, it was thought that by manipulating leptin and leptin-like chemicals, anorexic signals could be sent to the brain that would result in decreased eating. Many scientists investigated this possibility and found that, while leptin levels could be artificially increased, the hypothalamic-pituitary-adrenal axis developed resistance to the message, stopping the fullness signals.[11]

The same thing was found to happen with another fullness hormone, peptide YY 3–36 (PYY). This hormone is released when the stomach gets full, making it a "meal-stopping" hormone, as opposed to leptin, which is a more long-term appetite-suppressing hormone. Again, when PYY was injected into human subjects, their appetites were diminished initially, but the effect was soon lost.[12]

On the other hand, the same diminishing "desensitization" is not found with hunger hormones. Ghrelin, the main hunger hormone, discovered in 1999, also proved to potentially hold great promise in the world of medical weight management.[13] If ghrelin could increase appetite, it was thought that by decreasing ghrelin, appetite might also be decreased. Interestingly, this has been borne out to some degree. Because ghrelin is produced by gut mucosa when the stomach is empty, when part of the stomach is removed, as in classic gastric bypass patients, not as much ghrelin is produced. Many of these patients report slightly decreased appetites. However, there were two problems with lowering ghrelin levels to achieve weight loss. The first problem stemmed from the multiple roles ghrelin plays. Not only an orexigenic, meal-starting hormone, ghrelin is a growth hormone that plays a role in keeping the heart healthy. Lower ghrelin levels do not necessarily mean healthier patients. In fact, the other problem with ghrelin is that overweight people have lower levels than those at a normal weight.[14] While the exact reason is unknown, what is known is that 4 to 6 hours after a meal, ghrelin levels peak,

urging the individual to begin eating. As soon as the stomach is full, the ghrelin levels drop dramatically. The drop turns off a signal in the hypothalamus to trigger other orexigenic hormones like neuropeptide Y.[15] This rise and fall is healthy and useful in energy homeostasis and maintaining optimal cardiac health.

When ghrelin-induced hunger is ignored or overridden, and ghrelin levels remain high, other metabolic responses are elicited. In essence, extreme hunger sends out a "chemical mayday" response. Messages are sent to the thyroid to slow down, to the sympathetic nervous system to conserve energy, and to the liver and adipocytes to turn glycoproteins into fat cells.[8] The lessons learned from manipulating hunger and fullness hormones show us that:

- Humans are programmed to get hungry and get full. Honoring these signals leads to a balanced weight.
- When hunger and fullness are ignored, the biochemical response will err on the side of shoring up extra energy stores. This is presumably a way to prevent starvation, a more immediate threat to survival than obesity.

What Is Wrong with Current Weight Control Recommendations?

Current recommendations are calorie centric. This means that they rely on behavior to decrease Calories consumed and increase Calories expended. This approach has ignored the myriad of compensatory mechanisms, from both the psyche and the body, to resist the effects of famine. In essence, current weight management strategies have failed because they are not holistic. Evidence is showing us that humans are not an empty box to which Calories can be added and subtracted to arrive at a desired weight. To provide patients with an effective and holistic approach to eating and moving, homeostatic forces must guide our recommendations. As discussed earlier, disrupting homeostasis by telling people to cut back on calories and fat often sends metabolic messages that sabotage weight loss.[15] Recent discoveries show that extreme fat restriction causes the body to be a better fat creator.[16] In addition, without a balance of fat, excessive hunger results. This leads to excessive eating and emotional distress, either from the shame and frustration at weight gain, or discomfort from not fulfilling a basic physical need.

A calorie-centric view also does not take into account the role of different kinds of exercise. Ten thousand mindless steps may be overtraining for the individual who is sedentary. Overtraining increases cortisol levels, which increases hunger and decreases energy expenditure.[17] Interspersing short bursts of intense exercise with a movement-oriented day or week is more metabolically friendly and more helpful in achieving a healthy weight.

The Takeaway Message from Weight Homeostasis

The science behind energy homeostasis is one of the latest physiologic frontiers. The more we understand about the delicate biochemical balance between hunger and fullness, the greater our understanding about the errors in previous recommendations. The conclusion must be that the old standby "Eat less and exercise more" may not be as helpful as previously thought. Ultimately, it is true that weight is determined by how much energy comes in and how much goes out. What is also true is that there are forces increasing or decreasing calories that are not related to how much we eat or how much we move. If the recommendation to eat less results in ignoring hunger cues and delaying or skipping meals, the extra ghrelin will add weight through lipogenesis and reduce energy output by slowing thyroid and metabolism function.[18]

Like every other homeostatic system, ignoring the principles of weight homeostasis harms our health and our sense of physical and emotional well-being. In the hopes of staving off starvation, the hormonal hunger response keeps insulin levels high and triggers a resistance to the insulin.[19] And although not as intense (we cannot store oxygen), like air, hunger is triggered by baroreceptors, and extended food hunger is also painful and disquieting.

Holism and Homeostasis

A holistic approach to food and weight must honor the body's signals to maintain homeostasis. Neither the body, the psyche, nor the soul is nourished or put at ease when life-threatening messages are sent throughout the body and received by both the body and the mind. If holism requires a "whole" system approach, than the approach must have a foundation that is homeostasis-friendly. The homeostatic cues of hunger and fullness must be honored. The message to eat always and only when hungry is a way to achieve this. This is a strategy used currently by infants, toddlers, children, and even many normal-weight adults throughout the world today. Eating *always* when hungry prevents ghrelin levels from getting so high that metabolism is not disrupted. Eating *only* when hungry prevents eating more calories than the body needs. Eating always and only when hungry avoids getting too full, eating too much, and ultimately weighing too much.

What Went Wrong with This Innate Guidance System?

Like other organisms, early humans honored hunger by starting a meal and fullness by finishing. Early human hunters and gatherers, like their 20th-century descendants, were more successful in hunting and gathering when lean and lithe. Responding to homeostatic cues worked well for them. However, depending on the season and environment, they also faced times of feast and times of famine. After lean times, hunger hormones incited hyperphagia, which would have led to overeating, or feasting. Those of us in the 21st century who are food affluent can only imagine the relief and joy experienced by those who were finally eating after food had been scarce. There is something very reassuring about meeting physical needs and maintaining homeostasis. Like drinking cool water after a dehydrating race, or coming up for air after snagging an abalone 25 feet under water, eating is immensely gratifying after prolonged hunger. For the early human, whose emotional needs were met through relationships in tightly knit families and communities, and whose spiritual needs were met through moment-to-moment presence with nature, food was wonderful and good, but food was just food, like water was just water. It took the emergence of agricultural and class societies before food and weight had significance beyond satisfying a homeostatic need.

Prior to the 20th century, many of the emerging wealthy overindulged in food. Depending on the place, era, and position or role in society, extra weight was seen as a sign of health and affluence. At the same time, laborers around the world faced both harsh physical demands and marginal food supplies. For this reason, thinness was associated with being poor and, in many cases, plumpness was associated with being wealthy.

However, throughout the beginning to the mid-20th century, access to food supplies was increasing. Industrialization of agriculture in the West meant that even working classes could have plenty of food. However, this abundance was new. It is understandable that mothers born in times of food scarcity may still have seen extra weight as beneficial and big babies as healthy babies. Coming from a scarcity mentality, perhaps many of these mothers either consciously or unconsciously encouraged overeating "just in case." It takes more than one generation to transition out of plump as a sign of wealth, health, and beauty, to thin as desirable.

Nutrition Transition

In the United States, starting in the 1920s, it seemed that as soon as the working classes put on a few extra pounds, the wealthy classes opted to lose those pounds. The nutrition transition out of scarcity and into relative abundance resulted in the standard of beauty going from chubby to slender and slender to skinny over the next century. In the 1890s, advertisements for show girls were for 5′0″ and 135 pounds (a body mass index [BMI] of 26), by the 1930s, the desired female form lost curves and went down to a BMI of about 21. The ensuing decades saw the advent of fad diets and a dissemination of desired thinness by the wealthy all the way down to the working poor. The extreme thinness seen in runway models as role models for today's girls is mirrored in the epidemic of eating disorders. This unhealthy reality has even forced countries to legislate that models must have a BMI of greater than 18.

Implications of the Nutrition Transition

What happens to children born during the change from heavy as a sign of health and affluence to heaviness as a sign of weakness? Many recent immigrants, children, and grandchildren of the U.S. depression have a firsthand understanding of this plight. Food scarcity favors excess weight as an insurance against leaner times. Toddlers who grow fast and large are seen as robust. However, as they mature and socialize with others who have been influenced by the thinness ideal, they can experience a sense of self-loathing. This self-critical view has no easy remedy as excess weight in childhood is extremely resistant to loss[5] Childhood obesity creates extra fat cells as well as bigger fat cells and resistance to leptin, possibly leading to a higher "set point." Because of homeostatic forces, asking those children born from parents and grandparents of lean times to diet will most likely result in a higher postdieting weight.[20]

Yo-Yo Dieting and Self-Loathing: Not Only for the Nutrition Transitioners

Feasting was most likely the only nonhomeostatic way to eat in human's prehistory. Overriding fullness cues come from both physical prompting from high hunger hormone levels, as well as psychological security that extra food now may ward off insufficient supplies later. Wanting extra is natural, but only when food is scarce. The human body is programmed to have a healthy, balanced weight. Eating only and always when hungry promotes this and is possible when food supplies are adequate. However, because famine is more immediately life threatening than obesity, homeostasis will default to getting and storing energy. Because current cultural beliefs view excess weight as ugly and as a sign of weakness, for the first time in history individuals are choosing a self-imposed "famine." Never before have entire subpopulations chosen to override hunger cues when food supplies are plentiful.

Although overriding hunger seems logical to those wanting to cut back on calories to lose weight, it is anathema to body and soul. Despite this, large sections of the industrialized world judge themselves based on their ability to fight homeostatic urges. In addition to this negative psychological effect, there has been an epidemic rise in eating disorders. In much of the industrialized world, disordered eating is becoming the rule rather than the exception.

Homeostasis and the Psyche

The body is not the only part of the triangle calling out for homeostatic needs to be met. It turns out that the mind is geared to override decisions to deprive or restrain. In the mid-1980s, two researchers began examining the psychology behind restraint and overeating/bingeing.[21, 22] One study involved chocolate and restraint from eating it. In the study there were different types of eaters: chocolate lovers who had permission to indulge, individuals who were not fans of chocolate, and chocolate lovers who were not permitted to eat chocolate. In the end, the group that ate the most chocolate was the chocolate lovers who were restraining themselves from eating chocolate. The Herman and Polivy studies showed that inhibiting a need for food would result in the eventual disinhibition of that taboo.

Sleep and Bacteria Crucial to Healthy Weight

While the exact mechanisms are still being investigated, both a good night's sleep and healthy gut flora are also crucial in maintaining a healthy weight and a healthy metabolic profile. Perhaps it was always known that sleep deprivation decreased the amount of energy expended. Logically, a tired person feels lethargic and tends to be less physically active. However, this is only a part of the decrease in energy expenditure that comes from sleep deprivation. The other part involves biochemical reactions that actually send signals from the central nervous system to the sympathetic nervous system to slow down and conserve.[16] Lack of sleep is associated with increased belly fat, otherwise known as visceral fat.[23] Visceral fat in particular has been linked to diabetes and heart disease.[24]

Lack of sleep, however, causes other hormonal and biochemical reactions. Recent studies show that sleep deprivation leads to leptin resistance as well as increased cortisol levels and increased ghrelin levels, both of which lead to increased appetite.[25] Sleep deprivation can put an individual in a vicious circle. Nonhomeostatic eating behavior leads to an initial weight gain that can cause sleep apnea, which, in turn, leads to even greater weight gain through sleep deprivation mechanisms. Individuals can also face challenges to weight management by depriving themselves of sleep, gaining weight, becoming apneic, losing more sleep, and gaining more weight. In this way, they continue the vicious cycle.

Intestinal microbes also appear to play a role in maintaining a normal weight and a healthy metabolic profile. A healthy gut microbiota is created and sustained by diet, prebiotics, and probiotics. High-fat diets are associated with an increase in pro-obesity bacteria from the phylum firmuctes, whereas a diet with either moderate amounts of fat (41%) or low amounts (17%) is associated with the more lean-promoting bacteroides class. High levels of butyrate, a prebiotic produced by the fermentation of short fatty acid chains, is associated with leanness by promoting the growth of bacteria from the bacteroides family. Low levels of butyrate and other prebiotics, such as the *sacchyroides* species, are associated with the development and progression of obesity and its related metabolic disorders.[26] Finally, probiotics from the *lactobacillus* genus and the *bifidus* genus have been found to be supportive of a healthy gut and a healthy metabolic profile.[27]

The Lay Movement

The 1980s also saw the beginning of "intuitive eating" pioneers. Molly Groger's book, *Eating Awareness Training: The Natural Way to Permanent Weight Loss*, helped people who were compulsively overeating to match portion size with the level of hunger they had.[28] Readers were encouraged to gauge their hunger 4 to 6 hours after a meal, and if they were 5 on a scale of 1 to 10 then they were considered ideally hungry and should eat a fist-sized portion of the meal in front of them. Unlike the prescription fad diets found in women's magazines, this way of eating gave chronic dieters permission to eat. For those compulsive eaters, having to eat when ideally hungry provided them with guilt-free eating. Many noticed that when they had permission to eat, they did not eat as much.

Geneen Roth was another pioneer, providing workable solutions to guilt-ridden bingers. Her first book, *Feeding the Hungry Heart*, spoke to readers' conflict between the self-loathing that came from being unable to restrain themselves and the longing they had to enjoy food and life.[29] Believing that the relationship one has with food is the relationship one has with life, Roth launched a mission to revive the dreams and daily joys of chronic dieters by connecting a permission to eat with a permission to live.

Throughout the 1990s and 2000s, more and more lay authors spoke to readers' souls, asking them to stop beating themselves up just because they failed by abusing their bodies with deprivation.[30, 31]

Disordered eating is eating in contradiction to homeostatic cues. There are four ways to do this:

- Overriding hunger
  - Delaying meals
  - Ending meals while still hungry

- Overriding fullness
  - Eating past the point of fullness
  - Starting a meal while still full

While it is impossible to follow cues to begin and end meals 100% of the time, when cues are ignored most of the time, the body, mind, and spirit are threatened. The following case studies illustrate the emotional distress that goes along with disrupting physiologic homeostasis. Food, body image, and weight have become important in ways our early ancestors could not begin to understand. A holistic approach to caring for these four individuals is included.

Case Studies

Case Study 1

Nurse practitioner at Student Health. Katya is a 24-year-old college student presenting at Student Health because she is concerned about a recent, unplanned weight gain of 8 pounds over the last 3 months. The nurse practitioner finds Katya to have no thyroid problems, sleeping 8 hours or more a night, and a metabolic panel and physical exam that are all within normal limits. This leads the nurse practitioner to rule out organic causes for her weight gain. With a fervent request from Katya, she refers her to the Student Health nutritionist despite a BMI that is normal at 24.3.

Nutritionist at Student Health. During the 30-minute visit, after doing a 24-hour-recall, the nutritionist finds that Katya eats 5 or more servings of fruits and vegetables and adequate amounts of protein, which she consumes mostly in the form of protein-infused juices and smoothies. She discovers that while Katya is following the food pyramid recommendations with whole grains, vegetable-based protein and fat, and minimal sugary foods, Katya's average caloric intake hovers around 1,800 kilocalories (kcals) per day, which the nutritionist deems 300 kcals above her desired intake based on her 5'1" frame and her daily 50- to 75-minute workouts. The nutritionist recommends eliminating one of the fruit smoothies a day as it contains 300 to 400 Calories.

Student nurse researcher. Katya becomes an avid Calorie counter and has even given up her gluttonous days but has only lost 2 pounds in the last month. She is unhappy and feeling desperate. When she sees a flyer announcing a study in the School of Nursing to help people use health-promotion strategies to slim down and tone up, she calls the number and volunteers to be part of the study. The student nurse researcher is happy to enroll Katya into her study; however, she points out that she is a normal body weight. Katya says it is very hard for her to give up the calorie-rich smoothie the nutritionist recommended she eliminate from her diet. She complains that even though she counts her Calories and movement with a new smartphone application, she is not losing weight. To determine what stage she is in with regard to maintaining healthy habits, the student researcher gives her a 10-item quiz based on the Transtheoretical Model of Behavior Change: precontemplation, contemplation, preparation, action, maintenance, or relapse. After being told that she is in the maintenance phase, which is desirable, Katya leaves discouraged and signs up for another advertised weight loss program, Extreme Boot Camp.

Holistic weight control nurse. One month later, increasingly dispirited at not losing more than 2 pounds, even after boot camp and cutting out the smoothie, Katya finds an ad in the school newspaper explaining how intuitive eating can provide effortless weight control. Skeptical but desperate, she makes an appointment. The holistic nurse begins with motivational interviewing techniques, including probing questions, and discovers that Katya is an ex-gymnast from Eastern Europe. Katya explains that growing up in her country there were very few options to improve one's lifestyle, but because she was on the national gymnastics team, she could get a nice apartment for her whole family. She admits that it was very stressful having to practice long hours and master increasingly difficult routines; she also had to stay thin. Despite having a normal BMI she is disgusted by her flabby stomach and thighs and longs to be the 43 kg (105 pound) superstar she once was. Katya explains that her current strategy is to try to eat only one small meal a day, and then just eat high-fiber protein bars and protein smoothies to keep her weight down. She realizes that she is always a little hungry but prefers this to an overwhelming sense of guilt if she allows herself to get full. When asked why eating to satisfy a physical need would make her feel guilty, she explains, "Back in my country, my family depended on me. I was only 13, but I got us a good apartment and jobs for my father and brother. If I got fat, all that would go away. I could not let that happen." She further admitted that everyone was equally uneasy about her weight, watching her at meals and chastising her for eating any desserts or second helpings. She admitted feeling powerful and hopeful when

she got on the scale and had lost a kilo, and she still does.

The holistic nurse gives Katya the Sabotaging Beliefs Quiz (see **Exhibit 34-1**) on which she scores 50% in *using food as comfort*, 70% in *weight control as a metaphor for success*, 10% in *extra size as safety*, and 70% as a *rebellious eater*.

When asked if it was hard on her body to go without enough food, she stated that her body just had to get used to it. She also explained how she thought about food, shopping for food, or cooking/preparing food all day long. She described the guilt when she occasionally stuffed herself at parties and the ritualistic fasting she engaged in the entire day before the meal.

When asked if she could be a healthy weight if she ate enough food to satisfy her hunger, she wistfully said, "This will never be. Look, before I ate so much more than now (and grabbing a pinch of skin near her belly button) and this is what I have." The holistic nurse had her complete the Intuitive Weight Control application for the most recent typical day of eating, which found her to be a *deprivation grazer*, which meant that although she ate more than five meals or snacks a day, she was always a little hungry. She also filled out the application for 2 aberrant days in the previous week and was found to have been a *meal skipper* on Wednesday, putting her hunger level very high, and a *gluttonous eater* on Thursday, meaning that she got extremely full for at least two out of three or four meals.

Holistic physical analysis. In terms of homeostasis, most days Katya is overriding hunger cues by stopping eating while she is still hungry. On occasion, she will also skip meals but then overeat the following day. Despite being a normal BMI, she is at risk of metabolic syndrome and fatty liver. Both fasting and feasting cause the liver to turn free fatty acids into fat cells.[16] The lower blood glucose levels get, the more likely hyperglycemic hormones will cause the release of glycogen from the liver and excess glucose into the blood. The higher the glucose, the higher the insulin and ultimately the more likely to result in insulin resistance. Katya is also at risk of overtraining, which can occur with more than 20 hours of aerobic activity per week with no down days. Unrelenting, excessive daily

| EXHIBIT 34-1   Sabotaging Beliefs Quiz |

Directions: Without spending too much time on each question, choose the response that best fits your recollection.

	Not at all True (0 points)	Somewhat True (1 point)	Very Much True (2 points)	TOTAL
I don't deny myself anything when I'm upset.				
I eat more when I'm stressed or depressed.				
I feel ashamed if I overindulge.				
I feel safer knowing I can binge occasionally.				
If I have a whole box of cookies, I may eat them all.				
Add Score Section I				
Being slim increases people's expectations of me.				
Controlling your weight makes you more powerful.				
I'm always looking for new ways to slim down or stay slim.				
It isn't fair I have to struggle so hard to be slim.				
Losing weight/maintaining weight is painful; you just have to bite the bullet.				
Add Score Section II				
I think my mother/father was worried I'd be fat.				
I used to sneak food when I was a kid.				
Weight was important to my mother/father.				
Sometimes I would eat dessert before dinner.				
My mother/father made me feel guilty when I ate.				
Add Score Section III				
As a kid/baby I wouldn't always eat even when I was hungry.				
Big babies are healthy babies.				

(continues)

EXHIBIT 34-1 Sabotaging Beliefs Quiz (*continued*)				
	Not at all True (0 points)	**Somewhat True (1 point)**	**Very Much True (2 points)**	**TOTAL**
I felt vulnerable when I was smaller.				
I never let myself get too hungry.				
Somehow it just feels right to be extra full at the end of a meal.				
Add Score Section IV				

Copyright® Inner Resource, 2003

Results:

Section I: Using Food for Comfort

What's Going on with You: If you scored between 5 and 10 points in this category you most likely use food to soothe yourself. Whether it's stress or sadness, you view food as nurturing and soothing.

Why It's Bad: Physically, putting nourishment in your mouth when you're not hungry, means you are eating extra over and over again and that can mean extra weight. Once the weight is there, leptin insensitivity sets in and it's like you have a new set point. Your body is not receiving messages from fat cells that they exist. Your brain turns on the hunger hormones as though you didn't have any fat.

Psychologically, most of you who eat for emotional reasons feel remorse, guilt, and shame almost immediately after the cookie hits your lips.

How to Break Away from This Belief: In the realm of food and sustenance, true nourishment comes out of satisfying a physical need. Humans have felt true emotional highs feasting with friends and family. Eating enough to feel satisfied is nourishing and fulfilling. You might want to ask yourself if you give yourself permission to enjoy eating. Often, though eating starts out as a guilty pleasure, it devolves into a shameful habit.

To help shift the belief and behavior that follows, you may want to:

1. Imagine what it would be like to give yourself guilt-free permission to enjoy eating enough to be satisfied. Then try it.
2. Not make eating the only enjoyable thing you allow yourself to do on a daily basis. If you work so hard that your only free time is meals, then it's no wonder you prolong them. Try bringing a crossword, solitaire game, or book chapter to do for 10–15 minutes after eating a fist-sized portion of healthy and delicious food. If you're still hungry after that, then by all means eat some more (though chances are you won't be).
3. Try other ways to nourish yourself. Take a long bath, or get a massage. Watch something funny, or go dancing.
4. Find a friend or confidante with whom you can share your feelings, especially the ones of sadness, frustration, or loneliness. Sometimes people overeat to communicate their desperation with a loved one or spouse.

Section II: Weight Control as a Metaphor for Success

What's Going on with You: If you scored between 5 and 10 points in this category, you most likely are a chronic dieter, believing yourself especially powerful when you are staying slim or losing weight.

Why It's Bad: It may not seem like there's a downside to "slimming down," after all, most of us could stand to lose a few pounds. It is absolutely true that there are health benefits to being lean. However, dieting does not result in long-term leanness for anyone but a paltry few (2%). In fact, eating so little you feel hungry and deprived most likely results in rebound weight gain and many negative health effects. The huge surges in ghrelin turn off your thyroid, reduce your energy expenditure, and make it more likely for you to put on weight around your middle. Unfortunately, for 98% of us, chronic dieting results in extra weight overall, leptin

EXHIBIT 34-1   Sabotaging Beliefs Quiz (*continued*)

insensitivity, hyperinsulinemia, and glucose intolerance. None of these conditions can be cured by "dropping the weight" if it means depriving yourself. Bottom line: Chronic dieting bottoms out your metabolism and puts the rebound weight in places more likely to cause metabolic syndrome.

Psychologically, being addicted to losing weight can be a hard habit to quit. The exhilaration you feel overriding hunger and biting the bullet is a powerful motivator to going without. Indulging in previously forbidden foods after the diet can be equally rewarding until the pounds creep back on. But in your mind you probably believe, "No worries, I can take off the weight." Many of you spend huge amounts of your days strategizing on how to eat less, not trusting your bodies.

How to Break Away from This Belief: Unfortunately, knowing something is unhealthy to body and spirit doesn't make it an easier habit to break. IF you find your self-worth tied to your weight or ability to lose weight, this is indeed very sad. Even though it doesn't feel sad when you're successfully losing weight or convincing yourself you have NO unmet needs because you can numb yourself to hunger, you are missing out on part of your life. Try to do the "death bed" exercise. In this exercise you imagine yourself to have lived your life, and you are essentially "on your death bed." Write down the things you want to be known for, your contributions, your relationships, and your regrets. What most likely won't make the list of what brings you contentment is anything to do with the hours spent figuring out how to eat less while constantly thinking of food, or fantasizing about a life available only to those who go without and are unsatisfied. Ultimately, most naturally slim people enjoy eating and do not think about it unless they are shopping, cooking, or hungry. Focus on fitness and remember, like the cheetah at the San Diego Wild Animal Park, short bursts of effort are the best way to communicate to your body you need to be lean. Long, exhausting workouts tend to have the opposite effect, telling your body you are in danger and need to conserve calories.

Section III: Rebellious Eater

What's Going on with You: If you scored between 5 and 10 points in this category, you most likely see rebellion as a way to communicate to your loved ones that you suffered from their depriving you. Your parents may have wanted "only the best" for your health. However, parents are looked to as the source of nurturing, not the source of keeping you from sustenance. Often, restricting children, besides being unnecessary, has the opposite effect from what is intended. Toddlers forbidden to eat desserts eat much more in the absence of parental control than do toddlers who are allowed to eat sweets. Your mother or father may have also treated you differently than your siblings, making you feel the sting of injustice.

Why It's Bad: Regardless of how unfair it is to be denied the rewarding experience of eating delicious food, eating for any reason other than hunger will not lead to psychological and physical health. Reaching for a cookie before dinner just because you can doesn't mean it is a good thing to do. When your body's hungry, it wants protein, not sugar. Your blood glucose levels soar, then your insulin levels, causing your blood sugar to crash. Do this enough times and you may be tipping the scales in favor of hyperinsulinemia, insulin resistance, and prediabetes. Psychologically, it isn't very satisfying when you don't give your body what it craves.

How to Break Away from This Belief: Try noticing when you eat for reasons other than satisfying a hunger. Compare these moments to those when you are giving your body what it craves. Believe it or not, our bodies crave savory foods, rife with protein and micronutrients. Yes, your body may also crave sweets, but you will notice a chocolate chip cookie tastes much better after a small meal than in between meals and you will probably find you eat fewer sweets that way.

Regardless of the origins of your destructive food path (e.g., parents who were misguided or overtly neglectful), it probably would be beneficial to talk to friends, people in Overeaters Anonymous, or a therapist to sort out what you need to do to have the life you want.

Section IV: Extra Size as Safety

What's Going on with You: If you scored between 5 and 10 points in this category, you most likely find extra weight or size beneficial. There are many reasons why people find themselves in this category. Kids who might have been bullied by peers or parents may have longed, like Tom Hanks in *Big*, to be bigger. Bigger meaning safer. Children, especially girls, who were sexually abused may also find themselves wanting to obliterate their curves, and/or be big enough to resist unwanted violations. Or finally, extra food may be seen as insurance against lean times. People who grew up during the depression or in an area where there was famine or

(continues)

EXHIBIT 34-1   Sabotaging Beliefs Quiz (*continued*)

food scarcity may believe extra weight is healthy. Big babies are seen as healthy. Whether you are eating as a way to shore up extra reserves or to feel safer and more powerful, breaking free from this belief, though difficult, is much to your benefit.

Why It's Bad: Your body needs to be lean with just a bit in reserve. Your body does not need too much extra fat. You may not even be aware of it, but being smaller makes you less visible to your predators, a survival advantage. Only to a powerless child who has few choices is being an unhealthy weight an advantage, and then the advantage is psychological only (as discussed below). Your body is suffering from the results of excess poundage. Sustained excess weight makes you insensitive to leptin, turning off an important feedback loop telling your hypothalamus you have had enough. Too much truncal weight can disturb the metabolic balance of hormones and lead to prediabetes and diabetes. All in all, using your body as a shield or a reservoir is not necessary for protection and makes you vulnerable instead of resilient.

Psychologically, depending on extra flesh to keep you safe does not really feel all that good, does it? Abusing your body with too much food cannot really protect you. If you think of your body as a separate being, like a baby or a pet, you would feel badly if you took away their litheness, power, independence, and health.

How to Break Away from This Belief: This is a hard belief to overcome. But like all detrimental beliefs, transformation starts with noticing the belief behind the behavior. This in fact may be one of the hardest parts. You may not even acknowledge you have this belief. The belief may be buried under more immediate thoughts, like, "I don't think there is any advantage to being heavy. Ugh!" or "I hate my flab!" Society has taught us well. But deep below the surface a feeling may bubble up when you eat past the point of fullness that there is some advantage, however irrational, to being big. Many years ago, Oprah Winfrey had an episode on her show dealing with sexual abuse victims. Many people in the audience had extra weight on their frames. She asked her audience to close their eyes and go back in time and confront their abuser. She asked how that would feel. Many seemed strong enough to face their tormentor. However, when she asked them how they would feel if they weighed 50 pounds less, there was an audible gasp. In their powerless position as children, only physical size could give them the strength or invisibility to resist being violated.

So if you do not yet recognize your underlying belief that "size is safety," feel free to do this quick exercise. Take out a piece of paper, put at the top of the page in nice bold writing, "I can weigh 50 pounds less," and then right below it in much smaller writing, put in parentheses, "no I can't." Then set a timer for 4 minutes and just start listing all the reasons why you can't weigh 50, or 100, or 20 pounds less. Try not to even think about it. Just let your hand do the work.

Ultimately, you are an adult, with adult choices. You do not have to associate with predators, and you can store food on shelves and emergency kits in case of scarcity. Tae Kwon do and dating smarts are much more foolproof ways of staying safe than having a muffin top or a big derriere.

---

workouts increase stress hormone levels, impairing muscle formation and increasing hunger.[17]

Holistic emotional analysis. Psychologically, Katya is in a double bind. She feels powerful when she ignores hunger, but her constant lack makes her obsessed with food and always dissatisfied. For her, controlling weight is a metaphor for her success. Her self-esteem is linked to successfully and continually fighting her body's urges. This is a war that cannot be won. In trying to resolve it, Katya is using up energy and creativity and is giving up much in the way of relationships.

Holistic spiritual analysis. Spiritually, Katya may be seen as a "Hungry Ghost." She is, in essence, roaming the world unfulfilled, unsatisfied, and in constant need.

Holistic Caring Process

Body. In order to help Katya's body not suffer the famine/fasts she indulges in four to five times a month, she is urged to notice how hungry she is when she begins a meal and how full she gets when she stops eating. This is not an easy task for Katya, who as a chronic dieter. Hunger has been the enemy for so long that she has trained herself to be numbed to it. The nurse asks her to complete the water test, where she waits 4.5 to 6 hours after a meal, drinks a cold glass of water, and, if she feels the cold water coat her stomach, notes the feeling so that she can recognize what she feels as hunger in the future. Katya discovers, with the help of the nutritionist, that all foods are not created equal. She learns that liquid meals are not as satisfying as bulk meals and that high-nutrient foods such as avocado, blackberries, and kale can curb hunger and decrease cravings. Katya also learns that fasting and the lack of fiber she ends up with by drinking juices and smoothies instead of the whole fruit or vegetable is favoring an unhealthy phylum of bacteria to take over her gut. She is willing to switch from protein powder smoothies to real food such as lean meats, legumes, berries, greens, and occasional desserts. She learns to cook these in delicious ways and realizes that many of her cravings have subsided.

Mind. Katya is asked to journal sequential answers to the questions "What will happen if I eat as soon as I am ideally hungry?" and "What will happen if I eat until I am satisfied?" The immediate answer to both of these questions is "I'll get fat." When Katya questions, "What will happen if I gain weight?" she believes she would be weak, useless, and ineffective, and others would perceive her as disgusting, piggish, and unworthy. After a few weeks and with greater reflection, Katya finds, much to her surprise, that if she eats until she is ideally full she will also feel nourished and taken care of. Katya discovers that she is holding on to many harsh and conflicting beliefs. She makes a pact with the holistic nurse to notice how she feels with each snack or meal. She also agrees that these issues need to be addressed in therapy.

Spirit. To avoid reinventing the wheel, holistic nurses can refer patients to the plethora of self-help books and electronic applications that address psychophysiologic needs for sustenance and spiritual well-being. One of the foremost pioneers in this arena is Geneen Roth. In her book *Why Weight? A Guide to Ending Compulsive Eating*, there is an exercise that asks the reader to think about "if I had to do it over," originally popularized by Nadine Stair.[32] It is hoped that the answers will provoke Katya to look at the big picture of life's meaning and the smallness when weight becomes the whole world. Roth also points out that your relationship to food is your relationship to life, something that is beginning to resonate with Katya.

Case Study 2

Primary care physician visit. Al presents for his yearly visit to his primary care physician. He grimaces as he gets on the scale because he knows he has gained back a lot of the weight he lost last year. At 78 years of age and 5'10", Al got his weight down to 196; now, however, he is back up to 213 pounds. He promises to sign up again for water aerobics and go back on the treadmill every day for 30 minutes. He explains that he lost his willpower over the holidays, with the many parties, events, and get-togethers. The physician tells him that his health depends on his sticking to "his diet": "Don't you want to be around for your granddaughter's graduation?" She notes that his iPad application has all of the tools he needs to help him to slim down again. He just has to commit to following the recommended caloric intake. Based on his activity, she refers him to a nutritionist to help him develop meals that support his congestive heart failure, hypertension, and diabetes. However, she does not just stick to the talk about exercise and food. She ends the visit by ordering a sleep study. A week later the results show that Al is severely sleep deprived due to sleep apnea and restless leg syndrome. During the study he woke up 274 times during the 7.5 hours he was asleep.

Nutritionist. The very slim nutritionist points out to Al that his BMI went from overweight (28.1) to obese (30.4) in the last 6 months. A 24-hour recall shows that Al is eating 43% of his 2,340 daily calories in the form of fat, 20% as protein, and 37% in the form of carbohydrates. While Al is eating salad twice a day and using a light salad dressing, he admits that it does not taste like anything unless he uses three to four tablespoons of dressing and covers the salad in bacon bits or cheese. Al states that he only eats skinless chicken breasts or low-fat ground turkey in the main dishes that he or his wife cooks, but again he admits that the roughly 350-Calorie dinners leave him hungry before he turns in, so he will open the liverwurst and low-fat mayonnaise and make a sandwich late at night. He eats a high-fiber cereal for breakfast but discovers that he is eating two servings instead of one. He also adds applesauce, strawberry toppings, and sometimes whipped cream. The nutritionist recommends using the American Heart Association cookbook and doubling the 170- to 220-kcal recipes for lunch and dinner and not eat after 8:00 p.m. Al stops at the bookstore and looks for the cookbook. As he is searching, he notices another book on intuitive eating. After spending much of the evening reading this book, he calls the author to make an appointment at her nutrition consulting business.

Intuitive eating author. The intuitive eating nutritionist starts the session by asking probing questions. She learns that Al was born halfway through the depression, the son of a mother who grew up on a homesteading farm in the Midwest. While Al always had enough to eat in his middle-class home, his mother faced occasional food scarcity as her farmer father tried to eke out enough of a living on a rocky soil to feed and clothe nine children. Often, there was just barely enough food to feed the family of 11. However, when she was 15 she got a job working for a family in the city. For the first time in her life there was always enough food in this affluent family home. She went from scrawny to chubby in less than a year. While she felt better and safer with extra weight on, it was the end of the roaring twenties and her excess pounds did not serve her as she tried to fit in with the more affluent "townies." She started one fad diet after another, trying to slim down. Al remembers his mother either on a diet or off a diet, often relegating herself and her family to cottage cheese and tomato breakfasts for half the month and then indulging them in butter-laden au gratin potatoes and dessert the other half. Growing up as a skinny kid, Al did not need a 120-kcal breakfast. He tells the nutritionist that his father's side of the family ate much differently than his mother's. Father, aunts, and uncles all ate when they were hungry, stopped when they were full, and stayed slim their entire lives. No matter how delicious the food, when Thanksgiving or Christmas came around, these individuals ate slowly, savoring every bite, and ate just enough to be satisfied. Al appeared to be taking after them throughout his high school and even into his college years. However, a spell of unemployment after leaving the army sent him into his mother's world, where he imagined the boost to self-esteem he would feel after losing 5 pounds. In less than a month, through a crash diet and intense physical exercise, Al took 6.5 pounds off of his 174-pound, 5'10" frame. He got the next job he interviewed for. However, by the first-year anniversary at his new job, he had gained back not only the weight he had lost but another 8 pounds. Apparently, Al had adopted his mother's relationship to food: delicious delicacies that must be given up, no matter how difficult, in order to achieve that victorious feeling of weight loss. On the one hand, food was physically and emotionally lifesaving, but on the other it was a sign of weakness if he ate too much. Al ended up recreating his mother's life of yo-yo dieting. With each diet came rebound weight gain equal to or greater than the weight he was before reducing. Just like her, he was either on a diet or off a diet. These days, when Al is on a diet he exercises, using his NordicTrack ski machine, treadmill, rowing machine, or total gym. When he goes off his diet, he stops exercising and overeats in spectacular ways. Initially, he will eat double portions of diet food, and then he will give in completely to eating large portions of juicy steaks, cheesy potatoes, and bowls of ice cream.

Holistic physical analysis. Al's metabolic syndrome (hypertension, insulin resistance, obesity) was caused by his chronic dieting. Al weighed 174 pounds before his first diet, and his highest weight was 242 pounds. Homeostatic forces interpreted each crash diet as famine and reversed the life-threatening condition by increasing hunger and holding onto every Calorie. In diet mode, Al overrides hunger by delaying meals until very hungry and stopping meals while still hungry. Off of a diet, Al overrides fullness cues by eating past the point of fullness. According to the Intuitive Weight Control application, Al is afraid to not be full when he is off his diet, which means that for three out of four meals he gets very full. When he is on his diet, he becomes a *deprivation eater*, which means that he is very to extremely hungry when starting each of his three meals.

The effects of dieting on homeostasis has Al's body ramping up energy conservation, decreasing energy output of the sympathetic nervous system, and decreasing the amount of thyroxin secreted by the thyroid. In addition to this quasi-hibernation state, the liver sends messengers to the adipocytes to incorporate the free fatty acids, turning them into fat cells. When Al goes off his diet, he responds to high ghrelin levels with hyperphagia. Off a diet, his sympathetic nervous system kicks in, and his thyroid also wakes up. In splurging mode, excess glucose from overeating sends the same message to the liver so that free fatty acids continue to be turned into fat cells. Physically, as mentioned previously, both feast and famine result in the storing of fat. In addition to Al's behavior, his obstructive sleep apnea is helping keep weight on his body by increasing his cortisol and decreasing his leptin levels, which increase his hunger and cravings for fat. Also, sleep deprivation raises ghrelin levels. The result is additional hunger and more weight.

Holistic emotional analysis. Psychologically, Al thrives on both the success he feels overriding his bodily needs and the pleasure of giving into those same needs. Emotionally, at 78 he is also struggling with a shortened life expectancy due to congestive heart failure. This yo-yo dieting results in a high-risk cardiac metabolic profile.[33] While not a full-blown addiction, Al's feast-and-famine way of eating has milder versions of two of the three Cs a traditional addict is struggling with: *cravings*, can't *control*, and *continues* despite negative *consequences*. In Al's case, compulsively dieting and bingeing harken to both cravings and lack of control. Yo-yo dieting has negative health consequences, and yet, Al continues to do it. While in the beginning he was able to eat moderately after dieting, he currently can eat three portions of food despite the harm it causes his metabolic state. Al has lived through an era where weight gain after dieting was seen as a loss of willpower and the solution was to bite the bullet again. The health threats of yo-yo dieting are just beginning to be understood.[34]

Both overeating and undereating can be seen as a substance/process addiction, causing obesity and metabolic disturbance. Al scores 50% in *using food for comfort*, 70% in *weight control as a metaphor for success*, 20% as a *rebellious eater*, and 50% in *extra size as safety*.

Holistic spiritual analysis. While Al has no complaints, by losing control over his behavior and continuing to do something that is damaging, it is hard to be connected spiritually. Ultimately, fighting his body's powerful messages to begin and to stop eating, he may be missing some of the gentleness of the universe. By ignoring lifesaving cues, he is, in effect, punishing his body to serve his own attachment to the cycle of starving and splurging. Willfully depriving himself of eating can be seen as harsh as sleeping without covers, living without shelter, or even going without water or air for short periods. Spiritual health eschews asceticism; spiritual enlightenment is, at its root, holistic, focusing on comfort and consolation as an end reward.

Holistic Caring Process

Body. Going on another diet will not help Al in the long term. What will help Al is getting enough physical activity every day despite not being on a diet. Combining consistent exercise, a nutrient-rich diet to help with restless legs, and a CPAP machine for his sleep apnea are the most sustainable ways to improve cardiovascular health.[35] In addition to the CPAP machine, he gets a Fitbit activity tracker to help record his movements and sleep quality. He is encouraged not to count calories on his iPad application.

Mind. Al is very attached to the power he feels while he is losing weight, as well as to the nurturing sensation he feels when he is splurging. It is unlikely that he will want to reverse these habits in his golden years. Al signs up for the 11:00 a.m. daily water aerobics class, committing to 6 months. There he makes friends with the instructor and strikes up several more acquaintanceships with other aerobic goers. This plan supports two of the tenets of Social Cognitive Theory: (1) He is encouraged by *peers* and is bolstered by the camaraderie he feels going there, and (2) he believes that he has the skill set to accomplish this exercise; in other words, he feels a sense of *self-efficacy*. Choosing a form of physical activity supported by a health-promotion theory will make it easier for Al to continue physical activity during the times that he is "off a diet." His wife has also committed to going on evening walks with him, replacing the loner activity of the treadmill that Al has only found the impetus to go on when he is in his ascetic warrior state.

Spirit. Al considers himself an agnostic Catholic. He attends church once a month for the social aspect, "And I do feel closer to the goodness of humanity when I'm there." He denies having any unmet spiritual needs, and although his health has suffered from his yo-yo dieting, he is not unhappy with his lifestyle.

Case Study 3

Nurse midwife. Debbie is a 48-year-old mother of three teenage boys and is also a business owner. When she goes to her nurse midwife for her yearly physical, the midwife notices that she is 12 pounds heavier than last year and inquires about that. Debbie complains that her appetite has increased and she is getting night sweats that wake her up several times a night. She complains of fatigue and daytime sleepiness. The midwife orders a hormonal panel and discovers that Debbie is perimenopausal and the vaginal ultrasound is showing some luteal cysts. An at-home sleep study also shows that she is getting only about 5 hours of adequate sleep, with the other 3 being very restless and light. The midwife explains that progesterone coming from the luteal cysts is an appetite stimulant and that exercise and birth control pills can sometimes help balance hormones. The midwife orders a low-dose birth control pill to balance her hormones during perimenopause. She points out that strength training is also very helpful for perimenopausal and postmenopausal women because muscle mass tends to shrink during this time.

Physical trainer. Debbie signs up for a personal trainer at the local gym. For the first 3 weeks she is very motivated to subject herself to a grueling 45-minute workout of machine repetitions to strengthen most of the muscles of her body. She is starting to notice that the

night sweats are less frequent and she is sleeping a little more deeply. Her business is picking up, however, and she is having to wake up an hour earlier (5:45) just to get to work on time. By week 5 she has lost much of her motivation to wake up while it is dark, not see her kids, drive 15 minutes to the gym, change into gym clothes, work out for almost an hour, and then shower and change just to get to work on time. She calls her midwife and asks if she knows of a holistic weight expert who can help her be healthy *and* have a balanced life.

Holistic weight coach. Motivational interviewing uncovers that Debbie has struggled with her weight since childhood. Being a little chubby, Debbie went into puberty very early, having to wear a bra at age 9 and starting her period at 10, 2 years before any of her friends did. Not only did her maturing body make her feel like an outcast among her friends, it also made her feel sick and violated at family events. One of her uncles would examine her and make lewd comments about her changing body. Her mother and father dismissed their daughter's discomfort. They even laughed at some of her uncle's demeaning jokes. She found herself alone, feeling vulnerable and disgusting, and turned to food both as a coping mechanism and to make her feminine form blur into indistinct curves. However, the heavier she got, the more her mother tried to reverse the weight gain and began serving the entire family Weight Watchers meals and banishing desserts. Debbie would use her allowance to buy food that she would hide so that she could secretly binge at night before going to bed.

By the time Debbie went to college, she wore a size 16 on her 5′4″ frame. In college things started changing; she noticed feeling conflicted about her sexuality and her body. In this culture, sex was exciting, mutually satisfying, and forged a connection with another human being. Debbie wanted what her roommates had, but she felt unattractive. To make herself more sexually attractive, she began going to Weight Watchers, getting down to a size 12. Believing her metabolism to be shot, it was an uphill battle to lose those first 5 pounds. She did feel a boost to her self-esteem and continued the weight loss, with a goal of 20 more pounds.

When she dropped a whole size and saw her feminine curves return, she felt uneasy. Somewhat giddy that men might want her, she was also feeling that old vulnerability as her body became slimmer. Debbie fluctuated between a size 12 and a size 16 throughout college, marrying the first serious boyfriend she met her senior year. After the wedding her weight crept up to a size 16/18, where she has been ever since. Her husband, heavy himself at 230 pounds, has been okay with his wife's body. Debbie admits she that feels more comfortable in the bedroom at her current weight than she did in college at a size 12.

Holistic physical analysis. In terms of homeostasis, Debbie's forced overriding of hunger cues with her mother's meager rations sent her ghrelin levels soaring. This primed her body to become very efficient at conserving calories and converting them to fat. With the nightly binges she saturated her liver with lipids and glucose, making lipogenesis easy. In college, she overrode hunger cues by ending meals while still a little hungry and delaying them until she got very hungry. The difficulty Debbie has in losing weight comes from two physiologic forces. Being overweight throughout middle and high school induced a resistance to leptin, raising her set point to a heavier size, and the extended high levels of ghrelin throughout the day decreased her metabolism and energy expenditure and made her efficient at creating fat cells. Currently, thinking back to her last typical day of eating, Debbie turns out to be a *nighttime seesaw eater*, eating when hungry and stopping when full during the day but splurging in the night, having two meals and sometimes two desserts. While Debbie is not night bingeing, she is overeating at night. Part of this may stem from the fact that her breakfasts and lunches are more "Weight Watchers" style and not giving her enough food to satisfy her hunger, causing her to be ravenous at night. She overrides hunger by stopping both breakfast and lunch while still a little hungry. She overrides fullness by eating past the point of fullness and starting snacking while still slightly full.

Holistic emotional analysis. Psychologically, Debbie feels safer at a bigger size. This is a common way children can fend off undesired sexual attention or physical abuse. Her ability to give up bingeing relatively easily indicates that she is not addicted to overeating as much as overeating allows her to feel more comfortable sexually. She takes the Sabotaging Beliefs Quiz and scores 60% in *extra size as safety*, 40% in *using food as comfort*, 50% in *weight control as a metaphor for success*, and 60% as a *rebellious eater*.

Holistic spiritual analysis. Debbie feels a strong connection to God. While she does not believe every dictate of the Lutheran Church, she feels a holy presence in the church itself and enjoys going to services. She has been in therapy and touched on the violation she experienced at a vulnerable age, feeling that she has let it go. She has tried to repair the damage by ensuring that she is able to protect her own children. She loves her life and her family.

Holistic Caring Process

Body. Debbie may have increased her set point by both undereating and overeating, thereby causing a resistance to leptin. Without resistance, the central nervous system is apprised when extra fat cells are on board. Resistance to leptin means that appetite will stay high, as though there is a deficit in fat cells. Fortunately, this state of resistance does not have to exist long term. Recent studies show that exercise may help regain leptin sensitivity. It appears that short bursts of very intense exercise may be especially helpful. Sleep deprivation negatively affects weight in three ways: (1) It increases cortisol levels and ghrelin levels, (2) it increases hunger hormones, and (3) it decreases leptin levels. When Debbie finds out about the connection between sleep, weight, and health, she is very open to exercise that would let her sleep in. Consistent with the ecological model of health promotion, the holistic weight coach helps Debbie find a bike route to her office instead of interrupting her sleep. Debbie likes this approach as it has her getting in only 12 minutes later than if she drove. Despite the 6 minutes of intense pedaling during the first part of the ride, she can clean up at the sink and change into one of her work outfits that she brings in at the beginning of the week. On the weekends she takes a Zumba class.

Mind. While never having had therapy to deal with the inappropriate behavior of a predatory uncle, Debbie does seem reflective about its effect on her life. Her faith has helped her create the life she desires, especially ensuring that her sons are heard and taken care of. She does wonder, however, if there might be residual resentment, especially of her parents, whom she believes did not protect her, were in part to blame, and might be the recipients of her blame.

Case Study 4

Nurse midwife visit. Elvia is a 24-year-old recent immigrant from Mexico to Los Angeles who presents for her 25-week prenatal visit and brings her 2-year-old son, Brandon, with her. The nurse midwife notes that Elvia is gaining the recommended weight for gestational age. Her 2-year-old, however, looks to be almost 40 pounds. The midwife asks if she breastfed her first baby, and if she plans to breastfeed this one. Elvia says she plans to do both bottle and breast, but, with a more in-depth history, the midwife discovers that she tried breastfeeding her son but gave up after she got home from the hospital. She explains in Spanish, "My milk never came in." The daughter of subsistence farmers in Oaxaca, she came to the United States at the age of 19 to make a better life for herself and her future children. The midwife thinks that Elvia would be a perfect fit for the Breastfeed LA project and calls her friend who is on the board. Her friend enrolls Elvia in the study.

Breastfeed LA project coordinator. The project coordinator gets a full history from Elvia and learns that her mother, father, and all of her siblings are still in Mexico. The coordinator understands how important it is to have someone who has successfully breastfed be a support to help Elvia successfully nurse her baby. The coordinator discovers that Elvia has only her husband and a brother-in-law who is not yet married for support. She "knows" some people but only has one good friend. She has no close friends or family who have ever breastfed. She pulls out a sippy cup and hands it to her son, saying, "¿Quieres jugo de manzana, m'hijo?" (Do you want apple juice?). The coordinator asks Elvia about her son Brandon and learns that he was born in a small private hospital that was not designated as "baby-friendly." He was bottle fed the entire 2 days they were in the hospital. Elvia said she tried to breastfeed Brandon when she came home, but he could not latch on, and, although she tried to express her milk by hand, no milk came out. She explained that it was much easier just to bottle feed him, and that way also she could be sure he was getting enough. She used the bottles the hospital gave her and then bought formula with the WIC (Women, Infants, and Children supplemental nutrition program) coupons. During the interview, the project coordinator showed Elvia pictures of infants and toddlers at varying sizes. When asked to choose the healthiest children Elvia consistently chose babies in the 95th percentile of BMI and above. When asked to choose the healthiest food for age, she chose the bottle for babies less than 4 months and baby food for 4 months and above. During a structured interview on infant-centered feeding, Elvia revealed her distrust of her baby getting enough milk through breastfeeding. The reasons cited involved "not enough milk," "harder to get out," and "breast milk is not rich enough (thin and gray)."

Elvia believes that her 33-pound 2-year-old is at a healthy weight. A 24-hour recall for Brandon via his mother reveals that he receives more than 84% of his Calories in the form of fats, carbs, and sugars. Instead of water, Brandon drinks juice or soda, up to 600 kcals a day.

Holistic physical analysis. Elvia's newborn is at risk of overriding fullness cues as Brandon does. The extra Calories the future newborn will get if bottle fed will increase both the number and size of the fat cells, just as Brandon has both fat cell hypertrophy and hyperplasia. Low-income mothers are reluctant to throw out unused formula and tend to force the last few ounces into their babies.[36] Babies fed like this will get used to the feeling of being extra full and will regard this sensation as normal. Overfed children, like adults, will become resistant to leptin, and, if fed frequently enough, will miss out on the heart benefits of having ghrelin levels peak right before meals.

Holistic psychological analysis. Elvia went from subsistence farming in a small, tightly knit community to a large metropolis with few close relationships. She carries the sensibilities of a generation facing food scarcity, and she believes that extra fat on babies and toddlers is insurance against lean times. Soda and juice (seldom part of the daily fair in Oaxaca) are ways she shows love and abundance to her children. Fresh fruits and vegetables are more expensive than juices and Calorie-dense processed foods. She takes the Sabotaging Beliefs Quiz and scores 30% in *using food as comfort*, 0% in *weight control as a metaphor for success*, 50% in *extra size as safety*, and 20% as a *rebellious eater*. A very important difference between Elvia and Brandon is that Elvia was not bottle fed, or fed on schedule, helping her to eat based on homeostatic cues.

Holistic Caring Process

Body. For Elvia's future newborn, giving birth in a baby-friendly hospital, along with a lactation consultant, are all interventions in line with Social Cognitive Theory. Seeing peers who may have already achieved some success in their new country with healthy children will help Elvia embrace the benefits of breastfeeding. She is also referred to a La Leche group that meets at 11:00 a.m. on Fridays in a storefront church next to a Mexican market. At that meeting she will be exposed to Spanish-speaking women, both recent immigrants and first-generation Latinas from low- to middle-income groups. Social Cognitive Theory predicts that pro-breastfeeding peer groups will be more successful in educating her on the benefits of breastfeeding. Her future newborn will learn to stop when full and can carry this habit through adulthood as a naturally slim person.

Brandon has already gotten used to the feeling of overriding fullness and is probably resistant to leptin, so he may or may not be able to slim down naturally. Recommending dietary changes by increasing the quality of food must be done by peer counselors who are knowledgeable about the Southern Mexican diet. Identifying what Brandon's favorite foods are and helping Elvia find ways to prepare them with fewer fats and sugars would be helpful. Tacos al carbon, beans (at least part of the time not refried) and rice, tomatoes, and "sopa de albondigas" (made of low-fat ground turkey) are all valuable building blocks of a heart healthy, nutritious, and a culturally sensitive diet.

Coupling this approach with peer recommendations to save sugary drinks for special occasions may work together to prevent extra weight gain. However, because children are very resistant to long-term weight loss, and "dieting" can even increase weight gain in this group, focusing on lower weight as an outcome could be detrimental.[6] Focusing on fitness, however, would be optimal. Determining with Elvia whether the playgrounds near her urban Los Angeles home are safe enough to play in would be helpful. If not, investigating Head Start programs, or eventually a Boys and Girls Club or Police League afterschool sports program is recommended. As soon as Brandon starts kindergarten, Elvia must be aware that he can be enrolled in 2 hours of afterschool playground time for free. Encouraging Brandon's father to play soccer with him as he gets older would also be very beneficial.

Mind. Elvia comes from an area and an era of food scarcity, which has her mentality in the *prenutrition transition* mode, where excess weight is seen as a sign of health and affluence. Many low-income Mexicans are beginning to prefer a slimmer appearance for adults. However, embracing the Spartan eating habits and thin limbs of a toddler may run contrary to those brought up with a fear of food scarcity. Extra fat on youngsters is seen as protection. It may be very difficult to alter this view. Helping Brandon and the newborn by encouraging activity and breastfeeding may go a long way toward maintaining homeostasis. Helping Elvia establish friendships with women who eat based on homeostatic cues, and who have children who are a healthy weight, will help Elvia trust that enough (not extra) food is the best choice.

Spirit. Fortunately, Elvia's culture has provided a foundation for mindful eating. As Elvia makes her new home in a place with resources and options to thrive and not just survive, it is hoped that she will become more and more available to spiritual awakening and wholeness.

Holistic Caring Tips for All Nurses

Because of our background in honoring homeostasis and promoting holistic approaches to health threats, as nurses, we are the optimal champions of the new paradigm addressing weight control. A holistic approach to weight maintenance must honor the homeostasis and allow food to be nourishing to the psyche. It is extremely useful to understand several things.

1. Long-term weight loss is unlikely for all but a few people. Initial weight loss is probable, but the willpower required to override hunger cues may bode poorly for homeostasis overcompensation, leading to rebound weight gain.

2. Children are resistant to weight-loss intervention. Encouraging children to eat always and only when hungry is essential. Improving fitness and food quality are the only interventions that are evidence based. This is best done with ecological, social cognitive, and dissemination of innovation-based theoretical underpinnings.

3. Breastfeeding is the best way to support intuitive eating as an infant is programmed to eat when hungry until satisfied. Parents should be supported in the initiation of breastfeeding through baby-friendly hospitals, lactation specialists, and inexpensive rental of breast pumps. Breastfeeding also creates and supports healthy gut bacteria required for a lifetime of healthy weight. Parents should also be supported in their correct interpretation of their child's hunger and satiety, weight, and health.

4. Consciously, everyone knows it is better for their health to be a normal weight. Unconsciously, there may be reasons why people put and keep weight on. Motivational interviewing and the Sabotaging Beliefs Quiz may be helpful ways to uncover unconscious motivations in overriding homeostatic cues.

Intuitive Eating

When a chronic dieter begins to eat based on body cues, it is very easy to either undereat or overeat. The skill of knowing when you are hungry is sometimes forgotten when hunger has become the enemy. The exercise presented in **Exhibit 34-2** can help reawaken that innate experience we were all born with.

Mindful Eating

This way of eating is very nourishing to body, mind, and soul. It is also very foreign to the chronic dieter, who is often racked by guilt when

---

EXHIBIT 34-2   Tips to Help Your Patients Eat Healthier

Say YES to giving your body the right amount and type of food to be healthy.

The benefit of eating intuitively allows people to eat with a positive attitude. Instead of musing, "Oh no, I shouldn't eat because I'm so fat," the approach is positive: "I'm hungry. I should eat until I'm satisfied." When full, tell yourself, "I have had enough." Intuitive or homeostatic eating entails several key practices.

Key Practices of Ideal/Intuitive Eating

1. Begin a meal or snack when ideally hungry. *Ideally hungry* means hungry without hunger pangs or rumblings.
2. Eat until ideally satisfied. *Ideally satisfied* means that you will not be hungry again for 4 to 6 hours and have not gotten too full or "stuffed."
3. Choose what your body is craving from your favorite foods that are both delicious and healthy.

How to Know When You Are Hungry

The cold water test:

1. Four-and-one-half to 6 hours after eating a meal, drink a cold glass of water.
2. If you feel it coat the bottom of your stomach, then you are ideally hungry.

How to Know When You Are Full

The taste experiment:

1. When you become ideally hungry, provide yourself with a fist-sized portion of delicious, healthy food.
2. Close your eyes and notice flavors as you eat your portion.

EXHIBIT 34-2   Tips to Help Your Patients Eat Healthier (*continued*)

3. Stop and wait 10 minutes.
4. Put another bite of the same food in your mouth. Notice the flavors again. If the food does not taste as good this time as it did when you began, then you are probably full.

Get Some Help

1. There are many books and programs available to help people eat intuitively, from Geneen Roth[29, 32] to the Gabriel Method[37] to the Intuitive Weight Control application for smartphones and electronic devices. These resources explain the reasons to eat intuitively, describe what to expect when you go from dieting to eating intuitively, and provide tools to help you eat exactly what your body needs—no more, no less.
2. Instead of counting calories or keeping a food journal, keep a hunger/fullness log, noting how hungry you are when you begin each meal or snack and how full you get when you stop.
3. Find a group to support you in your lifestyle change and an activity you enjoy doing.

TABLE 34-1   Tips for Mindful Eating

Activities Associated with Eating	Mindful Questions to Be Fully Engaged
Holding, seeing, and touching	How does it look and feel?
Smelling	Which memories are evoked by the smell?
Placing	What does it feel like on your tongue?
Tasting	What does it taste like?
Swallowing	How does this experience satisfy?

Source: Data from: J. Kabat-Zinn, "Mindfulness for Beginners: Reclaiming the Present Moment and Your Life" Sounds True (Colorado, 2012).

eating "bad" foods. The best way to encourage mindful eating is to follow the simple (and yet not necessarily easy) steps recommended by Jon Kabat-Zinn, a pioneer in mindfulness meditation,[38] shown in **Table 34-1**.

Conclusion

Prevention

Preventing childhood and adult obesity must start prenatally. Especially for soon-to-be parents who come from areas of food scarcity, the message must be that babies know how much to eat, and healthy babies can be many sizes. Baby-friendly hospitals that promote breastfeeding are critical partners in the movement to have children and adults eat always and only when hungry throughout their lives.

Keeping in mind that health can be achieved at any size, we can "make peace" with our patients by taking weight loss off the table.[39] Metabolic disturbance caused by overeating and failed dieting can be corrected. For patients and clients struggling with metabolic illnesses, we must resist the urge to encourage weight loss. Instead, we must focus on what can restore homeostasis. This includes promoting the following:

- Eating always and only when hungry.
- Eating gut-friendly foods, including prebiotic and probiotic supplements.
- Getting enough good-quality sleep.
- Finding movement and exercise that can be done daily.

Promoting Health

From a homeostatic perspective, although we live in the 21st century, we have the psyches and bodies of our early human ancestors. From this perspective, it makes sense that any threat to health can tip the scales from maintaining leanness to overcompensating and shoring up

TABLE 34-2 Promoting Health		
Health-Promoting Activities	**Physically Reassuring**	**Psychologically Reassuring**
Sleep well	Less cortisol = less ghrelin = appetite decreased	More energy
Eat Intuitively		
Eat only when hungry	Excess Calories avoided	Less shame
Eat always when hungry	Excess ghrelin avoided = appetite decreased	Less fear
"Exercise"		
Move daily	More Calories burned	More stamina
More independence		
Include bursts of intense exercise	Leptin sensitivity increased = less adipose	More resilience
Eat Healthy Foods		
Eat whole foods, more fiber, prebiotics, and probiotics	More healthy gut bacteria = leptin sensitivity increased = less adipose	Less bloating
Avoid artificial preservatives and sweeteners	More regularity	Improved self-image
Include healthy fats	More nutrients absorbed	Satiety prolonged

energy stores (see **Table 34-2**). An unhealthy gut might prevent the absorption of key nutrients. A lack of sleep might impair the ability to secure and prepare food. On the other hand, adequate food supplies that allow us to eat always and only when hungry will promote leanness by sending homeostatic signals that remove the threat of famine from our physiologic lexicon. Other messages encouraging leanness can also come from the intense bursts of speed needed by our early human ancestors to catch the day's meal. This activity sent important messages that litheness, speed, and leanness were necessary.

Far from an empty box where Calories can be added and subtracted, the human organism is wired to protect energy stores if threatened. Embracing this reality and removing threats is at the foundation of a holistic approach to weight control. It is the new paradigm that is hoped will bring more health and less self-loathing to the next generation. This new paradigm contains two of the cornerstones of nursing practice: homeostasis and holism. Nurses can be at the forefront of championing this intuitive way of eating.

Directions for Future Research

1. Measure outcomes of patient satisfaction with intuitive eating techniques.
2. Examine various educational methods to teach eating only when hungry strategies.
3. Do children change their eating pattern when exposed to other children who use homeostatic cues for determining hunger?

Nurse Healer Reflections

After reading this chapter, the nurse healer will be able to answer or to begin the process of answering the following questions:

1. Am I aware of my own personal feelings toward hunger?
2. How can I begin to discuss homeostasis related to food with patients?

3. How can I introduce the homeostasis concept with colleagues to implement in patient care?

NOTES

1. Centers for Disease Control and Prevention, "Overweight and Obesity" (2013). www.cdc.gov /obesity/data/adult.html.

2. National Center for Health Statistics, *Health, United States, 2012: With Special Feature on Emergency Care* (Hyattsville, MD: National Center for Health Statistics, 2013).

3. B. M. Popkin, L. S. Adair, and S. W. Ng, "Global Nutrition Transition and the Pandemic of Obesity in Developing Countries," *Nutritional Reviews* 70, no. 1 (2012): 3–21.

4. J. A. Rivera, S. Barquera, F. Campirano, I. Campos, M. Safdie, and V. Tovar, "Epidemiological and Nutritional Transition in Mexico: Rapid Increase of Non-Communicable Chronic Diseases and Obesity," *Public Health Nutrition* 5, no. 1A (2002): 113–122.

5. D. Neumark-Sztainer, M. Wall, J. Haines, M. Story, and M. E. Eisenberg, "Why Does Dieting Predict Weight Gain in Adolescents? Findings from Project EAT-II: A 5-Year Longitudinal Study," *Journal of the American Dietetic Association* 107, no. 3 (2007): 448–455.

6. L. Ritchie, "Less Frequent Eating Predicts Greater BMI and Waist Circumference in Female Adolescents," *American Journal of Clinical Nutrition* 95, no. 2 (2012): 290–296.

7. L. Outland, "Bringing Homeostasis Back into Weight Control," *Journal of Obesity and Weight Loss Therapy* 2, no. 2 (2012): 115.

8. R. Nogueiras, M. H. Tschöp, and J. M. Zigman, "Central Nervous System Regulation of Energy Metabolism: Ghrelin Versus Leptin," *Annals of the New York Academy of Sciences* 1126 (2008): 14–19.

9. G. Hervey, "A Hypothetical Mechanism for the Regulation of Food Intake in Relation to Energy Balance," *Proceedings of the Nutrition Society* 28 (1969): 54A–55A.

10. J. M. Friedman and J. L. Halaas, "Leptin and the Regulation of Body Weight in Mammals," *Nature* 395, no. 6704 (1998): 763–770.

11. M. G. Myers Jr., R. L. Leibel, R. J. Seeley, and M. W. Schwartz, "Obesity and Leptin Resistance: Distinguishing Cause from Effect," *Trends in Endocrinology and Metabolism* 21, no. 11 (2010): 643–645.

12. D. Renshaw and R. L. Batterham, "Peptide YY: A Potential Therapy for Obesity," *Current Drug Targets* 6, no. 2 (2005): 171–179.

13. M. Kojima, H. Hosoda, Y. Date, M. Nakazato, H. Matsuo, and K. Kangawa, "Ghrelin Is a Growth-Hormone-Releasing Acylated Peptide from Stomach," *Nature* 402 (1999): 656–660.

14. E. S. Hanson and M. F. Dallman, "Neuropeptide Y (NPY) May Integrate Responses of Hypothalamic Feeding Systems and the Hypothalamo-Pituitary-Adrenal Axis," *Journal of Neuroendocrinology* 7, no. 4 (1995): 273–279.

15. D. S. Ludwig and M. I. Friedman, "Increasing Adiposity: Consequence or Cause of Overeating?" *Journal of the American Medical Association* 311, no. 21 (2014): 2167–2168.

16. M. Tschöp, D. L. Smiley, and M. L. Heiman, "Ghrelin Induces Adiposity in Rodents," *Nature* 407 (2000): 908–913.

17. M. B. Johnson and S. M. Thiese, "A Review of Overtraining Syndrome: Recognizing the Signs and Symptoms," *Journal of Athletic Training* 27, no. 4 (1992): 352–354.

18. D. Perez-Tilve, K. Heppner, H. Kirchner, S. H. Lockie, S. C. Woods, D. L. Smiley, M. Tschöp, et al., "Ghrelin-Induced Adiposity Is Independent of Orexigenic Effects," *Journal of the Federation of American Societies for Experimental Biology* 25, no. 8 (2011): 2814–2822.

19. L. da Conceição Antunes, M. N. da Jornada, J. L. Elkfury, K. C. Foletto, and M. C. Bertoluci, "Fasting Ghrelin but Not PYY Is Associated with Insulin-Resistance Independently of Body Weight in Wistar Rats," *Arquivos Brasileiros de Endocrinolgia e Metabolismo* 58, no. 4 (2014): 377–381.

20. A. E. Field, S. B. Austin, C. B. Taylor, S. Malspeis, B. Rosner, H. R. Rockett, M. W. Gillman, et al., "Relation Between Dieting and Weight Change Among Preadolescents and Adolescents," *Pediatrics* 112, no. 4 (2003): 900–906.

21. C. P. Herman and J. Polivy, "From Dietary Restraint to Binge Eating: Attaching Causes to Effects," *Appetite* 14, no. 2 (1990): 142–143.

22. J. Polivy, J. Coleman, and C. P. Herman, "The Effect of Deprivation on Food Cravings and Eating Behavior in Restrained and Unrestrained Eaters," *International Journal of Eating Disorders* 38, no. 4 (2005): 301–309.

23. K. G. Hairston, M. Bryer-Ash, J. M. Norris, S. Haffner, D. W. Bowden, and L. E. Wagenknecht, "Sleep Duration and Five-Year Abdominal Fat Accumulation in a Minority Cohort: The IRAS Family Study," *Sleep* 33, no. 3 (2010): 289–295.

24. J. C. Lovejoy, S. R. Smith, and J. C. Rood, "Comparison of Regional Fat Distribution and Health Risk Factors in Middle-Aged White and African American Women: The Healthy Transitions Study," *Obesity* 9, no. 1 (2001): 10–16.

25. K. Spiegel, E. Tasali, P. Penev, and E. Van Cauter, "Brief Communication: Sleep Curtailment

in Healthy Young Men Is Associated with Decreased Leptin Levels, Elevated Ghrelin Levels, and Increased Hunger and Appetite," *Annals of Internal Medicine* 141, no. 11 (2004): 846–850.

26. R. Jumpertz, D. S. Le, P. J. Turnbaugh, C. Trinidad, C. Bogardus, J. I. Gordon, and J. Krakoff, "Energy-Balance Studies Reveal Associations Between Gut Microbes, Caloric Load, and Nutrient Absorption in Humans," *American Journal of Clinical Nutrition* 94, no. 1 (2011): 58–65.

27. V. K. Ridaura, J. J. Faith, F. E. Rey, J. Cheng, A. E. Duncan, A. L. Kau, N. W. Griffin, et al., "Gut Microbiota from Twins Discordant for Obesity Modulate Metabolism in Mice," *Science* 341, no. 6150 (2013): 1241–1251.

28. M. Groger, *Eating Awareness Training: The Natural Way to Permanent Weight Loss* (New York: Simon & Schuster, 1985).

29. G. Roth, *Feeding the Hungry Heart: The Experience of Compulsive Eating* (New York: Plume, 1982).

30. E. Tribole and E. Resch, *Intuitive Eating: A Revolutionary Program That Works* (New York: St Martin's Press, 2003).

31. L. Outland and F. Rust, "Why Disrupt Homeostasis? Reasons Given for Not Eating When Hungry and Not Stopping When Full," *Holistic Nursing Practice* 27, no. 4 (2013): 239–245.

32. G. Roth, *Why Weight? A Guide to Ending Compulsive Eating* (New York: Plume, 1989).

33. S. Graci, G. Izzo, S. Savino, L. Cattani, G. Lezzi, M. E. Berselli, F. Balzola, et al., "Weight Cycling and Cardiovascular Risk Factors in Obesity," *International Journal of Obesity* 28, no. 1 (2004): 65–71.

34. J. P. Montani, A. K. Viecelli, A. Prévot, and A. G. Dulloo, "Weight Cycling During Growth and Beyond as a Risk Factor for Later Cardiovascular Diseases: The 'Repeated Overshoot' Theory," *International Journal of Obesity* 30, Suppl 4 (2006): S58–S66.

35. E. Shahar, C. W. Whitney, S. Redline, E. T. Lee, A. B. Newman, F. J. Nieto, G. T. O'Connor, et al., "Sleep-Disordered Breathing and Cardiovascular Disease: Cross-Sectional Results of the Sleep Heart Health Study," *American Journal of Respiratory and Critical Care Medicine* 163, no. 1 (2001): 19–25.

36. A. Singhal, K. Kennedy, J. Lanigan, M. Fewtrell, T. J. Cole, T. Stephenson, A. Elias-Jones, et al., "Nutrition in Infancy and Long-Term Risk of Obesity: Evidence from Two Randomized Controlled Trials," *American Journal of Clinical Nutrition* 92 (2010): 1133–1144.

37. J. Gabriel, *The Gabriel Method: The Revolutionary Diet-Free Way to Totally Transform Your Body* (New York: Atria Books, 2008).

38. J. Kabat-Zinn, *Mindfulness for Beginners: Reclaiming the Present Moment—and Your Life* (Boulder, CO: Sounds True, 2012).

39. L. Bacon, "End the War on Obesity: Make Peace with Your Patients," *Medscape General Medicine* 8, no. 4 (2006): 40.

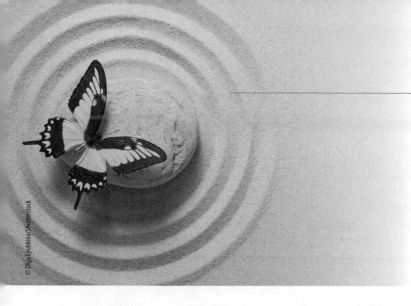

CHAPTER 35

Smoking Cessation

Christina Jackson

Nurse Healer Objectives

Theoretical

- Explore antecedents to smoking behavior.
- Analyze the mind–body responses to nicotine.
- Examine theoretical strategies for successful smoking cessation.

Clinical

- Interview a client who smokes and listen to the client's story, including reasons the client gives for starting and continuing smoking.
- Through the interview, try to gain insight into the client's readiness for change, and design interventions that correspond to the stages and processes of change as appropriate to the client.
- Recognize and use all opportunities to offer brief smoking cessation encouragement and advice to clients.

Personal

- If applicable, examine the effect of passive smoking on you and what changes you can facilitate in your environment.
- Consider your own coping mechanisms and how you can make changes for greater health.

- If you are a smoker, explore your need for healthier coping mechanisms, and identify habit breakers (behaviors) to become a successful nonsmoker.

Definitions

Habit breakers: New action behaviors that replace old "smoke signals" or triggers.

Quit line: A telephone smoking cessation resource available 7 days a week to support tobacco cessation efforts.

Smokefree.gov: A detailed online resource for information to support tobacco cessation efforts (for those trying to quit as well as for professionals who work with clients).

Smoke signals/triggers: Phenomena in the internal and external environment that create a desire to smoke.

Theory and Research

Many smokers who have achieved sobriety from drugs or alcohol might say that quitting smoking is an even more formidable challenge than quitting those other substances. In fact, nicotine is highly addictive for several reasons. It has powerful effects on brain function and the feel-good neurotransmitters dopamine, endorphins, and norepinephrine. It can both calm the user who is feeling anxious or stimulate the user who is feeling sluggish. What an ideal drug—and it is legal and does not alter level of consciousness or ability to function; in fact, many believe it enhances thinking and performance. An older nurse who sought smoking cessation treatment said, "I've always had 20 friends in this pack who have helped me any time I needed them. I will miss them dearly." Indeed, smokers have an emotional attachment to their drug of choice and have often bypassed the development of other (healthier) coping mechanisms because smoking became the default mode of adaptation.

It is likely most helpful to view tobacco use as a coping mechanism indicative of underlying issues in need of healing rather than viewing smoking as the chief problem in and of itself. Smokers often report starting the habit at a young age—even at 10 or 11 years—not only to impress peers but to cope with "stress." This is an indication of the plethora of adverse childhood events and traumas from which children must recover and heal. By viewing smoking as an attempt (albeit unhealthy) to handle the stresses and traumas of life, we can get a more complete picture of a holistic plan to support the cessation of tobacco use.

The Prevalence of Smoking and Its Health Consequences

With an estimated 42.1 million smokers in the United States (18.1% of adults 18 and older), it is thought that 480,000 premature deaths are caused annually because of smoking, and more than 41,000 of these deaths are thought to be due to secondhand smoke exposure.[1] Smoking-related illness in the United States accounts for more than $289 billion a year in direct healthcare costs and lost productivity. It is estimated that although 41% of smokers try to quit smoking each year, only 4.7% maintain abstinence for at least 3 months.[2] These statistics are sobering and underscore the need to focus on smoking *prevention*.

Currently, there are about 1.3 billion smokers in the world, 84% of whom live in developing countries.[3] Tobacco use is responsible for an estimated 5 million deaths worldwide each year and is projected to cause 10 million deaths per year by 2030.[4] Between direct healthcare costs and loss of productivity from smoking-related illness around the world, tobacco use is projected to cost governments more than $200 billion per year.[3]

Cigarette smoking (and secondhand smoke) contributes to four of the five leading causes of death per year in the United States, including lung cancer, coronary heart disease, chronic lung disease, and stroke. In May 2007, the state of Arizona put into effect a comprehensive statewide smoking ban. Research into the effect of this ban reveals significant reductions in hospital admissions for smoking-linked diagnoses, including acute myocardial infarction, angina, stroke, and asthma.[5] The American Heart Association and the American Stroke Association strongly recommend smoking cessation because of the direct correlation between smoking and both coronary artery disease and ischemic stroke.[6] It is estimated that tobacco is responsible for 85% of deaths caused by lung cancer.

As of 2012 data collection in the United States, 18.1% of adults are smokers (20.5% of men and 15.8% of women). And although rates of smoking have declined across all ethnic population groups in the United States between 2005 and 2012, smoking remains the leading cause of mortality and morbidity.[1] Multiple races (non-Hispanic) have the highest rates of smoking at 26.1%, followed by American Indians/Alaska Natives (21.8%), whites (19.7%), blacks (18.1%), Hispanics (12.5%), and Asians (10.7%). Most adult tobacco smokers become addicted during adolescence, and greater than 17% of those aged 18 to 24 are already smoking, with rates peaking between ages 25 to 44 (21.6%) then declining slightly in those 45 to 64 years old (19.5%) and tapering to 8.9% in those over 65.[1] Smoking rates are highest among those with a General Educational Development certificate (41.9%). Conversely, rates of smoking are lowest among adults with graduate degrees (5.9%). Adults who live below poverty levels also experience a high prevalence of tobacco use (27.9%).[1]

Women and Smoking

Though the use of tobacco by women in the United States was 6% in 1924, peaked at 33% in 1965, and is now down to 15.8% (including 11%

of pregnant women), it is estimated that 250 million women throughout the world smoke, and most of these are in developed countries. Women metabolize nicotine 15% faster than men, and if they use oral contraceptives, this rate increases to 40% faster than men. Using smoking to maintain a more ideal body weight and to manage negative mood states such as anxiety and depression are more common in women than in men. These negative mood states are associated with body image concerns in women, and fears of weight gain or unwelcomed mood can create barriers to smoking cessation in women. Research demonstrates that the cardiovascular risks of smoking are greater in women than in men, and the numbers of women who die from lung cancer are increasing faster in women than in men.[7]

In Europe, South Africa, and Australia, 20% to 45% of pregnant women smoke.[8] Smoking during pregnancy harms both mother and baby and is a leading cause of morbidity and mortality during the intrauterine and early childhood stages of life. These preventable problems include premature birth and miscarriages; implantation, placental, and membrane issues; and infant respiratory, cognitive, and behavioral issues.[8]

In the United States, 54.3% of women quit smoking during pregnancy, and 15.9% resumed after delivery with the highest prevalence in women aged 20 to 24 (25.5%), American Indians/Alaska Natives (40.1%), those with fewer than 12 years of education (24.5%), and those who had Medicaid coverage during pregnancy or delivery (24.3%).[9]

Marketing campaigns over the years have used glamorous imagery to promote cigarettes and offer "light" or low-tar alternatives that falsely claim safety advantages. Chronic obstructive pulmonary disease (COPD), once thought of as a predominately male disease, now kills more women than breast cancer, and the number of new cases of COPD in women is increasing three times faster than in men.[10] Growth and development of lung and airway tissue are different in males and females, and the airways of females are vulnerable to hormonal effects. Estrogen affects the metabolism of nicotine, and this also affects addiction and cessation in

women smokers. Healthcare providers tend to diagnose COPD more readily in men than in women, offering spirometry evaluation more often to men than to women, even in women with more severe dyspnea and cough.[10]

Smoking cessation should be a priority in women's health, and it should be geared toward the unique needs of females. For example, one study reported increased smoking relapse rates among women during the premenstrual (luteal, progesterone predominant) phase of the cycle. Another found no difference in relapse rates according to stage of menstrual cycle but did find the withdrawal symptoms of craving and anger to be the most frequently associated with relapse but only in women who quit during the follicular phase of the cycle. For many women, mood changes occur in the premenstrual phase that place them at risk for urges to smoke.[10]

Although some research shows increased difficulty for women to quit, other studies show women to have greater receptivity to smoking cessation. Women tend to be more afraid of weight gain as a result of cessation than male smokers do. Smoking cessation has been associated with increased body fat in several studies; however, one study also found an increase in functional muscle mass.[11] This potential for increased functional capacity in women who quit could be used as a motivator, especially when designing holistic approaches to cessation that include exercise and other lifestyle changes. In a study of female prisoners who participated in a group smoking cessation intervention with nicotine replacement, significant weight gain (net difference of 10 pounds) was experienced by abstainers when compared to continuing smokers. This effect did slow down at 1 year postintervention, however.[12] The fear of weight gain should be taken into account when designing cessation programs for women.

Various mood states such as depression and anxiety have been correlated with higher rates of exacerbation and hospitalization in patients with COPD and are more frequently seen in women. Among COPD patients with psychiatric comorbidity, 60% of women had psychiatric disorders as compared to 38% of men.[10] Although research on women and smoking is often contradictory, there is evidence that hormone fluctuation, physiology, mood, and differences in motivation play roles in smoking and cessation that make women different from men. Providers who inquire about these factors can assist women in preventing relapse.

Special Groups

Smoking prevalence is notably high among several groups in the United States including lesbian, gay, bisexual, and transgender individuals (LGBT), military service personnel and veterans, and those who are HIV (human immunodeficiency virus) positive.[13] Data collected between 2009 and 2010 reveal prevalence at 32.8% among LGBT, most likely due to the aggressive marketing of tobacco products to this population, along with the risk of stress from stigma and prejudice they may face.[13] Twenty-nine to 36% of veterans reported current smoking (by age group) versus 24% of those who had not served. Rates are even higher for those who have been deployed.[14] For those living with HIV, it is estimated that smoking prevalence is fully two times higher than among the general population. Because those with HIV can live longer, healthy lives, the health risks from smoking (including heart disease, stroke, COPD, pneumonia, and cancer) are serious concerns for this population.[15]

Hookah Smoking: An Emerging Threat

The smoking of flavored, sweetened, humidified tobacco in social "bar"-type settings has emerged as a concerning trend among U.S. youth. While legislated interventions aimed at limiting the marketing, affordability, and accessibility of cigarettes have reduced cigarette smoking in youth in recent years, smoking tobacco using a hookah (also referred to as a waterpipe, hubble bubble, goza, and nargile) is on the rise among teens and college-aged students. A recent survey found that 18.5% of 12th-grade students had smoked from a hookah in the past year.[16] Hookah lounges have proliferated and are exempted from smoke-free air laws. In addition, websites dedicated to promoting the use of hookahs are proliferating in the United States.[17] Dozens of websites sell hookah tobacco (called *shisha*, or *maassel*), and regulations against selling and

postal handling of tobacco products do not yet apply to shisha. "Expanded restrictions on credit processing for Internet purchases and on shipping tobacco products would make hookah smoking less accessible to youth."[16, p. 3]

The antecedents to youth hookah smoking are the same as for cigarette smoking, including social acceptance, having family and friends who smoke, and believing hookah smoking to be safe and nonaddictive. In fact, many youth believe that the health effects of hookah smoke are less dangerous than with cigarettes, but this is not true. The same toxins and risk for addiction are present in hookah smoke as in cigarette smoke and lead to cancer, respiratory illness, low birth weight, and periodontal disease.[16]

Environmental Tobacco Smoke

In addition to smoking cigarettes and inhaling smoke directly, there is also the problem of passive smoking (sometimes referred to as secondhand smoke), better known as environmental tobacco smoke (ETS). The ETS is a combination of smoke from the burning end of a cigarette, cigar, or pipe and the smoke exhaled from a smoker's lungs. This environmental perspective on exposure has now been expanded to include "thirdhand smoke," or the residual chemical contamination that remains in an environment (clinging to furniture, carpets, walls, and the like) even 24 hours after a cigarette has been extinguished. The ETS contains more than 4,000 highly toxic chemicals, such as formaldehyde, nitrogen oxide, acrolein, Group A carcinogens (asbestos), cadmium, nickel, and carbon monoxide. In addition, ETS contains a radioactive substance from tobacco leaves that has been subjected to high-phosphate fertilizers.[18]

Approximately 34,000 nonsmokers in the United States die each year due to heart disease caused by exposure to secondhand smoke. An estimated 7,300 lung cancer deaths occur annually among nonsmokers. Those nonsmokers who live or work in environments with secondhand smoke have a 20% to 30% increased risk of lung cancer. Children and adults exposed to ETS also have a greater risk for other illnesses, including respiratory tract infections, exacerbation of asthma, otitis media, and sudden infant death syndrome.[18] One study found higher rates of mental health disorders among adolescents and children exposed to ETS.[19]

Physiologic Responses to Smoking

Smoking and tobacco contribute directly to death. Yet deaths from smoking do not receive the same amount of attention from the news media as do airplane crashes, violence, and disease epidemics, situations resulting in far fewer deaths. Smoking causes more deaths, but these deaths take a very long time to develop; therefore, the significance of the problem is often minimized.

Over time, smoking strips the lungs of their normal defenses and completely paralyzes the natural cleansing processes. The early morning cough associated with smoking results from attempts by the bronchial cilia to clear the thick yellow or yellow-green mucus that accumulates in the air passage to an abnormal amount because toxic cigarette smoke interferes with the cilia's normal function. This cleansing action triggers the cough reflex. As exposure continues, the bronchi begin to thicken, which predisposes the person to bacterial and viral infections, asthma, emphysema, and cancer.[20]

Within seconds after the smoke is inhaled, irritating gases (e.g., formaldehyde, hydrogen sulfide, ammonia) begin to affect the eyes, nose, and throat. With each inhaled breath of smoke, carbon monoxide enters the bloodstream, and its concentration eventually rises to a level 4 to 15 times as high as that of a nonsmoker. The carbon monoxide passes immediately to the bloodstream, binding to the oxygen receptor sites and, thus, depleting the cells of oxygen. Hemoglobin, which normally carries oxygen throughout the body, becomes bound to the carbon monoxide and is converted to carboxyhemoglobin, which is unable to deliver oxygen to the cells. In addition, smoking increases platelet aggregation, allowing the blood to clot more easily.[2]

The constriction of tiny blood vessels decreases the delivery of oxygen to the skin and contributes to "smoker's face," where deep lines appear around the mouth, eyes, and center of the brow. The muscular puffing action also contributes to lines around the mouth. There is an established link between nicotine and erection problems in male smokers, and smoking is believed to be the leading cause of impotence in the United States today. Smoking also adversely affects fertility by decreasing sperm count and sperm motility. Female smokers are significantly more likely than nonsmoking females to be infertile, and heavy smoking amplifies this decline in fertility. Recent research demonstrates a clear correlation between smoking and gene expression (individual genes as well as entire networks of gene interaction) that corresponds to smoking-related pathologies including cancer, cell death, and immune response.[21]

Nicotine is the drug inhaled from cigarettes that quickly reaches the smoker's brain. As the average smoker takes an estimated 10 puffs per cigarette, a pack-a-day smoker gets about 200 puffs per day. Each nicotine "hit" goes directly to the lungs, and the nicotine-rich blood travels to the brain in approximately 7 seconds. As nicotine enters the brain, it acts as a "mood thermostat" and can help users to maintain a steady and pleasant sensation of psychological neutrality. Nicotine stimulates people when they are drowsy and calms them when they are tense; it affects cognitive processes of concentration and emotional states.[20]

The action of nicotine causes the brain to release norepinephrine, endorphins, corticosteroids, and dopamine.[3] The brain then adapts to accept these chemicals by increasing the number of nicotine receptors and becomes physically dependent on nicotine. Thus, the general level of arousal is adjusted up or down by introducing nicotine levels that allow the smoker to feel stimulated or relaxed. Nicotine has been described as being as addictive as cocaine and heroine and with similar development of tolerance that increases the desire for higher doses.[20] Unlike other powerful street drugs, however, nicotine does not interfere with the capacity to work and create, and it may actually enhance individuals' capabilities. The effects of nicotine are reached in a matter of seconds; the smoker experiences drug-induced contentedness, all in a legally sanctioned manner.

Norepinephrine controls arousal and alertness. Beta-endorphin, referred to as the brain's natural analgesic, can decrease pain and anxiety. Dopamine is part of the brain's pleasure center and also can decrease pain and anxiety. Smoking's "attention thermostat" effect is mediated through the brain's limbic system, where the major neurotransmitters are adrenaline and dopamine, both of which are influenced by nicotine. It appears that nicotine helps the smoker concentrate by promoting selective attention to important tasks, which increases learning and memory. Nicotine can enhance cognitive processes and reduce fatigue. In addition, nicotine can exert a sedating effect, reducing anxiety and inducing euphoria.[3] Continued smoking also prevents the unpleasant side effects of nicotine withdrawal, such as irritability, irrational mood changes, low energy levels, inability to feel stimulated, and increased sensitivity to light, touch, and sound.

The overall effect of smoking is a shift in brain chemistry that creates the mood needed for the situation at hand—that is, increased relaxation, alertness, or pleasure and decreased pain or anxiety. But, even though nicotine is a powerful and effective drug, concerned smokers can create and sustain new behaviors to achieve the same positive effects without the health risk to themselves or those around them. The physiologic dependency declines sharply in the first week of cessation; however, the behavioral or habitual pattern triggering the desire to smoke is more difficult to modify. Success in smoking cessation requires a plan of action and a great deal of body-mind-spirit self-care. A growing body of research underscores the fact that successful cessation plans must address any issues pertaining to mood disorders and focus on underlying or withdrawal-related depression. Although some smokers go it alone and quit "cold turkey," for many, smoking cessation is a process that can take time and a great deal of emotional and physical support. The hopeful reality is that cessation can be achieved by anyone who is motivated, open to addressing concomitant depression and anxiety, and willing to try a variety of strategies to find what works.

Cultural Considerations and Special Populations

Research supports the effectiveness of smoking cessation counseling and programming for people from all cultural backgrounds.[22, 23]

Resources must be linguistically appropriate and accessible, including for those with sensory impairments such as deafness or blindness. The Internet is a valuable resource for those with special needs of any kind and can link almost anyone to resources tailored to help with cessation. Those with mental illness (including psychosis) can benefit from cessation counseling and resources, but again, the mode of delivery must be accessible and tailored to accommodate special needs.[24] Smoking cessation in those with mental illness is also more complex because smoking is a pervasive behavior in most mental health environments, so triggers are difficult, if not impossible, to avoid. In addition, nicotine often calms and enhances well-being in a way that the other drugs persons with mental illness take do not. Motivation to quit among this population of clients is often a problem.

Native American tobacco users often have difficulty with smoking cessation because for them tobacco use is part of sacred ceremony. The deep cultural, spiritual, and social ties to smoking and tobacco can make addressing the addiction component more complex. Careful exploration of perceived benefits, motivation, and supportive resources is necessary to assist in quitting.

Smoking Cessation

Measuring Successful Cessation

Because smoking cessation is not an easy task, success is often measured in small increments. Smoking quit rates vary with the different approaches to cessation. Over the years, researchers have evaluated a variety of public and private multicomponent cessation programs, healthcare provider-directed counseling, and Internet-based and community-based programs.

Self-Quitters, Healthcare Provider Counseling, and Nurse Follow-Up Advice

There are conflicting data as to the best way to quit smoking. Research reports estimate 90% of successful quitters kick the habit on their own each year, and quit rates tend to be higher for those who quit on their own than for those who participated in a cessation program. Recent studies demonstrate that smokers who quit cold turkey are as likely to remain abstinent than were those who gradually decreased their daily consumption of cigarettes, switched to cigarettes with lower tar or nicotine, or used special filters or holders.[25] Recent research results indicate that those who use medications to support behavioral cessation efforts are more likely to be successful. All agree that the quitter must be motivated and ready to quit. Careful exploration of these factors with the client, and strategic support to bolster strengths and minimize challenges, can amplify chances of quitting.

Smokers who receive nonsmoking advice from their healthcare providers are nearly twice as likely to quit smoking than those who do not. In fact, even brief advice alone from a healthcare provider regarding the need for and benefits of smoking cessation is effective in promoting cessation, though not to the same degree as with behavioral support alone or in combination with pharmacotherapies.[25] Behavioral support consists of counseling over several sessions where clients are assisted in identifying their smoking history, motivation to quit, triggers to smoke, and exploring problem-solving strategies. Group behavioral support happens with others over several sessions. Research indicates that these approaches can double the chances of cessation when compared to self-help materials alone.[25]

A Cochrane review examined 14 studies involving more than 10,000 smokers that used motivational interviewing as an intervention (see Chapter 23). This focused, goal-directed interview lasts between 20 and 45 minutes and explores the smoking behavior from the client's perspective in a nonjudgmental manner, aiming to help him or her gain insight and formulate a quit plan. Usually, the client's readiness for making change is taken into consideration. Most of the studies also involved provision of self-help materials and telephone follow up. Participants receiving motivational interviewing had 23% improved success rates for quitting, with better results if they were offered by primary care providers or counselors and the interviews lasted longer than 20 minutes. In fact, for those who were offered motivational interviewing by their primary care providers, the success rate was three times higher than in those who received "usual care."[25] Details regarding specific content of the counseling were lacking in the study reports, making application difficult. A recent study reported no effect on cessation when motivational interviewing was added to the use of a nicotine patch in 430 homeless smokers.[26] Still, one could extrapolate Cochrane review findings to suggest that nurses could have a significant effect on smoking cessation using motivational interviewing. The skills needed to maximize this intervention include using open-ended questions and expressing understanding of the client's dilemma, attentive listening and empathy, and the ability to affirm and empower the client and to support self-efficacy.[7]

Healthcare providers and nurses have considerable opportunity to reach all demographic population subgroups. Most smokers see a healthcare provider at least once per year. Nurses working in hospitals regularly encounter patients who are smokers. These represent ideal opportunities for motivational interviewing, whereby the smoker is asked about the behavior, reminded of his or her inherent strengths, and given the opportunity to explore personal hopes and visions for his or her life. Cessation strategies that build on strengths may facilitate a move toward achieving these dreams.

The Tobacco Free Nurses (TFN) initiative was launched in 2003 as an effort to reduce smoking among nurses as well as to encourage nurses to become more involved in tobacco control efforts. The 5 As behavioral approach has been adopted by TFN and can be readily used by nurses and other healthcare providers during encounters with patients in any setting.[20] Key elements of this approach include the following:

Ask. Always ask about tobacco use during every patient encounter.

Advise. Provide any and all tobacco users with strong verbal encouragement to quit.

Assess. Determine motivation to quit and stage of readiness to make a change (based on the Transtheoretical Model of Change).

Assist. Provide counseling, refer to cessation resources, and arrange support.

Arrange. Plan follow-up visits to encourage ongoing abstinence or new attempts to quit.

Recent studies are lending less support to the 5 As approach (which is more planful and based on the Transtheoretical Model of Change) as compared to briefer approaches.[27] One approach is the AAA framework: *Ask* and record smoking status with each client healthcare encounter; clearly *advise* the patient of the benefits of cessation; and *act* on the patient's response by making immediate recommendations and referrals (including smokefree.gov resources, local quit line telephone support, lifestyle/nutrition/exercise coaching, and medication support, to name a few).[7] The ABC approach (*Ask, Brief* advice, and *Cessation* support) increases the likelihood of triggering quit attempts in a spontaneous, less-planned manner (thus acting on momentary desires to smoke) and includes behavioral and pharmacologic support. It is important that *everyone* who smokes should be advised to stop smoking, whether or not they express an interest and regardless of their readiness for change.[27]

Although the influence of healthcare provider advice varies, many smokers say that they would quit if urged to do so by a healthcare provider. For smoking interventions to become a routine part of healthcare practice, however, medical and nursing education must integrate smoking cessation strategies into the curriculum. While the dangers of tobacco use are included in most nursing (and medical) curricula, discreet and specific smoking cessation education skills are frequently absent. This content fits well into health-promotion content, and approaches such as ABC can easily be taught to all nursing students. Face-to-face behavioral support strategies, along with the basics of pharmacological support, should be included in any content. Research findings support the value and effectiveness of treatment and follow up by nurses and other healthcare providers.

Quit Lines

Initially developed with input from psychologists and available 7 days a week and (most often) 24 hours a day, telephone quit lines offer personal, convenient, accessible, and comprehensive support for those endeavoring to quit tobacco use.[28] Trained counselors are available to talk with callers about their readiness and motivation to quit, smoking triggers, support system, local referral resources, and more. These counselors can customize a quit plan with the client and are also available during a craving or to answer questions such as "I have redness under my nicotine patch. Is that normal?" Most states have quit lines, and most state departments of health can connect callers with a quit line. Most services are free of charge, including free medications such as nicotine replacement patches. When medication support is determined to be appropriate, a brief medical interview is conducted, and medications are sent through the mail. In some cases, a caller's healthcare provider must sign for the medications, as in the case of someone with a cardiac history or a pregnant caller. The quit line counselors also link individuals with local resources (such as smoking cessation support groups or local chapters of the 12-step program Nicotine Anonymous) and assist them in maximizing relevant benefits available through their health insurance. The American Cancer Society (1-866-784-8454) and American Lung Association (1-800-586-4872) have quit lines, and Great Start has a quit line for pregnant women (1-866-667-8278). All of these resources are easily explored on the Internet.

Pharmacologic Therapies in Support of Cessation

Seven medications have been shown to support long-term smoking cessation, including five forms of nicotine replacement therapy (NRT), which decreases intensity of withdrawal symptoms and the urge to smoke. Nicotine gum, lozenges, and the transdermal patch are available over the counter, and nicotine cartridge inhalers, nasal spray, and higher-dose patches are available by prescription.[29] There have been four major controversies regarding the use of NRT: (1) the use of NRT while a person continues to smoke; (2) how long to use NRT before weaning from the drug; (3) the recommended dose of the NRT product; and (4) misusing and abusing NRT, especially becoming addicted to over-the-counter gum. Many tobacco cessation experts believe that sufficient doses of NRT are needed for appropriate lengths of time to support cessation and that the risks of smoking far outweigh the risks of NRT. And, although NRT is expensive and carries with it the potential for adverse effects, many believe that the benefit is estimated to outweigh the risks. Use of NRT is thought to increase the rate of quitting by 50% to 70%.[30]

Combining forms of NRT (e.g., the patch with a faster-acting form) may increase efficacy, especially in heavy smokers, and result in comparable quit rates to that of some oral medications such as varenicline.[30] By using NRT, maintenance of nicotine levels is divorced from cigarettes, helping the smoker to break the emotional ties with smoking. The NRT does not release the client from the bad effects of nicotine, including nausea, dyspepsia, altered cardiac rhythms, dizziness, headache, and local irritations of the nose, mouth, and skin that vary with mode of delivery; however, recent Cochrane reviews support the safety and efficacy of NRT.[30] Approximately 25% of those using NRT experience adverse effects in the first 2 weeks of use, and 40% experience adverse effects within 2 to 3 months of use; however, these effects are usually described as mild and there does not seem to be an increased risk of heart attack in those using NRT.[30]

Because of nicotine's potentially dangerous side effects, NRT must be used with caution in cardiac patients and should not be used within 4 weeks of myocardial infarction.[29] Once a person quits smoking or tapers cigarette intake, NRT is started, used, tapered, and then discontinued over 2 to 3 months, depending on the route of delivery and needs of the user. Although NRT is a means for achieving short-term smoking cessation for nicotine-addicted individuals, it may not reduce relapse rates and is not a substitute for learning new and healthier coping behaviors. The NRT should be used in tandem with a smoking cessation program that addresses behavior and lifestyle changes.

Three oral drugs that are currently identified in Cochrane reviews as the best first-line cessation therapies due to efficacy and safety are bupropion SR (Zyban), varenicline (Chantix), and nortriptyline (Pamelor). Bupropion (an atypical antidepressant) and nortriptyline (a tricyclic antidepressant) are used to improve abstinence in smokers independent of a history of depression.[31] Cigarette smoking is closely associated with a history of depression that often predicts failure with cessation efforts.[32] Smoking cessation may also trigger the onset of depression as a serious nicotine withdrawal symptom in otherwise healthy individuals. This may be the result of removing a primary coping mechanism—the cigarettes—thus leaving the person vulnerable and without a way to cope with the many feelings that are likely to arise. Again, this reinforces the need for therapeutic support and behavioral and lifestyle modifications to be used along with any plan of pharmacotherapy. Clients who need psychotherapy should be referred to an appropriate professional.

Bupropion is contraindicated in those with seizure disorders, eating disorders, and those who take monoamine oxidase inhibitors (MAOIs). It is recommended to be taken for 12 months and may be taken concurrently with NRT. It often causes constipation. Varenicline is classified as a smoking deterrent that reduces cravings and withdrawal symptoms, prevents nicotine from binding to receptors, and lessens the satisfaction derived from smoking. Varenicline should not be used for clients with a prior diagnosis of depression; nor should it be used concurrently with NRT. Both bupropion and varenicline carry boxed warnings about increased risk for suicide, and frequent assessment for suicidal ideation is necessary.[31] Both drugs interfere with normal sleep patterns and can induce bizarre dreams. Both drugs have been associated with lessening weight gain in abstainers, though this effect is limited.[29]

Nortriptyline, a tricyclic antidepressant, is another drug that has shown efficacy for cessation. The mechanisms behind these antidepressants (bupropion and nortriptyline) are observed through their direct interactions with nicotine in the brain. When nicotine is inhaled through smoking or ingested through chewing tobacco it binds to receptors in the brain and causes release of the neurotransmitters dopamine and norepinephrine. These drugs mimic the neurochemical effects of nicotine on noradrenergic and dopaminergic systems in the brain, thus relieving withdrawal symptoms and alleviating a negative affect and depression.[32] Bupropion and nortriptyline are equally effective as NRT, and there seems to be little evidence that adding either of these medications to NRT provides any long-term benefit.[31]

Interestingly, a randomized clinical trial using St. John's wort showed that it did not attenuate withdrawal symptoms; nor did it increase smoking abstinence rates.[33]

Electronic Cigarettes

Also called e-cigarettes, these battery-powered devices are shaped like a cigarette and contain a cartridge with nicotine, flavoring, and an aerosolizing substance (usually propylene glycol). They deliver nicotine without the other harmful substances found in tobacco; however, researchers have found potentially harmful and carcinogenic substances in electronic cigarettes, prompting a call for further study. Currently unregulated by the Food and Drug Administration, these devices can be sold to minors and are used in public places. Surveys conducted by the manufacturers and Web sources for these devices have demonstrated the use of e-cigarettes as helpful for those who may be trying to quit regular tobacco use. To date, no independent studies have revealed these benefits. Side effects from using e-cigarettes include mouth and throat irritation, nausea, headache and vertigo.[34, 35]

Life Span Considerations

Recent research indicates that, although rates of smoking are decreasing overall in the adult population, they are increasing among youth.[36] A large body of research suggests that children with attention deficit hyperactivity disorder (ADHD) are more likely to start smoking in their teens when compared with non-ADHD peers.[37] It makes sense that they may seek tobacco as a way to self-medicate, given the positive physiologic effects of nicotine on focus and attention.

It is critical to identify teens in need of cessation counseling because this is when so many smokers become addicted. Providing smoking cessation counseling to adolescents may be different from working with adults. Facilitators of smoking programs aimed at youth must be able to connect in nonjudgmental ways with teens. Using schools as places where children and teens can learn about the risks of smoking by offering trained peer-led educational and cessation programs and the creative use of social media are examples of youth-friendly approaches being implemented.[38] Researchers looking at characteristics of smoking cessation success and failure among 55 teen girls found that the involvement of teachers and parents was very important to promote quitting, as were being in smoke-free environments.[36]

A study of 32 pregnant teens led to the development of an online tool aimed at education and increasing quit rates among teens. This tool, "Baby Be Smoke Free," was then piloted with 36 pregnant teens with positive results.[39] The concept of self-efficacy is very important because teens who perceive that they are capable of executing a cessation plan are more likely to make the attempt. Antecedents to self-efficacy include developmental stage, emotional support and past experiences with support, available resources, and preferred (healthy) coping strategies. In the absence of any of these conditions that would promote self-efficacy and therefore successful smoking cessation, nurses can facilitate strategic support and growth.[40]

In a meta-analysis of randomized controlled trials measuring effectiveness of pharmacologic therapies in adolescent smokers, results show no significant effects on abstinence rates. This study also reveals few adverse events resulting from the medications used. Increasing use of medications for cessation is seen in those over 12 years of age.[41]

When reviewing research on cessation in older smokers, it is clear that they derive significant health and financial benefits and that it is never too late to offer support and strategies to assist quit efforts. Doing so may also protect others from ETS.[42] Many older smokers (and their healthcare providers) may shy away from cessation because they think that the damage is already done, that it is not worth giving up one of few remaining life pleasures, or they do not know of appropriate resources. In reality, research on older smokers hospitalized with cardiovascular disease shows they can quit at high rates with proper support. With increased likelihood of hospitalizations in this age group, these times can provide opportunities for nurses to offer cessation encouragement using the AAA or ABC approaches.[7, 25] Additional support from medications can be an important adjunct and should be evaluated for safety in older adults on a case-by-case basis. As with any habit, the person who smokes must want to quit and must be ready to do so before he or she will be successful, but triggering more attempts may also favor a positive outcome.

Online and Social Network Resources as Cessation Support Mechanisms

Online resources to support cessation have burgeoned. The smokefree.gov website provides abundant resources for those who smoke, as well as for healthcare professionals.

A recent Cochrane review of 20 studies describing short- and long-term effectiveness of a variety of Internet-based interventions found that appropriately tailored content including frequent automated contact with users was most effective.[43] Interactive sites seemed the most effective, and one trial demonstrated cessation success was boosted if NRT was used along with the Internet resource. Many youth embrace online program formats, and these routes should be employed for youth smoking cessation programming and support. For example, smartphone applications and text messages are available that provide reminders, encouragement, and support for those who are trying to become or remain smoke free and are available through smokefree.gov.

Risks Associated with Quitting

Smoking cessation alters the physiology of the abstainer in powerful ways and may affect the metabolism of certain drugs that are being taken. Be aware that the client who is taking theophylline, clozapine, warfarin, insulin, or olanzapine while smoking may need to have dosage adjustments (most likely reductions) once he or she abstains from tobacco.[29]

Psychoemotional risks of cessation include a tendency toward depression, especially if other coping mechanisms and outlets for emotional issues are not facilitated and developed. The risk for suicide should be taken into account when assessing individuals who are abstaining, particularly if they are taking bupropion or varenicline.

Smokers may experience flu-like symptoms and/or cough as they withdraw from smoking and the body detoxifies itself. They also may experience feelings of loss. These are natural processes and are often dose related (varying with the amount smoked and duration of the habit) yet may be frightening to the smoker who does not know what to expect. Nutritious foods and appropriate supplements, fluids, and exercise can support healing and feelings of well-being as the former smoker goes through a process of detoxification.

Behavioral and Lifestyle Approaches to Smoking Cessation

Smoking cessation is stressful to the body, and careful planning and scrupulous self-care on the part of the quitter can help a great deal. The smoker may like the image of being "in training," as an athlete would be. Using a variety of preferred strategies in combination can bolster the client's ability to be successful.

Smoking Diary

Recording habits in a smoking diary increases self-awareness. Smoking is such a pervasive, automatic habit that it is helpful for clients to keep a smoking diary of when, where, how often, and which moods are associated with smoking. The client records the feelings associated with smoking and begins to think about new habits to replace these urges. Keeping such a record for several weeks before the quit date allows the client to identify patterns, and knowing the smoking triggers leads to permanent changes. To strengthen the new awareness, the client may record thoughts, feelings, urges, and observations about smoking. With each cigarette that is smoked, for example, the client should consider the following questions:

1. Which internal cues made me think that I needed a cigarette (e.g., breathing patterns, mouth watering, tense muscles, fidgety hands)?

2. Which external cues made me think that I needed a cigarette (e.g., talking on the phone, watching television, finishing eating, drinking alcohol, sitting down with friends)?

3. Now that I have smoked that cigarette, did I enjoy it?

Preparing for the Quit Date

Preparation for a quit date makes the process a reality. The desire to be a nonsmoker should build. Becoming smoke free requires preparation. The client should take the time to identify personal reasons for quitting, such as to reduce the risk of heart, lung, or circulatory disease; increase endurance and productivity; improve sense of smell and taste; increase self-esteem; be in control; or decrease the risk to family health from ETS. Once certain that it is time to quit, the client's goal is to be a nonsmoker in 5 days. The nurse may encourage the client to identify family members, friends, or a specific person who may want to join the effort as a quit-smoking partner. The client should tell significant people the quit date and solicit their support.

Preparing for Nicotine Withdrawal

Preparation for nicotine withdrawal facilitates the process of being a nonsmoker. There is no one best way to quit smoking. Some people are successful at quitting cold turkey and going through the nicotine withdrawal, with the worst part usually lasting 5 days or less. Many benefit from a gradual decrease of nicotine with the use of NRT. The client must decide which approach to try.

Preparing a Smoke-Free Environment

Creating a smoke-free body and environment can be a creative process for the client. During the first few nonsmoking days, the client rids the body of toxic waste left from the cigarettes by bathing, brushing teeth, drinking water, exercising, relaxing, imaging, resting, and ingesting good nutrition. A fresh nonsmoking living environment can be accomplished by placing clean filters in heating and cooling units and cleaning carpets, drapes, clothes, office, and car. Signs may be placed on the office door: "Thank you

for not smoking." The more energy that the client puts into these activities, the more likely the client will quit and become a permanent nonsmoker. The client should become aware of how quickly the senses of smell and taste increase and how disgusting the smell and taste of cigarettes become.

Identifying Smoking Triggers and Creating Habit Breakers

Identifying personal smoking triggers (smoke signals) and creating habit breakers can also be a creative process for the client. Becoming smoke free is directly related to minor changes in daily routines, referred to as habit breakers. Many ex-smokers report that the first 5 days of being smoke free are the hardest. Minor or major changes in daily activities can be less stressful if accompanied by a healing state of awareness. If the client should slip and fall back into old routines, these relapses can become learning situations. The client can identify negative self-talk or a stressful situation in which a new habit breaker may not have been used soon enough. The following events are the times when smoking is most likely:

Before starting the day:

- Getting out of bed
- Taking a bath or shower
- Eating breakfast
- Reading the newspaper
- Starting work or driving to work

Mornings:

- During telephone calls
- With coffee
- While driving
- During office work or housework
- In meetings
- During morning breaks
- Before, during, and after lunch

Afternoons:

- During telephone calls
- During office work or housework
- In meetings
- With coffee
- During afternoon breaks

- While completing and organizing your work for the next day
- While driving home or resting in late afternoon
- With alcohol

Evenings:

- Before, during, and after dinner
- If stressed or lonely
- With alcohol
- While relaxing, watching television, or out with family or friends
- While preparing for bed

It is helpful to create habit breakers for each of these events. Success with habit breakers requires commitment to identifying them, writing them down, creativity, and finding ways to personalize this list. For example, the client can take this list, divide a piece of paper into two columns, and write down new habit breakers:

Routine	Habit Breaker
Smoke cigarette upon awakening	Play relaxing music or shower on awakening
Two cups of coffee at breakfast	Hot tea instead of coffee at breakfast
Frequent lighting of cigarettes	Keep sugarless gum or natural licorice sticks nearby
Midmorning smoke break for energy	Eat an apple, drink water, take a walk
Smoking while driving in the car	Listen to music or an educational CD, think, breathe

Nutritional Counseling

Nutritional counseling should encourage the client to choose nutrient-dense foods. In general, vegetables, fruits, whole grains, and high-quality protein are essential. Nuts, seeds, vegetable juices, lots of good water to maintain generous hydration and flush out toxins, a high-potency multivitamin/mineral supplement with omega-3 fish oils, B supplement, vitamin C, and vitamin D are indicated. Avoidance of highly processed foods, sweets, and alcohol is helpful because these foods may dysregulate blood glucose and increase inflammation in the body, negatively affecting mood and increasing withdrawal symptoms and cravings. Miso soup is thought to cleanse the body of nicotine, and leafy greens, lemon juice, carrots, and celery promote alkalinity and decrease cravings. Green tea, white tea, and red (rooibos) tea contain valuable antioxidants and less caffeine and are also recommended. Chewing natural licorice sticks found in health food stores helps manage cravings as well as tactile and oral urges. Using licorice root chew sticks (not candy) is sometimes recommended and can be helpful but must be used in moderation because too much can lower potassium and raise blood pressure. Sugarless gum may help for the same reason.

Exercise

Exercise is a powerful ally in the effort to quit smoking. Regular exercise has been shown to reduce stress in the body and improve mood. Because these are key aspects of the motivation to smoke, as well as problematic issues during withdrawal, it is beneficial for the client to engage in a regular program of enjoyable movement at the highest level of vigor possible. This reduces cravings and mood disturbance, improves self-esteem, promotes self-concept as a person who engages in healthy behaviors (reinforcing identity as a nonsmoker), and reduces weight gain, a significant deterrent to smoking cessation (see Chapter 34).

Several large studies have demonstrated that those who engaged in regular, vigorous exercise were more likely to abstain from smoking, even at 12 months post quit date. Several smaller studies did not show significant improvement in abstinence in those who exercised; however, the frequency and intensity of exercise programs were not clearly described, or adherence was poor. Many smaller studies have demonstrated short-term benefits of exercise on cravings and withdrawal symptoms, including a yoga intervention.[44] A recent study examined the relationship between an 8-week (twice weekly) Vinyasa yoga practice on smoking cessation in 55 female participants. Those who used the yoga had better outcomes than the control group.[45]

Yoga postures that are particularly helpful for smoking cessation include spinal twists (seated and standing), back bends (seated and standing), Camel, Bridge, Bow, and Corpse poses. In general, the breathing, stretching, strengthening, and meditative aspects of yoga practice are of benefit to those seeking a release from addictive behaviors as these approaches may help the mindful quitter get from moment to moment without tobacco.

For the person becoming smoke free, an exercise program serves as a stress manager (as an alternative to smoking), helps with weight management, improves self-concept and esteem, and increases energy levels. If the client does not have an exercise program, the nurse offers assistance and helps the client decide which lifestyle patterns to approach first. It usually takes about 3 months for an exercise program to become a regular part of life, so the client may look for an exercise partner who is serious about exercising or being a nonsmoker.

Weight gain can be avoided. It occurs because the nonsmoker eats too much, lacks aerobic exercise, or consumes too much alcohol. If weight management is a challenge, it is helpful to set a target date for establishing and following an exercise program 2 to 3 months before the quit date. Then, as the client commits to quitting smoking, one component of an effective stress management program has already begun.

Client Bill of Rights

Clients engaged in smoking cessation should recite their bill of rights. They can be creative and add to this list:

I have a right to:
- Be smoke free in any situation
- Review my list of reasons to stop smoking frequently, particularly before any social gathering
- Ask others not to smoke in my home, office, or car
- Choose a network of people who will support me in my efforts to quit

- Avoid those who rob me of energy or motivation to stay smoke free
- Avoid environments and situations where people smoke
- Remind myself that cigarettes leave toxic substances in my body and in my environments, sometimes harming others
- Throw away all objects associated with smoking
- Keep sugarless gum and natural licorice sticks close at hand
- Practice my relaxation, imagery, and coping skills anywhere and at any time
- Seek healing for underlying emotional wounds revealed through my quit process
- Seek therapy to support new coping behaviors and address any underlying trauma
- Keep healthy beverages close by at work and at home
- Support legislation to protect nonsmokers from the dangers of passive smoking in public places

Integration of Rewards

The client should plan a reward at least every 5 to 7 days for having a smoke-free lifestyle. These rewards should continue as long as the client needs to be aware of new lifestyle habits. The client is considered smoke free when his or her habits are indeed nonsmoking behaviors. Continued use of the listed habit breakers always helps a client anticipate when smoke signals can surface and, thus, quickly take actions to prevent relapse.

Reinforcement of Positive Self-Talk

Feelings, moods, behaviors, and motivation affect physiologic changes. As the client learns to recognize the self-talk that sabotages his or her positive outlook, it is possible for the client to remain in control and not give in to the urge to smoke. Positive affirmations such as "I am feeling more free," "I am feeling in control," and "Every day I am getting healthier" can help the client be successful. The nurse can also assist with cognitive restructuring of automatic negative thoughts of those who are quitting (see Chapter 22). Negative rationalization must be recognized because it can gradually lead to doubt about the ability to change. The client may reframe negative statements, for example, changing "I've become more nervous since I quit smoking" to "I am noticing a change in my moods since quitting and I am adding a relaxation and imagery practice. This makes me feel much better than the short burst of nicotine energy." Similarly, negative thoughts must be identified and replaced with positive thoughts. For example, "I'll never get over this urge to smoke; I'll never be successful at breaking the habit" may be reframed as "Of course I can get over this urge. I am learning new coping strategies, and I can really imagine myself smoke free."

Journaling and Self-Reflection

Journal writing and self-reflection may help to get feelings up and out through the quit process rather than the client holding them in (see Chapter 14). Self-reflection can lead to self-awareness, and by journaling clients may identify changes they can make. For example, setting good boundaries in relationships can help to keep out "energy-draining people" and naysayers (those who may not support quit efforts), thus helping the former smoker stay on course with the quit plan. Staying away from other smokers, even loved ones, may be well worth the effort.

Breathing Techniques

Breathing is a powerful strategy to aid in smoking cessation. There are as many ways to breathe as there are smokers, but it is helpful to teach deep breathing exercises to soothe, energize, and calm the client. Breathing, like nicotine, can serve many purposes. The 4-2-8 count breath can be very helpful, and the counts can be varied to meet the needs of the individual client because breathing rhythm mimics smoking behavior. In this technique, the client breathes in slowly and fully to the count of 4, holds it for 2 counts, and then exhales slowly and fully to the count of 8. By repeating this pattern, the parasympathetic nervous system (the "rest and digest" response) is triggered.

Another breathing technique that may be helpful is the "Butt Kicking Breath" demonstrated online at www.sadienardini.com. To practice this technique, place hands on sides of ribcage, drop shoulders down away from ears,

inhale to the count of 4 through the nose, hold to the count of 2, exhale through pursed lips to the count of 8. Repeat, keeping shoulders down and adding abdominal contractions with the belly tucked in toward the spine.

Alternate nostril breathing can soothe and shift mood in a positive direction, therefore enhancing quit efforts. Clients can use the thumb and forefinger of one hand to alternately occlude one nostril and breathe fully in and out of the open nostril each time. Repeating for at least 12 cycles/switches elicits an effect. Online videos clearly demonstrate this technique.

Guided Imagery and Hypnosis

Hypnosis, a process that includes relaxation techniques, guided imagery, and suggestion, is often used in behavioral approaches to smoking cessation. A dearth of research evidence documents effectiveness of this strategy, yet anecdotal evidence abounds that hypnosis is effective, and it makes intuitive sense to harness the power of the mind–body connection to promote cessation. The imagery scripts that follow enable the nurse to begin working with a client using this process.

Guided imagery with suggestions (hypnosis) enhances the client's success at becoming smoke free. The nurse can use the following scripts to create a live session with the client or create a relaxation and imagery recording, or the nurse can provide the scripts to the client to make his or her own recording. The scripts help the client form correct biological images of being smoke free. They can be modified or expanded, depending on present habits and which new skills the client wishes to develop to break the nicotine habit. A relaxation exercise (see Chapter 11) may be used/recorded for 5 to 10 minutes to induce a relaxed and receptive state; then, the script for smoking cessation is used/recorded for 15 minutes. The nurse should encourage the client to listen to the tape daily or several times a day throughout the first week of cessation when physiologic withdrawal is occurring. Then, the client can listen every other day for a week, and then as often as needed thereafter.

Excellent smoking cessation guided imagery CDs and MP3 downloads created by therapist Belleruth Naparstek and marketed by Health

Journeys are available at www.healthjourneys .com. Physiologically correct, specific, and well constructed, these resources are readily available and reasonably priced.

Script: Introduction. [NAME], as your mind becomes clearer and clearer, feel it becoming more and more alert. Somewhere deep inside of you, a brilliant light begins to glow. Sense this happening. . . . The light grows brighter and more intense. . . . This is your mind–body communication center. Breathe into it. . . . Energize it with your breath. The light is powerful and penetrating, and a beam begins to grow from it. The beam shines into your body now as you prepare to focus on being smoke free. . . . In your relaxed state, affirm to yourself at your deep level of inner strength and knowing . . . that you are already becoming a nonsmoker. Say it over and over as you begin to see the words and feelings in every cell in your body. Feel your relaxed state deepen. You can get to this space anytime you wish. . . . All you have to do is give yourself the suggestion and stay with the suggestion as you move into your relaxed state. This is a skill that you will use repeatedly as you move into being smoke free.

Script: Quit date. You are at a place in time where smoking no longer suits you. It is no longer a comfortable behavior for you. Congratulate yourself on reaching this point in your life journey and for setting your quit date. You are aware of all of the resources available to help you quit. With your mind's eye now . . . see your calendar and experience yourself reading your quit date. With full intention to quit, mark your quit date on the calendar. Enlist the help of your family or a friend as you set your quit date. The process has begun.

Script: Cleansing your body and environment. It is now time to rid your body of toxins left from the cigarettes. Begin to cleanse your body. . . . Feel the toxins flowing out of your body as you increase the liquids you drink. Practice your deep breathing exercises,

---

remembering to exhale completely . . . enjoying this new awareness of how healthy your lungs will become with the cleansing and clearing of toxins. Experience your breath, skin, hair . . . fresh as a spring breeze. See yourself making your surroundings smoke free day by day. Notice the pleasant changes in your new, nonsmoking environment. . . . First, begin to notice how you are becoming more sensitive to smells. . . . Enjoy the freshness of your clothes, home, office, and car being free of smoke.

As you keep your records, become aware of your progress. Reward yourself regularly. Imagine you have had 5 smoke-free days. The worst of any withdrawal is over. What is your first reward going to be? Give yourself that reward!

As you continue to deepen your relaxation, inhale to the count of 4, hold to the count of 2, then exhale to the count of 8. Repeat to yourself the words "I am calm" as you exhale. Let your body experience these words in your own unique way.

Register this feeling throughout your body. Begin to increase your awareness of feeling good about being alive, to be conscious of beginning new habits . . . free of smoking.

Script: Triggers/smoke signals. Starting now, as a nonsmoker, reflect on your wonderful decision to release the habit of smoking . . . a habit that could cause illness and take away your energy and vitality. Get in touch with your smoke signals/smoking triggers. Is it a certain time of day, a person, a place, or a social gathering? As you bring them into awareness . . . rehearse in your mind the healthy behaviors you will use to replace the urges. . . . Is it drinking a glass of water, chewing sugar-free gum, going for a walk, listening to music, chewing on a toothpick, or taking a hot shower or bath? And as you think about smoking urges . . . those unconscious habits . . . you realize that, from now on, you will never unconsciously reach for a tobacco product again. . . . As a nonsmoker, you have simply lost the desire and urge to smoke. . . . You are very aware of your body, mind, and spirit. . . . You can hear your powerful inner voice repeating clear affirmations, . . . "I have stopped smoking . . . I am free of smoking . . . I feel strong and healthy . . . I can taste and smell fragrances. My cough has gone."

Hear your own voice saying, "I no longer crave a habit negatively affecting my health. I no longer unconsciously reach for a cigarette or smoke. This habit is diminishing steadily, and I can envision being completely free of this addiction. My mind–body is functioning in such a manner that I no longer crave tobacco. . . . I value my lungs and heart and care for them. I no longer place unnecessary strain on these organs so vital to life."

When you feel the urge to smoke, hear yourself saying, "Stop!" followed by inhaling to the count of 4, holding to the count of 2, and exhaling to the count of 8. Then, tell yourself, "Smoking no longer suits me. It is no longer a part of who I am. I am free." These words will become more powerful the more you say them. Feel a warm inner glow of healthy pride that grows every day. It fills you with warmth and a sense of freedom and control on deep levels of your being. Remember this message of freedom and pride is always with you . . . and you are no longer a smoker. That is behind you. Any feelings of loss have already been replaced by the stronger feelings of freedom, control, vitality, and hope.

Script: Nutritious eating and exercise. "As I stop smoking, I will not be excessively hungry or eat excessively. Because of my body-mind-spirit connection, I am free of my addiction. Because of increasing feelings of energy, I take any and all opportunities to move my body. I increase my exercise to three or four times a week for 20 minutes or longer. I am conscious of using deep breathing exercises regularly and any time I feel stressed or have a craving. I increase my fluid intake and chew sugar-free gum. I sleep soundly at night. My environment is fresh. Food tastes and smells wonderful. I have more money to use as I choose. I am in control at deeper levels of my being. I am free of smoking. I am free." You can access this inner wisdom any time that you wish. . . . All you have to do is get calm and easy, breathe deeply, and focus inward.

Script: Closure. Take a few slow, energizing breaths and, as you come back to full awareness of the room, know that you are on a body-mind-spirit journey, and whatever is right for you at this point in time is unfolding just as it should and that you have done your best, regardless of the outcome.

Prevention as the Best Protection from Smoking

Because smoking is highly addictive, it is best not to start in the first place. The average age of first use is 14.5 years, and approximately 40% of teens who smoke become addicted to nicotine.[3] With that knowledge, prevention efforts must start when children are young, with school-based programs beginning in later elementary and middle school years. An interesting study revealed that parents who quit smoking enhanced their children's negative attitudes toward smoking, especially if the parent quit before the child was in third grade. These parents are often actively engaged in relapse-prevention behaviors, and this has a protective and deterring effect on children.[46]

Evidence shows that tobacco control programs reduce smoking behavior, and that tobacco advertising and public health counter-advertising measures vie for the attention of youth. In the last two decades, improvements have been documented in terms of the prevalence of high school students who smoke. In 1991, the prevalence of high school student smoking was 27.5%, and by 1997 it had grown to 36.4%; however, the rate for teen smoking in the United States dropped to 19.5% in 2009.[47] These data support the findings of other studies that indicate youth smoking has reached its peak and is now in decline, though the rate of decline has slowed in recent years.

Factors that discourage smoking in youth include more aggressive school health policies and school-based prevention and cessation programs, strict restrictions on selling to minors, harnessing the power of media images and messages by having effective role models on television and in magazines, and strong counter-advertising campaigns that depict smoking and tobacco use in a negative light. In addition, measures that discourage smoking across the life span include high cigarette prices through taxation, smoking bans in public places, restricted access to tobacco products, and ongoing public education campaigns depicting the harmful health effects of tobacco.[3]

Unfortunately, the *Healthy People 2010* goal to reduce the high school smoking rate to 16% or less was not met. However, the Family Smoking Prevention and Tobacco Control Act (TCA) enacted in 2009 offers new opportunities for comprehensive reductions in tobacco use. By giving the Food and Drug Administration additional authority to regulate the tobacco industry, the TCA imposes specific marketing, labeling, and advertising requirements and establishes restrictions on youth access and promotional practices that are targeted toward youth. Evidence of this act may be seen in the new, gruesome pictures that are now included on cigarette packaging depicting the harmful consequences of smoking.

Research demonstrates that living farther away from stores that sell tobacco products enhances abstinence after a quit attempt.[48] Therefore, zoning restrictions in residential areas could be an effective means to bolster existing strategies aimed at reducing tobacco use. The regulation of tobacco products is an essential aspect of a comprehensive national tobacco prevention and control strategy that will strengthen the effect of the growing body of evidence-based interventions already in use.

Educating our youth and offering healthy strategies to cope with the stresses of life are likely the best ways to keep them away from cigarettes. Mindful exercise, such as yoga classes that include breathing and meditation, should be a part of this approach. Developing healthy coping behaviors begins early and sets the pattern for life.

Holistic Caring Process

Holistic Assessment

In preparing to use smoking cessation interventions, the nurse assesses the following parameters:

- The client's level of addiction to cigarettes
- The meaning of smoking to the client
- The client's attitudes and beliefs about successful and sustained smoking cessation
- The client's motivation to learn interventions to become a permanent nonsmoker
- The client's stage of change in terms of smoking cessation
- The client's eating patterns and exercise program
- The client's existing stress management strategies
- The client's support and encouragement from family and friends

Identification of Patterns/ Challenges/Needs

The patterns, challenges, and needs (see Chapter 8) compatible with smoking cessation interventions are as follows:

- Exchanging:
    - Altered circulation
    - Altered oxygenation

- Valuing:
    - Spiritual distress
    - Spiritual well-being

- Choosing:
    - Ineffective individual coping
    - Effective individual coping

- Moving: Self-care deficit
- Perceiving:
    - Disturbance in body image
    - Disturbance in self-esteem
    - Hopelessness

- Knowing: Knowledge deficit
- Feeling:
    - Anxiety
    - Fear

Outcome Identification

Table 35-1 guides the nurse in client outcomes, nursing prescriptions, and evaluation for successful smoking cessation.

TABLE 35-1 Nursing Interventions: Smoking Cessation		
Client Outcomes	**Nursing Prescriptions**	**Evaluation**
The client will demonstrate attitudes, beliefs, and behaviors that indicate the desire to be a nonsmoker.	Offer advice about the benefits of cessation. Determine the client's desire to be a nonsmoker.	The client demonstrated attitudes, beliefs, behaviors, and the desire to be a nonsmoker.
	Assist the client in setting realistic plans for being a nonsmoker by:	The client set a realistic plan and became a nonsmoker over 1 week as follows:
	▪ Establishing a quit date	▪ Focused on a quit-date goal and stopped use of cigarettes
	▪ Self-assessing bodymindspirit health to identify which areas need bolstering	▪ Cleansed body and environment of nicotine
	▪ Drawing up a nicotine withdrawal schedule	▪ Adhered to habit-breaker strategies
	▪ Cleansing self and environment of nicotine	▪ Kept a smoking, exercise, and food diary
	▪ Developing habit-breaker strategies	
	▪ Keeping a smoking diary	▪ Practiced relaxation and imagery daily
	▪ Practicing relaxation and imagery	▪ Integrated behavior changes daily
	▪ Assessing the support network	▪ Rewarded self for attaining goals
	▪ Integrating behavior changes	
	▪ Deciding on rewards for attaining goals	

Source: Data from "Stages of Change Model." AddictionInfo.org.

Therapeutic Care Plan and Interventions

Before the session:

- Spend a few moments to become mindfully present and to begin the session with the intention to facilitate healing.
- Gather any materials you will use during the session.
- Create a quiet place to begin guiding the client in smoking cessation strategies.

At the beginning of the session:

- Review the smoking diary if client has been keeping one. Explore the meaning of smoking patterns with the client. Elicit insight into changing behaviors.
- Establish pre-quitting strategies. Suggest that the client identify and combine the methods that can work best.
- Encourage the client to take a few days before the quit date to rid the body of toxins and to clean the house, office, and car of any evidence of cigarettes or odors.
- Advise attention to exercise and nutrition ahead of the quit date.
- Have the client establish the quit date and sign a contract that specifies the quit date.
- Encourage the client to call on family and friends on the first smoke-free days, particularly when confidence is low. Remind them that their support is very important.
- Encourage the client to practice small acts of control (such as delaying gratification). This enhances feelings of self-control and has been shown to enhance quit efforts.

During the session:

- Reinforce the quit date, and have the client imagine being smoke free in 5 days.
- Teach basic relaxation and imagery skills to shape mind–body changes for internal and external smoke-free images. These

images create a new self-perception and will enhance the client's success. Rhythmic breathing and progressive muscle relaxation are most helpful in teaching body-centered awareness and effective coping. Relaxation and imagery help the client to recognize and block triggers/smoke signals. Combine this practice with a stop-smoking CD once or twice a day.

- Teach the client to create specific imagery patterns (see Chapter 12):
  - *Active images.* Cleansing the body of nicotine and other toxins; finding a safe place that establishes a feeling of security and comfort; envisioning a protective bubble that receives what is needed from others and blocks out negative images, such as smoke signals.
  - *Process images.* People, events, and situations that trigger the desire to smoke. Have the client rehearse being in a situation where smoking normally occurs but now using a new behavior, such as breathing deeply, and saying, "I am calm" on exhalation or reaching for a glass of water.
  - *End-state images.* Being smoke free; accessing feelings of control and freedom.
- Have the client create strategies to break smoke signals and become smoke free—waking up and having a glass of water, reading the morning paper in a different room, taking a break and drinking water or juice, brushing teeth, talking on the telephone, and practicing relaxation and rhythmic breathing.
- Encourage the client to be patient in making this major lifestyle change and to remember that smoking is about self-protective control. The old, superficial (and unhealthy) sense of control must be replaced with a new, deeper (healthy) sense of control. Identify internal and external experiences as new health behaviors are being shaped. Some are easy to change; others take longer.
- Ask the client to become aware of new opportunities for being with family, friends, and self while being smoke free. Discuss options for new patterns of socializing.

- Discuss the people who form the client's support network. Who is supportive and energy giving? Who is energy draining? In which ways can social patterns change to support being smoke free? It can be helpful to identify who to reduce time with until new patterns of nonsmoking become stronger.

At the end of the session:

- Suggest that the client create a series of personal rewards—establishing a schedule that will be motivating. Perhaps having a reward after 5 smoke-free days, or having a small reward each day, with a larger reward after 5 days.
- Evaluate with the client the goals of behavior changes—reduction of smoking urges and development of new habit patterns.
- Encourage the client to make a list of anticipated high-risk situations and decide (in advance) ways to prevent a relapse. The most frequent high-risk situations are social situations, emotional upsets, home or work frustration, interpersonal conflict, driving, and relaxing after a meal. In general, when a person is hungry, angry or anxious, lonely or tired (HALT), vulnerability to addictive behaviors is heightened. Using the breathing techniques described in this chapter can help the client get through a craving or relapse-prone situation.
- Reinforce the fact that the client can avoid relapse. Having learned to recognize high-risk situations for relapse, the client can be ready quickly to use strategies to resist smoking temptations. Successful coping strategies must honor internal responses (mind–body feelings and thoughts) and action-oriented responses (action steps).
- Suggest that the client become a support person for someone else who is trying to become smoke free to decrease chances of relapse.
- Use the client outcomes that were established before the session to evaluate the session.
- Schedule a follow-up session.

Case Study (Implementation)

Case Study

Setting: Nurse-based wellness clinic smoking cessation program

Client: J. N., a 48-year-old interior designer, telling her story to the new clients after she has been smoke free for 5 years

Patterns/Challenges/Needs: Health maintenance related to engagement in strategies to remain smoke free

"You can call it midlife crisis or whatever; I just happened to wake up and tell myself that I'm worth a better state of health and mind. How did I do it? Lots of determination and reprogramming my mind with successful images. I never dreamed that I could be so successful at quitting smoking. I'd tried to quit on many occasions, but the reason I never was able to sustain change is that I had tried to quit before I really was ready to do so.

"I'd been smoking for 27 years, and I just got tired of my chronic cough and feeling tired. Other things began to happen also. My family and friends began to ask for nonsmoking sections in restaurants and gave me 3 months before they declared the house a nonsmoking house. They also placed a disgusting, ugly series of pictures of me smoking with a title on it saying, 'We Love You—Quit Smoking!' The first time I looked at the pictures, I burst into tears and heard their message loud and clear. I got in touch with why I began smoking in the first place as a teenager—I thought I looked important and glamorous. Those pictures certainly didn't convey that image.

"The last straw that really got my attention was when a friend and I were driving along with our windows down on a nice spring day. My friend said to me, 'Who do you think is smoking?' We could see no person smoking, but my friend could smell it. Sure enough, there was a smoker three cars in front of us in the left lane to us. I was driving, and, as we passed the car, smoke came in our window. I couldn't smell it even though I could see the smoke coming in the window.

"I really planned a ritual for my quit date for ending smoking—which has changed my life in many ways. I have now been smoke free for 5 years. Let me begin by saying that, in the previous 15 years, I had tried to quit smoking seven times; each time I was successful for 1 month at the longest, so I knew that it was possible. As I look back on it now, the reason that I didn't have any sustained change was that I didn't shape any new behaviors or thoughts.

"Let me share with you my rituals. I planned a 5-day period to be by myself to focus on shaping new behaviors. The reason I chose to stay at home was the importance of preparation and concentration of new thoughts and behaviors prior to my quit date.

"Prior to that special week, I began my 'detox' process. I decided to buy a new bright blue toothbrush, which I placed in a beautiful small wicker basket. I also placed this on the opposite side of where I usually kept my toothbrush. When brushing my teeth gently, frequently followed by a mouthwash, I was aware of repeating words to myself about cleansing and purifying. I used these same thoughts when I bathed. I would stand in the shower and concentrate on the water washing the toxins from my skin. For the internal removal of toxins, I increased my fluid intake of water and herb teas to six to eight glasses a day. Exercise also became part of my ritual. I would get up each day and start my morning with a 30-minute walk. On the walk, I used the time to see myself smoke free.

"Well, my home environment reeked of smoke and staleness. My drapes and fabric chairs and couches had not been cleaned in 16 years; my carpets in 8. I allowed myself the luxury of having them professionally cleaned. Not only did the house smell fresh, but all the colors were very fresh and seemed new. Air-conditioning filters were changed. I cleaned clothes that were well overdue. I aired the house.

"The biggest task was to gather all the cigarette packages throughout the house. They were in every room, and I had about three full cartons when I finally gathered them all up. This was really scary for me, because when I saw them all together, the thought that came to me was, 'I'm really addicted. There is no way I can break this habit.' Out of nowhere, this very loud, powerful voice blurted out, 'Yes, you can, and you have already begun.' I have never heard such volume from my own voice. It was as if it was a voice other than my own. Prior to that, I also removed all of the ashtrays and bought a beautiful door sign that read "Thank You For Not Smoking." When I placed it above the door bell, I felt this inner sensation of glee and energy. It was very affirming to me, and, from that moment on, there was no stopping my success. I really believed for the first time that I was going to be successful, and I felt an inner strength that I had never experienced before. I also received so much encouragement from my husband and two children when they came home that evening. I cleaned my car as well as I had the house.

"During this period of 1 week of cleaning my body, house, and car, I recorded my internal and external cues of why I smoked. It was when I was hungry, talking on the phone, when I was putting on my makeup in the morning, and after meals. During this time, I let myself smoke no more than three cigarettes a day—outside standing up. I concentrated on what a disgusting habit smoking was. As I focused on these messages to myself, I not only slowed down the smoking, I also didn't enjoy the cigarettes and found that it was really not as pleasant as in the past. I had tried this before, but my thoughts were also on how much I was going to miss the smoking and pleasure of the buzz from smoking. I was so aware of not really enjoying it as much as I used to.

"I well remember my quit date 5 years ago. It is so clear; it is as if I planned it just yesterday. The reason it seems so recent is that my preparation and commitment to stopping smoking spilled over into other areas in my life. Do I miss smoking? Frankly, I'll say yes. I have those urges on occasions. However, as I've integrated relaxation, imagery, and positive affirmations into my life, my commitment to being smoke free is stronger. I honor that inner voice that says, 'Light Up.' For me, what works best is to hear the message, honor that I heard it, but replace smoking with something that is always with me—the power of relaxed breathing. I also use a saying a friend taught me, which is "Avoid HALT": Avoid becoming too Hungry, too Angry, too Lonely, or too Tired. Time, commitment,

and believing in my success are part of every day for me. Quitting smoking is one of the hardest things I've ever done. I can't remember planning so well for any event in my life. I believed I could do it, and that is exactly what continued to happen."

Evaluation

With the client, the nurse determines whether the client outcomes for smoking cessation were achieved. See **Exhibit 35-1** for a useful model in helping patients achieve and maintain smoking cessation.

EXHIBIT 35-1   Strategies to Promote Cessation Based on Stage of Readiness for Change

The Transtheoretical Model of Change can assist the holistic nurse in understanding client readiness to make behavioral changes and in offering strategies appropriate to the client's perspective and concerns.

Precontemplation: Assess attitude about smoking cessation; offer presence.

Contemplation: Evaluate pros and cons of change; assist client in self-reflection ("Why do I want to smoke?" "Why do I want to quit smoking"); offer information.

Preparation: Explore past successes; provide guidance in creating a plan of action (set a quit date, communicate with friends and family about plans).

Action: Assist client with healthy coping behaviors to replace smoking; facilitate environmental and social patterns modification to support cessation; plan regular rewards for being smoke-free.

Maintenance: Continue positive reinforcement; explore, avoid, and modify triggers for relapse (hungry, angry, lonely, tired); identify and avoid tempting situations.

Termination: Reflect on new patterns and benefits of being smoke-free; reflect on ways in which client proactively addresses areas of vulnerability.

Source: AddictionInfo, "Stages of Change Model" (2015). http://www.addictioninfo.org/articles/11/1/Stages-of-Change-Model/Page1.html.

Conclusion

In becoming an ex-smoker, a client must understand that it is a gradual step-by-step process that requires learning new skills. Smoking cessation involves (1) recognizing smoking habits and triggers, (2) establishing habit breakers, (3) preparing for detoxification of the body and environment, (4) establishing a support network, (5) modifying behavior including using habit breakers and following good nutrition and exercise programs, (6) using medications and other resources as needed, and (7) addressing underlying emotional issues and mood disturbances to enhance healing and prevent relapse. The integration of these seven areas helps clients achieve new levels of self-awareness and increase the chance of being smoke free.

Directions for Future Research

1. Determine the nursing interventions that most effectively minimize stress and enhance emotional healing as clients begin a smoking cessation program.
2. Evaluate combinations of smoking cessation content and teaching methods to determine which are most effective in assisting a client in sustained smoking cessation.
3. Determine the nursing interventions that are most effective in helping a client explore underlying emotional issues to enhance cessation and prevent relapse.

Nurse Healer Reflections

After reading this chapter, the nurse healer will be able to answer or to begin a process of answering the following questions:

- Which rituals can I create or assist others in creating to detoxify and cleanse the body and environment of all traces of nicotine?
- Which underlying emotional issues need healing so that the client can let go of unhealthy behaviors?
- Which coping mechanisms and resources can be used to facilitate healing?
- What are specific process, end-state, and general healing images for teaching myself or others about releasing attachments to smoking and moving forward in being smoke free?

NOTES

1. Centers for Disease Control and Prevention, "Cigarette Smoking Among Adults—United States, 2005-2012," *Morbidity and Mortality Weekly Report* 63, no. 2 (2014): 29–34.
2. U.S. Department of Health and Human Services, *The Health Consequences of Smoking—50 Years of Progress: A Report of the Surgeon General* (Rockville, MD: U.S. Department of Health and Human Services, 2014).
3. R. G. Lande, E. Dunayevich, M. Lertzman, and S. Sharma, "Nicotine Addiction: Overview, Clinical Presentation, Treatment, and Follow Up," *Medscape* (2011). http://emedicine.medscape.com/article/287555.
4. N. Cobb, A. Graham, and D. Abrams, "Social Network Structure of a Large Online Community for Smoking Cessation," *American Journal of Public Health* 100, no. 7 (2010): 1282–1289.
5. M. Herman and M. Walsh, "Hospital Admissions for Acute Myocardial Infarction, Angina, Stroke, and Asthma After Implementation of Arizona's Comprehensive Statewide Smoking Ban," *American Journal of Public Health* 101, no. 3 (2011): 491–498.
6. L. B. Goldstein, C. D. Bushnell, R. J. Adams, L. J. Appel, L. T. Braun, S. Chaturvedi, M. A. Creager, et al., "Guidelines for the Primary Prevention of Stroke: A Guideline for Healthcare Professionals from the American Heart Association/American Stroke Association," *Stroke* 42, no. 2 (2011): 517–584.
7. N. Davies, "The Effect of Body Image and Mood on Smoking Cessation in Women," *Nursing Standard* 26, no. 25 (2012): 35–38.
8. G. Karatay, K. Gulumser, and O. Emiroglu, "The Effect of Motivational Interviewing on Smoking Cessation in Pregnant Women," *Journal of Advanced Nursing* 66, no. 6 (2010): 1328–1337.
9. Centers for Disease Control and Prevention, "Trends in Smoking Before, During, and After Pregnancy: Pregnancy Risk Assessment Monitoring System, United States, 40 Sites, 2000-2010," *Morbidity and Mortality Weekly Report* 62, no. 6 (2013): 1–19.
10. S. D. Rahmanian, P. T. Diaz, and M. E. Wewers, "Tobacco Use and Cessation Among Women:

Research and Treatment-Related Issues," *Journal of Women's Health* 20, no. 3 (2011): 349–357.

11. A. Kleppinger, M. D. Litt, A. M. Kenny, and C. A. Oncken, "Effects of Smoking Cessation on Body Composition in Postmenopausal Women," *Journal of Women's Health* 19, no. 9 (2010): 1651–1657.

12. K. L. Cropsey, L. A. McClure, D. O. Jackson, G. C. Villalobos, M. F. Weaver, and M. L. Stitzer, "The Impact of Quitting Smoking on Weight Among Women Prisoners Participating in a Smoking Cessation Intervention," *American Journal of Public Health* 100, no. 8 (2010): 1442–1448.

13. U.S. Department of Health and Human Services, "Lesbian, Gay, Bisexual, and Transgender Health" (2014). http://healthypeople.gov/2020 /topicsobjectives2020/overview.aspx?topicid=25.

14. Centers for Disease Control and Prevention, "QuickStats: Current Smoking Among Men Aged 25–64 Years, by Age Group and Veteran Status—National Health Interview Survey (NHIS), United States, 2007–2010," *Morbidity and Mortality Weekly Report* 61, no. 45 (2012): 929.

15. U.S. Department of Health and Human Services, "HIV and Smoking" (2014). www.aids.gov /hiv-aids-basics/staying-healthy-with-hiv-aids /taking-care-of-yourself/smoking-tobacco-use/.

16. D. S. Morris, S. C. Fiala, and R. Pawlak, "Opportunities for Policy Interventions to Reduce Youth Hookah Smoking in the United States," *Preventing Chronic Disease* 9 (2012): doi:10.5888/ pcd9.120082.

17. B. A. Primack, K. R. Rice, A. Shensa, M. V. Carroll, E. J. DePenna, R. Nakkash, and T. E. Barnett, "U.S. Hookah Tobacco Smoking Establishments Advertised on the Internet," *American Journal of Preventive Medicine* 42, no. 2 (2012): 150–156.

18. Centers for Disease Control and Prevention, "Vital Signs: Nonsmokers' Exposure to Secondhand Smoke—United States, 1999–2008," *Morbidity and Mortality Weekly Report* 59, no. 35 (2010): 1141–1146.

19. F. C. Bandiera, A. K. Richardson, D. J. Lee, J. P. He, and K. R. Merikangas, "Secondhand Smoke Exposure and Mental Health Among Children and Adolescents," *Archives of Pediatric and Adolescent Medicine* 165, no. 4 (2011): 332–338.

20. A. Porter, "The Role of the Advanced Practice Nurse in Promoting Smoking Cessation in the Adult Population," *MEDSURG Nursing* 22, no. 4 (2013): 264–268.

21. J. C. Charlesworth, J. E. Curran, M. P. Johnson, H. H. H. Göring, T. D. Dyer, V. P. Diego, J. W. Kent Jr., et al., "Transcriptomic Epidemiology of Smoking: The Effect of Smoking on Gene Expression in Lymphocytes," *BMC Medical Genomics* 3, no. 29 (2010): www.biomedcentral .com/1755-8794/3/29.

22. B. Borrelli, E. L. McQuaid, S. P. Novak, S. K. Hammond, and B. Becker, "Motivating Latino Caregivers of Children with Asthma to Quit Smoking: A Randomized Trial," *Journal of Consulting and Clinical Psychology* 78, no. 1 (2010): 34–43.

23. M. S. Webb, D. R. de Ybarra, E. A. Baker, I. M. Reis, and M. P. Carey, "Cognitive-Behavioral Therapy to Promote Smoking Cessation Among African American Smokers: A Randomized Clinical Trial," *Journal of Consulting and Clinical Psychology* 78, no. 1 (2010): 24–33.

24. K. N. Morrison and M. A. Naegle, "An Evidence-Based Protocol for Smoking Cessation for Persons with Psychotic Disorders," *Journal of Addictions Nursing* 21, nos. 2–3 (2010): 79–86.

25. O. Dogar and K. Siddiqi, "An Evidence Based Guide to Smoking Cessation Therapies," *Nurse Prescribing* 11, no. 11 (2013): 543–548.

26. K. S. Okuyemi, K. Goldade, G. L. Whembolua, J. L. Thomas, S. Eischen, B. Sewali, H. Guo, et al., "Motivational Interviewing to Enhance Nicotine Patch Treatment for Smoking Cessation Among Homeless Smokers: A Randomized Controlled Trial," *Addiction* 108, no. 6 (2013): 1136–1144.

27. G. Wong and G. Stokes, "Preparing Undergraduate Nurses to Provide Smoking Cessation Advice and Help," *Nursing Praxis in New Zealand* 27, no. 3 (2011): 21–30.

28. E. Lichtenstein, S. H. Zhu, and G. J. Tedeschi, "Smoking Cessation Quitlines: An Underrecognized Intervention Success Story," *American Psychologist* 65, no. 4 (2010): 252–261.

29. J. Feigenbaum, "Pharmacological Aids to Promote Smoking Cessation," *Journal of Addictions Nursing* 21, nos. 2–3 (2010): 87–97.

30. K. Cahill, S. Stevens, R. Perera, and T. Lancaster, "Pharmacological Interventions for Smoking Cessation: An Overview and Network Meta-Analysis," *Cochrane Database of Systematic Reviews* 5 (2013): doi:10.1002/14651858. CD009329. pub2.

31. J. R. Hughes, L. F. Stead, J. Hartmann-Boyce, K. Cahill, and T. Lancaster, "Antidepressants for Smoking Cessation," *Cochrane Database of Systematic Reviews* 1 (2014): doi:10.1002/14651858. CD000031.pub4.

32. R. Bränström, C. Penilla, E. J. Pérez-Stable, and R. F. Muñoz, "Positive Affect and Mood Management in Successful Smoking Cessation," *American Journal of Health Behaviors* 34, no. 5 (2010): 553–562.

33. A. Sood, J. O. Ebbert, K. Prasad, I. T. Croghan, B. Bauer, and D. R. Schroeder, "A Randomized

Clinical Trial of St. John's Wort for Smoking Cessation," *Journal of Alternative and Complementary Medicine* 16, no. 7 (2010): 761–767.

34. Centers for Disease Control and Prevention, "Notes from the Field: Electronic Cigarette Use Among Middle and High School Students—United States, 2011–2012," *Morbidity and Mortality Weekly Report* 62, no. 35 (2013): 729–730.

35. L. E. Odum, K. A. O'Dell, and J. S. Schepers, "Electronic Cigarettes: Do They Have a Role in Smoking Cessation?" *Journal of Pharmacy Practice* 25 (2012): 611–614.

36. J. A. Kim, C. Y. Lee, E. S. Lim, and G. S. Kim, "Smoking Cessation and Characteristics of Success and Failure Among Female High-School Smokers," *Japan Journal of Nursing Science* 10, no. 1 (2013): 68–78.

37. K. Flory, P. S. Malone, and D. A. Lamis, "Childhood ADHD Symptoms and Risk for Cigarette Smoking During Adolescence: School Adjustment as a Potential Mediator," *Psychology of Addictive Behaviors* 25, no. 2 (2011): 320–329.

38. C. Voogd, "Young People Friendly Smoking Prevention and Cessation Services," *British Journal of School Nursing* 9, no. 1 (2014): 17–20.

39. S. Hill, D. Young, A. Briley, J. Carter, and B. Lang, "Baby Be Smoke Free: Teenage Smoking Cessation Pilot," *British Journal of Midwifery* 21, no. 7 (2013): 485–491.

40. J. B. Bricker, J. Liu, B. A. Comstock, A. V. Peterson, K. A. Kealey, and P. M. Marek, "Social Cognitive Mediators of Adolescent Smoking Cessation: Results from a Large Randomized Intervention Trial," *Psychology of Addictive Behaviors* 24, no. 3 (2010): 436–445.

41. Y. Kim, S. K. Myung, Y. J. Jeon, E. H. Lee, C. H. Park, H. G. Seo, and B. Y. Huh, "Effectiveness of Pharmacologic Therapy for Smoking Cessation in Adolescent Smokers: Meta-Analysis of Randomized Controlled Trials," *American Journal of Health-System Pharmacists* 68, no. 3 (2011): 219–226.

42. N. Rowa-Dewar and D. Ritchie, "Smoking Cessation for Older People: Neither too Little nor too Late," *British Journal of Community Nursing* 15, no. 12 (2010): 578–582.

43. M. Civljak, L. F. Stead, J. Hartmann-Boyce, A. Sheikh, and J. Car, "Internet-Based Interventions for Smoking Cessation," *Cochrane Database Systematic Review* 9 (2010): doi:10.1002/14651858.CD007078.pub4.

44. B. C. Bock, J. L. Fava, R. Gaskins, K. M. Morrow, D. M. Williams, E. Jennings, B. M. Becker, et al., "Yoga as a Complementary Treatment for Smoking Cessation in Women," *Journal of Women's Health* 21, no. 2 (2012): 240–248.

45. B. C. Bock, K. M. Morrow, D. M. Williams, G. Tremont, R. B. Gaskins, E. Jennings, J. Fava, et al., "Yoga as a Complementary Treatment for Smoking Cessation: Rationale, Study Design and Participant Characteristics of the Quitting-in-Balance Study," *BMC Complementary and Alternative Medicine* 10 (2010): 14.

46. C. M. Wyszynski, J. B. Bricker, and B. A. Comstock, "Parental Smoking Cessation and Child Daily Smoking: A 9-Year Longitudinal Study of Mediation by Child Cognitions About Smoking," *Health Psychology* 30, no. 2 (2011): 171–176.

47. Centers for Disease Control and Prevention, "Cigarette Use Among High School Students—United States, 1991–2009," *Morbidity and Mortality Weekly Report* 59, no. 26 (2010): 797–801.

48. L. R. Reitzel, E. K. Cromley, Y. Li, Y. Cao, R. D. Mater, C. A. Mazas, L. Cofta-Woerpel, et al., "The Effect of Tobacco Outlet Density and Proximity on Smoking Cessation," *American Journal of Public Health* 101, no. 2 (2011): 315–320.

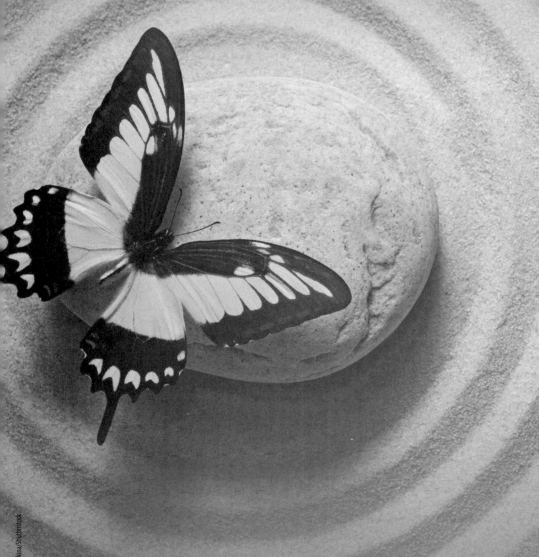

Advanced Concepts

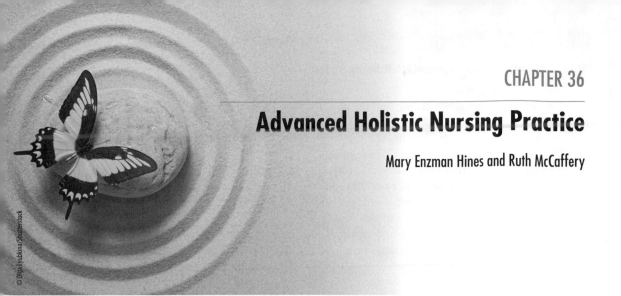

CHAPTER 36

Advanced Holistic Nursing Practice

Mary Enzman Hines and Ruth McCaffery

It has been predicted that the greatest advance in the next decade will not come from technology but from our deeper understanding of what it means to be human, spiritual beings.

—Aburdene, 2007[1]

Nurse Healer Objectives

Theoretical

- Explore the worldview, theories, and models embraced by advanced holistic nurses.
- Discuss the theories and research supporting holistic and integrative care.
- Explore patient-centered care and its components.
- Examine the growth of integrative care models in the U.S. healthcare system.

Clinical

- Explicate the foci of care for advanced holistic nurses.
- Analyze the Consensus Model and its potential effect on advanced holistic nurses.
- Define the key benefits of certification for advanced holistic nurses.
- Analyze the complementary aspects of holistic and integrative care related to patient-centered treatment.
- Define holistic entrepreneurial nursing and discuss its relevance in today's complex healthcare system.

Personal

- Create an integrative/healing model for advanced nursing practice.
- Identify entrepreneurial skills for developing integrative/holistic independent practice.
- Examine areas where you will need assistance to develop a viable holistic/integrative practice and how to obtain resources for the development of this practice.
- Develop short- and long-tern goals for implementing and sustaining an advanced holistic nursing practice.

Definitions

Advanced practice holistic nurses: A unique group of nurses weaving a tapestry of bio-psycho-social-spiritual-cultural elements to promote healing within self and others. As advanced practice holistic nurses engage in this healing process, it is a journey of changing and evolving of self and others.

APHN-BC: A certified advanced holistic nurse who synthesizes multiple sources of knowledge and therapies, including patient self-knowledge, when prescribing holistic treatments; develops holistic care plans co-created by partnering with the patient; and prescribes pharmacologic agents based on current knowledge of pharmacology and physiology, clinical indicators, age, holistic status/needs, results of diagnostic labs, and the person's beliefs, values, and choices. Certified advanced practice holistic nurses have the skills and education to evaluate and analyze the therapeutic effects, possible side effects, and interactions of all prescribed treatments; provide patients with information about cost and expected outcomes of planned treatment and integrative options; partner with others to create an interprofessional plan that focuses on safe, effective, holistic outcomes; document collaborative discussions, including holistic plan changes, communications, and rationale; and document referrals, including provisions for continuity of holistic care.[2]

Business plan: A detailed plan setting out the objectives of a business, the strategy and tactics planned to achieve them, and the expected profits.

Certification: Offers employers, healthcare organizations, and patients validation that certified advanced practice holistic nurses possess the specialty knowledge, skills, and experience to effectively deliver safe, quality care that promotes optimal health and wellness outcomes and maintains a detailed set of standards of practice that validate these professional competencies.[2]

Consensus Model for APRN regulation: Provides guidance for the licensure, accreditation, certification, and education of APRNs.[3] In this document, the APRN is defined as a nurse who has completed a graduate-level education program in preparation for one of four recognized APRN roles; passed a national certification examination and remains certified; acquired advanced clinical knowledge and skills; gained practice building on the competencies of registered nurses demonstrating greater knowledge, increased complexity of skills and interventions, and greater role autonomy; prepared to assume responsibility and accountability for health promotion and/or maintenance and assessment, diagnosis, and management of patient problems, including prescription of pharmacologic and nonpharmacologic interventions; performed sufficient clinical experience to reflect the intended license; and obtained a license to practice as an APRN in one of the four following roles: certified registered nurse anesthetist, certified nurse midwife, clinical nurse specialist, and certified nurse practitioner. The Consensus Model also classifies key requirements for APRN education.

Current Procedural Terminology (CPT) codes: These codes describe medical, surgical, and diagnostic services and are designed to communicate uniform information about medical services and procedures for financial and analytical purposes.

Entrepreneur: An individual who exercises initiative by organizing a venture to take benefit of an opportunity and, as the decision maker, decides what, how, and how much of a good or service will be produced. According to economist Joseph Alois Schumpeter (1883–1950), entrepreneurs are not necessarily motivated by profit but regard it as a standard for measuring achievement or success.

Integrative health care: An approach characterized by a high degree of collaboration and communication among health professionals. What makes integrative health care unique is the sharing of information among team members while keeping the patient at the center of care and decision making. The plan of care for each patient addresses biological, psychological, spiritual, and social needs. The interdisciplinary healthcare team includes a diverse group of members (e.g., physicians, nurses, psychologists, social workers, and occupational and physical therapists), depending on the needs of the patient.

Patient-focused care: Embraces a disease treatment model and views the patient from a systems approach and the person-centered view of practice.[4]

Person-centered care: Puts the patient at the center of care and partners with patients in more meaningful ways.[4]

Praxis: The synthesis of thoughtful reflection, caring, and action within a theory- and research-driven practice.[5]

The Evolving Role of the Advanced Practice Holistic Nurse

In the 21st century, significant demographic, economic, social, and environmental changes have affected individual and population-based health care. Complex health conditions plaguing individuals today require greater skills and knowledge for advanced practice nurses (APNs). In an era of increasingly sophisticated healthcare technology and technical demands, APNs must preserve efforts to provide humanistic, compassionate, and holistic care.[6]

Recent developments, including the Institute of Medicine's report, *The Future of Nursing: Leading Change, Advancing Health*,[7] and the 2010 healthcare reform, Patient Protection and Affordable Care Act (PPACA),[8] provide APNs and advanced practice registered nurses (APRNs) with opportunities to deliver care and contribute to roles leading to change in the healthcare landscape. With the passage of the PPACA, the focus of national and international health care will shift from disease management and cure to wellness, health promotion, and disease prevention. Clearly, a movement is occurring to ensure that APNs are allowed to practice to their full potential.

Today, virtually every discussion of healthcare reform begins with multiple concerns: the rising cost of health care, an expanding aging population, the role of advanced technology in healthcare documentation and monitoring, and the rising numbers of uninsured Americans.[9] Reforming health care to address these challenges requires a well-educated and informed nursing workforce.[10] With millions of Americans now gaining access to health care, there is an appreciation for the roles of APRNs in meeting the critical healthcare needs of this population, as well as an increased mindfulness of the barriers that currently prevent many APRNs from delivering care.[11, 12]

Over the past 35 years, holistic nursing as an organized nursing specialty has gained momentum in its pursuit to define the future of nursing and health care. Initiated as a different way of viewing the metaparadigm of nursing, holistic nurses provide a complementary way of practicing professional nursing that is consistent with the shift in the nations' healthcare views (see www.ahna.org). Holistically caring for humankind as mental, emotional, and spiritual beings has gained popularity in health care.[13] Holistic nursing is the art and science of caring for the whole person. It is based on the belief that dynamic mind-body-spirit interactions are ongoing and influence a person's ability to grow and heal. Holistic nurses aim to promote health and wellness as they facilitate their patients' growth and healing. Health is a perception of wellness, as well as a quality of life. Holistic nurses work with people in all settings and at all phases of life. Their primary goal is to facilitate people to live their lives as fully as possible, in all situations.[11]

Complementary modalities are increasing in popularity, and advanced practice holistic nurses (APHNs) integrate holistic therapies into everyday care for both self and patient. Approximately 40% of individuals are seeking and using complementary modalities, holistic approaches to stress management, and holistic treatment plans in addition to their allopathic care.[14] Holistic care expands the experiences of the APRN and the patient. Holistic care is changing the way the APRN experiences practice and health care.

Advanced practice nurses using a holistic approach to health care embrace a worldview that emphasizes healing as always possible, no matter what the individual's situation.[15] In the healing process, patients draw on an inner strength with a goal to reach something that is intangible. One of the greatest challenges for holistic APNs is focusing on healing within a healthcare system that predominately embraces a reductionistic view of health care. Advanced practice nurses can meet these challenges by expanding caring, healing approaches informed by research, education, and practice (praxis).[5] "To create a caring environment and engender an atmosphere of respect and compassion, nurses need to understand what caring is, how to be caring, and the impact of caring and noncaring on others."[16, p. 19] Praxis is the synthesis of thoughtful reflection, caring, and action within a theory- and research-driven practice.[5] Holistic APNs are a unique group of nurses weaving a tapestry of bio-psycho-social-spiritual-cultural elements to promote healing within self and others. As holistic APNs engage in this healing process, it is a journey of changing and evolving of self and others.[17-19]

Practicing as an advanced holistic nurse (AHN) in any nursing role and setting, whether in acute care, primary care, or academia, the AHN's greatest influence is contributing to patient-centered care and a whole-person approach based on a holistic philosophy of caring/healing. Advanced holistic nurses of any degree level are finding great satisfaction in providing care by embracing a holistic approach. Advanced holistic nurses graduating from programs with holistic conceptual frameworks and philosophies are uniquely prepared to take a leadership role in the promotion of health and wellness, prevention of illness and complications with individuals, and advancement of the health and well-being of society. Advanced holistic nurses who do not graduate from a holistically based education program can further expand their knowledge through courses available in university and continuing education platforms.

The American Holistic Nurses Association (AHNA) in collaboration with the American Nurses Association (ANA) published *Holistic Nursing: Scope and Standards of Practice, Second Edition*, which defines the scope of holistic nursing practice and the expected level of care provided by basic and advanced holistic nurses.[20] Based on a philosophy that nursing is an art and a science, with the primary purpose of providing holistic care for the whole person, the scope and standards of holistic nursing practice support five core values:

1. Holistic Philosophy, Theory, and Ethics
2. Holistic Caring Process
3. Holistic Communication, Therapeutic Healing Environment, and Cultural Diversity
4. Holistic Education and Research
5. Holistic Nurse Self-Reflection and Self-Care

Currently, the American Holistic Nurses Certification Corporation (AHNCC) provides certification for advanced holistic nurses (AHN-BC) and advanced practice holistic nurses (APHN-BC).[2]

Defining Advanced Practice Registered Nurses

Various definitions exist for APRNs. The practice of AHNs focuses on facilitating healing, health, and wellness in the holistic person throughout the lifespan.[20] Advanced holistic nurses honor the individual's subjective experience about health, health beliefs, and values. Embracing a holistic worldview, nurses become a therapeutic partner with individuals, families, communities, and populations by drawing on nursing knowledge, theories, research, expertise, intuition, and creativity and incorporating the roles of clinician, educator, consultant, coach, partner, role model, and advocate. Holistic nursing practice encourages peer review of professional practice in various clinical settings and provides care based on current professional standards, laws, and regulations governing nursing practice.[20] Advanced holistic nurses embrace a holistic, person-centered approach to health care. Key elements in the scope of practice in patient care for holistic APRNs are summarized in **Exhibit 36-1**. *Holistic Nursing: Scope and Standards of Practice, Second Edition*, further elaborates the competencies of advanced holistic nursing practice.[20]

The dominant model for APRN practice, supporting the conventional model of health care (patient-centered), is recognized by the American Academy of Colleges of Nursing, who endorsed a *Consensus Model for APRN Regulation: Licensure, Accreditation, Certification and Education* in 2008.[3] In this document, the APRN is defined as a nurse who has:

1. Completed a graduate-level education program in preparation for one of four recognized APRN roles
2. Passed a national certification examination and remains certified
3. Acquired advanced clinical knowledge and skills
4. Gained practice building on the competencies of registered nurses demonstrating greater knowledge, increased complexity of skills and interventions, and greater role autonomy
5. Prepared to assume responsibility and accountability for health promotion and/ or maintenance and assessment, diagnosis,

---

EXHIBIT 36-1   Exemplar Competencies of the Advanced Practice Holistic Nurse in Patient Care

1. Collects comprehensive data pertinent to the healthcare consumer's health and situation
2. Analyzes data to determine the diagnosis or the issues by synthesizing data or information to identify patterns and variances with a life content
3. Identifies expected outcomes for a plan individualized for consumer care by partnering with the client and/or healthcare provider, setting realistic time frames for achieving outcomes, and documenting outcomes
4. Develops a plan that prescribes strategies and alternatives to attain expected outcomes
5. Implements identified plan
6. Coordinates care within nursing and across the interprofessional team
7. Provides clients with information regarding their health and wellness
8. Provides consultation to influence the identified plan, enhance the abilities of others, and effect change
9. Evaluates the progress of the caring process

Source: Reproduced from ANA/AHNA Scopes and Standards of Holistic Nursing, 2013.[20]

---

and management of patient problems, including prescription of pharmacologic and nonpharmacologic interventions

6. Performed sufficient clinical experience to reflect the intended license

7. Obtained a license to practice as an APRN in one of the four following roles: certified registered nurse anesthetist, certified nurse midwife, clinical nurse specialist, and certified nurse practitioner (see **Table 36-1**)

TABLE 36-1   Consensus Model of Advanced Practice Registered Nurse Roles

Role	Description
Certified Nurse Midwife (CNM)	The CNM provides a full range of primary health services to women throughout the life span, including gynecological care, family planning services, preconception care, prenatal and postpartum care, childbirth, and care of the newborn.
Clinical Nurse Specialist (CNS)	The CNS has a unique APRN role to integrate care across the continuum and throughout three spheres of influence: patient, nurse, and system. The three spheres are overlapping and interrelated, but each sphere possesses a distinctive foci. In each sphere, the primary goal is continuous improvement of patient outcomes and nursing care. Key elements of CNS practice are to create environments through mentoring and system change that empower nurses to develop caring, evidence-based practices to alleviate patient distress, facilitate ethical decision making, and respond to diversity.
Certified Nurse Practitioner (CNP)	The CNP provides care along the wellness–illness continuum as a dynamic process in which direct primary and acute care is provided across settings. The CNP is a member of the health delivery system, practicing autonomously in areas as diverse as family, pediatrics, internal medicine, geriatrics, and women's health care.
	The CPN is prepared to diagnose and treat patients with undifferentiated symptoms as well as those with established diagnoses. This can be primary or acute-care focused depending on the CPN's preparation.
Certified Registered Nurse Anesthetist (CRNA)	The CRNA is prepared to provide the full spectrum of patients' anesthesia care and anesthesia-related care for individuals across the life span, whose health status may range from healthy through all recognized levels of acuity, including persons with immediate, severe, or life-threatening illnesses or injury. The care is provided in diverse settings including hospitals, obstetrical delivery rooms, pain management centers, and ambulatory surgical centers.

Source: Reproduced from AACN (2008). Consensus Model for APRN Regulation: Licensure, Accreditation, Certification & Education. APRN Consensus Work Group & the National Council of State Boards of Nursing APRN Advisory Committee. http://www.aacn.nche.edu/education-resources/APRNReport.pdf.[3]

Advanced practice registered nurses are educated in one of four roles and in at least one of six population foci: family/individual across the life span, adult-gerontology, pediatrics, neonatal, women's health/gender related, or psychiatric-mental health. In addition, APRNs may further specialize in practice beyond the role and population focus, including but not limited to oncology, orthopedics, nephrology, palliative care, pain management, cardiology, and gastroenterology (see **Figure 36-1**). Specifically, the three criteria for APRN status require (1) the nurse to select one of four specified roles (CNA, CNM, CNS, CNP), (2) a specific population, and (3) a formal education that includes three courses to acquire knowledge specific to these roles (advanced assessment, advanced pathophysiology, and advanced pharmacology).

Graduate nurses have also expanded roles into specialties including informatics, public health, administration, and education. Like APRNs, these roles have gained importance in providing high-quality care in the reformed healthcare system. The distinction between these roles and specialties and the four APRN roles is the focus on direct care to individuals.[21] Furthermore, these additional roles do not require regulatory licensure beyond the RN.

The Consensus Model

The model for APRN regulation is the result of the APRN Consensus Work Group and the National Council of State Boards of Nursing APRN Advisory Committee dialogue.[3] The

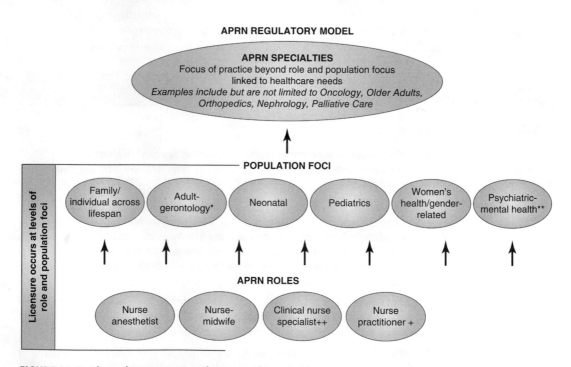

FIGURE 36-1 Advanced Practice Registered Nurse Regulatory Model

*The population focus *adult-gerontology* encompasses the young adult to the older adult, including the frail elderly. Advanced practice registered nurses educated and certified in the adult-gerontology population are educated and certified across both areas of practice and will be titled Adult-Gerontology CNP or CNS. In addition, all APRNs in any of the four roles providing care to the adult population (e.g., family or gender specific) must be prepared to meet the growing needs of the older adult population. Therefore, the education program should include didactic and clinical education experiences necessary to prepare APRNs with these enhanced skills and knowledge.

**The population focus *psychiatric-mental health* encompasses education and practice across the life span.

Source: Reproduced from AACN (2008). Consensus Model for APRN Regulation: Licensure, Accreditation, Certification & Education. APRN Consensus Work Group & the National Council of State Boards of Nursing APRN Advisory Committee. http://www.aacn.nche.edu/education-resources/APRNReport.pdf.[3]

APRN Joint Dialogue Group recommended the APRN Regulatory Model for the licensure, accreditation, certification, and education of APRNs. Advanced practice registered nurse regulations identify four essential components—licensure, accreditation, certification, and education—giving rise to the acronym LACE. The model states that, for successful implementation, all four of the following elements must be present and working together to ensure appropriate regulations:[21]

1. **L**icensure is the granting of authority to practice. The model requires state boards of nursing to license APRNs as independent practitioners.
2. **A**ccreditation is the formal review and approval by a recognized agency of the educational degree or certificate program in graduate nursing. The model requires accreditation standards and processes to assess APRN education programs to ensure that the APRN core, roles, and population core competencies are met and to monitor education programs throughout the accreditation period.
3. **C**ertification is the formal recognition of the knowledge, skills, and experience identified by standards within the profession. Certifiers, accredited by a national certification body, are required to follow established testing and psychometrically based standards for an APRN exam. In addition, provisions ensure competence and maintenance of certification and participate in ongoing relationships and transparency to state boards of nursing.
4. **E**ducation is the formal preparation of the APRN within a graduate program granting a graduate degree or graduate certificate. Advanced practice registered nurse education programs/tracks must be accredited by a nursing accrediting organization recognized by the U.S. Department of Education and/or the Council for Higher Education Accreditation, be preapproved and preaccredited prior to the admission of students, and ensure that graduates are eligible for national certification and licensure.

APRN Education

The Consensus Model classifies key requirements for APRN education. These requirements include recommendations for formal education with a graduate degree or postgraduate certificate awarded by an accredited academic institution. Academic institutions have also ensured that curricula comply with the model requirements for the 3 xPs: three separate comprehensive graduate courses (the APRN core) in advanced pathophysiology, advanced health assessment, and advanced pharmacology. Although there is a future recommendation that the entry level to APRN practice be the doctor of nursing practice (DNP), there presently is no consensus about this requirement.[22] Many education institutions are converting both postmaster's and bachelor of science in nursing programs to DNP programs to move this recommendation forward by 2015.

APRN Specialties

Preparation in specialty practice, an option for APRNs, represents a focused area of preparation and practice beyond the APRN role. Criteria for defining specialties as an APRN is informed by the ANA criteria for recognition as a nursing specialty and encompasses areas including but not exclusive of palliative care, cardiology, pulmonary, oncology, nephrology, and pain management. A family nurse practitioner could specialize in nephrology, a pediatric nurse practitioner could specialize in pain management, and a clinical nurse specialist could specialize in palliative care. State licensing boards do not regulate APRNs at this level of specialization, but certification in a specialty area of practice is strongly recommended.[21]

Implementation of the Consensus Model

The implementation of the Consensus Model has met with opposition. Because state nursing board laws and regulations continue to vary, there has been a tendency to focus on those that will require careful analysis of each state's laws and regulations to determine which revisions are necessary. However, not all laws and regulations are legal or regulatory. The implementation of educational requirements continues to vary from state to state, specifically the work required to meet the 3 Ps in advanced practice.[21] An interdependence of licensure, accreditation, certification, and education will require a sequential implementation. After the Joint Dialogue Group agreed on the APRN Consensus Model, the LACE Network was formed as an implementation team. The APRN LACE Network is collaboratively working to produce a structure and process for implementation of these recommendations.[23] Stakeholders are now developing documents for clarifying the issues posed in the model. The American College of Nurse-Midwives, the Accreditation Commission for Midwifery Education, and the American Midwifery Certification Board recently published a white paper, *Midwifery in the United States and the Consensus Model for APRN Regulation.*[24] Several other specialty organizations are responding to the Consensus Model in a similar way, including the National Association of Clinical Nurse Specialists (NACNS) and the National Organization of Nurse Practitioner Faculties (NONPF). Concerns have been voiced about the LACE Network focus on nurse practitioners (NPs) as the major role described for the APRN and the "vanishing" role of CNSs in some institutions secondary to the lack of certifications for CNSs in specialty and community settings.[2, 12]

The differences between an APRN in conventional medicine and a holistic APRN are summarized in **Table 36-2**. The AHNCC has responded to the Consensus Model by stating that this document would clearly limit the scope and practice of AHNs.

Daley addressed the current transformation in health care and the nurse's worldview of practice and identified two dominant worldviews that are clearly present in the healthcare landscape: patient-focused care that embraces a disease treatment model and views the patient from a systems approach and the person-centered view of practice.[4] As Daley shared:

> Supported by a growing body of evidence, *person-centered care* is now widely

acknowledged as a central factor related to improving quality and reducing cost of care. There is a clear difference between "person-focused" and "person-centered" care, and I believe that while it's safe to say that today's health care to a large extent is person focused, we have much work to do to make care person-centered.[4]

Daley clearly differentiated the two divergent views and contends that nursing needs to put the patient at the center of care and partner with patients in "more meaningful ways." "We [nurses] have long understood that respect and relationship between the nurse and individual—not simply proximity and knowledge—are what engender trust and contribute to more positive individual experiences and better health outcomes."[4]

Paradoxically, the current major regulation initiative by nursing, the Consensus Model designed to position APRNs to provide leadership in the present healthcare transformation, does not consider the differences in worldview in the formulation of the guidelines.[26] The current Consensus Model emphasizes person-focused care and hinders person-centered care. In the Consensus Model, the role of the holistic APN will be considered an add-on specialty that forces education programs to adapt to person-focused care dedicated to the management of health/disease conditions rather than person-centered care that emphasizes health, wellness, and healing. This has the potential to create a barrier to those who practice advanced practice holistic nursing.[11] The Consensus Model also requires that APHNs (AHN-BC and APHN-BC) take traditional courses (e.g., select 3 Ps) to acquire formal education based on precepts, knowledge, and skills associated with a *reductionistic view* of health care before acquiring knowledge, skills, and experience consistent with the competencies essential to advanced practice holistic nursing (e.g., courses in pharmacology, psychoneuroimmunology, nutritional supplements, herbal and homeopathic remedies, and integrative health practices).[2]

TABLE 36-2   Comparison of Currently Recognized Clinical Nurse Specialists and Advanced Holistic Nurses Description of Population, Setting, Subspecialty, Type of Care, and Type of Health Concern

	Advanced Practice Registered Nurses Currently Recognized by the Consensus Model	Advanced Practice Holistic Nurses as Either AHN-BC or APHN-BC
Description	Experts in subspecialty, type of care, and/or problem focus who work in any setting where their role is mandated, needed, or incorporated into a system. *Person-focused care*	Experts in holism, healing, health promotion, and illness prevention who work in any setting where a nurse–client professional relationship exists. *Person-centered care*
Population	Pediatrics, adult-geriatrics, women's health/gender related, family, neonatal, psychiatric-mental health.	The population of advanced holistic nursing consists of all persons who want or need to be facilitated with healing, health, or growth that results in mind-body-spirit synchrony and integration.
Setting	Critical care, emergency room, doctor's office, private practice settings.	Holistic nurses practice in any setting where nurse and client establish a professional partnership.
Disease of medical subspecialty	Diabetes, oncology, renal, cardiology, pulmonary, gastroenterology.	Not applicable for holistic nurses. Holistic nurses are concerned with the integration of mind-body-spirit of all persons, including those who have a chronic or acute medical problem or disease. Although some holistic nurses work with a population of individuals with diabetes or oncology problems (and may have advanced education in this area), their focus is on the entire person's need.
Type of care	Psychiatric, rehabilitation, primary care, acute care.	Holistic nursing embraces all nursing that has the enhancement of healing the whole person from birth to death — and all age groups from infant to elder — as its goal. This means viewing the whole person and his or her needs in their entirety with integration as the goal. The holistic nurse creates a caring, healing space within herself or himself that allows the nurse to be an instrument of healing; shares authenticity of unconditional presence that helps to remove the barriers to the healing process; facilitates another person's growth (body-mind-emotion-spirit-energetic-environment connections); and assists with maintaining wellness, recovery from illness, or transition to peaceful death.
Type of problem or practice focus	Pains, wounds, stress, chronic medical problems, etc.	Holistic nurses are concerned with their client's health and well-being needs, problems, and/or conditions.
Licensure/ certification	Certified by the American Nurses Credentialing Center or other specialty credentialing centers (e.g., National Association of Pediatric Nurse Practitioners). Examination is based on specialty advanced practice competencies.	Certified by the American Holistic Nurses Credentialing Corporation. Examination is based on holistic nursing advanced practice competencies.

Source: Reproduced from AHNCC Position on Consensus Model (2013)[11] and NACNS Clinical Nurse Specialist's Statement on Consensus Model Implementation (2012).[25]

Education Programs for Advanced Practice Nurses

Graduate nursing programs integrate a world-view and conceptual framework that direct the development of their curriculum. This curriculum is accredited by higher education nursing certifying groups, either the Commission on Collegiate Nursing Education or the National League for Nursing Accrediting Commission. Most graduate programs follow the *patient-focused* approach to APN education, supporting the process presented in the Consensus Model (see Figure 36-1). Specialty organizations, such as NONPF and NACNS, work closely with nursing schools and colleges to develop curricula that will prepare APN students for the certification exam by specialty certifying bodies in a population focus, including the American Association of Nurse Practitioners, AHNCC, the American Nurses Credentialing Center, which has both population-based NP certification and CNS certification in some specialty populations, and the Pediatric Nursing Certification Board. According to the Consensus Model and the NCSBN, APRN education must include the following components:[3]

1. Formal education with a graduate degree or postgraduate certification (either post-master's or postdoctoral) that is granted by an academic institution and accredited by nursing or nursing-related accrediting organizations recognized by the U.S. Department of Education and/or the Council for Higher Education Accreditation.
2. Awarded preapproval, preaccreditation, or accreditation prior to admitting students, be comprehensive, and be at the graduate level.
3. Prepare the graduate to practice in one of four identified APRN roles (CNS, CNM, NP, CNA); prepare the graduate with the core competencies for one of the APRN roles across at least one of the six population foci (adult-gerontology, pediatrics, neonatal, women's health/gender related, family, psychiatric-mental health).
4. Minimally include three separate graduate-level courses (referred to as the 3 Ps or APRN core) in advanced physiology/pathophysiology, including principles that apply across the life span; advanced health assessment, including assessment of all human systems, advanced assessment techniques, concepts, and approaches; and advanced pharmacology, including pharmacodynamics, pharmacokinetics, and pharmacotherapeutics of all broad categories of drugs. In addition, content specific to the role and population should be included in other role and population didactics and clinical courses; include a basic understanding of decision making in the identified role; prepare the graduate to assume responsibility and accountability for health promotion and/or maintenance, specifically assessment, diagnosis, and management of patient problems, including the use and prescription of pharmacologic and non-pharmacologic agents/interventions; and ensure that clinical and didactic coursework is comprehensive and sufficient to prepare graduates with the skills to practice in an APRN role and population focus.

Advanced Holistic Nursing Education

Nursing, a person-centered profession, has embraced two paradigms.[27-29] First described as models of holism versus wholism[30] then as the simultaneity and totality paradigms,[29] nursing has been split between traditional and holistic approaches to health care. These paradigms differ in how the nurse views the world: Nurses who use art and science in the development of a nursing profession and carry out the role and responsibilities of nursing or embrace nursing as a traditional science employ a systems model as their guide, and nurses who practice according to a holistic or simultaneity paradigm to view health as a sense of well-being, a quality of life.[28] These nurses focus on "protecting, promoting, and optimizing health and wellness; assisting healing; preventing illness and injury; alleviating suffering; and supporting people to find peace, comfort, harmony, and balance."[20]

The nurse's professional activities are designed to comfort and empower the patient, facilitate patients in find meaning and purpose in life experiences, foster growth and healing when needed, and transcend with grace and peace when the time occurs. Holistic nurses also mentor and provide leadership and guidance for colleagues and interprofessional team members embracing holistic health care.[28] Hills and Watson devote an entire book to describing a caring curriculum for undergraduate and graduate holistic nursing programs.[31] Promoting caring within advanced practice education, Enzman Hines provides a holistic framework for graduate education for an advanced practice program that provides the core elements of a holistic advanced practice curriculum.[32]

The AHNCC first started credentialing holistic nurses in 1997 and has since moved into credentialing AHNs through a national certification process. The AHNCC Board of Directors provides specific guidelines for nursing programs. Most nursing programs are based on a mixture of paradigms, while others are based on a simultaneity (holistic) paradigm. The AHNCC contends that these conclusions were validated by reviewing hundreds of qualitative assessments submitted by candidates for certification.[33] Many nurses prepared in the totality paradigm, or a program mixed with both paradigms, have a desire to practice holistically. As a result, after graduation, these nurses will need to seek continuing education to assist them in gaining the knowledge and skills to practice as a holistic nurse. The nurses who attend programs based on the holistic/simultaneity paradigm graduate prepared to practice as holistic nurses and are advocates of the principles of holistic nursing,[20] providing leadership for holism in the healthcare system. The AHNCC developed an Endorsement Program for nursing to support the simultaneity paradigm and provide programs in holistic undergraduate and advanced practice.[33] Endorsed programs in holistic nursing provide a curriculum consistent with the AHNA core values and prepare graduates to practice within the AHNA scope and standards of holistic nursing,[20] employ faculty certified as holistic nurses who support the simultaneity

paradigm, and advertise the school or college as one that prepares holistic nurses qualified to sit for AHNCC certification as a basic or advanced practice nurse. A list of current AHNCC-endorsed programs is found in **Table 36-3**.

Endorsed holistic nursing education programs have a school or college philosophy that reflects the AHNA's philosophy of nursing and code of ethics and core values. The school's or college's mission statements reflect goals consistent with preparing nurses based on *Holistic Nursing: Scope and Standards of Practice, Second Edition*.[20] Both the philosophy and mission must be consistent with the level of the program being endorsed. The curriculum outline and all courses include course descriptions and objectives that evidence holistic nursing as a thread running throughout the program. A single elective course in the program is not sufficient. Course content, threaded throughout the program, provides the knowledge and skills needed to practice holistic nursing at the appropriate level and demonstrates how the student is prepared to practice holistic nursing. Concepts such as presence, intentionality, unconditional acceptance (of the human), self-care, and other key holistic nursing concepts must be evident in the course content, descriptions, and practice experiences.[33] The lead faculty teaching the courses must be certified by AHNCC as either an AHN-BC or APHN-BC.

The Value of the Certification Process for AHN-BC and APHN-BC

Changes in the social and professional environment of nursing over the past two decades have moved holistic nursing into mainstream health care and resulted in a call for national certification of holistic nurses.[34] The AHNCC assumed the responsibility for this certification in 1997 and has expanded the certification for registered nurses to three levels: (1) the diploma/associate degree nurse (HN-BC), (2) the baccalaureate degree nurse (HNB-BC) and the nurse with a graduate degree preparing the APN as an advanced holistic nurse (AHN-BC), and (3) the advanced practice holistic nurse (APHN-BC). The AHN-BC is able to demonstrate

TABLE 36-3   American Holistic Nurses Credentialing Corporation Endorsed Programs for Holistic Nursing

Name of Institution	Holistic Programs Endorsed
Capitol University Department of Nursing Columbus, Ohio	**Undergraduate** Baccalaureate Accelerated Bachelor of science completion **Graduate** Master of science in nursing programs
Eastern University Department of Nursing St. Davids, Pennsylvania	RN-BSN and second-degree programs
Florida Atlantic University Boca Raton, Florida	**Undergraduate** Baccalaureate BSN program Accelerated BSN RN-BSN **Graduate** MSN DNP PhD
Metropolitan State University St. Paul, Minnesota	**Undergraduate** Baccalaureate program **Graduate** Entry-level master of science
Massachusetts General Hospital Institute of Health Professionals Boston, Massachusetts	Postgraduate certificate of advanced mind body spirit nursing Certificate of completion in mind body spirit nursing
New York University New York, New York	Holistic nurse practitioner
Northern New Mexico College Espanola, New Mexico	RN to BSN completion program
Quinnipiac University Hamden, Connecticut	Baccalaureate and master's programs
University of Texas at Brownsville and Texas Southmost College Brownsville, Texas	Baccalaureate program

TABLE 36-3 American Holistic Nurses Credentialing Corporation Endorsed Programs for Holistic Nursing (*continued*)	
Name of Institution	**Holistic Programs Endorsed**
University of Texas Medical Branch	Baccalaureate program
Galveston School of Nursing	Generic and flexible option program
Galveston, Texas	
Western Michigan University	Baccalaureate program
Bronson School of Nursing	
Kalamazoo, Michigan	
Xavier University	Baccalaureate program
School of Nursing	RN to MSN and MIDAS programs
Cincinnati, Ohio	

Source: Reproduced from AHNCC

expertise in the basic practice of holistic nursing and performs the competences of AHNs (see Table 36-3). Advanced practice holistic nurses practicing in the educational setting, as holistic life coaches, and in entrepreneurial practice settings often seek this certification. In addition, the APHN holding the credential APHN-BC has obtained and demonstrated competencies in advanced knowledge of pharmacology, psychoneuroimmunology, nutritional supplements, herbal and homeopathic remedies, and integrative health practices to plan and prescribe care consistent with patient needs, health issues, and problems. The APHN-BC also synthesizes multiple sources of knowledge and therapies, including patient self-knowledge, when prescribing holistic treatments; develops holistic care plans co-created by partnering with the patient; and prescribes pharmacologic agents based on current knowledge of pharmacology and physiology, clinical indicators, age, holistic status/needs, results of diagnostic labs, and the person's beliefs, values, and choices. In addition, the APHN-BC evaluates and analyzes the therapeutic effects, possible side effects, and interactions of all prescribed treatments; provides patients with information about cost and expected outcomes of planned treatment and integrative options; partners with others to create an interprofessional plan that focuses on safe, effective, holistic outcomes; documents collaborative discussions, including holistic plan changes, communications, and rationale; and documents referrals, including provisions for continuity of holistic care.[2]

Why Should an Advanced Holistic Nurse Become Certified?

Professional nursing certification for AHN-BC and APHN-BC has established the importance of holistic nursing as a specialty. Certification assures employers, healthcare organizations, and patients that certified AHNs possess the specialty knowledge, skills, and experience to effectively deliver safe, quality care that promotes optimal health and wellness outcomes.[2] Certification maintains a detailed set of standards of practice that ensure these professional competencies. Credentialing and certification provide consumers increased choices when selecting healthcare providers, identify the level of care provided to patients, and assist in the evaluation of educational preparation of potential providers.[18]

Who Are Certified Advanced Holistic Nurses?

Certified AHNs and APHNs integrate caring, healing, person-centered care, the dynamics of holism, and unity into an approach to practice. Person-centered care supports the essential stance that the patient is the primary source of information and the patient's self-knowledge must be a key consideration in care. Thus, APHNs consider the patient's worldview as essential data. Input from many AHNs reveals that nursing is not only a profession but also a calling and a way of being in the world.[19] Advanced holistic nurses do the healing work in health care and understand the importance of caring, healing environments, relationship-centered care, presence, intention, and the human spirit in healing. Advanced practice holistic nurses identify opportunities for expanding practice.[10] The AHNCC defines holistic nursing as all nursing practice that cares for the person as an integrated, holistic human being, inseparable and integral to the environment.[33] Holistic nurses recognize and honor the belief systems of others and have increased awareness of the interconnectedness of all living beings within the global community.[18] "Holistic nursing practice is the science, art, and the 'creative fire' where holistic nurses uncover, recover, support and celebrate the creative self."[35, p. 15]

The AHNCC certification examinations for the AHN-BC and APHN-BC test the individual nurse's knowledge of advanced practice. Ongoing certification requires nurses to show evidence of continued efforts to enhance knowledge of advanced holistic nursing through continuing education. Once certified, APHNs will be challenged to become lifelong learners, enhancing and expanding their knowledge of holistic nursing.

A Definition of Integrative Health Care

Integrative health care is a practice where the care provider and patient are both empowered partners in an effort to best address the patient's unique conditions and needs.[36] Andrew Weil first coined the term *integrative medicine* as a way of providing health care that meets the needs of patients and families. When describing types of integrative health care, holistic nursing and advanced holistic nursing practice cannot be overlooked. It has been noted that while integrative care is varied in its approach, there is a common thread of holism that puts the patient at the center of decision making.[37] While integrative care is a method of care delivery, holistic care is a philosophy that views the patient as whole, taking into consideration the complete person: physically, environmentally, and psychologically. To describe the two concepts in practice, the idea of holism leads one to create an integrative method of healthcare delivery. In 2009, the U.S. Senate held a conference to discuss improving the nation's health care. The following statement came from the conclusion of that conference: "The overarching recommendation is to create a Wellness Initiative for the Nation focused on promotion of health through lifestyle change and integrative health practices."[38]

The integrative healthcare trend is growing among providers and healthcare systems across the United States.[39] Driving factors in the growth of integrative healthcare practices include increased consumer knowledge in the area of health care, consumers' desire to participate in health decision making, and the popularity of alternative and complementary therapies. Consumers perceive benefits from integrative healthcare services and are interested in emerging evidence that these benefits are real and meaningful.[40]

The World Health Organization defines integrative care as "The management and delivery of health services so that clients receive a continuum of preventive and curative services, according to their needs over time and across different levels of the health system."[41, p. 4] In this definition, the idea of integrative health emphasizes the need to address and manage immediate health problems as well as the deeper causes of the disease or illness. A second important aspect of this definition is the need to foster the development of healthy behaviors and skills for effective self-care that patients can use throughout their lives.

To create a working definition, U.S. providers have broadly defined integrative health care as providing whole-person-focused, patient- and family-centered care across all levels of the healthcare system.[36] The key theme in the delivery of integrative health care is the person at the center of all treatment decision making, goals, and outcome development and his or her ability to choose therapy options. Some healthcare providers have questioned the ability of patients to choose what is best for themselves; however, the role of the holistic nurse and other providers in integrative care is one of educating the patient on options and outcomes, allowing them to choose what meets their needs best. Obtaining health care is a complex and often overwhelming prospect, and the integrative and holistic provider must be a navigator and advocate for the patient's wishes and needs.

Focusing on the educational role of the integrative healthcare provider, the Consortium of Academic Health Centers for Integrative Medicine defines integrative health care as offering care that "reaffirms the relationship between practitioner and patient."[42] Salerno has defined integrative health as

> a focus on all stages and aspects of an individual's care, placing the patient at the center and making individuals responsible for and involved in their own health. The physical, mental, social, spiritual, cultural, environmental, and other states of being must be considered to ensure that patients receive the highest quality and most comprehensive and coordinated care possible.[43]

Understanding and monitoring all of these aspects of comprehensive patient-centered care requires a whole-person approach and an ability to build patient trust and confidence that their voice will be heard. While all of these definitions of integrative health have slight variations, the main themes are patient centeredness, health promotion, and holism.

Integrative care is not concentrated on medical care alone but rather on healing and a team-oriented approach to promoting an active and healthy life for patients as they define it. As holistic nurses focus on whole-person care and holism as a practice perspective, it is essential that holistic nursing be involved in the development and implementation of integrative health care and provide evidence of the effectiveness of many different types of therapies to meet individual patient needs.

The concepts within integrative health care and holistic nursing care are different; however, they are both important for optimal patient care and positive patient outcomes. Holistic nursing can be practically defined as a way of being with a person in a caring and healing manner. Holistic nurses are focused on coming to know and being authentically present with the person in mind, body, and spirit within his or her personal environment and culture. In the practice of holistic nursing there is consideration of economic, physical, social, emotional, and spiritual aspects of the person and how these aspects affect the person's response to illness or life struggles when caring for them.[45]

Integrative health care is about creating a healthcare setting where the patient and healthcare provider interact to determine what is best for the patient using traditional and nontraditional treatments and therapies. In the integrative healthcare model, physical, emotional, mental, social, cultural, spiritual, and environmental aspects of the person are evaluated, keeping the patient at the center of all decision-making and treatment options. This moves health care away from a disease-oriented model where the healthcare provider simply makes decisions and arranges treatments without regard for patient and family wishes. While holistic care and integrative health care are similar and blend together, they are not the same and may be mutually exclusive. This means that holistic nurses can practice within an integrative healthcare setting and provide the added benefit of a holistic way of being with patients. For the purposes of this chapter, integrative health care will be discussed with the understanding that this care is provided in a holistic fashion.

Ring and colleagues acknowledge that true integrative health care is informed by evidence and makes use of many different types of therapies and therapeutic approaches from many different disciplines in order to achieve optimal health and healing for patients.[46] One of the drawbacks to integrative health is that scientific evidence is limited for many of the therapies that are used. In many instances, a lack of reliable data makes it difficult for people to make informed decisions about using integrative healthcare therapies. The outcomes and effects of many complementary and alternative therapies are not easily measured using randomized controlled trials, which are the gold standard of Western medicine. Clinical trials of complementary and alternative therapies can be costly and are prone to design and feasibility issues as well as small sample sizes.[14] To overcome some of the difficulties involved in uncovering the evidence that supports the use of complementary and alternative therapies, Verhoef and colleagues have endorsed whole-systems research as a better way to uncover evidence on the complex range of modalities in integrative health care.[47] Many complementary and alternative therapies have potential synergistic effects that require an innovative evaluative approach to providing evidence. This type of holistic research encompasses a mixed methods approach and is often used in the area of complementary and alternative therapies, allowing for a fuller understanding of how these therapies affect the whole person.

Holism, in the context of integrative health care, creates a practice of viewing the patient in a holistic manner, including evaluating environmental and cultural aspects of health. Each patient has a unique system of health beliefs that guide their intuitive ideas about health promotion and disease prevention as well as tertiary care when disease is present. These unique beliefs support the use of complementary and alternative therapies. In the integrative healthcare setting, the healthcare provider acts as a teacher and mentor by making the patient aware of the existing evidence, as a negotiator in the planning of treatments, as a partner co-creating the healthcare plan, and as a nonjudgmental advocate for decisions made by the patient. The Bravewell Collaborative established several outcome measures and concepts that define and explicate integrative health. **Exhibit 36-2** provides a declaration for a new medicine that outlines the values and beliefs of integrative

---

EXHIBIT 36-2   Declaration for a New Medicine

- We value the treatment of the individual in a holistic manner and the fulfillment of the needs of mind, body, and spirit.

- We recognize the sacred and healing nature of the relationships between patients and healthcare providers and acknowledge that humanism, compassion, and caring are central to health and healing.

- We believe that the empowered patient is responsible and that a person's emotions, trauma, and stress levels directly affect the risk and course of disease.

- We will work for a healthcare system that supports healing relationships and recognizes that, in order to be healing and empowering, healers themselves must be restored and whole.

- We will support truly integrative medicine that offers the highest standards of excellence in a full and complete array of evidence-based care modalities.

- We embrace the spiritual dimension of life and acknowledge the importance of context and intention in the healing process for patients, caregivers, and healers.

- We acknowledge that the risks of many serious illnesses, such as cancer, cardiovascular disease, and diabetes, can be reduced with scientifically based nutrition, exercise, and mind–body interventions.

- We believe in giving voice to the patient, in the openness of healers, and in honest and supportive communications among all members of the healthcare community.

- We will support the efforts of healers to develop the integrity and spiritual qualities, which are as important as medical knowledge and technical skills to the process of healing.

- We dedicate ourselves to the change necessary to bring about the new medicine in an optimal healing environment.

Source: Reproduced from Bravewell Collaboration http://www .bravewell.org/integrative_medicine/[48]

---

healthcare providers. **Exhibit 36-3** provides the patient's bill of rights in integrative health care.

Many of the concepts that integrative healthcare groups consider integrative have long been the focus of holistic nursing. It is essential that holistic nurses who have practiced in

EXHIBIT 36-3   Integrative Health Care Patient's Bill of Rights

As an individual, you have:

- The right to person-centered care.
- The right to receive health care that addresses the wholeness of who you are — body, mind, and spirit — in the context of community.
- The right to a healthcare system that focuses on prevention and wellness.
- The right to be empowered as the responsible, central actor in your own healing.
- The right to education about self-care that includes access to scientifically based nutrition, exercise, and mind–body interventions.
- The right to a healing relationship with your healthcare provider that is grounded in humanism, compassion, and caring.
- The right to speak openly and honestly with your healthcare provider and, in return, to experience honest and supportive communications from all members of the healthcare community.
- The right to a healthcare environment that recognizes that, to be healing and empowering, healthcare providers themselves must seek to be restored and whole.
- The right to embrace the spiritual dimension in the context of your health care.
- The right to healthcare providers who understand that integrity and spiritual qualities are as important as medical knowledge and technical skills in the process of healing.
- The right to truly integrative medicine that is supported by rigorous scientific research, maintains the highest standards of excellence, and offers a full and complete array of care modalities.
- The right to healing even when there is no cure.
- The right to be whole.

Source: Reproduced from Bravewell Collaboration http://www.bravewell.org/integrative_medicine/[49]

these modalities are seen as alternative or complementary. The common thread throughout the idea of integrative health care is the focus on holism: treating the patient as whole and complete in each moment, developing a collaborative relationship with each patient, and putting the patient at the center of decision making. Collaboration between practitioner and patient enables this wholeness to be apparent and allows the evolution of patterns that can lead the patient to a higher level of health and well-being. There is an increasing demand among patients and families for an integrative healthcare approach using alternative and complementary therapies in addition to traditional medicines.

Public demand for integrative health care and the ability to choose alternative and complementary therapies has continued to increase over the last decade.[14] According to the National Center for Complementary and Integrative Health, approximately 38% of adults (about 4 in 10) and approximately 12% of children (about 1 in 9) in the United States are using some form of complementary and alternative medicine, and these numbers are expected to grow rapidly over the next decades. Adult women and those with higher levels of education and income are the highest consumers of these therapies. The types of therapies used most often include deep breathing exercises, massage therapy, and yoga.[14] In 2006, the number of hospitals offering complementary and alternative services increased to about 20%.[50] This increase is largely due to patient interest in the types of therapies promoting the concept of integrative healthcare delivery, where the patient is in charge of decision making rather than the clinician. Creating healing environments within hospitals has been a focus for many, and the effects of the physical environment on the healing process and well-being is increasingly relevant for patients and families as well as healthcare staff.[51] Providing a healing, quiet, and peaceful environment in the hospital setting can reduce falls and medical errors as well as enhance privacy, comfort, and patient control.[51] Bazuin and Cardon found that creating a quieter environment in the critical care unit that includes family and friends as well as windows and natural light provides a sense of balance and safety for patients, family, and

this integrative way for years involve the unfolding of a truly unique and patient-centered care delivery system.

Integrative health care incorporates a large group of modalities. In Western health care staff.[52] Providing holistic health care for patients focuses on the relationship between healthcare provider and patient as the preeminent factor in creating positive outcomes.[39]

Personalization of health care for each patient emphasizes an integrative approach that includes engaging the patient as an informed and empowered care partner. An integrative approach in health care is a natural outflow of holistic nursing. Holistic nurses have always focused on treating the whole person and family, considering all aspects of the whole person. Integrative health care emphasizes the use of evidence-based personalized therapeutic approaches and health promotion and disease prevention to optimize health and well-being across the life span. Integrative care uses "best evidence" from medicine as well as alternative and complementary care. Integrative health has commonly been described in the literature as treating the mind, body, and spirit of each patient. Holistic nurses do not consider these three aspects of the person as separate and needing individual attention but instead view them as holographic, representative of the whole, not separate attributes. Providers of true integrative health care view the patient as the center of care; the patient's mind, body, and spirit are inseparable, an integrated whole.

Although integrative health care has been discussed as a model for delivering primary care for many years, more recently it has become a transformative change to healthcare systems. Many healthcare providers and systems are offering patients a wider choice of therapies and services to promote health and well-being. Patients are increasingly well informed and desire to participate and guide decision making about their own health and health care. To be most effective, integrative health care must ensure that the full spectrum of opportunities for prevention is made available to patients. These opportunities include clinical, behavioral, social, spiritual, and environmental-based therapies. Integrative care considers all of the elements of an individual's care, including an individual's conditions, needs, and circumstances.

Let us imagine what a truly integrative and holistic healthcare system looks like. The following is an exemplar:

Jane Worthington has been experiencing headaches for the past month that have begun to interfere with her daily activities and her life at home with her family. The headaches begin at any time of the day and often last for many hours. She has tried over-the-counter remedies such as Tylenol and ibuprofen without relief. The headaches can bring on nausea and dizziness at times, and she is having trouble sleeping because of the pain. Jane has experienced no changes in vision, but she does have neck pain at times with the headaches. She has been to her primary care provider who has not been able to diagnose the cause of her headaches: a CT scan was negative for brain lesion, her sinuses were normal, and her spinal X-ray showed no spinal problems. Jane has been reading about an integrative healthcare practice in her area and, because they advertise patient-centered care and the use of alternative and complementary therapies to relieve problems, she decides to make an appointment.

When Jane arrives at the office she is asked to complete the usual forms for insurance, but no health history forms are given to her. Instead, she is taken to a pleasant room where a nurse asks her about her health history, her life, her job, and her health beliefs and ideas about what she wants from her visits to the care center. The nurse asks Jane about the coping skills she uses when problems arise and about her spiritual beliefs. She also asks Jane about her living and working environments both in terms of physical requirements and stress level. Jane states that she has a very stressful job that requires at least 8 to 10 hours a day. She has two teenage children who need her guidance and a husband. She tells the nurse practitioner (a holistic advanced practice nurse) that she began having the headaches about 1 year ago. At that time she would get a headache about once a month, but now she gets headaches almost every day. The headaches start at the base of her head and radiate up into her head. She has no problems with light or sound but sometimes she has such pain with the headaches that she gets nauseous. Jane sometimes has a glass or two of red wine with dinner but that only seems to increase the likelihood of headaches the next day.

Jane was sent to have blood work and a cervical spinal X-ray and given a follow-up appointment in 2 days. The integrative team, made up of a nurse practitioner, physician, physical therapist, and nutritionist, meet to discuss her case. They propose a program including nutrition counseling and diet review to remove triggers for the headaches, massage and yoga to reduce muscle tension (if the cervical spine is not injured), meditation and training in mindfulness to reduce stress levels, and medication to manage the pain when the headaches appear. Jane returns in 2 days. Her cervical spine X-rays are normal and her blood work is normal, except that her thyroid levels are elevated. After a discussion with the integrative team, Jane agrees to the plan that now includes thyroid hormone replacement. She is not sure about the meditation and mindfulness stress reduction but is willing to "give them a try." She will return to the office in 2 weeks to reevaluate her therapies to determine if her goal of reduced headaches is reached.

In 2 weeks Jane returns to the office and states that she feels much better. She has reviewed her diet history with the nutritionist and adjusted her diet in ways that were recommended. Jane is enthusiastic about these dietary changes and states that in her discussion with the nutritionist she was given choices and options to still eat the foods she enjoys. Jane really liked the yoga and massage, is sleeping better, and is more relaxed after work

and no longer drinks red wine to help her cope. The meditation and mindful stress reduction sessions are somewhat challenging for her at this time. She finds it hard to "shift" from a fast-paced work setting to being still and quiet; however, the instructor has given her some exercises to do on her way to the session that are helping her to calm her mind and prepare. Jane is willing to keep going to these classes for now and will report on her progress. Her most important goal has been reached. In the last 2 weeks she has had only one headache, and she used the visualization she learned in mindfulness stress reduction to relieve the pain and the headache went away quickly. Jane states that she is very happy that her headaches are gone and she did not need "medication" but could work on the problem with her team and resolve the headaches in a natural way.

Integrative health care uses a holistic approach to patient care and is a growing reality in the United States. Cost-effective, integrative health puts patients in charge of their own health, allowing them and their provider/team to be active partners in care. Holistic nurses are at the forefront of initiatives to promote integrative health. Creating a healthcare system that values the whole person and empowers each patient to make decisions based on health beliefs and a sense of wholeness will move our entire healthcare system away from a disease-oriented model to a wellness model.

Envisioning a Holistic Framework for Independent Practice

Traditionally, all nurses have worked for hospitals or doctors and have not seen themselves as entrepreneurs. This is changing, and nurse entrepreneurs in all areas of care are considering opening their own businesses. Businesses owned and operated by nurses include home care, staffing, care navigation, wound care, nurse practitioner care in the home, and holistic services.

Entrepreneurial nurses across all healthcare settings are a positive force for a wider scope of practice to fill the gaps in health care. Nurses who establish their own business use nursing and holistic visions and values, expanding the human influence and use of whole-person knowledge and skill in health care.[53]

Entrepreneurial nurses focus on innovation and evidence-based interventions, effectiveness, and efficiency, leading to change and modernization of health systems.[54] Holistic entrepreneurial nurses fulfill a leadership role that focuses on health and well-being rather than disease. Able to develop new ideas and creative strategies combined with specialists' skills and knowledge, holistic nurses create new and exciting products and services to improve the health of patients and provide a meaningful and satisfying professional opportunity for nurses.

The World Health Organization has reviewed the use of nurses in health care across the globe and found that they are underdeployed and that their knowledge and services are underutilized.[41] A paucity of research is available to provide practical guidelines for entrepreneurial nursing while barriers to practice remain. One of the barriers to entrepreneurial nursing historically begins with nursing education that has focused on acceptance, standardization, and prescription rather than on innovation and leadership.[55] As U.S. health care changes rapidly, it shifts the focus to a team approach on health, health promotion, and disease prevention. This system is poised for innovation and creativity that directly effects health care.

Scala has an entrepreneurial nursing practice that focuses on Reiki services, and she presents the following five tips for owning a successful healthcare business:[56]

1. *Get help.* Learn to set up and manage a website, promote your brand using social selling, or dabble in video and audio creation for advertising. There are business coaches who can keep you on course. Using a coach, a support system, and even a team can help to start and grow a healthcare business.
2. *Get focused.* Get clear right from the start on what your business will provide and where your skills are best used. How do you want

your business to be modeled? The clearer you are with your work, the better your business will function.
3. *Get organized.* Be prepared to work long hours, especially at first, but also ensure that you balance your work–life, even as a nurse entrepreneur. The best way to ensure that work does not take over your life is to stay organized.
4. *Get connected.* If your potential clients and customers do not know about you, they cannot come to your business. You need to stay social, keep up with your networks, and create meaningful collaborations. Here is where quality connections create more value than sheer numbers alone. Identify which social media platform works for you and focus on one thing at a time.
5. *Get confident.* Everything is energy. Believe in and adhere to spiritual, universal, and energetic laws. If you do not believe in yourself and your value, guess what? Neither will anyone else. They can feel what you are sending out, even if your words say otherwise. It is the "vibe" that people pick up on. Do what you can to own your success.

Starting a business can be an exciting prospect, although beginning an independent practice requires a great deal of work and patience. Wearing two hats, that of a business person and that of a provider, requires effort and a focus on patient satisfaction/outcomes as well as financial outcomes. Even small practices that start in a home or shared space are businesses that require ongoing care. Whether you are billing insurance companies or getting paid at the time of the patient's visit, it is important to implement a business model in order for your practice to survive and thrive. You will be required to work long hours; however, owning your own business allows you to design your practice and practice goals, work flexible hours, and practice in a way that will attract patients and create a practice that is well reimbursed.

One of the first steps is to determine the structure of your business. Will it be a sole proprietorship, partnership, or corporation? Do not think that because you are the only employee of your business or that you are small that it is unnecessary to think about these issues. There are benefits and drawbacks to these business types, both financially and legally. It is a good idea to consult an attorney to help you decide. Many areas have a small business organization that provides free or low-cost assistance for decision making. The following are some definitions that can begin your thinking along these lines:

- *Sole proprietorship*. This is usually the least costly and easiest way to start a practice. It means that you are the practitioner and the sole owner at the same time. You form it by filing a business or practice name certificate with your local county clerk's office. With a sole proprietorship, you own everything and reap all of the profits. However, you are also financially and legally responsible for all debts and liabilities that occur while you are in practice. If something happens in your practice that results in harm to another person, your business assets *and* your personal assets (i.e., personal checking and savings accounts, deferred savings plans) are equally at risk. Strengths include the ease and low cost of start-up: You have complete control and earn 100% of the profits, and it is easy to dissolve your business if needed. Limitations include the risk to business and personal assets in the event of legal problems. Also, this type of practice may limit your potential for future funding from banks (i.e., lines of credit, obtaining future funding).
- *Partnership*. There are several types of partnerships: general partnerships, limited partnerships, and partnerships with limited liability. Basically, you have a business partner (or several) with whom you share the costs, risks, and profits of your business. General partnerships tend to be fairly even, cut down the middle with equal shares of the business. A limited partnership is one in which partners limit liabilities to the extent of available investments and therefore have limited input into most management decisions. Some strengths of partnerships include the ease of establishing the business (use legal documents;

partnerships sealed with handshakes typically lead to trouble down the line); the ease of funding the business because more people are involved; and the benefit of partners providing different skillsets, which can round out a practice. Limitations include the fact that all partners are jointly responsible for the actions (if one partner does something illegal or wrong, *all* partners are responsible); all profits and losses must be shared and some benefits may not be legally deductible from business income on tax returns (such as medical insurance); and the partnership can end abruptly upon the withdrawal or death of a partner.

- *Corporations*. Incorporating your business makes your personal assets exempt from any liability that might arise from your practice. You can incorporate quickly and easily with the help of an experienced attorney. But there are different kinds of corporations, such as C or S corporations. Each has special tax benefits that would be best explained by an accountant. An S corporation is very similar to a sole proprietorship but with more protection of your personal assets. A limited liability company (or LLC) is also very similar to a sole proprietorship regarding income, and it offers increased risk protection. Advantages to incorporating include limited liability for the corporation's debts or judgments against it and the ability of corporations to deduct the cost of fringe benefits such as medical insurance, individual retirement accounts, and 401Ks. Limitations include increased time, money, and energy to incorporate; the close monitoring of corporations by federal, state, and local agencies; and the possibility that the venture will result in overall higher taxes.[57]

Whichever structure you choose, you will need to obtain a business license. This allows you to own and operate a business within your city or town. A business license is usually not difficult to acquire, and an application can be filed at your city hall. A small fee may be required, and you will be required to renew this license annually.

As you take these first steps toward becoming a nurse entrepreneur, it may be necessary to access many different community partners. Beginning a business can be a daunting task, but if you have the right team, right support, and right ideas, you can do it.

Creating a Business Plan

Business plans typically contain three major elements: organizational plan, marketing plan, and financial plan. The organizational segment describes the management team (i.e., partners, management matrix). The marketing section discusses who may use the service and which product is offered by the business. The financial statement contains the numbers that illustrate how the project is expected to operate over the initial start-up period. An executive summary is recommended that outlines key points and introduces the business plan. This section is often what gains further examination of the business plan.[58] The executive summary must include a clear and concise outline of the services and products. **Exhibit 36-4** outlines the key elements of the executive summary, and **Exhibit 36-5** contains an actual executive summary of a proposed business.

While the components of a business plan are essentially the same in all organizations, the templates may vary. An example of a business plan template can be found at www.hced.co.uk /download/Business%20Plan%20Template.doc; however, there are many templates available for this purpose. The process of writing a business plan, coupled with knowledge of macro systems of health care, can result in ensuring success in initiating and operating a successful program or business. The ability to innovate as well as develop an entrepreneurial proposal and solid business plan will prepare nurses to have a strong voice in the financial and business world.[59]

Financing and Sustaining a Practice

Nurse practitioners are competent healthcare providers who deliver valuable, cost-effective health care. As the general public, government, and insurers recognize the benefits of utilizing NPs, the demand for service will increase. Developing business savvy and carefully planning a practice-based business future can bolster confidence and predict success. No medical care venture ever succeeds without confident, enthusiastic leadership around a mission that will attract patients. But this rosy outlook can become a liability, especially when dealing with financial projections.

Nurses have not had financial preparation and do not always understand the importance of the financial structure required to sustain a practice. Obtaining financial capital to start a business is the first step in any planning. Proper financial projections include money to purchase equipment and hire personnel and enough operating capital to sustain the practice until it becomes profitable. The amount of funding needed before beginning or opening a practice depends on the type of practice and the business plan. Many financial advisors note the importance of determining the predicted need and increasing that amount by 25% to 50%. Capitalization can come from family, a bank, or some combination of these. The first step is developing a working budget for the first year of operation within the business plan.

As a general rule, estimate the amount of money needed to open a practice and then double it to be sure there is enough. Also estimate the time that it will take the practice to become profitable and double that time as a reasonable

---

EXHIBIT 36-4   Executive Summary

The executive summary is a one- to two-page document that summarizes the opportunity and importance of the proposed business and contains the following elements:

- Description of the present situation and summary of existing conditions, also termed a *gap analysis*
- Description of the new program or proposed solution
- Presentation of options
- Market analysis
- Implementation plan
- Timeline and schedule
- Evaluation plan
- Financials

Source: Data from Mary Hines and Ruth McCafferty

EXHIBIT 36-5   Sample Executive Summary

National healthcare reform, a shortage of primary care physicians, and shifting health are delivery models that are the driving force behind the establishment of alternative care models to meet the increasing demand for healthcare services. The Institute of Medicine's 2010 *Future of Nursing* report recommendation to improve access to health care includes allowing advanced practice registered nurses (APRNs) to function to the full extent of their education and training, including the establishment of autonomous practice. The establishment of retail-based clinics is but one outgrowth of that trend. In the state of Colorado, APRNs are allowed to set up an autonomous practice including the provision of health care, the evaluation and treatment of minor acute illness, and the monitoring of stable chronic conditions. Recent advances in insurance company and Medicaid reimbursement has helped to make the reality of nurse practitioner-based clinics financially feasible. These factors, as well as a desire to give back to the community we serve, provide the foundation upon which we have created Integrative Pediatrics of Colorado, LLC.

Integrative Pediatrics of Colorado (IPC) is a nurse-practitioner owned and operated primary care practice serving children and families of all income levels. We will specialize in the integration of holistic and conventional healthcare approaches in caring for the unique needs of children. IPC will exemplify the primary care medical home model with a philosophy of care rooted in holism. We feel that by embracing each person as a unique and unified being, encompassing mind, body, and spirit, and providing cutting-edge, caring, primary care services, we will achieve our key practice goals of:

- Providing high-quality, cost-effective, specialized, holistic primary care to children and families in a medical home model

- Increasing access to integrative pediatric care in a medically underserved area

- Recruiting and maintaining a creative, caring, quality staff that exemplifies a philosophy of caring

- Providing a supportive environment for parents to explore complementary approaches to health care for their child

- Participating in research and utilizing evidence-based practice guidelines to support new knowledge and growth in pediatric health care

- Providing clinical preceptor experiences for advanced practice nursing students in collaboration with area universities and colleges

- Developing a loyal customer base where children receive medical care from birth to college

- Including an onsite retail component, making available to our clients at low cost plant- and botanical-based preparations, common prescriptive medications used in pediatrics, and over-the-counter medications and remedies.

The owners of IPC are three APRNs (Mary Enzman Hines, Jennifer Gaughan, Clare Huber-Navin) with more than 60 years of combined experience in pediatrics. The mission and vision of IPC will be supported by a caring, conscientious, efficient staff and will include a collaborative relationship with a physician and a network of specialist providers, including those who practice both conventional and complementary modalities.

The purpose of the following business plan portfolio is to highlight the structure and operational approach of IPC, explore evidence to support a need for such services, review a market analysis, provide financial statements, provide a timeline, discuss legal implications, and introduce owners and staff. IPC owners are proposing a small business loan agreement with your organization in the amount of $XXXXXX. With these funds, IPC will achieve start-up goals and create a sustainable, profitable, and unique pediatric practice, allowing us to pay back the loan in 5 to 7 years.

Source: Data from Mary Hines and Ruth McCafferty. *Note:* The contents of this executive summary are not to be copied without express permission of the authors.

---

estimate for repaying loans. Some of the costs to consider include the following:

- *Equipment.* Equipment can include office rental computers, phones, refrigerator, medical equipment, and supplies. Durable equipment companies and medical supply companies supply office furniture and exam room equipment. Second-hand medical equipment can be found through brokers or advertisements in nursing and medical journals.

- *Salaries.* Salaries can include providers (including your own salary), medical assistants, receptionist, biller/insurance coder, and office manager. Coders and office managers can make or break a practice financially. If the APN takes on these responsibilities at first, make sure all of the rules of coding are understood so that over- or undercoding does not pose a problem financially or legally. Remember that coding translates into money. Knowledge of laws and statutes regulating a healthcare practice as well as the components of human resources management are essential for independent practice. These laws govern how employees must be treated and paid, and they protect the rights of the employees in the workplace.

- *Treatment costs.* These cost include test kits for CLIA-waived (Clinical Laboratory Improvement Amendment) tests such as urine analysis and strep tests.
- *Insurance.* This encompasses general business liability insurance and malpractice insurance.
- *Apply for grants and foundation funding* to enable the practice to have foreign language interpreters. Reaching out to the United Way may be an additional funding source.
- *Seek funding for health insurance benefits* for practice providers and staff.
- *Maintain a relationship with key professionals* outside of the healthcare field to support a private practice. Relationships with bankers, attorneys, and accountants will make financial dealings less complex.

Some of these costs may be reduced, shifted, or avoided by focusing the practice on home visits. In a home visit practice, office rental and many other equipment costs will not be required; however, travel costs such as gas, care expenses, and insurance will need to be included. When thinking about starting a practice, consider creating a niche that will bring in patients to the practice, such as a holistic weight loss clinic, a stress reduction clinic, and an acupuncture/acupressure or a holistic pain reduction clinic. Consider being open during times that are convenient for working people, such as evenings and weekends, to attract patients. Consider having day care services or health navigation services (even if patients must pay for these services) to increase accessibility to patients and families. Offer services within the practice setting, such as massage, yoga, or tai chi, that make the practice a "one stop" for patients. Determine what services will cost and whether the practice will be a cash-only practice or if insurance will be accepted.

If the practice will accept insurance, make a very detailed investigation of which insurance plans or payer plans will be accepted, how much each of these payers pay for services provided, how fast they pay, and whether they accept this practice on their insurance panel. Medicare is the largest U.S. insurer, and many other insurance companies follow Medicare rules. As an APRN you may bill the Medicare program directly for services using a national provider identifier (NPI) or an employer's or contractor's NPI. The NPI is a unique 10-digit identification number issued to U.S. healthcare providers by the Centers for Medicare and Medicaid Services. It is important to know exactly which reimbursement levels will be received for services rendered. There is a set amount for each type of visit, treatment, and follow up based on diagnosis and therapy. Payment is made only on an assignment basis, which means that payment will be the Medicare-allowed amount as payment in full, and the APRN may not bill or collect from the beneficiary any amount other than unmet copayments, deductibles, and/or coinsurance. Services are paid at 85% of the Medicare Physician Fee Schedule amount. Medicaid reimbursement is similar, and in the pediatric population reimbursements are similarly differential for the APRN billing (85% of the Physician Fee Schedule).

Understanding and in some cases pursuing reimbursement for APN services may be key to survival for an independent nurse-run practice. To be prepared to adequately and successfully have an independent practice, APRNs must be competent clinicians but also well versed in the business/financial constructs for providing care. Understanding the key concepts of APRN definitions, Medicare/Medicaid billing regulations, private insurance regulations, credentialing for privileges in the healthcare setting, inpatient versus outpatient billing issues, the use of Current Procedural Terminology codes, and other topics as defined by the specific setting in which the APRN works is critical for success.[60] Billing to various third-party payers can be accomplished with a variety of medical management software; however, the challenge is the monitoring of claims submitted, tracking the date and amount of payments received, and resubmitting denied claims.

Getting the advice of professionals before developing a business plan or attempting to raise capital is a safe and reasonable step to ensure sustainability of an independent practice. Speak with an accountant who is an expert in financial management to determine how much money may be needed and how long it will be before the business turns a profit. The accountant's ability to assist depends on accurate assessments made in the business plan, the market for provided services, a willingness to work hard, and a tolerance to hang in there until the business becomes profitable. Speaking to others in a successful practice venture who have become independent entrepreneurs would be very helpful to avoid financial pitfalls. Johnson & Johnson offers a resource on the nurse entrepreneur at www.discovernursing.com/specialty /nurse-entrepreneur. The National Nurses in Business Association website (https://nnbanow .com/) provides valuable information, and the Nurse Entrepreneur website (www.nursing entrepreneurs.com) shares knowledge about opening a business and connecting nurse entrepreneurs in discussions about critical issues.

Federal, state, and local governments offer a wide range of financing programs and grants to help small businesses start and grow their operations. These programs include low-interest loans, venture capital, and scientific and economic development grants. Banks receive monies from the federal government to loan to small business start-up companies. If the services offered in the practice are sufficiently unique and interesting to the community in which the business will be located, it may be possible to obtain grants and loans from within the community itself. Finally, there are personal funds and family loans that are often used to start a business; however, be sure to have all aspects of the loan, including repayment schedules, in writing to avoid problems later.

Starting an independent nursing practice is not easy, but, for the right individual, it is the opportunity of a lifetime to make a difference and to become successful. It requires a lot of work, strength, and perseverance, as well as help from many others in the community and around the country. Holistic nurses are well positioned to offer independent services in a variety of settings that are unique and desired by many, including complementary therapies such as yoga, meditation, Healing Touch, diet therapy, and others. Starting a business as a solo practitioner or with a group of like-minded individuals can be a rewarding and thrilling opportunity if the right steps are taken to ensure sustainability and success.

Conclusion

Advanced holistic nursing as an organized nursing specialty has gained momentum in its pursuit to define the future of nursing and health care. Initiated as a different way of viewing the metaparadigm of nursing, advanced holistic nurses provide a complementary way of practicing professional nursing that is consistent with the shift in the nation's healthcare views. One of the greatest challenges for the future roles of holistic APNs is focusing on healing within a healthcare system that predominately embraces a reductionistic view of health care. Advanced practice holistic nurses can meet these challenges by expanding caring, healing approaches informed by research, education, and practice (praxis). Certification provides reassurance to employers, healthcare organizations, and patients that AHNs possess the specialty knowledge, skills, and experience to effectively deliver safe, quality care that promotes optimal health and wellness outcomes.[2]

In December 2014, the National Center for Complementary Medicine changed its name to the National Center for Complementary and Integrative Health. This provides a clear and strong message that integrative health care with the patient at the center of decision making is the way of the future. The focus on integrative health care provides an impetus for holistic nurses to become more active as healthcare providers using integrative therapies and care principals. Preparing nurses to become entrepreneurs can only strengthen the profession and allow holistic nurses who have the desire to move into more independent practices and become substantive members of the healthcare team.

Directions for Future Research

1. Examine the benefits of having certified advanced holistic nurses providing care in our healthcare system.
2. Analyze the outcomes of caring, healing practices for advanced holistic nurses.
3. Compare and contrast the outcomes of care provided by certified advanced holistic nurses and advanced practice nurses following the traditional medical model.
4. Investigate the successes of students graduating from holistic nursing programs.
5. Evaluate patient ratings of care provided by advanced holistic nurses.
6. Describe and explicate the patient experience of integrative/healing care.
7. Measure outcomes and patient satisfaction in independent advanced holistic nursing practice.
8. Evaluate outcomes such as decreases in chronic disease burden, improvements in health and well-being, and health promotion in patient populations by advanced practice nurses embracing holistic and integrated therapies and demonstrating the value of these therapies to individuals and society as a whole.
9. Investigate outcomes within established payer and reimbursement models for integrative/holistic services.
10. Explore patient satisfaction with integrative/holistic care (e.g., Do patients follow the care plan more systematically when they feel as though they have been a part of the plan development? How does that affect health outcomes?).
11. Examine the barriers faced by advanced practice nurse entrepreneurs from state legislatures, insurance companies, and other groups and how these barriers have been overcome by those who have created successful businesses.
12. Determine the satisfaction of nurse entrepreneurs with their work life and how they plan to encourage others to start independent practices.

Nurse Healer Reflections

After reading this chapter, the nurse healer will be able to answer or to begin the process of answering the following questions:

- How can I apply patient-centered care to advanced holistic practice?
- What are the barriers to establishing an advanced holistic nursing practice?
- How does certification enhance my advanced holistic nursing practice?
- Which entrepreneurial skills do I possess and how will these enhance my ability to establish an independent practice?
- Which business skills do I possess and which resources do I need to establish an independent advanced holistic practice?

NOTES

1. P. Aburdene, *Megatrends 2010: The Rise of Conscious Capitalism* (Charlottesville, VA: Hampton Roads, 2007).
2. American Holistic Nurses Credentialing Corporation, "Core Essentials for the Practice of Advanced Holistic Nursing AHN-BC and APHN-BC" (December 2012). www.ahncc.org/images/Final_HN_ADVANCED_ESSENTIALS,_DEC,_2012.pdf.
3. APRN Consensus Work Group and National Council of State Boards of Nursing APRN Advisory Committee, "Consensus Model for APRN Regulation: Licensure, Accreditation, Certification and Education" (July 7, 2008). www.aacn.nche.edu/education-resources/APRNReport.pdf.
4. K. A. Daley, "Person-Centered Care—What Does It Actually Mean?" *The American Nurse* 44, no. 6 (2012): 3.
5. M. Enzman Hines, "Reflective Practice: How We Know What We Know," *Beginnings* 29, no. 2 (2009): 3–5.
6. M. Driessnack, "Remember Me: Mask Making with Chronically and Terminally Ill Children," *Holistic Nursing Practice* 18, no. 4 (2004): 211–214.
7. Institute of Medicine, *The Future of Nursing: Leading Change, Advancing Health* (Washington, DC: National Academies Press, 2010).

8. United States Senate, "Patient Protection and Affordable Care Act" (January 5, 2010). https://democrats.senate.gov/pdfs/reform/patient-protection-affordable-care-act-as-passed.pdf.

9. J. Rother and R. Lavizzo-Mourey, "Addressing the Nursing Workforce: A Critical Element for Health Reform," *Health Affairs* 28, no. 4 (2009): 620–624.

10. M. Enzman Hines, "Holistic Nursing and Healthcare Reform: Challenges and Opportunities," *Beginnings* 32, no. 4 (2012): 4–7.

11. American Holistic Nurses Credentialing Corporation, "A Position Statement on the APRN Consensus Model" (March 12, 2013). http://ahncc.org/images/A_POSITION_STATEMENT,_APRN_for_NCSBN,_FINAL.pdf.

12. M. M. Libster, D. Shields, and L. Evers, "APRN-Voices: Holes in the Historical Fabric of American Nursing," *Clinical Nurse Specialist* (forthcoming).

13. L. Sessanna, "Teaching Holistic Child Health Promotion Using Watson's Theory of Human Science and Human Care," *Journal of Pediatric Nursing* 18, no. 1 (2003): 64–68.

14. National Center for Complementary and Integrative Health, "The Use of Complementary and Alternative Medicine in the United States" (December 2008). https://nccih.nih.gov/news/camstats/2007/camsurvey_fs1.htm.

15. N. C. Frisch, "Standards for Holistic Nursing Practice: A Way to Think About Our Care That Includes Complementary and Alternative Modalities," *Online Journal of Issues in Nursing* 6, no. 2 (2001): 4–9.

16. J. Hunt, "Feminism and Nursing," *The Nursing Monograph* (1998): 17–22.

17. M. Enzman Hines, D. Wind Wardell, J. Engebretson, R. Zahourek, and M. C. Smith, "Holistic Nurses' Stories of Healing Another," *Journal of Holistic Nursing* 32, no. 3 (2014): 1–19.

18. L. Sharoff, "Exploring Nurses' Perceived Benefits of Utilizing Holistic Modalities for Self and Clients," *Holistic Nursing Practice* 22, no. 1 (2008): 15–24.

19. M. C. Smith, R. Zahourek, M. Enzman Hines, J. Engebretson, and D. Wind Wardell, "Holistic Nurses' Stories of Personal Healing," *Journal of Holistic Nursing* 31, no. 3 (2013): 173–187.

20. American Holistic Nurses Association and American Nurses Association, *Holistic Nursing: Scope and Standards of Practice*, 2nd ed. (Silver Spring, MD: Nursesbooks.org, 2013): 1.

21. L. Summers, "Coming to a Consensus About APRN Regulation," *Nursing Management* 42, no. 12 (2011): 10–14.

22. American Association of Colleges of Nursing, *The Essentials of Doctoral Education for Advanced Nursing Practice* (Washington, DC: American Association of Colleges of Nursing, 2006).

23. American Association of Colleges of Nursing, "Update on the LACE Network and Implementation of the APRN Consensus Model" (October 2012). www.aacn.nche.edu/members-only/meeting-highlights/2012/LACE-APRN-Report.pdf.

24. American College of Nurse-Midwives, Accreditation Commission for Midwifery Education, and American Midwifery Certification Board, "Midwifery in the United States and the Consensus Model for APRN Regulation" (2014). www.midwife.org/ACNM/files/ccLibraryFiles/Filename/000000001458/LACE_White_Paper_2011.pdf.

25. National Association of Clinical Nurse Specialists, "Statement on the APRN Consensus Model Implementation" (January 12, 2012). www.nacns.org/docs/NACNSConsensusModel.pdf.

26. National Council of State Boards of Nursing, "APRN Consensus Model" (August 19, 2010). www.ncsbn.org/APRN_Consensus_Model_FAQs_August_19_2010.pdf.

27. W. K. Cody, "Of Life Immense in Passion, Pulse, and Power: Dialoguing with Whitman and Parse—A Hermeneutic Study," in *Illuminations: The Human Becoming Theory in Practice and Research*, R. R. Parse (Sudbury, MA: Jones and Bartlett, 1999): 269–307.

28. H. Erickson, ed., *Exploring the Interface Between the Philosophy and Discipline of Holistic Nursing: Modeling and Role-Modeling at Work* (Cedar Park, TX: Unicorns Unlimited, 2010).

29. R. R. Parse, *Nursing Science: Major Paradigms, Theories, and Critiques* (Philadelphia: Saunders, 1987).

30. H. Erickson and M. A. Swain, "A Model for Assessing Potential Adaptation to Stress," *Research in Nursing and Health* 5, no. 2 (1982): 93–101.

31. M. Hills and J. Watson, *Creating a Caring Science Curriculum: An Emancipatory Pedagogy for Nursing* (New York: Springer, 2011).

32. M. Enzman Hines, "Caring in Advance Practice Education: A New View of the Future," in *Creating a Caring Science Curriculum: An Emancipatory Pedagogy for Nursing*, M. Hills and J. Watson (New York: Springer, 2011): 203–216.

33. American Holistic Nurses Credentialing Corporation, "Endorsement Program" (n.d.). www.ahncc.org/endorsementprogram.html.

34. H. Erickson, "Holistic Nurses' Examinations: Past, Present, Future," *Journal of Holistic Nursing* 27, no. 3 (2009): 186–202.

35. B. M. Dossey, "Holistic Nursing: From Florence Nightingale's Historical Legacy to 21st-Century Global Nursing," *Alternative Therapies in Health and Medicine* 16, no. 5 (2010): 14–16.

36. The Bravewell Collaborative, *Integrative Medicine: Improving Health Care for Patients and Health Care Delivery for Providers and Payors* (Minneapolis, MN: The Bravewell Collaborative, 2010).

37. D. Van Sant-Smith, "Supporting the Integrative Health Care Curriculum in Schools of Nursing," *Holistic Nursing Practice* 28, no. 5 (2014): 312–315.

38. Committee on Health, Education, Labor, and Pensions, "Principles of Integrative Health: A Path to Healthcare Reform," *Senate Hearing 111-387* (February 23, 2009). www.gpo.gov /fdsys/pkg/CHRG-111shrg47760/html/CHRG-111shrg47760.htm.

39. M. J. Kreitzer, B. Kligler, and W. C. Meeker, "Health Professions Education and Integrative Health Care" (February 2009). www.iom.edu /˜/media/Files/Activity%20Files/Quality /IntegrativeMed/Health%20Professions%20 Education%20and%20Integrative%20Health Care.pdf.

40. National Center for Complementary and Integrative Health, "Complementary, Alternative, or Integrative Health: What's In a Name?" (July 2014). https://nccih.nih.gov/health/whatiscam.

41. World Health Organization, "Integrated Health Services: What and Why?" *Technical Brief No. 1* (May 2008). www.who.int/healthsystems/service _delivery_techbrief1.pdf.

42. Consortium of Academic Health Centers for Integrative Medicine, "CAHCIM Leadership" (2014). www.imconsortium.org/about/home .cfm.

43. J. Salerno, "Integrative Medicine: A Movement Whose Time Has Come," *The Bravewell Collaborative* (2012). www.bravewell.org /integrative_medicine/.

44. A. Weil, "Balanced Living" (2015). www.drweil .com/drw/u/ART02054/Andrew-Weil-Integrative -Medicine.html.

45. N. A. Klebanoff and D. Hess, "Holistic Nursing: Focusing on the Whole Person," *American Nurse Today* 8, no. 10 (2013): 2.

46. M. Ring, M. Brodsky, T. Low Dog, V. Sierpina, M. Bailey, A. Locke, M. Kogan, et al., "Developing and Implementing Core Competencies for Integrative Medicine Fellowships," *Academic Medicine* 89, no. 3 (2014): 421–428.

47. M. J. Verhoef, G. Lewith, C. Ritenbaugh, H. Boon, S. Fleishman, and A. Leis, "Complementary and Alternative Medicine Whole Systems Research: Beyond Identification of Inadequacies of the RCT," *Complementary Therapies in Medicine* 13, no. 3 (2005): 206–212.

48. The Bravewell Collaborative, "Declaration for a New Medicine" (2012). www.bravewell .org/integrative_medicine/declaration_for_a _new_medicine/.

49. The Bravewell Collaborative, "The Patient's Bill of Rights" (2012). www.bravewell.org /integrative_medicine/patient_rights/.

50. L. Knutson, P. J. Johnson, A. Sidebottom, and A. Fyfe-Johnson, "Development of a Hospital-Based Integrative Healthcare Program," *Journal of Nursing Administration* 43, no. 2 (2013): 101–107.

51. E. R. C. M. Huisman, E. Morales, J. van Hoof, and H. S. M. Kort, "Healing Environment: A Review of the Impact of Physical Environmental Factors on Users," *Building and Environment* 58 (2012): 70–80.

52. D. Bazuin and K. Cardon, "Creating Healing Intensive Care Unit Environments: Physical and Psychological Considerations in Designing Critical Care Areas," *Critical Care Nursing Quarterly* 34, no. 4 (2011): 259–267.

53. A. Wilson, N. Whitaker, and D. Whitford, "Rising to the Challenge of Health Care Reform with Entrepreneurial and Intrapreneurial Nursing Initiatives," *Online Journal of Issues in Nursing* 17, no. 2 (2012): 5–10.

54. P. Raine, "Promoting Breast-Feeding in a Deprived Area: The Influence of a Peer Support Initiative," *Health and Social Care in the Community* 11, no. 6 (2003): 463–469.

55. F. Robinson, "Nurse Entrepreneurs," *Practice Nurse* 36, no. 5 (2008): 11–12.

56. E. Scala, *Nursing from Within: A Fresh Alternative to Putting Out Fires and Self-Care Workarounds* (Elizabeth Scala, 2014).

57. R. Harrison, "Establish and Optimize Your Own Holistic Business" (n.d.). www.bewholebewell .com/documents/EstablishandOptimizeHolistic Business.pdf.

58. J. J. Baker and R. W. Baker, *Health Care Finance: Basic Tools for Nonfinancial Managers*, 4th ed. (Burlington, MA: Jones & Bartlett Learning, 2014).

59. K. T. Waxman and M. Barter, "Entrepreneurial Leadership: Innovation and Business Acumen," in *Financial and Business Management for the Doctor of Nursing Practice*, ed. K. T. Waxman (New York: Springer, 2013): 241–259.

60. Wound Care Society, "Reimbursement of Advanced Practice Registered Nurse Services: A Fact Sheet," *Journal of Wound, Ostomy and Continence Nursing* 39, no. 2S (2012): S7–S16.

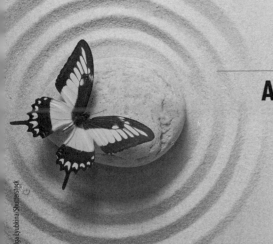

CHAPTER 37

Advancing Integrative Health and Well-Being Practice

Karen M. Avino

Nurse Healer Objectives

Theoretical

- Identify the holistic core values used in nursing practice.
- Compare and contrast the various interventions used.
- Articulate potential changes in practice that can result in a new outcome.

Clinical

- Develop your abilities to integrate new holistic nursing interventions.
- Experiment with integrating the core values of holistic nursing to create an optimal healing environment.

Personal

- Examine the significance of patient stories to your professional practice.
- Create opportunities to enhance your practice with holistic core values and interventions.

The Sharing of Professional Experiences

The sharing of experiences of patient encounters, self-care activities, various creative nursing interventions, and methods of working with patients are critical to advancing nursing practice. Working in traditional healthcare settings, nurses may not be exposed to interventions that can be approached by integrating the healing arts with technical competence. Those of us who have been fortunate enough to have been exposed to a community of holistic nurses have learned through role modeling and formal or continuing education the ways of knowing patient needs and the methods to use to reach the ultimate outcome of healing.

Some of the holistic core values used by nurses on a daily basis are obvious and some are less so. Therefore, documenting through case studies the path chosen is critical to envision the real-life context of human nature. This case study chapter relies on the gracious gifts from fellow nurses who shared the lived experience of distinctive and caring moments. Exploring how nurses' actions, interventions, or recommendations can shape an experience, and, likewise, how a patient can influence the nurse, is invaluable. It is through interpretation and refection on the case that insight into patient care can be understood at a deeper level.

The hope is that the following case studies will reflect a process of telling a story in its complexity, yet describe the unique ability of holistic nurses to create an environment for healing. We are grateful to all nurses, at all levels, who value the complex relationships of health, illness, and wellness and weave together both the scientific foundations and the art of nursing in their practice.

Case Studies

Integrative Nurse Coaching: Stress Reduction in Nursing Students Using HeartMath

Holistic nurse: Karen Avino, EdD, MSN, RN, AHN-BC, HWNC-BC

Place of employment: University of Delaware, Newark, Delaware

Specialty: Integrative nurse coach, HeartMath® Certified Trainer, Reiki Master, stress management instructor

Holistic modality specialization: HeartMath® system, energy medicine, guided imagery, meditation

Setting. A School of Nursing faculty member teaching a sophomore-level Health: Promotion and Vulnerability course. It is well known that nursing students experience stress and anxiety in nursing school and the better they can manage this, the more successful they will be in school.

As the holistic nurse teaching stress management techniques, students frequently visit my office. As a nurse coach, I work with students using various integrative techniques to help build resilience.

Session 1: 1.5 Hours

Patient. B. G. is a 20-year-old female who moved to the United States from the Philippines as a child. The session began with the patient crying while telling her story. She is the middle child in a traditional family, with one older sister and one younger sister. She is a sophomore nursing student who transferred into the nursing program this semester from the School of Education. Her parents thought nursing would be a better career, as she would be able to find employment more easily. B. G. has been seen as the "smartest" child of her family and has received a scholarship to attend the university. She will lose the scholarship if her grades do not stay above a 3.2 grade point average.

B. G. is experiencing anxiety about her grades this semester, as she has never received anything other than an A. She states that her grades are in the B to C range following midterm exams. She is crying as she verbalizes her grades and states that she is not sure she has made the right decision to transfer into the nursing program. She has also verbalized that her parents recently moved to another state and she no longer has any family close by. She is unsure if she should transfer to a school in the state where they now live, or if she made the right decision for nursing as a career. She does not want to talk with her parents or older sister about the situation so as not to worry her family members. When asked what she needs help with, she says she cannot focus on studying and feels overwhelmed.

B. G. denies any medication or drug or alcohol use. She presently does not use any methods to relax or reduce anxiety. She states that she cries frequently and for long periods of time (about 30 minutes), after which she is unable to focus on her schoolwork.

Holistic interventions. Because B. G. has already attended classroom sessions on stress and coping and learned interventions such as guided imagery and breathing techniques, HeartMath® techniques were introduced to provide immediate feedback on the level of heart coherence—a mind–body state directly associated with improved health and cognitive functioning that allows for a sense of inner balance and happiness.[3] When B. G. is in a state of balance she is more able to tap into her natural intuitive guidance to solve her own problems. The Depletion to Renewal Plan® was explained and completed. She placed herself in the upper-left quadrant of feeling anxious and overwhelmed. Her goal is to be able to feel more love and appreciation.

Heart Rate Variability Assessment

With the emWave® Pro set at challenge level one, the ear sensor is applied. No feedback noted. Resting for 2 minutes and 30 seconds her heart rate variability (HRV) was about 30 beats per minute (BPM) and her heart rate (HR) was 85 BPM. Coherence ratio: 70% low, 13% medium, and 17% high. B. G. was still tearful, and I felt she was already in stress recall. I decided to conduct the full baseline assessment at the next visit.

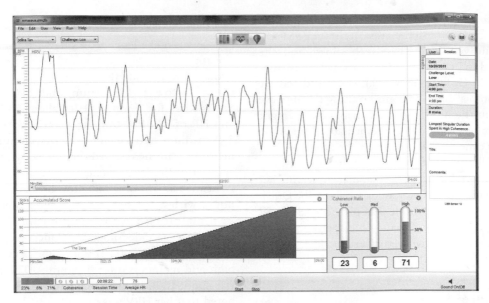

The Quick Coherence® technique is ideal for college students to help reduce anxiety. I addressed her stress in the moment and taught the Neutral and Quick Coherence® technique to begin the focus on her breath. The breathing worked very well. The Quick Coherence® technique revealed a change in rhythm. I observed a steady climb of the accumulated score for 5.5 minutes upon adding the positive attitude feeling. Breathing coherence ratios reached 23% low, 6% medium, and 71% high. The HRV was normal for her age, about 30 BMP. B. G. was excited to see her high coherence rate score and realized that this would help her to be able to focus on her studies and improve her information retention and recall.

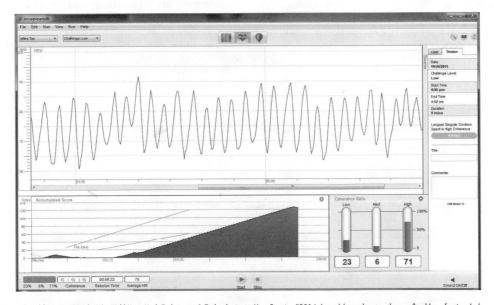

Plan. B. G. was instructed in the use of the emWave® Personal Stress Reliever (PSR), a mobile version of this technology, and she agreed to practice two times per day for 10 minutes. B. G. felt this was all she could achieve within her day. She plans on using the emWave PSR in the morning upon arising and at night before bed. She was concerned about finding a quiet time to practice this as she does not want her fellow students to question her about it. She is comfortable with her roommate observing her using the PSR. A handout describing the Quick Coherence® technique was provided. She will focus on the one-day-at-a-time approach to her schoolwork. She will return in 1 week.

Session 2: 1 Hour

B. G. reports that she is feeling better. She used the emWave PSR daily and two times daily on most days. She did not keep a log. She reports that she likes being able to control her emotions and finds the green light "her reward for being positive." She states that she has decided to stay in the nursing program and not move to another state to be with her family. She did not talk to her parents about her dilemma and is okay with her decision. She wants to continue learning some techniques to help her improve her grades and her ability to focus on tasks.

Heart Rate Variability Assessment

emWave Pro challenge level one with ear sensor applied. No feedback noted. Resting HRV about 23 BPM and HR of 70 BPM. Coherence ratio: 0% low, 85% medium, and 14% high. Stress recall for 1 minute: HRV about 23 BPM and HR of 78 BPM. Coherence ratio: 65% low, 34% medium, and 2% high. The first minute of neutral breathing revealed the following coherence ratio: 39% low, 53% medium, and 8% high; BPM with an HR of 65. Shallow breathing was noted with a few occasional deeper breaths. At 4 minutes a positive emotion was introduced in the guided imagery. Coherence ratio improved to 26% low, 22% medium, and 52% high and maintained for 4 minutes. The HRV was about 15 BMP, and HR was 65 BMP. It was noted that her HRV was much lower than during the first session.

I was curious what positive emotion she chose, as I would have liked to see a better response. She envisioned going to be with her family for Thanksgiving, but it also made her upset that she would have to leave. We discussed what other vision or place gave her a sense of calm. She described a dream she frequently has with a woman dressed in white taking her through a beautiful forest and revealing new things to her from behind a white sheet. She stated that she imagined things visually

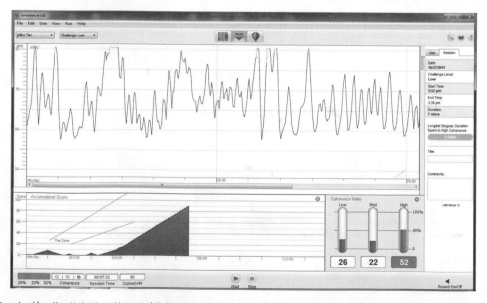

Source: Reproduced from HeartMath LLC. "Add HeartMath Techniques & Technologies to Your Practice." 2014, http://www.heartmath.com/health-professionals/

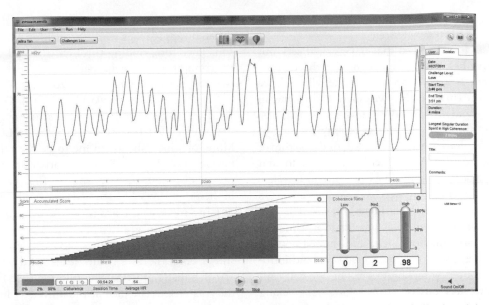

Source: Reproduced from HeartMath LLC. "Add HeartMath Techniques & Technologies to Your Practice."2014, http://www.heartmath.com/health-professionals/

and not in words or other symbols. We talked about finding a visual symbol that had meaning to her as a focal point or reminder throughout the day to practice the breathing. Once we changed her positive emotion, there was marked improvement in the coherence ratio: 0% low, 2% medium, and 98% high; HR 64 BPM, HRV 30 BPM. She was "amazed at the difference" and also described physically feeling different.

The sixth breath assessment taken earlier in the visit for 1 minute revealed a coherence ratio of 0% low, 0% medium, and 100% high; HR 71 BPM and HRV 22 BPM.

I then introduced the Garden Game, but it was the Child's Heart Visualizer games that are within the emWave Pro technology[3] that helped her to maintain and visually see the "zone." She said it was "powerful to be able to push out the positive emotion to the world." The energy

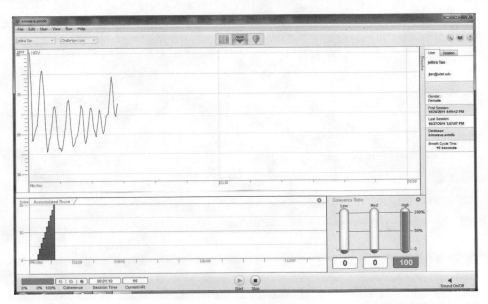

Source: Reproduced from HeartMath LLC. "Add HeartMath Techniques & Technologies to Your Practice."2014, http://www.heartmath.com/health-professionals/

shown changes color from red, blue, and green based on heart coherence.

Plan. It was agreed that B. G. would seek out tutoring help for the courses needed through the Student Nurse Organization. She will practice using the emWave PSR twice daily so that she can understand and visually see when she is in the "zone" and using the correct positive emotion to bring her into coherence. She will find a picture or symbol of calm that will become a focal point and remind her to practice. She will return in 1 week.

Evaluation. There were some valuable lessons learned for both the student and me. The student demonstrated great potential for using the HeartMath® methodologies and showed positive outcomes. I will continue to see B. G. and introduce some new techniques to her. We will continue to work on visualizing taking tests, talking with her parents about concerns, and taking a positive approach to studying without feeling overwhelmed. B. G. is eager to continue the sessions.

Reflections. My use of HeartMath® techniques and the technology have grown with personal practice as well as with clients. I have found that different approaches work for each unique person. Therefore, finding through trial and error the connection that helps patients to understand how to get in and maintain the "zone" is key.

Within 6 months of working with B. G., she went on to develop a registered student organization called CALM: Caring About Living More, of which she asked me to be the faculty adviser. For 2 years, B. G. led other students campus-wide on their journey to find balance in their daily lives. She studied, led, and brought outside meditation programs to campus for students. Upon graduation, she received the Holistic Nursing Award given to a student who shows potential as a future leader and visionary of holistic practice. She told me that I was the reason she remained at the university in the nursing program, and I told her that she was the reason I continue to teach. She has since passed the National Council Licensure Examination and is working and considering a graduate degree in mental health nursing where she

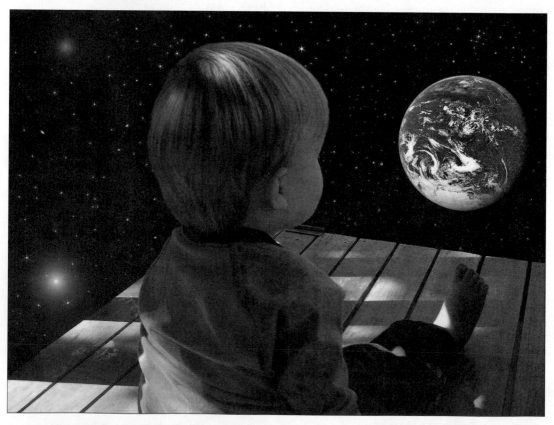

Source: © Jeff Davies/Cubby House/Shutterstock

can incorporate integrative therapies. I cannot wait to see what she does next.

NOTES

1. P. Ratanasiripong, N. Ratanasiripong, and D. Kathalae, "Biofeedback Intervention for Stress and Anxiety Among Nursing Students: A Randomized Controlled Trial," *ISRN Nursing* 2012 (2012): doi:10.5402/2012/827972.

2. P. Ratanasiripong, K. Sverduk, J. Prince, and D. Hayashino, "Biofeedback and Counseling for Stress and Anxiety Among College Students," *Journal of College Student Development* 53, no. 5 (2012): 742–749.

3. HeartMath, "Add HeartMath Techniques and Technologies to Your Practice" (2014). www .heartmath.com/health-professionals/.

Mental Health Nursing: Holistic Interventions in Cancer Care

Holistic nurse: Marjorie S. Anderson, MS, RN, PMHCNS-BC, QTTT

Place of employment: Private practice consultant, Ohio Heart of Healing, Inc., Columbus, Ohio

Nursing specialty: Mental health, holistic nursing

Holistic modality specialization: Therapeutic touch, reflexology

Setting. A tertiary care setting in a large teaching hospital with continuous care following discharge and during outpatient care. This was a case involving a patient whose worldview was very pragmatic and conventional until receiving a diagnosis of cancer. Then her worldview shifted gradually to one that was more holistic and healing rather than focused on surviving. This case is interesting due to the transformative experience of the patient and her family over time. The most challenging aspect of this case was managing the side effects of the treatment regimen. Her anticipated life span was about 6 months postdiagnosis. Yet with all of the holistic modalities assisting her with the side effects of treatment and her will to live, she was able to exceed those expectations and lived almost 2 years longer.

Patient. Jenny was a woman in her mid-50s experiencing abdominal cancer stage 4 at diagnosis. Prior to diagnosis, she was very active physically, contributing greatly in her family and workplace as well as in the community. She had one son, finishing his junior year in high school. Her primary wish was "to live long enough to see him graduate from high school."[1] She also stated, "I want everything I can get to make me better: surgery, chemo, radiation, and all that your [mental health] team can offer as well." Her surgery occurred immediately following diagnosis. Postoperatively, her primary concern was, "I don't want to lose my ability to think clearly. Will you check on me often and let me know if I start to do that?" Chemotherapy began a few weeks after surgery. She was hospitalized multiple times due to nausea, vomiting, and dehydration, along with decreased white blood cell counts. In a conventional setting, she presented with multiple nursing diagnoses. From a holistic perspective, the primary diagnoses included imbalanced nutrition: less than body requirements, with diarrhea and nausea; disturbed energy field, with fatigue and impaired comfort; disturbed personal identity, risk for impaired parenting; and death anxiety, readiness for enhanced spiritual well-being.

Holistic interventions. Our team implemented multiple holistic interventions over the almost 2-year treatment period. Each intervention was selected based on the specific needs of the patient at the time. Interventions included therapeutic touch, a holistic, evidence-based therapy that incorporates the intentional and compassionate use of universal energy to promote balance and well-being;[2] reflexology, the use of alternating pressure applied to the reflexes within the reflex maps of the body located on the feet, hands, or ears;[3] bibliotherapy, the use of reading materials for help in solving personal problems; counseling and psychotherapy, primarily brief cognitive therapy; and music therapy, an expressive art form designed to help the individual move into harmony and balance. However, these were just the pegs on which to hang the healing relationship experienced by Jenny, her family, and her healthcare team.

Reflections. As I reflect on the outcomes of these encounters with Jenny, our team learned as much from Jenny as she learned from us. She taught us the importance of each team member identifying one's self and role in her care each day and acknowledging her by name. She taught us the importance of presence and physical contact. She stated, "When you come in and touch my arm, I already start to relax and feel safe." The healing relationship was a dual relationship. There was reciprocity in our caring for one another. I was deeply moved by her will to live, her continued efforts with chemotherapy, and her decision to move into home hospice. She reached out to family and friends who loved her just as her caregivers reached out to her. Our team continues to use these authentic and compassionate approaches with our patients each day.

As Jenny reflected on her care, she stated that therapeutic touch was useful for relaxation prior to chemotherapy, so she received this at the start of each chemotherapy treatment. Yet receiving reflexology on her feet during chemotherapy was most effective in decreasing her nausea, vomiting, and diarrhea after chemotherapy. Our team provided foot reflexology each chemotherapy session to prevent the side effects and reduce the potential for dehydration. In the early phase of her treatment, she requested information about Ayurveda medicine, and she was given a book to read to learn more on the topic. Jenny's life, struggles, and optimism through her illness and final transition illustrated the transformative nature of healing relationships.

During each visit, Jenny received a cognitive assessment and we assured her, "You are still thinking clearly." With the counseling sessions, which occurred along with the integrative modalities, we explored ways to include her son as well as her husband in decision-making processes. Initially, Jenny was hesitant to include her son as she did not want "to ruin his senior year." Yet she found that as she included him, the whole family experienced healing. For example, her husband and son were able to talk about their hopes and fears with her and make decisions about hospice care together. Her faith tradition was very important to Jenny, so she was encouraged to incorporate music, especially "Amazing Grace," while at home alone to boost her spirits. She reported singing this song "almost every day and it really helps." Various team members saw her once each week during her outpatient chemotherapy regimen and daily while hospitalized. The team met periodically to discuss treatment approaches and Jenny's progress. As her physical health deteriorated over time, we offered Jenny the Hand-Heart Connection as a way of offering hope and compassionate comfort during her transitional period.[1] Her death was peaceful, and family and close friends surrounded her.

NOTES

1. C. Fanslow-Brunjes, *Using the Power of Hope to Cope with Dying: The Four Stages of Hope* (Fresno, CA: Quill Driver Books, 2008).

2. D. Krieger, *Therapeutic Touch as Transpersonal Healing* (New York: Lantern Books, 2002).

3. B. Kunz and K. Kunz, *Reflexology: Health at Your Fingertips* (New York: DK, 2003).

Medical-Surgical Nursing: Holistic Care of the Dying

Holistic nurse: Abby Robin, MSN, RN, Holistic CNS

Place of employment: Westchester Medical Center, Valhalla, New York

Nursing specialty: Medical intensive care unit

Holistic modality specialization: Reiki, therapeutic touch, meditation and imagery, chair yoga

Setting. Jane was admitted to the medical intensive care unit of a large trauma center after she had undergone a pericardial window and what was hoped to be a lifesaving surgery to remove the malignant mass over her sternum. However, the mass was more extensive than previously believed and both the cardiothoracic surgeons and her oncologist felt that the only humane way to continue caring for Jane would be to allow her a dignified death.

Patient. Jane was in her 60s and had a history of breast cancer with a malignancy to her sternum. It was the day before I cared for her that she had undergone the surgery. Postoperatively, she remained intubated and comfortably sedated. She was unable to follow commands but otherwise had no neurologic deficits. Her blood pressure was being maintained on two vasopressors, her left breast was hardened with an orange peel appearance on the left lateral side, and a chest tube remained to her left posterior lung.

Early in the day, Jane's cousin was present at her bedside, at which point the oncologist spoke to her for a prolonged period. While I usually attend meetings of this kind, I was unable to due to the care of my other critically ill patient. After completing care for my other patient, I spoke with the oncologist and was notified of the family's decision to withdraw care. Withdrawal of life-sustaining care is common within my unit; however, this was a challenge because her cousin was no longer present. This would be the first time one of my patients would die without a loved one being physically present.

After I started Jane on a morphine drip and removed her ventilator and vasopressors, she appeared anxious. She became tachypnic, tachycardic, appeared fearful, and was unable to make her needs known. Even though elevated and/or irregular heart rate and respirator rates are common in dying patients, it was her appearance that was upsetting to me. Along with the medical team, I attempted to alleviate her pain and anxiety with morphine and Ativan. Because she persisted without any significant changes, I decided to use this opportunity to share my Reiki practice with her.

Holistic interventions. I created a healing environment by playing soft music and dimming the lights. I also positioned her in the bed for optimal comfort. As I practiced Reiki with Jane, by placing one hand on her forehead and the other on her chest, I repeated my intention for peace, comfort, and the healing life force to travel where it was most needed.[1] Almost immediately after making my connection with her, I felt the heat of her energy. I remained for 2 to 3 minutes at a time as my other patient required my presence as well.

After some time, Jane's breathing and heart rate slowed as her face softened. The heat from her head and chest eased. As her body accepted the healing life force, she surrendered to death. Being present and able to share Reiki with Jane during one of her most vulnerable times brought me a sense of peace. Together, in mutual process, I was able to assist Jane as she passed.

Reflections. Sometimes I think the word *caring* is specific to nurses and nurse healers. Caring requires choice, patience, respect, positive caring intentions, sensitivity to the patient and family, and gaining trust. Caring is both an art and a science.[2] It is no coincidence that nurses say that they "cared for" or took "care of" a patient. As I cared for Jane, she also cared for me.

NOTES

1. C. Jackson and C. Latini, "Touch and Hand-Mediated Therapies," in *Holistic Nursing: A Handbook for Practice*, 6th ed., eds. B. M. Dossey and L. Keegan (Burlington, MA: Jones & Bartlett Learning, 2013): 417–438.
2. Watson Caring Science Institute, "Caring Science Defined" (2013). http://watsoncaring science.org/about-us/caring-science-definitions -processes-theory/.

Pediatric Nursing: Holistic Interventions with New Parents

Holistic nurse: Jennifer Gaughan, MS, APRN, CPNP

Place of employment: Rocky Mountain Pediatrics, Lakewood, Colorado

Nursing specialty: Certified pediatric nurse practitioner

Holistic modality specialization: Caritas coach certification, Reiki Master

Setting. Working in a hectic pediatric primary care office presents challenges in creating caring, holistic connections with patients and families in short, definitive appointment slots. It is common in allopathic medicine to follow a standardized approach to achieve healthcare goals set forth by the leading medical professional organizations. The same medical goals can be achieved while creating caring, healing relationships between patients, families, and practitioners by integrating wisdom traditions, complementary approaches, and trust and hope. The following is an exemplar of a holistic healing approach to advanced holistic care.

Patient. Three-day-old Lilly presents with her parents Jane and David for her first well-baby visit. Lilly is jaundiced. Jane is nervous, as she was instructed to follow up no later than 24 hours after being discharged from the hospital to ensure Lilly's bilirubin level was not too high. Ten minutes late for the appointment, Lilly was whisked through the vital signs, the parents were asked to quickly undress Lilly for a naked weight, and they were placed in a room to wait for the nurse practitioner. Feeling a bit rushed, I noted that the birth records had not arrived yet, and I had 10 minutes left to ensure that Lilly was "doing well." I stopped at the door, pausing to center myself, take a deep breath, and enter quietly with a smile. Gently extending a hand to Jane and David, I wished them congratulations on their beautiful new baby girl. Both parents were obviously stressed, tired, and anxious about the first visit. The bilirubin level upon leaving the hospital was elevated, and Lilly had lost a few ounces of weight. Jane stated that Lilly was latching on well to the breast but that "her milk hadn't come in yet." She had two lactation consultation sessions in the hospital that gave conflicting advice that left her feeling uncertain, and, as a result, with breastfeeding difficulties. One lactation consultant recommended a breast shield for inverted nipples. Even after using the breast shield, Lilly was still having trouble latching on. Physicians at the hospital had urged Jane to feed Lilly formula if her milk had not come in after 48 hours. "That way Lilly doesn't need to stay in the hospital under those lights," Jane explained.

I relaxed my posture and said, "I'd like to start today by explaining my role and allowing some time for you to ask any questions about Lilly. Let's talk about what is going well and what is hard for you right now." Jane and David looked at one another and said, "Well, how is she doing? We just want to know if she is eating enough. Are her bilirubin levels okay?" It was obvious that the pressure and focus on negative possibilities for Lilly's first few days of life were of concern. Jane and David were not settling in as new parents easily. They had experienced less than a full day at home before having to bring her "to a germ-infested place" to find out if Lilly was doing well or needed phototherapy.

As a holistic nurse, it is important to deeply listen to the situation to provide care that views the person and family in their wholeness.

I wanted to share with this family that everything would be okay, explore their backgrounds, and establish trust and rapport. In addition, I wanted to identify their goals and dreams for Lilly. It is easy to overlook these viewpoints in a typical medical model focused on time, productivity, and profit. I asked questions about Jane's hopes for breastfeeding to determine the level of commitment. How did she feel about formula feeding? Was she worried about Lilly? I was also concerned about her stress level and if Jane had any history of depression. Other unanswered questions included: Does Jane have to return to work soon? Does David want to help with feedings? What can I do to support their specific parenting style? Is Jane eating well and drinking enough? Are both Lilly and Jane getting adequate sleep? Does David have any time to bond with Lilly? and How does he want to help? These questions are more inclusive of a holistic approach rather than an interviewing style to establish a relationship. In contrast, the questions in the electronic health record guide the visit in a different direction: How many ounces of formula is the infant taking? How many hours apart? How many wet diapers? Does the infant lift her head? Did the baby get hepatitis B vaccine in the hospital? and Did she pass the hearing screen?

Jane explained that she did not want to use formula; she really wanted to breastfeed for the benefits of bonding and allergy and infectious disease prevention. During the visit, Lilly was agitated, fussing, and hungry. Jane kept trying to bounce, rock, shush, and swaddle Lilly, although she was aware that Lilly wanted to eat. I shared with Jane, "Feel free to feed her while we finish up the visit." Jane hesitated, "It takes a really long time. Are you sure?" I responded, "Absolutely, take your time. In fact, if you breastfeed her while I take blood for the bilirubin level, it will help provide some pain relief and comfort."[1] Encouraging Jane that her innate bond with Lilly would be enhanced by breastfeeding was important. Jane seemed proud that she could provide some comfort. David acted surprised because they had brought a bottle of formula "just in case" they needed to feed Lilly in the waiting room. Jane said she felt awkward breastfeeding in front of people. I explained that this is a common feeling in new mothers and if she focused on the fact that breastfeeding is natural and healthy it might help. I explained the benefits of breastfeeding as preventing ear infections, improving bonding, and balancing hormones and immunity. "In fact, breast milk is the best nutrition for Lilly." It took Lilly a few minutes to get a good latch. Then Jane relaxed back into her chair. We talked about stress reduction, and, while pumping, to focus on the love and gratitude for Lilly. I also suggested that Jane could try having David help hold Lilly while she nursed so he could participate. In answering Jane's questions about breast milk production, we discussed the benefits of using mother's milk tea, fenugreek seed, or goat's rue tincture to increase breast milk.[2] Time for questions was allowed while Lilly nursed and being gentle and present with the family. The visit flowed and was productive by following the cues of the parents, although not in a particular order supported by the electronic health record. Through focusing on creating a welcoming, healing environment, the beginnings of a co-created, helping, trusting relationship with the family began. I gave Jane and David praise for being committed to breastfeeding and the instinctual ability to provide for their baby. I suggested waiting before beginning to offer formula to treat the bilirubin level. I recommended that they "get some sunshine with Lilly. Expose Lilly's whole backside to the sun while you position her on Jane's bare chest. The oxytocin and endorphins from the sunny snuggle can help you produce more breast milk too." The parents were encouraged to call with any questions or if they felt concerned about not providing formula as others may suggest.

Questions about spiritual practices, socioeconomic status, and family support were assessed. Instead of trying to achieve an agenda of clicking boxes in the electronic health record and getting through the sea of anticipatory guidance, following the parents' cues allowed for a gentle exam. Positive thinking, rest, rehabilitation, bonding, and nesting are the goals until the next visit the following week.

Holistic interventions. The typical allopathic model for the newborn visit is to ensure that weight loss is not excessive, validate physical health and safety, promote infectious disease prevention, manage newborn hyperbilirubinemia, evaluate feeding practices, and assess whether the infant is stooling and urinating normally. A holistic approach allows for a richer view of the infant's environment and provides the opportunity to engage in open-ended dialogue between parents and practitioner. Encouraging breastfeeding during a painful procedure or lab draw for pain relief highlights how integrating healing practices into everyday primary care occurs. Holistic interventions exemplified in this reflective story include motivational support and strategies by asking questions focused on wellness and prevention to assess the cultural, psychosocial, and mind–body realms. Recommending complementary approaches for improving breast milk production, addressing stress, and educating about available herbal preparations reveal how healing modalities are linked as holistic and integrative approaches in primary practice.

Reflections. Regular follow up with consistent providers is helpful to establish continued caring relationships between patients, families, and practitioners. Scheduling follow-up visits according to established guidelines is recommended; however, holistic approaches allow for identifying and managing the most pressing issues in a caring way while focusing on education, motivation, prevention, and wholeness. The follow-up visit at 2 weeks of age revealed that Jane was successful and exclusively breastfeeding Lilly with David's support. Lilly's bilirubin level was normal, and Jane was becoming comfortable with Lilly's patterns for care. This holistic partnership supported the family to develop strong bonds.

NOTES

1. L. Gray, L. W. Miller, B. L. Phillip, and E. M. Blass, "Breastfeeding Is Analgesic in Healthy Newborns," *Pediatrics* 109, no. 4 (2002): 590–593.

2. C. Turkyılmaz, E. Onal, I. M. Hirfanoglu, O. Turan, E. Koç, E. Ergenekon, and Y. Atalay, "The Effect of Galactagogue Herbal Tea on Breast Milk Production and Short-Term Catch-Up of Birth Weight in the First Week of Life," *Journal of Alternative and Complementary Medicine* 17, no. 2 (2011): 139–142.

Midwifery Nursing: Lifestyle Coaching in Gynecological Care

Holistic nurse: Kathleen D. McCarthy, CNM, MSN, RScP

Place of employment: The Birth Center: Holistic Women's Health Care, LLC, Wilmington, Delaware

Nursing specialty: Nurse midwife

Holistic modality specialization: Holistic coaching, nutritional guidance, meditation

Setting. A freestanding birth center that provides full-scope nurse midwifery services. This case involves a patient who is a mother of two teen boys. She is recently divorced and works as a nonprofit attorney. When she presented for care she was anxious and teary eyed. She felt like her life was swirling out of control. She was busy focusing on the day-to-day aspects of her life with little time for enjoyment or reflection. She felt stuck. She was able to move forward with some coaching.

Patient. Katie is a woman in her late 40s who presented for her annual exam with complaints of insomnia, hot flashes, anxiety attacks, and weight gain. Katie was "on the run" most days of the week and gave little attention to health and well-being behaviors. In order to assess which areas of Katie's life needed attention or redirection, the Circle of Life worksheet was completed.[1] Katie chose three areas on which to focus: spirituality, physical activity, and home cooking. Katie also described experiencing periods of insomnia.

Holistic interventions. For the insomnia, Katie was emailed the handout "Want a Good Night's Sleep? Then Never Do These Things Before Bed."[2] She was encouraged to download and listen each night to "Super Sleep," a Hemi-Sync audio product.[3] Hemi-Sync uses audio-guidance technology to blend and sequence the brain to various states ranging from deep relaxation or sleep to expanded states of awareness.

I reinforced that many of Katie's symptoms will decrease or dissipate with diet and lifestyle changes. For home cooking, Katie agreed to have at least three healthy meals per week and, for her "on-the-go days," healthy snacks. We reviewed healthy meal and snack choices.

For exercise, Katie agreed to walk three times per week and resume yoga once a week. For spirituality, Katie chose a simple breath work technique (inhale for 4 seconds, hold, and then exhale for 4 seconds), 10 minutes per day, 3 times weekly. We planned a follow-up visit in 4 weeks.

Reflections. At the next visit, Katie reported that she was in a much better place. She was sleeping well, felt much less anxious, and was experiencing fewer hot flashes. The biggest revelation to Katie was that she no longer felt stuck. She expressed that she "felt liberated by that thought." It was very helpful to Katie to identify the areas in her life where she was blossoming and the areas that needed her attention. She recognized that she had the power to move forward.

Katie, by nature, was an overachiever; therefore, she had started meditating for 20 minutes most days of the week, had returned to walking and yoga, and had managed to cook healthy meals three to four times weekly.

Katie was excited and glowing. Her energy was bountiful. I have found that Katie and many other women in my practice feel stuck in a "life" rut. Once they are able to see a way out they become liberated and empowered.

NOTES

1. J. Rosenthal, *Integrative Nutrition: Feed Your Hunger for Health and Happiness* (New York: Integrative Nutrition, 2008): 165.
2. J. Mercola, "Want a Good Night's Sleep? Then Never Do These Things Before Bed" (October 2, 2010). http://articles.mercola.com/sites/articles/archive/2010/10/02/secrets-to-a-good-night-sleep.aspx.
3. Monroe Products, "How Hemi-Sync Works" (2014). www.hemi-sync.com/hemi-sync-technology/how-hemi-sync-works/.

Holistic Family Nurse Practitioner: Use of Supplements in Primary Care

Holistic nurse: Mary Helming, PhD, APRN, FNP-BC, AHN-BC

Place of employment: Quinnipiac University School of Nursing, Hamden, Connecticut

Nursing specialty: Family nurse practitioner

Holistic modality specialization: Spirituality in health, integrative health care

Setting. This patient case represents a typical patient in an internal medicine practice caring for patients from adolescence to geriatrics. The setting is in a rural community in Connecticut. Clinicians in this practice are open to the use of integrative health. Therefore, many of the patients come to this practice because they favor integrative modalities as well.

Patient. Mrs. K is a 52-year-old woman who is new to this practice. She heard through friends that the physician and nurse practitioners in this office are willing to treat patients using complementary and alternative modalities. Because her past physician did not believe in integrative medicine, she decided to change practices. Her first appointment is for a complete physical exam. Per the usual practice, she had routine lab work drawn 2 weeks before the appointment with a holistic nurse practitioner.

Holistic interventions. Mrs. K has avoided routine care for the past 3 years because her brother died as a result of a medical error. She then began to distrust the traditional medical establishment. Centering myself, I began her history and physical examination review with intentionality for her best outcome.

Medical History

- *Past medical history* is significant for a subtotal hysterectomy at age 40 for uterine fibroids, and she has never been placed on hormone therapy. Her history is also positive for Lyme disease twice, with doxycycline treatment both times.
- *Family history* is positive for early heart disease; her father died of a myocardial infarction (MI) at age 52 and her paternal uncle has survived two MIs. There is also a family history of breast cancer in her maternal grandmother and her maternal aunt.
- *Social history.* She is a past cigarette smoker for 10 years, one pack per day. She smoked from age 16 to 26. Alcohol intake is one glass of wine per week average when out to dinner. Married to second husband for 19 years and has two children ages 21 and 26, both out of the house.
- *Patient medications.* Over-50 women's daily multivitamin, calcium and vitamin D, and Protonix 40 mg/day for chronic dyspepsia.
- *Allergies.* None known.

Review of Systems

- *Skin.* She complains of increasingly dry skin. Denies rashes, changes in nevi.
- *Head, eyes, ears, nose, and throat.* She complains of occipital headaches occurring about once per week, band-like, without associated gastrointestinal symptoms, dizziness, or etiology. Relieved with ibuprofen 400 mg normally. Headaches have worsened since patient took on a new job in an insurance company. Wears glasses for reading. Last eye exam was 4 years ago.
- *Chest.* No complaints of dyspnea, wheeze, or cough.
- *Cardiac.* No chest pain, palpitations, or history of murmur.
- *Abdomen.* She still gets occasional heartburn with certain foods, such as pizza and orange juice, especially if she eats them later at night. Denies nausea, diarrhea, and melena. Admits to periodic constipation for which she takes no treatment except increasing her fiber foods. No rectal pain.
- *Breast.* She denies breast pain, mass, or nipple discharge. Decided against getting mammograms over the past 5 years because she is worried about radiation exposure.
- *Genitourinary.* She sees a gynecologist on average every 3 to 4 years. Because she had a subtotal hysterectomy, she feels that she does not need routine examinations anymore. She complains of increasing urinary incontinence when she sneezes or coughs. Denies polyuria and dysuria.
- *Musculoskeletal.* She complains of intermittent low back pain when she "overdoes" work. Denies sciatica or leg paresthesias. Improves with rest. She does not take any medications for this because she is afraid of upsetting her gastrointestinal tract with anti-inflammatories.

- *Neurologic.* Denies numbness, weakness, or paresthesias.
- *Endocrine.* No polydipsia or polyuria but does have polyphagia. Also complains of periodic night sweats and some mood lability.

Physical Exam

- *Vital signs.* Blood pressure, left arm, sitting 162/88; blood pressure, right arm, sitting 156/86; pulse: 84, regular; respirations: 16; temperature: 97.6; height: 5′6″; weight: 202 pounds; body mass index 30 to 34.9 range, obesity level 1; skin: dryness apparent on forearms and distal extremities with mild scaling, no lesions.
- *Head, eyes, ears, nose, and throat.* Pupils equal, round, and react to light and accommodation; optic discs normal; sclerae clear; tympanic membranes gray, no erythema; oropharynx: no lesions, dentition fair, some fillings apparent; no significant adenopathy; thyroid: no goiter palpated and no masses palpable.
- *Chest.* Clear to auscultation and percussion.
- *Cardiac.* S1S2 normal, S4 audible. Grade II/VI systolic ejection murmur heard left sternal border, supine and seated the same. Carotids: no bruits.
- *Abdomen.* Soft positive bowel sounds, no hepatosplenomegaly but mild tenderness over epigastric area, without rebound or referred pain.
- *Breast.* No masses palpable, right breast larger than left, slight nipple deviation right breast to right side, no nipple discharge.
- *Musculoskeletal.* Mild pain bilateral lumbosacral paravertebral muscles. Negative straight leg raise, seated, and supine. No scoliosis but marginal kyphosis apparent. No joint deformities. Muscle strength 5+/5+.
- *Neurologic.* Alert and oriented to person, place, and time; distal tendon reflexes 2+/2+ throughout, normal plantar reflex. Cranial nerves II–XII within normal limits.
- *Gynecological/rectal.* Deferred to gynecologist.

Laboratory Results

- Complete blood count within normal limits.
- Comprehensive metabolic panel: normal except blood glucose slightly elevated at 113 mg/dl fasting.
- Lipid profile: total cholesterol elevated at 238 mg/dl; HDL cholesterol low at 45 mg/dl, LDL cholesterol elevated at 137 mg/dl; triglycerides elevated at 172 mg/dl.
- Thyroid functions: thyroid-stimulating hormone slightly elevated at 4.2mIU/L; no other tests done.
- Urinalysis: trace proteinuria.

Assessment

1. Mild hypertension likely
2. Hyperlipidemia
3. Elevated blood glucose
4. Chronic dyspepsia
5. Constipation: periodic, with dry skin and elevated thyroid-stimulating hormone: possible new hypothyroidism
6. Systolic murmur, unknown whether new or old
7. Positive family history of early coronary artery disease
8. Positive family history of breast cancer
9. Potential for stress/tension headaches at work
10. Health maintenance issues

Holistic approach. Speaking with Mrs. K, she was very surprised and upset to learn about her laboratory abnormalities. The last time she had lab work at least 4 years ago, she did not know of any abnormalities, and her old record is unavailable. Using skills to create a therapeutic relationship, I assessed Mrs. K's understanding of her risk factors and her knowledge about her potential problems. She has no medical background, so she needs health education to be given in a nonthreatening and calm approach. As a nurse practitioner, I provided a healing environment for Mrs. K by allowing her to verbalize her upset feelings and her sense of shock at the noted abnormalities. I gave her adequate space and time, without rushing, to take in the news.

Mrs. K was very averse to using pharmaceutical medications to treat any potential disorders, especially because of her brother's death due to a medical error that involved an adverse reaction to a pharmaceutical drug. She was adamant that she wanted to use "all natural" treatments for any problems that were identified. We began a discussion of how she could *begin* to address these newly identified health problems in some natural ways.

Sensitive to her need to control this situation with making decisions for her own health, I worked with Mrs. K to come to a good solution. Here is the plan we devised together to allow the patient to be involved in her holistic care.

Holistic plan. Some items are not discussed until the 6-week revisit due to not wanting to overload Mrs. K with information and make her fearful or anxious.

1. Begin a regimen of red yeast rice, standardized dose, 300-mg capsules, two per day for 8 weeks to decrease her cholesterol.[1] If successful, the cycle may be repeated twice more for 8 weeks at a time. Because her liver function tests are now normal, she can begin this treatment. However, she must return for repeat liver function tests in 6 weeks because red yeast rice is actually the same as a statin drug (e.g., atorvastatin or pravastatin) and it can raise liver function tests and myalgias just as a statin drug can.

2. Begin taking fish oil 2000 mg/day to decrease triglycerides.[2] It is also useful for cardiac health, especially with her family history of early heart disease.

3. Begin taking coenzyme Q10 100 mg/day to avoid mitochondrial energy depletion with statin (red yeast rice) and also for general heart health.

4. Go to a holistic nutritionist to help deal with hypertension, hyperlipidemia, and elevated blood sugar from a nutritional standpoint. Needs to work on decreasing her sodium intake, monitoring her caffeine intake, and watching her carbohydrate intake. Start with a diet diary to bring to the nutritionist. Also needs weight reduction plan done in a holistic manner, with slow, gradual weight loss.

5. Plan hemoglobin A1C test with next lab testing in 6 weeks to see if Mrs. K actually is diabetic or may have metabolic syndrome (elevated blood pressure [BP], elevated blood glucose 100 to 125 mg/dl, obesity, and elevated triglycerides may suggest metabolic syndrome, or prediabetes). Test ALT and AST, retest fasting blood glucose, and add free T4 thyroid test to determine if Mrs. K may truly have hypothyroidism.

6. Recheck BP twice per week at her local pharmacy, which has an electronic BP monitor, or purchase her own BP equipment. Measure BP at different times of day to see if it elevates just with stress. Call every week with BP measurements. Begin education on what hypertension is and how it can sometimes be managed, especially early on, with lifestyle changes.

7. Obtain electrocardiogram (ECG) today as well as past medical records to check old ECG and past lab tests for comparison.

8. Continue on Protonix 40 mg daily for chronic dyspepsia. Prescription given for 90 days with one refill. Discussed lifestyle management to decrease breakthrough dyspepsia/heartburn symptoms with food. Includes raising head of bed with adjustable bed or wedge pillow to decrease nocturnal reflux, which causes risk for Barrett's esophagus, a precancerous condition. Decrease food intake at night; do not eat 3 hours before lying down. Avoid high-acidity foods or supplement with a calcium antacid tablet after eating such foods. Avoid tight clothing with belts, chocolate, and irritating foods, and decrease caffeine. Give Mrs. K occult blood testing stool cards to make certain there is no occult blood from chronic dyspepsia. Encourage her to schedule a colonoscopy and possible endoscopy as she is over 50 years old, the time when she should begin periodic gastrointestinal screening. Give her the names of several gastroenterologists to select from.

9. Explore stress management options to decrease BP and her apparent tension headaches at work. Evaluate if this helps

her back pain, which is often stress associated. Discuss a variety of holistic stress reduction modalities, such as meditation, deep breathing, guided imagery, and yoga. Consider beginning a slow walking program with 10 minutes every other day. Eat a protein snack in the late afternoon to decrease headaches late in the day.

10. Due to her positive family history of breast cancer, discuss the importance of mammograms, ask the patient why she is declining mammograms and what she knows about the amount of radiation; softly explain the risks with hereditary breast cancer as she has two females on her mother's side with breast cancer history.

11. For her 6-week return visit for labs and BP, check positive family history of coronary artery disease (CAD); monitor BP and, if lifestyle management options do not decrease it and if stress is determined not to be the main factor, Mrs. K may need to start a pharmaceutical agent to reduce her BP so as to reduce her CAD risk. Compare new ECG with old ECG to ensure that there are no changes. Emphasize that she can use lifestyle management and herbs or supplements as long as they are working to decrease her lipids. Look for existence of past murmur when past medical records are obtained. If there is no history of past murmur, Mrs. K should have an echocardiogram to determine if there are any valvular issues with possible cardiologist referral, depending on the results.

12. For her 6-week return visit discuss gynecologic health maintenance. Mrs. K needs to have a pelvic exam because she still has her ovaries and she needs a vulvar exam and possible vaginal Pap smear. Even though she has her ovaries, she is menopausal by age and may be experiencing ovarian hormonal decline. She had declined estrogen replacement after her partial hysterectomy because she still had her "natural hormones," but with some night sweats, mood lability, and the fact that she is 52, she may be in ovarian menopause. At a later point in time, so as not to overload Mrs. K with information, I will discuss integrative

menopausal options. Black cohosh and soy preparations will not be recommended to Mrs. K because she has a family history of breast cancer, and these agents are estrogenic, possibly increasing her risk of breast cancer. Many other natural menopause agents are not considered as useful as soy or black cohosh.

13. For her 6-week return visit, discuss osteoporosis screening with a bone density test, or have the gynecologist order this. This is the prime time to test as she appears to be early menopausal.

Mrs. K reports that although she is concerned about her potential and actual health problems, she is pleased to have switched to a practice where her nurse practitioner and physician will allow her the chance to use herbal medications and supplements and focus on lifestyle and stress management before taking prescription pharmaceuticals. She stated that she feels calmer than she thought she would because she feels she was listened to and respected. She is happy to stay in this practice.

NOTES

1. D. Rakel, *Integrative Medicine*, 3rd ed. (Philadelphia: Saunders, 2012): 233.
2. M. T. Murray and J. Pizzorno, *The Encyclopedia of Natural Medicine*, 3rd ed. (New York: Atria, 2012).

Family Nurse Practitioner: Therapeutic Touch in Older Adults

Holistic nurses: Denise Coppa, PhD, FNP-C, PNP-BC; Mary Grace Amendola, PhD, RN

Place of employment: University of Rhode Island, Hasbro Children's Hospital Pediatric Clinic; Rhode Island Free Clinic, Rutgers University College of Nursing

Nursing specialty: Family and pediatric nurse practitioner in primary care, nurse practitioner educator

Holistic modality specialization: Therapeutic touch

Setting. The distinguishing characteristic of this case is the fact that the two authors had entered into a mentorship relationship so that the second author could work toward the Therapeutic Touch International Associates' credential "Qualified Therapeutic Touch Practitioner." The client was a well, gregarious 98-year-old resident (referred to as A. B.) of an assisted living facility, who was skeptical of the therapeutic touch (TT) process but agreed to "try it out" to "help" the mentoree. He had hypertension with minimal kidney function, but both were well controlled with medication. His medical history included a large but stable abdominal aortic aneurysm, macular degeneration, and partial deafness.

The mentor arranged the first meeting. A. B. greeted the mentoree and said, "I will do anything to help." Before the TT treatment, A. B. asked me if I spoke Italian, and I answered him in my Neapolitan dialect, "Si', parlo Italiano" ("Yes, I speak Italian."). A. B. also spoke the same dialect so we chatted for a bit in Italian and then proceeded with the TT treatment. This was a perfect example of an essential component to establish a rapport between the TT provider and the client.

Holistic interventions. Because this was a mentorship relationship, TT was the sole modality used so that the mentoree could focus on the TT process. The TT treatment was explained to the client in detail. The process was demonstrated by the TT provider performing it on herself, showing him how the hands would pass over the surface of his skin, without touching it, beginning from the head down to the feet, on both sides. The actual treatment started with a centering exercise, during which the provider "goes to a deep place within" to enable her to focus on this client. Permission to touch, if necessary, on specific areas of the body that needed hand contact to the skin was obtained. For example, if blockage to the arm was detected, then one hand would be placed on top of the shoulder while the other hand would be touching the arm in a downward movement, releasing the energy out through the fingers.

Critical to the TT process is for the healer to establish an intent to heal, streaming from a compassionate demeanor. In this case, compassion was expressed by "sending thoughts of peace and happiness" from the centered

orientation. Assessment is the next step in the process, distinguishing TT from other common energy modalities. The healer passed her hands over A. B.'s entire body, approximately three to five inches away. Her palms were in a downward position, using long, sweeping, flowing movements. A mental note of his energy fields' imbalance was made. Irregularities, such as "tingling" and areas of "warmness" manifested as imbalances in the field. Based on this assessment, the healer proceeded to "treat" with the intent to reestablish balance and symmetry of the field.

In this particular treatment, the types of treatment techniques include unruffling, light, feather-like movements extending from the patient's midline to the periphery and from head to toe. This technique is effective in "smoothing" irregularities. It can also be used to assist in the reintegration of the field near the end of a treatment. Visualizing the color blue was also used in this treatment to repattern the field. In the areas assessed as "warm," coolness was used as a healing technique as well. In TT, the law of opposites is utilized to recreate symmetry of the field closest to the client's physical body.[1]

In TT, reassessment is simultaneous with the healing process. The healer, in this case, purposively visualized the patient's field as being rebalanced. When the sensations of imbalance were felt to be diminished, the patient also appeared to lower his shoulders and move down into the chair. He stated, "I feel relaxed." The healer then ended the treatment by gently holding his feet with the intent of "grounding" the energy. This encourages the energy to move to the ground.[2]

Evaluation. The patient reported that he "felt relaxed." In addition, the healer had taken his blood pressure and pulse prior to the treatment. She was able to document a decrease in both of these vital signs at the conclusion of the treatment. Most important, the patient slept for an extended period of time after each treatment, which was not typical for this patient. A. B. was treated weekly during a 2-month period. During that time, the client was noticeably more relaxed, with little expression of anxiety, which had been his usual demeanor on many occasions. Each treatment ended in deep relaxation, and the client was able to articulate his profound level of "a peaceful feeling" after the treatments. During the last 2 weeks of his life, the healer conducted TT treatments to ease his passing. It was a peaceful, calm, and painless death. The treatments appeared to have a synergistic effect, each one fostering a deeper relaxation response, evidenced by how long he "napped" after these sessions, as evidenced by the staff at the assisted living facility.

Reflections. One of the most profound lessons learned from this longitudinal case study was that, in older adults, TT can be an effective modality to aid relaxation and sleep, decrease anxiety, and ultimately assist the client to make a peaceful end-of-life transition. This is very useful to nurse practitioners when working with older adults in long-term care facilities.

NOTES

1. D. Coppa, "The Internal Process of Therapeutic Touch," *Journal of Holistic Nursing* 26, no. 1 (2008): 17–24.
2. D. Krieger, *Therapeutic Touch Inner Workbook* (Santa Fe, NM: Bear & Co., 1997).

Family Nurse Practitioner: Stress Reduction in Early Pregnancy

Holistic nurse: Karen M. Myrick, DNP, APRN, FNP-BC, ANP-BC

Place of employment: Quinnipiac University, Pro-Health Physicians, Avon, Connecticut

Nursing specialty: Family and adult nurse practitioner

Holistic modality specialization: Biofeedback, therapeutic communication, aromatherapy

Setting. Family nurse practitioners, working in primary care, encounter a variety of patients. The patients cared for range from birth to senescence and from healthy to very ill. The scope of care can also vary greatly, from a well visit to an anaphylactic reaction, and may incorporate multiple patient variables that must all be taken into consideration. There are patients who are common and similar, and there are patients who are unique and will never be forgotten. A patient

with a variable to be considered, and who was unforgettable, was Mrs. M. The patient was a G6P0, 38-year-old woman presenting with a cough and a newly confirmed pregnancy after four rounds of in vitro fertilization who needed to be listened to, completely understood, and helped.

Patient. Mrs. M presented with a cough with a duration of 7 days. The cough began with an upper respiratory infection, described by a mild sore throat, clear rhinorrhea, and a hacking cough. The cough was productive of clear sputum, worse with lying down, and was now interrupting sleep. She had no associated symptoms, no shortness of breath or fever. No recent travel, no rashes or lesions.

On physical examination, Mrs. M's vital signs were within normal limits at 98.4 (temporal), 80, 14, and 114/70. Her tympanic membranes were normal without effusion, sinuses had no tenderness to palpation, eyes were clear, nose had swollen turbinates, mild erythema, and clear mucoid discharge. Throat had 1+ tonsils without exudate, mild erythema in the posterior pharynx, and a cobblestone appearance. Heart was a normal rate and rhythm, and there were no murmurs. Lungs were clear to auscultation bilaterally, no rhonchi or wheezes.

The general appearance of Mrs. M was concerning. She made little eye contact, spoke very quickly, sighed frequently, and rolled her eyes often. It was a challenge to obtain a history, and it felt as though she was bothered by the physical examination.

When the diagnosis of pharyngitis was given, Mrs. M groaned, and then asked what the treatment would be. The treatment plan was outlined and included rest, increasing oral fluids, a mucolytic, humidified air, nasal saline, and return if not better.

After a long period of silence, Mrs. M asked if we could prescribe the cough medicine she had last year. Looking up the medication, I noted a cough medicine that included a narcotic was prescribed for pneumonia. The cough medicine was a pregnancy category C and not recommended in pregnancy. After an explanation of the class of medication and the contraindication in pregnancy, and the indications for a narcotic antitussive were reviewed, Mrs. M was again silent for a period of time. The silence was awkward, and she did not make eye contact. I asked if she had any questions, and she answered no. She looked away and began to cry.

Holistic interventions. Realizing the difficulty of the situation, and becoming more in touch with my own potential wholeness to assist this patient, I decided how to best intervene for the situation. Therapeutic silence and being present were employed. Initially, I chose to be still and silent. After that pause, I made a box of tissues available to Mrs. M's reach and paused as I handed them to her, taking the opportunity to hold her hand. She flinched initially, and then grasped tightly as she began to sob. The therapeutic touch seemed to allow Mrs. M to connect with me, and me with her, in a deeper and more effective relationship.

In the minute that occurred after the touch, she began to speak in a trembling voice, stating, "I am sorry." She continued, "I have been so anxious since I found out I am pregnant. I have had six losses and cannot bear to deal with another. I stay awake at night, worrying not only about when, but how, I will lose this baby. I know this is not rational, and that is why I thought about the cough medicine. You see, this was the only thing that has ever really made me sleep deeply, and I thought if I had this cold, and the cough was bad enough, you would prescribe that for me."

Evaluation. I acknowledged her apology and her admission of the rationale for wanting the cough medication. We spoke at length about her anxiety and how this was normal, especially in her current situation. We discussed several methods to help her deal with this symptom, which did not include a narcotic antitussive. She was familiar with biofeedback and thought this may be very beneficial to her at this time. She also welcomed the suggestion of lavender on her pillow as an aromatherapy agent. The plan was made to have her follow up in 1 week with me to evaluate the methods and their effectiveness.

Upon return, Mrs. M was doing much better. She had begun to work on her biofeedback mechanisms and was focusing on her thoughts and feelings about a viable pregnancy. She was practicing deep breathing, and we discussed thought redirection. The lavender was working well, and, in combination with the biofeedback, she was able to rest for several hours at night, peacefully.

Reflections. Mrs. M. went on to deliver a 36-week, healthy baby boy, 6 pounds and 15 ounces, 20 inches long. It is unknown if the biofeedback and complementary interventions contributed to a healthy pregnancy outcome, but it is known that it is important to measure stress during pregnancy, as it can affect the length of gestation.[1] Without a holistic approach to care, the emotional state of the mother may not have been discovered, but using presence and deep listening allowed for a healing environment.

NOTES

1. H. J. Cole-Lewis, T. S. Kershaw, V. A. Earnshaw, K. A. Yonkers, H. Lin, and J. R. Ickovics, "Pregnancy-Specific Stress, Preterm Birth, and Gestational Age Among High-Risk Young Women," *Health Psychology* 33, no. 9 (2014): 1033–1045.

Family Nurse Practitioner: Knowing in Patient Care

Holistic nurse: Kathleen Gareth, RN, MSN, FNP

Place of employment: Center for Integrative Health, Medoptions, Wilmington, Delaware

Nursing specialty: Family nurse practitioner, holistic nursing

Holistic modality specialization: Energy medicine, homeopathy, integrative medicine

Setting. This is an interesting case because of the sudden and unexpected results that were obtained. The case used Reiki and Healing Touch I techniques. The outcome was challenging for the spouse, whose belief system did not incorporate any alternative healing therapies. Normally, healing occurs over several sessions and such dramatic results are not usual in a first session and especially after only one session. I did not see the spouse during the remaining 6 months of his wife's life. Because he did not bring up the energy session after that time, I honored his privacy and did not approach the subject with him. I do know that family leave was an issue because he had planned to take

2 weeks off, but it ultimately turned into 6 months. I do not know if or how he integrated what happened during this session into his belief system.

Patient. B. T. was a 69-year-old female diagnosed with cancer. She had gone through all of the conventional cancer treatments and was no longer responding to them. She had recently been placed on hospice care. Due to pain, she was not sleeping well, she was on bed rest due to weakness, and her life expectancy was about 2 weeks. Because the spouse and I were both members of the same community group, I offered to give her a Reiki session with the intention of helping her sleep. Her spouse had taken family leave to help with hospice care. Though the husband was a conventionally trained healthcare worker, he agreed to the Reiki session after checking with his wife.

Due to the wife's condition, I made a home visit. I entered the bedroom quietly and saw a frail older female who was awake, alert, and oriented. She was in a much weakened state. I asked if I could place crystals on her to enhance the healing and she agreed. I explained what I would be doing and then started the session using traditional Reiki hand positions and added specific techniques as I was guided. During the session, I had heightened awareness that this patient had not decided whether she was ready yet to let go of life. With this knowledge, the session became more about helping B. T. make this difficult decision. My intention changed from just wanting to help with sleep to using the energy to open her up to her highest good and allowing that decision to manifest. Many Reiki practitioners find that as they work with the Reiki energy they develop or experience intuitive or psychic abilities. These abilities manifest differently in each person. Some practitioners claim to see or hear things, but I am a knower.[1] I just know things that I have no other logical way of knowing. It does not manifest at every session, but it does with most. The information that comes to me is something that will help the patient work through an issue.

The entire session for B. T. lasted about an hour, and she slept through the entire session. By the end of the session, I knew that she would be alive longer than expected. I told the spouse before I left that I had picked up her reluctance

to leave just yet and that the session became about giving her that choice. The next morning B. T. woke up and got out of bed but, due to being deconditioned, she fell but was not hurt. As the days progressed, she continued to increase ambulation, her appetite picked up, and she lived for approximately another 6 months. She died quickly and peacefully with her husband at her side. Her last days overall were comfortable and allowed her to do some of her favorite things, such as working in her garden.

During the time she was alive I offered another session but was not asked back. I do not know if this was due to the unexpected results that may have caused an uncomfortable reaction for her husband, a conventionally trained healthcare worker. Each person reacts in different ways when they are confronted with something that goes against their basic belief system.

I do not think that another session would have prolonged B. T.'s life any longer. I feel that the outcome obtained is exactly what was best for the patient and, it is hoped, for the spouse. I feel that an emotional/spiritual healing occurred; whether this couple realized that fully, I do not know.

Holistic interventions. In this situation there was only one session of Reiki given, which is not normally the case with most clients. Typically, many sessions over time are given to provide continued healing. Reiki is one form of energy healing, and, like many practitioners, I am also trained in more than one form of energy healing such as Healing Touch. Both of these modalities use techniques to balance the chakras, smooth the aura, and ground the patient.[2] Reiki also uses specific hand positions. Other techniques were also used that were personally guided to me. I also used crystals placed on the chakras and in the hands. Crystals have their own energy and are used to enhance the session.

Evaluation. The results from this healing are not usual. Healing results are not predictable. Many factors affect a healing, but most important are the patient's needs. Healing occurs when sacred space is created and universal energy is allowed to flow into that space through the practitioner.

Reiki energy is accepted or received by patients in a time frame that is best for them. Occasionally, there are dramatic changes, as in this healing. Forcing a healing may actually cause the recipient to block the energy. The patient (recipient) is the one who directs where the energy flows. The healer is a conduit or a channel for the energy to flow through. The practitioner uses intention, which is always for the highest good of the patient.[3]

Reflections. This case demonstrated unexpected but powerful results that surprised me and made me realize at a deeper level how important and sacred this work really is. All healing work is sacred, but we tend to forget that in the rushing around and task orientation of our practice. All forms of healing, including conventional medicine, have their dramatic stories. Unfortunately, healing from alternative medicine is traditionally disregarded or claimed as spontaneous remission. It is important to remember that there is more to a healing than can be measured by our current scientific, empirical techniques.

NOTES

1. M. M. Archibald, "The Holism of Aesthetic Knowing in Nursing," *Nursing Philosophy* 13, no. 3 (2012): 179–188.
2. J. Mentgen and M. J. T. Bulbrook, *Healing Touch: Healing Touch Level I Notebook* (Carrboro: North Carolina Center for Healing Touch, 2001).
3. B. A. Brennan, *Hands of Light: A Guide to Healing Through the Human Energy Field* (New York: Bantam Books, 1988).

Mental Health Nursing: A Story of Lingering Presence

Holistic nurse: Dorothy Larkin, PhD, RN

Place of employment: College of New Rochelle School of Nursing, Holistic Nursing Master's CNS Program

Nursing specialty: Holistic nursing, psychiatric mental health nursing, brief solution-focused psychotherapy, meaningful dialogue, therapeutic touch, Reiki, reflexology, aromatherapy, relaxation techniques, imagery, meditation

Holistic modality specialization: Ericksonian hypnosis

Setting. Thirty-three years ago, I taught my friend Debbie hypnosis for labor and delivery. Approximately 15 years ago I taught her husband Tom hypnosis for smoking cessation.

Debbie and I have seen one another every few years and, when together, we talk about hypnosis. I offered both Debbie and Tom sporadic hypnotherapeutic inductions for augmenting their health and well-being.

Holistic interventions. Three years ago, Tom was in a near fatal snowmobile accident. The next time we visited, about 1 year after Tom's accident, Debbie recounted how she integrated the naturalistic/utilization approach[1] and conversationally provided interspersed therapeutic suggestions[2-4] to help Tom come off of the ventilator and manage his pain.

I asked Debbie to share her story for this case study. The following is her verbatim description. Please note her use of present tense language as this experience is still very alive for her. It is a story of how the "lingering presence"[5, 6] of an initial holistic nursing intervention can continue to therapeutically benefit individuals over time.

Tom lies in intensive care under an induced coma with all body functions, except his heart, being run mechanically. His regular doctor leaves for the night, intending to pull the ventilator out and replace it with a trach the next morning. With all of Tom's ribs broken in multiple places, the doctor doesn't believe me that he could breathe on his own when brought out of his coma. He said Tom would find himself in intense pain. The night doctor came in at 9:00 and listens to my thoughts. "We'll give it a try."

While Tom is still "under," I start to do intentional talk. "You need to breathe regularly when the ventilator tube comes out and you are no longer in a coma. You are a runner and have always concentrated on your breath. You just ran the Leadville marathon 2 months ago at an altitude of 10,000 to 13,500 feet. Your breathing was as critical to you then as it is now." (I audibly breathe in and out, in and out, in Tom's ear, with my hand resting on his chest, and pace my words: "In and out, in and out.")

"When you come out of your coma, you will feel pain—intense pain in your chest. I want you to recognize that pain and then concentrate to turn it off through your breath . . . in with the healing, out with the pain. Breathing in and out, in and out. . . . Remember when Dorothy taught me self-hypnosis for birthing all three of our children and I didn't need pain medication? You were my coach each time, helping me concentrate on breathing and shutting off the pain. That's what you need to do now.

"Remember your experience of control and conquer when you quit smoking with the help of self-hypnosis? You were successful then as you will be now." (Breathing in his ear while my hand lies gently on his chest.) Breathing in and out, in and out . . .

"Control the pain with your mind, concentrate on your breath. You can do this. The doctor will bring you out of the coma, he will stop the Versed and give you morphine. You will be conscious again, which you have not been since the night of the snowmobile accident. That was a month ago. I will be here for you, acting as your coach, and love you as you did for me birthing our children.

"You can do this: Breathing regularly . . . in and out, in and out . . .

"Okay, Doc, I do believe he's ready." After 40 or more minutes of talking with Tom, the night doctor takes him out of his induced coma and pulls out the ventilator tube. Tom panics for a second, looks in my eyes, and we breathe together with my hand on his chest. "In and out," I say. "Concentrate on your breath. Turn off the pain, breathe in and out . . ." He does. Success. The doctor waits for an hour to make sure he doesn't need to intubate him again. Success.

Another two weeks and Tom is out of intensive care and into a rehabilitation facility. He has made a full recovery and has experienced the birth of his four grandchildren. He is a lucky man with great willpower. He overcame a head injury with bleeding in the brain, multiple breaks of each rib, two punctured lungs, a broken scalpula, and a hematoma on his right bun cheek down his leg.

He learned to walk, think, and function normally within a mysteriously short time. He is my hero! (Story as told by Debora Jackson-Bliss.)

Reflections. When a holistic nurse hears subjective stories from clients that the health patterning modalities you taught many years ago continue to be used, and that they are able to cater the modality to the health needs of the moment, that is the ultimate outcome to teaching that could be achieved.

NOTES

1. M. H. Erickson, "Naturalistic Techniques of Hypnosis," in *The Nature of Hypnosis and Suggestion*, Vol. 4, ed. E. L. Rossi (New York: Irvington, 1980): 168–176.
2. M. H. Erickson, "The Interspersal Hypnotic Technique for Symptom Correction and Pain Control," in *The Nature of Hypnosis and Suggestion*, Vol. 4, ed. E. L. Rossi (New York: Irvington, 1980): 262–278.
3. D. Larkin, "Therapeutic Suggestion," in *Relaxation and Imagery: Tools for Therapeutic Communication and Intervention*, ed. R. P. Zahourek (Philadelphia: W. B. Saunders, 1988): 84–100.
4. D. M. Larkin, "Principles of Therapeutic Suggestions (Part 1) and Clinical Applications of Therapeutic Suggestions (Part II)," *EXPLORE: The Journal of Science and Healing* 10, no. 6 (2014): 330–388.
5. R. R. Parse, *The Human Becoming School of Thought: A Perspective for Nurses and Other Health Professionals* (Thousand Oaks, CA: Sage, 1998).
6. R. R. Parse, *Community: A Human Becoming Perspective* (Sudbury, MA: Jones and Bartlett, 2003).

Pediatric Nurse Practitioner: Therapeutic Touch in Neonates

Holistic nurse: Denise Coppa, PhD, FNP-C, PNP-BC

Place of employment: University of Rhode Island, coordinator of Family Nurse Practitioner Program; nurse practitioner at Teen Tot Clinic, Hasbro Children's Hospital

Nursing specialty: Pediatric and family nurse practitioner

Holistic modality specialization: Therapeutic touch

Setting. Multiple patient encounters occurred in the normal newborn nursery at a local hospital that has approximately 11,000 deliveries per year. All babies were the product of term pregnancies and exhibited no signs of illness or distress during these encounters. I was the family nurse practitioner (FNP) student preceptor in the nursery and the course professor for the Pediatric Physical Assessment course. The nurseries typically had a census of 10 to 20 newborns, from the ages of 2 hours to 4 days. On any given clinical day, there would be five FNP students assigned to the nursery to conduct a physical examination on specific newborns. The main challenge in this setting was the fact that many of the babies cried incessantly while the FNP students were attempting to examine them. It made listening to hearts, lungs, and bowel sounds particularly challenging.

Holistic interventions. The modality chosen by the nurse practitioner in this situation was therapeutic touch (TT), a goal-directed therapy. In this case of mild chaos (all babies crying at once), the goal was to "calm" the environment and the babies. In effect, when this goal was attained, the students attempting to examine the babies became visibly less anxious about the clinical assignment. A study I conducted demonstrated that the TT process was slightly different in children compared to adults.[1] Centering, or calming and focusing prior to attempting to "treat" the child, was the same first step while treating adults or children. For the nurse practitioner (NP), centering in a busy newborn nursery can be entered into upon arrival with the goal of calming the environment.

Second in the process is the assessment. While this is conceptually identical in adults and children, as are the treatment methods, in children, typically only one hand is used to scan the field. This, as opposed to two hands used in adults, tends not to "overwhelm" the baby,

energetically. During the assessment, slight imbalances in the energy field closest to the infant's body were detected in the hands of the NP. Most often, the field was perceived as "congested" or "electrically charged."

The TT treatment then ensued but was administered using only one hand over the body, gently. Because the babies were well, smoothing and unruffling were the only treatment strategies needed to produce results. The entire time the NP was using her right hand in the "treatment" phase, her left hand was gently holding the baby's feet to encourage "grounding" of the field. Lastly, the child's field was reassessed. The entire treatment takes 2 to 3 minutes.

Reflections. In most cases, the babies first became quiet and appeared hypervigilant of their environments. Their eyes opened wide and they seemed slightly "stunned." The TT in all cases helped the babies to quiet, which, in turn, allowed the students to conduct a complete physical examination.

NOTES

1. D. Coppa. "The Internal Process of Therapeutic Touch," *Journal of Holistic Nursing* 26, no. 1 (2008): 17–24.

Nurse Healer Reflections

After reading this chapter, the nurse will be able to answer or to begin a process of answering the following questions:

- In what way do these case studies influence my practice?
- Which holistic interventions can I consider for use in my practice?
- What would I like to learn more about to enhance my practice?
- Which research approaches can be used to scientifically examine the interventions and patient outcomes?

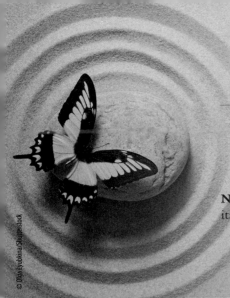

Index

Note: Page numbers followed by *e*, *f*, and *t* indicate material in exhibits, figures, and tables respectively.

T